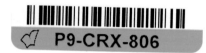

ADVANCES IN CELL AGING AND GERONTOLOGY

VOLUME 11

Mechanisms of Cardiovascular Aging

ADVANCES IN CELL AGING AND GERONTOLOGY
VOLUME 11

Mechanisms of Cardiovascular Aging

Volume Editor:

Tory Hagen
Biochemistry and Biophysics
Linus Pauling Institute
Oregon State University
Corvallis, OR
USA

2002

ELSEVIER
Amsterdam – Boston – London – New York – Oxford – Paris
San Diego – San Francisco – Singapore – Sydney – Tokyo

ELSEVIER SCIENCE B.V.
Sara Burgerhartstraat 25
P.O. Box 211, 1000 AE Amsterdam, The Netherlands

First edition 2002

Library of Congress Cataloging in Publication Data
Mechanisms of cardiovascular aging / volume editor, Tory Hagen.--1st ed.
    p.; cm. -- (Advances in cell aging and gerontology, ISSN 1566-3124; v. 11)
   Includes bibliographical references and index.
   ISBN 0-444-51159-8 (alk. paper)
   1. Cardiovascular system--Pathophysiology. 2. Cardiovascular system--Aging. I.
Hagen, Tory. II. Series.
   [DNLM: 1. Cardiovascular Diseases--etiology. 2. Aging--physiology. 3.
Cardiovascular Diseases--physiopathology. WG 120 M486 2002]
   QP86 .A34 vol. 11
   [RC669.9]
   612.6'7 s--dc21
   [616.1'07]   2002029425
A catalog record from the Library of Congress has been applied for.

British Library Cataloging in Publication Data
A catalogue record from the British Library has been applied for.

ISBN: 0 444 51159 8
Series ISSN: 1566-3124

⊗ The paper used in this publication meets the requirements of ANSI/NISO Z39.48-1992 (Permanence of Paper).
Printed in The Netherlands.

TABLE OF CONTENTS

PREFACE

During the last fifty years there has been a marked increase in mean human lifespan, largely due to the conquering of many pathogen-borne diseases, better prenatal care and improved clinical management of chronic diseases. Aside from accidents and rare inherited disorders, relatively few deaths occur before the age of 65 in developed countries. While we are living longer, an increasing concern is that the quality of life, or healthspan, has not concomitantly increased along with lifespan. Age itself is the leading risk factor for cardiovascular diseases of all types; other chronic diseases such as cancer and senile dementias also markedly increase with age. The mechanisms underlying the aging process as well as that for age-related chronic diseases have been intensely studied; however, significant gaps in knowledge still remain. In particular, little is known about how the aging process affects disease progression and outcome. A case in point is cardiovascular diseases (CVD), which include loss of vasomotor function, athero- and arterio-sclerosis, hypertension, congestive heart failure and stroke. Together these pathologies comprise the leading causes of permanent disability, hospitalization and death for individuals over the age of 65 in the United States. Direct healthcare costs for congestive heart failure alone are currently estimated to exceed 18 billion dollars per annum and future costs will undoubtedly rise along with the aging of the "baby-boom" generation. Thus, there is a critical need to assess both the age-associated causes leading to CVD as well as determine the current state of knowledge on preventative regimens designed to slow or modulate disease progression. Much of the investigation in this important field is focused on the molecular and cellular basis of CVD, and this issue of Advances in Cell Aging and Gerontology provides a timely review of this field.

The book begins with a chapter by Wolk and Somers who eloquently overview both the mechanisms leading to phenotypic manifestations of cardiovascular diseases as well as features of the aging cardiovascular system that may predispose the elderly to risk for CVD. Both genetic and humoral factors associated with cardiac function and vessel compliance are concisely reviewed. This chapter serves as a springboard into others that provide in depth discussions of these topics. The book is divided into three general aspects, which discuss factors that contribute to 1) atherosclerosis; 2) vascular endothelial dysfunction/vessel compliance, and 3) oxidative stress and myocardial decay.

For atherosclerosis, the chapters by Yamashita and Krishnaswamy individually discuss how cholesterol and cytokines affect disease progression, respectively. Other chapters by Drs. Lüscher and Taddei explore endothelial dysfunction and subsequent loss of vasomotor tone. These authors place a particular emphasis on mechanisms contributing to loss of endothelial-derived nitric oxide signaling and its consequences for increased hypertension. The chapter by Fujishima further explores age-related alterations in vessel compliance that contribute to increased hypertension. Finally, Dr. Emily Wilson provides one of the only reviews available on how aging affects the extracellular matrix and contributes to altered vascular smooth muscle function.

The contribution of oxidants to cardiovascular decay is also prominently featured. Dr. Charles Hoppel and coworkers review the role of mitochondrial decline and cardiovascular disease while Dr. St. Clair examines how superoxide/superoxide dismutase imbalance may significantly contribute to a number of cardiovascular pathologies of aging. Also included is an excellent chapter by Dr. Rifkind summarizing age-related changes in red blood cell physiology.

Additionally, a strength of this book is its discussions summarizing current thought on how diet may modulate cardiovascular decay. The chapter by Marco Cattaneo discusses the evidence that folate modulates homocysteine, thus lowering risk for atherosclerosis. May and Burk also examine how selenium, vitamin C and vitamin E contribute to cardiovascular health. These chapters are further augmented with two additional ones by the editors which review emerging findings suggesting that dietary antioxidants and caloric restriction may effectively slow or prevent disease progression during adult life.

Thus, this book concisely summarizes the current knowledge related to the major aspects contributing to cardiovascular dysfunction in the elderly as well as potential ways of maintaining or improving human cardiovascular healthspan. It is our hope that the information provided will not only act as a review of the current knowledge related to CVD and aging, but will also spur further research designed to improve quality of life in the elderly.

HAGEN
Editor

**Advances in
Cell Aging and
Gerontology**

Overview of cardiovascular aging

Robert Wolk and Virend K. Somers*

*Division of Hypertension and Division of Cardiology, Department of Medicine, Mayo Clinic,
200 First St. SW, Rochester, MN 55905, USA*

Contents

Abbreviations

PON1	paraoxonase1
APOE	apolipoprotein E
LDL	low-density lipoprotein

* Corresponding author. Mayo Foundation, St. Mary's Hospital, DO-4-350, 1216 Second St. SW,
Rochester, MN 55902, USA. Tel.: +1-507-2551144; fax: +1-507-2557070.
  E-mail address: somers.virend@mayo.edu (V.K. Somers).

Advances in Cell Aging and Gerontology, vol. 11, 1–22

TNFalpha	tumor necrosis factor alpha
IGF-I	insulin-like growth factor I
REM	rapid eye movement
HRV	heart rate variability
SERCA	sarcoplasmic reticulum Ca^{+2} ATPase
NO	nitric oxide
EDHF	endothelium-derived hyperpolarizing factor

1. Aging and the cardiovascular disease burden

Aging is widely conceived as a progressive loss of function, with increasing morbidity and mortality accompanying advancing age. The aging process may be defined by objective quantitative markers, such as functional and cognitive capacities and co-existent diseases. In this context, successful aging is thought of as a state of overall disease-free physical and mental well being. However, qualitative aspects of aging, although not well defined, are an important part of the aging process (von Faber et al., 2001). These markers (such as social contacts, motivations, expectations, the perception of fitness, etc.) reflect adaptation to objectively measured physical limitations inherent to old age. The focus of this overview will be on the mechanisms and characteristics of age-related cardiovascular impairment and the clinical consequences thereof, taking into consideration that cardiovascular aging is not always quantifiable, and is often inferred from surrogates such as reduced exercise tolerance and overt cardiac and vascular disease.

Over the past decades, we have observed a major demographic shift with a dramatic rise in the number and proportion of the elderly population. This trend is likely to continue, with the number of citizens over 65 years of age in the USA projected to be $\sim$70 million by the year 2030 (Population Division, US Census Bureau). These increased numbers will result in a magnified cardiovascular disease burden in the aged population. Over 80% of coronary disease occurs in the elderly, the prevalence rising from 4.5% in 50-year-old men to almost 30% in people in their 70s (Kelly, 1997) (Fig. 1). The incidence of heart failure is 15% in people in their 80s (vs. 1–2% in 40- and 50-year-olds) and that of hypertension is over 30% in the aged population (Kelly, 1997). The morbidity and mortality of cardiovascular diseases in a burgeoning elderly population will impact substantially on health care resources. Hence there is a compelling need to understand better both the mechanisms of cardiovascular aging and the pathophysiological processes underlying cardiovascular diseases in the elderly.

Normal aging is characterized by specific age-related changes in cardiovascular structure and function. These changes may be accelerated by diseases such as hypertension, heart failure, atherosclerosis and diabetes, the prevalence of which are greater in the elderly population. The process of cardiovascular aging is often marked by age-related acute cardiovascular events (such as myocardial infarction or stroke), which further affect the aging process. This overview will focus on the mechanisms and cardiovascular consequences of "normal" aging.

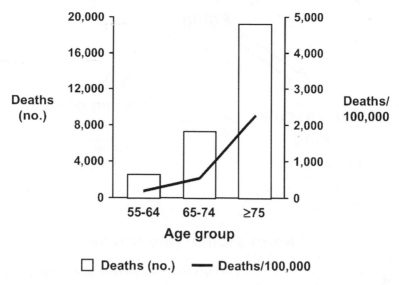

Fig. 1.   Total number of deaths and mortality rate from coronary heart disease in various age groups (adapted with permission from Kelly, 1997).

2. Mechanisms affecting phenotypic manifestations of cardiovascular aging

The process of cardiovascular aging and the determinants thereof are complex. The phenotype is dynamic and governed by various age-related processes that directly affect cells and tissues of the cardiovascular system. In addition, aging of other non-cardiovascular systems (neuroendocrine, respiratory, etc.) can modify the process of cardiovascular aging and contribute to the overall clinical phenotype (Fig. 2). In this section, we will address the most important influences on the manifestations of cardiovascular aging, ranging from basic genetic and cellular mechanisms to behavioral determinants.

2.1. *Genetics*

Longevity is familial. Members of long-lived families tend to live longer. Experimental studies suggest that genes can determine life span, and that longevity is a polygenic trait. Although most studies used relatively simple, invertebrate, short-lived organisms, many human homologs of the longevity genes have been identified or are being sought. Some examples are *age-1*, *daf-2* or *clk* mutations in nematodes (Finch and Tanzi, 1997) or the yeast *RAS2* gene, which encodes a homolog of the mammalian signal transduction protein c-H-ras (Jazwinski, 1998). The common denominator for many mutations associated with a longer life span is increased resistance to stress. Unfortunately, these phenomena are difficult to study because of the complexity of gene–gene and gene–environment interactions during development. Therefore, there is still a large gap between identification of certain molecular or cellular defects and our understanding of their effects on human aging.

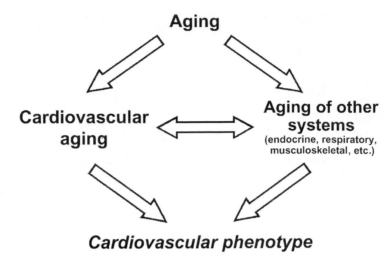

Fig. 2. Interactions between cardiovascular and non-cardiovascular systems in determining the phenotype of the aged cardiovascular system.

Although genetic factors have an influence on the aging process, it has been
calculated that the heritability of the human life span is relatively modest, accounting
for less than 35% of its variance (Herskind et al., 1996; Finch and Tanzi, 1997). On
the other hand, rather than individual longevity genes, certain genetic variants can
likely modify the aging process. These gene variants can alter some metabolic
pathways, thereby influencing interactions with environmental factors that affect the
process of aging. Variation in the serum paraoxonase1 (PON1) gene, the PON1-192
polymorphism, is such an example (Senti et al., 2001). PON1 activity decreases as a
function of age only in subjects homozygous for the Q allele. In addition, advancing
age increases the risk of myocardial infarction mainly in subjects with the low-
activity QQ genotype (Senti et al., 2001).

The French centenarian study of human subjects has attracted great interest
(Schachter et al., 1994). In this study, the apoE4 and apoE2 isoforms of the apolipoprotein E (APOE) gene were associated with shorter and longer life span,
respectively. Similar results were obtained in a Finnish population (Louhija et al.,
1994). The apoE4 allele of APOE is thought to promote premature atherosclerosis,
whereas the apoE2 allele has been associated with types III and IV hyperlipidemia.
In Italian centenarians, the frequency of apoB with low tandem repeats (apoB-
VNTR) was found to be 50% of that in young controls (De Benedictis et al., 1997).
Also, the high frequency of the HinfI(+/+) polymorphism of the apo A-IV gene
(accompanied by low levels of low-density lipoprotein (LDL) cholesterol and higher
concentrations of Lp(a)) has been associated with longevity (Pepe et al., 1998).

De Benedictis et al. (1999) compared mitochondrial DNA population pools
between older and younger individuals. The frequency of a particular genotype (the J
haplogroup) was higher in centenarians than in younger individuals, suggesting that

mitochondrial DNA inherited variability may play a role in aging and longevity. Also, centenarians appear to have a higher frequency of the 4G allele of the plasminogen activator inhibitor 1 gene (Mannucci et al., 1997), as well as certain alleles of the major histocompatibility complex (Caruso et al., 2000).

2.2. *Oxidative stress*

Free radicals and their biology represent one of the most popular theories to explain aging (Bunker, 1992; Muscari et al., 1996). Reactive oxygen species are constantly produced in biological systems as a normal part of aerobic metabolism. The body protects itself against oxidative damage by using various anti-oxidant, free radical scavenger systems (such as superoxide dismutase, catalase, and glutathione). Many reactive oxygen particles escape this defense system to damage critical targets such as DNA. Permanent damage is prevented by a process of constant and efficient repair. Fig. 3 illustrates the fine balance between free radical generating and scavenging systems in human physiology and pathophysiology.

There is evidence to suggest that the aging process is associated with an imbalance between production and removal of free radicals. The increase in oxidative stress may result both from an increase in the generation of free radicals and from a

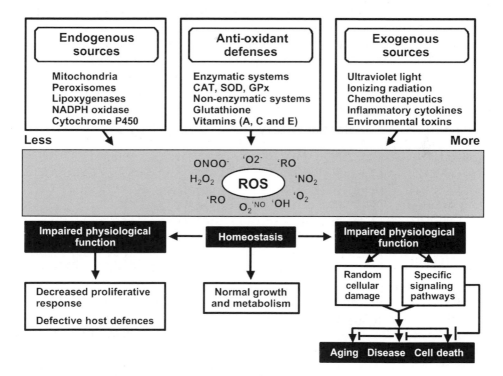

Fig. 3. The sources and biological responses to reactive oxygen species (ROS) (adapted with permission from Finkel and Holbrook, 2000).

decrease in the activity of anti-oxidative enzymes. Both these mechanisms play a role in the process of cardiovascular aging. Age-related mitochondrial damage increases the level of oxidative stress, which in turn further impairs mitochondrial function and, thereby, increases the amount of oxidative stress (a positive feed-back loop) (Cottrell and Turnbull, 2000; Van Remmen and Richardson, 2001). Toxins in the environment (including bacterial and viral infections) may activate a variety of free radical generating systems, leading to tissue damage. These detrimental effects are exacerbated by age-related changes in the immune system and augmented systemic inflammatory responses (Brod, 2000; Saito and Papaconstantinou, 2001).

On the other hand, free radical scavenger enzymes are depleted in the cardio-vascular system at an older age. In a recent study in human subjects, the anti-oxidant protection of intracranial arteries (glutathione peroxidase, superoxide dismutase, catalase) markedly decreased with age (Fig. 4), coinciding with a rapid acceleration of atherogenesis in elderly subjects (D'Armiento et al., 2001). In another experimental study, cardiac concentrations of glutathione peroxidase and superoxide dismutase decreased significantly with age in the rat heart (Abete et al., 1999). In addition, older hearts were more susceptible to the detrimental effects of hydrogen peroxide. Taken together, these results suggest that aging hearts are intrinsically more susceptible to free radical-induced damage.

As a consequence of these processes, the amount of oxidative stress increases as an organism ages, allowing progressive cellular damage to occur (Sastre et al., 2000). Most cellular components are known to be susceptible to damage by free radicals. Oxidation of proteins and carbohydrates may result in fragmentation and cross-linking, with a subsequent loss of function (Bunker, 1992). Membrane lipid

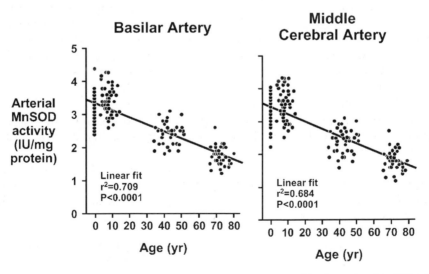

Fig. 4.   Activity of the oxygen-radical scavenger manganese superoxide dismutase (Mn-SOD) in the human basilar and middle cerebral arteries (adapted with permission from D'Armiento et al., 2001).

peroxidation may cause a loss of integrity of plasma and intracellular organelle membranes. Free radical-induced DNA cross-linking leads to somatic mutations and the production of defective gene products. Importantly, all these changes are accompanied by an impairment of a variety of cellular repair systems. There is evidence to suggest that species with longer life spans have more efficient repair mechanisms.

An important factor involved in cessation of cell proliferation in normal human cells is the absence of telomerase activity with a consequent erosion of chromosomal telomeres (Bodnar et al., 1998). Oxidative stress increases the rate of telomere shortening (due to single strand DNA breaks) in human fibroblasts, and this effect can be reversed by free radical scavengers (Serra et al., 2000; von Zglinicki et al., 2000). Interestingly, the shorter telomere length has been associated with vascular aging and increased stiffness of large arteries in humans (Chang and Harley, 1995; Benetos et al., 2001). The syndrome of progeria (which accelerates some features of the aging process) is characterized, among other abnormalities, by telomere shortening and premature atherosclerosis (Martin and Oshima, 2000).

It has to be emphasized that, in spite of rapid progress in this area, it is still uncertain whether free radicals influence aging and life span directly or simply play a role in the development of associated cardiovascular diseases. These two processes are likely interrelated.

2.3. *Apoptosis*

Apoptosis is a complex and highly regulated process, whereby injured or aging cells are removed from the body. This programmed cell death goes on continuously throughout life and plays an important regulatory role in normal tissue development. Advanced age is associated with dysregulation of apoptosis, with changes in the levels of proteins and other factors that regulate this process (Joaquin and Gollapudi, 2001). This may lead to significant loss of cells in various tissues of the cardiovascular system, with consequent impairment of cardiac and vascular function.

Mitochondrial dysfunction may be an important trigger in age-related apoptosis (Pollack and Leeuwenburgh, 2001; Van Remmen and Richardson, 2001). Specifically, activation of apoptotic mechanisms is caused by mitochondrial oxidative stress, alterations in mitochondrial turnover and a decline in mitochondrial energy production. As discussed above, the amount of oxygen-free radicals and oxidative stress increase with aging.

A number of other factors are also involved in apoptosis. The sympathetic nervous system (noradrenaline), the renin-angiotensin system, cytokines (such as tumor necrosis factor alpha [TNFalpha]), insulin-like growth factor I (IGF-I), calcium overload, etc. may be implicated. Notably, all of these are affected by aging.

2.4. *Neuroendocrine aging*

Age-related changes in the neuroendocrine system can indirectly influence cardiovascular physiology as well as the process of aging itself, thereby affecting the phenotypic features of the aging cardiovascular system (Fig. 2). Some of the most important aspects of this process are addressed below.

Impaired glucose tolerance is common in the aged population. Approximately 40% of individuals aged 65–74 years and 50% of those older than 80 years have impaired glucose tolerance or diabetes mellitus (Lamberts et al., 1997; Perry, 1999). This results from an impairment of insulin secretion by the pancreatic beta cells and from an increase in peripheral insulin resistance. The latter is related to poor diet, physical inactivity, age-related changes in body composition, as well as changes in growth hormone, cortisol, sex hormones and catecholamines (see below). Hyperglycemia leads to aging of the cardiovascular system via increased oxidative stress, potentiated DNA injury and non-enzymatic glycosylation of proteins (Monnier and Cerami, 1981; Fukagawa et al., 1999). In fact, tissue accumulation of glycosylation products occurs with aging even in the absence of hyperglycemia. The role of hyperglycemia in myocardial, microvascular and macrovascular pathology (Duckworth, 2001), and the relationship between insulin resistance and cardiovascular morbidity (Cefalu, 2001; Smiley et al., 2001) are well established.

Growth hormone (and hence IGF-I) secretion decreases with age (Lamberts et al., 1997; Perry, 1999). This decrease has been associated with reduced exercise capacity and increased cardiovascular and cerebrovascular risk, related to increased body fat, hyperlipidemia, structural and functional cardiac abnormalities (e.g. thinning of cardiac walls, reduced diastolic filling), as well as vascular changes (e.g. increased intima/media thickness and more frequent occurrence of atheromatous plaques) (Colao et al., 2001).

The secretion of sex hormones decreases or ceases with age, leading to abrupt menopause in women and more gradual andropause in men. In both sexes, changes in gonadal hormone concentrations affect cardiovascular physiology and confer an increased cardiovascular risk. This increased risk is related to dyslipidemia and atherosclerosis, changes in the regulation of vascular tone (including alterations in central sympathetic neural control) or abnormalities of ventricular relaxation.

Adrenal function is also affected by the aging process. Glucocorticoid secretion and plasma levels increase in older individuals (Van Cauter et al., 1996; Yen and Laughlin, 1998) and may contribute to the cardiovascular effects of aging. Baseline secretion of epinephrine from the adrenal medulla decreases markedly with age. Plasma epinephrine concentrations do not change, however, because of a reduction in epinephrine clearance (Seals and Esler, 2000). Although epinephrine secretion from the adrenal gland is reduced, the release of epinephrine from the heart may be increased (Seals and Esler, 2000).

Plasma norepinephrine (the main neurotransmitter released from post-ganglionic sympathetic nerve endings) also increases with aging (Seals and Esler, 2000). Although norepinephrine measurements in plasma can be affected by age-related changes in catecholamine clearance, measurements of muscle sympathetic nerve activity or tissue catecholamine spillover also confirm that there is an overall increase in the activity of the sympathetic nervous system in the healthy elderly (Fig. 5). This age-related increase in sympathetic activity may be caused by impairment of the arterial or cardiopulmonary baroreflex or by an elevated central sympathetic drive

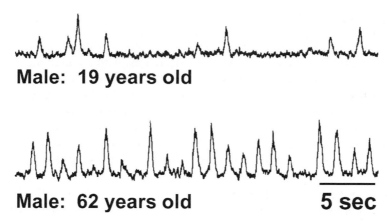

Male: 19 years old

Male: 62 years old   **5 sec**

Fig. 5.   Effects of age on muscle sympathetic nerve activity (MSNA).

(associated with increased forebrain noradrenergic activity) (Seals and Esler, 2000). Also, it has been suggested that the increase in sympathetic activity may be markedly accelerated during or after menopause (Matsukawa et al., 1998). Interestingly, although baseline serum concentrations of epinephrine and norepinephrine increase with aging, there may be a relative decrease in the release of stimulated catecholamines (Mazzeo et al., 1997; Kerckhoffs et al., 1998).

These autonomic effects of aging are accompanied by changes at the adrenoceptor level. Most notably, elevated catecholamine levels may lead to desensitization and decreased responsiveness of alpha- and beta-adrenoceptors (Kelly and O'Malley, 1984; Jones et al., 2001).

2.5. *Dyslipidemia*

Age-related increase in atherosclerosis (see below) may be explained in part by an increase in the plasma concentration of the atherogenic LDLs that occurs with increasing age (Green et al., 1985). The increase in LDL levels in the elderly is accentuated by reduced LDL clearance from the circulation, possibly due to a reduced hepatic LDL receptor expression and enhanced glycosylation of LDLs (Ericsson et al., 1991; Reaven et al., 1999), as well as a number of other factors, including those related to neuroendocrine abnormalities discussed earlier. The increase in LDL cholesterol with age is frequently associated with higher triglyceride levels and insulin resistance. Dyslipidemia is common in elderly people even when they remain active and consume a low fat Mediterranean diet.

Oxidative stress may also relate importantly to atherosclerosis. The oxidized form of LDL may affect endothelial function, alter vasomotor tone and initiate the cascade of atherosclerosis. As discussed, oxidative stress increases with age. Moreover the susceptibility of LDL to oxidation is enhanced in the elderly, with a consequent increase in the accumulation of oxidation products (including oxidized LDL) in the vascular wall (Reaven et al., 1999).

R. Wolk and V. K. Somers

2.6. *Sleep*

Normal aging is associated with characteristic changes in sleep architecture. Slow-wave sleep (stages 3 and 4 of NREM sleep) decreases, with a simultaneous increase in the number and duration of awakenings (Bliwise, 1994). These changes occur relatively early, during transition from young to midlife adulthood. Rapid eye movement (REM) sleep seems to be relatively preserved, but then decreases between mid and late adulthood (44–83 years), with concomitant sleep fragmentation and a decrease in the amount of total sleep (Fig. 6) (Van Cauter et al., 2000). Recent evidence suggests a temporal association between the decrease in deep slow-wave sleep and a reduction in growth hormone secretion (Van Cauter et al., 2000). Also, the decrease in REM sleep seems to coincide with an increase in nocturnal cortisol release (Van Cauter et al., 2000). These effects are similar to those seen with normal neuroendocrine aging and may have implications for cardiovascular aging, as described earlier in this chapter.

The prevalence of sleep apnea also increases with age. A number of mechanisms have been implicated to explain this phenomenon, such as increased body weight, chemoreflex abnormalities and changes in the properties of upper airway muscles

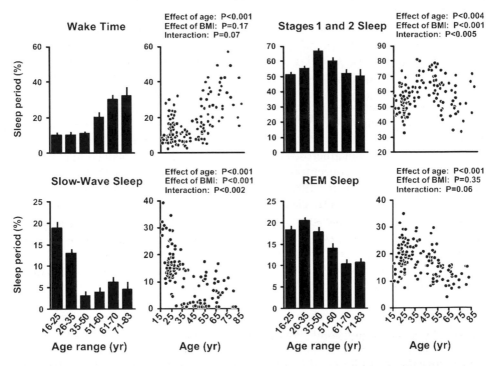

Fig. 6. Percentages of sleep period spent in wake, stages 1 and 2, slow-wave sleep, and REM sleep as a function of age. Means (SEM) for each age group are shown in the left panels and individual data are plotted in the right panels (adapted with permission from Van Cauter et al., 2000).

(Krieger et al., 1997; Oliven et al., 2001). The contribution of sleep apnea to cardiovascular pathophysiology in the elderly includes increased oxidative stress, systemic inflammation, abnormalities of endothelial function, increased coagulability and elevated sympathetic activity (Narkiewicz et al., 1998; Phillips et al., 1999; Kato et al., 2000a; Schulz et al., 2000; Mohsenin, 2001; Shamsuzzaman et al., 2002). Whether these maladaptive responses to sleep apnea contribute to cardiovascular risk through acceleration of the processes that characterize aging itself is not clear. Nevertheless, these effects of sleep apnea per se may contribute to cardiovascular phenotypic abnormalities and the morbidity of old age, by facilitating the development of atherosclerosis, hypertension, stroke or heart failure.

An important component of the age-related decrease in sleep quality is sleep deprivation, a very common problem affecting quality of life and perhaps cardiovascular function. Voluntary sleep curtailment is also becoming more and more frequent. This sleep debt has been shown to have detrimental effects on carbohydrate metabolism and endocrine function even in young men, leading to decreased glucose tolerance, lower thyrotropin concentration and elevated cortisol (Spiegel et al., 1999). In healthy humans, sleep deprivation results in higher blood pressures (Kato et al., 2000b). These metabolic, neuroendocrine and hemodynamic changes are similar to those associated with aging, suggesting the intriguing possibility that sleep debt can actually contribute to premature (endocrine) aging and to the occurrence of age-related pathologies.

Whether chronic sleep loss influences longevity is at this time controversial. Kripke et al. (2002) have recently reported that people who sleep 8 h or more have significantly higher mortality than those who sleep 6 h or less. Risk was also increased in those sleeping less than $4\frac{1}{2}$ h. "Insomnia" was not associated with excess mortality risk. Some other observational reports suggest that daytime siesta may be also associated with increased mortality in the elderly (Bursztyn et al., 1999, 2002). These intriguing and somewhat counter-intuitive results need to be confirmed and a causal relationship between longer sleep duration and mortality has to be demonstrated.

2.7. *Lifestyle*

Lifestyle factors (such as smoking, diet, caloric intake or physical activity) have important influences on cardiovascular aging. Interventions based on these behavioral factors (such as caloric restriction or increased physical activity) may have beneficial effects on the process of cardiovascular aging. These issues will be addressed in more detail in other chapters of this book.

3. Clinical features of the aging cardiovascular system

The age-related pathophysiological changes described above have functional consequences at different levels of the cardiovascular system. The major effects of the aging process on the cardiovascular phenotype are discussed below.

3.1. *Heart rate*

Resting heart rate decreases slightly or remains unchanged in older individuals. However, the maximal heart rate response to exercise is reduced by ~25%. The causes include a decrease in the number of sinus node cells, a loss/decreased responsiveness of the beta-adrenoceptors, or a vagal neuropathy (Lombardi et al., 1997; Lakatta, 1999). Significant reductions in heart rate variability (HRV) as well as in the complexity of heart rate (based on chaos theory) have been consistently noted in elderly individuals (Lipsitz and Goldberger, 1992; Lombardi et al., 1997). The effects of age on heart rate and heart rate variance at rest and during head-up tilt are shown in Fig. 7.

3.2. *Cardiac electrophysiology*

The cardiac conduction system is affected by aging. The number of pacemaker cells in the sinus node diminishes (see above), together with degenerative changes in the atrio-ventricular node and the Purkinje system. All these changes predispose to rhythm and conduction disturbances, such as sick sinus syndrome or atrio-ventricular block. Interestingly, an increase in the electrocardiographic P-R interval has been associated with cardiovascular morbidity and mortality in the elderly (Bernstein et al., 1997). One specific consequence of aging of the atrio-ventricular node is the occurrence of atrio-ventricular nodal tachycardias (Crijns and Van Gelder, 1997).

Another type of arrhythmia commonly observed in the elderly population is atrial fibrillation, which results from dilatation and degeneration of the atria. It is more frequent in elderly patients with underlying structural heart disease.

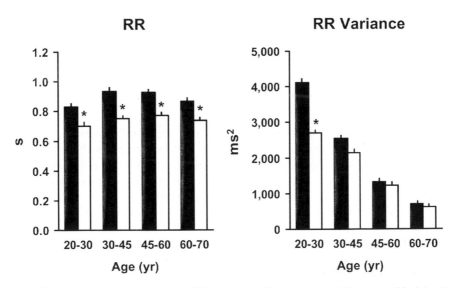

Fig. 7.   Effects of age on mean heart rate (RR interval) and heart rate variance at rest (black bars) and during 90° head-up tilt (empty bars) (adapted with permission from Lombardi et al., 1997).

Ventricular arrhythmias (ranging from ventricular premature beats to non-sustained ventricular tachycardia) are also more frequent in the elderly. As with atrial fibrillation, the occurrence of ventricular arrhythmias is often related to the presence of underlying cardiovascular disease. However, their prognostic value in healthy aged individuals is uncertain (Podrid, 1997).

3.3. *Ventricular function*

Although aging myocardium is characterized by a loss of myocytes (due to apoptosis or necrosis), ventricular mass is slightly increased or unchanged. This is due to reactive cellular hypertrophy in response to myocyte loss (Olivetti et al., 1991). Sometimes the process of reactive hypertrophy is asymmetric (not uniform), changing the shape of the ventricular cavity and the outflow tract, which may lead to hemodynamic instability during periods of altered ventricular loading. The myocyte loss is accompanied by varying degrees of amyloid deposition and continuing production of collagen by fibroblasts, which leads to an increase in stiffness and a decrease in ventricular compliance.

These structural effects of aging are accompanied by functional changes in myocytes. Most notably, intracellular calcium regulation is impaired consequent on changes in the Na–Ca exchanger (Koban et al., 1998) or the sarcoplasmic reticulum Ca^{2+} ATPase (SERCA) with age (Lakatta, 1993). A decrease in the cardiac SERCA 2a isoform leads to lower levels of SERCA 2a protein and impaired myocardial function (mainly diastolic dysfunction). Diminished myocardial contraction velocity seen with aging may be related to changes in the expression of various myosin heavy chain isoforms (Lakatta, 1999). Another important factor that modifies mechanical performance of the aged heart is prolongation of cellular action potential (due to changes in the magnitude or gating of membrane ion channels). Importantly, age-related desensitization of cardiac adrenoceptors and their second messenger systems (as discussed earlier) decreases contractile responses of the heart to adrenergic stimulation (Xiao et al., 1994). Altered myocardial energy metabolism and reduced mitochondrial ATP production also play a role.

All these structural and functional effects of aging influence the hemodynamic performance of the heart. Cardiac output at rest remains unchanged (Lakatta, 1993, 1999). Contractile force of the aged heart is not markedly affected at rest and the increase in afterload is compensated for by myocardial hypertrophy. The heart rate and inotropic response to exercise are blunted, but cardiac output during exercise is relatively preserved through the Frank–Starling mechanism (with an increase in end-diastolic volume).

A hallmark of the aging heart is prolonged myocardial contraction and relaxation, related to changes in intracellular calcium homeostasis. Left ventricular end-diastolic pressure is increased both at rest and during exercise, with a reduction in early-phase diastolic filling. The latter falls linearly with age at a rate of 6–7% per decade (Schulman, 1999) and is thought to reflect diastolic dysfunction. In the absence of other underlying cardiovascular diseases, a minority of elderly patients (perhaps those with more severe age-related changes) develop clinical diastolic heart failure (i.e. heart failure with normal or increased ejection fraction) (Schulman, 1999). Progression from diastolic dysfunction to diastolic heart failure may be accelerated during tachycardia (reduced diastolic filling time) and with intravascular volume depletion or overload. Overall, diastolic dysfunction is responsible for over 50% of heart failure cases in the elderly (Senni et al., 1998; Vasan et al., 1999).

3.4. *Vascular changes*

3.4.1. *Compliance*

Degenerative changes similar to those in the myocardium (cell loss, fibrosis, etc.) occur also in the vascular wall. Large arteries dilate with medial thickening. A decrease in the elastin/collagen ratio reduces vascular compliance (distensibility), thereby increasing pulse wave velocity and leading to systolic hypertension with a wide pulse pressure. Hypertrophy of resistance arteries has also been reported. Fig. 8 demonstrates interactions between arterial and cardiac changes that occur during the aging process.

3.4.2. *Endothelial function*

Important functional changes occur in the endothelial and smooth muscle cells of the vascular system, although many of these age-related changes are confined to specific vascular beds. Impairment of endothelium-dependent vasodilatation has been well documented in humans. Most notably, aging decreases both basal and

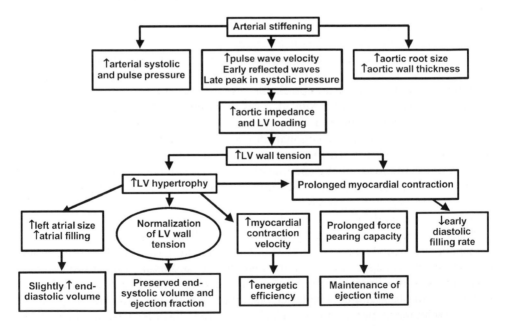

Fig. 8.   Structural and functional effects of age-related arterial and cardiac alterations (adapted with permission from Lakatta, 1999).

stimulated release of nitric oxide (NO) (Gerhard et al., 1996; Marin and Rodriguez-Martinez, 1999; Andrawis et al., 2000; Taddei et al., 2000, 2001), suggesting that aging causes dysfunction of the NO system and influences NO-mediated relaxation. This effect of aging may be related to increased oxidative stress (causing NO breakdown in the presence of reactive oxygen species), a decrease in NO synthesis, changes in second messenger systems (G protein, cGMP) or changes at the receptor level. Impaired access of NO to smooth muscle cells (due to vascular wall thickening) has also been proposed.

The release of another vasodilator by the endothelium, the endothelium-derived hyperpolarizing factor (EDHF), is also impaired by aging (Urakami-Harasawa et al., 1997). In addition, the aging process increases the release of some vasoconstrictor mediators, such as endothelin or cyclooxygenase products (thromboxane A2, prostaglandin H2) (Luscher et al., 1992; Matz et al., 2000; Stewart et al., 2000), although the sensitivity to endothelin may decrease, especially in small resistance arteries. Also, the production of prostacyclin (an endothelial vasodilator) may be actually increased (Ishihata et al., 1999). Overall, it seems that aging alters the production of and/or the sensitivity to endothelium-derived relaxing and constricting factors in favor of vasoconstriction.

Endothelium-independent vasomotion is also affected by aging. This is mainly due to cellular desensitization to beta- and, possibly, alpha-adrenergic stimulation, occurring at the level of the receptors themselves as well as at downstream intracellular levels. In some vascular beds, decreased relaxation in response to calcitonin gene-related peptide or nitroprusside has been reported (Marin and Rodriguez-Martinez, 1999).

3.4.3. *Atherosclerosis*

A very important aspect of aging of the vascular system is atherosclerosis. It is related to many of the factors mentioned above, such as oxidative stress, endothelial dysfunction, hyperlipidemia, hypertension, neuroendocrine changes, etc. Not surprisingly, therefore, atherosclerotic changes in blood vessels arc almost universally present in the elderly population. Atherosclerosis of the vascular wall leads to further impairment of vascular function and is the single main cause of increased morbidity and mortality in the elderly. The most devastating sequelae of progressing atherosclerosis are myocardial infarction and stroke. The exact causes and mechanisms of age-related atherosclerosis will be discussed in more detail in other chapters.

3.4.4. *Isolated systolic hypertension*

One consequence of thickening and hardening of the artery wall with aging is a change in the hemodynamic profile. Population studies have revealed a compelling and consistent difference in the age-related changes in systolic and diastolic blood pressures. This dichotomy is illustrated in Fig. 9 and demonstrates that, after the age of 50–59 years, there is a progressive and marked increase in systolic blood pressure, whereas diastolic blood pressure declines (Burt et al., 1995). This age-related differential effect on systolic and diastolic pressures holds true for both men and women. The clinical consequence is that the vast majority of hypertension in the

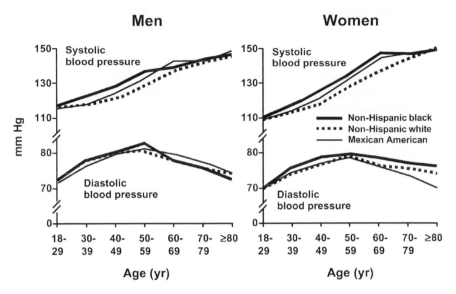

Fig. 9.   Changes in systolic and diastolic blood pressures with age in the US population (adapted with permission from Burt et al., 1995).

elderly consists of isolated systolic hypertension (Wilking et al., 1988) (Fig. 10), which is strongly linked to an increase in acute cardiac and vascular events. Treatment of isolated systolic hypertension elicits an early and sustained decrease in acute cardiovascular presentations (The SHEP Cooperative Research Group, 1991; Staessen et al., 1997).

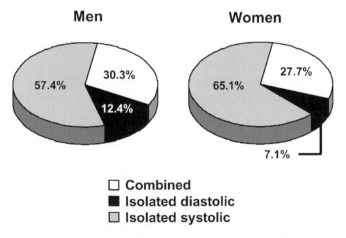

Fig. 10.   Distribution of hypertension among Framingham heart study elderly aged 65–89 years (adapted with permission from Wilking et al., 1988).

3.5. *Orthostatic intolerance*

In healthy young people, the immediate decrease in blood pressure and cardiac filling pressure that occurs after standing leads to carotid and cardiopulmonary baroreceptor unloading, resulting in sympathetic activation, with peripheral vasoconstriction and increased heart rate and cardiac output. These reflex autonomic mechanisms stabilize and maintain blood pressure during standing. Malfunction in one or more of these reflex mechanisms and vascular responses has been implicated in orthostatic hypotension, which is especially common in the elderly (Applegate et al., 1991; Rutan et al., 1992). The mechanisms of orthostatic intolerance in the elderly include cardiac dysfunction, autonomic dysfunction, impaired baroreceptor function, attenuated vascular responses or reduced intravascular volume. Autonomic dysfunction and orthostatic intolerance in the elderly may lead to decreased physical activity, and decreased activity may predispose to autonomic dysfunction. Orthostatic hypotension in the elderly may increase cardiovascular risk (i.e. the more marked the blood pressure fall on standing, the greater the cardiovascular risk) (Rose et al., 2000). It is possible, therefore, that this component of aging of neurocirculatory and vasoconstrictor control mechanisms may contribute to eventual cardiovascular events.

4. Conclusions

Aging is a complex and poorly understood process that represents the integrated effect of multiple interrelated mechanisms. It is clear that advancing age is accompanied by unequivocal changes in cardiac and vascular structure and function and predisposition to the development of acute and chronic cardiovascular diseases (such as hypertension, coronary artery disease, stroke, heart failure, and orthostatic hypotension). Aging also predisposes to co-existing medical conditions, which may influence the process of cardiovascular aging. Reduced activity due to arthritis, for example, may further accelerate the progression of cardiovascular aging, and vice versa. Hypertension causes "premature aging" of endothelial function. On the other hand, both morbidity and mortality are dramatically increased when the aging process is associated with hypertension. This is also true for diabetes, heart failure, etc.

It is not known whether the cardiovascular pathology represents an inevitable eventual consequence of "physiologic aging" or whether the development of cardiovascular disease is in fact the result of the interaction between behavioral, environmental, and other influences disrupting the "physiologic aging" process. What is known is that the mechanisms involved in aging are very often those that also contribute to cardiovascular diseases even in young individuals. Whether interventions targeted at interrupting these mechanisms will attenuate age-related changes in cardiovascular structure and function, and hence delay the development of cardiac and vascular disease, is not clear.

Research on aging has already changed dramatically our approach to the clinical management of cardiovascular diseases in the elderly. For example, recent dogma held that "normal" systolic blood pressure in older patients should be 100 + age mm Hg.

On the contrary, it is now recognized that systolic blood pressure greater than 140 mm Hg in the elderly confers increased cardiovascular risk, which is strikingly reduced by lowering systolic blood pressure (Guidelines Subcommittee, 1999). An analogous situation is also evident in the treatment of hyperlipidemia. In contrast to past acceptance of high cholesterol in older people as part of "normal aging", we now find that it is in the old patient with dyslipidemia in whom the benefit of pharmacologic intervention is most striking (Kagansky et al., 2001). Therapeutic interventions of proven cardiac and vascular benefit, such as lipid lowering and anti-hypertensive therapy, may have even greater benefits in elderly than in young individuals, in part because acute cardiac and vascular events occur earlier and more frequently in old as compared to young subjects.

The altered physiology of the aged myocardium and vasculature affects the clinical course, prognosis and medical treatment of various cardiovascular diseases. Further research in this area holds great promise for ameliorating disease and improving quality of life in the aging population. Understanding the mechanisms of physiologic aging and age-associated disease processes, and identifying appropriate therapeutic strategies, may yield the greatest cost benefit in the practice of 21st century medicine.

References

Abete, P., Napoli, C., Santoro, G., Ferrara, N., Tritto, I., Chiariello, M., Rengo, F., Ambrosio, G., 1999. Age-related decrease in cardiac tolerance to oxidative stress. J. Mol. Cell Cardiol. 31, 227–236.

Andrawis, N., Jones, D.S., Abernethy, D.R., 2000. Aging is associated with endothelial dysfunction in the human forearm vasculature. J. Am. Geriatr. Soc. 48, 193–198.

Applegate, W.B., Davis, B.R., Black, H.R., Smith, W.M., Miller, S.T., Burlando, A.J., 1991. Prevalence of postural hypotension at baseline in the Systolic Hypertension in the Elderly Program (SHEP) cohort. J. Am. Geriatr. Soc. 39, 1057–1064.

Benetos, A., Okuda, K., Lajemi, M., Kimura, M., Thomas, F., Skurnick, J., Labat, C., Bean, K., Aviv, A., 2001. Telomere length as an indicator of biological aging: the gender effect and relation with pulse pressure and pulse wave velocity. Hypertension 37, 381–385.

Bernstein, J.M., Frishman, W.H., Chang, C.J., 1997. Value of ECG P-R and Q-Tc interval prolongation and heart rate variability for predicting cardiovascular morbidity and mortality in the elderly: the Bronx Aging Study. Cardiol. Elderly 5, 31–41.

Bliwise, D.L., 1994. Normal aging. In: Kryger, M.H., Roth, T., Dement, W.C. (Eds.), Principles and Practice of Sleep Medicine. WB Saunders, Philadelphia, pp. 26–39.

Bodnar, A.G., Ouellette, M., Frolkis, M., Holt, S.E., Chiu, C.P., Morin, G.B., Harley, C.B., Shay, J.W., Lichtsteiner, S., Wright, W.E., 1998. Extension of life-span by introduction of telomerase into normal human cells. Science 279, 349–352.

Brod, S.A., 2000. Unregulated inflammation shortens human functional longevity. Inflamm. Res. 49, 561–570.

Bunker, V.W., 1992. Free radicals, antioxidants and ageing. Med. Lab. Sci. 49, 299–312.

Bursztyn, M., Ginsberg, G., Hammerman-Rozenberg, R., Stessman, J., 1999. The siesta in the elderly: risk factor for mortality? Arch. Intern. Med. 159, 1582–1586.

Bursztyn, M., Ginsberg, G., Stessman, J., 2002. The siesta and mortality in the elderly: effect of rest without sleep and daytime sleep duration. Sleep 25, 187–191.

Burt, V.L., Whelton, P., Roccella, E.J., Brown, C., Cutler, J.A., Higgins, M., Horan, M.J., Labarthe, D., 1995. Prevalence of hypertension in the US adult population. Results from the Third National Health and Nutrition Examination Survey, 1988–1991. Hypertension 25, 305–313.

Caruso, C., Candore, G., Romano, G.C., Lio, D., Bonafe, M., Valensin, S., Franceschi, C., 2000. HLA, aging, and longevity: a critical reappraisal. Hum. Immunol. 61, 942–949.

Cefalu, W.T., 2001. Insulin resistance: cellular and clinical concepts. Exp. Biol. Med. 226, 13–26.

Chang, E., Harley, C.B., 1995. Telomere length and replicative aging in human vascular tissues. Proc. Natl. Acad. Sci. USA 92, 11190–11194.

Colao, A., Marzullo, P., Di Somma, C., Lombardi, G., 2001. Growth hormone and the heart. Clin. Endocrinol. 54, 137–154.

Cottrell, D.A., Turnbull, D.M., 2000. Mitochondria and ageing. Curr. Opin. Clin. Nutr. Metab. Care 3, 473–478.

Crijns, H.J.G.M., Van Gelder, I.C., 1997. Age-related changes in electrophysiology of the atrioventricular node and electrocardiographic manifestations. Cardiol. Elderly 5, 3–8.

D'Armiento, F.P., Bianchi, A., de Nigris, F., Capuzzi, D.M., D'Armiento, M.R., Crimi, G., Abete, P., Palinski, W., Condorelli, M., Napoli, C., 2001. Age-related effects on atherogenesis and scavenger enzymes of intracranial and extracranial arteries in men without classic risk factors for atherosclerosis. Stroke 32, 2472–2480.

De Benedictis, G., Falcone, E., Rose, G., Ruffolo, R., Spadafora, P., Baggio, G., Bertolini, S., Mari, D., Mattace, R., Monti, D., Morellini, M., Sansoni, P., Franceschi, C., 1997. DNA multiallelic systems reveal gene/longevity associations not detected by diallelic systems. The APOB locus. Hum. Genet. 99, 312–318.

De Benedictis, G., Rose, G., Carrieri, G., De Luca, M., Falcone, E., Passarino, G., Bonafe, M., Monti, D., Baggio, G., Bertolini, S., Mari, D., Mattace, R., Franceschi, C., 1999. Mitochondrial DNA inherited variants are associated with successful aging and longevity in humans. FASEB J. 13, 1532–1536.

Duckworth, W.C., 2001. Hyperglycemia and cardiovascular disease. Curr. Atheroscler. Rep. 3, 383–391.

Ericsson, S., Eriksson, M., Vitols, S., Einarsson, K., Berglund, L., Angelin, B., 1991. Influence of age on the metabolism of plasma low density lipoproteins in healthy males. J. Clin. Invest. 87, 591–596.

Finch, C.E., Tanzi, R.E., 1997. Genetics of aging. Science 278, 407–411.

Finkel, T., Holbrook, N.J., 2000. Oxidants, oxidative stress and the biology of ageing. Nature 408, 239–247.

Fukagawa, N.K., Li, M., Liang, P., Russell, J.C., Sobel, B.E., Absher, P.M., 1999. Aging and high concentrations of glucose potentiate injury to mitochondrial DNA. Free Radic. Biol. Med. 27, 1437–1443.

Gerhard, M., Roddy, M.A., Creager, S.J., Creager, M.A., 1996. Aging progressively impairs endothelium-dependent vasodilation forearm resistance vessels of humans. Hypertension 27, 849–853.

Green, M.S., Heiss, G., Rifkind, B.M., Cooper, G.R., Williams, O.D., Tyroler, H.A., 1985. The ratio of plasma high-density lipoprotein cholesterol to total and low-density lipoprotein cholesterol: age-related changes and race and sex differences in selected North American populations. The Lipid Research Clinics Program Prevalence study. Circulation 72, 93–104.

Guidelines Subcommittee, 1999. 1999 World Health Organization – International Society of Hypertension guidelines for the management of hypertension. J. Hypertens. 17, 151–183.

Herskind, A.M., McGue, M., Holm, N.V., Sorensen, T.I., Harvald, B., Vaupel, J.W., 1996. The heritability of human longevity: a population-based study of 2872 Danish twin pairs born 1870–1900. Hum. Genet. 97, 319–323.

Ishihata, A., Katano, Y., Nakamura, M., Doi, K., Tasaki, K., Ono, A., 1999. Differential modulation of nitric oxide and prostacyclin release in senescent rat heart stimulated by angiotensis II. Eur. J. Pharmacol. 382, 19–26.

Jazwinski, S.M., 1998. Genetics of longevity. Exp. Gerontol. 33, 773–783.

Joaquin, A.M., Gollapudi, S., 2001. Functional decline in aging and disease: a role for apoptosis. J. Am. Geriatr. Soc. 49, 1234–1240.

Jones, P.P., Shapiro, L.F., Keisling, G.A., Jordan, J., Shannon, J.R., Quaife, R.A., Seals, D.R., 2001. Altered autonomic support of arterial blood pressure with age in healthy men. Circulation 104, 2424–2429.

Kagansky, N., Levy, S., Berner, Y., Rimon, E., Knobler, H., 2001. Cholesterol lowering in the older population: time for reassessment? Q. J. Med. 94, 457–463.

Kato, M., Roberts-Thomson, P., Phillips, B.G., Haynes, W.G., Winnicki, M., Accurso, V., Somers, V.K., 2000a. Impairment of endothelium-dependent vasodilatation of resistance vessels in patients with obstructive sleep apnea. Circulation 102, 2607–2610.

Kato, M., Phillips, B.G., Sigurdsson, G., Narkiewicz, K., Pesek, C.A., Somers, V.K., 2000b. Effects of sleep deprivation on neural circulatory control. Hypertension 35, 1173–1175.

Kelly, D.T., 1997. Disease burden of cardiovascular disease in the elderly. Coron. Artery Dis. 8, 667–669.

Kelly, J., O'Malley, K., 1984. Adrenoceptor function and aging. Clin. Sci. 66, 509–515.

Kerckhoffs, D.A., Blaak, E.E., Van Baak, M.A., Saris, W.H., 1998. Effect of aging on β-adrenergically mediated thermogenesis in men. Am. J. Physiol. 274, E1075–E1079.

Koban, M.U., Moorman, A.F.M., Holtz, J., Yacoub, M.H., Boheler, K.R., 1998. Expressional analysis of the cardiac Na–Ca exchanger in rat development and senescence. Cardiovasc. Res. 37, 405–423.

Krieger, J., Sforza, E., Boudewijns, A., Zamagni, M., Petiau, C., 1997. Respiratory effort during obstructive sleep apnea. Role of age and sleep state. Chest 112, 875–884.

Kripke, D.F., Garfinkel, L., Wingard, D.L., Klauber, M.R., Marler, M.R., 2002. Mortality associated with sleep duration and insomnia. Arch. Gen. Psychiatry 59, 131–136.

Lakatta, E.G., 1993. Cardiovascular regulatory mechanisms in advanced age. Physiol. Rev. 73, 413–467.

Lakatta, E.G., 1999. Cardiovascular aging research: the next horizons. J. Am. Geriatr. Soc. 47, 613–625.

Lamberts, S.W.J., van den Beld, A.W., van der Lely, A.-J., 1997. The endocrinology of aging. Science 278, 419–424.

Lipsitz, L.A., Goldberger, A.L., 1992. Loss of "complexity" and aging. Potential applications of fractals and chaos theory to senescence. JAMA 267, 1806–1809.

Lombardi, F., Malliani, A., Pagani, M., 1997. Age-related changes in heart rate including sympathetic and parasympathetic tone. Cardiol. Elderly 5, 14–17.

Louhija, J., Miettinen, H.E., Kontula, K., Tikkanen, M.J., Miettinen, T.A., Tilvis, R.S., 1994. Aging and genetic variation of plasma apolipoproteins: relative loss of the apolipoprotein E4 phenotype in centenarians. Arterioscler. Thromb. 14, 1084–1089.

Luscher, T.F., Tanner, F.C., Dohi, Y., 1992. Age, hypertension and hypercholesterolaemia alter endothelium-dependent vascular regulation. Pharmacol. Toxicol. 70, S32–S39.

Mannucci, P.M., Mari, D., Merati, G., Peyvandi, F., Tagliabue, L., Sacchi, E., Taioli, E., Sansoni, P., Bertolini, S., Franceschi, C., 1997. Gene polymorphisms predicting high plasma levels of coagulation and fibrinolysis proteins. A study in centenarians. Arterioscler. Thromb. Vasc. Biol. 17, 755–759.

Marin, J., Rodriguez-Martinez, M.A., 1999. Age-related changes in vascular responses. Exp. Gerontol. 34, 503–512.

Martin, G.M., Oshima, J., 2000. Lessons from human progeroid syndromes. Nature 408, 263–266.

Matsukawa, T., Sugiyama, Y., Watanabe, T., Kobayashi, F., Mano, T., 1998. Gender difference in age-related changes in muscle sympathetic nerve activity in healthy subjects. Am. J. Physiol. 275, R1600–R1604.

Matz, R.L., de Sotomayor, M.A., Schott, C., Stoclet, J.C., Andriantsitohaina, R., 2000. Vascular bed heterogeneity in age-related endothelial dysfunction with respect to NO and eicosanoids. Br. J. Pharmacol. 131, 303–311.

Mazzeo, R.S., Rajkumar, C., Jennings, G., Esler, M., 1997. Norepinephrine spillover at rest and during submaximal exercise in young and old subjects. J. Appl. Physiol. 82, 1869–1874.

Mohsenin, V., 2001. Sleep-related breathing disorders and risk of stroke. Stroke 32, 1271–1278.

Monnier, V.M., Cerami, A., 1981. Nonenzymatic browning in vivo: possible process for aging of long-lived proteins. Science 211, 491–493.

Muscari, C., Giaccari, A., Giordano, E., Clo, C., Guarnieri, C., Caldarera, C.M., 1996. Role of reactive oxygen species in cardiovascular aging. Mol. Cell Biochem. 160/161, 159–166.

Narkiewicz, K., van de Borne, P.J., Montano, N., Dyken, M.E., Phillips, B.G., Somers, V.K., 1998. Contribution of tonic chemoreflex activation to sympathetic activity and blood pressure in patients with obstructive sleep apnea. Circulation 97, 943–945.

Oliven, A., Carmi, N., Coleman, R., Odeh, M., Silbermann, M., 2001. Age-related changes in upper airway muscles morphological and oxidative properties. Exp. Gerontol. 36, 1673–1686.

Olivetti, G., Melissari, M., Capasso, J.M., Anversa, P., 1991. Cardiomyopathy of the aging human heart: myocyte loss and reactive cellular hypertrophy. Circ. Res. 68, 1560–1568.

Pepe, G., Di Perna, V., Resta, F., Lovecchio, M., Chimienti, G., Colacicco, A.M., Capurso, A., 1998. In search of a biological pattern for human longevity: impact of apo A-IV genetic polymorphisms on lipoproteins and the hyper-Lp(a) in centenarians. Atherosclerosis 137, 407–417.

Perry III, H.M., 1999. The endocrinology of aging. Clin. Chem. 45, 1369–1376.

Phillips, B.G., Narkiewicz, K., Pesek, C.A., Haynes, W.G., Dyken, M.E., Somers, V.K., 1999. Effects of obstructive sleep apnea on endothelin-1 and blood pressure. J. Hypertens. 17, 61–66.

Podrid, P.J., 1997. Arrhythmias in the elderly subject. Cardiol. Elderly 5, 18–21.

Pollack, M., Leeuwenburgh, C., 2001. Apoptosis and aging: role of the mitochondria. J. Gerontol. A Biol. Sci. Med. Sci. 56, B475–B482.

Population Division, Population Projections Branch. US Census Bureau Website. http://www.census.gov/population/www/projections/popproj.html

Reaven, P.D., Napoli, C., Merat, S., Witztum, J.L., 1999. Lipoprotein modification and atherosclerosis in aging. Exp. Gerontol. 34, 527–537.

Rose, K.M., Tyroler, H.A., Nardo, C.J., Arnett, D.K., Light, K.C., Rosamond, W., Sharrett, A.R., Szklo, M., 2000. Orthostatic hypotension and the incidence of coronary heart disease: the Atherosclerosis Risk in Communities study. Am. J. Hypertens. 13, 571–578.

Rutan, G.H., Hermanson, B., Bild, D.E., Kittner, S.J., LaBaw, F., Tell, G.S., 1992. Orthostatic hypotension in older adults. The Cardiovascular Health Study. CHS Collaborative Research Group. Hypertension 19, 508–519.

Saito, H., Papaconstantinou, J., 2001. Age-associated differences in cardiovascular inflammatory gene induction during endotoxic stress. J. Biol. Chem. 276, 29307–29312.

Sastre, J., Pallardo, F.V., Garcia de la Asuncion, J., Vina, J., 2000. Mitochondria, oxidative stress and aging. Free Radic. Res. 32, 189–198.

Schachter, F., Faure-Delanef, L., Guenot, F., Rouger, H., Froguel, P., Lesueur-Ginot, L., Cohen, D., 1994. Genetic associations with human longevity at the *APOE* and *ACE* loci. Nat. Genet. 6, 29–32.

Schulman, S.P., 1999. Cardiovascular consequences of the aging process. Cardiol. Clin. 17, 35–49.

Schulz, R., Mahmoudi, S., Hattar, K., Sibelius, U., Olschewski, H., Mayer, K., Seeger, W., Grimminger, F., 2000. Enhanced release of superoxide from polymorphonuclear neutrophils in obstructive sleep apnea. Impact of continuous positive airway pressure therapy. Am. J. Respir. Crit. Care Med. 162, 566–570.

Seals, D.R., Esler, M.D., 2000. Human aging and the sympathoadrenal system. J. Physiol. 528, 407–417.

Senni, M., Tribouilloy, C.M., Rodeheffer, R.J., Jacobsen, S.J., Evans, J.M., Bailey, K.R., Redfield, M.M., 1998. Congestive heart failure in the community: a study of all incident cases in Olmsted County, Minnesota, in 1991. Circulation 98, 2282–2289.1

Senti, M., Tomas, M., Vila, J., Marrugat, J., Elosua, R., Sala, J., Masia, R., 2001. Relationship of age-related myocardial infarction risk and Gln/Arg 192 variants of the human paraoxonase1 gene: the REGICOR study. Atherosclerosis 156, 443–449.

Serra, V., Grune, T., Sitte, N., Saretzki, G., von Zglinicki, T., 2000. Telomere length as a marker of oxidative stress in primary human fibroblast cultures. Ann. NY Acad. Sci. 908, 27–30.

Shamsuzzaman, A.S., Winnicki, M., Lanfranchi, P., Wolk, R., Kara, T., Accurso, V., Somers, V.K., 2002. Elevated C-reactive protein in patients with obstructive sleep apnea. Circulation 105, 2462–2464.

Smiley, T., Oh, P., Shane, L.G., 2001. The relationship of insulin resistance measured by reliable indexes to coronary artery disease risk factors and outcomes – a systematic review. Can. J. Cardiol. 17, 797–805.

Spiegel, K., Leproult, R., Van Cauter, E., 1999. Impact of sleep debt on metabolic and endocrine function. Lancet 354, 1435–1439.

Staessen, J.A., Fagard, R., Thijs, L., Celis, H., Arabidze, G.G., Birkenhager, W.H., Bulpitt, C.J., de Leeuw, P.W., Dollery, C.T., Fletcher, A.E., Forette, F., Leonetti, G., Nachev, C., O'Brien, E.T., Rosenfeld, J., Rodicio, J.L., Tuomilehto, J., Zanchetti, A., 1997. Randomised double-blind comparison of placebo and active treatment for older patients with isolated systolic hypertension. The Systolic Hypertension in Europe (Syst-Eur) Trial Investigators. Lancet 350, 757–764.

Stewart, K.G., Zhang, Y., Davidge, S.T., 2000. Aging increases PGHS-2-dependent vasoconstriction in rat mesenteric arteries. Hypertension 35, 1242–1247.

Taddei, S., Galetta, F., Virdis, A., Ghiadoni, L., Salvetti, G., Franzoni, F., Giusti, C., Salvetti, A., 2000. Physical activity prevents age-related impairment in nitric oxide availability in elderly athletes. Circulation 101, 2896–2901.

Taddei, S., Virdis, A., Ghiadoni, L., Salvetti, G., Bernini, G., Magagna, A., Salvetti, A., 2001. Age-related reduction of NO availability and oxidative stress in humans. Hypertension 38, 274–279.

The SHEP Cooperative Research Group, 1991. Prevention of stroke by antihypertensive drug treatment in older persons with isolated systolic hypertension: final results of the Systolic Hypertension in the Elderly Program (SHEP). JAMA 265, 3255–3264.

Urakami-Harasawa, L., Shimokawa, H., Nakashima, M., Egashira, K., Takeshita, A., 1997. Importance of endothelium-derived hyperpolarizing factor in human arteries. J. Clin. Invest. 100, 2793–2799.

Van Cauter, E., Leproult, R., Kupfer, D.J., 1996. Effects of gender and age on the levels and circadian rhythmicity of plasma cortisol. J. Clin. Endocrinol. Metab. 81, 2468–2473.

Van Cauter, E., Leproult, R., Plat, L., 2000. Age-related changes in slow wave sleep and REM sleep and relationship with growth hormone and cortisol levels in healthy men. JAMA 284, 861–868.

Van Remmen, H., Richardson, A., 2001. Oxidative damage to mitochondria and aging. Exp. Gerontol. 36, 957–968.

Vasan, R.S., Larson, M.G., Benjamin, E.J., Evans, J.C., Reiss, C.K., Levy, D., 1999. Congestive heart failure in subjects with normal versus reduced left ventricular ejection fraction: prevalence and mortality in a population-based cohort. J. Am. Coll. Cardiol. 33, 1948–1955.

von Faber, M., Bootsma-van der Wiel, A., van Exel, E., Gussekloo, J., Lagaay, A.M., van Dongen, E., Knook, D.L., van der Geest, S., Westendorp, R.G., 2001. Successful aging in the oldest old: who can be characterized as successfully aged? Arch. Intern. Med. 161, 2694–2700.

von Zglinicki, T., Pilger, R., Sitte, N., 2000. Accumulation of single-strand breaks is the major cause of telomere shortening in human fibroblasts. Free Radic. Biol. Med. 28, 64–74.

Wilking, S.V.B., Belanger, A., Kannel, W.B., D'Agostino, R.B., Steel, K., 1988. Determinants of isolated systolic hypertension. JAMA 260, 3451–3455.

Xiao, R.-P., Spurgeon, H.A., O'Connor, F., Lakatta, E.G., 1994. Age-associated changes in β-adrenergic modulation on rat cardiac excitation–contraction coupling. J. Clin. Invest. 94, 2051–2059.

Yen, S.S.C., Laughlin, G.A., 1998. Aging and the adrenal cortex. Exp. Gerontol. 33, 897–910.

**Advances in
Cell Aging and
Gerontology**

Lipoprotein metabolism and molecular pathogenesis of atherosclerosis

Naohiko Sakai*, Makoto Nishida, Yuji Matsuzawa and Shizuya Yamashita

Department of Internal Medicine and Molecular Science, Graduate School of Medicine, Osaka University, 2-2 B5, Yamadaoka, Suita, Osaka 565-0871, Japan

Contents

---

*Corresponding author. Tel.: +81-6-6879-3732; fax: +81-6-6879-3739.
E-mail address: naosakai@imed2.med.osaka-u.ac.jp (N. Sakai).

Advances in Cell Aging and Gerontology, vol. 11, 23–77

24

Abbreviations

ABCA1	ATP-binding cassette transporter A1
ACAT	acyl-coenzyme A:cholesterol acyltransferase
AGE	advanced glycation product
apo	apoprotein or apolipoprotein
ATP	adenosine triphosphate
AcLDL	acetylated LDL
CAD	coronary artery disease
CCR2	CC chemokine receptor 2
CE	cholesteryl ester(s)
CETP	cholesteryl ester transfer protein
CRP	C-reactive protein
CS-1	connecting segment 1
CXCR2	CXC chemokine receptor 2
EC	endothelial cell
ELAM	endothelial leukocyte adhesion molecule
eNOS	endothelial NO synthase
ER	endoplasmic reticulum
FH	familial hypercholesterolemia
GM-CSF	granulocyte/macrophage colony-stimulating factor
HDL	high-density lipoprotein
HDL-C	HDL cholesterol
HETE	hydroxyeicosatetraenoic acid
HL	hepatic lipase
HMG-CoA	3-hydroxy-3-methylglutaryl coenzyme A
ICAM-1	intercellular adhesion molecule
IDL	intermediate-density lipoprotein
IFN-γ	interferon-γ
IL	interleukin
iNOS	inducible NO synthase

LCAT	lecithin:cholesterol acyltransferase
LDL	low-density lipoprotein
LDL-C	LDL cholesterol
LO	lipoxygenase
Lp (a)	lipoprotein (a)
LPL	lipoprotein lipase
LPS	lipopolysaccharide
MARCO	macrophage receptor with collagenous structure
M-CSF	macrophage colony-stimulating factor
MCP-1	monocyte chemoattractant protein-1
MPO	myeloperoxidase
MTP	microsomal triglyceride transfer protein
NF-κB	nuclear factor-κB
NO	nitric oxide
OxLDL	oxidized LDL
PAI-1	plasminogen activator inhibitor-1
PDGF	platelet-derived growth factor
PPAR-γ	peroxisome proliferator-activated receptor-γ
RCT	reverse cholesterol transport
S1P	site-1 protease
S2P	site-2 protease
SCAP	SREBP cleavage-activating protein
SMC	smooth muscle cell
SR	scavenger receptor
SR-A	scavenger receptor class A
SR-BI	scavenger receptor class B type I
SREBP	sterol regulatory element binding protein
TG	triglyceride(s)
TGF-β	transforming growth factor-β
TNF-α	tumor necrosis factor-α
VCAM-1	vascular cell adhesion molecule
VLA4	very late antigen 4
VLDL	very low-density lipoprotein

1. Introduction

Atherosclerotic diseases, represented by coronary artery diseases (CAD) and strokes, have become one of the leading causes of death in most industrialized countries (Epstein, 1996). As a result of the increasing age of the population and decreased mortality, the prevalence of atherosclerotic diseases will increase in the elderly population. The development of atherosclerotic lesions starts even during the second and third decades of life, and the earliest type of lesion, the fatty streak, may be common even in infants and young children (Napoli et al., 1997). Therefore, it appears unlikely to be able to prevent initial lesion formation. However, the progression of intermediate atherosclerotic lesions to more advanced plaques and the development of vulnerable plaques can be slowed down, with interventions based on the current knowledge of the pathogenesis of atherosclerosis. Recent rapid advances in morphological analyses, cell and molecular biology, and genetic engineering of mice have demonstrated that atherosclerosis is not simply an inevitable degenerative consequence of aging, but rather a form of chronic inflammation resulting from interaction between modified lipoproteins, monocyte-derived macrophages, T lymphocytes, and the normal cellular elements of the arterial wall (Ross, 1999; Lusis, 2000).

The original "response to injury" hypothesis for atherogenesis first proposed in the 1980s (Ross, 1986) is now modified, and the most recent version of this hypothesis emphasizes endothelial dysfunction rather than denudation as an initiation factor (Ross, 1993). In this concept, elevated levels of plasma cholesterol and/or other risk factors are considered injurious agents that cause endothelial dysfunction. A series of inflammatory responses of arterial wall cells occur subsequent to the endothelial dysfunction. These responses involve secretion of various kinds of cytokines, chemokines, vasoactive molecules, growth factors, some enzymes, and extracellular matrix, expression of adhesion molecules, induction of cell migration, cell proliferation, cell transformation, and also apoptosis, finally resulting in the formation of atherosclerotic plaques. Nevertheless, atherosclerosis is characterized by the accumulation of lipids and fibrous elements in the large arteries, indicating an important pathological role of lipid and lipoprotein metabolism in atherogenesis. In this chapter, a molecular pathogenesis of atherosclerosis is discussed, especially relating to lipid and lipoprotein metabolisms.

2. Pathology of atherosclerosis

2.1. *Morphological alterations of normal arteries by aging*

Morphological changes of arteries have long been studied to widen our understanding of the mechanism of atherosclerosis. In general, the intima is thin, consists of loose connective tissue and glycosaminoglycans, containing few cells in children and young adults. The accumulation of glycosaminoglycans, elastic fibrils, small collagen bundles, smooth muscle cells (SMCs) and macrophages renders the intima thick with age. The process of atherosclerosis increases exponentially with age. Because the degree of atherosclerosis differs in different regions of arterial trees, it is important to know the structure and age-related changes of normal arterial trees (Bouissou et al., 1989).

Arteries are classified into elastic and muscular types by the composition of their media. Elastic-type arteries include the aorta, brachiocephalic trunk, and prescalenic subclavian, common carotid, internal mammary, and pulmonary arteries. The common iliac, extrascalenic subclavian, axillary, external carotid, coronary, and renal arteries are classified as muscular-type arteries. In the elastic-type arteries, the media is made up of parallel elastic layers, which increase in number from birth to young adult. The SMCs are surrounded by glycosaminoglycans and a small quantity of collagen in elastic-type arteries. Aging causes intimal thickening by accumulation of glycosaminoglycans and lysis of several elastic layers. These changes mean the corresponding layers of the media become part of the intima. The medial elastic layers are increasingly separated by accumulated glycosaminoglycans and collagen fibers. The artery becomes fibrous, and sometimes shows musculo-elastic or muco-elastic alterations according to the content accumulated. Proliferation of SMCs in the internal part of the media causes musculo-elastic changes, and large accumulation of glycosaminoglycans results in muco-elastic alterations.

In muscular-type arteries, the media becomes fibrous and atrophic, because the SMCs disappear and are replaced by fibroblast-like cells that produce collagens. Hyalinization of the medial layer is sometimes observed, following plasma infiltration and resulting in a homogeneous, eosinophilic media, which may become calcified (Mönckeberg's medial sclerosis).

2.2. *Classification of atherosclerotic lesions*

The classification of atherosclerotic lesions has been of interest in the study of the progression of atherosclerosis. The recent classification of atherosclerotic lesions proposed by the American Heart Association (Stary et al., 1992, 1994, 1995) is summarized in Table 1. Type I and Type II are referred to as "early lesions", Type III lesions as "intermediate lesions", and Types IV through VI as "advanced lesions". Advanced lesions are characterized by structural changes of the vascular wall that early lesions do not have.

In the initial (Type I) lesion, the intima contains atherogenic lipoprotein and scattered macrophages and foam cells. The changes are more marked in portions of

Table 1
Classification of atherosclerotic lesions

Nomenclature	Main histology	Main growth mechanism	Earliest onset	Clinical correlation
Type I (initial) lesion	Isolated macrophage foam cell	Growth mainly by lipid accumulation	From first decade	Clinically silent
Type II (fatty streak) lesion	Mainly intracellular lipid accumulation			
Type III (intermediate) lesion	Type II changes and small extracellular lipid pools		From third decade	
Type IV (atheroma) lesion	Type II changes and core of extracellular lipid			Clinically silent or overt
Type V (fibroatheroma) lesion	Lipid core and fibrotic layer, or multiple lipid cores and fibrotic layers (Va), or mainly calcified (Vb), or mainly fibrotic (Vc)	Accelerated smooth muscle and collagen increase	From fourth decade	
Type VI (complicated) lesion	Surface defect, hematoma–hemorrhage, thrombus	Thrombosis, hematoma		

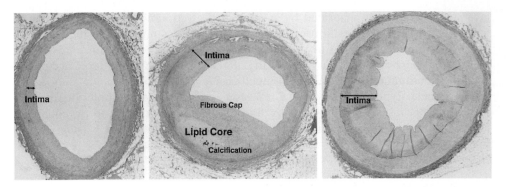

Fig. 1. Hematoxylin–eosin staining of normal and atherosclerotic coronary arteries. The left panel demon-strates a normal coronary artery. The center and the right panels show eccentric and diffuse intimal thick-ening lesions. The core lesion of the eccentric intimal thickening contains extracellular lipids and macrophages that are covered with a fibrous cap. The diffuse intimal thickening lesion mainly consists of smooth muscle cells and fibrous tissue. In this lesion, there is excessive proliferation of smooth muscle cells.

arteries with adaptive intimal thickening, which are present in everyone from birth. Type II lesions, including fatty streak lesions, consist of layers of macrophage foam cells and lipid-laden SMCs. Type III is the intermediate stage between Type II and Type IV (atheroma, a lesion that is potentially symptom-producing). Besides the change of Type II, Type III lesions contain scattered extracellular lipid droplets, preceding the larger and more disruptive core of extracellular lipid that characterizes Type IV lesions. Type V lesions, typically Type Va lesions, have a lipid core covered with thick layers of fibrous connective tissue. If fissure, hematoma, or thrombus is observed in this type, the lesion is termed Type VI. Some Type V lesions are largely calcified (Type Vb), and some consist mainly of fibrous connective tissue and little accumulated lipid (Type Vc).

A normal coronary artery is depicted in the left panel of Fig. 1. The center panel shows an atherosclerotic plaque of Type V that may rupture in the future. On the other hand, age-related intimal thickening, shown in the right panel, does not cause clinical complications if the lesion does not exhibit an excessive proliferation of SMCs or a considerable lipid deposition.

3. Lipoprotein abnormalities as a risk factor for atherosclerosis

3.1. Hypercholesterolemia

Epidemiological studies over the past 50 years have revealed numerous risk fac-tors for atherosclerosis (Table 2). These risk factors can be grouped into factors with an important genetic component and those that are largely environmental. The common forms of CAD result from the combination of an unhealthy environment, genetic susceptibility, and increased lifespan. The relative abundance of the different plasma lipoproteins appears to be of primary importance, as raised levels of

Table 2
Risk factors for development of atherosclerosis
_____

Factors with a significant genetic component
  Aging
  Male gender
  Family history
  Lipoprotein metabolism disorder
    Elevated levels of LDL, VLDL, remnant, Lp (a)
    Decreased levels of HDL
  Diabetes mellitus
  Hypertension
  Elevated levels of homocysteine
  Elevated levels of hemostatic factors
    Fibrinogen, platelet, von Willebrand factor, factor VII
  Genetic defects
    Hutchinson–Gilford syndrome
    Werner's syndrome

Environmental factors
  Smoking
  Non- or heavy alcohol intake
  Reduced exercise and physical activity
  Obesity
  Visceral fat accumulation (metabolic syndrome due to insulin resistance)
  High-fat diet
  Infection (*Chlamydia pneumoniae*, cytomegalovirus)
_____

atherogenic lipoproteins are a prerequisite for most forms of the disease. Elevated levels of serum cholesterol, especially those of low-density lipoprotein (LDL) cholesterol, are probably unique in being sufficient to drive the development of atherosclerosis in humans and animals, even in the absence of other known risk factors (Kannel et al., 1971; Iso et al., 1989; Sytkowski et al., 1990; Frohlich et al., 2001). It is exceedingly rare to have clinically significant lesions if plasma cholesterol levels are below 150 mg/dl in humans (Schonfeld, 1995). Multiple clinical trials have established the efficacy of lowering cholesterol in both primary and secondary prevention of CAD. Thus, while atherosclerosis is a complex and multifactorial disease, there can be no doubt now that elevated plasma cholesterol levels play a dominant role (The 4 S Study Group, 1994; The LIPID Study Group, 1998; Shepherd et al., 1995; Sacks et al., 1996; Downs et al., 1998). On the other hand, even among individuals with the same cholesterol levels, there is great disparity in the expression of clinical disease (Goldbourt and Neufeld, 1986). Therefore, other factors should be also taken into consideration, even though hypercholesterolemia is important in approximately 50% of patients with cardiovascular disease.

    The most cogent illustration of the causal relation between high plasma cholesterol levels and coronary atherosclerosis is familial hypercholesterolemia (FH). The primary defect in FH is a mutation in the gene specifying the receptor for plasma LDL (Hobbs et al., 1992). Located on the surfaces of cells in the liver and other organs, the LDL receptor binds LDL and facilitates its uptake by receptor-mediated endocytosis and its delivery to lysosomes, where the LDL is degraded and its cholesterol is released for metabolic use. When LDL receptors are deficient, the rate of removal of LDL from plasma declines, and the level of LDL rises in inverse proportion to receptor number. The excess of plasma LDL is deposited in scavenger cells and other cell types, which produces xanthomas and atheromas. As a consequence, cardiac atherosclerosis involving the supravalvular aorta and the coronary arteries is rapidly progressive, leading to angina pectoris, myocardial infarction, or sudden death before age 30 in homozygous individuals (Goldstein et al., 2001).

The disorder of the lipid or lipoprotein metabolism plays an important role in any stage of atherosclerosis, including initiation, progression, and complication. The accumulation of lipids and fibrous elements within the arterial wall, intracellularly and extracellularly, is undoubtedly one of the characteristics of the process of atherosclerosis. A recent hypothesis is that atherosclerosis is a form of chronic inflammation resulting from interaction between modified lipoproteins, monocyte-derived macrophages, T cells, and the normal cellular elements of the arterial wall (Ross, 1993; Glass and Witztum, 2001). LDL retained in the arterial wall and subsequently modified, especially oxidized, is a trigger of this series of inflammatory processes. Hypercholesterolemia also renders the plaque susceptible to rupture, resulting in thrombus formation that causes clinically important complications.

3.2. Hypertriglyceridemia

The contribution of elevated plasma triglyceride (TG) levels as a risk factor for atherosclerosis has been elusive. A major reason is that TG-rich lipoproteins are very heterogeneous in size, properties, origin, and metabolic fate. Therefore, the relation of hypertriglyceridemia to atherosclerosis depends on the elevated TG-rich lipoprotein species in the plasma.

Studies have consistently shown an inverse relationship between lipoprotein particle size and the capacity of the lipoprotein to enter the arterial wall. As such, certain TG-rich lipoproteins are atherogenic, whereas others are not. For example, large chylomicrons and very low-density lipoproteins (VLDLs) are not considered as proatherogenic because they cannot penetrate the arterial intima to initiate the atherosclerosis. However, the atherogenic potential of the subset of TG-rich lipoproteins known as remnant lipoproteins has been studied since the early 1980s (Kameda et al., 1984).

Remnant lipoproteins are products of the lipolytic degradation of TG-rich lipoproteins produced by the liver (VLDL) and the intestine (chylomicrons) that are reduced in size, partially depleted of TG, and enriched with cholesteryl esters (CEs). A considerable body of evidence indicates that remnant lipoproteins enriched in CEs and apo E are particularly atherogenic (Krauss, 1998; Hodis, 1999). The atherogenicity of remnant lipoproteins is often discussed with relation to postprandial hyperlipidemia. A number of reports point to an association between impaired metabolism of postprandial TG-rich lipoproteins and the presence or development of CAD (Karpe, 1999).

A mechanistic hypothesis linking the postprandial generation of TG-rich lipoprotein remnants to the development of atherosclerosis was formulated about 20 years ago by Zilversmit (1979). TG-rich lipoproteins may contribute to lesion progression, plaque rupture, and clinical coronary events through a variety of mechanisms. TG-rich lipoproteins are susceptible to peroxidative damage, can be taken up by macrophages directly without oxidative modification to produce foam cells, and are intimately associated with the clotting and fibrinolytic pathways, thus linking atherosclerosis and thrombosis (Karpe, 1999; Havel, 2000). In addition to the atherogenicity of TG-rich lipoprotein remnants, increased levels of small, dense LDL, reduced high-density lipoprotein (HDL) cholesterol levels (high TG–low HDL dyslipidemic state), as well as insulin resistance often accompany hypertriglyceridemia and are all considered proatherogenic (see Section 3.4).

A recent meta-analysis has also clearly shown that plasma TG levels are an independent risk factor for CAD (Hokanson and Austin, 1996). The most compelling evidence for this relation has come from clinical trials, the Bezafibrate Coronary Atherosclerosis Intervention Trial (Ericsson et al., 1996) and the Lopid Coronary Angiographic Trial (Frick et al., 1997). Results from these randomized serial coronary angiographic clinical trials that tested bezafibrate and gemfibrozil, respectively, support the growing evidence for the relationship between TG-rich lipoproteins and atherosclerosis. In these trials, a reduction in TG with essentially no change in LDL cholesterol (LDL-C) levels resulted in a reduction in the progression of coronary artery atherosclerosis in both native arteries and aortocoronary bypass grafts to a similar degree as did LDL-C lowering with the HMG-CoA reductase inhibitors. These studies suggest that TG-rich lipoprotein reduction by fibric acid derivatives results in the reduction of atherosclerosis progression, indicating the significant role of TG-rich lipoproteins in atherogenesis.

3.3. *Hypoalphalipoproteinemia*

Numerous clinical and epidemiological studies have demonstrated the inverse and independent association between HDL-cholesterol (HDL-C) and the risk of CAD (Miller and Miller, 1975; Gordon et al., 1977; Miller, 1980; Castelli et al., 1986; Abbott et al., 1988; Genest et al., 1999). It has been calculated that every 1 mg/dl increase in HDL is associated with a 2–3% lower risk of CAD. To date, it is confirmed that a low level of HDL-C is an important cardiovascular risk factor. HDLs exert various potentially antiatherogenic properties (Genest et al., 1999; Stein and Stein, 1999; von Eckardstein and Assmann, 2000). Reverse cholesterol transport (RCT) describes the metabolism and an important antiatherogenic function of HDL, namely, the HDL-mediated efflux of cholesterol from non-hepatic cells and its subsequent delivery to the liver and steroidogenic organs, in which it is used for the synthesis of lipoproteins, bile acids, vitamin D, and steroid hormones (Glomset, 1968; Fielding and Fielding, 1995; von Eckardstein et al., 2001). Distortion of RCT can favor the deposition of cholesterol within the arterial wall and thereby contribute to the development of atherosclerosis. Therefore, modulation of HDL metabolism and the RCT system might be an important target for antiatherosclerotic drug therapy (see Section 4.5).

3.4. Importance of multiple risk factor syndrome

Though the pathogenesis of atherosclerosis is complicated, substantial efforts have been made to identify and treat independent risk factors and to prevent atherosclerotic disease. Recently, the "multiple risk factor syndrome," in which multiple risks, including glucose intolerance, dyslipidemia, and hypertension, are clustered in each individual, has been recognized as a common basis of atherosclerotic disease in the industrialized countries. These include the Metabolic Syndrome X or "Syndrome X" as proposed by Reaven (Reaven and Hoffman, 1987) and the deadly quartet proposed by Kaplan (1989). Insulin resistance is believed to play a key role in the multiple risk factor syndrome. Environmental factors such as high dietary intake and low physical activity may be factors leading to the multiple risk factor syndrome through accumulation of intra-abdominal visceral fat. Recently, one of the candidate genes for multiple risk factor syndrome, CD36, has been identified in spontaneous hypertensive rats and humans (see Section 6.3).

Obesity is one of the most common risk factors for atherosclerotic diseases. Previous studies have demonstrated that the fat distribution, rather than total fat mass, is more closely related to the severity of obesity-related metabolic complications. The classification based on the amount of intra-abdominal visceral fat is most appropriate for predicting the association of obesity-related metabolic complications. In fact, a number of clinical studies have demonstrated the contribution of visceral fat accumulation to the development of metabolic disorders, including glucose intolerance and hyperlipidemia (Fujioka et al., 1987; Matsuzawa et al., 1987). Visceral fat accumulation is associated with not only quantitative change in serum lipid and lipoprotein but also qualitative changes in lipoproteins, such as the appearance of small, dense LDL particles, which may be related to the high TG and low HDL dyslipidemic state found in visceral fat obesity (Depres, 1991). In addition, visceral fat accumulation is often associated with insulin resistance or a hyperinsulinemic state. As a consequence of these metabolic disorders with insulin resistance, visceral fat accumulation has causative effects on CAD. Thus, visceral fat obesity is characterized by high-risk obesity with multiple complications, including insulin resistance and disorders of glucose and lipid metabolism and hypertension (Matsuzawa et al., 2002).

Interestingly, visceral fat accumulation is related to the development of both metabolic disorders and circulatory disorders even in normal-weight subjects (Nakamura et al., 1994; Matsuzawa et al., 1995). Thus, a disease entity, "visceral fat syndrome," is proposed for those with visceral fat accumulation associated with glucose intolerance, hyperlipidemia, and hypertension, irrespective of absolute body weight. Visceral fat obesity, or the visceral fat syndrome, coincides with the Metabolic Syndrome X or the deadly quartet, which is susceptible to atherosclerosis by the clustering of plural risk factors. In these syndromes, insulin resistance may be involved in various disorders, but visceral fat accumulation may be upstream of insulin resistance and may contribute to the onset of morbidity independent of insulin resistance.

More recently, it was demonstrated that adipocytes synthesize and secrete biologically active molecules, such as complements or cytokines. Adipose tissues not only act as an organ for energy storage, but also act as an endocrine organ or an organ that secretes cytokines, and these molecules are named "adipocytokines" (Matsuzawa et al., 2002). Adiponectin is an atheroprotective molecule secreted from adipocytes, and its decreased levels are associated with CAD (Maeda et al., 1996; Ouchi et al., 2001). Plasminogen activator inhibitor-1 (PAI-1) is also secreted from adipocytes, especially from visceral fat, and increased PAI-1 levels are associated with visceral fat obesity, which may accelerate the development of atherosclerosis (Shimomura et al., 1996). Thus, visceral fat accumulation enhances the development of atherosclerosis through its association with the multiple risk factor syndrome and its secretion of molecules related to atherogenesis.

4. Metabolic pathways of plasma lipoproteins

4.1. *Structure and classification of plasma lipoproteins*

The current knowledge of the process of lipid transport in the blood owes much to discoveries of major gene mutations affecting the apolipoproteins, the key enzymes and transfer proteins that control lipid transport, and cellular receptors that recognize specific apolipoproteins. Despite extraordinary advances during the past decade, the basis of much of the variation in lipoprotein concentrations among humans remains poorly understood. However, the primary structure of almost all the proteins that direct the processes of lipid transport in plasma is now known.

To make the most appropriate and effective clinical choices for patients at risk of cardiovascular disease, a basic understanding of the metabolism of the plasma lipoproteins, and the major lipids that they transport, cholesterol and TGs, is of primary importance. Because the metabolism of the plasma lipoproteins is highly interrelated, one must consider each of the lipoproteins and their subclasses to optimize the complete lipid profile, rather than focusing on only one or two lipo-proteins, as was common in the past.

The lipoproteins normally present in plasma vary widely in size, but virtually all but the smallest appear to be microemulsions (Edelstein et al., 1979; Gotto et al., 1986). Lipoprotein particles are thus spherical and contain a central core of non-polar lipids (primarily TGs and CEs) and a surface monolayer of polar lipids (primarily phospholipid and unesterified cholesterol) and protein moieties called apoproteins or apolipoproteins. Most of the apoproteins (A-I, A-II, A-IV, C-I, C-II, C-III and E) have amphipathic (detergent-like) properties. With the exception of the apoprotein (apo) B, the apoproteins, together with unesterified cholesterol, have appreciable water stability and can be exchanged readily between lipoprotein particles or with other lipid surfaces in the blood circulation. Phospholipids and the non-polar lipids have little potential for exchange, and are transferred between lipoproteins by specific transfer proteins.

The density of lipoprotein particles is inversely related to their size, reflecting the relative contents of low-density, non-polar core lipid, and high-density surface protein. Based on density and certain compositional and functional properties, the lipoproteins are usually separated into several classes (Havel and Kane, 2001). The two largest classes contain mainly TGs in their cores. These are the chylomicrons, secreted from absorptive enterocytes, in which the B apoprotein is primarily or exclusively apo B-48 (Chan et al., 1997), and the VLDLs, secreted by hepatocytes, which contain apo B-100. The B apoproteins (B-100 and B-48) are by far the largest of the apoproteins and the products of a single gene. LDL, HDL_2, and HDL_3 contain mainly CEs in their cores. The mature forms of these particles are not secreted directly from cells but rather are produced by metabolic processes within the blood plasma. LDL is mainly produced as the end product of the metabolism of VLDL. Components of HDL are secreted with chylomicrons and VLDL, as well as independently as HDL precursors (nascent HDL). Intermediate-density lipoproteins (IDLs), which contain appreciable amounts of both TGs and CEs in their core, are produced during the conversion of VLDL to LDL. Lipoprotein (a), Lp (a), is present in highly variable amounts in plasma. It is composed of a particle of LDL complexed via disulfide bonding to a large, polymorphic glycoprotein, apo (a) (Utermann, 2001).

LDL, VLDL, and Lp (a) are the three major apo B-containing lipoproteins found in blood. Elevated blood levels of these lipoproteins as well as IDL can promote atherosclerosis. When these lipoproteins cross over the endothelial cell barrier, enter the vessel wall, and are retained in proteoglycans, they can become oxidized, and then are taken up by macrophages, resulting in the formation of foam cells. The apoprotein component of Lp (a), apo (a), can also promote thrombosis by interfering with the conversion of plasminogen to plasmin on the surface of endothelial cells (Utermann, 2001). HDL is considered to have atheroprotective roles by inhibiting oxidation of LDL and cholesterol removal from lipid-laden macrophages in a process known as reverse cholesterol transport (von Eckardstein et al., 2001). Chylomicron and its remnant, chylomicron remnant, are lipoproteins that transfer dietary or exogenous lipid. Recent studies emphasize the atherogenic property of chylomicron remnants in relation to postprandial hyperlipidemia (Parks, 2001; Ginsberg and Illingworth, 2001).

4.2. *LDL receptor pathway and cellular cholesterol homeostasis*

Familial hypercholesterolemia results from a mutation that affects the structure and function of LDL receptor on cell surfaces (see Section 3.1). The disorder is characterized clinically by a lifelong elevation in the concentration of LDL-cholesterol in blood, leading to premature CAD, pathologically by cholesterol deposits that form xanthomas, arcus corneae, and coronary atherosclerotic plaques, and genetically by autosomal dominant inheritance (Goldstein et al., 2001).

Using cultured fibroblasts from homozygous FH to define the basic biochemical defect, Brown and Goldstein, in the 1970s (Brown et al., 1975), discovered the cell-surface LDL receptor and demonstrated that FH is caused by mutations in the gene specifying this receptor. The LDL receptor is a member of an expanding gene family, most of which bind lipoproteins through apo E. The LDL receptor binds apo B-100 as well as apo E, and thus mediates the endocytosis of partially catabolized VLDL, IDL, and LDL. Like other receptors that mediate macromolecular endocytosis, the

LDL receptor is a transmembrane protein. The lipoprotein particles bound to the receptor via apo B-100 or apo E are endocytosed via coated pits on the plasma membrane. The lipoproteins dissociate from the receptor in the acidic internal environment of endosomes and are eventually catabolized in secondary lysosomes (Goldstein et al., 2001; Goldstein and Brown, 2001).

The cholesterol derived from the lysosomal hydrolysis of LDL's cholesteryl esters mediates a sophisticated system of feedback control that stabilizes the intracellular cholesterol concentration. First, this cholesterol suppresses the activity of 3-hydroxy-3-methylglutaryl coenzyme A reductase (HMG-CoA reductase), the rate-limiting enzyme in cholesterol biosynthesis, thereby turning off cholesterol synthesis in the cell. Second, the cholesterol activates a cholesterol-esterifying enzyme called acyl-coenzyme A:cholesterol acyltransferase (ACAT), so that excess cholesterol can be stored as cholesteryl esters. Third, the cholesterol turns off the synthesis of the LDL receptor, preventing further entry of LDL, thereby protecting cells against an overaccumulation of cholesterol (Goldstein et al., 2001).

The receptor separates from the endosome in prelysosomal compartments and recycles to the cell surface. The number of LDL receptors in cells is tightly regulated by the availability of cholesterol. Excess cellular cholesterol inhibits the proteolytic release from the endoplasmic reticulum (ER) of soluble domains of transcription factors called sterol regulatory element binding proteins (SREBPs), which down-regulate transcription of the LDL receptor and cholesterol biosynthetic enzymes (Yokoyama et al., 1993). These events contribute to the maintenance of cellular cholesterol concentrations within narrow limits.

The SREBPs are unique among transcription factors because they are membrane-bound molecules whose activity is controlled by sterol-regulated proteolysis (Brown et al., 2000). Accumulation of cholesterol suppresses the proteolytic release of the transcriptionally active amino-terminal fragment of SREBP from the membrane-bound precursor. In response to cellular demand for cholesterol, the precursor is cleaved sequentially at two locations to release the soluble transcription factor domain that then translocates to the nucleus to stimulate the transcription of target genes. The first cleavage, which is directly regulated by sterols, occurs at site-1 within the luminal loop. This cleavage is carried out by a membrane-bound, subtilisin-like serine protease termed site-1 protease (S1P) (Sakai et al., 1998; Brown and Goldstein, 1999). Cleavage of SREBP by S1P absolutely requires the activity of SREBP cleavage-activating protein (SCAP) (Rawson et al., 1999). After site-1 cleavage, the intermediate form of SREBP remains bound to the membrane by virtue of its single remaining membrane-spanning domain. Site-2 protease (S2P), a large, hydrophobic, integral membrane protein with the characteristics of a zinc metallo-protease, cleaves the intermediate form of SREBP at site-2 (Rawson et al., 1997). This second cleavage releases the soluble, transcriptionally active amino-terminal domain of SREBP, which then translocates to the nucleus and mediates the increased transcription of target genes. The most recent studies revealed that SCAP escorts SREBP from the ER to the Golgi, where cleavage at site-1 occurs, in response to cellular cholesterol demand and serves as a sterol sensor for the SREBP pathway (DeBose-Boyd et al., 1999; Nohturfft et al., 2000). In the presence of sterols, the

SCAP/SREBP complex is retained in the ER owing to interaction between the sterol-sensing domain of SCAP and an unidentified ER protein, resulting in the inhibition of cleavage at site-1 (Yang et al., 2000).

4.3. *Transport of hepatic or endogenous fat*

TG-rich VLDL is synthesized and secreted from the liver, a process that requires apo B-100. The assembly of lipids and apo B-100 takes place in ER by the action of the microsomal triglyceride transfer protein (MTP), a causative gene product of abetalipoproteinemia (Olofsson et al., 1999; Kang and Davis, 2000). In plasma, the TG in VLDL is hydrolyzed into free fatty acids and glycerol by lipoprotein lipase (LPL) with its cofactor, apo C-II (Goldberg and Merkel, 2001). This hydrolysis results in the production of smaller VLDL remnants and, ultimately, IDLs, the final remnant particles. Some of the IDL particles are removed from circulation via LDL receptors on the surface of the liver, with apo E as a ligand (Eisenberg and Sehayek, 1995; Chappell and Medh, 1998). The TGs in IDL can be hydrolyzed further by hepatic lipase (HL) to produce the final product, LDL (Santamarina-Fojo and Haudenschild, 2000). LDL is normally removed by LDL receptor-mediated uptake, mainly by the liver. The retention of LDL in the circulation and vascular wall renders it susceptible to modification. The most important LDL modification is oxidation by 12/15-lipoxygenase (LO) (Witztum and Steinberg, 2001; Gaut and Heinecke, 2001). These modified or oxidized LDLs can be recognized and taken up through scavenger receptors (SRs), such as SR-A and CD36, expressed on the surface of macrophages (Boullier et al., 2001; Febbraio et al., 2001; Linton and Fazio, 2001). Because the negative feedback mechanism does not work for SR-mediated uptake of modified lipoproteins, continuous intake of these lipoproteins results in the formation of foam cells.

4.4. *Transport of dietary or exogenous fat*

The metabolic route of dietary lipids such as TG and cholesterol from the intestine to the liver and the peripheral tissues is referred to as the exogenous pathway of lipoprotein removal. Dietary fats absorbed by the small intestine are reconstituted into chylomicrons in the intestinal epithelium (Goldstein et al., 2001). Chylomicrons are TG-rich lipoproteins synthesized to transport dietary fat and fat-soluble vitamins, and contain primarily apo B-48 and apo A-I. The apo B-48 is a truncated form of apo B-100 produced by tissue-specific editing of the apo B-100 mRNA (Chan et al., 1997; Davidson and Shelness, 2000). Apo B-48 is a major apoprotein component found only on lipoproteins in the exogenous pathway. Chylomicrons get into intestinal lymphatic capillaries after synthesis, pass through the network of mesenteric lymphatic vessels into the thoracic duct, and finally drain into the systemic blood circulation. In the thoracic lymph duct, chylomicrons acquire apo C-II and apo E. During circulation in the blood, chylomicrons are exposed to lipolysis and apoprotein exchange, resulting in conversion into chylomicron remnants (Havel, 1994; Karpe and Hamsten, 1995). Chylomicron remnants are the intermediate metabolites of chylomicrons, enriched with CE and apo E (Eisenberg and Sehayek, 1995; Chappell and Medh, 1998), and finally removed from the circulation by the liver through receptor-mediated uptake (Cooper, 1997).

A delayed removal of chylomicron remnants may promote atherogenesis. In normal patients, postprandial TG levels return to baseline within 8–10 h after an intake of dietary fat. In contrast, patients with CAD have been found to have both higher elevations of postprandial TG after a fat load and a delayed return of the TG to baseline, due to a slowed removal of chylomicron remnant particles (Patsch et al., 1992; Parks, 2001; Ginsberg and Illingworth, 2001). A diet low in total fat and saturated fats therefore remains important in patients with CAD to decrease the amount of dietary fat that must be cleared through the exogenous lipoprotein pathway and reduce the consequent elevation in chylomicron remnant particles.

4.5. *Reverse cholesterol transport and HDL metabolism*

4.5.1. *Reverse cholesterol transport*

A schematic representation of RCT and HDL metabolism is shown in Fig. 2. In this process, HDL takes up cholesterol from peripheral tissues and the cholesterol is esterified by lecithin:cholesterol acyltransferase (LCAT) on HDL (Glomset, 1968; Santamarina-Fojo et al., 2000). The produced CE is then transferred by plasma cholesteryl ester transfer protein (CETP) to apo B-containing lipoproteins (Yamashita et al., 2000, 2001). These apo B-containing lipoproteins are finally catabolized via the hepatic LDL receptor, resulting in the delivery of HDL-derived cholesterol to the liver. Alternatively, the HDL obtains apo E in the plasma or tissue, and this apo E-containing HDL is taken up directly by the liver through the LDL receptor or remnant receptor (Yamashita et al., 1990). Recent findings show that the CE moiety of HDL is selectively taken up by the liver via scavenger receptor class B type I (SR-BI) (Acton et al., 1996; Krieger, 2001). The HDL, enriched with TG after the CETP-mediated transfer of CE, is hydrolyzed by hepatic lipase and gets smaller for further cholesterol efflux from the cells (Rye et al., 1999; von Eckardstein et al., 2001). In heterogeneous HDL particles, the preβ-migrating HDL subclass may have a very potent antiatherogenic function (Castro and Fielding, 1988; Barrans et al., 1996; Thuren, 2000). Thus, HDL serves as a shuttle that transports excess cholesterol from tissue to the liver for its excretion in the RCT system.

The first step of RCT is the interaction between HDL and peripheral cells such as macrophages and fibroblasts. This step is postulated to include aqueous diffusion, lipid-free apoprotein membrane microsolubilization, and SR-BI-mediated cholesterol flux (Ji et al., 1997; Rothblat et al., 1999; Fidge, 1999). A key insight into the molecular mechanisms responsible for cholesterol efflux resulted from studies of patients with Tangier Disease. Tangier Disease is a genetic deficiency of HDL characterized by an absence of plasma HDL and accumulation of CE in the reticuloendothelial system, with splenomegaly and enlargement of the tonsils and lymph nodes (Hoffman and Fredrickson, 1965). It had been known that HDL-mediated cholesterol efflux, as well as intracellular lipid trafficking and turnover, is impaired in Tangier fibroblasts and macrophages. Several different approaches led to the

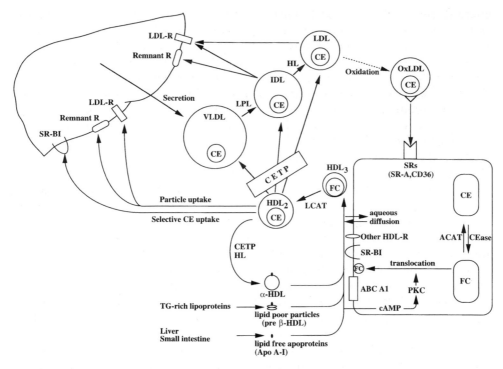

Fig. 2. Reverse cholesterol transport and HDL metabolism. ABCA1, ATP-binding cassette transporter
A1; ACAT, acyl-coenzyme A:cholesterol acyltransferase; CE, cholesteryl ester; CEase, cholesteryl esterase; CETP, cholesteryl ester transfer protein; FC, free cholesterol; HDL-R, HDL receptor; HL, hepatic
lipase; LCAT, lecithin:cholesterol acyltransferase; LPL, lipoprotein lipase; OxLDL, oxidized LDL;
PKC, protein kinase C; SR, scavenger receptor; SR-A, scavenger receptor class A; SR-BI, scavenger receptor class B type I.

identification of null mutations in ABCA1, encoding a member of the ATP-binding
cassette family of transporters, as the cause of Tangier disease (Bodzioch et al., 1999;
Brooks-Wilson et al., 1999; Lawn et al., 1999; Rust et al., 1999). This identification
demonstrated that ABCA1 mediates the first step of RCT: the transfer of cellular
cholesterol and phospholipids to lipid-poor apoproteins, mainly to apo A-I, which is
the major apoprotein of HDL. The efflux of phospholipids and cholesterol to apo A-
I synthesizes the original HDL particles. The low HDL levels seen in Tangier disease
are mainly due to an enhanced catabolism of HDL precursors containing cholesterol
poor, phospholipid- and apo A-I-rich particles (Schaefer et al., 1978). Variability in
ABCA1 expression and function due to more subtle mutations may account for at
least some of the variability of HDL levels in human populations.

ABC transporters constitute a large family of proteins present in many different
organisms, which translocate many different substrates to various compartments
(Klein et al., 1999). ABCA1 is the founding member of the ABCA superfamily
(Broccardo et al., 1999), and its identification has led to the discovery of additional

transporters, bringing the total number of ABCAs so far to 11. Amino acid alignment in combination with hydropathy analysis of the ABCA subfamily members reveals striking features unique to this subgroup of ABC transporters: first, a highly conserved hydrophobic region at the N-terminus and second, a large segment between the first ATP-binding cassette and the second transmembrane domain. The latter, the so-called regulatory domain (Luciani et al., 1994), is separated into two halves of similar size by an extra hydrophobic region. At least 14 highly conserved hydrophobic domains are predicted for the full-length ABCA proteins from hydropathy plots (Zhao et al., 2000).

With several other putative functions, ABCA1 is definitely a key player in cholesterol and phospholipid efflux from the cells, the first step of RCT (Schmitz and Langmann, 2001). Although mechanistic details remain to be defined, in vitro studies indicate that ABCA1 mediates the transport of cholesterol from cells to HDL acceptors. ABCA1 expression is sensitive to the intracellular cholesterol level in macrophages (Langmann et al., 1999; Schmitz et al., 2000; Klucken et al., 2000). Fibroblasts from human patients with Tangier disease or ABCA1 knockout mice display a nearly complete absence of apo A-I-dependent efflux of choline-phospholipids and cholesterol, suggesting that the cotransport of both lipid classes is facilitated by ABCA1 (Orso et al., 2000; Hamon et al., 2000). It is also unclear what mechanisms are involved in the process whereby ABCA1 targets specific pools of excess cellular cholesterol for secretion (Slotte et al., 1987). As one possible mechanism, the binding of apo A-I to ABCA1 or its partner protein may stimulate translocation of intracellular cholesterol and phospholipids from Golgi to plasma-membrane ABCA1 by a signal-responsive vesicular transport pathway. As another possibility, ABCA1-containing vesicles travel to intracellular lipid deposits, ABCA1 pumps lipids into the vesicle lumen, and the vesicles transport their lipid cargo back to the plasma membrane (Takahashi and Smith, 1999; Santamarina-Fojo et al., 2001).

Once the free cholesterol has been taken up from peripheral cells by HDL, it is esterified to CEs by LCAT. This esterification of free cholesterol keeps the concentration gradient of free cholesterol between HDL surface and cell surface monolayer, maintaining the continuous aqueous diffusion of cholesterol from cells to HDL (Glomset, 1968). The formed CE moiety in the core of HDL is then transported to the liver in the blood circulation. The final step of RCT, uptake of HDL-derived cholesterol to the liver, consists of three different pathways. In the first pathway, the CE is transferred by CETP from HDL to apo B-containing lipoproteins (VLDL, IDL, and LDL) in exchange for TG (Yamashita et al., 2000, 2001). These apo B-containing lipoproteins, which received cholesterol from HDL, are in turn taken up by the liver through LDL receptors and remnant receptors, resulting in the delivery of HDL-derived cholesterol to the liver. The finding that human CETP deficiency is associated with marked hyperalphalipoproteinemia (HDL-C > 100 mg/dl) indicates that this pathway is predominant in humans (Sakai et al., 1991). In the second pathway, HDL may be taken up directly as whole particles by the liver through the interaction between apo E and remnant receptors and/or LDL receptors (Yamashita et al., 1990). The last, and most dominant one in rodents, is selective uptake of HDL-CE mediated by the recently identified HDL receptor, SR-BI.

The HDL receptor SR-BI belongs to the growing CD36 family of proteins. Acton et al. (1996) made the key discovery that selective cholesterol uptake from HDL is mediated by this receptor, and characterized SR-BI as the first authentic HDL receptor. Since then, a series of in vitro and in vivo experiments have established that SR-BI is a physiologically and pathophysiologically relevant receptor for HDL metabolism (Trigatti et al., 2000; Silver and Tall, 2001). The selective uptake of HDL-CE by SR-BI accounts for ~50% of total HDL-CE clearance in rodents, which do not express CETP (Pittman and Steinberg, 1984; Glass et al., 1985). Even in rabbits that do express the CETP-mediated pathway for HDL-CE metabolism, selective CE uptake from HDL to cells accounts for approximately 20% of total HDL-CE (Goldberg et al., 1991).

Consistent with the major role of the liver in selective HDL cholesterol uptake, the highest absolute amount of tissue SR-BI protein expression is found in the liver. In addition, SR-BI is highly expressed in steroidogenic tissues (Landschulz et al., 1996), which are the sites with the highest specific activity for selective HDL cholesterol uptake in rodents. This pathway is an important source of cholesterol for storage and steroid hormone synthesis in steroidogenic tissues. SR-BI is concentrated in caveolae at least in some cells (Babitt et al., 1997), suggesting that these may be the sites of selective uptake on the cell surface. In fact, recent studies indicate that HDL-CEs taken up by the SR-BI-mediated pathway are rapidly and reversibly incorporated into plasma membrane caveolae, followed by irreversible internalization of cholesterol into intracellular compartments (Graf et al., 1999).

Although the precise mechanisms of SR-BI-mediated selective HDL-CE uptake are not yet clear, SR-BI does not mediate the endocytosis and degradation of bound lipoproteins, unlike the LDL receptors (Acton et al., 1996). Instead, HDL binds to SR-BI expressed on the cell surface, its cholesterol is transferred to the cell, and the cholesterol-depleted HDL particle is released from the cell surface, so that SR-BI binding results in the uptake of only the lipid portion of the lipoprotein particle. The selective HDL cholesterol uptake pathway appears to involve reversible incorporation of HDL-CE into the plasma membrane, followed by a step in which cholesterol molecules are irreversibly internalized (Knecht and Pittman, 1989; Rinninger et al., 1993) through a non-lysosomal non-endocytic pathway (Sparrow and Pittman, 1990; Delamatre et al., 1993). Interestingly, SR-BI may also be involved in HDL-dependent cholesterol efflux from the cells (Rothblat et al., 1999) and the uptake of non-lipoprotein cholesterol into the cells (Stangl et al., 1998; Hauser et al., 1998).

The physiologic importance of the SR-BI receptor for RCT is suggested by studies of mice in which the levels of SR-BI were manipulated in vivo by either over-expression of the gene in the liver using adenovirus-mediated gene transfer or transgenic approaches. Overexpression of SR-BI in the liver resulted in a profound reduction in the level of HDL (cholesterol and apo A-I) and increased cholesterol in hepatic bile (Wang et al., 1998; Sehayek et al., 1998; Ueda et al., 1999). The role of SR-BI in HDL metabolism in vivo was further assessed in mice by introducing targeted mutations in its gene (Rigotti et al., 1997; Varban et al., 1998). A lack of

SR-BI expression in homozygous SR-BI knockout mice results in an over twofold increase in total cholesterol levels, mostly as a result of increased cholesterol in HDL particles (Rigotti et al., 1997). The direct measurement of selective clearance and tissue uptake of HDL-C demonstrated that reduced levels of SR-BI were accompanied by apparent reductions in the plasma clearance of HDL-CE and hepatic selective uptake of HDL-C (Varban et al., 1998; Ji et al., 1999). This supports the idea that the increased size and cholesterol content of HDL in the absence of SR-BI in SR-BI knockout mice is caused by impaired RCT. Therefore, SR-BI appears to be essential for normal murine HDL metabolism through the selective HDL-C uptake pathway. As a consequence of its key role in controlling lipoprotein metabolism and HDL-mediated RCT, SR-BI activity exhibits antiatherogenic properties. Studies of atherosclerosis in several models of SR-BI overexpression or ablation show that SR-BI can be atheroprotective in mice (Trigatti et al., 1999; Krieger and Kozarsky, 1999; Arai et al., 1999; Kozarsky et al., 2000). However, it is still unclear to what extent the SR-BI-mediated selective uptake of HDL-CE and direct uptake of whole HDL particles by the liver contribute in the RCT system in humans.

4.5.2. *Other antiatherogenic effects of HDL*

It has been argued that the inverse relationship between CAD and HDL may not reflect a cause and effect in spite of the clear clinical and epidemiological demonstrations (de Backer et al., 1998; Hergenc et al., 1999; Bobak et al., 1999). Low HDL-C levels are often associated with other atherogenic metabolic abnormalities, such as elevated TG levels, insulin resistance, and small dense LDL (Despres and Marette, 1994; Hergenc et al., 1999). However, experimental observations make a compelling argument that HDL and its major apoprotein moiety, apo A-I, have direct antiatherogenic and vascular protective effects. In addition to RCT, several biological actions are postulated to contribute to the beneficial antiatherogenic effects of HDL and apo A-I. Although the precise mechanisms are still under investigation, those actions expand on antioxidant effects (Hayek et al., 1995; Toikka et al., 1999; Mackness et al., 2000), antiinflammatory effects (Hamilton et al., 1993; Cockerill et al., 1995; Xia et al., 1999), scavenging of toxic phospholipids such as lysophosphatidylcholine (lysoPC) (Matsuda et al., 1993; Nilsson et al., 1998), protection of endothelial function (Zeiher et al., 1994; Kinlay et al., 2001), antithrombotic (Naqvi et al., 1999; Griffin et al., 1999) and profibrinolytic effects (Saku et al., 1985), and reduced lipoprotein retention (Saxena et al., 1993; Williams and Tabas, 1998).

5. Modification of atherogenic lipoproteins

5.1. *Oxidation hypothesis*

The first observable change in the artery wall following the feeding of a high-fat, high-cholesterol diet is the accumulation of lipoprotein particles and their aggregates in the intima at sites of lesion predilection. The "response-to-retention" hypothesis of atherogenesis emphasizes the subendothelial retention of cholesterol-rich, atherogenic lipoproteins within the arterial wall (Boren et al., 1998; Williams and

Tabas, 1998). Once retained, these lipoproteins are modified and provoke a cascade of responses that lead to disease in a previously non-lesional artery. This hypothesis specifically addresses the mechanism for the link between blood lipids and disease and the pathological observation of atherosclerosis. The accumulation is greater when levels of circulating LDL are raised, and both the transport and retention of LDL are increased in the preferred sites for lesion formation. LDL diffuses passively through endothelial cell junctions, and its retention in the vessel wall seems to involve interactions between the apo B and matrix proteoglycans (Boren et al., 1998). In addition to LDL, other apo B-containing lipoproteins, namely Lp (a) and remnants, can accumulate in the intima and promote atherosclerosis (Utermann, 2001).

Native LDL is not taken up by macrophages rapidly enough to generate foam cells, because macrophages lose LDL receptors as they differentiate from monocytes after recruitment in the vessel walls (Goldstein et al., 1979). Then, it was proposed that LDL is somehow "modified" within or on the vessel wall. Modifications of LDL include oxidization, glycation (in diabetes), aggregation, association with pro-teoglycans, or incorporation into an immune complex. One of the modifications most significant for early lesion formation is lipid oxidation as a result of exposure to the oxidative waste of vascular cells. Such modifications initially give rise to "minimally oxidized" or "minimally modified" LDL (mmLDL) species that have proinflammatory activity but may not be sufficiently modified to be recognized by macrophage scavenger receptors (Navab et al., 1996; Itabe et al., 1996; Palinski et al., 1996; Holvoet et al., 1998). This "oxidation hypothesis" has been a central focus of investigation on the pathogenesis of the atherosclerotic process for almost 20 years. This hypothesis states that the oxidative modification of LDL, or other lipoproteins, is central, if not obligatory, to the atherogenic process. The important corollary is that inhibition of such oxidation should reduce the progression of atherosclero-sis, independent of reduction of other risk factors, such as elevated LDL levels (Steinberg et al., 1989; Witztum, 1994; Chisolm and Steinberg, 2000).

The original interest in oxidized LDL (OxLDL) stemmed from two basic sets of observations. The first was that OxLDL was cytotoxic to endothelial and other cells and thus could directly cause damage to arterial cells (Hessler et al., 1983; Kinlay et al., 2001). The second observation was that uptake of native LDL by macrophages occurred at a sufficiently low rate to prevent foam cell formation, but uptake of OxLDL was unregulated and led to macrophage foam cell formation (Heinecke et al., 1984; Steinbrecher et al., 1984). However, it is now abundantly clear that OxLDL, with its many oxidatively modified lipids and degradation products, con-tributes to the pathophysiology of both the initiation and progression of the atherosclerotic lesion by many mechanisms, including its proinflammatory, immu-nogenic, and cytotoxic properties (Navab et al., 1996). Products of OxLDL contribute to monocyte and T cell recruitment, directly or indirectly via induction of chemokines and endothelial cell adhesion molecules. They alter the gene expression of vascular cells, leading to growth factor and cytokine stimulation, and they are cytotoxic. Because oxidation of LDL generates many "neo-self determinants" that induce an active immune response, there is, in turn, a both humoral and cellular response that affects the progression of the atherosclerotic lesion in complex ways (Libby et al., 1999). Indeed, the notion that oxidation of LDL is a driving force in atherosclerosis fits in nicely with the widely held notion that atherosclerosis is a chronic inflammatory process.

It should also be appreciated that not only LDL but also other apo B-100-containing lipoproteins are also oxidized, such as IDL, which may also play similar roles. In addition, oxidative modification of other structures in the artery wall, such as cell membranes (Chang et al., 1999) and matrix proteins (O'Brien et al., 1996), may also have important biological effects.

5.2. *Evidence for the presence of OxLDL in vivo*

The following data suggest that OxLDL exists in vivo, that the oxidation hypothesis is highly relevant to the pathogenesis of lesion formation, and that the oxidation hypothesis should be applicable in humans as well.

Using antibodies against oxidized lipids and apo B, it is possible to show extensive immunostaining of essentially all atherosclerotic tissue in experimental animals and humans (Esterbauer et al., 1990; Horkko et al., 1999). OxLDL has been recovered from atherosclerotic lesions of both rabbits and humans and shown to be comparable to LDL oxidized in vitro by structural, immunological, and biological properties (Yla-Herttuala et al., 1989). A variety of oxidized lipids have been shown to be present in atherosclerotic plaques in animals and humans (Hulten et al., 1996; Pratico et al., 1997). Of great interest, oxidized lipids, such as hydroxy-eicosatetraenoic acids (HETEs), were significantly elevated in unstable atherosclerotic plaques obtained from endarterectomy samples (Mallat et al., 1999). Similarly, such oxidized lipids are also present in human plasma (Pratico et al., 1998; Bjorkhem et al., 1999). Autoantibodies directed against oxidation-specific epitopes of OxLDL are found in the plasma of humans and also in human atherosclerotic plaques, where they are part of immune complexes. In general, the titers of such autoantibodies are increased in populations at risk for CAD and in many studies have been shown to correlate with various clinical manifestations of atherosclerotic disease and to prospectively predict an increased risk for the development of carotid artery disease as well as myocardial infarction (Yla-Herttuala, 1998). In some studies, the susceptibility of circulating LDL to ex vivo oxidative modification has correlated with the extent of atherosclerosis or with rates of progression of atherosclerosis in human subjects. There are an increasing number of studies demonstrating that very mildly oxidized LDL can be demonstrated in the plasma of animals and humans, using both physical and immunological techniques (Sevanian et al., 1996). Several data demonstrate not only that mmLDL is present in the circulation, but that it appears to accumulate at a greater rate in animals or subjects with increased rates of atherogenesis (Itabe et al., 1996; Palinski et al., 1996; Holvoet et al., 1998).

Finally, the most compelling feature in support of the oxidation hypothesis is the direct demonstration that treatment of hypercholesterolemic animal models with a variety of antioxidants leads to the suppression of atherogenesis. Most of the successful studies have used powerful synthetic antioxidants, such as probucol or probucol analogs (Kita et al., 1987; Sasahara et al., 1994; Parker et al., 1995). However, probucol did not protect murine models in the initial studies reported and even seemed to increase the extent of lesion formation, suggesting some sort of toxicity peculiar to the mouse (Zhang et al., 1997; Bird et al., 1998; Cynshi et al., 1998).

Another line of evidence suggesting that antioxidants decrease atherosclerosis by inhibiting the oxidation of LDL comes from studies in which human LDL was injected into rats (Calara et al., 1998). Using a monoclonal antibody that exclusively recognized human apo B, it was shown that apo B appeared in rat aortas within 6 h. Shortly thereafter appeared oxidation-specific epitopes that colocalized with the apo B. When this experiment was repeated in rats using LDL enriched with probucol, the human apo B appeared in the aorta with the same time sequence, but this time the appearance of oxidation-specific epitopes was greatly reduced. In a recent dramatic experiment in humans, iodinated LDL was injected into patients undergoing carotid endarterectomy and demonstrated the appearance of radioactivity in macrophage foam cells in the removed specimens (Iuliano et al., 2000). No accumulation of radioactivity occurred in atherosclerotic plaques after the injection of radiolabeled albumin. In several other patients, pretreated for 4 weeks with 900 mg/d of vitamin E, there was an almost complete suppression of radiolabeled LDL uptake by macrophages.

5.3. *Mechanisms of LDL oxidation*

There are many postulated mechanisms by which LDL could become oxidized within the artery wall. One mechanism that has now gained strong support is that the enzyme 12/15-LO initiates the "seeding" of LDL with hydroperoxides, leading to the subsequent initiation of lipid peroxidation. The resultant changes render the OxLDL proinflammatory and lead to its subsequent enhanced uptake by macrophages. Evidence to support this hypothesis includes the observations that both mRNA and protein of 15-LO (the homologous enzyme in rabbits and humans) are found in atherosclerotic lesions of rabbits and humans, but not in normal arteries (Yla-Herttuala et al., 1990), that stereospecific products of the LO reaction can be found in lesions, consistent with enzymatic oxidation (Folcik et al., 1995; Kuhn et al., 1997), and that treatment of hypercholesterolemic rabbits with specific inhibitors of 15-LO reduces the progression of atherosclerosis (Sendobry et al., 1997; Bocan et al., 1998). Recent studies showed that crossing 12/15-LO-deficient mice into apo E-deficient mice caused a dramatically reduced extent of early lesions (Cyrus et al., 1999). In a further study, plasma levels of F_2-isoprostanes, non-enzymatic breakdown products resulting from lipid peroxidation of arachidonic acid, were highly correlated with the extent of lesion formation, and autoantibodies to epitopes of OxLDL were also strongly correlated to lesion area as well as to isoprostane levels (Cyrus et al., 2001). Furthermore, overexpression of 15-LO in endothelium led to an enhancement of atherosclerosis in LDL receptor-negative mice (Harats et al., 2000). However, in contrast is a report that macrophage-specific overexpression of 15-LO led to protection against atherosclerosis in cholesterol-fed rabbits (Shen et al., 1996).

It is likely that in vivo there are many mechanisms, other than LO, which oxidize LDL within the artery wall (Gaut and Heinecke, 2001). These may include myeloperoxidase (MPO), metal ions, superoxide, and reactive nitrogen species.

Nitric oxide (NO) is also a potent oxidant produced by both endothelial cells and macrophages that appears to exert both atherogenic and protective effects, dependent on its source of production. The vasodilator function of NO produced by endothelial NO synthase (eNOS) is protective, as deletion of the eNOS gene in the background of apo E deficiency results in hypertension and increased atherosclerosis (Knowles et al., 2000). In contrast, NO produced via the much higher capacity inducible NO synthase (iNOS) in macrophages serves antimicrobial functions based on its potent oxidative properties. Evidence that iNOS contributes to LDL oxidation in vivo has recently been provided by studies demonstrating that apo E-deficient mice lacking iNOS develop less atherosclerosis, although this was not observed by Knowles et al., and that inhibitors of iNOS decrease atherosclerosis in rabbits (Behr-Roussel et al., 2000; Detmers et al., 2000). In contrast, disruption of the gene encoding gp91-phox required for phagocyte NADPH oxidase activity, another potential contributor to LDL oxidation, did not reduce the development of atherosclerosis (Kirk et al., 2000). Degradation of biologically active lipids within OxLDL also appears to determine atherosclerosis susceptibility, as disruption of the gene encoding serum paraoxonase, an esterase/peroxidase carried on HDL that degrades oxidized phospholipids, resulted in increased lesion development (Shih et al., 2000).

5.4. *Role of OxLDL in atherogenesis*

The modification of LDL can range from "minimal" modification (mmLDL), in which the LDL particle can still be recognized by LDL receptors (Navab et al., 1996), to extensive oxidation, in which the apo B component is fragmented and lysine residues are covalently modified with reactive breakdown products of oxidized lipids. Such particles are not bound by the LDL receptor, but rather by several so-called scavenger receptors expressed on macrophages and SMCs. While LDL is protected from oxidation in the plasma compartment, it is thought to become susceptible to enzymatic and non-enzymatic modifications when retained by extracellular matrix proteins in the artery wall (Schwenke and Carew, 1989; Williams and Tabas, 1998). A large number of proinflammatory and proatherogenic properties have been ascribed to mmLDL and OxLDL and their components, and these are summarized in Table 3.

5.5. *Foam cell formation*

The development of macrophage foam cells that contain massive amounts of CEs is a hallmark of both early and late atherosclerotic lesions. One of the reasons that there has been so much interest in OxLDL is that it has unregulated uptake by macrophages, leading to CE accumulation and foam cell formation. This uptake occurs by way of macrophage scavenger receptors, such as the SR-As and CD36. Apo E knockout mice have been reported to develop severe atherosclerotic plaques

Table 3
Potential mechanisms by which OxLDL may influence atherogenesis

1. *Effect of OxLDL on foam cell formation*
    Further oxidation
        Increased expression of PLA2 and MPO in macrophages
    Induction of scavenger receptors
        Increased expression of SR-A, CD36 and SR-D in macrophages
        Rapid and unregulated uptake leading to massive cholesterol accumulation
2. *Effect of OxLDL on monocytes/macrophages*
    Adhesion and infiltration of monocytes/macrophages
        Increased expression of ICAM1, VCAM-1, E-selectin and fibronectin in ECs
        Increased expression of MCP-1 in ECs
    Proliferation/differentiation of monocytes/macrophages
        Increased expression of M-CSF in ECs
3. *Effect of OxLDL on smooth muscle cells (SMCs)*
    Migration of SMCs
        Increased expression of PDGF in ECs, SMCs and macrophages
    Proliferation of SMCs
        Increased expression of bFGF in ECs and SMCs
4. *Effect of OxLDL on thrombosis*
    Adhesion and aggregation of platelets
        Increased expression of PGI2 and prostaglandins
        Decreased expression of NO
    Procoagulant activity
        Increased expression of TF
        Decreased expression of thrombomodulin and protein C
    Fibrinolytic activity
        Decreased expression of PAI-1
5. *Induction of proinflammatory genes*
    Increased expression of NF-κB, AP-1, IL-8, TNF-α and TGF-β
6. *Induction of apoptosis and necrosis*
    Cytotoxicity of lysoPC and oxysterol
7. *Induction of vasoconstriction*
    Increased expression of endothelin
    Decreased expression of NO
8. *Plaque instability*
    Increased expression of MMP-9
    Decreased expression of TIMP-1

(Plump et al., 1992; Zhang et al., 1992). In contrast, apo E-deficient mice with gene-targeted deletion of either the SR-A (Suzuki et al., 1997) or CD36 (Febbraio et al., 2000) have a marked reduction in the extent of lesion development. While it is possible that there are other explanations for the inhibition of atherogenesis, these data are consistent with the more likely possibility that the beneficial effect of scavenger receptor deletion is due to decreased uptake of OxLDL and diminished foam cell formation.

OxLDL-derived cholesterol brought into the macrophage via scavenger receptors consists of free cholesterol as well as CEs that are hydrolyzed in lysosomes. Free cholesterol has a number of potential metabolic fates, including esterification by

ACAT1 and storage in the lipid droplets that characterize foam cells (Chang et al., 2001). CEs within lipid droplets can, in turn, be hydrolyzed by neutral cholesteryl ester hydrolases (e.g., hormone-sensitive lipase), generating free cholesterol for incorporation into membranes and transport out of the cells. Membrane incorporation of excess cholesterol inhibits the proteolytic activation of the SREBP transcription factors required for cholesterol biosynthesis and LDL receptor expression (Brown and Goldstein, 1999) (see Section 4.2). While this prevents further accumulation of cholesterol via these pathways, it does not alter cholesterol uptake via scavenger receptors or via phagocytic mechanisms. Thus, mechanisms mediating cholesterol efflux are critical for the maintenance of cholesterol homeostasis in the macrophages. Disruption of ACAT-1 results in marked systemic abnormalities in lipid homeostasis in hypercholesterolemic apo E-deficient and LDL-R-deficient mice, leading to extensive deposition of free cholesterol in skin and brain (Accad et al., 2000; Yagyu et al., 2000). ACAT-1 deficiency did not prevent development of atherosclerosis in these models, but reduced the lipid and macrophage content of lesions. Although these alterations could result in more stable lesions, the systemic lipid abnormalities observed in ACAT-1-deficient mice suggest that therapeutic inhibition of ACAT-1 could have detrimental effects.

The macrophage has two potential mechanisms for disposing of excess cholesterol: enzymatic modification to more soluble forms and efflux via membrane transporters. The enzyme cholesterol 27-hydroxylase is expressed in macrophages at relatively high levels and could potentially play a role in cholesterol excretion by converting it to the more soluble 27-OH-cholesterol (Bjorkhem, 1992). The major mechanism for cholesterol efflux, however, is likely to be via membrane transporters, with HDL serving as the primary extracellular acceptor (see Section 4.5). There is also evidence that macrophages may contribute directly to the availability of extracellular cholesterol acceptors through secretion of apo E (Linton et al., 1995), which is capable of contributing to the formation of HDL particles.

The balance between cholesterol intake via scavenger receptors and cholesterol efflux regulates cholesterol accumulation in macrophages. As seen in patients with Tangier disease, macrophages can be transformed to foam cells despite low levels of plasma LDL-C, when HDL levels are extremely low and/or RCT or cholesterol efflux is impaired for some reasons.

6. Scavenger receptors

6.1. *Classification of scavenger receptors*

Scavenger receptors were first described for macrophages as alternative receptors to the LDL receptor in the uptake of (excessive) cholesterol and lipid, leading to the development of foam cells. According to a proposal by Krieger (1997) and recently extended by Greaves et al. (1998), the members are classified as follows (Fig. 3) (Linton and Fazio, 2001; Krieger, 2001; Febbraio et al., 2001): SR class A consists of SR-AI, SR-AII, SR-AIII, and the macrophage receptor with collagenous structure

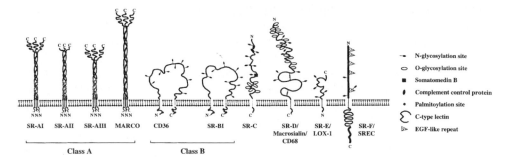

Fig. 3. Classification and proposed structures of scavenger receptors (Terpstra et al., 2000). EGF denotes epidermal growth factor.

(MARCO); class B consists of SR-BI and CD36; and class C contains only the *Drosophila* SR-C. Class D, E, and F receptors have only recently been identified, and none of these show any structural similarity with class A, B, or C receptor. Among these, SR-A and CD36 play a pivotal role in the process of macrophage taking up modified LDL, resulting in foam cell formation.

Most SRs bind a variety of polyanionic ligands. SR classes A and B are expressed in atherosclerotic plaques and are involved in the development of lipid-laden foam cells. SRs are particularly involved in the removal of modified (e.g., oxidized, gly-cosylated) lipoproteins. Some of the SRs, such as CD36 and SR-BI, bind (in addition to the modified lipoproteins) native lipoproteins, such as HDL and LDL. In addition, SRs have been implicated in adhesion, the clearance of dying cells (apoptotic cells) and advanced glycation products (AGE), and host defense against bacterial infection (Terpstra et al., 2000).

6.2. Scavenger receptor class A (SR-A)

SR-A is expressed by tissue macrophages, aortic endothelial cells, liver sinusoidal endothelial cells, and Kupffer cells (Naito et al., 1992; Hughes et al., 1995; Daugherty et al., 1997). This class of scavenger receptor includes SR-AI, SR-AII, and SR-AIII, which are all products of the same gene, and MARCO (Elomaa et al., 1995). SR-AI and SR-AII are the first molecules cloned as scavenger receptors in 1990 (Kodama et al., 1990; Rohrer et al., 1990). There seems to be no major difference between SR-AI and SR-AII in ligand binding. SR-AIII was recently identified as an alternative splice product that is not expressed on the plasma membrane (Gough et al., 1998), and may negatively regulate the ligand binding and membrane localization of SR-AI/SR-AII. SR-AI forms a homotrimeric structure and consists of intracellular transmembrane, α-helical coiled coil, and collagenous and C-terminal cysteine-rich domains. SR-AII is different from SR-AI in lacking cysteine-rich domain.

Macrophages increase their expression of SR-A during differentiation from monocytes. Freshly isolated monocytes and macrophages express low levels of

SR-A, but mRNA and protein levels rapidly increase during culture (de Vries et al., 1999). SR-A is highly expressed in macrophage-derived foam cells in atherosclerotic plaques in humans (Matsumoto et al., 1990; Naito et al., 1992; Hiltunen et al., 1998; de Vries et al., 1999). SMCs within atherosclerotic plaques have been reported to highly express SR-A (Li et al., 1995), suggesting the contribution of this type of SR in transforming SMCs into lipid-laden foam cells during atherogenesis. Macrophage colony-stimulating factor (M-CSF) (de Villiers et al., 1994) and phorbol esters induce monocyte differentiation into macrophages and increase the functional expression of SR-A, whereas tumor necrosis factor (TNF)-α (van Lenten and Fogelman, 1992; Hsu et al., 1996), transforming growth factor (TGF)-β (Bottalico et al., 1991), granulocyte/macrophage colony-stimulating factor (GM-CSF) (van der Kooij et al., 1996), and interferon (IFN)-γ (Fong et al., 1990; Geng and Hansson, 1992) decrease its expression. On human macrophages, the expression of SR-A decreases after stimulation with lipopolysaccharide (LPS) (van Lenten and Fogelman, 1992). Expression of SR-A is also increased by some of its own ligands, such as minimally and highly oxidized LDL (Han and Nicholson, 1998; Yoshida et al., 1998), the process of which enables the unregulated accumulation of lipid in macrophages, leading to foam cell formation.

The potential role of SR-AI/AII in atherosclerotic plaque formation was confirmed in a study with apo E and SR-A double knockout mice (Suzuki et al., 1997). Apo E and SR-A double knockout mice have been shown to develop 58% smaller atherosclerotic lesions compared with apo E knockout mice, in spite of a 46% higher level of plasma cholesterol. Similar findings were reported in LDL receptor/SR-A double knockout mice with more modest reduction ($\sim$20%) in plaque formation (Sakaguchi et al., 1998). However, SR-A deficiency in apo E3 Leiden transgenic mice, another mouse model that shows hyperlipidemia and high susceptibility to diet-induced atherosclerosis, results in the development of significantly more severe lesions (de Winther et al., 1999). Peritoneal macrophages from SR-A knockout mice showed 80% less uptake of acetylated LDL (AcLDL), another chemically modified LDL, and 30% less uptake of OxLDL (Lougheed et al., 1997; Terpstra et al., 1997). Thus, there are apparently other receptors expressed in the macrophages that are able to compensate in part for the absence of SR-A in the SR-A knockout mice. Surprisingly, SR-A knockout mice and wild-type mice did not differ in in vivo clearance rates of modified LDL (Van Berkel et al., 1998; Suzuki et al., 1997; Ling et al., 1997).

Another scavenger receptor in this class, MARCO, shows structural features very similar to those of SR-AI. MARCO, like SR-A, forms a homotrimeric structure and is expressed on the plasma membrane of macrophages. Although its ligands include AcLDL, it is unclear that MARCO recognizes OxLDL, glycated LDL, and apoptotic cells (Elomaa et al., 1995).

6.3. *CD36*

CD36 was previously known as the OKM5 antigen, platelet glycoprotein IV, or GP88. CD36 belongs to the SR-B superfamily and is expressed in mammary epithelial cells, adipocytes, platelets, erythrocyte precursors, monocyte/macrophages, and microvascular endothelial cells. Ligands of CD36 include native and modified lipoproteins, anionic phospholipids, thrombospondin, collagen, apoptotic cells, and *Plasmodium falciparum*-infected red blood cells (Febbraio et al., 2001). The expression cloning technique with fluorescently labeled OxLDL for selecting OxLDL binding proteins showed murine CD36 as a candidate SR (Endemann et al., 1993). CD36-transfected 293 cells bound, internalized, and degraded OxLDL with a binding affinity of $\sim$1.5 µg/ml. Moreover, human CD36-deficient monocytes and macrophages showed $\sim$40% reduction in OxLDL uptake and degradation and less CE accumulation when incubated with OxLDL (Nozaki et al., 1995; Hughes et al., 1995). Thus, CD36 was established as a new member of the SR family. It was also suggested that OxLDL bound to CD36 by its lipid moiety (Nicholson et al., 1995). With the use of chimeric constructs of murine and human CD36, amino acid residues 155 to 183 were shown to be the OxLDL binding domain (Puente Navazo et al., 1996). The binding domain for OxLDL does not coincide with the binding domain for thrombospondin, collagen, or *P. falciparum*-infected erythrocytes, suggesting that there may be a different mechanism for regulating lipoprotein binding. A recent report has shown that not only modified lipoproteins but also native LDL, VLDL, and HDL bind to CD36 (Calvo et al., 1998). CD36 shares this broad recognition of lipoproteins with SR-BI, another member of the SR-B class (Calvo et al., 1997). Several recent reports showed that CD36 mRNA and protein expression increased after the incubation of cells with minimally or fully oxidized LDL. Interestingly, one of the constituents of OxLDL, an oxidized lipid, is a ligand for peroxisome proliferator-activated receptor-γ (PPAR-γ), which increases the expression of CD36 (Nagy et al., 1998; Tontonoz et al., 1998). Thus, uptake of OxLDL through SRs could stimulate its own uptake by activating PPAR-γ and increasing the expression of CD36. There was a 76.5% decrease in aortic tree lesion area (Western diet) and a 45% decrease in aortic sinus lesion area (normal chow) in the CD36/apo E double knockout mice when compared with apo E knockout mice. It is also noted that CD36 may be the first identified molecule responsible for the cause of metabolic multiple risk factor syndrome associated with insulin resistance (Aitman et al., 1999; Pravenec et al., 2001; Miyaoka et al., 2001).

SR-A and CD36 are definitely implicated as key players in the pathogenesis of atherosclerosis. However, these two SRs explain only two-thirds of the binding and degradation capacities of OxLDL in monocytes/macrophages (Nozaki et al., 1995). As other SRs continue to be found, the more precise mechanisms that lead to uptake of modified LDL and resultant formation of foam cells will be clarified. These may contribute to the development of novel therapeutic strategies.

7. Endothelial dysfunction and fatty streak formation

7.1. *Endothelial dysfunction and atherosclerosis*

Endothelial dysfunction has been implicated in the pathogenesis and clinical course of all known cardiovascular diseases and is associated with future risk of adverse cardiovascular events. It is well accepted that endothelial dysfunction occurs in response to cardiovascular risk factors and precedes the development of athero-sclerosis (Ross, 1999; Lusis, 2000; Glass and Witztum, 2001). The endothelium, with its intercellular tight junctional complexes, functions as a selectively permeable barrier between blood and subendothelial tissues. In addition, the vascular endo-thelium produces a number of vasoactive substances that not only regulate vaso-motor tone, but also are involved in the regulation of inflammation in the vessel wall and the balance of thrombotic/thrombolytic factors at the lumen–wall interface. Possible "injurious agents" that cause endothelial dysfunction include elevated and modified LDL (Navab et al., 1996; Griendling and Alexander, 1997), free radicals caused by cigarette smoking, hypertension, and diabetes mellitus, elevated plasma homocysteine concentrations, infectious microorganisms such as herpes viruses or *Chlamydia pneumoniae*, fluid shear stress, and combinations of these or other factors. The endothelial dysfunction that results from the injury leads to compensatory responses that alter the normal homeostatic properties of the endothelium. Thus, the different forms of injury increase the adhesiveness of the endothelium with respect to leukocytes or platelets, as well as its permeability. These changes induce the adhesion of monocytes/macrophages and T cells, and the retention of atherogenic lipo-proteins in the arterial wall, leading to the initial lesion of atherosclerosis. The injury also induces the endothelium to have procoagulant instead of anticoagulant prop-erties and to form vasoactive molecules, cytokines, and growth factors (Kinlay et al., 2001).

Lipids (particularly LDL-C) and oxidant stress play a major role in impairing endothelial functions, by reducing the bioavailability of NO and by activating endothelial proinflammatory signaling pathways such as nuclear factor kappa B (NF-κB). These activated inflammatory responses include upregulation of adhesion molecules, increased chemokine secretion and leukocyte adherence, increased cell permeability, enhanced LDL oxidation, platelet activation, cytokine elaboration, and vascular SMC proliferation and migration. Endothelial cells play an active role in the recruitment of inflammatory cells into the vessel wall, by producing cytokines and expressing cellular adhesion molecules that capture monocytes/macrophages and T cells and assist their passage into the subendothelial space (Kinlay et al., 1998). The NF-κB signal transduction pathway is a particularly important regulator of the transcription of a number of proinflammatory genes, including those that lead to the expression of adhesion molecules (Barnes and Karin, 1997). NF-κB is redox sensitive and activated by the degradation of its inhibitory component Iκ-Bα, a process that is accelerated by OxLDL cholesterol (Li et al., 2000; Cominacini et al., 2000) and prevented by antioxidants (Li et al., 2000). Since exogenous (Peng et al., 1995b; Khan et al., 1996; Usui et al., 2000) and endogenous (Boger et al., 2000) inhibitors of endothelium-derived NO also activate NF-κB, the coronary risk factors that reduce the bioavailability of endothelium-derived NO thus activate NF-κB partly by this mechanism.

Biomechanical forces on the endothelium, including low shear stress from dis-turbed blood flow, also activate the endothelium, increasing vasomotor dysfunction and promoting inflammation by upregulating proatherogenic genes. Fatty streaks and atherosclerosis tend to develop at areas of low shear stress. These typically occur at branch points on the opposite side of the flow divider, and downstream of stenoses, where disturbances in laminar flow result in recirculation eddies, flow separation, and oscillatory flows. In addition, lipid-independent pathways of endothelial cell activation are increasingly recognized, and may provide new therapeutic targets. Endothelial vasoconstrictors, such as endothelin, antagonize endothelium-derived vasodilators and contribute to endothelial dysfunction. AGEs are formed in diabetes, and these promote inflammation via specific receptors on endothelial cells.

The finding that endothelial function can change rapidly in response to altered levels of plasma LDL-C clearly demonstrated that elevated levels of LDL-C itself are injurious to endothelium. LDL apheresis, which dramatically lowers LDL, improves myocardial blood flow (Mellwig et al., 1998) and peripheral endothelium-dependent vasomotor function (Tamai et al., 1997), and reduces soluble cellular adhesion molecules (Sampietro et al., 1997) over several hours. Vasomotor function can improve over a period of weeks with LDL lowering, using oral HMG-CoA reductase inhibitors (statins) (Dupuis et al., 1999; Mullen et al., 2000). Such studies provide mechanisms that may explain the therapeutic benefit of a rapid and intensive reduction in LDL-C in patients with advanced atherosclerosis or unstable coronary syndrome (Pitt et al., 1999).

HDL-C, a protective risk factor for cardiovascular diseases, has opposing effects on the endothelium. Elevated HDL prevents endothelial vasomotor dysfunction (Zeiher et al., 1994), and therapies that increase "functional" HDL may improve endothelial vasomotor function independent of LDL-C (Evans et al., 2000). HDL also reduces the expression of adhesion molecules by the endothelium (Cockerill et al., 2001), but probably through NF-κB-independent pathways.

7.2. Recruitment of monocytes/macrophages and fatty streak formation

Pathological studies have revealed a defined series of changes in the vessel during atherogenesis, fatty streak formation, fibrous cap formation, and advanced complicated lesion formation. Although the recruitment of monocytes to the arterial wall and their subsequent differentiation into macrophages may initially serve a protective function by removing cytotoxic and proinflammatory OxLDL particles or apoptotic cells, progressive accumulation of macrophages and their uptake of OxLDL ultimately leads to the development of atherosclerotic lesions. The recruitment of monocytes to lesion-prone sites or large arteries is regulated by cell adhesion molecules that are expressed on the surface of ECs in response to inflammatory stimuli and mmLDL. mmLDL stimulates the overlying ECs to produce adhesion molecules, chemotactic proteins such as MCP-1, and growth factors such as M-CSF, resulting in the recruitment of monocytes to the vessel wall. OxLDL has other effects, such as inhibiting the production of NO, an important mediator of vasodilation and expression of endothelial leukocyte adhesion molecules (ELAMs). Among EC adhesion molecules likely to be important in the recruitment of leukocytes are

ICAM-1, P-selectin, E-selectin, PCAM-1 and VCAM-1. Important adhesion molecules on monocytes include β2 integrin, VLA-4, and PCAM-1.

The first step in adhesion, the "rolling" of leukocytes along the endothelial surface, is mediated by selectins that bind to carbohydrate ligands on leukocytes. Adherent monocytes migrate into the subendothelial space and differentiate into macrophages. The role of M-CSF in the migration, proliferation, and differentiation of monocytes/macrophages and resultant atherosclerosis was confirmed by the reduced atherosclerotic lesions in spontaneous M-CSF null mice with apo E-deficient genetic background (Smith et al., 1995; Qiao et al., 1997). Several cell adhesion molecules have been suggested to play roles in macrophage recruitment. One of the first to be implicated was VCAM-1, based on its increased expression on endothelial cells over lesion-prone areas, its preferential recruitment of monocytes, and its pattern of regulation by proinflammatory stimuli (Cybulsky and Gimbrone, 1991). Studies confirming a role of VCAM-1 in atherosclerosis in the mouse have been complicated by the fact that systemic deletion of the VCAM-1 gene results in early embryonic lethality. E-selectin and P-selectin appear to play quantitative roles in monocyte entry based on a 40–60% decrease in atherosclerosis in apo E-deficient mice lacking both genes (Dong et al., 1998). Similarly, gene deletion of ICAM-1 resulted in small but significant reductions in monocyte recruitment to atherosclerotic lesions in apo E-deficient mice (Collins et al., 2000). Chronic delivery of a peptidomimetic corresponding to the connecting segment 1 (CS-1) domain of fibronectin 1, which blocks the function of the adhesion molecule VLA-4 on the leukocyte surface, reduced lipid accumulation in C57BL/6J mice fed an atherogenic diet (Shih et al., 1999). Together, these findings suggest that many cell adhesion molecules contribute to the recruitment of monocytes and T cells to the atherosclerotic lesion. Neutrophils, which normally contribute to most inflammatory responses, are notably absent in lesions, although the mechanisms leading to their exclusion remain to be defined.

Migration of monocytes into the artery wall is likely to be stimulated in part by OxLDL, which can directly attract monocytes (Steinberg et al., 1989) and can also induce the expression of chemotactic molecules by endothelial cells, such as monocyte chemotactic protein 1 (MCP-1) (Navab et al., 1996). Intriguingly, monocyte expression of CCR2, the receptor for MCP-1, is stimulated by hypercholesterolemia and monocytes derived from hypercholesterolemic patients exhibit increased chemotactic responses to MCP-1 (Han et al., 1999). Disruption of the MCP-1 or CCR2 genes markedly reduces the development of atherosclerosis in apo E−/− or apo B-overexpressing mice, respectively (Boring et al., 1998; Gu et al., 1998; Gosling et al., 1999). Interleukin (IL)-8, which is present in human atherosclerosis lesions, may also play a role in monocyte-macrophage trafficking. Although a clear homolog of IL-8 has not been established in the mouse, reconstitution of the hematopoietic system of LDL R-deficient mice with bone marrow cells lacking CXCR2, one of two high-affinity receptors for IL-8 and other CXC chemokines, resulted in significantly less atherosclerosis than in mice reconstituted with wild-type bone marrow cells (Boisvert et al., 1998). In concert, these findings suggest that inhibition of macrophage chemotaxis mediated by MCP-1 and/or interference with CXCR-2 activity may be of therapeutic benefit.

8. Fibrous cap and advanced, complicated lesion formation

8.1. *Migration of smooth muscle cells and fibrous cap formation*

Fatty streaks are characterized by the accumulation of macrophage-derived foam cells but are not clinically significant. As fatty streaks progress to intermediate and advanced lesions, they tend to form a fibrous cap that walls off the lesion from the lumen. This represents a type of healing or fibrous response to the injury. The fibrous cap covers a mixture of leukocytes, lipid, and debris, which may form a necrotic core. The fibrous cap with recurrent events of microthrombosis, reabsorption, and healing can evolve into an advanced complicated lesion and often-calcified plaque, one that may itself cause significant stenosis, and produce symptoms of stable angina pectoris. The fibrous cap lesions expand at their shoulders by means of continued leukocyte adhesion and entry caused by the same factors as those described above (see Section 7.2). The principal factors associated with macrophage accumulation include M-CSF, MCP-1, and OxLDL. The necrotic core represents the results of apoptosis and necrosis, increased proteolytic activity, and lipid accumulation. The fibrous cap forms as a result of increased activity of platelet-derived growth factor (PDGF), TGF-β, IL-1, TNF-α, and osteopontin and of decreased connective tissue degradation.

Fibrous plaques are characterized by a growing mass of extracellular lipid, mostly cholesterol and its ester, and by the accumulation of SMCs and SMC-derived extracellular matrix. The transition from the relatively simple fatty streak to the more complex lesion is characterized by the immigration of SMCs from the medial layer of the artery wall past the internal elastic lamina and into the intimal, or subendothelial, space. Intimal SMCs may proliferate and take up modified lipo-proteins, contributing to foam cell formation, and synthesize extracellular matrix proteins that lead to the development of the fibrous cap (Ross, 1999; Paulsson et al., 2000). Recent studies have shown that the interaction of CD40 with its ligand CD40L (CD154) makes an important contribution to the development of advanced lesions (Schonbeck et al., 2000). This interaction was first recognized as being essential to major immune reactions involving T and B cells, but it is now clear that CD40 is also expressed on macrophages, ECs, and SMCs. The engagement of CD40 and CD40L results in the production of inflammatory cytokines, matrix-degrading proteases, and adhesion molecules. Studies using CD40L-null mice or neutralizing antibodies to CD40L have shown that disruption of the interaction results in smaller lesions that are less inflammatory and more fibrous (Schonbeck et al., 2000). Cytokines and growth factors secreted by macrophages and T cells are important for SMC migration and proliferation, and extracellular matrix production. Several risk factors seem to contribute to the development of fibrous lesions, including elevated homocysteine, hypertension, and hormones. Homocysteine is toxic to endothelium and is prothrombotic, and it increases collagen production (Majors et al., 1997) and proliferation of SMC (Gerhard and Duell, 1999), and decreases the availability of NO (Upchurch et al., 1997). Some of the effects of raised blood pressure on athero-sclerosis seem to be mediated by components of the renin–angiotensin pathway, such as angiotensin II. In addition to causing hypertension by its vasoconstrictor action, it can contribute to atherogenesis by stimulating SMC growth and the production of extracellular matrix. It can augment IL-6, MCP-1 elaboration by human SMCs in culture. Angiotensin II also alters fibrinolytic balance by augmenting PAI-1 expression. In addition, activation of the renin–angiotensin system also spurs the production of reactive oxygen species from vascular cells. It increases SMC lipoxygenase activity as well, which can increase inflammation and the oxidation of LDL.

Several reports have shown a correlation between the incidence of atherosclerosis and the presence of at least two types of infectious microorganisms, herpesviruses and *Chlamydia pneumoniae* (Libby et al., 1997; Jackson et al., 1997). Both organisms have been identified in atheromatous lesions in coronary arteries and in other organs obtained at autopsy. Increased titers of antibodies to these organisms have been used as a predictor of further adverse events in patients who have had a myocardial infarction. On the basis of in vitro studies, a plausible mechanism for this correlation is stimulation of SMC migration by the virus-coded chemokine receptor US28 (Streblow et al., 1999). However, prospective and well-controlled seroepidemiological studies have failed to support a consistent link between infections and coronary events. Cytomegalovirus infection is also associated with inactivation of the p53 protein, and p53-null mice exhibited increased SMC proliferation and accelerated atherosclerosis (Guevara et al., 1999).

8.2. *Advanced complicated lesion formation*

Continued inflammation results in increased numbers of macrophages and lymphocytes, both of which emigrate from the blood and multiply within the lesion. Activation of these cells leads to the release of hydrolytic enzymes, cytokines, chemokines, and growth factors, which can induce further damage and eventually lead to focal necrosis. Thus, cycles of accumulation of mononuclear cells, migration and proliferation of SMCs, and formation of fibrous tissue lead to further enlargement and restructuring of the lesion, so that it becomes covered by a fibrous cap that surrounds a core of lipid and necrotic tissue, a so-called advanced, complicated lesion. Plaques can become increasingly complex, with calcification, ulceration at the luminal surface, and hemorrhage from small vessels that grow into the lesion from the media of the blood vessel wall. Analysis of human atherosclerosis suggests that the evolution of advanced plaques may involve repetitive cycles of microhemorrhage and thrombosis.

Continued exposure to M-CSF permits macrophages to survive in vitro and possibly to multiply within the lesions. In contrast, inflammatory cytokines such as IFN-γ activate macrophages and, under certain circumstances, induce them to undergo programmed cell death (apoptosis). The death of foam cells leaves behind a growing mass of extracellular lipids and other cell debris. If this occurs in vivo, macrophages may become involved in the necrotic cores characteristic of advanced, complicated lesions. Replication of monocyte-derived macrophages and T cells is as important as that of SMCs in atherosclerotic lesions.

Studies of human and animal models of atherosclerosis suggest that programmed cell death plays a quantitatively important role in the formation of the necrotic core

(Martinet and Kockx, 2001; Panini and Sinensky, 2001). Apoptosis of macrophages and vascular SMCs appears to result from cell–cell interactions and the local cytokine environment within the arterial wall, involving the actions of pro- and anti-apoptotic proteins that include death receptors, protooncogenes, and tumor suppressor genes. Oxidized sterols present in OxLDL also appear to promote apoptosis and necrosis in lesions (Colles et al., 1996). Necrosis of macrophages and SMC-derived foam cells leads to the formation of a necrotic core and accumulation of extracellular cholesterol. The release of oxidized and insoluble lipid from necrotic cells undoubtedly contributes to the formation of the "gruel" characteristic of advanced lesions.

9. Plaque instability, rupture, thrombosis and acute coronary syndrome

Although advanced lesions can grow sufficiently large to block blood flow, the most important clinical complication is an acute occlusion due to the formation of a thrombus or blood clot, resulting in myocardial infarction or stroke. Pathological studies suggest that the development of thrombus-mediated acute coronary events depends principally on the composition and vulnerability of a plaque rather than the severity of stenosis. The plaque ruptures associated with acute myocardial infarction generally occur at the shoulder regions of the plaque and are more likely to occur in lesions with thin fibrous caps, a relatively high concentration of lipid-filled macrophages within the shoulder region, and large necrotic cores (Davies et al., 1993; Lee and Libby, 1997). The characteristics of vulnerable or unstable plaques are shown in Table 4.

At the shoulder of the plaque, monocytes continue to enter, accumulate, differentiate, and undergo activation and apoptosis. Thinning of the fibrous cap is

Table 4
Characteristics of vulnerable or unstable plaques

Structural
Thin fibrous cap
Large lipid core
High circumferential mechanical stress

Cellular
Abundant macrophage-derived foam cells
Accumulation of T cells
Paucity of vascular SMCs
Existence of local inflammation

Functional
Expression of active inflammatory markers
Expression of cytokines
Expression of matrix-degrading proteases
Decreased synthesis of extracellular matrix
Induction of apoptosis and necrosis
Production of procoagulant (tissue factor) and antifibrinolytic (PAI-1) factors

---

apparently due to the continuing influx and activation of macrophages, which release metalloproteinases and other proteolytic enzymes to cause degradation of the matrix at these sites. These enzymes include matrix metalloproteinases, including interstitial collagenases and gelatinases, and certain elastolytic cathepsins, including the sulfhydryl-dependent proteinases cathepsins S and K. The degradation of the matrix can lead to hemorrhage from the vasa vasorum or from the lumen of the artery and result in thrombus formation and occlusion of the artery. Thus, macrophage secretion of matrix metalloproteinases and neovascularization contribute to weakening of the fibrous plaque. In fact, matrix metalloproteinases secreted by macrophages have been detected in regions of plaque rupture and are suggested to influence plaque stability by degrading extracellular matrix proteins (Galis et al., 1994; Carmeliet, 2000). Plaque rupture exposes blood components to tissue factor, initiating coagulation, the recruitment of platelets, and the formation of a thrombus. Macrophage accumulation may be associated with increased concentrations of both fibrinogen and C-reactive protein (CRP), two markers of inflammation thought to be early signs of atherosclerosis.

The protective fibrous cap, far from being fixed and static, actually can undergo continuous and dynamic remodeling and displays considerable metabolic activity (Libby, 2001). The balance between synthetic and degradative processes regulates the levels of collagen and elastin in the structure, which confer biomechanical strength on the fibrous cap. This balance is closely controlled by inflammatory mediators, such as IFN-γ, which can inhibit de novo synthesis of interstitial collagen by SMC (Amento et al., 1991). The plaque's SMC population also influences the level of extracellular matrix, because these cells repair and maintain the all-important collagenous matrix of the fibrous cap. Sites of fatal thrombosis, where plaques fail mechanistically and rupture, typically have few SMCs and, indeed, have thin and friable fibrous caps because of the lack of collagen (Davies et al., 1993; van der Wal et al., 1994). This SMC loss in the atherosclerotic lesion results from apoptosis triggered by inflammatory stimuli such as cytokines and fas ligand, factors overexpressed in atherosclerotic plaques (Geng et al., 1997). Apoptosis of macrophages and SMCs may not only be important in determining the ability of lesions to undergo regression, but may also influence plaque stability, as such lipids in the necrotic core are suggested to increase the potential for thrombosis (Bennett, 1999).

Endothelial dysfunction may also contribute to the mechanism of coronary thromboses. In some cases, occlusive thrombi arise not from fracture of the fibrous cap but from superficial erosion of the endothelial layer (van der Wal et al., 1994; Farb et al., 1996). ECs, like SMCs, may undergo apoptosis in response to inflammatory mediators (Slowik et al., 1997). Membrane type I matrix metalloproteinase, secreted by ECs, can activate matrix metalloproteinase-2, a type IV collagenase, resulting in local thrombosis at the superficial erosive site. One important function of ECs, an anticoagulant property, may also be disturbed in response to inflammatory mediators and bacterial products such as endotoxin. Endothelial expression of the procoagulant molecule, tissue factor, and fibrinolytic PAI-1 can vary in the presence of inflammatory mediators and may underlie thrombosis in situ. Vasospasm, caused by decreased production of NO and increased release of superoxide anion (O_2^-), may also contribute to impaired arterial flow in the presence of inflammation (Ohara et al., 1993). Other roles of NO, impairment of platelet aggregation and antiin-flammatory effect mediated by augmenting production of the inhibitor of NF-κB, may also be impaired, causing thromboses. (De Caterina et al., 1995; Peng et al., 1995a; Thurberg and Collins, 1998).

10. Prevention of atherosclerotic cardiovascular diseases by antihyperlipidemic drugs

10.1. *Stabilization of the plaque by lipid lowering therapy*

A consistent body of evidence from large clinical trials has established beyond doubt that lipid lowering can reduce the incidence of coronary events and stroke in a broad spectrum of individuals. Curiously, lipid lowering produces only modest improve-ments in the luminal caliber of fixed atherosclerotic lesions. The event reduction is more prominent in secondary prevention trials than in primary prevention. In addition, a significant reduction in clinical cardiovascular events was seen as early as 6 months in the West of Scotland Coronary Prevention Study (WOSCOPS) (Shepherd et al., 1995). These findings suggest that qualitative changes in plaques, rather than improvements in the degree of stenosis, must contribute importantly to the striking reduction in clinical events produced by lipid lowering. Lipid lowering not only yields an increased level of interstitial collagen in the atherosclerotic intima, but also decreases the thrombotic potential of the lesion. Such improvements in features of plaques asso-ciated with stability or reduced thrombogenicity occur both with dietary and statin-induced lipid lowering and with lesions resulting from either dietary or endogenous hypercholesterolemia (Aikawa et al., 2001).

In view of the central role of inflammation in the pathophysiology of these events, lipid lowering can be thought to act as an antiinflammatory intervention. Con-siderable experimental data show that lipid lowering results in decreased levels of inflammatory cells and inflammatory mediators (Aikawa et al., 1998; Bustos et al., 1998), reduced levels of collagenolytic enzymes and tissue factor (Aikawa et al., 1999), decreased expression of VCAM-1, and less abundant plexus of microvessels. A significant decline in the levels of CRP shown in lipid lowering with pravastatin in the Cholesterol and Recurrent Events (CARE) study supports the hypothesis that lipid lowering can reduce inflammation (Ridker et al., 1999). These qualitative changes in the atheroma should yield a more stable plaque, one less likely to cause thrombosis if it were to rupture.

10.2. *Pleiotropic effects of statins*

HMG-CoA reductase inhibitors or statins block the rate-limiting step of choles-terol biosynthesis. The overall clinical benefits observed with statin therapy appear to be greater than what might be expected from changes in lipid profile alone, suggesting that the beneficial effects of statins may extend beyond their effects on serum cholesterol levels. Indeed, recent experimental and clinical evidence indicates some of the cholesterol-independent or "pleiotropic" effects of statins. These effects involve improvement or restoration of endothelial function (Bourcier and Libby, 2000; Kureishi et al., 2000; Rikitake et al., 2001; Essig et al., 1998; Hernandez-Perera et al., 1998), attenuation of SMC proliferation (Laufs et al., 1999), reduction in expression of matrix metalloproteinases (Aikawa et al., 2001; Fukumoto et al., 2001) and tissue factors (Colli et al., 1997), and decreasing oxidative stress (Laufs et al., 1998) and vascular inflammation (Vaughan et al., 2000). These effects of statins in concert may stabilize atherosclerotic plaque. Many of these pleiotropic effects of statins are mediated by their ability to block the synthesis of important isoprenoid intermediates, which serve as lipid attachments for a variety of intracellular signaling molecules. In particular, the inhibition of small GTP-binding proteins, Rho, Ras, and Rac, whose proper membrane localization and function are dependent on iso-prenylation, may play an important role in mediating the direct cellular effects of statins on the vascular wall (Takemoto and Liao, 2001). Although the statins have non-lipid effects, it is uncertain how important they are in the doses used in clinical practice compared with the lipid-mediated effects of these drugs. The study of non-lipid effects may lead to the development of drugs with more potent actions on these non-lipid pathways that could supplement current therapeutic approaches.

11. Conclusion

Effective drugs for lowering cholesterol and high blood pressure have been developed. In particular, the statins lower levels of atherogenic lipoproteins and dramatically decrease clinical events and mortality from atherosclerosis. Never-theless, heart disease and stroke remain by far the most common causes of death in industrialized countries, and new weapons, particularly agents that block disease at the level of the vessel wall or that raise antiatherogenic HDL, are expected.

Atherosclerosis is clearly an inflammatory disease and does not result simply from the accumulation of lipids. Multiple steps in the atherogenic process could theore-tically serve as the basis for intervention, including steps that control LDL levels and LDL oxidation, monocyte recruitment, scavenger receptor expression, and RCT. Molecules involved in this pathogenic process of atherosclerosis, such as enzymes, adhesion molecules, cytokines, and nuclear factors, can be a target for therapeutic intervention. As discussed above, over the past decade, a number of promising new targets have been identified, including 15-LO, MCP-1, M-CSF, TNF-α, NF-κB, Iκ-B, estrogen receptors, PPARs, and the CD40–CD40L system.

In addition to blocking the development and/or progression of atherosclerosis, it may be possible and desirable to achieve significant regression of established atherosclerotic lesions. HDL and RCT are the only well-understood protective system against atherosclerosis in vivo. The identification of CETP, SR-BI, and ABCA1 in addition to LCAT, LPL, HL, and ACAT presents exciting new oppor-tunities for enhancing RCT. It has also become clear that HDLs are functionally very heterogeneous. For example, CETP-deficient patients present with marked hyperalphalipoproteinemia, but they are not protected against atherosclerotic diseases. Thus, rather than attempting to increase levels of HDL, it is more productive to focus on the activity of HDL in RCT. Other functional properties of HDL, such as its antioxidant activity, also need to be taken into consideration.

The most critical clinical aspects of atherosclerosis are plaque rupture and thrombosis. Recent findings have established the importance of qualitative aspects of plaques as decisive determinants of their propensity to cause acute complication. Understanding the mechanism(s) of plaque rupture and delineation of novel strategies to stabilize lesions by protecting them from rupture represents a major goal of vascular biologists and clinical cardiologists. In addition, considerable interest exists in developing diagnostic tools to identify plaques most vulnerable to rupture in order to direct therapy in a timely and effective fashion.

Despite advances in our understanding and intervention with regard to cardiovascular risk, much remains to be done. Further inroads into reduction of cardiovascular risk may well emerge as we begin to apply our recently acquired knowledge of the role that inflammation plays in atherosclerosis and plaque stability. In all likelihood, future basic research, including the application of functional genomics, will teach us new lessons about atherosclerosis and its complications and show the path to further ways to limit this disease.

Acknowledgments

The authors thank Cathy Knapper, Atsuko Ohya and Chiaki Ikegami for their technical assistance. Supported in part by Grant-in-Aid for Scientific Research (No. 11557054 and No. 12670666) to N.S. from the Ministry of Education, Science, Sports and Culture in Japan.

References

Abbott, R.D., Wilson, P.W., Kannel, W.B., Castelli, W.P., 1988. High density lipoprotein cholesterol, total cholesterol screening, and myocardial infarction. The Framingham Study. Arteriosclerosis 8, 207–211.

Accad, M., Smith, S.J., Newland, D.L., Sanan, D.A., King Jr., L.E., Linton, M.F., Fazio, S., Farese Jr., R.V., 2000. Massive xanthomatosis and altered composition of atherosclerotic lesions in hyperlipidemic mice lacking acyl CoA:cholesterol acyltransferase 1. J. Clin. Invest. 105, 711–719.

Acton, S., Rigotti, A., Landschulz, K.T., Xu, S., Hobbs, H.H., Krieger, M., 1996. Identification of scavenger receptor SR-BI as a high density lipoprotein receptor. Science 271, 518–520.

Aikawa, M., Rabkin, E., Okada, Y., Voglic, S.J., Clinton, S.K., Brinckerhoff, C.E., Sukhova, G.K., Libby, P., 1998. Lipid lowering by diet reduces matrix metalloproteinase activity and increases collagen content of rabbit atheroma: a potential mechanism of lesion stabilization. Circulation 97, 2433–2444.

Aikawa, M., Voglic, S.J., Sugiyama, S., Rabkin, E., Taubman, M.B., Fallon, J.T., Libby, P., 1999. Dietary lipid lowering reduces tissue factor expression in rabbit atheroma. Circulation 100, 1215–1222.

Aikawa, M., Rabkin, E., Sugiyama, S., Voglic, S.J., Fukumoto, Y., Furukawa, Y., Shiomi, M., Schoen, F.J., Libby, P., 2001. An HMG-CoA reductase inhibitor, cerivastatin, suppresses growth of macrophages expressing matrix metalloproteinases and tissue factor in vivo and in vitro. Circulation 103, 276–283.

Aitman, T.J., Glazier, A.M., Wallace, C.A., Cooper, L.D., Norsworthy, P.J., Wahid, F.N., Al-Majali, K.M., Trembling, P.M., Mann, C.J., Shoulders, C.C., Graf, D., St Lezin, E., Kurtz, T.W., Kren, V.,

Pravenec, M., Ibrahimi, A., Abumrad, N.A., Stanton, L.W., Scott, J., 1999. Identification of Cd36 (Fat) as an insulin-resistance gene causing defective fatty acid and glucose metabolism in hypertensive rats. Nat. Genet. 21, 76–83.

Amento, E.P., Ehsani, N., Palmer, H., Libby, P., 1991. Cytokines and growth factors positively and negatively regulate interstitial collagen gene expression in human vascular smooth muscle cells. Arterioscler. Thromb. 11, 1223–1230.

Arai, T., Wang, N., Bezouevski, M., Welch, C., Tall, A.R., 1999. Decreased atherosclerosis in heterozygous low density lipoprotein receptor-deficient mice expressing the scavenger receptor BI transgene. J. Biol. Chem. 274, 2366–2371.

Babitt, J., Trigatti, B., Rigotti, A., Smart, E.J., Anderson, R.G., Xu, S., Krieger, M., 1997. Murine SR-BI, a high density lipoprotein receptor that mediates selective lipid uptake, is N-glycosylated and fatty acylated and colocalizes with plasma membrane caveolae. J. Biol. Chem. 272, 13242–13249.

Barnes, P.J., Karin, M., 1997. Nuclear factor-kappaB: a pivotal transcription factor in chronic inflammatory diseases. N. Engl. J. Med. 336, 1066–1071.

Barrans, A., Jaspard, B., Barbaras, R., Chap, H., Perret, B., Collet, X., 1996. Pre-beta HDL: structure and metabolism. Biochim. Biophys. Acta 1300, 73–85.

Behr-Roussel, D., Rupin, A., Simonet, S., Bonhomme, E., Coumailleau, S., Cordi, A., Serkiz, B., Fabiani, J.N., Verbeuren, T.J., 2000. Effect of chronic treatment with the inducible nitric oxide synthase inhibitor N-iminoethyl-L-lysine or with L-arginine on progression of coronary and aortic atherosclerosis in hypercholesterolemic rabbits. Circulation 102, 1033–1038.

Bennett, M.R., 1999. Apoptosis of vascular smooth muscle cells in vascular remodelling and atherosclerotic plaque rupture. Cardiovasc. Res. 41, 361–368.

Bird, D.A., Tangirala, R.K., Fruebis, J., Steinberg, D., Witztum, J.L., Palinski, W., 1998. Effect of probucol on LDL oxidation and atherosclerosis in LDL receptor-deficient mice. J. Lipid Res. 39, 1079–1090.

Bjorkhem, I., 1992. Mechanism of degradation of the steroid side chain in the formation of bile acids. J. Lipid Res. 33, 455–471.

Bjorkhem, I., Diczfalusy, U., Lutjohann, D., 1999. Removal of cholesterol from extrahepatic sources by oxidative mechanisms. Curr. Opin. Lipidol. 10, 161–165.

Bobak, M., Hense, H.W., Kark, J., Kuch, B., Vojtisek, P., Sinnreich, R., Gostomzyk, J., Bui, M., von Eckardstein, A., Junker, R., Fobker, M., Schulte, H., Assmann, G., Marmot, M., 1999. An ecological study of determinants of coronary heart disease rates: a comparison of Czech, Bavarian and Israeli men. Int. J. Epidemiol. 28, 437–444.

Bocan, T.M., Rosebury, W.S., Mueller, S.B., Kuchera, S., Welch, K., Daugherty, A., Cornicelli, J.A., 1998. A specific 15-lipoxygenase inhibitor limits the progression and monocyte-macrophage enrichment of hypercholesterolemia-induced atherosclerosis in the rabbit. Atherosclerosis 136, 203–216.

Bodzioch, M., Orso, E., Klucken, J., Langmann, T., Bottcher, A., Diederich, W., Drobnik, W., Barlage, S., Buchler, C., Porsch-Ozcurumez, M., Kaminski, W.E., Hahmann, H.W., Oette, K., Rothe, G., Aslanidis, C., Lackner, K.J., Schmitz, G., 1999. The gene encoding ATP-binding cassette transporter 1 is mutated in Tangier disease. Nat. Genet. 22, 347–351.

Boger, R.H., Bode-Boger, S.M., Tsao, P.S., Lin, P.S., Chan, J.R., Cooke, J.P., 2000. An endogenous inhibitor of nitric oxide synthase regulates endothelial adhesiveness for monocytes. J. Am. Coll. Cardiol. 36, 2287–2295.

Boisvert, W.A., Santiago, R., Curtiss, L.K., Terkeltaub, R.A., 1998. A leukocyte homologue of the IL-8 receptor CXCR-2 mediates the accumulation of macrophages in atherosclerotic lesions of LDL receptor-deficient mice. J. Clin. Invest. 101, 353–363.

Boren, J., Olin, K., Lee, I., Chait, A., Wight, T.N., Innerarity, T.L., 1998. Identification of the principal proteoglycan-binding site in LDL. A single-point mutation in apo-B100 severely affects proteoglycan interaction without affecting LDL receptor binding. J. Clin. Invest. 101, 2658–2664.

Boring, L., Gosling, J., Cleary, M., Charo, I.F., 1998. Decreased lesion formation in CCR2−/− mice reveals a role for chemokines in the initiation of atherosclerosis. Nature 394, 894–897.

Bottalico, L.A., Wager, R.E., Agellon, L.B., Assoian, R.K., Tabas, I., 1991. Transforming growth factor-beta 1 inhibits scavenger receptor activity in THP-1 human macrophages. J. Biol. Chem. 266, 22866–22871.

Bouissou, H., Pieraggi, M.T., Julian, M., 1989. Age-related morphological changes of the arterial wall. In: Camilleri, J.P., Berry, C.L., Fiessinger, J.N., Bariéty, J. (Eds.), Diseases of Arterial Wall. Springer-Verlag, New York, pp. 71–78.

Boullier, A., Bird, D.A., Chang, M.K., Dennis, E.A., Friedman, P., Gillotre-Taylor, K., Horkko, S., Palinski, W., Quehenberger, O., Shaw, P., Steinberg, D., Terpstra, V., Witztum, J.L., 2001. Scavenger receptors, oxidized LDL, and atherosclerosis. Ann. N. Y. Acad. Sci. 947, 214–222.

Bourcier, T., Libby, P., 2000. HMG CoA reductase inhibitors reduce plasminogen activator inhibitor-1 expression by human vascular smooth muscle and endothelial cells. Arterioscler. Thromb. Vasc. Biol. 20, 556–562.

Broccardo, C., Luciani, M., Chimini, G., 1999. The ABCA subclass of mammalian transporters. Biochim. Biophys. Acta 1461, 395–404.

Brooks-Wilson, A., Marcil, M., Clee, S.M., Zhang, L.H., Roomp, K., van Dam, M., Yu, L., Brewer, C., Collins, J.A., Molhuizen, H.O., Loubser, O., Ouelette, B.F., Fichter, K., Ashbourne-Excoffon, K.J., Sensen, C.W., Scherer, S., Mott, S., Denis, M., Martindale, D., Frohlich, J., Morgan, K., Koop, B., Pimstone, S., Kastelein, J.J., Genest, J., Hayden, M.R., 1999. Mutations in ABC1 in Tangier disease and familial high-density lipoprotein deficiency. Nat. Genet. 22, 336–345.

Brown, M.S., Goldstein, J.L., 1999. A proteolytic pathway that controls the cholesterol content of membranes, cells, and blood. Proc. Natl. Acad. Sci. U. S. A. 96, 11041–11048.

Brown, M.S., Faust, J.R., Goldstein, J.L., 1975. Role of the low density lipoprotein receptor in regulating the content of free and esterified cholesterol in human fibroblasts. J. Clin. Invest. 55, 783–793.

Brown, M.S., Ye, J., Rawson, R.B., Goldstein, J.L., 2000. Regulated intramembrane proteolysis: a control mechanism conserved from bacteria to humans. Cell 100, 391–398.

Bustos, C., Hernandez-Presa, M.A., Ortego, M., Tunon, J., Ortega, L., Perez, F., Diaz, C., Hernandez, G., Egido, J., 1998. HMG-CoA reductase inhibition by atorvastatin reduces neointimal inflammation in a rabbit model of atherosclerosis. J. Am. Coll. Cardiol. 32, 2057–2064.

Calara, F., Dimayuga, P., Niemann, A., Thyberg, J., Diczfalusy, U., Witztum, J.L., Palinski, W., Shah, P.K., Cercek, B., Nilsson, J., Regnstrom, J., 1998. An animal model to study local oxidation of LDL and its biological effects in the arterial wall. Arterioscler. Thromb. Vasc. Biol. 18, 884–893.

Calvo, D., Gomez-Coronado, D., Lasuncion, M.A., Vega, M.A., 1997. CLA-1 is an 85-kD plasma membrane glycoprotein that acts as a high-affinity receptor for both native (HDL, LDL, and VLDL) and modified (OxLDL and AcLDL) lipoproteins. Arterioscler. Thromb. Vasc. Biol. 17, 2341–2349.

Calvo, D., Gomez-Coronado, D., Suarez, Y., Lasuncion, M.A., Vega, M.A., 1998. Human CD36 is a high affinity receptor for the native lipoproteins HDL, LDL, and VLDL. J. Lipid Res. 39, 777–788.

Carmeliet, P., 2000. Proteinases in cardiovascular aneurysms and rupture: targets for therapy? J. Clin. Invest. 105, 1519–1520.

Castelli, W.P., Garrison, R.J., Wilson, P.W., Abbott, R.D., Kalousdian, S., Kannel, W.B., 1986. Incidence of coronary heart disease and lipoprotein cholesterol levels. The Framingham Study. J. Am. Med. Assoc. 256, 2835–2838.

Castro, G.R., Fielding, C.J., 1988. Early incorporation of cell-derived cholesterol into pre-beta-migrating high-density lipoprotein. Biochemistry 27, 25–29.

Chan, L., Chang, B.H., Nakamuta, M., Li, W.H., Smith, L.C., 1997. Apobec-1 and apolipoprotein B mRNA editing. Biochim. Biophys. Acta 1345, 11–26.

Chang, M.K., Bergmark, C., Laurila, A., Horkko, S., Han, K.H., Friedman, P., Dennis, E.A., Witztum, J.L., 1999. Monoclonal antibodies against oxidized low-density lipoprotein bind to apoptotic cells and inhibit their phagocytosis by elicited macrophages: evidence that oxidation-specific epitopes mediate macrophage recognition. Proc. Natl. Acad. Sci. U. S. A. 96, 6353–6358.

Chang, T.Y., Chang, C.C., Lin, S., Yu, C., Li, B.L., Miyazaki, A., 2001. Roles of acyl-coenzyme A:cholesterol acyltransferase-1 and -2. Curr. Opin. Lipidol. 12 (3), 289–296.

Chappell, D.A., Medh, J.D., 1998. Receptor-mediated mechanisms of lipoprotein remnant catabolism. Prog. Lipid Res. 37, 393–422.

Chisolm, G.M., Steinberg, D., 2000. The oxidative modification hypothesis of atherogenesis: an overview. Free Radic. Biol. Med. 28, 1815–1826.

Cockerill, G.W., Rye, K.A., Gamble, J.R., Vadas, M.A., Barter, P.J., 1995. High-density lipoproteins inhibit cytokine-induced expression of endothelial cell adhesion molecules. Arterioscler. Thromb. Vasc. Biol. 15, 1987–1994.

Cockerill, G.W., Huehns, T.Y., Weerasinghe, A., Stocker, C., Lerch, P.G., Miller, N.E., Haskard, D.O., 2001. Elevation of plasma high-density lipoprotein concentration reduces interleukin-1-induced expression of E-selectin in an in vivo model of acute inflammation. Circulation 103, 108–112.

Colles, S.M., Irwin, K.C., Chisolm, G.M., 1996. Roles of multiple oxidized LDL lipids in cellular injury: dominance of 7 beta-hydroperoxycholesterol. J. Lipid Res. 37, 2018–2028.

Colli, S., Eligini, S., Lalli, M., Camera, M., Paoletti, R., Tremoli, E., 1997. Vastatins inhibit tissue factor in cultured human macrophages. A novel mechanism of protection against atherothrombosis. Arterioscler. Thromb. Vasc. Biol. 17, 265–272.

Collins, R.G., Velji, R., Guevara, N.V., Hicks, M.J., Chan, L., Beaudet, A.L., 2000. P-Selectin or intercellular adhesion molecule (ICAM)-1 deficiency substantially protects against atherosclerosis in apolipoprotein E-deficient mice. J. Exp. Med. 191, 189–194.

Cominacini, L., Pasini, A.F., Garbin, U., Davoli, A., Tosetti, M.L., Campagnola, M., Rigoni, A., Pastorino, A.M., Lo Cascio, V., Sawamura, T., 2000. Oxidized low density lipoprotein (ox-LDL) binding to ox-LDL receptor-1 in endothelial cells induces the activation of NF-kappaB through an increased production of intracellular reactive oxygen species. J. Biol. Chem. 275, 12633–12638.

Cooper, A.D., 1997. Hepatic uptake of chylomicron remnants. J. Lipid Res. 38, 2173–2192.

Cybulsky, M.I., Gimbrone Jr., M.A., 1991. Endothelial expression of a mononuclear leukocyte adhesion molecule during atherogenesis. Science 251, 788–791.

Cynshi, O., Kawabe, Y., Suzuki, T., Takashima, Y., Kaise, H., Nakamura, M., Ohba, Y., Kato, Y., Tamura, K., Hayasaka, A., Higashida, A., Sakaguchi, H., Takeya, M., Takahashi, K., Inoue, K., Noguchi, N., Niki, E., Kodama, T., 1998. Antiatherogenic effects of the antioxidant BO-653 in three different animal models. Proc. Natl. Acad. Sci. U. S. A. 95, 10123–10128.

Cyrus, T., Witztum, J.L., Rader, D.J., Tangirala, R., Fazio, S., Linton, M.F., Funk, C.D., 1999. Disruption of the 12/15-lipoxygenase gene diminishes atherosclerosis in apo E-deficient mice. J. Clin. Invest. 103, 1597–1604.

Cyrus, T., Pratico, D., Zhao, L., Witztum, J.L., Rader, D.J., Rokach, J., FitzGerald, G.A., Funk, C.D., 2001. Absence of 12/15-lipoxygenase expression decreases lipid peroxidation and atherogenesis in apolipoprotein e-deficient mice. Circulation 103, 2277–2282.

Daugherty, A., Cornicelli, J.A., Welch, K., Sendobry, S.M., Rateri, D.L., 1997. Scavenger receptors are present on rabbit aortic endothelial cells in vivo. Arterioscler. Thromb. Vasc. Biol. 17, 2369–2375.

Davidson, N.O., Shelness, G.S., 2000. Apolipoprotein B: mRNA editing, lipoprotein assembly, and presecretory degradation. Annu. Rev. Nutr. 20, 169–193.

Davies, M.J., Richardson, P.D., Woolf, N., Katz, D.R., Mann, J., 1993. Risk of thrombosis in human atherosclerotic plaques: role of extracellular lipid, macrophage, and smooth muscle cell content. Br. Heart J. 69, 377–381.

de Backer, G., de Bacquer, D., Kornitzer, M., 1998. Epidemiological aspects of high density lipoprotein cholesterol. Atherosclerosis 137 (Suppl.), S1–S6.

De Caterina, R., Libby, P., Peng, H.B., Thannickal, V.J., Rajavashisth, T.B., Gimbrone Jr., M.A., Shin, W.S., Liao, J.K., 1995. Nitric oxide decreases cytokine-induced endothelial activation. Nitric oxide selectively reduces endothelial expression of adhesion molecules and proinflammatory cytokines. J. Clin. Invest. 96, 60–68.

de Villiers, W.J., Fraser, I.P., Hughes, D.A., Doyle, A.G., Gordon, S., 1994. Macrophage-colony-stimulating factor selectively enhances macrophage scavenger receptor expression and function. J. Exp. Med. 180, 705–709.

de Vries, H.E., Buchner, B., van Berkel, T.J., Kuiper, J., 1999. Specific interaction of oxidized low-density lipoprotein with macrophage-derived foam cells isolated from rabbit atherosclerotic lesions. Arterioscler. Thromb. Vasc. Biol. 19, 638–645.

de Winther, M.P., Gijbels, M.J., van Dijk, K.W., van Gorp, P.J., Suzuki, H., Kodama, T., Frants, R.R., Havekes, L.M., Hofker, M.H., 1999. Scavenger receptor deficiency leads to more complex atherosclerotic lesions in APOE3Leiden transgenic mice. Atherosclerosis 144, 315–321.

DeBose-Boyd, R.A., Brown, M.S., Li, W.P., Nohturfft, A., Goldstein, J.L., Espenshade, P.J., 1999. Transport-dependent proteolysis of SREBP: relocation of site-1 protease from Golgi to ER obviates the need for SREBP transport to Golgi. Cell 99, 703–712.

Delamatre, J.G., Carter, R.M., Hornick, C.A., 1993. Evidence that a neutral cholesteryl ester hydrolase is responsible for the extralysosomal hydrolysis of high-density lipoprotein cholesteryl ester in rat hepatoma cells (Fu5AH). J. Cell Physiol. 157, 164–168.

Depres, J.P., 1991. Obesity and lipid metabolism: relevance of body fat distribution. Curr. Opin. Lipidol. 2, 5–15.

Despres, J.P., Marette, A., 1994. Relation of components of insulin resistance syndrome to coronary disease risk. Curr. Opin. Lipidol. 5, 274–289.

Detmers, P.A., Hernandez, M., Mudgett, J., Hassing, H., Burton, C., Mundt, S., Chun, S., Fletcher, D., Card, D.J., Lisnock, J., Weikel, R., Bergstrom, J.D., Shevell, D.E., Hermanowski-Vosatka, A., Sparrow, C.P., Chao, Y.S., Rader, D.J., Wright, S.D., Pure, E., 2000. Deficiency in inducible nitric oxide synthase results in reduced atherosclerosis in apolipoprotein E-deficient mice. J. Immunol. 165, 3430–3435.

Dong, Z.M., Chapman, S.M., Brown, A.A., Frenette, P.S., Hynes, R.O., Wagner, D.D., 1998. The combined role of P- and E-selectins in atherosclerosis. J. Clin. Invest. 102, 145–152.

Downs, J.R., Clearfield, M., Weis, S., Whitney, E., Shapiro, D.R., Beere, P.A., Langendorfer, A., Stein, E.A., Kruyer, W., Gotto Jr., A.M., 1998. Primary prevention of acute coronary events with lovastatin in men and women with average cholesterol levels: results of AFCAPS/TexCAPS. Air Force/Texas Coronary Atherosclerosis Prevention Study. J. Am. Med. Assoc. 279, 1615–1622.

Dupuis, J., Tardif, J.C., Cernacek, P., Theroux, P., 1999. Cholesterol reduction rapidly improves endothelial function after acute coronary syndromes. The RECIFE (reduction of cholesterol in ischemia and function of the endothelium) trial. Circulation 99, 3227–3233.

Edelstein, C., Kezdy, F.J., Scanu, A.M., Shen, B.W., 1979. Apolipoproteins and the structural organization of plasma lipoproteins: human plasma high density lipoprotein-3. J. Lipid Res. 20, 143–153.

Eisenberg, S., Sehayek, E., 1995. Remnant particles and their metabolism. Baillieres. Clin. Endocrinol. Metab. 9, 739–753.

Elomaa, O., Kangas, M., Sahlberg, C., Tuukkanen, J., Sormunen, R., Liakka, A., Thesleff, I., Kraal, G., Tryggvason, K., 1995. Cloning of a novel bacteria-binding receptor structurally related to scavenger receptors and expressed in a subset of macrophages. Cell 80, 603–609.

Endemann, G., Stanton, L.W., Madden, K.S., Bryant, C.M., White, R.T., Protter, A.A., 1993. CD36 is a receptor for oxidized low density lipoprotein. J. Biol. Chem. 268, 11811–11816.

Epstein, F.H., 1996. Cardiovascular disease epidemiology: a journey from the past into the future. Circulation 93, 1755–1764.

Ericsson, C.G., Hamsten, A., Nilsson, J., Grip, L., Svane, B., de Faire, U., 1996. Angiographic assessment of effects of bezafibrate on progression of coronary artery disease in young male postinfarction patients. Lancet 347, 849–853.

Essig, M., Nguyen, G., Prie, D., Escoubet, B., Sraer, J.D., Friedlander, G., 1998. 3-Hydroxy-3-methylglutaryl coenzyme A reductase inhibitors increase fibrinolytic activity in rat aortic endothelial cells. Role of geranylgeranylation and Rho proteins. Circ. Res. 83, 683–690.

Esterbauer, H., Dieber-Rotheneder, M., Waeg, G., Striegl, G., Jurgens, G., 1990. Biochemical, structural, and functional properties of oxidized low-density lipoprotein. Chem. Res. Toxicol. 3, 77–92.

Evans, M., Anderson, R.A., Graham, J., Ellis, G.R., Morris, K., Davies, S., Jackson, S.K., Lewis, M.J., Frenneaux, M.P., Rees, A., 2000. Ciprofibrate therapy improves endothelial function and reduces postprandial lipemia and oxidative stress in type 2 diabetes mellitus. Circulation 101, 1773–1779.

Farb, A., Burke, A.P., Tang, A.L., Liang, T.Y., Mannan, P., Smialek, J., Virmani, R., 1996. Coronary plaque erosion without rupture into a lipid core. A frequent cause of coronary thrombosis in sudden coronary death. Circulation 93, 1354–1363.

Febbraio, M., Podrez, E.A., Smith, J.D., Hajjar, D.P., Hazen, S.L., Hoff, H.F., Sharma, K., Silverstein, R.L., 2000. Targeted disruption of the class B scavenger receptor CD36 protects against atherosclerotic lesion development in mice. J. Clin. Invest. 105, 1049–1056.

Febbraio, M., Hajjar, D.P., Silverstein, R.L., 2001. CD36: a class B scavenger receptor involved in angiogenesis, atherosclerosis, inflammation, and lipid metabolism. J. Clin. Invest. 108, 785–791.

Fidge, N.H., 1999. High density lipoprotein receptors, binding proteins, and ligands. J. Lipid Res. 40, 187–201.

Fielding, C.J., Fielding, P.E., 1995. Molecular physiology of reverse cholesterol transport. J. Lipid Res. 36, 211–228.

Folcik, V.A., Nivar-Aristy, R.A., Krajewski, L.P., Cathcart, M.K., 1995. Lipoxygenase contributes to the oxidation of lipids in human atherosclerotic plaques. J. Clin. Invest. 96, 504–510.

Fong, L.G., Fong, T.A., Cooper, A.D., 1990. Inhibition of mouse macrophage degradation of acetyl-low density lipoprotein by interferon-gamma. J. Biol. Chem. 265, 11751–11760.

Frick, M.H., Syvanne, M., Nieminen, M.S., Kauma, H., Majahalme, S., Virtanen, V., Kesaniemi, Y.A., Pasternack, A., Taskinen, M.R., 1997. Prevention of the angiographic progression of coronary and vein-graft atherosclerosis by gemfibrozil after coronary bypass surgery in men with low levels of HDL cholesterol. Lopid Coronary Angiography Trial (LOCAT) Study Group. Circulation 96, 2137–2143.

Frohlich, J., Dobiasova, M., Lear, S., Lee, K.W., 2001. The role of risk factors in the development of atherosclerosis. Crit. Rev. Clin. Lab. Sci. 38, 401–440.

Fukumoto, Y., Libby, P., Rabkin, E., Hill, C.C., Enomoto, M., Hirouchi, Y., Shiomi, M., Aikawa, M., 2001. Statins alter smooth muscle cell accumulation and collagen content in established atheroma of watanabe heritable hyperlipidemic rabbits. Circulation 103, 993–999.

Galis, Z.S., Sukhova, G.K., Lark, M.W., Libby, P., 1994. Increased expression of matrix metalloproteinases and matrix degrading activity in vulnerable regions of human atherosclerotic plaques. J. Clin. Invest. 94, 2493–2503.

Gaut, J.P., Heinecke, J.W., 2001. Mechanisms for oxidizing low-density lipoprotein. Insights from patterns of oxidation products in the artery wall and from mouse models of atherosclerosis. Trends Cardiovasc. Med. 11, 103–112.

Genest Jr., J., Marcil, M., Denis, M., Yu, L., 1999. High density lipoproteins in health and in disease. J. Invest. Med. 47, 31–42.

Geng, Y.J., Hansson, G.K., 1992. Interferon-gamma inhibits scavenger receptor expression and foam cell formation in human monocyte-derived macrophages. J. Clin. Invest. 89, 1322–1330.

Geng, Y.J., Henderson, L.E., Levesque, E.B., Muszynski, M., Libby, P., 1997. Fas is expressed in human atherosclerotic intima and promotes apoptosis of cytokine-primed human vascular smooth muscle cells. Arterioscler. Thromb. Vasc. Biol. 17, 2200–2208.

Gerhard, G.T., Duell, P.B., 1999. Homocysteine and atherosclerosis. Curr. Opin. Lipidol. 10, 417–428.

Ginsberg, H.N., Illingworth, D.R., 2001. Postprandial dyslipidemia: an atherogenic disorder common in patients with diabetes mellitus. Am. J. Cardiol. 88, 9H–15H.

Glass, C., Pittman, R.C., Civen, M., Steinberg, D., 1985. Uptake of high-density lipoprotein-associated apoprotein A-I and cholesterol esters by 16 tissues of the rat in vivo and by adrenal cells and hepatocytes in vitro. J. Biol. Chem. 260, 744–750.

Glass, C.K., Witztum, J.L., 2001. Atherosclerosis. The road ahead. Cell 104 (4), 503–516.

Glomset, J.A., 1968. The plasma lecithins:cholesterol acyltransferase reaction. J. Lipid Res. 9, 155–167.

Goldberg, D.I., Beltz, W.F., Pittman, R.C., 1991. Evaluation of pathways for the cellular uptake of high density lipoprotein cholesterol esters in rabbits. J. Clin. Invest. 87, 331–346.

Goldberg, I.J., Merkel, M., 2001. Lipoprotein lipase: physiology, biochemistry, and molecular biology. Front. Biosci. 6, D388–D405.

Goldbourt, U., Neufeld, H.N., 1986. Genetic aspects of arteriosclerosis. Arteriosclerosis 6, 357–377.

Goldstein, J.L., Brown, M.S., 2001. Molecular medicine. The cholesterol quartet. Science 292, 1310–1312.

Goldstein, J.L., Ho, Y.K., Basu, S.K., Brown, M.S., 1979. Binding site on macrophages that mediates uptake and degradation of acetylated low density lipoprotein, producing massive cholesterol deposition. Proc. Natl. Acad. Sci. U. S. A. 76, 333–337.

Goldstein, J.L., Hobbs, H.H., Brown, M.S., 2001. Familial hypercholesterolemia. In: Scriver, C.R., Beaudet, A.L., Sly, W.S., Valle, D. (Eds.), The Metabolic Bases of Inherited Disease, 8th ed., vol. 2. McGraw-Hill, New York, pp. 2863–2913.

Gordon, T., Castelli, W.P., Hjortland, M.C., Kannel, W.B., Dawber, T.R., 1977. High density lipoprotein as a protective factor against coronary heart disease. The Framingham Study. Am. J. Med. 62, 707–714.

Gosling, J., Slaymaker, S., Gu, L., Tseng, S., Zlot, C.H., Young, S.G., Rollins, B.J., Charo, I.F., 1999. MCP-1 deficiency reduces susceptibility to atherosclerosis in mice that overexpress human apolipoprotein B. J. Clin. Invest. 103, 773–778.

Gotto Jr., A.M., Pownall, H.J., Havel, R.J., 1986. Introduction to the plasma lipoproteins. Meth. Enzymol. 128, 3–41.

Gough, P.J., Greaves, D.R., Gordon, S., 1998. A naturally occurring isoform of the human macrophage scavenger receptor (SR-A) gene generated by alternative splicing blocks modified LDL uptake. J. Lipid Res. 39, 531–543.

Graf, G.A., Connell, P.M., van der Westhuyzen, D.R., Smart, E.J., 1999. The class B, type I scavenger receptor promotes the selective uptake of high density lipoprotein cholesterol ethers into caveolae. J. Biol. Chem. 274, 12043–12048.

Greaves, D.R., Gough, P.J., Gordon, S., 1998. Recent progress in defining the role of scavenger receptors in lipid transport, atherosclerosis and host defence. Curr. Opin. Lipidol. 9, 425–432.

Griendling, K.K., Alexander, R.W., 1997. Oxidative stress and cardiovascular disease. Circulation 96, 3264–3265.

Griffin, J.H., Kojima, K., Banka, C.L., Curtiss, L.K., Fernandez, J.A., 1999. High-density lipoprotein enhancement of anticoagulant activities of plasma protein S and activated protein C. J. Clin. Invest. 103, 219–227.

Gu, L., Okada, Y., Clinton, S.K., Gerard, C., Sukhova, G.K., Libby, P., Rollins, B.J., 1998. Absence of monocyte chemoattractant protein-1 reduces atherosclerosis in low density lipoprotein receptor-deficient mice. Mol. Cell. 2, 275–281.

Guevara, N.V., Kim, H.S., Antonova, E.I., Chan, L., 1999. The absence of p53 accelerates atherosclerosis by increasing cell proliferation in vivo. Nat. Med. 5, 335–339.

Hamilton, K.K., Zhao, J., Sims, P.J., 1993. Interaction between apolipoproteins A-I and A-II and the membrane attack complex of complement. Affinity of the apoproteins for polymeric C9. J. Biol. Chem. 268, 3632–3638.

Hamon, Y., Broccardo, C., Chambenoit, O., Luciani, M.F., Toti, F., Chaslin, S., Freyssinet, J.M., Devaux, P.F., McNeish, J., Marguet, D., Chimini, G., 2000. ABC1 promotes engulfment of apoptotic cells and transbilayer redistribution of phosphatidylserine. Nat. Cell Biol. 2, 399–406.

Han, J., Nicholson, A.C., 1998. Lipoproteins modulate expression of the macrophage scavenger receptor. Am. J. Pathol. 152, 1647–1654.

Han, K.H., Han, K.O., Green, S.R., Quehenberger, O., 1999. Expression of the monocyte chemoattractant protein-1 receptor CCR2 is increased in hypercholesterolemia. Differential effects of plasma lipoproteins on monocyte function. J. Lipid Res. 140, 1053–1063.

Harats, D., Shaish, A., George, J., Mulkins, M., Kurihara, H., Levkovitz, H., Sigal, E., 2000. Overexpression of 15-lipoxygenase in vascular endothelium accelerates early atherosclerosis in LDL receptor-deficient mice. Arterioscler. Thromb. Vasc. Biol. 20, 2100–2105.

Hauser, H., Dyer, J.H., Nandy, A., Vega, M.A., Werder, M., Bieliauskaite, E., Weber, F.E., Compassi, S., Gemperli, A., Boffelli, D., Wehrli, E., Schulthess, G., Phillips, M.C., 1998. Identification of a receptor mediating absorption of dietary cholesterol in the intestine. Biochemistry 37, 17843–17850.

Havel, R.J., 1994. Postprandial hyperlipidemia and remnant lipoproteins. Curr. Opin. Lipidol. 5, 102–109.

Havel, R.J., 2000. Remnant lipoproteins as therapeutic targets. Curr. Opin. Lipidol. 11, 615–620.

Havel, R.J., Kane, J.P., 2001. Introduction: structure and metabolism of plasma lipoproteins. In: Scriver, C.R., Beaudet, A.L., Sly, W.S., Valle, D. (Eds.), The Metabolic Bases of Inherited Disease, 8th ed., vol. 2. McGraw-Hill, New York, pp. 2705–2716.

Hayek, T., Oiknine, J., Dankner, G., Brook, J.G., Aviram, M., 1995. HDL apolipoprotein A-I attenuates oxidative modification of low density lipoprotein: studies in transgenic mice. Eur. J. Clin. Chem. Clin. Biochem. 33, 721–725.

Heinecke, J.W., Rosen, H., Chait, A., 1984. Iron and copper promote modification of low density lipoprotein by human arterial smooth muscle cells in culture. J. Clin. Invest. 74, 1890–1894.

Hergenc, G., Schulte, H., Assmann, G., von Eckardstein, A., 1999. Associations of obesity markers, insulin, and sex hormones with HDL-cholesterol levels in Turkish and German individuals. Atherosclerosis 145, 147–156.

Hernandez-Perera, O., Perez-Sala, D., Navarro-Antolin, J., Sanchez-Pascuala, R., Hernandez, G., Diaz, C., Lamas, S., 1998. Effects of the 3-hydroxy-3-methylglutaryl-CoA reductase inhibitors, atorvastatin and simvastatin, on the expression of endothelin-1 and endothelial nitric oxide synthase in vascular endothelial cells. J. Clin. Invest. 101, 2711–2719.

Hessler, J.R., Morel, D.W., Lewis, L.J., Chisolm, G.M., 1983. Lipoprotein oxidation and lipoprotein-induced cytotoxicity. Arteriosclerosis 3, 215–222.

Hiltunen, T.P., Luoma, J.S., Nikkari, T., Yla-Herttuala, S., 1998. Expression of LDL receptor, VLDL receptor, LDL receptor-related protein, and scavenger receptor in rabbit atherosclerotic lesions: marked induction of scavenger receptor and VLDL receptor expression during lesion development. Circulation 97, 1079–1086.

Hobbs, H.H., Brown, M.S., Goldstein, J.L., 1992. Molecular genetics of the LDL receptor gene in familial hypercholesterolemia. Hum. Mutat. 1, 445–466.

Hodis, H.N., 1999. Triglyceride-rich lipoprotein remnant particles and risk of atherosclerosis. Circulation 99, 2852–2854.

Hoffman, H.N., Fredrickson, D.S., 1965. Tangier disease (familial high density lipoprotein deficiency). Clinical and genetic features in two adults. Am. J. Med. 39 (4), 582–593.

Hokanson, J.E., Austin, M.A., 1996. Plasma triglyceride level is a risk factor for cardiovascular disease independent of high-density lipoprotein cholesterol level: a meta-analysis of population-based prospective studies. J. Cardiovasc. Risk. 3, 213–219.

Holvoet, P., Vanhaecke, J., Janssens, S., Van de Werf, F., Collen, D., 1998. Oxidized LDL and malondialdehyde-modified LDL in patients with acute coronary syndromes and stable coronary artery disease. Circulation 98, 1487–1494.

Horkko, S., Bird, D.A., Miller, E., Itabe, H., Leitinger, N., Subbanagounder, G., Berliner, J.A., Friedman, P., Dennis, E.A., Curtiss, L.K., Palinski, W., Witztum, J.L., 1999. Monoclonal autoantibodies specific for oxidized phospholipids or oxidized phospholipid–protein adducts inhibit macrophage uptake of oxidized low-density lipoproteins. J. Clin. Invest. 103, 117–128.

Hsu, H.Y., Nicholson, A.C., Hajjar, D.P., 1996. Inhibition of macrophage scavenger receptor activity by tumor necrosis factor-alpha is transcriptionally and post-transcriptionally regulated. J. Biol. Chem. 271, 7767–7773.

Hughes, D.A., Fraser, I.P., Gordon, S., 1995. Murine macrophage scavenger receptor: in vivo expression and function as receptor for macrophage adhesion in lymphoid and non-lymphoid organs. Eur. J. Immunol. 25, 466–473.

Hulten, L.M., Lindmark, H., Diczfalusy, U., Bjorkhem, I., Ottosson, M., Liu, Y., Bondjers, G., Wiklund, O., 1996. Oxysterols present in atherosclerotic tissue decrease the expression of lipoprotein lipase messenger RNA in human monocyte-derived macrophages. J. Clin. Invest. 97, 461–468.

Iso, H., Jacobs Jr., D.R., Wentworth, D., Neaton, J.D., Cohen, J.D., 1989. Serum cholesterol levels and six-year mortality from stroke in 350,977 men screened for the multiple risk factor intervention trial. N. Engl. J. Med. 320, 904–910.

Itabe, H., Yamamoto, H., Imanaka, T., Shimamura, K., Uchiyama, H., Kimura, J., Sanaka, T., Hata, Y., Takano, T., 1996. Sensitive detection of oxidatively modified low density lipoprotein using a monoclonal antibody. J. Lipid Res. 37, 45–53.

Iuliano, L., Mauriello, A., Sbarigia, E., Spagnoli, L.G., Violi, F., 2000. Radiolabeled native low-density lipoprotein injected into patients with carotid stenosis accumulates in macrophages of atherosclerotic plaque: effect of vitamin E supplementation. Circulation 101, 1249–1254.

Jackson, L.A., Campbell, L.A., Schmidt, R.A., Kuo, C.C., Cappuccio, A.L., Lee, M.J., Grayston, J.T., 1997. Specificity of detection of *Chlamydia pneumoniae* in cardiovascular atheroma: evaluation of the innocent bystander hypothesis. Am. J. Pathol. 150, 1785–1790.

Ji, Y., Jian, B., Wang, N., Sun, Y., Moya, M.L., Phillips, M.C., Rothblat, G.H., Swaney, J.B., Tall, A.R., 1997. Scavenger receptor BI promotes high density lipoprotein-mediated cellular cholesterol efflux. J. Biol. Chem. 272, 20982–20985.

Ji, Y., Wang, N., Ramakrishnan, R., Sehayek, E., Huszar, D., Breslow, J.L., Tall, A.R., 1999. Hepatic scavenger receptor BI promotes rapid clearance of high density lipoprotein free cholesterol and its transport into bile. J. Biol. Chem. 274, 33398–33402.

Kameda, K., Matsuzawa, Y., Kubo, M., Ishikawa, K., Maejima, I., Yamamura, T., Yamamoto, A., Tarui, S., 1984. Increased frequency of lipoprotein disorders similar to type III hyperlipoproteinemia in survivors of myocardial infarction in Japan. Atherosclerosis 51, 241–249.

Kang, S., Davis, R.A., 2000. Cholesterol and hepatic lipoprotein assembly and secretion. Biochim. Biophys. Acta 1529, 223–230.

Kannel, W.B., Castelli, W.P., Gordon, T., McNamara, P.M., 1971. Serum cholesterol, lipoproteins, and the risk of coronary heart disease. The Framingham study. Ann. Intern. Med. 74, 1–12.

Kaplan, N.M., 1989. The deadly quartet. Upper-body obesity, glucose intolerance, hypertriglyceridemia, and hypertension. Arch. Intern. Med. 149, 1514–1520.

Fujioka, S., Matsuzawa, Y., Tokunaga, K., Tarui, S., 1987. Contribution of intra-abdominal fat accumulation to the impairment of glucose and lipid metabolism in human obesity. Metabolism 36, 54–59.

Karpe, F., 1999. Postprandial lipoprotein metabolism and atherosclerosis. J. Intern. Med. 246, 341–355.

Karpe, F., Hamsten, A., 1995. Postprandial lipoprotein metabolism and atherosclerosis. Curr. Opin. Lipidol. 6, 123–129.

Khan, B.V., Harrison, D.G., Olbrych, M.T., Alexander, R.W., Medford, R.M., 1996. Nitric oxide regulates vascular cell adhesion molecule 1 gene expression and redox-sensitive transcriptional events in human vascular endothelial cells. Proc. Natl. Acad. Sci. U. S. A. 93, 9114–9119.

Kinlay, S., Selwyn, A.P., Libby, P., Ganz, P., 1998. Inflammation, the endothelium, and the acute coronary syndromes. J. Cardiovasc. Pharmacol. 32 (Suppl. 3), S62–S66.

Kinlay, S., Libby, P., Ganz, P., 2001. Endothelial function and coronary artery disease. Curr. Opin. Lipidol. 12, 383–389.

Kirk, E.A., Dinauer, M.C., Rosen, H., Chait, A., Heinecke, J.W., LeBoeuf, R.C., 2000. Impaired superoxide production due to a deficiency in phagocyte NADPH oxidase fails to inhibit atherosclerosis in mice. Arterioscler. Thromb. Vasc. Biol. 20, 1529–1535.

Kita, T., Nagano, Y., Yokode, M., Ishii, K., Kume, N., Ooshima, A., Yoshida, H., Kawai, C., 1987. Probucol prevents the progression of atherosclerosis in Watanabe heritable hyperlipidemic rabbit, an animal model for familial hypercholesterolemia. Proc. Natl. Acad. Sci. U. S. A. 84, 5928–5931.

Klein, I., Sarkadi, B., Varadi, A., 1999. An inventory of the human ABC proteins. Biochim. Biophys. Acta 1461, 237–262.

Klucken, J., Buchler, C., Orso, E., Kaminski, W.E., Porsch-Ozcurumez, M., Liebisch, G., Kapinsky, M., Diederich, W., Drobnik, W., Dean, M., Allikmets, R., Schmitz, G., 2000. ABCG1 (ABC8), the human homolog of the *Drosophila* white gene, is a regulator of macrophage cholesterol and phospholipid transport. Proc. Natl. Acad. Sci. U. S. A. 97, 817–822.

Knecht, T.P., Pittman, R.C., 1989. A plasma membrane pool of cholesteryl esters that may mediate the selective uptake of cholesteryl esters from high-density lipoproteins. Biochim. Biophys. Acta 1002, 365–375.

Knowles, J.W., Reddick, R.L., Jennette, J.C., Shesely, E.G., Smithies, O., Maeda, N., 2000. Enhanced atherosclerosis and kidney dysfunction in eNOS(−/−)Apoe(−/−) mice are ameliorated by enalapril treatment. J. Clin. Invest. 105, 451–458.

Kodama, T., Freeman, M., Rohrer, L., Zabrecky, J., Matsudaira, P., Krieger, M., 1990. Type I macrophage scavenger receptor contains alpha-helical and collagen-like coiled coils. Nature 343, 531–535.

Kozarsky, K.F., Donahee, M.H., Glick, J.M., Krieger, M., Rader, D.J., 2000. Gene transfer and hepatic overexpression of the HDL receptor SR-BI reduces atherosclerosis in the cholesterol-fed LDL receptor-deficient mouse. Arterioscler. Thromb. Vasc. Biol. 20, 721–727.

Krauss, R.M., 1998. Atherogenicity of triglyceride-rich lipoproteins. Am. J. Cardiol. 81, 13B–17B.

Krieger, M., 1997. The other side of scavenger receptors: pattern recognition for host defense. Curr. Opin. Lipidol. 8, 275–280.

Krieger, M., 2001. Scavenger receptor class B type I is a multiligand HDL receptor that influences diverse physiologic systems. J. Clin. Invest. 108, 793–797.

Krieger, M., Kozarsky, K., 1999. Influence of the HDL receptor SR-BI on atherosclerosis. Curr. Opin. Lipidol. 10, 491–497.

Kuhn, H., Heydeck, D., Hugou, I., Gniwotta, C., 1997. In vivo action of 15-lipoxygenase in early stages of human atherogenesis. J. Clin. Invest. 99, 888–893.

Kureishi, Y., Luo, Z., Shiojima, I., Bialik, A., Fulton, D., Lefer, D.J., Sessa, W.C., Walsh, K., 2000. The HMG-CoA reductase inhibitor simvastatin activates the protein kinase Akt and promotes angiogenesis in normocholesterolemic animals. Nat. Med. 6, 1004–1010.

Landschulz, K.T., Pathak, R.K., Rigotti, A., Krieger, M., Hobbs, H.H., 1996. Regulation of scavenger receptor, class B, type I, a high density lipoprotein receptor, in liver and steroidogenic tissues of the rat. J. Clin. Invest. 98, 984–995.

Langmann, T., Klucken, J., Reil, M., Liebisch, G., Luciani, M.F., Chimini, G., Kaminski, W.E., Schmitz, G., 1999. Molecular cloning of the human ATP-binding cassette transporter 1 (hABC1): evidence for sterol-dependent regulation in macrophages. Biochem. Biophys. Res. Commun. 257, 29–33.

Laufs, U., La Fata, V., Plutzky, J., Liao, J.K., 1998. Upregulation of endothelial nitric oxide synthase by HMG CoA reductase inhibitors. Circulation 97, 1129–1135.

Laufs, U., Marra, D., Node, K., Liao, J.K., 1999. 3-Hydroxy-3-methylglutaryl-CoA reductase inhibitors attenuate vascular smooth muscle proliferation by preventing rho GTPase-induced down-regulation of p27(Kip1). J. Biol. Chem. 274, 21926–21931.

Lawn, R.M., Wade, D.P., Garvin, M.R., Wang, X., Schwartz, K., Porter, J.G., Seilhamer, J.J., Vaughan, A.M., Oram, J.F., 1999. The Tangier disease gene product ABC1 controls the cellular apolipoprotein-mediated lipid removal pathway. J. Clin. Invest. 104, R25–R31.

Lee, R.T., Libby, P., 1997. The unstable atheroma. Arterioscler. Thromb. Vasc. Biol. 17, 1859–1867.

Li, D., Saldeen, T., Romeo, F., Mehta, J.L., 2000. Oxidized LDL upregulates angiotensin II type 1 receptor expression in cultured human coronary artery endothelial cells: the potential role of transcription factor NF-kappaB. Circulation 102, 1970–1976.

Li, H., Freeman, M.W., Libby, P., 1995. Regulation of smooth muscle cell scavenger receptor expression in vivo by atherogenic diets and in vitro by cytokines. J. Clin. Invest. 95, 122–133.

Libby, P., 2001. Current concepts of the pathogenesis of the acute coronary syndromes. Circulation 104, 365–372.

Libby, P., Egan, D., Skarlatos, S., 1997. Roles of infectious agents in atherosclerosis and restenosis: an assessment of the evidence and need for future research. Circulation 96, 4095–4103.

Libby, P., Hansson, G.K., Pober, J.S., 1999. Atherogenesis and inflammation. In: Chein, K.R. (Ed.), Molecular Basis of Cardiovascular Disease. W.B. Saunders, Philadelphia, pp. 349–366.

Ling, W., Lougheed, M., Suzuki, H., Buchan, A., Kodama, T., Steinbrecher, U.P., 1997. Oxidized or acetylated low density lipoproteins are rapidly cleared by the liver in mice with disruption of the scavenger receptor class A type I/II gene. J. Clin. Invest. 100, 244–252.

Linton, M.F., Fazio, S., 2001. Class A scavenger receptors, macrophages, and atherosclerosis. Curr. Opin. Lipidol. 12, 489–495.

Linton, M.F., Atkinson, J.B., Fazio, S., 1995. Prevention of atherosclerosis in apolipoprotein E-deficient mice by bone marrow transplantation. Science 267, 1034–1037.

Lougheed, M., Lum, C.M., Ling, W., Suzuki, H., Kodama, T., Steinbrecher, U., 1997. High affinity saturable uptake of oxidized low density lipoprotein by macrophages from mice lacking the scavenger receptor class A type I/II. J. Biol. Chem. 272, 12938–12944.

Luciani, M.F., Denizot, F., Savary, S., Mattei, M.G., Chimini, G., 1994. Cloning of two novel ABC transporters mapping on human chromosome 9. Genomics 21, 150–159.

Lusis, A.J., 2000. Atherosclerosis. Nature 407, 233–241.

Mackness, M.I., Durrington, P.N., Mackness, B., 2000. How high-density lipoprotein protects against the effects of lipid peroxidation. Curr. Opin. Lipidol. 11, 383–388.

Maeda, K., Okubo, K., Shimomura, I., Funahashi, T., Matsuzawa, Y., Matsubara, K., 1996. cDNA cloning and expression of a novel adipose specific collagen-like factor, apM1 (AdiPose Most abundant Gene transcript 1). Biochem. Biophys. Res. Commun. 221, 286–289.

Majors, A., Ehrhart, L.A., Pezacka, E.H., 1997. Homocysteine as a risk factor for vascular disease. Enhanced collagen production and accumulation by smooth muscle cells. Arterioscler. Thromb. Vasc. Biol. 17, 2074–2081.

Mallat, Z., Nakamura, T., Ohan, J., Leseche, G., Tedgui, A., Maclouf, J., Murphy, R.C., 1999. The relationship of hydroxyeicosatetraenoic acids and F2-isoprostanes to plaque instability in human carotid atherosclerosis. J. Clin. Invest. 103, 421–427.

Martinet, W., Kockx, M.M., 2001. Apoptosis in atherosclerosis: focus on oxidized lipids and inflammation. Curr. Opin. Lipidol. 12, 535–541.

Matsuda, Y., Hirata, K., Inoue, N., Suematsu, M., Kawashima, S., Akita, H., Yokoyama, M., 1993. High density lipoprotein reverses inhibitory effect of oxidized low density lipoprotein on endothelium-dependent arterial relaxation. Circ. Res. 72, 1103–1109.

Matsumoto, A., Naito, M., Itakura, H., Ikemoto, S., Asaoka, H., Hayakawa, I., Kanamori, H., Aburatani, H., Takaku, F., Suzuki, H., et al., 1990. Human macrophage scavenger receptors: primary structure, expression, and localization in atherosclerotic lesions. Proc. Natl. Acad. Sci. U. S. A. 87, 9133–9137.

Matsuzawa, Y., Fujioka, S., Tokunaga, T., Tarui, S., 1987. A novel classification: visceral fat obesity and subcutaneous fat obesity. In: Berry, V.E.M., Blondheim, S.H., Shafrir, E. (Eds.), Recent Advances in Obesity Research. John Libbey & Co. Ltd., London, pp. 92–96.

Matsuzawa, Y., Shimomura, I., Nakamura, T., Keno, Y., Kotani, K., Tokunaga, K., 1995. Pathophysiology and pathogenesis of visceral fat obesity. Obes. Res. 3, 187S–194S.

Matsuzawa, Y., Funahashi, T., Nakamura, T., 2002. Molecular mechanism of vascular disease in metabolic syndrome X. J. Diabetes Complic. 16, 17–18.

Mellwig, K.P., Baller, D., Gleichmann, U., Moll, D., Betker, S., Weise, R., Notohamiprodjo, G., 1998. Improvement of coronary vasodilatation capacity through single LDL apheresis. Atherosclerosis 139, 173–178.

Miller, G.J., 1980. High density lipoproteins and atherosclerosis. Annu. Rev. Med. 31, 97–108.

Miller, G.J., Miller, N.E., 1975. Plasma-high-density-lipoprotein concentration and development of ischaemic heart-disease. Lancet 1, 16–19.

Miyaoka, K., Kuwasako, T., Hirano, K., Nozaki, S., Yamashita, S., Matsuzawa, Y., 2001. CD36 deficiency associated with insulin resistance. Lancet 357, 686–687.

Mullen, M.J., Wright, D., Donald, A.E., Thorne, S., Thomson, H., Deanfield, J.E., 2000. Atorvastatin but not L-arginine improves endothelial function in type I diabetes mellitus: a double-blind study. J. Am. Coll. Cardiol. 36, 410–416.

Nagy, L., Tontonoz, P., Alvarez, J.G., Chen, H., Evans, R.M., 1998. Oxidized LDL regulates macrophage gene expression through ligand activation of PPARgamma. Cell 93, 229–240.

Naito, M., Suzuki, H., Mori, T., Matsumoto, A., Kodama, T., Takahashi, K., 1992. Coexpression of type I and type II human macrophage scavenger receptors in macrophages of various organs and foam cells in atherosclerotic lesions. Am. J. Pathol. 141, 591–599.

Nakamura, T., Tokunaga, K., Shimomura, I., Nishida, M., Yoshida, S., Kotani, K., Islam, A.H., Keno, Y., Kobatake, T., Nagai, Y., et al., 1994. Contribution of visceral fat accumulation to the development of coronary artery disease in non-obese men. Atherosclerosis 107, 239–246.

Napoli, C., D'Armiento, F.P., Mancini, F.P., Postiglione, A., Witztum, J.L., Palumbo, G., Palinski, W., 1997. Fatty streak formation occurs in human fetal aortas and is greatly enhanced by maternal hypercholesterolemia. Intimal accumulation of low density lipoprotein and its oxidation precede monocyte recruitment into early atherosclerotic lesions. J. Clin. Invest. 100, 2680–2690.

Naqvi, T.Z., Shah, P.K., Ivey, P.A., Molloy, M.D., Thomas, A.M., Panicker, S., Ahmed, A., Cercek, B., Kaul, S., 1999. Evidence that high-density lipoprotein cholesterol is an independent predictor of acute platelet-dependent thrombus formation. Am. J. Cardiol. 84, 1011–1017.

Navab, M., Berliner, J.A., Watson, A.D., Hama, S.Y., Territo, M.C., Lusis, A.J., Shih, D.M., Van Lenten, B.J., Frank, J.S., Demer, L.L., Edwards, P.A., Fogelman, A.M., 1996. The Yin and Yang of oxidation in the development of the fatty streak. A review based on the 1994 George Lyman Duff Memorial Lecture. Arterioscler. Thromb. Vasc. Biol. 16, 831–842.

Nicholson, A.C., Frieda, S., Pearce, A., Silverstein, R.L., 1995. Oxidized LDL binds to CD36 on human monocyte-derived macrophages and transfected cell lines. Evidence implicating the lipid moiety of the lipoprotein as the binding site. Arterioscler. Thromb. Vasc. Biol. 15, 269–275.

Nilsson, J., Dahlgren, B., Ares, M., Westman, J., Hultgardh Nilsson, A., Cercek, B., Shah, P.K., 1998. Lipoprotein-like phospholipid particles inhibit the smooth muscle cell cytotoxicity of lysophosphatidylcholine and platelet-activating factor. Arterioscler. Thromb. Vasc. Biol. 18, 13–19.

Nohturfft, A., Yabe, D., Goldstein, J.L., Brown, M.S., Espenshade, P.J., 2000. Regulated step in cholesterol feedback localized to budding of SCAP from ER membranes. Cell 102, 315–323.

Nozaki, S., Kashiwagi, H., Yamashita, S., Nakagawa, T., Kostner, B., Tomiyama, Y., Nakata, A., Ishigami, M., Miyagawa, J., Kameda-Takemura, K., et al., 1995. Reduced uptake of oxidized low density lipoproteins in monocyte-derived macrophages from CD36-deficient subjects. J. Clin. Invest. 96, 1859–1865.

O'Brien, K.D., Alpers, C.E., Hokanson, J.E., Wang, S., Chait, A., 1996. Oxidation-specific epitopes in human coronary atherosclerosis are not limited to oxidized low-density lipoprotein. Circulation 94, 1216–1225.

Ohara, Y., Peterson, T.E., Harrison, D.G., 1993. Hypercholesterolemia increases endothelial superoxide anion production. J. Clin. Invest. 91, 2546–2451.

Olofsson, S.O., Asp, L., Boren, J., 1999. The assembly and secretion of apolipoprotein B-containing lipoproteins. Curr. Opin. Lipidol. 10, 341–346.

Orso, E., Broccardo, C., Kaminski, W.E., Bottcher, A., Liebisch, G., Drobnik, W., Gotz, A., Chambenoit, O., Diederich, W., Langmann, T., Spruss, T., Luciani, M.F., Rothe, G., Lackner, K.J., Chimini, G., Schmitz, G., 2000. Transport of lipids from golgi to plasma membrane is defective in tangier disease patients and Abc1-deficient mice. Nat. Genet. 24, 192–196.

Ouchi, N., Kihara, S., Arita, Y., Nishida, M., Matsuyama, A., Okamoto, Y., Ishigami, M., Kuriyama, H., Kishida, K., Nishizawa, H., Hotta, K., Muraguchi, M., Ohmoto, Y., Yamashita, S., Funahashi, T., Matsuzawa, Y., 2001. Adipocyte-derived plasma protein, adiponectin, suppresses lipid accumulation and class A scavenger receptor expression in human monocyte-derived macrophages. Circulation 103, 1057–1063.

Palinski, W., Horkko, S., Miller, E., Steinbrecher, U.P., Powell, H.C., Curtiss, L.K., Witztum, J.L., 1996. Cloning of monoclonal autoantibodies to epitopes of oxidized lipoproteins from apolipoprotein E-deficient mice. Demonstration of epitopes of oxidized low density lipoprotein in human plasma. J. Clin. Invest. 98, 800–814.

Panini, S.R., Sinensky, M.S., 2001. Mechanisms of oxysterol-induced apoptosis. Curr. Opin. Lipidol. 12, 529–533.

Parker, R.A., Sabrah, T., Cap, M., Gill, B.T., 1995. Relation of vascular oxidative stress, alpha-tocopherol, and hypercholesterolemia to early atherosclerosis in hamsters. Arterioscler. Thromb. Vasc. Biol. 15, 349–358.

Parks, E.J., 2001. Recent findings in the study of postprandial lipemia. Curr. Atheroscler. Rep. 3, 462–470.

Patsch, J.R., Miesenbock, G., Hopferwieser, T., Muhlberger, V., Knapp, E., Dunn, J.K., Gotto Jr., A.M., Patsch, W., 1992. Relation of triglyceride metabolism and coronary artery disease. Studies in the postprandial state. Arterioscler. Thromb. 12, 1336–1345.

Paulsson, G., Zhou, X., Tornquist, E., Hansson, G.K., 2000. Oligoclonal T cell expansions in atherosclerotic lesions of apolipoprotein E-deficient mice. Arterioscler. Thromb. Vasc. Biol. 20, 10–17.

Peng, H.B., Libby, P., Liao, J.K., 1995a. Induction and stabilization of I kappa B alpha by nitric oxide mediates inhibition of NF-kappa B. J. Biol. Chem. 270, 14214–14219.

Peng, H.B., Rajavashisth, T.B., Libby, P., Liao, J.K., 1995b. Nitric oxide inhibits macrophage-colony stimulating factor gene transcription in vascular endothelial cells. J. Biol. Chem. 270, 17050–17055.

Pitt, B., Waters, D., Brown, W.V., van Boven, A.J., Schwartz, L., Title, L.M., Eisenberg, D., Shurzinske, L., McCormick, L.S., 1999. Aggressive lipid-lowering therapy compared with angioplasty in stable coronary artery disease. Atorvastatin versus Revascularization Treatment Investigators. N. Engl. J. Med. 341, 70–76.

Pittman, R.C., Steinberg, D., 1984. Sites and mechanisms of uptake and degradation of high density and low density lipoproteins. J. Lipid Res. 25, 1577–1585.

Plump, A.S., Smith, J.D., Hayek, T., Aalto-Setala, K., Walsh, A., Verstuyft, J.G., Rubin, E.M., Breslow, J.L., 1992. Severe hypercholesterolemia and atherosclerosis in apolipoprotein E-deficient mice created by homologous recombination in ES cells. Cell 71, 343–353.

Pratico, D., Iuliano, L., Mauriello, A., Spagnoli, L., Lawson, J.A., Rokach, J., Maclouf, J., Violi, F., FitzGerald, G.A., 1997. Localization of distinct F2-isoprostanes in human atherosclerotic lesions. J. Clin. Invest. 100, 2028–2034.

Pratico, D., Tangirala, R.K., Rader, D.J., Rokach, J., FitzGerald, G.A., 1998. Vitamin E suppresses iso-prostane generation in vivo and reduces atherosclerosis in ApoE-deficient mice. Nat. Med. 4, 1189–1192.

Pravenec, M., Landa, V., Zidek, V., Musilova, A., Kren, V., Kazdova, L., Aitman, T.J., Glazier, A.M., Ibrahimi, A., Abumrad, N.A., Qi, N., Wang, J.M., St Lezin, E.M., Kurtz, T.W., 2001. Transgenic res-cue of defective Cd36 ameliorates insulin resistance in spontaneously hypertensive rats. Nat. Genet. 27, 156–158.

Puente Navazo, M.D., Daviet, L., Ninio, E., McGregor, J.L., 1996. Identification on human CD36 of a domain (155–183) implicated in binding oxidized low-density lipoproteins (Ox-LDL). Arterioscler. Thromb. Vasc. Biol. 16, 1033–1039.

Qiao, J.H., Tripathi, J., Mishra, N.K., Cai, Y., Tripathi, S., Wang, X.P., Imes, S., Fishbein, M.C., Clinton, S.K., Libby, P., Lusis, A.J., Rajavashisth, T.B., 1997. Role of macrophage colony-stimulating factor in atherosclerosis: studies of osteopetrotic mice. Am. J. Pathol. 150, 1687–1699.

Rawson, R.B., Zelenski, N.G., Nijhawan, D., Ye, J., Sakai, J., Hasan, M.T., Chang, T.Y., Brown, M.S., Goldstein, J.L., 1997. Complementation cloning of S2P, a gene encoding a putative metalloprotease required for intramembrane cleavage of SREBPs. Mol. Cell. 1, 47–57.

Rawson, R.B., DeBose-Boyd, R., Goldstein, J.L., Brown, M.S., 1999. Failure to cleave sterol regulatory element-binding proteins (SREBPs) causes cholesterol auxotrophy in Chinese hamster ovary cells with genetic absence of SREBP cleavage-activating protein. J. Biol. Chem. 274, 28549–28556.

Reaven, G.M., Hoffman, B.B., 1987. A role for insulin in the aetiology and course of hypertension? Lancet 2, 435–437.

Ridker, P.M., Rifai, N., Pfeffer, M.A., Sacks, F., Braunwald, E., 1999. Long-term effects of pravastatin on plasma concentration of C-reactive protein. The Cholesterol and Recurrent Events (CARE) Investiga-tors. Circulation 100, 230–235.

Rigotti, A., Trigatti, B.L., Penman, M., Rayburn, H., Herz, J., Krieger, M., 1997. A targeted mutation in the murine gene encoding the high density lipoprotein (HDL) receptor scavenger receptor class B type I reveals its key role in HDL metabolism. Proc. Natl. Acad. Sci. U. S. A. 94, 12610–12615.

Rikitake, Y., Kawashima, S., Takeshita, S., Yamashita, T., Azumi, H., Yasuhara, M., Nishi, H., Inoue, N., Yokoyama, M., 2001. Anti-oxidative properties of fluvastatin, an HMG-CoA reductase inhibitor, contribute to prevention of atherosclerosis in cholesterol-fed rabbits. Atherosclerosis 154, 87–96.

Rinninger, F., Jaeckle, S., Pittman, R.C., 1993. A pool of reversibly cell-associated cholesteryl esters involved in the selective uptake of cholesteryl esters from high-density lipoproteins by Hep G2 hepa-toma cells. Biochim. Biophys. Acta 1166, 275–283.

Rohrer, L., Freeman, M., Kodama, T., Penman, M., Krieger, M., 1990. Coiled-coil fibrous domains med-iate ligand binding by macrophage scavenger receptor type II. Nature 343, 570–572.

Ross, R., 1986. The pathogenesis of atherosclerosis—an update. N. Engl. J. Med. 314 (8), 488–500.

Ross, R., 1993. The pathogenesis of atherosclerosis: a perspective for the 1990s. Nature 362, 801–809.

Ross, R., 1999. Atherosclerosis—an inflammatory disease. N. Engl. J. Med. 340, 115–126.

Rothblat, G.H., de la Llera-Moya, M., Atger, V., Kellner-Weibel, G., Williams, D.L., Phillips, M.C., 1999. Cell cholesterol efflux: integration of old and new observations provides new insights. J. Lipid Res. 40, 781–796.

Rust, S., Rosier, M., Funke, H., Real, J., Amoura, Z., Piette, J.C., Deleuze, J.F., Brewer, H.B., Duverger, N., Denefle, P., Assmann, G., 1999. Tangier disease is caused by mutations in the gene encoding ATP-binding cassette transporter 1. Nat. Genet. 22, 352–355.

Rye, K.A., Clay, M.A., Barter, P.J., 1999. Remodelling of high density lipoproteins by plasma factors. Atherosclerosis 145, 227–238.

Sacks, F.M., Pfeffer, M.A., Moye, L.A., Rouleau, J.L., Rutherford, J.D., Cole, T.G., Brown, L., Warnica, J.W., Arnold, J.M., Wun, C.C., Davis, B.R., Braunwald, E., 1996. The effect of pravastatin on coron-ary events after myocardial infarction in patients with average cholesterol levels. Cholesterol and Recurrent Events Trial Investigators. N. Engl. J. Med. 335, 1001–1009.

Sakaguchi, H., Takeya, M., Suzuki, H., Hakamata, H., Kodama, T., Horiuchi, S., Gordon, S., van der Laan, L.J., Kraal, G., Ishibashi, S., Kitamura, N., Takahashi, K., 1998. Role of macrophage scavenger receptors in diet-induced atherosclerosis in mice. Lab. Invest. 78, 423–434.

Sakai, J., Rawson, R.B., Espenshade, P.J., Cheng, D., Seegmiller, A.C., Goldstein, J.L., Brown, M.S., 1998. Molecular identification of the sterol-regulated luminal protease that cleaves SREBPs and controls lipid composition of animal cells. Mol. Cell. 2, 505–514.

Sakai, N., Matsuzawa, Y., Hirano, K., Yamashita, S., Nozaki, S., Ueyama, Y., Kubo, M., Tarui, S., 1991. Detection of two species of low density lipoprotein particles in cholesteryl ester transfer protein deficiency. Arterioscler. Thromb. 11, 71–79.

Saku, K., Ahmad, M., Glas-Greenwalt, P., Kashyap, M.L., 1985. Activation of fibrinolysis by apolipoproteins of high density lipoproteins in man. Thromb. Res. Suppl. 39, 1–8.

Sampietro, T., Tuoni, M., Ferdeghini, M., Ciardi, A., Marraccini, P., Prontera, C., Sassi, G., Taddei, M., Bionda, A., 1997. Plasma cholesterol regulates soluble cell adhesion molecule expression in familial hypercholesterolemia. Circulation 96, 1381–1385.

Santamarina-Fojo, S., Haudenschild, C., 2000. Role of hepatic and lipoprotein lipase in lipoprotein metabolism and atherosclerosis: studies in transgenic and knockout animal models and somatic gene transfer. Int. J. Tissue React. 22, 39–47.

Santamarina-Fojo, S., Lambert, G., Hoeg, J.M., Brewer Jr., H.B., 2000. Lecithin–cholesterol acyltransferase: role in lipoprotein metabolism, reverse cholesterol transport and atherosclerosis. Curr. Opin. Lipidol. 11, 267–275.

Santamarina-Fojo, S., Remaley, A.T., Neufeld, E.B., Brewer Jr., H.B., 2001. Regulation and intracellular trafficking of the ABCA1 transporter. J. Lipid Res. 42, 1339–1345.

Sasahara, M., Raines, E.W., Chait, A., Carew, T.E., Steinberg, D., Wahl, P.W., Ross, R., 1994. Inhibition of hypercholesterolemia-induced atherosclerosis in the nonhuman primate by probucol. I. Is the extent of atherosclerosis related to resistance of LDL to oxidation? J. Clin. Invest. 94, 155–164.

Saxena, U., Ferguson, E., Bisgaier, C.L., 1993. Apolipoprotein E modulates low density lipoprotein retention by lipoprotein lipase anchored to the subendothelial matrix. J. Biol. Chem. 268, 14812–14819.

Schaefer, E.J., Blum, C.B., Levy, R.I., Jenkins, L.L., Alaupovic, P., Foster, D.M., Brewer Jr., H.B., 1978. Metabolism of high-density lipoprotein apolipoproteins in Tangier disease. N. Engl. J. Med. 299, 905–910.

Schmitz, G., Langmann, T., 2001. Structure, function and regulation of the ABC1 gene product. Curr. Opin. Lipidol. 12, 129–140.

Schmitz, G., Kaminski, W.E., Orso, E., 2000. ABC transporters in cellular lipid trafficking. Curr. Opin. Lipidol. 11, 493–501.

Schonbeck, U., Sukhova, G.K., Shimizu, K., Mach, F., Libby, P., 2000. Inhibition of CD40 signaling limits evolution of established atherosclerosis in mice. Proc. Natl. Acad. Sci. U. S. A. 97, 7458–7463.

Schonfeld, G., 1995. The hypobetalipoproteinemias. Annu. Rev. Nutr. 15, 23–34.

Schwenke, D.C., Carew, T.E., 1989. Initiation of atherosclerotic lesions in cholesterol-fed rabbits. I. Focal increases in arterial LDL concentration precede development of fatty streak lesions. Arteriosclerosis 9, 895–907.

Sehayek, E., Ono, J.G., Shefer, S., Nguyen, L.B., Wang, N., Batta, A.K., Salen, G., Smith, J.D., Tall, A.R., Breslow, J.L., 1998. Biliary cholesterol excretion: a novel mechanism that regulates dietary cholesterol absorption. Proc. Natl. Acad. Sci. U. S. A. 95, 10194–10199.

Sendobry, S.M., Cornicelli, J.A., Welch, K., Bocan, T., Tait, B., Trivedi, B.K., Colbry, N., Dyer, R.D., Feinmark, S.J., Daugherty, A., 1997. Attenuation of diet-induced atherosclerosis in rabbits with a highly selective 15-lipoxygenase inhibitor lacking significant antioxidant properties. Br. J. Pharmacol. 120, 1199–1206.

Sevanian, A., Hwang, J., Hodis, H., Cazzolato, G., Avogaro, P., Bittolo-Bon, G., 1996. Contribution of an in vivo oxidized LDL to LDL oxidation and its association with dense LDL subpopulations. Arterioscler. Thromb. Vasc. Biol. 16, 784–793.

Shen, J., Herderick, E., Cornhill, J.F., Zsigmond, E., Kim, H.S., Kuhn, H., Guevara, N.V., Chan, L., 1996. Macrophage-mediated 15-lipoxygenase expression protects against atherosclerosis development. J. Clin. Invest. 98, 2201–2208.

Shepherd, J., Cobbe, S.M., Ford, I., Isles, C.G., Lorimer, A.R., MacFarlane, P.W., McKillop, J.H., Packard, C.J., 1995. Prevention of coronary heart disease with pravastatin in men with hypercholesterolemia. West of Scotland Coronary Prevention Study Group. N. Engl. J. Med. 333, 1301–1307.

Shih, D.M., Xia, Y.R., Wang, X.P., Miller, E., Castellani, L.W., Subbanagounder, G., Cheroutre, H., Faull, K.F., Berliner, J.A., Witztum, J.L., Lusis, A.J., 2000. Combined serum paraoxonase knockout/apolipoprotein E knockout mice exhibit increased lipoprotein oxidation and atherosclerosis. J. Biol. Chem. 275, 17527–17535.

Shih, P.T., Brennan, M.L., Vora, D.K., Territo, M.C., Strahl, D., Elices, M.J., Lusis, A.J., Berliner, J.A., 1999. Blocking very late antigen-4 integrin decreases leukocyte entry and fatty streak formation in mice fed an atherogenic diet. Circ. Res. 84, 345–351.

Shimomura, I., Funahashi, T., Takahashi, M., Maeda, K., Kotani, K., Nakamura, T., Yamashita, S., Miura, M., Fukuda, Y., Takemura, K., Tokunaga, K., Matsuzawa, Y., 1996. Enhanced expression of PAI-1 in visceral fat: possible contributor to vascular disease in obesity. Nat. Med. 2, 800–803.

Silver, D.L., Tall, A.R., 2001. The cellular biology of scavenger receptor class B type I. Curr. Opin. Lipidol. 12, 497–504.

Slotte, J.P., Oram, J.F., Bierman, E.L., 1987. Binding of high density lipoproteins to cell receptors promotes translocation of cholesterol from intracellular membranes to the cell surface. J. Biol. Chem. 262, 12904–12907.

Slowik, M.R., Min, W., Ardito, T., Karsan, A., Kashgarian, M., Pober, J.S., 1997. Evidence that tumor necrosis factor triggers apoptosis in human endothelial cells by interleukin-1-converting enzyme-like protease-dependent and -independent pathways. Lab. Invest. 77, 257–267.

Smith, J.D., Trogan, E., Ginsberg, M., Grigaux, C., Tian, J., Miyata, M., 1995. Decreased atherosclerosis in mice deficient in both macrophage colony-stimulating factor (op) and apolipoprotein E. Proc. Natl. Acad. Sci. U. S. A. 92, 8264–8268.

Sparrow, C.P., Pittman, R.C., 1990. Cholesterol esters selectively taken up from high-density lipoproteins are hydrolyzed extralysosomally. Biochim. Biophys. Acta 1043, 203–210.

Stangl, H., Cao, G., Wyne, K.L., Hobbs, H.H., 1998. Scavenger receptor, class B, type I-dependent stimulation of cholesterol esterification by high density lipoproteins, low density lipoproteins, and nonlipoprotein cholesterol. J. Biol. Chem. 273, 31002–31008.

Stary, H.C., Blankenhorn, D.H., Chandler, A.B., Glagov, S., Insull Jr., W., Richardson, M., Rosenfeld, M.E., Schaffer, S.A., Schwartz, C.J., Wagner, W.D., Wissler, R.W., 1992. A definition of the intima of human arteries and of its atherosclerosis-prone regions: a report from the Committee on Vascular Lesions of the Council on Arteriosclerosis, American Heart Association. Special report. Circulation 85, 391–405.

Stary, H.C., Chandler, A.B., Glagov, S., Guyton, J.R., Insull Jr., W., Rosenfeld, M.E., Schaffer, A., Schwartz, C.J., Wagner, W.D., Wissler, R.W., 1994. A definition of initial, fatty streak, and intermediate lesions of atherosclerosis: a report from the Committee on Vascular Lesions of the Council on Arteriosclerosis, American Heart Association. Special report. Arterioscler. Thromb. 14, 840–856.

Stary, H.C., Chandler, A.B., Dinsmore, R.E., Fuster, V., Glagov, S., Insull Jr., W., Rosenfeld, M.E., Schwartz, C.J., Wagner, W.D., Wissler, R.W., 1995. A definition of advanced types of atherosclerotic lesions and a histological classification of atherosclerosis: a report from the Committee on Vascular Lesions of the Council on Arteriosclerosis, American Heart Association. Circulation 92, 1355–1374.

Stein, O., Stein, Y., 1999. Atheroprotective mechanisms of HDL. Atherosclerosis 144, 285–301.

Steinberg, D., Parthasarathy, S., Carew, T.E., Khoo, J.C., Witztum, J.L., 1989. Beyond cholesterol. Modifications of low-density lipoprotein that increase its atherogenicity. N. Engl. J. Med. 320, 915–924.

Steinbrecher, U.P., Parthasarathy, S., Leake, D.S., Witztum, J.L., Steinberg, D., 1984. Modification of low density lipoprotein by endothelial cells involves lipid peroxidation and degradation of low density lipoprotein phospholipids. Proc. Natl. Acad. Sci. U. S. A. 81, 3883–3887.

Streblow, D.N., Soderberg-Naucler, C., Vieira, J., Smith, P., Wakabayashi, E., Ruchti, F., Mattison, K., Altschuler, Y., Nelson, J.A., 1999. The human cytomegalovirus chemokine receptor US28 mediates vascular smooth muscle cell migration. Cell 99, 511–520.

Suzuki, H., Kurihara, Y., Takeya, M., Kamada, N., Kataoka, M., Jishage, K., Ueda, O., Sakaguchi, H., Higashi, T., Suzuki, T., Takashima, Y., Kawabe, Y., Cynshi, O., Wada, Y., Honda, M., Kurihara, H., Aburatani, H., Doi, T., Matsumoto, A., Azuma, S., Noda, T., Toyoda, Y., Itakura, H., Yazaki, Y., Kodama, T., et al., 1997. A role for macrophage scavenger receptors in atherosclerosis and susceptibility to infection. Nature 386, 292–296.

Sytkowski, P.A., Kannel, W.B., D'Agostino, R.B., 1990. Changes in risk factors and the decline in mortality from cardiovascular disease. The Framingham Heart Study. N. Engl. J. Med. 322, 1635–1641.

Takahashi, Y., Smith, J.D., 1999. Cholesterol efflux to apolipoprotein AI involves endocytosis and resecretion in a calcium-dependent pathway. Proc. Natl. Acad. Sci. U. S. A. 96, 11358–11363.

Takemoto, M., Liao, J.K., 2001. Pleiotropic effects of 3-hydroxy-3-methylglutaryl coenzyme a reductase inhibitors. Arterioscler. Thromb. Vasc. Biol. 21, 1712–1719.

Tamai, O., Matsuoka, H., Itabe, H., Wada, Y., Kohno, K., Imaizumi, T., 1997. Single LDL apheresis improves endothelium-dependent vasodilatation in hypercholesterolemic humans. Circulation 95, 76–82.

Terpstra, V., Kondratenko, N., Steinberg, D., 1997. Macrophages lacking scavenger receptor A show a decrease in binding and uptake of acetylated low-density lipoprotein and of apoptotic thymocytes, but not of oxidatively damaged red blood cells. Proc. Natl. Acad. Sci. U. S. A. 94, 8127–8131.

Terpstra, V., van Amersfoort, E.S., van Velzen, A.G., Kuiper, J., van Berkel, T.J., 2000. Hepatic and extrahepatic scavenger receptors: function in relation to disease. Arterioscler. Thromb. Vasc. Biol. 20, 1860–1872.

The LIPID Study Group, 1998. Prevention of cardiovascular events and death with pravastatin in patients with coronary heart disease and a broad range of initial cholesterol levels. N. Engl. J. Med. 339, 1349–1357.

The 4S Study Group, 1994. Randomised trial of cholesterol lowering in 4444 patients with coronary heart disease: the Scandinavian Simvastatin Survival Study (4 S). Lancet 344, 1383–1389.

Thurberg, B.L., Collins, T., 1998. The nuclear factor-kappa B/inhibitor of kappa B autoregulatory system and atherosclerosis. Curr. Opin. Lipidol. 9, 387–396.

Thuren, T., 2000. Hepatic lipase and HDL metabolism. Curr. Opin. Lipidol. 11, 277–283.

Toikka, J.O., Ahotupa, M., Viikari, J.S., Niinikoski, H., Taskinen, M., Irjala, K., Hartiala, J.J., Raitakari, O.T., 1999. Constantly low HDL-cholesterol concentration relates to endothelial dysfunction and increased in vivo LDL-oxidation in healthy young men. Atherosclerosis 147, 133–138.

Tontonoz, P., Nagy, L., Alvarez, J.G., Thomazy, V.A., Evans, R.M., 1998. PPARgamma promotes monocyte/macrophage differentiation and uptake of oxidized LDL. Cell 93, 241–252.

Trigatti, B., Rayburn, H., Vinals, M., Braun, A., Miettinen, H., Penman, M., Hertz, M., Schrenzel, M., Amigo, L., Rigotti, A., Krieger, M., 1999. Influence of the high density lipoprotein receptor SR-BI on reproductive and cardiovascular pathophysiology. Proc. Natl. Acad. Sci. U. S. A. 96, 9322–9327.

Trigatti, B., Rigotti, A., Krieger, M., 2000. The role of the high-density lipoprotein receptor SR-BI in cholesterol metabolism. Curr. Opin. Lipidol. 11, 123–131.

Ueda, Y., Royer, L., Gong, E., Zhang, J., Cooper, P.N., Francone, O., Rubin, E.M., 1999. Lower plasma levels and accelerated clearance of high density lipoprotein (HDL) and non-HDL cholesterol in scavenger receptor class B type I transgenic mice. J. Biol. Chem. 274, 7165–7171.

Upchurch Jr., G.R., Welch, G.N., Fabian, A.J., Freedman, J.E., Johnson, J.L., Keaney Jr., J.F., Loscalzo, J., 1997. Homocyst(e)ine decreases bioavailable nitric oxide by a mechanism involving glutathione peroxidase. J. Biol. Chem. 272, 17012–17017.

Usui, M., Egashira, K., Tomita, H., Koyanagi, M., Katoh, M., Shimokawa, H., Takeya, M., Yoshimura, T., Matsushima, K., Takeshita, A., 2000. Important role of local angiotensin II activity mediated via type 1 receptor in the pathogenesis of cardiovascular inflammatory changes induced by chronic blockade of nitric oxide synthesis in rats. Circulation 101, 305–310.

Utermann, G., 2001. Lipoprotein (a). In: Scriver, C.R., Beaudet, A.L., Sly, W.S., Valle, D. (Eds.), The Metabolic Bases of Inherited Disease, 8th ed., vol. 2. McGraw-Hill, New York, pp. 2753–2787.

Van Berkel, T.J., Van Velzen, A., Kruijt, J.K., Suzuki, H., Kodama, T., 1998. Uptake and catabolism of modified LDL in scavenger-receptor class A type I/II knock-out mice. Biochem. J. 331, 29–35.

van der Kooij, M.A., Morand, O.H., Kempen, H.J., van Berkel, T.J., 1996. Decrease in scavenger receptor expression in human monocyte-derived macrophages treated with granulocyte macrophage colony-stimulating factor. Arterioscler. Thromb. Vasc. Biol. 16, 106–114.

van der Wal, A.C., Becker, A.E., van der Loos, C.M., Das, P.K., 1994. Site of intimal rupture or erosion of thrombosed coronary atherosclerotic plaques is characterized by an inflammatory process irrespective of the dominant plaque morphology. Circulation 89, 36–44.

van Lenten, B.J., Fogelman, A.M., 1992. Lipopolysaccharide-induced inhibition of scavenger receptor expression in human monocyte-macrophages is mediated through tumor necrosis factor-alpha. J. Immunol. 148, 112–116.

Varban, M.L., Rinninger, F., Wang, N., Fairchild-Huntress, V., Dunmore, J.H., Fang, Q., Gosselin, M.L., Dixon, K.L., Deeds, J.D., Acton, S.L., Tall, A.R., Huszar, D., 1998. Targeted mutation reveals a central role for SR-BI in hepatic selective uptake of high density lipoprotein cholesterol. Proc. Natl. Acad. Sci. U. S. A. 95, 4619–4624.

Vaughan, C.J., Gotto Jr., A.M., Basson, C.T., 2000. The evolving role of statins in the management of atherosclerosis. J. Am. Coll. Cardiol. 35, 1–10.

von Eckardstein, A., Assmann, G., 2000. Prevention of coronary heart disease by raising high-density lipoprotein cholesterol? Curr. Opin. Lipidol. 11, 627–637.

von Eckardstein, A., Nofer, J.R., Assmann, G., 2001. High density lipoproteins and arteriosclerosis. Role of cholesterol efflux and reverse cholesterol transport. Arterioscler. Thromb. Vasc. Biol. 21, 13–27.

Wang, N., Arai, T., Ji, Y., Rinninger, F., Tall, A.R., 1998. Liver-specific overexpression of scavenger receptor BI decreases levels of very low density lipoprotein ApoB, low density lipoprotein ApoB, and high density lipoprotein in transgenic mice. J. Biol. Chem. 273, 32920–32926.

Williams, K.J., Tabas, I., 1998. The response-to-retention hypothesis of atherogenesis reinforced. Curr. Opin. Lipidol. 9, 471–474.

Witztum, J.L., 1994. The oxidation hypothesis of atherosclerosis. Lancet 344, 793–795.

Witztum, J.L., Steinberg, D., 2001. The oxidative modification hypothesis of atherosclerosis: does it hold for humans? Trends Cardiovasc. Med. 11, 93–102.

Xia, P., Vadas, M.A., Rye, K.A., Barter, P.J., Gamble, J.R., 1999. High density lipoproteins (HDL) interrupt the sphingosine kinase signaling pathway. A possible mechanism for protection against atherosclerosis by HDL. J. Biol. Chem. 274, 33143–33147.

Yagyu, H., Kitamine, T., Osuga, J., Tozawa, R., Chen, Z., Kaji, Y., Oka, T., Perrey, S., Tamura, Y., Ohashi, K., Okazaki, H., Yahagi, N., Shionoiri, F., Iizuka, Y., Harada, K., Shimano, H., Yamashita, H., Gotoda, T., Yamada, N., Ishibashi, S., 2000. Absence of ACAT-1 attenuates atherosclerosis but causes dry eye and cutaneous xanthomatosis in mice with congenital hyperlipidemia. J. Biol. Chem. 275, 21324–21330.

Yamashita, S., Sprecher, D.L., Sakai, N., Matsuzawa, Y., Tarui, S., Hui, D.Y., 1990. Accumulation of apolipoprotein E-rich high density lipoproteins in hyperalphalipoproteinemic human subjects with plasma cholesteryl ester transfer protein deficiency. J. Clin. Invest. 86, 688–695.

Yamashita, S., Hirano, K., Sakai, N., Matsuzawa, Y., 2000. Molecular biology and pathophysiological aspects of plasma cholesteryl ester transfer protein. Biochim. Biophys. Acta 1529, 257–275.

Yamashita, S., Sakai, N., Hirano, K., Ishigami, M., Maruyama, T., Nakajima, N., Matsuzawa, Y., 2001. Roles of plasma lipid transfer proteins in reverse cholesterol transport. Front. Biosci. 6, D366–D387.

Yang, T., Goldstein, J.L., Brown, M.S., 2000. Overexpression of membrane domain of SCAP prevents sterols from inhibiting SCAP.SREBP exit from endoplasmic reticulum. J. Biol. Chem. 275, 29881–29886.

Yla-Herttuala, S., 1998. Is oxidized low-density lipoprotein present in vivo? Curr. Opin. Lipidol. 9, 337–344.

Yla-Herttuala, S., Palinski, W., Rosenfeld, M.E., Parthasarathy, S., Carew, T.E., Butler, S., Witztum, J.L., Steinberg, D., 1989. Evidence for the presence of oxidatively modified low density lipoprotein in atherosclerotic lesions of rabbit and man. J. Clin. Invest. 84, 1086–1095.

Yla-Herttuala, S., Rosenfeld, M.E., Parthasarathy, S., Glass, C.K., Sigal, E., Witztum, J.L., Steinberg, D., 1990. Colocalization of 15-lipoxygenase mRNA and protein with epitopes of oxidized low density lipoprotein in macrophage-rich areas of atherosclerotic lesions. Proc. Natl. Acad. Sci. U. S. A. 87, 6959–6963.

Yokoyama, C., Wang, X., Briggs, M.R., Admon, A., Wu, J., Hua, X., Goldstein, J.L., Brown, M.S., 1993. SREBP-1, a basic-helix–loop–helix–leucine zipper protein that controls transcription of the low density lipoprotein receptor gene. Cell 75, 187–197.

Yoshida, H., Quehenberger, O., Kondratenko, N., Green, S., Steinberg, D., 1998. Minimally oxidized low-density lipoprotein increases expression of scavenger receptor A, CD36, and macrosialin in resident mouse peritoneal macrophages. Arterioscler. Thromb. Vasc. Biol. 18, 794–802.

Zeiher, A.M., Schachlinger, V., Hohnloser, S.H., Saurbier, B., Just, H., 1994. Coronary atherosclerotic wall thickening and vascular reactivity in humans. Elevated high-density lipoprotein levels ameliorate abnormal vasoconstriction in early atherosclerosis. Circulation 89, 2525–2532.

Zhang, S.H., Reddick, R.L., Piedrahita, J.A., Maeda, N., 1992. Spontaneous hypercholesterolemia and arterial lesions in mice lacking apolipoprotein E. Science 258, 468–471.

Zhang, S.H., Reddick, R.L., Avdievich, E., Surles, L.K., Jones, R.G., Reynolds, J.B., Quarfordt, S.H., Maeda, N., 1997. Paradoxical enhancement of atherosclerosis by probucol treatment in apolipoprotein E-deficient mice. J. Clin. Invest. 99, 2858–2866.

Zhao, L.X., Zhou, C.J., Tanaka, A., Nakata, M., Hirabayashi, T., Amachi, T., Shioda, S., Ueda, K., Inagaki, N., 2000. Cloning, characterization and tissue distribution of the rat ATP-binding cassette (ABC) transporter ABC2/ABCA2. Biochem. J. 350, 865–872.

Zilversmit, D.B., 1979. Atherogenesis: a postprandial phenomenon. Circulation 60, 473–485.

Cytokines and the pathogenesis
of atherosclerosis

Guha Krishnaswamy*, Daniel Dube,
Mark Counts and David S. Chi

*Department of Internal Medicine, Divisions of Allergy and Immunology and Cardiology,
P.O. Box 70622, East Tennessee State University, Johnson City, TN 37614-0622, USA*

Contents

*Corresponding author. *E-mail addresses*: krishnas@etsu.edu, krishnaswamy.guha@mtn-home.va.-gov (G. Krishnaswamy).

This research was supported by NIH grants AI-43310 and HL-63070, State of Tennessee Grant 20233, Amgen, Inc., the Rondal Cole Foundation Grant, RDC grant (ETSU), and the Cardiovascular Research Institute (ETSU).

Abbreviations

PCI	percutaneous coronary intervention
PTCA	percutaneous transluminal coronary angioplasty
CABG	coronary artery bypass grafting
HDL	high density lipoprotein
VCAM-1	vascular cell adhesion molecule-1
ICAM-1	intercellular cell adhesion molecule-1
MCP-1	monocyte chemotactic protein-1
gro-α	growth related oncogene-α
RANTES	regulated upon activation normal T cell expressed and secreted
IL-1 β	interleukin-1 β
TNF-α	tumor necrosis factor α
IL-6	interleukin-6
CRP	C-reactive protein
GM-CSF	granulocyte/monocyte colony stimulating factor
M-CSF	monocyte colony stimulating factor
G-CSF	granulocyte colony stimulating factor
NF-κB	nuclear factor kappa B
ACE-1	angiotensin converting enzyme-1
TGF-β	transforming growth factor β
TRADD	TNF-α receptor-associated death domain
OSM	oncostatin M
SAA	serum amyloid A
IFN$-\gamma$	interferon-γ
TC	total cholesterol
TG	triglycerides
VEGF	vascular endothelial growth factor
SMC	smooth muscle cells
EC	endothelial cells
HDC	histidine decarboxylase
PDGF	platelet-derived growth factor
CMV	cytomegalovirus

TIMP-1	tissue inhibitor of metalloprotease-1
MMP	matrix metalloprotease
CAD	coronary artery disease
HAART	highly active anti-retroviral therapy

1. Introduction: epidemiology and disease classification of atherosclerosis

This chapter reviews the role of cytokines in the inflammatory response seen in atherosclerosis and its potential relevance to therapeutic strategies for coronary artery disease.

Throughout the world today, the economic and social toll of atherosclerotic cardiovascular disease is enormous (Smith et al., 1999). While cardiovascular disease accounted for less than 10% of all deaths worldwide in 1900, today almost half of all deaths in the developed world and 25% of all deaths in the developing world are attributable to cardiovascular disease. It is estimated that by the year 2020 cardio-vascular disease will claim 25 million lives annually and that coronary heart disease will surpass infectious disease as the world's number one cause of death accounting for at least one in every three deaths. Coronary heart disease often kills and disables people in their most productive years. In 1999, coronary heart disease was responsible for $53 billion in direct medical care costs and $47 billion in indirect medical care costs. It is estimated that more than 12 million people in the United States have coronary heart disease. Each year in the United States, coronary heart disease accounts for about 650,000 new myocardial infarctions and 450,000 recurrent myocardial infarctions.

1.1. *Atherosclerosis: clinical manifestations*

Atherosclerosis manifests with a focal-on-diffuse pattern of disease and affects various regions of the circulation preferentially. Distinct clinical manifestations depend on the particular circulatory bed involved. For example, atherosclerosis of the coronary arteries commonly causes angina pectoris and myocardial infarction. Atherosclerosis of the central nervous system arterial supply is a common cause of stroke and transient ischemic attack. Atherosclerosis in the peripheral circulation causes intermittent claudication and gangrene and can jeopardize limb viability. The renal circulation is at risk from renal artery stenosis as well as from atheroembolic disease. Mesenteric ischemia can result from involvement of the splanchnic circu-lation (Ward et al., 2000).

1.2. *Arterial remodeling: clinical consequences*

The evolution of the atherosclerotic plaque involves a complex balance between cell proliferation and cell death, extracellular matrix production and remodeling and ingress and egress of lipoproteins and leukocytes. It also involves calcification and neovascularization processes. Multiple signals (which are often competing) trigger these various cellular events. There are clear links between atherosclerotic risk factors and the behavior of intrinsic vascular wall cells and infiltrating leukocytes. Arterial remodeling during atheroma formation is a clinically important feature of atheroma formation. The plaque usually grows outwardly during the initial phases of atheroma development. Affected vessels increase in diameter at the area of the lesion in a process described as compensatory enlargement or outward vascular remodeling. In this way, the growing atheroma is delayed from encroaching upon the vessel lumen, and inward or constrictive remodeling is known to occur (Ward et al., 2000).

It is now clear that many lesions that cause acute coronary syndromes arise from atherosclerotic plaques that have no hemodynamic significance prior to their rupture. Indeed, on coronary angiography, these lesions may appear as mild luminal irregularities or may be completely inapparent. It is this type of "hemodynamically insignificant" plaque that often is unstable and ruptures. The rupture occurs most frequently at the "proximal shoulder region" which corresponds to the point of maximum hemodynamic stress and is mediated partially by elaboration of inflammatory mediators, cytokines and metalloproteinases (Kullo et al., 1998). Rupture of the plaque's fibrous cap exposes the lipid-rich core containing tissue factor to the coagulation factors in the blood generating immediate intraluminal thrombus formation (Fig. 2). Should the thrombus be transient or partially occlusive, the spectrum of clinical consequences ranges from an asymptomatic noninjurious event to an acute coronary syndrome of unstable angina or non-ST segment elevation myocardial infarction. Totally occlusive thrombi may be completely asymptomatic in the setting of adequate protection by endogenous collateral vessels (induced by angiogenesis) or by previous bypass grafting or may result in acute coronary syndromes or sudden cardiac death. The pathogenesis of this process involves an interaction between risk factors and cellular elements of the vascular system.

1.3. Atherosclerosis: management options

There are a variety of factors known to be associated with increased risk of atherosclerosis of the coronary arteries, that can cause an inflammatory insult to the vascular tissue and that need to be addressed (Fig. 1). These include hypertension, diabetes mellitus, cigarette smoking, hypercholesterolemia, a family history of premature coronary artery disease, obesity, post-menopausal status, low high-density cholesterol, elevated low-density cholesterol, elevated triglycerides, sedentary lifestyle, hyperhomocystinemia, age and gender (Fig. 1). Some of these risk factors are potentially modifiable (e.g., smoking cessation, glycemic control, blood pressure management, weight loss, cholesterol lowering, exercise) and some of these risk factors are nonmodifiable (e.g., age, gender, family history).

Approaches to therapy are outlined in Fig. 2. Fundamental lifestyle modifications together with appropriate pharmacotherapy with strict patient adherence are necessary to reduce the risk of adverse cardiac events (Fig. 2,1). Cardiovascular drugs such as the statins, beta blockers and angiotensin converting enzyme inhibitors act partially by modulating the cytokine-inflammatory axis (Fig. 2,2,3).

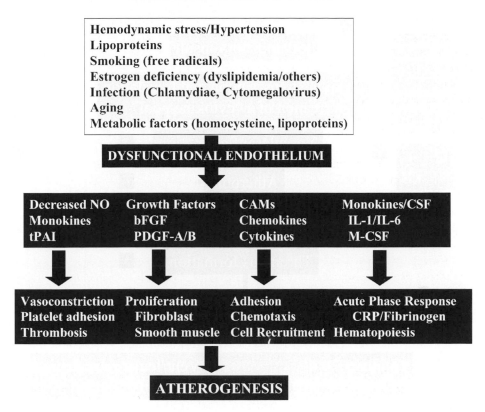

Fig. 1. Role of endothelium in induction of atherosclerosis. In the currently accepted paradigm of atherogenesis, various stimuli such as lipoproteins, infection and smoking lead to endothelial dysfunction followed by the expression of various cell adhesion molecules (CAMS), cytokines, colony stimulating factors (CSF) and altered production of nitric oxide (NO) and tissue plasminogen activator inhibitor (tPAI) leading to a variety of effects that lead to atherosclerosis. CRP = C reactive protein.

Revascularization by the use of percutaneous coronary intervention (PCI) in patients with ischemic coronary artery disease is widespread and rapidly expanding (Fig. 2,4). Balloon percutaneous transluminal coronary angioplasty (PTCA) expands the coronary lumen by stretching and tearing the atherosclerotic plaque and redistributing atherosclerotic plaque along the longitudinal axis (Fig. 2,4). Coronary stents are endoluminal metal scaffolds and are often placed after PTCA or in some cases initially as the primary intervention. Endoluminal thrombosis has largely been overcome with the aggressive use of thrombolytic and anti-platelet pharmacotherapies (Fig. 2,5). Neointimal hyperplasia in response to vessel wall injury caused by intracoronary stent placement may result in new tissue growth through the stent struts. Known as "in-stent restenosis", this process remains the bane of interventional cardiology complicating the course of up to 40% of all the patients who receive stents. Revascularization in the form of coronary artery bypass grafting (CABG) surgery is commonly performed in patients with a significant burden of

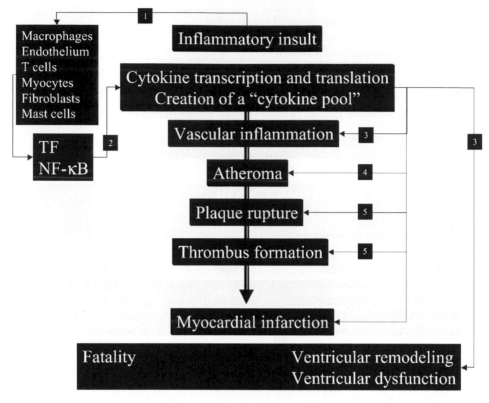

Fig. 2. Demonstrating the central role for cytokines in orchestrating the vascular inflammatory response. Cascade of events following inflammatory insult resulting in cellular activation, activation of transcription factors (TF) such as NF-kappaB (NF-κB) and the formation of an atheroma that leads to plaque rupture and an acute myocardial infarct. Myocardial infarction can be fatal or lead to ventricular dysfunction and remodeling, a process also mediated by cytokines. Numbers represent potential sites of therapeutic intervention: fundamental lifestyle modifications (1); drugs such as the statins, beta blockers and angiotensin converting enzyme inhibitors act partially by modulating the cytokine-inflammatory axis (2,3); Revascularization procedures (4); endoluminal thrombosis has largely been overcome with the aggressive use of thrombolytic and anti-platelet pharmacotherapies (5).

hemodynamically flow-limiting coronary artery disease affecting one or more vessels in a form not amenable to percutaneous intervention. Elderly patients with significant angina who are not candidates for CABG may be candidates for transmyocardial revascularization in an effort to improve symptoms. Patients with end-stage cardiomyopathy may be considered for cardiac transplant.

2. Atherosclerosis as an inflammatory disease

Recent data suggest that atherosclerosis is a chronic, inflammatory fibroproliferative disease involving the blood vessel (Schmitz et al., 1998). Early concepts of atherosclerosis suggested a rather bland role for lipoproteins in the disorder. Now it is becoming increasingly clear that the immune response is invoked in athero-sclerosis. The blood vessel wall in atherosclerosis is composed of infiltrating cells, many of which are activated. Macrophages, T cells, foam cells, mast cells, endo-thelial cells and myofibroblasts can all participate in atheromatous inflammation (Kelley et al., 2000a,b; Ross, 1999). This is important to keep in mind as a better understanding of the inflammatory response as it pertains to atherosclerosis and the definition of molecular targets pivotal to atherogenesis could lead to the generation of novel therapeutic agents for the disease. The following section will discuss briefly the cellular components of the atheromatous blood vessel and their potential role in creating the cytokine milieu that leads to the accelerated development of athero-sclerotic heart disease.

2.1. *Cellular biology of the inflammatory response*

Studies of the atheromatous plaque have demonstrated the inflammatory nature of the disease. Inflammatory cells are often seen infiltrating the plaques. Several groups have concentrated on the study of T lymphocytes. Schmitz et al. (1998) commented on the accumulation of CD4+ T cells and macrophages in the ather-omatous plaque, the expression of class II MHC molecules as well as cell–cell contact signaling molecules such as CD40 and CD40 L, molecules pivotal to mononuclear activation and function. Circulating mononuclear cells bearing the phenotype CD14 (dim) and CD16a (FcγRIIIa)-positive, correlate positively with cholesterol levels and negatively with high-density lipoprotein (HDL) levels (Schmitz et al., 1998). In a study of 691 patients under 40 years of age, Stary (1990) demonstrated intimal macrophages and foam cells as early as infancy and with later involvement of smooth muscle cells, T cells, mast cells and plasma cells. All these cells when acti-vated are capable of expressing inflammatory cytokines and can contribute to the "cytokine pool". Of pivotal importance to atherogenesis is endothelial dysfunction (LaRosa, 1998; Ross, 1999). Endothelial activation by a variety of risk factors such as infection, hypertension, diabetes mellitus, cigarette smoke or elevated homo-cysteine levels can lead to a sequence of changes resulting in increased aggregability of platelets and leukocytes, and the secretion of proinflammatory cytokines, che-mokines and growth factors. Fig. 1 demonstrates the effects of risk factors on endothelial function and expression of cytokines and chemokines that can regulate vascular inflammatory responses. Endothelium-dependent inflammation can result in migration of and proliferation of vascular smooth muscle cells leading to arterial wall thickening and vascular remodeling (Ross, 1997; Ross, 1999). T cells and macrophages infiltrate the lesions from peripheral blood and on activation, can produce a plethora of growth factors and cytokines that further compound the inflammatory process. Fig. 2 demonstrates the relationship between the inflamma-tory cytokine pool created as a result of injury and various biological, consequential processes leading ultimately to atherothrombotic disease and myocardial infarction. Cytokines could be potentially involved in every part of this process and the fasci-nating possibility is the likelihood that drug therapy can effectively modulate this inflammatory process, as discussed later.

The response to injury hypothesis was put forward in the early 1970s by Russell Ross and colleagues (Ross, 1997). According to this hypothesis, atherosclerosis is a chronic, inflammatory, fibroproliferative response to multiple stimuli. With chronicity of this insult, this response may become excessive, leading to the manifestation of disease. The possibility that control of genes that lead to elaboration of various cytokines and growth factors incriminated in this exuberant response may lead to amelioration of the disease has led to exciting insights into the molecular biology of atherosclerosis (Ross, 1993a).

2.2. *Mechanisms regulating atherogenesis*

In the earliest stages of atherosclerosis, normal resting endothelial cells undergo activation by various factors outlined in Fig. 1, including atherogenic lipids (low-density lipoproteins), smoking, infection (*Chlamydia pneumoniae* and cytomegalovirus), hypertension, homocysteine and diabetes mellitus. The dysfunctional and/or activated endothelium expresses genes for various molecules involved in the immune response (Krishnaswamy et al., 1999a; Ross, 1999). These include adhesion molecules (CAMs such as vascular cell adhesion molecule-1 [VCAM-1] and intercellular adhesion molecule-1 [ICAM-1]) and chemokines (such as monocyte chemotactic protein-1 [MCP-1], growth-related oncogene-alpha [gro-α], Regulated Upon Activation Normal T Cell Expressed and Secreted [RANTES]) that regulate cellular trafficking and the processes involved in mononuclear recruitment to the vascular wall (Krishnaswamy et al., 1999a). Other cytokines such as the monokines, interleukin-1 beta (IL-1 β), tumor necrosis factor alpha (TNF-α) and interleukin-6 (IL-6) activate the acute phase response characterized by hepatic synthesis of complement proteins, C-reactive Protein (CRP) and fibrinogen. These cytokines also make the endothelial surface more adhesive (by inducing CAMs) and procoagulant. Growth factors made by endothelial cells such as transforming growth factor beta (TGF-β) and platelet-derived growth factors A and B (PDGF-A and B) can alter the function of smooth muscle cells and fibroblasts. Colony stimulating factors made by endothelium such as granulocyte macrophage colony stimulating factor (GM-CSF), macrophage colony stimulating factor (M-CSF) and granulocyte colony stimulating factor (G-CSF), modulate hematopoiesis and modulate macrophage function and activation. As demonstrated in Fig. 2, orchestrated evolution of the inflammatory response can lead to atheroma formation culminating in plaque rupture and coronary thrombotic disease with a fatal consequence or development of ischemic cardiomyopathy (Kelley et al., 2000a,b; Ross, 1993b; Ross, 1999). Fig. 3 shows the potential interactions between the cytokines in atherosclerosis. These interactions are discussed in greater detail in later sections.

2.2.1. *Pivotal role for nuclear factor kappa-B in atherosclerosis*
A transcription factor of pivotal importance to the development of the inflammatory response is nuclear factor kappaB (NF-κB) (Krishnaswamy, 2001). This is a redox-sensitive transcription factor that regulates the expression of a battery of

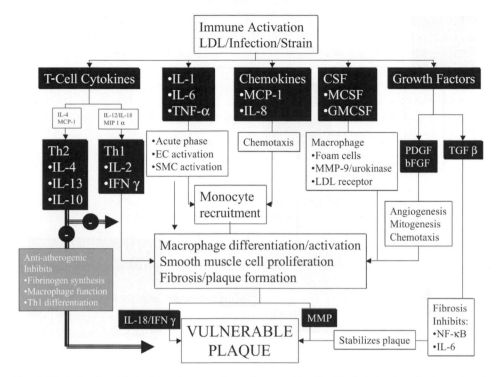

Fig. 3. The role of and interactions between the various cytokine families in induction of atherosclerosis and generation of a vulnerable plaque. Th1 cytokines, acute phase response cytokines, chemokines such as MCP-1 (monocyte chemotactic protein-1) and IL-8, colony stimulating factors such as M-CSF (macrophage colony stimulating factor) and GM-CSF (granulocyte macrophage colony stimulating factor) as well as growth factors such as PDGF (platelet-derived growth factor) and bFGF (basic fibroblast growth factor) have proatherogenic effects. IL-18 and IFN γ (interferon gamma) assist in plaque destabilization. On the other hand, Th2 cytokines such as IL-4 and IL-10 have anti-atherogenic effects while TGF-β (transforming growth factor beta) inhibits nuclear factor kappaB (NF-κB), IL-6 synthesis and stabilizes plaque by synthesis of collagen. MMP = matrix metalloproteinases; LDL = low density lipoprotein; SMC = smooth muscle cell; EC = endothelial cell.

cytokine genes that regulate inflammation (Fig. 4). Several factors are capable of inducing NF-κB activation and include hypoxemia, reactive oxygen intermediates, bacterial infection (Ebnet et al., 1997), bacterial endotoxin, viral infection, thrombin (Maruyama et al., 1997), inflammatory cytokines such as IL-1 and TNF-α (Krishnaswamy et al., 1999a; Krishnaswamy, 2001) and linoleic acid (Henning et al., 1996). NF-κB, in turn, regulates genes involved in both innate and adaptive immunity. These include the adhesion molecules (ICAM-1 and VCAM-1) (Shu et al., 1993), cytokines such as IL-1 and IL-6 (Scheinman et al., 1995) and inducible nitric oxide synthase. IL-1 and IL-6 can, in turn, induce acute phase protein synthesis from the liver, thereby compounding the inflammatory process.

The NF-κB family consists of the proteins p50, p52, p65 (RelA), c-Rel and RelB which exist as dimers within the cytoplasm of the cell coupled to an inhibitory

G. Krishnaswamy et al.

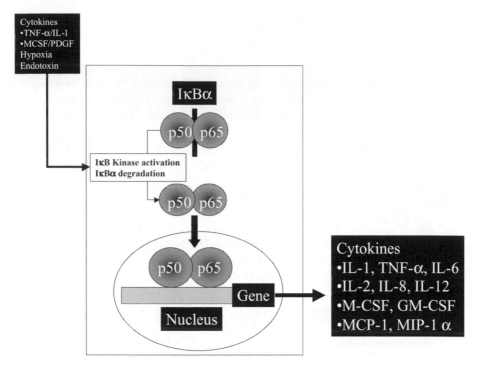

Fig. 4. Mechanisms of nuclear factor kappaB (NF-κB) activation. In the resting stage of the cell, inactive NF-κB is present in the cytoplasm complexed to an inhibitory protein (the most abundant form being IκBα). Following cellular activation, IκBα is phosphorylated by an IκB-specific kinase, IKK, resulting in its ubiquination and proteosomal degradation. This results in the liberation of free NF-κB (activated NF-κB) which then undergoes nuclear translocation and binding to specific κB-recognition sites on the promoters of target genes. This results in the expression of inflammatory cytokine and adhesion molecule genes, upon which vascular inflammation depends.

protein called IκBα. This latter protein maintains the dimers in an inactive state. Following cellular activation, IκBα is phosphorylated and undergoes ubiquination and proteolytic degradation. This is mediated by an IκB kinase (IKK) as shown in Fig. 4. This process results in the activation of NF-κB that subsequently translocates to the nucleus, binds to consensus sequences on the promoter of the specific genes mentioned above leading to their transcription (Adcock, 1997; Barnes, 1997; Scheinman et al., 1995). Hence, activation of NF-κB can have profound consequences on vascular inflammation and atherogenesis. Moreover, NF-κB is also important for cell survival and the activation of this ubiquitous transcription factor may prevent cell death from occurring (de Martin et al., 1999; Mattson et al., 2000). Obara et al. (2000) showed, e.g., that inhibition of NF-κB induces apoptosis in vascular smooth muscle cells. This could be significant therapeutically by modulating the survival of an important cell source for atherogenic cytokines.

There is evolving data that NF-κB activation can be pivotal to atherosclerosis (Brand et al., 1997a; Collins, 1993; Navab et al., 1995). First, recent studies have shown that NF-κB is expressed in atheromatous tissue and in the plaque. Utilizing a monoclonal antibody that recognizes the IκB binding site on the p65 component of NF-κB, Brand and colleagues demonstrated the presence of activated NF-κB in macrophages, smooth muscle cells and endothelium of atherosclerotic lesions of patients (Brand et al., 1996). Blood vessels from healthy individuals expressed only minimal amounts on quiescent NF-κB that was present mainly in the cytosol and not yet translocated to the nucleus. Since NF-κB modulates expression of adhesion molecules such as VCAM-1 as well as chemotactic cytokines such as MCP-1, mononuclear adhesion and emigration into vascular tissue is facilitated (Fig. 4). Second, NF-κB is inducible in endothelial cells and macrophages by such diverse stimuli as infection with *Chlaymydia pnemunoniae* (Molestina et al., 2000), lipo-proteins (Brand et al., 1997b; Dichtl et al., 1999) and linoleic acid (Henning et al., 1996). Finally, drugs effective in atherosclerotic heart disease such as the angiotensin converting enzyme inhibitors (ACE-I), salicylates and the statins act by modulating nuclear translocation of NF-κB (Bustos et al., 1998a; Hernandez-Presa et al., 1998; Pierce et al., 1996).

3. Cell–cell interactions in atherosclerosis: effects on cytokine generation

Atherogenic cytokines or atheroprotective cytokines can be generated by many cell types. While the predominant sources of these cytokines in the milieu of an atherosclerotic lesion are usually the endothelium, mononuclear cells and T lym-phocytes, many other cell types such as mast cells, smooth muscle cells and fibro-blasts may also have contributory roles. More importantly, these various cell types can contribute to a "cytokine pool" and vigorous cell–cell interactions can lead to further amplification of cytokine generation (Fig. 2). A molecule of pivotal importance to this cell–cell interaction is CD40 (Fig. 5), which interacts with CD40 ligand. CD40 ligand is a transmembrane protein (CD154) that was originally described on T cells. Subsequently it has been demonstrated on many other cell types including mast cells, endothelium, smooth muscle cells, B cells, platelets and on macrophages (Grewal and Flavell, 1997; Grewal and Flavell, 1998; Hernandez-Presa et al., 1998). This molecule can ligate CD40 on mononuclear cells and T cells, leading to elaboration of chemokines (MCP-1, RANTES, IL-8), inflammatory cytokines (IL-1, IL-2, IL-6, IL-8, IL-10, TNF-α, IFN γ and TGF-β) and metallo-proteinases (MMP-1, -2, -3, -9, -11, -13) (Grewal and Flavell, 1997; Grewal and Flavell, 1998). These mediators can lead to atherogenesis and modulate plaque rupture. Hence, inhibition of a CD40—CD40 L interaction may have profound consequences for atherogenesis. CD40 L is expressed by vascular endothelial cells, smooth muscle cells and by macrophages in atherosclerotic tissue (Mach et al., 1997). The cells expressing CD40 L in tissue also coexpressed CD40, allowing cell–cell interactions and cytokine signaling to occur. Accordingly, studies by Mach et al. (1998) have demonstrated that inhibition of cell–cell contact signaling using an anti-CD40 ligand antibody in mice inhibited the development of atherosclerosis. The atheromas of treated mice had fewer macrophages and T cells infiltrating the

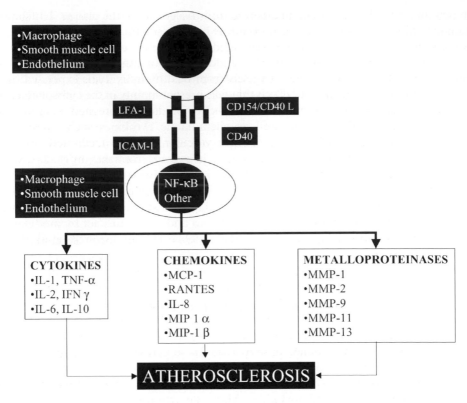

Fig. 5. Role of cell surface molecules in cell–cell interactions and cytokine transcription. The major role of the CD40–CD40 L (CD154) interactions as well as selected cell adhesion molecules (intercellular adhesion molecule-1 [ICAM-1] and lymphocyte function-associated antigen-1 [LFA-1]) is shown. Cell–cell interactions via these molecules result in transcription factor activation and transcription of key atherogenic cytokines, chemokines and metalloproteinases that can mediate and orchestrate atherosclerotic inflammation.

atheromatous lesions (Mach et al., 1998). Similarly, interactions between other cell surface molecules such as CAMs and cytokine-cytokine-receptor molecules can amplify inflammatory responses (Fig. 5).

4. Role of cytokines in atherosclerosis

Five categories of cytokines are discussed in the following sections: the cytokines regulating acute phase responses, T helper cell cytokines, colony stimulating factors, selected growth factors and chemokines.

4.1. *Acute phase response cytokines: mononuclear recruitment*

The monokines, IL-1 β, TNF-α and IL-6, constitute a cytokine set that mediates the acute phase response in inflammation. IL-1 is typical of a pleiotropic and redundant cytokine-meaning one cytokine with many biological actions and shared activities with the other cytokines in the group, such as TNF-α and IL-6. Interleukin-1 is produced by a variety of cell types including monocytes, macrophages, fibroblasts, endothelial cells, T and B lymphocytes, vascular smooth muscle and mast cells (Borish and Rosenwasser, 1996). Two isoforms have been described – IL-1 α and IL - 1 β. The former is mostly cell-associated and the latter secreted. The molecules have about 20% homology but share the same receptor and possess very similar properties. IL-1 mediates its actions by binding to the IL-1 receptor, of which two types have been described - type I and type II. Signaling by the IL-1 receptor is mediated through a cytosolic domain on these proteins termed the toll/IL-1 receptor domain. Gene expression is activated via several intermediary steps including the recruitment of proteins, MyD88, IL-1 receptor-associated kinase (IRAK) (Kanakaraj et al., 1998) and TRAF-6 promoting activation of an I-κB kinase that, in turn, activates NF-κB (Kopp et al., 1999).

In an immunohistochemical study of atherosclerotic plaques from iliac arteries of cynomolgus monkeys, expression of both IL-1 α and IL-1 β was found in foam cells and microvascular endothelium, while only expression of IL-1 α was detected in adherent leukocytes and vascular SMCs (VSMCs) (Moyer et al., 1991). The expression of both IL-1 α and IL-1 β was also detected in the aortic tissue from rabbits fed an atherogenic diet (Clinton et al., 1991). These results indicate that endothelium and VSMCs, in conjunction with macrophages, serve as a localized source of IL-1 proteins which modify vascular function and contribute to the pathogenesis of atherosclerotic vascular disease.

TNF-α is an important mediator of the inflammatory response. Like IL-1, it is produced by many cell types including mast cells, macrophages, T cells and fibroblasts. Besides contributing to the inflammatory response, it also has cytotoxic effects for many transformed cells. It shares induction of collagenases and the acute phase response with IL-1. TNF-α binds to two types of receptors, TNFR type I and TNFR type II, which are both members of the TNFR superfamily. The type I receptor has a death domain that recruits an adapter protein, TNF-α receptor-associated death domain (TRADD). TRADD, in turn, recruits the Fas-associated death domain that activates caspases leading to DNA fragmentation and cell death. TNF-α interaction with its receptor may also be associated with NF-κB activation, a molecule that inhibits apoptosis (Obara et al., 2000; Wang et al., 1998). The role of the type II receptor is incompletely understood at this point in time. TNF-α can potentiate oxidative stress and disruption of calcium homeostasis in vascular endothelial cells, and may thereby cause dysfunction and even death of these cells (Toborek et al., 1996, 1997; Herbst et al., 1999).

IL-1 has many biological effects, some of which it shares with TNF-α and IL-6. These include the acute phase response that is characterized by fever, weight loss, leukocytosis and elaboration of the acute phase proteins, fibrinogen, serum amyloid A protein and complement (Fig. 3). IL-1 can induce T-cell proliferation and induces fever by production of PGE_2 by the hypothalamus. IL-1 in conjunction with TNF-α activates endothelial cells and other cell types to express adhesion molecules and secrete atherogenic cytokines such IL-8, GM-CSF and MCP-1 (Krishnaswamy et al.,

1998; Stanford et al., 2000). Macrophages activated with LDL secrete IL-1 and TNF-α (Madej et al., 1998). IL-1, in turn, activates inducible nitric oxide synthase gene expression and nitrite secretion by vascular smooth muscle cells (Ikeda et al., 1998). IL-1 β also activates vascular endothelial growth factor expression in macrophages (Kuzuya, 1998). IL-1 β levels are elevated in patients with hypertension, and may thereby predispose these patients to accelerated atherogenesis (Dalekos et al., 1997). IL-1 and TNF-α can also induce ICAM-1 and VCAM-1 expression by smooth muscle cells, enhance mononuclear adhesion to smooth muscle (Thorne et al., 1996; Wang et al., 1994) and induce production of IL-11 by vascular smooth muscle (Taki et al., 1999). IL-1 enhances metalloproteinase (gelatinase) expression by vascular smooth muscle cells (Galis et al., 1995). This could contribute to smooth muscle cell migration, weakening of the fibrous cap and plaque rupture.

IL-1 and C-reactive protein (CRP) in the presence of serum have been shown to induce the expression of adhesion molecules, such as ICAM-1, VCAM-1 and E-selectin, in human endothelial cells, suggesting CRP may play a direct role in promoting the inflammatory component of atherosclerosis (Pasceri et al., 2000). Using a PCR-based method for quantifying the recruitment of monocytes to mouse atherosclerotic lesions in vivo, a recent study reported that intraperitoneal injection of a combination of TNF-α and IL-1 β more than doubled the rate of monocyte recruitment into developing lesions (Kim et al., 2000).

Recently, an intravital microscopy technique has been developed for direct observation of leukocyte–endothelium interactions in the mouse cremaster muscle (Thorlacius et al., 1997) and the mouse aorta (Eriksson et al., 2000). In untreated vessels, leukocyte–endothelium interactions virtually have not been observed. However, local or systemic treatment with IL-1 β and TNF-α induced conclusive leukocyte rolling and adhesion, compatible with normal blood flow and wall shear rate. Using antibodies to adhesion molecules, the investigators showed that cytokine-induced leukocyte rolling was found to be critically dependent on P-selectin and in some cases modulated by both E-selectin and alpha(4) integrin. In addition, atherectomy specimens had significantly greater P-selectin expression on endothelial cells from patients with unstable angina, which also had elevated levels of IL-6, than from patients with stable angina (Tenaglia et al., 1997). These studies directly provide the evidence of in vivo induction of monocyte recruitment by acute phase response cytokines.

IL-1 β and TNF-α are detectable in atherosclerotic plaque. Tipping and Hancock (1993) however, showed that TNF-α rather than IL-1 β is the dominant monokine expressed in macrophages obtained from atheromatous plaques. In the atheromatous plaque, it appears likely that macrophages, endothelial and vascular smooth muscle cells may be the main sources for IL-1 β (Moyer et al., 1991). Both IL-1 α and IL-1 β are also expressed by foam cells within the plaque (Moyer et al., 1991). Of interest to atherogenesis and inflammation, IL-1 and TNF-α activate CD40 L expression on vascular endothelial cells, smooth muscle cells and macrophages (Mach et al., 1997). TNF-α mRNA is also detectable by in situ hybridization within the arterial plaque (Wilcox et al., 1994). Both IL-1 β and TNF-α can activate NF-κB and may be involved in apoptotic pathways (Obara et al., 2000). Increased expression of TNF-α, fibronectin and IL-1 β has been detected in restenotic lesion, suggesting that an immune-inflammatory reaction probably contributes to neointimal formation and may represent a form of wound healing and repair secondary to mechanical injury (Clausell et al., 1995).

In vivo data have shown association of secretory sphingomyelinase (S-SMase) with subendothelial lipoprotein aggregation and macrophage foam cell formation. Cytokines, such as IL-1 β and TNF-α, have been shown not only to induce the secretion of S-SMase in cultured endothelial cells but also increase two- to threefold the S-SMase in LPS-injected mice (Wong et al., 2000). The data suggest a possibility that local stimulation of S-SMase may contribute to the effects of inflammatory cytokines in atherosclerosis.

IL-6 is a multifunctional cytokine elaborated by T and B cells, mast cells, bone marrow stromal cells, fibroblasts and macrophages (Hirano, 1998; Krishnaswamy et al., 1997; Krishnaswamy et al., 1998; Krishnaswamy et al., 1999a). IL-6 appears to regulate T and B cell function, hematopoiesis and the acute phase response. Both IL-1 β and TNF-α can induce IL-6 expression from many cell types. Thrombin and angiotensin induce IL-6 production from vascular cells (Kranzhofer et al., 1999). IL-6 by binding to its receptor induces acute phase protein synthesis in the liver and leads to amplification of the inflammatory state (Hirano, 1998). The IL-6 receptor consists of an IL-6 alpha (IL-6R α) chain and a signal transduction unit, gp130 (Hirano, 1998). IL-6 binds to IL-6 R and the IL-6/IL-6 R complex, then binds two gp130 molecules to form a homodimer that leads to tyrosine phosphorylation of gp130 followed by signal transduction, characterized by activation of Src family of kinases (Hallek et al., 1997). Other cytokines such as oncostatin M (OSM), leukemia inhibitory factor (LIF) and IL-11 share the gp130 signaling unit, again an example of receptor promiscuity in the immune response. Mice lacking the IL-6 gene fail to mount an immune response to obligate intracellular bacteria and have a severely impaired acute phase response (Kopf et al., 1994). On the other hand, mice injected with recombinant IL-6 developed atherosclerotic lesions and had elevated levels of fibrinogen and inflammatory cytokines (Huber et al., 1999). IL-6 has also been shown to increase endothelial permeability in vitro (Maruo et al., 1992). In addition, C reactive protein (CRP), a marker of the acute phase response, is often elevated in ischemic heart disease suggestive of a functional role for IL-6 in the disease (Plutzky, 2001). The acute phase response mediated by IL-6, characterized by elevated CRP levels, increased plasma viscosity, elevated fibrinogen levels and platelet numbers all predispose to the accelerated atherosclerosis. Moreover, circulating IL-6 stimulates the hypothalamo-pituitary-adrenal axis and thereby is associated with hypertension, central obesity and insulin resistance (Yudkin et al., 2000).

Elevated levels of IL-6 are detectable in acute coronary syndromes, stable angina pectoris as well as acute myocardial infarction (Biasucci et al., 1999; Gabriel et al., 2000). Elevated levels of IL-6 are also detected in occluded, thrombosed coronary arteries (Kato et al., 1999). Rus et al. (1996a) showed expression of IL-6 and IL-8 in endarterectomy samples, with larger concentrations present in fibrous plaque as opposed to the intima. Studies have also demonstrated a relationship between elevated IL-6 levels and myocardial infarction in healthy men (Ridker et al., 2000). In atherosclerotic plaques, IL-6 often colocalizes with angiotensin I, angiotensin II and angiotensin converting enzyme in CD68+ve macrophages (Schieffer et al., 2000). Macrophages and smooth muscle cells also express IL-6 within plaques (Yudkin et al., 2000). By RT-PCR, 30–40-fold elevation of IL-6 mRNA is present within the atherosclerotic plaque (Seino et al., 1994). Taken together, these data suggest an important role for IL-6 in atherosclerosis.

Serum amyloid A (SAA) family of acute phase reactants has been detected by immunoblot analysis in the culture medium of human aortic smooth muscle cells (HASMC) and has been shown to modulate the inflammatory process and lipid synthesis. The expression of SAA mRNA in HASMC was upregulated by corticoid hormones including dexamethasone (Dex), corticosterone, and to a less extent by IL-1, which is known to upregulate extrahepatic SAA expression in other cell system. Thus, it is possible that some of the SAA protein can originate from smooth muscle cells and participate in the formation of atherosclerotic plaques (Kumon et al., 2001). In addition, it has been reported that amyloid proteins can disrupt endothelial cell function and induce apoptosis of these cells (Blanc et al., 1997).

4.2. T helper cytokines and macrophage/endothelial activation

4.2.1. Th1 and Th2 responses

Activated lymphocytes infiltrate atherosclerotic plaques and their function and role is being actively studied. Mature T lymphocytes, expressing CD2 and CD3, derive from thymus and differentiate into helper T cells (Th) and cytotoxic T cells (T_C). T_C cells also express CD8. Activated T_C cells are cytotoxic to tumor cells, virus infected cells and allografts. Th cells express an extra membrane protein called CD4, and produce a variety of cytokines which play a role in activation and proliferation of B cells, T cells and macrophages, in inflammatory processes, as well as in stimulating hematopoiesis. Some cytokines and mediators that act between leukocytes are called interleukins. There are two types of Th cells: Th1 cells produce mainly IFN-γ, IL-2, IL-18 and lymphotoxin (LT), while Th2 cells primarily synthesize IL-4, IL-5, IL-9, IL-10 and IL-13 (Anderson and Coyle, 1994; Essayan et al., 1997; Paul and Seder, 1994). Both subtypes are capable of expressing cytokines such as GM-CSF and IL-3. Cytokines such as IL-4 enhance the development of Th2 cells while IL-12, IL-18 and interferon alpha (IFN α) regulate Th1 development (Essayan et al., 1999; Ricci et al., 1997). Also of interest, IFN γ inhibits Th2 development while IL-4 inhibits Th1 development. These are summarized in Table 1.

IFN-γ is of immunological importance because it induces macrophage activation, increases expression of MHC molecules and antigen presenting components and promotes immunoglobulin (Ig) class switching. IL-2 promotes T-cell proliferation, while IL-4 induces B cell activation and growth, and/or immunoglobulin isotype switching to IgE. IL-13 has functions similar to IL-4 while IL-3 acts in early hematopoiesis. IL-5 is involved in eosinophil growth and differentiation (Borish and Rosenwasser, 1996).

It has been demonstrated that the T-cell population in atherosclerotic lesions is heterogeneous, but the most dominant T cell by far is Th0 cytokine profile producing

Table 1
Role of selected cytokines in atherogenesis

Cytokine category	Cytokine members	Primary cell sources	Relevance to atherosclerosis
APR	IL-1 α/β/IL-6/TNF-α*	Mast cells, macrophages	• EC activation, cytokine synthesis, permeability
		T cells, endothelium	• Acute phase response-CRP, fibrinogen
			• Cellular recruitment-mono-cytes, T cells
			• Induces procoagulant state
Th1	IL-2*	T cells	• Growth/activation of plaque T cells
	IFN γ*	T cells, NK cells	• Enhances plaque Th1 cell differentiation
			• Inhibits Th2 differentiation
			• MHC II induction, macro phage activation
			• Plaque instability
Th2	IL-4**	T cells, mast cells	• Enhances Th2 development
			• Inhibits plaque Th1 differentiation
			• Inhibits of macrophage function
			• Inhibits fibrinogen synthesis
	IL-10**	T cells, monocytes	• Inhibits Th1 cytokine synthesis
		Macrophages	• Inhibits macrophage function, adhesion
			• Inhibits fibrinogen synthesis
Others	IL-12*	B cells, dendritic cells	• Proliferation/differentiation of Th1 subset
		Macrophages	• Enhances IFN γ and MCP-1 production
	IL-18*	Monocytes, macrophages	• Increased IFN γ and GM-CSF production
			• Plaque instability
			• Synergizes with IL-12 in Th1 differentiation

*proatherogenic; **anti-atherogenic; APR = acute phase response cytokines; CRP = C reactive protein.

both IFN-γ and IL-4 (81% of cloned T cells). Moreover, the production of IFN-γ was dominant in the majority of these clones. The dominant secretion of IFN-γ by T-cell clones suggests an important role for plaque T cells in modulating the growth and differentiation of other cells, such as macrophages and smooth muscle cells (SMCs) in atherosclerotic plaques (de Boer et al., 1999). Uyemara et al. (1996) demonstrated abundant expression of transcripts for IFN γ and IL-12 (Th1) but diminished expression of the transcript for IL-4 (Th2) in atheromatous plaques, suggesting a trend towards Th1 predominance in the lesions. Porphyromonas gingivalis-specific T-cell lines also have been established from atherosclerotic lesions from two patients with a periodontal disease. T-cell lines were found to be a mixture of CD4+ and CD8+ T-cells producing IFN-γ, IL-4 and IL-10 (Choi et al., 2001). In addition, the cytokine ratio of IFN-γ to IL-4 was found to be significantly higher in the high-cholesterol diet mice than that in the standard chow group, suggesting the presence of a predominantly Th1-type immune response in atherosclerosis (Mori et al., 2000). Recently, elevated plasma levels of TNF-α and IFN-γ have been detected in patients with hyperlipoproteinemia IIb and atherosclerosis. In addition, lowering plasma levels of total cholesterol (TC), triglycerides (TG) and low-density lipoproteins (LDL) by treatment of fibrates reduced plasma levels of TNF-α and IFN-γ in patients with hyperlipoproteinemia IIb (Madej et al., 1998). The results that decreased levels of TC, TG and LDL correlated with the reduced levels of proinflammatory cytokines are in agreement with in vitro findings that LDL can activate macrophages and T lymphocytes to produce TNF-α and IFN-γ, respectively.

The expression of IL-2 has been detected in 40–50% of analogous plaques in ischemic heart disease (Arbustini et al., 1991). It appears that IL-2 may be involved in heart disease. Using Southern blot analysis, it has been demonstrated that CD3$^+$ lymphocytes isolated from atherosclerotic carotid arterial specimens expressed IL-3 and IL-2 receptor alpha-chain transcripts, indicating that in this context, the activated T lymphocytes may release IL-3. In addition, ss-IL-3-transducing subunit was detected both on cultured SMCs and on endothelial cells and SMCs within atheroma. Finally, IL-3 was found to stimulate vascular endothelial growth factor (VEGF) gene transcription (Brizzi et al., 2001). These data suggest that IL-3, expressed by activated T lymphocytes infiltrating early and advanced atherosclerotic plaques, may sustain the atherosclerotic process either directly by activating SMC migration and proliferation, or indirectly via VEGF production.

In vitro, IL-4 has been reported to induce oxidative stress and upregulate the expression of VCAM-1 gene in human umbilical vein endothelial cells (EC) at transcriptional levels via activation of SP-1 transcription factor (Lee et al., 2001). Blockade of the CD40–CD154 pathway can inhibit CD4+ T-cell activation but is unable to prevent immune responses mediated by CD8+ T cells. In the absence of CD8+ T cells, inhibition of the CD40–CD154 pathway is insufficient to prevent the development of transplant arteriosclerosis (Ensminger et al., 2000). Using CD8+ T cells depleted CD40 (−/−) mice to study mechanisms of transplant arteriosclerosis in the absence of the CD40 pathway, Ensminger et al. (2001) reported that the number of eosinophils infiltrating the graft was markedly increased, which correlated with augmented intragraft production of IL-4. Treatment of the recipients with anti-IL4 resulted in significant reduction of eosinophil infiltration into the graft and the level of intimal proliferation. This suggests that elevated intragraft IL-4 production results in an eosinophil infiltrate causing transplant arteriosclerosis. In addition, atherosclerotic lesions can be induced in rabbits and mice immunized with heat shock protein 65 (HSP65). Fatty streak formation in IL-4 knockout mice immunized with HSP65 was significantly reduced when compared with lesions in wild-type mice (George et al., 2000a). However, using an IL-4 transgenic knockout, Mottram et al.

(1998) showed IL-4 deficiency did not alter vascular thickening in transplant arteriosclerosis, and George et al. (2000b) reported that deficiency in IL-4 did not affect early atherosclerosis in mice fed a high-cholesterol diet. This may be due to alternative pathways being activated to compensate in IL-4 knockout mice.

Mast cells have been documented in the atherosclerotic plaques to produce proinflammatory cytokines and mediators such as histamine. RT-PCR and immunohistochemical staining revealed that the gene of the histidine decarboxylase (HDC), which generates histamine from histidine, was expressed in monocytes/macrophages and T cells in the arterial intima. IL-4 has been shown to inhibit the expression of the HDC gene, but upregulate expression of the LOX-1 gene of an oxidized lipid scavenger receptor family of macrophages (Higuchi et al., 2001). These findings suggest that histamine synthesized in the arterial wall participates in the initiation and progression of atherosclerosis and that IL-4 can act as an important inhibitory and/or stimulatory factor in the function of monocytes/macrophages modulated by histamine in relation to the process of atherosclerosis.

4.2.2. *Other interleukins*

There has been no evidence that IL-7 or IL-9 may have a role in atherosclerosis. Both IL-4 and IL-13 downregulate fibrinogen biosynthesis and hence may play a role in dampening atherothrombotic disease (Vasse et al., 1996). IL-10 is detectable in human atherosclerotic plaques (Mallat et al., 1999a). IL-10 has several anti-atherogenic effects including inhibition of adhesion of LDL-activated monocytes to endothelium and downregulation of fibrinogen biosynthesis (Pinderski Oslund et al., 1999; Tedgui and Mallat, 2001; Vasse et al., 1996). IL-10 deficient mice fed an atherogenic diet appear to be prone to atherosclerosis (Mallat et al., 1999b). IL-10 expression has also been linked to diminished cell death and decreased expression of nitric oxide synthase (Mallat et al., 1999a). IL-11 is a cytokine that influences megakaryocyte and macrophage progenitor cell growth. It has been associated with thrombocytosis in humans (Araneda et al., 2001). Human vascular smooth muscle cells have been demonstrated to express IL-11 in response to IL-1α and this cytokine may play a role in atherosclerosis (Taki et al., 1999). IL-12 enhances Th1 cell development as stated earlier and IL-12 and IL-10 may have counter-regulatory influences on the development of atherosclerotic lesions. The balance between IL-10 and IL-12 may contribute to the degree of immune/inflammatory injury observed in atherosclerosis (Uyemura et al., 1996).

IL-15 shares many biological properties with IL-2, assisting in the chemotaxis, activation and recruitment of T cells (Wuttge et al., 2001). IL-15 also enhances the development and activation of natural killer (NK) cells. There is evidence that both mouse and human atherosclerotic lesions express IL-15 (Wuttge et al., 2001). IL-15 is found primarily in lipid-rich plaques in association with oxidized LDL-positive macrophages (Houtkamp et al., 2001). Plaque-derived T cells were found to be very responsive to IL-15, suggesting that IL-15 could provide an alternative route for T-cell activation in atherosclerosis (Houtkamp et al., 2001).

IL-16 is a proinflammatory cytokine that appears to require CD4 antigen for its activity (Center et al., 1997). IL-16 can be produced by fibroblasts, T cells and mast cells in the atherosclerotic lesion, though its expression is yet to be demonstrated in plaque tissue (Center et al., 1997; Rumsaeng et al., 1997; Sciaky et al., 2000). IL-16 is chemotactic for CD4+ cells, and has been shown to induce IL-2 receptor expression and HLA-DR expression on T cells. Its exact role in atherosclerosis is unknown.

IL-18 is a proatherogenic cytokine that has also been detected in atheromatous plaque. It is a macrophage-derived cytokine of importance to host defense against intracellular bacteria such as Mycobacterium tuberculosis (Sugawara, 2000). It may be of pivotal importance to atherosclerosis as it has been shown to activate IFN γ production by T cells (Sugawara, 2000). IL-18 acts like and in synergy with IL-12 and promotes Th1 cell development. Plaque macrophages obtained from atherosclerotic tissue express IL-18 (Mallat et al., 2001a). Vulnerable plaques were also shown to overexpress IL-18 (Mallat et al., 2001a). Inhibition of IL-18 in a murine model of atherosclerosis was associated with decreased lesion development and inflammatory cell infiltration of plaques (Mallat et al., 2001b). Of the other interleukins, neither IL-14 nor IL-17 has been shown to have any association with atherosclerosis at this point in time.

4.3. *Colony stimulating factors: macrophage activation/foam cell formation*

Two hematopoietic growth factors have been shown to be of significance to atherosclerosis – granulocyte macrophage colony stimulating factor (GM-CSF) and macrophage colony stimulating factor (M-CSF).

4.3.1. *Role of M-CSF*

M-CSF, also known as colony stimulating factor-1 (CSF-1) and macrophage and granulocyte inducer, is a survival, growth, differentiating and activation factor for macrophages (Flanagan and Lader, 1998). The cell sources for this cytokine include lymphocytes, monocytes, fibroblasts, epithelial cells, endothelial cells, smooth muscle and osteoblasts. M-CSF binds to CD115, the M-CSF receptor, identical to the product of the *c-fms* proto-oncogene, related to other receptors in this regard such as c-kit and receptor for platelet-derived growth factor (PDGF) (Inaba et al., 1992). These receptors have tyrosine kinase activity and also activate G proteins and may be expressed not only on macrophages but also on vascular smooth muscle cells (Inaba et al., 1992).

The pivotal role for this cytokine in atherosclerosis was demonstrated in the osteopetrosis (op/op) mouse which lacks M-CSF due to structural changes in the M-CSF gene (Ando et al., 1997). Mice deficient in M-CSF are protected from atherosclerosis (de Villiers et al., 1998). Atherosclerosis was induced in these mice either by feeding a high fat/high-cholesterol diet or by crossing these mice with ApoE-deficient mice. M-CSF deficiency in either case led to decreased levels of atherosclerosis (Ando et al., 1997). Homozygosity for the op mutation abolished atherosclerosis while heterozygosity for the mutation greatly diminished lesion size. Lipid levels were increased in the op/op mutants and hence these effects may have been related to altered levels of monocytes, tissue macrophages or M-CSF levels. Rajavashisth et al. (1998) utilized an LDL-receptor deficient mouse model and demonstrated that the op/op mutation diminishes the development of athero-sclerosis. These investigators showed that mice heterozygous or homozygous for the op/op mutation had significantly smaller lesion size compared to control mice. In the heterozygotes, a reduction of M-CSF levels by twofold was associated with a reduction in atheroma size by almost a 100-fold. M-CSF may enhance scavenger receptor expression (Ando et al., 1997; de Villiers et al., 1994) as well as low-density lipoprotein receptor-related protein on macrophages (LRP) (Watanabe et al., 1994).

Smooth muscle cells expressed from atherosclerotic lesions in an experimental rabbit model demonstrate M-CSF binding and tyrosine phosphorylation (Inaba et al., 1992). Both endothelium and smooth muscle cells in culture express M-CSF in response to bacterial lipopolysaccharide, IL-1 α and TNF-α (Clinton et al., 1992). M-CSF allows monocyte transformation into foam cells (Clinton et al., 1992) as measured by the accumulation of scavenger receptor and apolipoprotein mRNA in cultured macrophages. M-CSF also enhances production of MMP-9 and uroki-nase in a time- and concentration-dependent manner from monocytes and in vitro-derived foam cells (Tojo et al., 1999). Probucol, an inhibitor of atherosclerosis, decreased M-CSF levels and adhesion molecule expression in a rabbit model of accelerated atherosclerosis, while MCP-1 levels remained unaltered (Fruebis et al., 1997). This study provides one explanation for the efficacy of probucol in athero-sclerosis and again confirming a more significant role for M-CSF over MCP-1 in atherogenesis. To determine whether M-CSF is expressed in vivo in atherosclerotic plaques, Rosenfeld et al. (1992) analyzed atheromatous plaques of rabbits and humans using in situ hybridization. M-CSF expression was seen extensively in multiple cell types in fatty streaks, suggesting that this cytokine is expressed in vivo. Endothelial cells, smooth muscle cells and foam cells express M-CSF in vivo in rabbit models of atherosclerosis (Ruan et al., 1995). Clinton et al. (1992) also described M-CSF expression in intimal smooth muscle cells and macrophages in atheromatous lesions from rabbits.

4.3.2. *Role of GM-CSF*

GM-CSF is a pleuripotential growth and survival factor for hematopoietic cells. It activates eosinophils and allows growth of endothelial cells, erythroid cells, megakaryocytes as well as T cells. The GM-CSF receptor is a complex of two chains – an alpha chain and a promiscuous beta chain that is shared with IL-3 and IL-5 receptor alpha chains. The exact role of GM-CSF in atherogenesis is unclear. However, as it is a hematopoietic factor for macrophage-lineage cells, it may be involved in foam cell generation. Besides IL-1 and TNF-α, oxidized LDL activates GM-CSF expression from vascular cells and from macrophages in a protein kinase C (PKC)-dependent manner and may have an autocrine and/or paracrine effect on these cells (Sakai et al., 2000). Human vascular smooth muscle cells release GM-CSF after activation with IL-1 β, a process negatively regulated by cyclooxygenase-2 (COX2) (Stanford et al., 2000). Studies by Plenz et al. (1999a) have shown that in early atherogenesis, smooth muscles and endothelial cells were the principal sited of

GM-CSF expression. In advanced lesions, macrophages also expressed the cytokine. GM-CSF has also been shown to enhance transcription for collagen VIII (Plenz et al., 1999b), in conjunction with PDGF and TGF-β1 (Plenz et al., 1999a). Significant upregulation of GM-CSF is seen in atherosclerotic lesions compared to undiseased arteries suggesting an important but as yet undefined role for this cytokine in atherogenesis (Plenz et al., 1997). Moreover, fatty acid composition and the ratio of palmitic to linoleic acid levels in women are related to circulating GM-CSF levels (Fernandez-Real et al., 2001).

4.4. *Growth factors*

Several growth factors may play important roles in atherosclerosis. Transforming growth factor β (TGF-β) is a pleiotropic cytokine involved in tissue remodeling, fibrosis and angiogenesis (Cohen et al., 1997). Three isoforms are present in humans and these proteins have been described as members of a superfamily. It is produced by endothelial cells, macrophages, Th3-type T cells and by mast cells (Inobe et al., 1998). It inhibits cell growth and has been shown to be a switch factor for IgA (Cohen et al., 1997). It may act by inhibiting NF-κB/RelA activation (Arsura et al., 1996). The TGF-β family may play many essential roles in atherosclerosis (McCaffrey, 2000). TGF-β induces collagen synthesis by vascular smooth muscle cells (Amento et al., 1991). This may contribute to plaque stability. TGF-β1 inhibits cholesteryl ester accumulation in macrophages by inhibiting activity and expression of LDL and scavenger receptors and lipoprotein lipase (Argmann et al., 2001). In mice, inhibition of TGF-β accelerates atherosclerosis development and induces unstable plaque formation (Mallat et al., 2001c). There are also data to support a role for TGF-β in inducing synthesis of another anti-atherogenic cytokine, IL-10 (D'Orazio and Niederkorn, 1998; Maeda et al., 1995). TGF-β may also inhibit IL-6 synthesis by endothelial cells, a pivotal proatherogenic cytokine (Chen and Manning, 1996). Endoglin, a TGF-β receptor-associated protein, is expressed in atherosclerotic plaques (Conley et al., 2000). TGF-β1 levels are diminished in patients with coronary atherosclerosis (Grainger et al., 1995). Formation of lipid lesions on blood vessels may be accelerated by dietary fat in combination with low levels of TGF-β1 expression (Grainger et al., 2000). TGF-β1 has been shown to inhibit metalloproteinase (MMP-12) production from macrophages, a factor essential for plaque disruption (Feinberg et al., 2000).

On the other hand, TGF-β may induce production of MCP-1, a proatherogenic chemokine (Takeshita et al., 1995). Recent data also suggest that the various isoforms of TGF-β (−1, −2, −3) may be involved in calcification and bone formation in atherosclerotic plaque (Lindemann and Rumberger, 1993). TGF-β1 may be responsible for the fibrosis and vascular remodeling seen after arterial injury, as occurring following angioplasty procedures (Lindner, 2001). These data suggest many pleiotropic functions for TGF-β in atherosclerotic cardiovascular disease.

Platelet-derived growth factor (PDGF) is produced by vascular smooth muscle cells, fibroblasts, endothelial cells and mast cells. It is a mitogen for vascular smooth muscle cells and connective tissue cells. It is also chemotactic for fibroblasts, smooth muscle cells and monocytes. It is secreted as a dimer of disulfide-linked A and B chains (PDGF-AA, PDGF-BB or PDGF-AB). In endothelial cells, PDGF is induced by cyclical strain, shear stress and biomechanical forces (Resnick et al., 1997; Resnick and Gimbrone, 1995; Sumpio et al., 1998). Glucose (Mizutani et al., 1995), angiotensin (Okuda et al., 1996), thrombin (Shimizu et al., 2000) and adhesion of monocytes to endothelium (Funayama et al., 1998) also induce PDGF expression in different cell types. A shear stress element is present on the promoter of PDGF that mediates expression of the growth factor in endothelial cells (Resnick et al., 1997). Atherosclerotic lesions demonstrate strong staining for both PDGF and for TGF-β (Evanko et al., 1998) and it is likely that inflammatory cytokines and growth factors form a vicious loop that promotes atherosclerosis progression (Libby et al., 1992, Misiakos et al., 2001). At least in some studies of human plaque tissue, endothelial cells and smooth muscle cells are the major sites of PDGF expression (Wilcox et al., 1994). PDGF has been shown to activate NF-κB and produce sustained increases in oncogene expression, explaining its role in cell growth and vascular inflammatory processes (Inaba et al., 1995; Olashaw et al., 1992).

Another growth factor of interest to atherosclerosis is basic fibroblast growth factor (bFGF). The fibroblast growth factors are a family of multifunctional proteins that modulate cell proliferation, differentiation and angiogenesis. The FGFs have sequence homology with several proto-oncogenes in humans. In atherosclerosis, vascular remodeling and plaque formation may be modulated by bFGF. It is induced in smooth muscle cells by chlamydial infection (Rodel et al., 2000) and may mediate nicotine-induced smooth muscle proliferation (Cucina et al., 2000). Basic FGF has been administered safely in humans as implants in order to induce therapeutic angiogenesis, and gene transfer of this factor to vascular cells may be possible in the future (Lewis et al., 1997; Sellke et al., 1998).

4.5. *Chemokines*

There is evolving information that chemokines play a pivotal role in atherogenesis (Boring et al., 1998; Krishnaswamy et al., 1999a; Luster, 1998; Plutzky, 2001). The chemokines are chemotactic cytokines that are primarily involved in inflammatory cell recruitment to tissue. However, recent data suggest that these mediators may have many other biological effects (Luster, 1998). The chemokines have been traditionally classified into four groups – CC, C, CXC and CXXC, based on the relative position of the cysteine residues. In the α-chemokines, e.g., the first two cysteine residues are separated by a single amino acid (CXC), whereas in the β-chemokines, the two cysteine residues are adjacent to each other (CC). The α-chemokines containing the sequences, glutamic acid-leucine-arginine, are predominantly chemotactic for neutrophils while those lacking this sequence are chemotactic for lymphocytes. The C chemokine, lymphactin, has only two cysteine residues in the molecule, while fractalkine, a CXXC chemokine, has three amino acid residues separating the first two cysteines. Chemokines bind to chemokine receptors and many have been characterized. The CXC chemokines bind to CXCR, while the CC chemokines bind to CCR, leading to signal transduction and biological activity.

Table 2 summarizes the chemokines of interest to atherosclerosis. Since the recruitment of monocytes to the vascular wall is an early event in atherosclerosis, it is likely that chemokines such as IL-8 and MCP-1 play important roles in this regard (Fig. 3).

4.5.1. *Role of MCP-1*

In LDL-receptor knockout mice, hypercholesterolemia rapidly triggers expression of MCP-1 in resident intimal macrophages that leads to the recruitment of more macrophages expressing MCP-1, leading to an amplification of the inflammatory response (Kowala et al., 2000). Aiello et al. (1999) demonstrated the importance of MCP-1 in the accelerated development of atherosclerosis in apolipoprotein E-deficient mice. These investigators transplanted bone marrow cells from either mice overexpressing a murine MCP-1 transgene (on a background of apoE-deficiency) or from control mice into irradiated apoE-knockout mice. MCP-1 was

Table 2
Role of chemokines in atherosclerosis

Chemokine	Class	Source	Functions	Relevance to atherosclerosis
MCP-1	CC	Macrophages	Recruitment of monocytes and	• Cellular recruitment
		Fibroblasts	T cells Th2	• CCR2 knockout mice do
		Endothelium	development	not develop atherosclerosis
		Mast cells		• NF-κB regulated chemokine
		Smooth muscle		• Induced by chlamydiae, CMV, homocysteine and LDL
				• Increased tissue factor expression
MIP-1α	CC	Macrophages	Chemoattractant Th1 development	• Cellular recruitment
				• Differentiation of plaque Th1 cells?
MIPI-1β	CC	Monocytes	Chemoattractant for	• Inflammation
		Macrophages	CD8+ T cells and	• Cellular recruitment
		Endothelium	monocytes	
		Mast cells		
		T and B cells		
RANTES	CC	Endothelium	Chemoattractant for	• Cellular recruitment
		Platelets	monocyte, T cells,	• Vascular inflammation
		T cells	eosinophils	
IL-8	CXC	Macrophages	Chemottractant for	• Induced by thrombin,
		Endothelium	Neutrophil and naive	IL-1, cholesterol, strain
		Fibroblast	T cells	• Monocyte recruitment
		Mast cells		• Angiogenesis
				• Chemotactic for vascular smooth muscle cells
				• Inhibits expression of TIMP-1

CCR2 = chemokine receptor-2; CMV = cytomegalovirus; LDL = low density lipoprotein; TIMP-1 = tissue inhibitor of metalloproteinase-1.

detectable in vascular tissue and the mice demonstrated enhanced lipid staining, increased lipid oxidation and increased cell surface staining for macrophage markers (Aiello et al., 1999). Reckless et al. (1999) demonstrated the pivotal importance of MCP-1 in macrophage recruitment. Both the apoE-deficient mouse and C57BL/6 mice develop lipid lesions when fed a high fat diet, but the lesions in apoE-deficient mice are devoid of macrophages. The investigators demonstrated that both the types of mice expressed similar numbers of adhesion molecules (VCAM-1, ICAM-1) and the inflammatory cytokines, TNF-α and MIP-1 α. However, lesions from the apoE-deficient mice demonstrated no MCP-1 whereas heavy expression of this chemokine was observed in lesions of the C57BL/6 mice (Reckless et al., 1999). In a more intriguing study, Boring et al. (1998) developed mice deficient in the receptor for MCP-1, CCR2 and crossed these mice with the apoE-deficient mice which develop accelerated atherosclerosis. CCR deficiency decreased lesion formation in the apoE-deficient mice providing evidence that chemokines are of pivotal importance to atherogenesis (Boring et al., 1998). Cytomegalovirus (CMV) has been linked to atherosclerosis and MCP-1 may be involved in this process. For example, serum from CMV-infected mice induces MCP-1 in endothelial cells, a process probably mediated by interferon gamma (Rott et al., 2001). *Chlamydia pneumoniae*, recently linked to the development of atherosclerosis, also activates MCP-1 expression in endothelial cells in an NF-κB-dependent manner (Molestina et al., 2000). Homocysteine, a risk factor for accelerated atherosclerosis, induces nuclear translocation of NF-κB and MCP-1 and IL-8 transcription and secretion in vascular smooth muscle cells (Desai et al., 2001). Similarly, oxidized or modified lipoproteins have been shown to be potent inducers of the chemokines, IL-8 and MCP-1 in vascular cells, such as smooth muscle or endothelium, in vitro (Klouche et al., 2000; Maeno et al., 2000). Other stimuli such as cyclical strain and leptin are capable of inducing MCP-1 expression by various vascular cells (Bouloumie et al., 1999; Jiang et al., 1999). On the contrary, estrogens downregulate MCP-1 expression in vascular smooth muscle cells, explaining their anti-atherogenic effects (Seli et al., 2001).

Chemokine expression may be linked to other aspects of atherosclerosis, including T helper cytokine synthesis and the nitric oxide axis. Of interest, mice with the receptor for MCP-1 (CCR2) deleted not only had retarded development of atherosclerosis but also had lower production of interferon gamma, a potent macrophage activator (Peters and Charo, 2001). This suggested a link between Th1/Th2 cytokine regulation and the chemokines. In fact, the enhancement of Th2 cytokines by MCP-1 and of Th1 cytokines by MIP-1 α has been shown at a clonal level and is well recognized (Karpus et al., 1997). In one study, rats were fed with L-NAME that inhibits nitric oxide generation. These rats developed mononuclear infiltration, intimal thickening and perivascular fibrosis, all features of advancing atherosclerosis (Koyanagi et al., 2000). MCP-1 was expressed in vascular endothelial cells and monocytes in vascular lesions. However, when injected with an anti-MCP-1 antibody, monocyte recruitment as well as intimal thickening was greatly diminished but perivascular fibrosis remained unaffected (Koyanagi et al., 2000). This study suggests a role for chemokines in vascular inflammation and a possible role for other mediators, such as the growth factors for fibrosis. Besides mononuclear recruitment, alteration of smooth muscle differentiation and function may also be a property of MCP-1 (Denger et al., 1999). Other investigators have suggested that MCP-1 may increase tissue factor expression in smooth muscle and mononuclear cells suggesting a procoagulant role (Ernofsson and Siegbahn, 1996, Schecter et al., 1997).

4.5.2. *Role of IL-8*

IL-8 is a β- (or CXC) chemokine that binds to a distinct receptor, CXCR2 (Luster, 1998). It has been typically considered to be chemotactic to neutrophils. However, recent studies suggest that this chemokine may play a role in athero-sclerosis (Boisvert et al., 2000; Shin et al., 2002). IL-8 is expressed by macrophages in arterial plaque and may play a proatherogenic role (Boisvert et al., 2000). IL-8 is a potent chemotactic factor for neutrophils and basophils (Graves and Jiang, 1995). It also has chemotactic activity for certain subsets of lymphocytes and is a potent angiogenetic factor (Graves and Jiang, 1995; Koch et al., 1992; Norrby, 1996). IL-8 has been shown to be chemotactic for vascular smooth muscle cells (Yue et al., 1993). IL-8 can be secreted by a variety of cell types within the atheromatous plaque, including macrophages, smooth muscle cells, mast cells, eosinophils, lymphocytes and endothelium (Table 2) (Krishnaswamy et al., 1997; Yamashita et al., 1999). Neutrophils, basophils, eosinophils and lymphocytes express the CXCR1 and 2 receptors that mediate biological functions of this cytokine (Moller et al., 1993; Petering et al., 1999; Yamashita et al., 1999). IL-8 is stated to be an angiogenetic factor in the coronary vasculature (Simonini et al., 2000). IL-8 is induced by various stimuli including the monokines, IL-1 and TNF-α (Graves and Jiang, 1995; Krishnaswamy et al., 1998), HIV tat protein (Hofman et al., 1999), homocysteine (Desai et al., 2001), thrombin (Ludwicka-Bradley et al., 2000), cholesterol loading (Wang et al., 1996a), glucose (Temaru et al., 1997), histamine (Jeannin et al., 1994), IL-15 (Badolato et al., 1997), shear stress (Kato et al., 2001), mast cell tryptase (Cairns and Walls, 1996; Compton et al., 1998), platelet and mononuclear cell contact with endothelial cells in culture (Lukacs et al., 1995) and modified lipo-proteins (Brand et al., 1997b; Woenckhaus et al., 1998). Like MCP-1, induction of IL-8 transcription appears to require translocation of NF-κB to the nucleus (Brand et al., 1997b; Yamashita et al., 1999). There is evidence for dysregulated production of IL-8 in atheromatous tissue. Macrophages from atheromatous plaque tissue produce IL-8 (Apostolopoulos et al., 1996, Liu et al., 1997). Rus et al. (1996b) demonstrated IL-8 gene expression in atheromatous blood vessels. Foam cells in plaque tissue and macrophages loaded with LDL express IL-8 (Wang et al., 1996b). Moreover, using reverse transcriptase polymerase chain reaction and immunhis-tochemistry, Frostegard et al. (1999) showed dominance of Th1 cytokines, GM-CSF and IL-8 in endarterectomy tissue. IL-8 inhibits expression of the tissue inhibitor of metalloproteinase-1 (TIMP-1) and may explain the inhibitory effect of oxidized LDL on reduction of TIMP-1 in macrophages (Shin et al., 2002). This process can assist in the vascular accumulation of macrophages.

IL-8, which induces the migration and proliferation of endothelial cells and smooth muscle cells, is a potent angiogenic factor that may play a role in athe-rosclerosis. IL-8 expression was significantly elevated in directional coronary atherectomy (DCA) samples compared with internal mammary artery samples (IMA). When angiogenic activity of the homogenates from these samples was tested using the rat cornea micropocket assay and cultured cells, the in vivo corneal neovascular response and the in vitro proliferation of cultured cells were markedly positive with DCA samples, but not with IMA samples (Simonini et al., 2000). Many other cytokines such as vascular endothelial growth factor and basic fibroblast growth factor may have angiogenic effects in atherosclerosis and have been discussed earlier.

4.5.3. *Role of other chemokines*

The role of other chemokines in atherosclerosis is less clear. RANTES is a CC chemokine that binds to the chemokine receptors, CCR1, CCR3, CCR5 and CCR9. RANTES is produced by lymphocytes and mononuclear cells. It induces chemotaxis of monocytes, memory T cells and eosinophils. It also releases histamine from basophils. Recent data suggest that RANTES is an inhibitor of macrophage trophic strain of HIV. A recent study demonstrated that thrombin-stimulated platelets cause RANTES deposition on endothelium and allow monocyte arrest and recruitment (von Hundelshausen et al., 2001). RANTES is also expressed in transplant-related atherosclerotic lesions and is seen mainly in endothelium, macrophages, myofibro-blasts and lymphocytes (Pattison et al., 1996). Wilcox et al. (1994) found 5% of plaque cells expressed mRNAs for RANTES using in situ hybridization techniques. Thus, RANTES may play a role in monocyte recruitment and development of the cellular infiltrate in atherosclerosis. Macrophage inflammatory protein-1 beta (MIP-1 β) is another monocyte- and lymphocyte-derived molecule of the CC chemokine family and is chemotactic for monocytes, T cells and natural killer cells. Both MIP-β and its receptor, CCR5, have been detected in smooth muscle cells and macrophages in atheromatous lesions (Schecter et al., 2000).

5. Other effects of cytokines in atherosclerosis

Cytokines elaborated in response to vascular inflammation and mononuclear infiltration of the vessel wall can also influence other processes of importance to atherosclerosis. Smooth muscle activation, modulation of nitric oxide axis and effects on the coagulation system are examples of such effects. The vulnerable or unstable plaque is also an expression of cytokine-mediated destabilization that leads to rupture and thrombotic complications associated with atherosclerotic cardio-vascular disease. These effects are summarized below.

5.1. *Cytokines and smooth muscle cell modulation and nitric oxide*

Cytokines can modulate smooth muscle function. For example, in vitro pre-incubation of smooth muscle cells (SMCs) with both TNF-α and IL-1 β caused a significant increase in VCAM-1 and ICAM-1 expression and a more than ninefold increase in monocyte adhesion (Thorne et al., 1996). Another adhesion molecule, CD44, which participates in extracellular matrix binding, lymphocyte activation, cell migration and tumor metastasis, was induced in the neointima of allografted vessels of mice with transplant-associated arteriosclerosis and colocalized with a subset of proliferating vascular smooth muscle cells (VSMC). In the study of the molecular mechanisms regulating CD44 expression, Foster et al. (1998) reported that IL-1 β induced a fivefold increase in cell surface CD44 expression in SMC and suggested that regulation of CD44 gene expression by IL-1 β may contribute to SMC phenotypic modulation in the pathogenesis of arteriosclerosis.

Inflammatory cytokines are known to induce inducible NO synthase (iNOS) in the vascular smooth muscle. In vitro, IL-1 β induced nitric oxide production by VSMCs. Addition of TNF-α further enhanced IL-1 β-induced nitric oxide by VSMCs (Ikeda et al., 1998). In an in vivo study using a porcine model, it was reported that iNOS was absent in the normal coronary artery, whereas it was highly expressed one day after the in vivo local application of IL-1 β and thereafter downregulated during 14 d of the study period. In contrast, endothelial NOS (eNOS) was well maintained throughout the study period. Two weeks later, hyperconstric-tive responses to intracoronary serotonin and neointimal formation were noted at the IL-1 β-treated site, and both responses were significantly greater at the site cotreated with NOS inhibitors, either *n*-nitro-L-arginine methylester or amino-guanidine. These data indicate that iNOS is transiently induced in vivo in response to local inflammation and that NO produced by iNOS exerts an inhibitory effect against the cytokine-induced proliferative/vasospastic changes of the coronary artery in vivo (Fukumoto et al., 1997a). The same group of researchers also shows that IL-1 α and TNF-α had a similar ability to induce coronary arteriosclerosis-like changes and hyperconstrictive responses (Fukumoto et al., 1997b).

The exact role of nitric oxide on smooth muscle function is unclear. It is known that prolonged incubation of a coculture of vascular SMC (VSMC) and endothelial cells with IL-1 induced large amounts of NO release and cytotoxicity in VSMC. In addition, the DNA synthesis in cocultured EC was also found to be stimulated. The concentration of basic fibroblast growth factor in the supernatant of the coculture was increased and correlated with the degree of cytotoxicity in VSMC. Since supernatant from IL-1-treated VSMC culture stimulated DNA synthesis in EC alone, these results indicate that NO released from IL-1-stimulated VSMC induces VSMC death and release of basic fibroblast growth factor, which then stimulated adjacent EC proliferation and contributes to the formation of atherosclerotic pla-ques (Fukuo et al., 1995). Hence, a role for cytokine-mediated nitric oxide genera-tion and growth factor synthesis may allow a novel loop to function in these inflamed blood vessels.

Cytokines may also facilitate apoptotic pathways in smooth muscle and other cells. It has been demonstrated that SMCs bear Fas, markers of apoptosis, in advanced atherosclerotic plaques. The same plaques also contain macrophages and T lymphocytes, cells capable of expressing Fas ligand, a molecule that potentiates cell death by ligating Fas. In vitro, IFN γ, TNF-α and IL-1 β have been shown to increase expression of Fas in SMCs. These inflammatory cytokine-primed SMCs were readily programmed to die by treatment with anti-Fas antibody. These results suggest that activation of the Fas apoptosis pathway contributes to the induction of SMC death during atherogenesis and provides a role for inflammatory cytokines in promoting cell death process related to vascular remodeling and plaque rupture (Geng et al., 1997).

5.2. *Cytokines and the coagulation cascade*

Serum fibrinogen and fibrin degradation products have been found to be high in patients who had arterial surgery, and fibrinolysis has been depressed, suggesting high plasma fibrinogen may be an important risk factor for the development of athero-sclerosis (Martin-Paredero et al., 1998). Platelet volume and mass were found to be increased in patients with hypertension who had atherosclerotic renal artery stenosis, suggesting that increased platelet volume may contribute to the development of the disease (Bath et al., 1994). Acute phase response cytokines such as IL-1, TNF-α and IL-6 may be responsible for elevating fibrinogen levels and activating coagulation mechanisms. In studying the pathophysiologic role of TNF-α in vascular diseases, Cimminiello et al. (1994) found that the levels of TNF-α, tissue plasminogen activator (tPA) and von Willebrand factor (vWF) were significantly higher in occlusive vascular diseases. These results, showing correlationship between TNF-α, and vWF and tPA, suggest that TNF-α may affect endothelial cell function by inducing procoagulant changes. On the other hand, IL-4, IL-10 and IL-13, which protect vessel walls from monocyte injuries leading to atherosclerosis, downregulated in vitro IL-6-induced fibrinogen biosynthesis in hepatocytes (Vasse et al., 1996). Thus, cytokines, depending on their concentration and prevalence, may have potentiating or inhibitory effects on the coagulation cascade.

5.3. *Cytokines and the vulnerable plaque*

A major complication of atherosclerosis is the vulnerable plaque. Vulnerable plaques do not cause high-grade stenosis but nevertheless are associated with acute coronary syndromes, unstable angina, myocardial infarction and/or sudden death. Vulnerable plaques have a thin fibrous cap and demonstrate a core composed of lipids and inflammatory cells (Kolodgie et al., 2001). Inflammatory infiltration of the plaque by T lymphocytes, macrophages and mast cells leads to elaboration of cytokines and metalloproteinases (Krishnaswamy et al., 1999b; Kullo et al., 1998). This leads to plaque destabilization and potential rupture (Kullo et al., 1998). In the unstable plaque, activated T cells secrete interferon gamma (IFN γ). IFN γ inhibits collagen and elastin synthesis by smooth muscle cells and also activates macrophages to elaborate metalloproteinases that allow breakdown of matrix protein (Libby, 2001). Mast cell-derived tumor necrosis factor (TNF) may serve a similar role in activating metalloproteinases (Kaartinen et al., 1998). Kaartinen et al. (1998) demonstrated that plaques contain TNF-α-positive macrophages and MMP-9 (92 kD gelatinase) expressing macrophages, suggesting a relationship. Other factors such as MCP-1, macrophage colony stimulating factor (M-CSF) and interleukin-1 (IL-1) are all capable of macrophage activation and are detectable in plaque tissue (Libby, 2001). The mast cell is capable of expressing many of these factors and the role of mast cell-derived products in atherogenesis has been reviewed by us in some detail (Kelley et al., 2000a,b). Thus, interactions between cell types leading to metalloproteinase activation leads to matric protein breakdown and plaque instability.

Unstable angina occurs when atherosclerotic plaque ruptures. Increased levels of IL-6 have been demonstrated in unstable angina compared to stable angina. However, at 1-month follow-up after percutaneous coronary interventions, it was reported that there were no longer any significant differences between the levels of IL-6 in patients with unstable angina versus patients with stable angina and healthy control subjects (Yazdani et al., 1998). This suggests that IL-6 levels may correlate with the instability of atheromatous plaques and that the decrease of IL-6 levels after percutaneous coronary interventions may represent plaque reendothelialization and stabilization.

IL-18, a potent proinflammatory cytokine, is also highly expressed in human carotid atherosclerotic plaques. IL-18 receptor was also upregulated in plaque macrophages and endothelial cells, suggesting potential biological effects. Moreover, significantly higher levels of IL-18 mRNA were found in unstable than in stable plaques (Mallat et al., 2001a). These data suggest a role for IL-18 in atherosclerotic plaque destabilization leading to acute ischemic syndromes. In addition, in vivo electrotransfer of expression-plasmid DNA encoding for murine IL-18 binding protein (IL-18 BP), the endogenous inhibitor of IL-18, has been demonstrated to prevent fatty streak development in the aorta of apoE knockout mice and slows progression of advanced atherosclerotic plaques in the aortic sinus (Mallat et al., 2001b). Furthermore, transfection with the IL-18 BP plasmid induced profound changes in plaque composition leading to a stable plaque phenotype. Thus, IL-18 inhibitors appear to reduce plaque development and promote plaque stability.

The elaboration of metalloproteinases leads to alteration of stability of the fibrous cap leading to plaque rupture and subsequent thrombosis. Matrix metalloproteinases (MMPs) are expressed in atherosclerotic plaques, where in their active form, they may contribute to vascular remodeling and plaque disruption. Membrane type 1 MMP (MT1-MMP), a novel transmembrane MMP that activates pro-MMP-2 (gelatinase A), has been shown to be expressed by SMCs and macrophages in human atherosclerotic plaques. The expression of MT1-MMP in these cells was increased two- to fourfold after exposure to IL-1α and TNF-α (Rajavashisth et al., 1999). Thus, activation of SMCs and macrophages by proinflammatory cytokines may influence extracellular matrix remodeling and unstable plaque in atherosclerosis by regulating MT1-MMP expression. Vulnerable plaques can be identified by various techniques including intravascular ultrasonography, electron-beam computerized tomography, magnetic resonance imaging or angioscopy (Kullo et al., 1998). Current approaches to therapy of atherosclerotic cardiovascular disease include attempts towards plaque stabilization.

6. Cytokine gene polymorphisms and atherosclerosis

Recent molecular studies of human disease have attempted to correlate the occurrence of specific polymorphisms in cytokine genes with diseases such as asthma and coronary atherosclerosis. Functional single nucleotide polymorphisms in the genes of cytokines are associated with disease severity and phenotype. It is likely that over the course of the next few years, many more such studies will be available to determine whether specific gene loci and/or polymorphisms within pivotal cytokine genes are associated with either severity or incidence of coronary atherosclerosis. Koch et al. (2001) studied polymorphisms of IL-10, TNF α and TNF β genes in patients with coronary artery disease (CAD) and control individuals with no evidence of CAD. In their study of six different polymorphisms of the genes encoding IL-10, TNF α and TNF β, no correlations with risk of myocardial infarctions or angiographically demonstrable CAD were found (Koch et al., 2001). In another study, however, polymorphisms within the gene encoding TGF-β1 were found to correlate with early occurrence of coronary vasculopathy following cardiac transplantation (Densem et al., 2000). Keso et al. (2001) analyzed polymorphisms within the genes for TNF-α (TNFA) and TNF-β (TNFB) and found strong correlations between the TNFA and TNFB genotypes but no correlation with the frequency of old or recent myocardial infarction, coronary thrombosis or coronary stenosis in men with the different genotypes. However, patients with the TNFA22 or TNFB11 genotypes tended to have more fibrous lesions and calcifications in their coronary arteries. These researchers concluded that TNFA or TNFB polymorphisms were unlikely to contribute to atherosclerosis progression (Keso et al., 2001).

7. Modulation of atherogenic cytokines by exercise

Exercise has a beneficial effect on the development of atherosclerosis in conjunction with control of other conventional risk factors such as dyslipidemia, hypertension and diabetes mellitus. Exercise training enhances insulin sensitivity, improves glucose tolerance, decreases triglyceride and LDL levels while increasing HDL levels. Studies in our laboratories have also demonstrated influences of exercise on production of atherogenic cytokines (Smith et al., 1999). In a study of 43 subjects at risk of developing ischemic heart disease, Smith et al. (1999) found that 6 months of moderate-intensity exercise caused a greater than 50% reduction in peripheral blood mononuclear production of atherogenic cytokines, IFN γ, TNF-α and IL-1 β and also a significant increase in the production of atheroprotective cytokines, TGF-β, IL-4 and IL-10. This was accompanied by reductions in CRP levels. IFN γ is a typical Th1 cytokine while TNF-α is a mononuclear cell-derived cytokine. Both cytokines are capable of inducing endothelial and macrophage activation. These cytokines can thereby contribute to atherogenesis by activating mononuclear infiltration and foam cell formation. IFN γ has also been shown to weaken plaque stability by inhibiting TGF-β production altering fibrous cap structure (Libby, 2000; Libby, 2001). Exercise in our study was shown to enhance the production of the atheroprotective cytokines, IL-4, IL-10 and TGF-β. IL-4 been shown to inhibit IFN γ production and allow differentiation of T helper cells to a Th2 phenotype (Miossec, 1993). IL-4 also inhibits production of the atherogenic cytokines, TNF-α, IL-1, IL-6 and IL-8 (Miossec, 1993). Both IL-4 and IL-10 inhibit synthesis of fibrinogen (Vasse et al., 1996). Moreover, IL-10 has been shown to have anti-atherogenic properties both in vitro and in vivo (Pinderski Oslund et al., 1999). Thus, exercise, by enhancing release of atheroprotective T-cell-derived cytokines, prevents endothelial activation and thereby prevents the chain of events leading to atherosclerosis.

8. HIV-associated accelerated atherogenesis

With the advent of more effective therapies for human immunodeficiency virus infection (HIV), HIV-infected patients are living longer and cardiovascular disease is becoming more obvious in this population. In fact, patients with HIV infection represent one of the most rapidly developing groups with cardiovascular disease globally (Kelley et al., 2000a,b; Krishnaswamy et al., 2000). It is likely that HIV infection itself, opportunistic infections, secreted viral proteins such as gp120 or tat (transactivator of viral transcription), and cytokines elaborated during the course of HIV infection of the immune system all contribute to pathogenesis of these disorders. Accelerated atherosclerosis and vasculopathy are recognized complications of HIV infection. With the advent of highly active antiretroviral therapy (HAART), dyslipidemia, lipodystrophy and endothelial dysfunction are evolving problems (Krishnaswamy et al., 2000).

Endothelial activation in HIV can occur as a result of direct infection of endothelial cells by the virus (Chi et al., 2000; Poland et al., 1995). More likely mechanisms are activation of endothelial cells by tat protein and by the monokines, IL-1 and TNF-α (Chi et al., 2000). Zidovetzki et al. (1998) demonstrated expression of IL-6 in brain endothelial cells following activation by tat protein. The induction of IL-6 transcription was associated with activation of intracellular signaling pathways including protein kinase C and protein kinase A. HIV infection can also be associated with secretion of metalloproteinases associated with plaque stability (Weeks, 1998). Tat protein activates monocyte production of IL-1, TNF-α, IL-6, IL-8 and metalloproteinases, further compounding vascular inflammatory responses and endothelial activation (Lafrenie et al., 1997). Hence, by various mechanisms mediated by atherogenic cytokine production, HIV infection may be associated with accelerated atherogenesis.

9. Pharmacological manipulation of proatherogenic cytokines

The observation that inflammation is core to the mechanisms of atherosclerosis has raised the possibility of manipulating the cytokine networks, growth factors, transcription factors and intracellular metabolic pathways involved in the control of atherogenesis. The prospects that some novel transcription factors e.g., NF-κB are common mediators of disparate signaling pathways increase the possibility of controlling the inflammatory processes involved in atherogenesis. One surprising theme to emerge from the rapid explosion of knowledge on atherogenesis is the observation that many traditional cardiovascular drugs e.g., statins, β-blockers, salicylates and the ACE inhibitors function by interference with expression of proatherogenic cytokines (Plutzky, 2001). This contradicts previously held hypotheses which predominantly emphasized the hemodynamic effects of these medications. Future trends in cardiac pharmacology are likely to focus on manipulating the cytokine networks, replacement of vascular growth factors, or defective genes.

9.1. *Effects of standard cardiovascular drugs on the cytokine axis*

Lovastatin and simvastatin, inhibitors of HMG CoA reductase, produce a dose-dependent inhibition of MCP-1 production by mononuclear cells and endothelial cells in response to lipopolysaccharide and/or IL-1 β (Romano et al., 2000). The addition of mevalonate overrode this inhibitory effect of the statins suggesting a mevalonate-dependence on chemokine synthesis. Using a mouse air pouch model to study inflammatory cell recruitment in vivo, the same group also demonstrated that these drugs inhibited leukocyte recruitment and MCP-1 secretion into the exudate (Romano et al., 2000). Cerivastatin, another HMG CoA inhibitor, also inhibited the production of proatherogenic cytokines (MCP-1 and IL-8) from alveolar macrophages and human umbilical vein endothelial in response to chlamydial infection (Kothe et al., 2000). Atorvastatin was recently shown to inhibit neointimal inflammation, NF-κB activation and MCP-1 expression in a rabbit model of atherosclerosis (Bustos et al., 1998b). ACE inhibitors, like the statins, have anti-inflammatory effects and modulate the cytokine axis. For example, a study by Hernandez-Presa et al. (1997) demonstrated inhibition of MCP-1 production, NF-κB activation and macrophage infiltration in a rabbit model of atherosclerosis by the ACE-inhibitor drug, quinapril. In another study, the same group also showed inhibition of IL-8, MCP-1 and PDGF expression in vascular tissues and diminished NF-κB activation in a rabbit model of accelerated atherosclerosis (Hernandez-Presa et al., 1998). ACE-inhibitors also diminish expression of the lectin-like oxidized LDL receptor-1 (LOX-1) on endothelial cells, thereby decreasing the potential to develop atherosclerosis (Morawietz et al., 1999). It is of interest that LOX-1 expression on endothelial cells is regulated by angiotensin II (AT II) acting through the angiotensin receptor and losartan, the AT-II receptor blocker, decreases this expression.

Aspirin, an inhibitor of cyclooxygenase (COX), is used as an anti-platelet agent in coronary artery disease. Ikonomidis et al. (1999) demonstrated that aspirin decreases CRP levels as well as circulating cytokines, MCP-1 and IL-6, following six weeks of therapy. Aspirin also elevates levels of TGF b1, a growth factor that has beneficial effects in atherosclerosis and is responsible for plaque stability (Grainger et al., 1995). Besides inhibition of COX, salicylates also inhibit nuclear translocation of the ubiquitous transcription factor, NF-κB, that appears essential for atherogenesis to progress. They appear to do so by inhibiting IκBα phosphorylation and subsequent degradation (Pierce et al., 1996).

β adrenergic receptor stimulation via the catecholamines is a crucial regulator of immune responses, perhaps essential to the stress response. In one study, T cells cultured in the presence of epinephrine developed into Th1-type cells, producing IFN γ, a cytokine incriminated in atherosclerosis and plaque instability (Swanson et al., 2001). Infusion of isoprenaline, a beta adrenergic agonist in humans, is associated with significant elevations in IL-6, probably derived from adipocytes (Mohamed-Ali et al., 2000). Accordingly, the use of β blockers in patients with angina pectoris is associated with lower levels of IL-6 and CRP (Doo et al., 2001). Other studies of patients with cardiac disease treated with β blockers have demonstrated decreased levels of TNF-α, soluble IL-2 receptor and in one study, IL-10 (Gullestad et al., 2001a; Ohtsuka et al., 2001).

9.2. *Novel immunomodulatory and cytokine-directed therapies*

Given the inflammatory basis of atherosclerosis and the availability of mechanistic paradigms involving adhesion molecules, cytokines and transcription factors in the development of an atheromatous plaque, it is possible to design specific drugs that inhibit these mediators. This field is in its infancy in regard to clinical studies and randomized trials. Nevertheless, there are data to suggest a role for angiogenic cytokines in coronary artery disease (Isner, 1996). Of the various cytokines with angiogenic potential, basic fibroblast growth factor and vascular endothelial growth factor have been the most promising. Clinical trials with angiogenic cytokines in patients with advanced coronary artery disease have shown improved exercise tolerance, reduction in symptoms and improved ventricular function (Freedman and Isner, 2002). Other therapeutic strategies may include the use of intravenous immunoglobulin (Gullestad et al., 2001b), thalidomide, pentoxifylline, rapamycin or cyclosporine (Wasowska et al., 1997), TNF-α antagonists (such as Etanercept), chemokine inhibitors or chemokine receptor antagonists, and the use of recombinant cytokines (IL-10) or cytokine antagonists (such as IL-1 receptor antagonist) (Damas et al., 2001). More clinical trials and studies are needed to determine efficacy, toxicity and dosing for many of these immunomodulators before they can be included in routine therapy for atherosclerosis.

10. Conclusions

In summary, the global burden of atherosclerotic cardiovascular disease is enormous and continues to grow larger as the population ages resulting in a wide spectrum of clinical disease over a variety of vascular beds (and their respective organ systems) thereby generating tremendous diagnostic and treatment costs and very significant morbidity and mortality throughout the world. A better understanding of the basic mechanisms involved in the pathophysiology of atherosclerosis is essential for the development of new preventative strategies and diagnostic and treatment modalities. It is abundantly clear that the inflammatory process plays a central role in the atherosclerotic process and that cytokines, interleukins, colony stimulating factors and growth factors play a central role in the modulation of the inflammatory process. It is also likely that current therapeutic strategies, including drugs and exercise, have profound modulatory effects on the generation of cardiotoxic and proatherogenic cytokines. In the future, targeted approaches to inhibiting specific cytokines or signal transducing molecules using monoclonal antibodies or gene/molecular therapeutic approaches may be possible for what is essentially a systemic disease.

Therefore, the ability to understand and modulate the mechanisms involved in the inflammatory process holds great promise to suggest novel targets for future intervention and thereby reduce the burden of and achieve improved outcomes in atherosclerotic cardiovascular disease.

References

Adcock, I.M., 1997. Transcription factors as activators of gene transcription: AP-1 and NF-kappa B. Monaldi Arch Chest Dis. 52, 178–186.

Aiello, R.J., Bourassa, P.A., Lindsey, S., Weng, W., Natoli, E., Rollins, B.J., Milos, P.M., 1999. Monocyte chemoattractant protein-1 accelerates atherosclerosis in apolipoprotein E-deficient mice. Arterioscler. Thromb. Vasc. Biol. 19, 1518–1525.

Amento, E.P., Ehsani, N., Palmer, H., Libby, P., 1991. Cytokines and growth factors positively and negatively regulate interstitial collagen gene expression in human vascular smooth muscle cells. Arterioscler. Thromb. 11, 1223–1230.

Anderson, G.P., Coyle, A.J., 1994. TH2 and 'TH2-like' cells in allergy and asthma: pharmacological perspectives. Trends Pharmacol. Sci. 15, 324–332.

Ando, M., Gafvels, M., Bergstrom, J., Lindholm, B., Lundkvist, I., 1997. Uremic serum enhances scavenger receptor expression and activity in the human monocytic cell line U937. Kidney Int. 51, 785–792.

Apostolopoulos, J., Davenport, P., Tipping, P.G., 1996. Interleukin-8 production by macrophages from atheromatous plaques. Arterioscler. Thromb. Vasc. Biol. 16, 1007–1012.

Araneda, M., Krishnan, V., Hall, K., Kalbfleisch, J., Krishnaswamy, G., Krishnan, K., 2001. Reactive and clonal thrombocytosis: proinflammatory and hematopoietic cytokines and acute phase proteins. South Med. J. 94, 417–420.

Arbustini, E., Grasso, M., Diegoli, M., Pucci, A., Bramerio, M., Ardissino, D., Angoli, L., De Servi, S., Bramucci, E., Mussini, A., 1991. Coronary atherosclerotic plaques with and without thrombus in ischemic heart syndromes: a morphologic, immunohistochemical, and biochemical study. Am. J. Cardiol. 68, 36B–50B.

Argmann, CA., Van Den Diepstraten, C.H., Sawyez, C.G., Edwards, J.Y., Hegele, R.A., Wolfe, B.M., Huff, M.W., 2001. Transforming growth factor-beta1 inhibits macrophage cholesteryl ester accumulation induced by native and oxidized VLDL remnants. Arterioscler. Thromb. Vasc. Biol. 21, 2011–2018.

Arsura, M., Wu, M., Sonenshein, G.E., 1996. TGF beta 1 inhibits NF-kappa B/Rel activity inducing apoptosis of B cells: transcriptional activation of I kappa B alpha. Immunity 5, 31–40.

Badolato, R., Ponzi, A.N., Millesimo, M., Notarangelo, L.D., Musso, T., 1997. Interleukin-15 (IL-15) induces IL-8 and monocyte chemotactic protein 1 production in human monocytes. Blood 90, 2804–2809.

Barnes, P.J., 1997. Nuclear factor-kappa B. Int. J. Biochem. Cell Biol. 29, 867–870.

Bath, P.M., Missouris, C.G., Buckenham, T., MacGregor, G.A., 1994. Increased platelet volume and platelet mass in patients with atherosclerotic renal artery stenosis. Clin. Sci. (London) 87, 253–257.

Biasucci, L.M., Liuzzo, G., Fantuzzi, G., Caligiuri, G., Rebuzzi, A.G., Ginnetti, F., Dinarello, C.A., Maseri, A., 1999. Increasing levels of interleukin (IL)-1Ra and IL-6 during the first 2 days of hospitalization in unstable angina are associated with increased risk of in-hospital coronary events. Circulation 99, 2079–2084.

Blanc, E.M., Toborek, M., Mark, R.J., Henning, B., Mattson, M.P., 1997. Amyloid beta-peptide induces cell monolayer albumin permeability, impairs glucose transport, and induces apoptosis in vascular endothelial cells. J. Neurochem. 68, 1870–1881.

Boisvert, W.A., Curtiss, L.K., Terkeltaub, R.A., 2000. Interleukin-8 and its receptor CXCR2 in athero-sclerosis. Immunol. Res. 21, 129–137.

Boring, L., Gosling, J., Cleary, M., Charo, I.F., 1998. Decreased lesion formation in CCR2–/– mice reveals a role for chemokines in the initiation of atherosclerosis. Nature 394, 894–897.

Borish, L., Rosenwasser, L.J., 1996. Update on cytokines. J. Allergy Clin. Immunol. 97, 719–733.

Bouloumie, A., Marumo, T., Lafontan, M., Busse, R., 1999. Leptin induces oxidative stress in human endothelial cells. FASEB J. 13, 1231–1238.

Brand, K., Eisele, T., Kreusel, U., Page, M., Page, S., Haas, M., Gerling, A., Kaltschmidt, C., Neumann, F.J., Mackman, N., Baeurele, P.A., Walli, A.K., Neumeier, D., 1997b. Dysregulation of monocytic nuclear factor-kappa B by oxidized low-density lipoprotein. Arterioscler. Thromb. Vasc. Biol. 17, 1901–1909.

Brand, K., Page, S., Rogler, G., Bartsch, A., Brandl, R., Knuechel, R., Page, M., Kaltschmidt, C., Baeuerle, P.A., Neumeier, D., 1996. Activated transcription factor nuclear factor-kappa B is present in the atherosclerotic lesion. J. Clin. Invest. 97, 1715–1722.

Brand, K., Page, S., Walli, A.K., Neumeier, D., Baeuerle, P.A., 1997a. Role of nuclear factor-kappa B in atherogenesis. Exp. Physiol. 82, 297–304.

Brizzi, M.F., Formato, L., Dentelli, P., Rosso, A., Pavan, M., Garbarino, G., Pegoraro, M., Camussi, G., Pegoraro, L., 2001. Interleukin-3 stimulates migration and proliferation of vascular smooth muscle cells: a potential role in atherogenesis. Circulation 103, 549–554.

Bustos, C., Hernandez-Presa, M.A., Ortego, M., Tunon, J., Ortega, L., Perez, F., Diaz, C., Hernandez, G., Egido, J., 1998b. HMG-CoA reductase inhibition by atorvastatin reduces neointimal inflammation in a rabbit model of atherosclerosis. J. Am. Coll. Cardiol. 32, 2057–2064.

Bustos, C., Hernandez-Presa, M.A., Ortego, M., Tunon, J., Ortega, L., Perez, F., Diaz, C., Hernandez, G., Egido, J., 1998a. HMG-CoA reductase inhibition by atorvastatin reduces neointimal inflammation in a rabbit model of atherosclerosis. J. Am. Coll. Cardiol. 32, 2057–2064.

Cairns, J.A., Walls, A.F., 1996. Mast cell tryptase is a mitogen for epithelial cells. Stimulation of IL-8 pro-duction and intercellular adhesion molecule-1 expression. J. Immunol. 156, 275–283.

Center, D.M., Kornfeld, H., Cruikshank, W.W., 1997. Interleukin-16. Int. J. Biochem. Cell. Biol. 29, 1231–1234.

Chen, C.C., Manning, A.M., 1996. TGF-beta 1, IL-10 and IL-4 differentially modulate the cytokine-induced expression of IL-6 and IL-8 in human endothelial cells. Cytokine 8, 58–65.

Chi, D.S., Henry, J., Kelley, J., Thorpe, R., Smith, J.K., Krishnaswamy, G., 2000. The effects of HIV infection on endothelial function. Endothelium 7, 223–242.

Choi, J., Chung, S.W., Kim, S.J., Kim, S.J., 2001. Establishment of Porphyromonas gingivalis-specific T-cell lines from atherosclerosis patients. Oral Microbiol. Immunol. 16, 316–318.

Cimminiello, C., Arpaia, G., Toschi, V., Rossi, F., Aloisio, M., Motta, A., Bonfardeci, G., 1994. Plasma levels of tumor necrosis factor and endothelial response in patients with chronic arterial obstructive disease or Raynaud's phenomenon. Angiology 45, 1015–1022.

Clausell, N., de Lima, V.C., Molossi, S., Liu, P., Turley, E., Gotlieb, A.I., Adelman, A.G., Rabinovitch, M., 1995. Expression of tumour necrosis factor alpha and accumulation of fibronectin in coronary artery restenotic lesions retrieved by atherectomy. Br. Heart J. 73, 534–539.

Clinton, S.K., Fleet, J.C., Loppnow, H., Salomon, R.N., Clark, B.D., Cannon, J.G., Shaw, A.R., Dinarello, C.A., Libby, P., 1991. Interleukin-1 gene expression in rabbit vascular tissue in vivo. Am. J. Pathol. 138, 1005–1014.

Clinton, S.K., Underwood, R., Hayes, L., Sherman, M.L., Kufe, D.W., Libby, P., 1992. Macrophage col-ony-stimulating factor gene expression in vascular cells and in experimental and human atherosclero-sis. Am. J. Pathol. 140, 301–316.

Cohen, M.D., Ciocca, V., Panettieri Jr., R.A., 1997. TGF-beta 1 modulates human airway smooth-muscle cell proliferation induced by mitogens. Am. J. Respir. Cell. Mol. Biol. 16, 85–90.

Collins, T., 1993. Endothelial nuclear factor-kappa B and the initiation of the atherosclerotic lesion. Lab. Invest. 68, 499–508.

Compton, S.J., Cairns, J.A., Holgate, S.T., Walls, A.F., 1998. The role of mast cell tryptase in regulating endothelial cell proliferation, cytokine release, and adhesion molecule expression: tryptase induces expression of mRNA for IL-1 beta and IL-8 and stimulates the selective release of IL-8 from human umbilical vein endothelial cells. J. Immunol. 161, 1939–1946.

Conley, B.A., Smith, J.D., Guerrero-Esteo, M., Bernabeu, C., Vary, C.P., 2000. Endoglin, a TGF-beta receptor-associated protein, is expressed by smooth muscle cells in human atherosclerotic plaques. Atherosclerosis 153, 323–335.

Cucina, A., Sapienza, P., Corvino, V., Borrelli, V., Mariani, V., Randone, B., Santoro, D.L., Cavallaro, A., 2000. Nicotine-induced smooth muscle cell proliferation is mediated through bFGF and TGF-beta 1. Surgery 127, 316–322.

D'Orazio, T.J., Niederkorn, J.Y., 1998. A novel role for TGF-beta and IL-10 in the induction of immune privilege. J. Immunol. 160, 2089–2098.

Dalekos, G.N., Elisaf, M., Bairaktari, E., Tsolas, O., Siamopoulos, K.C., 1997. Increased serum levels of interleukin-1beta in the systemic circulation of patients with essential hypertension: additional risk factor for atherogenesis in hypertensive patients? J. Lab. Clin. Med. 129, 300–308.

Damas, J.K., Gullestad, L., Aukrust, P., 2001. Cytokines as new treatment targets in chronic heart failure. Curr. Control Trials Cardiovasc. Med. 2, 271–277.

de Boer, O.J., van der Wal, A.C., Verhagen, C.E., Becker, A.E., 1999. Cytokine secretion profiles of cloned T cells from human aortic atherosclerotic plaques. J. Pathol. 188, 174–179.

de Martin, R., Schmid, J.A., Hofer-Warbinek, R., 1999. The NF-kappaB/Rel family of transcription factors in oncogenic transformation and apoptosis. Mutat. Res. 437, 231–243.

de Villiers, W.J., Fraser, I.P., Gordon, S., 1994. Cytokine and growth factor regulation of macrophage scavenger receptor expression and function. Immunol. Lett. 43, 73–79.

de Villiers, W.J., Smith, J.D., Miyata, M., Dansky, H.M., Darley, E., Gordon, S., 1998. Macrophage phenotype in mice deficient in both macrophage-colony-stimulating factor (op) and apolipoprotein E. Arterioscler. Thromb. Vasc. Biol. 18, 631–640.

Denger, S., Jahn, L., Wende, P., Watson, L., Gerber, S.H., Kubler, W., Kreuzer, J., 1999. Expression of monocyte chemoattractant protein-1 cDNA in vascular smooth muscle cells: induction of the synthetic phenotype: a possible clue to SMC differentiation in the process of atherogenesis. Atherosclerosis 144, 15–23.

Densem, C.G., Hutchinson, I.V., Cooper, A., Yonan, N., Brooks, N.H., 2000. Polymorphism of the transforming growth factor-beta 1 gene correlates with the development of coronary vasculopathy following cardiac transplantation. J. Heart Lung Transplant 19, 551–556.

Desai, A., Lankford, H.A., Warren, J.S., 2001. Homocysteine augments cytokine-induced chemokine expression in human vascular smooth muscle cells: implications for atherogenesis. Inflammation 25, 179–186.

Dichtl, W., Nilsson, L., Goncalves, I., Ares, M.P., Banfi, C., Calara, F., Hamsten, A., Eriksson, P., Nilsson, J., 1999. Very low-density lipoprotein activates nuclear factor-kappaB in endothelial cells. Circ. Res. 84, 1085–1094.

Doo, Y.C., Kim, D.M., Oh, D.J., Ryu, K.H., Rhim, C.Y., Lee, Y., 2001. Effect of beta blockers on expression of interleukin-6 and C-reactive protein in patients with unstable angina pectoris. Am. J. Cardiol. 88, 422–424.

Ebnet, K., Brown, K.D., Siebenlist, U.K., Simon, M.M., Shaw, S., 1997. Borrelia burgdorferi activates nuclear factor-kappa B and is a potent inducer of chemokine and adhesion molecule gene expression in endothelial cells and fibroblasts. J. Immunol. 158, 3285–3292.

Ensminger, S.M., Spriewald, B.M., Sorensen, H.V., Witzke, O., Flashman, E.G., Bushell, A., Morris, P.J., Rose, M.L., Rahemtulla, A., Wood, K.J., 2001. Critical role for IL-4 in the development of transplant arteriosclerosis in the absence of CD40–CD154 costimulation. J. Immunol. 167, 532–541.

Ensminger, S.M., Spriewald, B.M., Witzke, O., Morrison, K., van Maurik, A., Morris, P.J., Rose, M.L., Wood, K.J., 2000. Intragraft interleukin-4 mRNA expression after short-term CD154 blockade may trigger delayed development of transplant arteriosclerosis in the absence of CD8+ T cells. Transplantation 70, 955–963.

Eriksson, E.E., Werr, J., Guo, Y., Thoren, P., Lindbom, L., 2000. Direct observations in vivo on the role of endothelial selectins and alpha(4) integrin in cytokine-induced leukocyte–endothelium interactions in the mouse aorta. Circ. Res. 86, 526–533.

Ernofsson, M., Siegbahn, A., 1996. Platelet-derived growth factor-BB and monocyte chemotactic protein-1 induce human peripheral blood monocytes to express tissue factor. Thromb. Res. 83, 307–320.

Essayan, D.M., Krishnaswamy, G., Huang, S.K., 1997. Immunologic investigations of T-cell regulation of human IgE antibody secretion and allergic responses. Methods 13, 69–78.

Essayan, D.M., Krishnaswamy, G., Oriente, A., Lichtenstein, L.M., Huang, S.K., 1999. Differential regulation of antigen-induced IL-4 and IL-13 generation from T lymphocytes by IFN-alpha. J. Allergy Clin. Immunol. 103, 451–457.

Evanko, S.P., Raines, E.W., Ross, R., Gold, L.I., Wight, T.N., 1998. Proteoglycan distribution in lesions of atherosclerosis depends on lesion severity, structural characteristics, and the proximity of platelet-derived growth factor and transforming growth factor-beta. Am. J. Pathol. 152, 533–546.

Feinberg, M.W., Jain, M.K., Werner, F., Sibinga, N.E., Wiesel, P., Wang, H., Topper, J.N., Perrella, M.A., Lee, M.E., 2000. Transforming growth factor-beta 1 inhibits cytokine-mediated induction of human metalloelastase in macrophages. J. Biol. Chem. 275, 25766–25773.

Fernandez-Real, J.M., Vayreda, M., Casamitjana, R., Gonzalez-Huix, F., Ricart, W., 2001. Circulating granulocyte-macrophage colony-stimulating factor and serum fatty acid composition in men and women. Metabolism 50, 1479–1483.

Flanagan, A.M., Lader, C.S., 1998. Update on the biologic effects of macrophage colony-stimulating factor. Curr. Opin. Hematol. 5, 181–185.

Foster, L.C., Arkonac, B.M., Sibinga, N.E., Shi, C., Perrella, M.A., Haber, E., 1998. Regulation of CD44 gene expression by the proinflammatory cytokine interleukin-1beta in vascular smooth muscle cells. J. Biol. Chem. 273, 20341–20346.

Freedman, S.B., Isner, J.M., 2002. Therapeutic angiogenesis for coronary artery disease. Ann. Intern. Med. 136, 54–71.

Frostegard, J., Ulfgren, A.K., Nyberg, P., Hedin, U., Swedenborg, J., Andersson, U., Hansson, G.K., 1999. Cytokine expression in advanced human atherosclerotic plaques: dominance of pro-inflammatory (Th1) and macrophage-stimulating cytokines. Atherosclerosis 145, 33–43.

Fruebis, J., Gonzalez, V., Silvestre, M., Palinski, W., 1997. Effect of probucol treatment on gene expression of VCAM-1, MCP-1, and M-CSF in the aortic wall of LDL receptor-deficient rabbits during early atherogenesis. Arterioscler. Thromb. Vasc. Biol. 17, 1289–1302.

Fukumoto, Y., Shimokawa, H., Ito, A., Kadokami, T., Yonemitsu, Y., Aikawa, M., Owada, M.K., Egashira, K., Sueishi, K., Nagai, R., Yazaki, Y., Takeshita, A., 1997b. Inflammatory cytokines cause coronary arteriosclerosis-like changes and alterations in the smooth-muscle phenotypes in pigs. J. Cardiovasc. Pharmacol. 29, 222–231.

Fukumoto, Y., Shimokawa, H., Kozai, T., Kadokami, T., Kuwata, K., Yonemitsu, Y., Kuga, T., Egashira, K., Sueishi, K., Takeshita, A., 1997a. Vasculoprotective role of inducible nitric oxide synthase at inflammatory coronary lesions induced by chronic treatment with interleukin-1beta in pigs in vivo. Circulation 96, 3104–3111.

Fukuo, K., Inoue, T., Morimoto, S., Nakahashi, T., Yasuda, O., Kitano, S., Sasada, R., Ogihara, T., 1995. Nitric oxide mediates cytotoxicity and basic fibroblast growth factor release in cultured vascular smooth muscle cells. A possible mechanism of neovascularization in atherosclerotic plaques. J. Clin. Invest. 95, 669–676.

Funayama, H., Ikeda, U., Takahashi, M., Sakata, Y., Kitagawa, S., Takahashi, Y., Masuyama, J., Furukawa, Y., Miura, Y., Kano, S., Matsuda, M., Shimada, K., 1998. Human monocyte–endothelial cell interaction induces platelet-derived growth factor expression. Cardiovasc. Res. 37, 216–224.

Gabriel, A.S., Ahnve, S., Wretlind, B., Martinsson, A., 2000. IL-6 and IL-1 receptor antagonist in stable angina pectoris and relation of IL-6 to clinical findings in acute myocardial infarction. J. Intern. Med. 248, 61–66.

Galis, Z.S., Muszynski, M., Sukhova, G.K., Simon-Morrissey, E., Libby, P., 1995. Enhanced expression of vascular matrix metalloproteinases induced in vitro by cytokines and in regions of human atherosclerotic lesions. Ann. NY Acad. Sci. 748, 501–507.

Geng, Y.J., Henderson, L.E., Levesque, E.B., Muszynski, M., Libby, P., 1997. Fas is expressed in human atherosclerotic intima and promotes apoptosis of cytokine-primed human vascular smooth muscle cells. Arterioscler. Thromb. Vasc. Biol. 17, 2200–2208.

George, J., Mulkins, M., Shaish, A., Casey, S., Schatzman, R., Sigal, E., Harats, D., 2000b. Interleukin (IL)-4 deficiency does not influence fatty streak formation in C57BL/6 mice. Atherosclerosis 153, 403–411.

George, J., Shoenfeld, Y., Gilburd, B., Afek, A., Shaish, A., Harats, D., 2000a. Requisite role for interleukin-4 in the acceleration of fatty streaks induced by heat shock protein 65 or Mycobacterium tuberculosis. Circ. Res. 86, 1203–1210.

Grainger, D.J., Kemp, P.R., Metcalfe, J.C., Liu, A.C., Lawn, R.M., Williams, N.R., Grace, A.A., Schofield, P.M., Chauhan, A., 1995. The serum concentration of active transforming growth factor-beta is severely depressed in advanced atherosclerosis. Nat. Med. 1, 74–79.

Grainger, D.J., Mosedale, D.E., Metcalfe, J.C., Bottinger, E.P., 2000. Dietary fat and reduced levels of TGFbeta1 act synergistically to promote activation of the vascular endothelium and formation of lipid lesions. J. Cell. Sci. 113, 2355–2361.

Graves, D.T., Jiang, Y., 1995. Chemokines, a family of chemotactic cytokines. Crit. Rev. Oral Biol. Med. 6, 109–118.

Grewal, I.S., Flavell, R.A., 1997. The CD40 ligand. At the center of the immune universe? Immunol. Res. 16, 59–70.

Grewal, I.S., Flavell, R.A., 1998. CD40 and CD154 in cell-mediated immunity. Annu. Rev. Immunol. 16, 111–135.

Gullestad, L., Aass, H., Fjeld, J.G., Wikeby, L., Andreassen, A.K., Ihlen, H., Simonsen, S., Kjekshus, J., Nitter-Hauge, S., Ueland, T., Lien, E., Froland, S.S., Aukrust, P., 2001b. Immunomodulating therapy with intravenous immunoglobulin in patients with chronic heart failure. Circulation 103, 220–225.

Gullestad, L., Ueland, T., Brunsvig, A., Kjekshus, J., Simonsen, S., Froland, S.S., Aukrust, P., 2001a. Effect of metoprolol on cytokine levels in chronic heart failure–a substudy in the Metoprolol Controlled-Release Randomised Intervention Trial in Heart Failure (MERIT-HF). Am. Heart J. 141, 418–421.

Hallek, M., Neumann, C., Schaffer, M., Danhauser-Riedl, S., von Bubnoff, N., de Vos, G., Druker, B.J., Yasukawa, K., Griffin, J.D., Emmerich, B., 1997. Signal transduction of interleukin-6 involves tyrosine phosphorylation of multiple cytosolic proteins and activation of Src-family kinases Fyn, Hck, and Lyn in multiple myeloma cell lines. Exp. Hematol. 25, 1367–1377.

Henning, B., Toborek, M., Joshi-Barve, S., Barger, S.W., Barve, S., Mattson, M.P., McClain, C.J., 1996. Linoleic acid activates nuclear transcription factor-kappa B (NF-kappa B) and induces NF-kappa B-dependent transcription in cultured endothelial cells. Am. J. Clin. Nutr. 63, 322–328.

Herbst, U., Toborek, M., Kaiser, S., Mattson, M.P., Hennig, B., 1999. 4-Hydroxynonenal induces dysfunction and apoptosis of cultured endothelial cells. J. Cell. Physiol. 181, 295–303.

Hernandez-Presa, M., Bustos, C., Ortego, M., Tunon, J., Renedo, G., Ruiz-Ortega, M., Egido, J., 1997. Angiotensin-converting enzyme inhibition prevents arterial nuclear factor-kappa B activation, monocyte chemoattractant protein-1 expression, and macrophage infiltration in a rabbit model of early accelerated atherosclerosis. Circulation 95, 1532–1541.

Hernandez-Presa, M.A., Bustos, C., Ortego, M., Tunon, J., Ortega, L., Egido, J., 1998. ACE inhibitor quinapril reduces the arterial expression of NF- kappaB-dependent proinflammatory factors but not of collagen I in a rabbit model of atherosclerosis. Am. J. Pathol. 153, 1825–1837.

Higuchi, S., Tanimoto, A., Arima, N., Xu, H., Murata, Y., Hamada, T., Makishima, K., Sasaguri, Y., 2001. Effects of histamine and interleukin-4 synthesized in arterial intima on phagocytosis by monocytes/macrophages in relation to atherosclerosis. FEBS Lett. 505, 217–222.

Hirano, T., 1998. Interleukin 6 and its receptor: ten years later. Int. Rev. Immunol. 16, 249–284.

Hofman, F.M., Chen, P., Incardona, F., Zidovetzki, R., Hinton, D.R., 1999. HIV-1 tat protein induces the production of interleukin-8 by human brain-derived endothelial cells. J. Neuroimmunol. 94, 28–39.

Houtkamp, M.A., Der Wal, A.C., de Boer, O.J., Der Loos, C.M., de Boer, P.A., Moorman, A.F., Becker, A.E., 2001. Interleukin-15 expression in atherosclerotic plaques: an alternative pathway for T-cell activation in atherosclerosis? Arterioscler. Thromb. Vasc. Biol. 21, 1208–1213.

Huber, S.A., Sakkinen, P., Conze, D., Hardin, N., Tracy, R., 1999. Interleukin-6 exacerbates early atherosclerosis in mice. Arterioscler. Thromb. Vasc. Biol. 19, 2364–2367.

Ikeda, U., Maeda, Y., Funayama, H., Hojo, Y., Ikeda, M., Minota, S., Kano, S., Shimada, K., 1998. Monocyte-vascular smooth muscle cell interaction enhances nitric oxide production. Cardiovasc. Res. 37, 820–825.

Ikonomidis, I., Andreotti, F., Economou, E., Stefanadis, C., Toutouzas, P., Nihoyannopoulos, P., 1999. Increased proinflammatory cytokines in patients with chronic stable angina and their reduction by aspirin. Circulation 100, 793–798.

Inaba, T., Gotoda, T., Harada, K., Shimada, M., Ohsuga, J., Ishibashi, S., Yazaki, Y., Yamada, N., 1995. Induction of sustained expression of proto-oncogene c-fms by platelet-derived growth factor, epidermal growth factor, and basic fibroblast growth factor, and its suppression by interferon-gamma and macrophage colony-stimulating factor in human aortic medial smooth muscle cells. J. Clin. Invest. 95, 1133–1139.

Inaba, T., Yamada, N., Gotoda, T., Shimano, H., Shimada, M., Momomura, K., Kadowaki, T., Motoyoshi, K., Tsukada, T., Morisaki, N., 1992. Expression of M-CSF receptor encoded by c-fms on smooth muscle cells derived from arteriosclerotic lesion. J. Biol. Chem. 267, 5693–5699.

Inobe, J., Slavin, A.J., Komagata, Y., Chen, Y., Liu, L., Weiner, H.L., 1998. IL-4 is a differentiation factor for transforming growth factor-beta secreting Th3 cells and oral administration of IL-4 enhances oral tolerance in experimental allergic encephalomyelitis. Eur. J. Immunol. 28, 2780–2790.

Isner, J.M., 1996. Therapeutic angiogenesis: a new frontier for vascular therapy. Vasc. Med. 1, 79–87.

Jeannin, P., Delneste, Y., Gosset, P., Molet, S., Lassalle, P., Hamid, Q., Tsicopoulos, A., Tonnel, A.B., 1994. Histamine induces interleukin-8 secretion by endothelial cells. Blood 84, 2229–2233.

Jiang, M.J., Yu, Y.J., Chen, Y.L., Lee, Y.M., Hung, L.S., 1999. Cyclic strain stimulates monocyte chemotactic protein-1 mRNA expression in smooth muscle cells. J. Cell. Biochem. 76, 303–310.

Kaartinen, M., van der Wal, A.C., van der Loos, C.M., Piek, J.J., Koch, K.T., Becker, A.E., Kovanen, P.T., 1998. Mast cell infiltration in acute coronary syndromes: implications for plaque rupture. J. Am. Coll. Cardiol. 32, 606–612.

Kanakaraj, P., Schafer, P.H., Cavender, D.E., Wu, Y., Ngo, K., Grealish, P.F., Wadsworth, S.A., Peterson, P.A., Siekierka, J.J., Harris, C.A., Fung-Leung, W.P., 1998. Interleukin (IL)-1 receptor-associated kinase (IRAK) requirement for optimal induction of multiple IL-1 signaling pathways and IL-6 production. J. Exp. Med. 187, 2073–2079.

Karpus, W.J., Lukacs, N.W., Kennedy, K.J., Smith, W.S., Hurst, S.D., Barrett, T.A., 1997. Differential CC chemokine-induced enhancement of T helper cell cytokine production. J. Immunol. 158, 4129–4136.

Kato, H., Uchimura, I., Nawa, C., Kawakami, A., Numano, F., 2001. Fluid shear stress suppresses interleukin 8 production by vascular endothelial cells. Biorheology 38, 347–353.

Kato, K., Matsubara, T., Iida, K., Suzuki, O., Sato, Y., 1999. Elevated levels of pro-inflammatory cytokines in coronary artery thrombi. Int. J. Cardiol. 70, 267–273.

Kelley, J., Chi, D.S., Henry, J., Stone, W.L., Smith, J.K., Krishnaswamy, G., 2000a. HIV- and cocaine-induced cardiovascular disease: pathogenesis and clinical implications. Cardiovascular Reviews and Reports XXI, 365–370.

Kelley, J.L., Chi, D.S., Abou-Auda, W., Smith, J.K., Krishnaswamy, G., 2000b. The molecular role of mast cells in atherosclerotic cardiovascular disease. Mol. Med. Today 6, 304–308.

Keso, T., Perola, M., Laippala, P., Ilveskoski, E., Kunnas, T.A., Mikkelsson, J., Penttila, A., Hurme, M., Karhunen, P.J., 2001. Polymorphisms within the tumor necrosis factor locus and prevalence of coronary artery disease in middle-aged men. Atherosclerosis 154, 691–697.

Kim, C.J., Khoo, J.C., Gillotte-Taylor, K., Li, A., Palinski, W., Glass, C.K., Steinberg, D., 2000. Polymerase chain reaction-based method for quantifying recruitment of monocytes to mouse atherosclerotic lesions in vivo: enhancement by tumor necrosis factor-alpha and interleukin-1 beta. Arterioscler. Thromb. Vasc. Biol. 20, 1976–1982.

Klouche, M., Rose-John, S., Schmiedt, W., Bhakdi, S., 2000. Enzymatically degraded, nonoxidized LDL induces human vascular smooth muscle cell activation, foam cell transformation, and proliferation. Circulation 101, 1799–1805.

Koch, A.E., Polverini, P.J., Kunkel, S.L., Harlow, L.A., DiPietro, L.A., Elner, V.M., Elner, S.G., Strieter, R.M., 1992. Interleukin-8 as a macrophage-derived mediator of angiogenesis (see comments). Science 258, 1798–1801.

Koch, W., Kastrati, A., Bottiger, C., Mehilli, J., von Beckerath, N., Schomig, A., 2001. Interleukin-10 and tumor necrosis factor gene polymorphisms and risk of coronary artery disease and myocardial infarction. Atherosclerosis 159, 137–144.

Kolodgie, F.D., Burke, A.P., Farb, A., Gold, H.K., Yuan, J., Narula, J., Finn, A.V., Virmani, R., 2001. The thin-cap fibroatheroma: a type of vulnerable plaque: the major precursor lesion to acute coronary syndromes. Curr. Opin. Cardiol. 16, 285–292.

Kopf, M., Baumann, H., Freer, G., Freudenberg, M., Lamers, M., Kishimoto, T., Zinkernagel, R., Bluethmann, H., Kohler, G., 1994. Impaired immune and acute-phase responses in interleukin-6-deficient mice. Nature 368, 339–342.

Kopp, E., Medzhitov, R., Carothers, J., Xiao, C., Douglas, I., Janeway, C.A., Ghosh, S., 1999. ECSIT is an evolutionarily conserved intermediate in the Toll/IL-1 signal transduction pathway. Genes Dev. 13, 2059–2071.

Kothe, H., Dalhoff, K., Rupp, J., Muller, A., Kreuzer, J., Maass, M., Katus, H.A., 2000. Hydroxy-methylglutaryl coenzyme A reductase inhibitors modify the inflammatory response of human macrophages and endothelial cells infected with Chlamydia pneumoniae. Circulation 101, 1760–1763.

Kowala, M.C., Recce, R., Beyer, S., Gu, C., Valentine, M., 2000. Characterization of atherosclerosis in LDL receptor knockout mice: macrophage accumulation correlates with rapid and sustained expression of aortic MCP-1/JE. Atherosclerosis 149, 323–330.

Koyanagi, M., Egashira, K., Kitamoto, S., Ni, W., Shimokawa, H., Takeya, M., Yoshimura, T., Takeshita, A., 2000. Role of monocyte chemoattractant protein-1 in cardiovascular remodeling induced by chronic blockade of nitric oxide synthesis. Circulation 102, 2243–2248.

Kranzhofer, R., Schmidt, J., Pfeiffer, C.A., Hagl, S., Libby, P., Kubler, W., 1999. Angiotensin induces inflammatory activation of human vascular smooth muscle cells. Arterioscler. Thromb. Vasc. Biol. 19, 1623–1629.

Krishnaswamy, G., 2001. Treatment strategies for bronchial asthma: an update. Hosp. Pract. (Off Ed.) 36, 25–35.

Krishnaswamy, G., Chi, D.S., Kelley, J., 1999b. Vulnerable plaque. Ann. Intern. Med. 131, 392–393.

Krishnaswamy, G., Chi, D.S., Kelley, J.L., Sarubbi, F., Smith, J.K., Peiris, A., 2000. The cardiovascular and metabolic complications of hiv infection. Cardiol. Rev. 8, 260–268.

Krishnaswamy, G., Kelley, J., Yerra, L., Smith, J.K., Chi, D.S., 1999a. Human endothelium as a source of multifunctional cytokines: molecular regulation and possible role in human disease. J. Interferon Cytokine Res. 19, 91–104.

Krishnaswamy, G., Lakshman, T., Miller, A.R., Srikanth, S., Hall, K., Huang, S.K., Suttles, J., Smith, J.K., Stout, R., 1997. Multifunctional cytokine expression by human mast cells: regulation by T cell membrane contact and glucocorticoids. J. Interferon Cytokine Res. 17, 167–176.

Krishnaswamy, G., Smith, J.K., Mukkamala, R., Hall, K., Joyner, W.L.Y., Chi, D.S., 1998. Multifunctional cytokine expression by human coronary endothelium and regulation by monokines and glucocorticoids. Microvasc. Res. 55, 189–200.

Kullo, I.J., Edwards, W.D., Schwartz, R.S., 1998. Vulnerable plaque: pathobiology and clinical implications. Ann. Intern. Med. 129, 1050–1060.

Kumon, Y., Suehiro, T., Hashimoto, K., Sipe, J.D., 2001. Dexamethasone, but not IL-1 alone, upregulates acute-phase serum amyloid A gene expression and production by cultured human aortic smooth muscle cells. Scand. J. Immunol. 53, 7–12.

Kuzuya, M., 1998. Effect of inflammatory cytokines and oxidized low density lipoprotein on vascular endothelial growth factor expression in macrophage. Nippon Ronen Igakkai Zasshi 35, 268–272.

Lafrenie, R.M., Wahl, L.M., Epstein, J.S., Yamada, K.M., Dhawan, S., 1997. Activation of monocytes by HIV-Tat treatment is mediated by cytokine expression. J. Immunol. 159, 4077–4083.

LaRosa, J.C., 1998. Atherogenesis and its relationship to coronary risk factors. Clinical Cornerstone 1, 3–11.

Lee, Y.W., Kuhn, H., Hennig, B., Neish, A.S., Toborek, M., 2001. IL-4-induced oxidative stress upregulates VCAM-1 gene expression in human endothelial cells. J. Mol. Cell. Cardiol. 33, 83–94.

Lewis, B.S., Flugelman, M.Y., Weisz, A., Keren-Tal, I., Schaper, W., 1997. Angiogenesis by gene therapy: a new horizon for myocardial revascularization? Cardiovasc. Res. 35, 490–497.

Libby, P., 2000. Coronary artery injury and the biology of atherosclerosis: inflammation, thrombosis, and stabilization. Am. J. Cardiol. 86, 3–8.

Libby, P., 2001. What have we learned about the biology of atherosclerosis? The role of inflammation. Am. J. Cardiol. 88, 3J–6J.

Libby, P., Schwartz, D., Brogi, E., Tanaka, H., Clinton, S.K., 1992. A cascade model for restenosis. A special case of atherosclerosis progression. Circulation 86, III47–III52.

Lindemann, A., Rumberger, B., 1993. Vascular complications in patients treated with granulocyte colony-stimulating factor (G-CSF). Eur. J. Cancer 29A, 2338–2339.

Lindner, V., 2001. Vascular repair processes mediated by transforming growth factor-beta. Z. Kardiol. 90 (Suppl. 3), 17–22.

Liu, Y., Hulten, L.M., Wiklund, O., 1997. Macrophages isolated from human atherosclerotic plaques produce IL-8, and oxysterols may have a regulatory function for IL-8 production. Arterioscler. Thromb. Vasc. Biol. 17, 317–323.

Ludwicka-Bradley, A., Tourkina, E., Suzuki, S., Tyson, E., Bonner, M., Fenton, J.W., Hoffman, S., Silver, R.M., 2000. Thrombin upregulates interleukin-8 in lung fibroblasts via cleavage of proteolytically activated receptor-I and protein kinase C-gamma activation. Am. J. Respir. Cell. Mol. Biol. 22, 235–243.

Lukacs, N.W., Strieter, R.M., Elner, V., Evanoff, H.L., Burdick, M.D., Kunkel, S.L., 1995. Production of chemokines, interleukin-8 and monocyte chemoattractant protein-1, during monocyte: endothelial cell interactions. Blood 86, 2767–2773.

Luster, A.D., 1998. Chemokines–chemotactic cytokines that mediate inflammation. N. Engl. J. Med. 338, 436–445.

Mach, F., Schonbeck, U., Sukhova, G.K., Atkinson, E., Libby, P., 1998. Reduction of atherosclerosis in mice by inhibition of CD40 signalling. Nature 394, 200–203.

Mach, F., Schonbeck, U., Sukhova, G.K., Bourcier, T., Bonnefoy, J.Y., Pober, J.S., Libby, P., 1997. Functional CD40 ligand is expressed on human vascular endothelial cells, smooth muscle cells, and macrophages: implications for CD40–CD40 ligand signaling in atherosclerosis. Proc. Natl. Acad. Sci. USA 94, 1931–1936.

Madej, A., Okopien, B., Kowalski, J., Zielinski, M., Wysocki, J., Szygula, B., Kalina, Z., Herman, Z.S., 1998. Effects of fenofibrate on plasma cytokine concentrations in patients with atherosclerosis and hyperlipoproteinemia IIb. Int. J. Clin. Pharmacol. Ther. 36, 345–349.

Maeda, H., Kuwahara, H., Ichimura, Y., Ohtsuki, M., Kurakata, S., Shiraishi, A., 1995. TGF-beta enhances macrophage ability to produce IL-10 in normal and tumor-bearing mice. J. Immunol. 155, 4926–4932.

Maeno, Y., Kashiwagi, A., Nishio, Y., Takahara, N., Kikkawa, R., 2000. IDL can stimulate atherogenic gene expression in cultured human vascular endothelial cells. Diabetes Res. Clin. Pract. 48, 127–138.

Mallat, Z., Besnard, S., Duriez, M., Deleuze, V., Emmanuel, F., Bureau, M.F., Soubrier, F., Esposito, B., Duez, H., Fievet, C., Staels, B., Duverger, N., Scherman, D., Tedgui, A., 1999b. Protective role of interleukin-10 in atherosclerosis. Circ. Res. 85, e17–e24.

Mallat, Z., Corbaz, A., Scoazec, A., Besnard, S., Leseche, G., Chvatchko, Y., Tedgui, A., 2001a. Expression of interleukin-18 in human atherosclerotic plaques and relation to plaque instability. Circulation 104, 1598–1603.

Mallat, Z., Corbaz, A., Scoazec, A., Graber, P., Alouani, S., Esposito, B., Humbert, Y., Chvatchko, Y., Tedgui, A., 2001b. Interleukin-18/interleukin-18 binding protein signaling modulates atherosclerotic lesion development and stability. Circ. Res. 89, E41–E45.

Mallat, Z., Gojova, A., Marchiol-Fournigault, C., Esposito, B., Kamate, C., Merval, R., Fradelizi, D., Tedgui, A., 2001c. Inhibition of transforming growth factor-beta signaling accelerates atherosclerosis and induces an unstable plaque phenotype in mice. Circ. Res. 89, 930–934.

Mallat, Z., Heymes, C., Ohan, J., Faggin, E., Leseche, G., Tedgui, A., 1999a. Expression of interleukin-10 in advanced human atherosclerotic plaques: relation to inducible nitric oxide synthase expression and cell death. Arterioscler. Thromb. Vasc. Biol. 19, 611–616.

Martin-Paredero, V., Vadillo, J., Diaz, J., Espinosa, A., Berga, C., Segura, J., Sanchez, J., Barbod, A., Villaverde, C., Richard, C.M., 1998. Fibrinogen and fibrinolysis in blood and in the arterial wall: its role in advanced atherosclerotic disease. Cardiovasc. Surg. 6, 457–462.

Maruo, N., Morita, I., Shirao, M., Murota, S., 1992. IL-6 increases endothelial permeability in vitro. Endocrinology 131, 710–714.

Maruyama, I., Shigeta, K., Miyahara, H., Nakajima, T., Shin, H., Ide, S., Kitajima, I., 1997. Thrombin activates NF-kappa B through thrombin receptor and results in proliferation of vascular smooth muscle cells: role of thrombin in atherosclerosis and restenosis. Ann. NY Acad. Sci. 811, 429–436.

Mattson, M.P., Culmsee, C., Yu, Z., Camandola, S., 2000. Roles of nuclear factor kappaB in neuronal survival and plasticity. J. Neurochem. 74, 443–456.

McCaffrey, T.A., 2000. TGF-betas and TGF-beta receptors in atherosclerosis. Cytokine Growth Factor Rev. 11, 103–114.

Miossec, P., 1993. (Anti-inflammatory properties of interleukin-4) Proprietes anti-inflammatoires de l'interleukine 4. Rev. Rhum. Ed. Fr. 60, 119–124.

Misiakos, E.P., Kouraklis, G., Agapitos, E., Perrea, D., Karatzas, G., Boudoulas, H., Karayannakos, P.E., 2001. Expression of PDGF-A, TGFb and VCAM-1 during the developmental stages of experimental atherosclerosis. Eur. Surg. Res. 33, 264–269.

Mizutani, M., Okuda, Y., Suzuki, S., Sawada, T., Soma, M., Yamashita, K., 1995. High glucose increases platelet-derived growth factor production in cultured human vascular endothelial cells and preventive effects of eicosapentaenoic acids. Life Sci. 57, L31–L35.

Mohamed-Ali, V., Bulmer, K., Clarke, D., Goodrick, S., Coppack, S.W., Pinkney, J.H., 2000. beta-Adrenergic regulation of proinflammatory cytokines in humans. Int. J. Obes. Relat. Metab. Disord. 24 (Suppl. 2), S154–S155.

Molestina, R.E., Miller, R.D., Lentsch, A.B., Ramirez, J.A., Summersgill, J.T., 2000. Requirement for NF-kappaB in transcriptional activation of monocyte chemotactic protein 1 by Chlamydia pneumoniae in human endothelial cells. Infect. Immun. 68, 4282–4288.

Moller, A., Lippert, U., Lessmann, D., Kolde, G., Hamann, K., Welker, P., Schadendorf, D., Rosenbach, T., Luger, T., Czarnetzki, B.M., 1993. Human mast cells produce IL-8. J. Immunol. 151, 3261–3266.

Morawietz, H., Rueckschloss, U., Niemann, B., Duerrschmidt, N., Galle, J., Hakim, K., Zerkowski, H.R., Sawamura, T., Holtz, J., 1999. Angiotensin II induces LOX-1, the human endothelial receptor for oxidized low-density lipoprotein. Circulation 100, 899–902.

Mori, Y., Kitamura, H., Song, Q.H., Kobayashi, T., Umemura, S., Cyong, J.C., 2000. A new murine model for atherosclerosis with inflammation in the periodontal tissue induced by immunization with heat shock protein 60. Hypertens. Res. 23, 475–481.

Mottram, P.L., Raisanen-Sokolowski, A., Glysing-Jensen, T., Stein-Oakley, A.N., Russell, M.E., 1998. Cardiac allografts from IL-4 knockout recipients: assessment of transplant arteriosclerosis and peripheral tolerance. J. Immunol. 161, 602–609.

Moyer, C.F., Sajuthi, D., Tulli, H., Williams, J.K., 1991. Synthesis of IL-1 alpha and IL-1 beta by arterial cells in atherosclerosis. Am. J. Pathol. 138, 951–960.

Navab, M., Fogelman, A.M., Berliner, J.A., Territo, M.C., Demer, L.L., Frank, J.S., Watson, A.D., Edwards, P.A., Lusis, A.J., 1995. Pathogenesis of atherosclerosis. Am. J. Cardiol. 76, 18C–23C.

Norrby, K., 1996. Interleukin-8 and de novo mammalian angiogenesis. Cell Prolif. 29, 315–323.

Obara, H., Takayanagi, A., Hirahashi, J., Tanaka, K., Wakabayashi, G., Matsumoto, K., Shimazu, M., Shimizu, N., Kitajima, M., 2000. Overexpression of truncated IkappaBalpha induces TNF-alpha-dependent apoptosis in human vascular smooth muscle cells. Arterioscler. Thromb. Vasc. Biol. 20, 2198–2204.

Ohtsuka, T., Hamada, M., Hiasa, G., Sasaki, O., Suzuki, M., Hara, Y., Shigematsu, Y., Hiwada, K., 2001. Effect of beta-blockers on circulating levels of inflammatory and anti-inflammatory cytokines in patients with dilated cardiomyopathy. J. Am. Coll. Cardiol. 37, 412–417.

Okuda, Y., Adrogue, H.J., Nakajima, T., Mizutani, M., Asano, M., Tachi, Y., Suzuki, S., Yamashita, K., 1996. Increased production of PDGF by angiotensin and high glucose in human vascular endothelium. Life Sci. 59, 1455–1461.

Olashaw, N.E., Kowalik, T.F., Huang, E.S., Pledger, W.J., 1992. Induction of NF-kappa B-like activity by platelet-derived growth factor in mouse fibroblasts. Mol. Biol. Cell 3, 1131–1139.

Pasceri, V., Willerson, J.T., Yeh, E.T., 2000. Direct proinflammatory effect of C-reactive protein on human endothelial cells. Circulation 102, 2165–2168.

Pattison, J.M., Nelson, P.J., Huie, P., Sibley, R.K., Krensky, A.M., 1996. RANTES chemokine expression in transplant-associated accelerated atherosclerosis. J. Heart Lung Transplant 15, 1194–1199.

Paul, W.E., Seder, R.A., 1994. Lymphocyte responses and cytokines. Cell 76, 241–251.

Petering, H., Gotze, O., Kimmig, D., Smolarski, R., Kapp, A., Elsner, J., 1999. The biologic role of interleukin-8: functional analysis and expression of CXCR1 and CXCR2 on human eosinophils. Blood 93, 694–702.

Peters, W., Charo, I.F., 2001. Involvement of chemokine receptor 2 and its ligand, monocyte chemoattractant protein-1, in the development of atherosclerosis: lessons from knockout mice. Curr. Opin. Lipidol. 12, 175–180.

Pierce, J.W., Read, M.A., Ding, H., Luscinskas, F.W., Collins, T., 1996. Salicylates inhibit I kappa B-alpha phosphorylation, endothelial- leukocyte adhesion molecule expression, and neutrophil transmigration. J. Immunol. 156, 3961–3969.

Pinderski Oslund, L.J., Hedrick, C.C., Olvera, T., Hagenbaugh, A., Territo, M., Berliner, J.A., Fyfe, A.I., 1999. Interleukin-10 blocks atherosclerotic events in vitro and in vivo. Arterioscler. Thromb. Vasc. Biol. 19, 2847–2853.

Plenz, G., Koenig, C., Reichenberg, S., Robenek, H., 1999b. Colony stimulating factors modulate the transcription of type VIII collagen in vascular smooth muscle cells. Atherosclerosis 144, 25–32.

Plenz, G., Koenig, C., Severs, N.J., Robenek, H., 1997. Smooth muscle cells express granulocyte-macrophage colony-stimulating factor in the undiseased and atherosclerotic human coronary artery. Arterioscler. Thromb. Vasc. Biol. 17, 2489–2499.

Plenz, G., Reichenberg, S., Koenig, C., Rauterberg, J., Deng, M.C., Baba, H.A., Robenek, H., 1999a. Granulocyte-macrophage colony-stimulating factor (GM-CSF) modulates the expression of type VIII collagen mRNA in vascular smooth muscle cells and both are codistributed during atherogenesis. Arterioscler. Thromb. Vasc. Biol. 19, 1658–1668.

Plutzky, J., 2001. Inflammatory pathways in atherosclerosis and acute coronary syndromes. Am. J. Cardiol. 88, 10K–15K.

Poland, S.D., Rice, G.P., Dekaban, G.A., 1995. HIV-1 infection of human brain-derived microvascular endothelial cells in vitro. J. Acquir. Immune Defic. Syndr. Hum. Retrovirol. 8, 437–445.

Rajavashisth, T., Qiao, J.H., Tripathi, S., Tripathi, J., Mishra, N., Hua, M., Wang, X.P., Loussararian, A., Clinton, S., Libby, P., Lusis, A., 1998. Heterozygous osteopetrotic (op) mutation reduces atherosclerosis in LDL receptor-deficient mice. J. Clin. Invest. 101, 2702–2710.

Rajavashisth, T.B., Xu, X.P., Jovinge, S., Meisel, S., Xu, X.O., Chai, N.N., Fishbein, M.C., Kaul, S., Cercek, B., Sharifi, B., Shah, P.K., 1999. Membrane type 1 matrix metalloproteinase expression in human atherosclerotic plaques: evidence for activation by proinflammatory mediators. Circulation 99, 3103–3109.

Reckless, J., Rubin, E.M., Verstuyft, J.B., Metcalfe, J.C., Grainger, D.J., 1999. Monocyte chemoattractant protein-1 but not tumor necrosis factor-alpha is correlated with monocyte infiltration in mouse lipid lesions. Circulation 99, 2310–2316.

Resnick, N., Gimbrone Jr., M.A., 1995. Hemodynamic forces are complex regulators of endothelial gene expression. FASEB J. 9, 874–882.

Resnick, N., Yahav, H., Khachigian, L.M., Collins, T., Anderson, K.R., Dewey, F.C., Gimbrone Jr., M.A., 1997. Endothelial gene regulation by laminar shear stress. Adv. Exp. Med. Biol. 430, 155–164.

Ricci, M., Matucci, A., Rossi, O., 1997. Source of IL-4 able to induce the development of TH2-like cells. Clin. Exp. Allergy 27, 488–500.

Ridker, P.M., Rifai, N., Stampfer, M.J., Hennekens, C.H., 2000. Plasma concentration of interleukin-6 and the risk of future myocardial infarction among apparently healthy men. Circulation 101, 1767–1772.

Rodel, J., Woytas, M., Groh, A., Schmidt, K.H., Hartmann, M., Lehmann, M., Straube, E., 2000. Production of basic fibroblast growth factor and interleukin 6 by human smooth muscle cells following infection with Chlamydia pneumoniae. Infect. Immun. 68, 3635–3641.

Romano, M., Diomede, L., Sironi, M., Massimiliano, L., Sottocorno, M., Polentarutti, N., Guglielmotti, A., Albani, D., Bruno, A., Fruscella, P., Salmona, M., Vecchi, A., Pinza, M., Mantovani, A., 2000. Inhibition of monocyte chemotactic protein-1 synthesis by statins. Lab. Invest. 80, 1095–1100.

Rosenfeld, M.E., Yla-Herttuala, S., Lipton, B.A., Ord, V.A., Witztum, J.L., Steinberg, D., 1992. Macrophage colony-stimulating factor mRNA and protein in atherosclerotic lesions of rabbits and humans. Am. J. Pathol. 140, 291–300.

Ross, R., 1993b. Rous-Whipple Award Lecture. Atherosclerosis: a defense mechanism gone awry. Am. J. Pathol. 143, 987–1002.

Ross, R., 1993a. The pathogenesis of atherosclerosis: a perspective for the 1990s. Nature 362, 801–809.

Ross, R., 1997. Cellular and molecular studies of atherogenesis. Atherosclerosis 131 (Suppl.), S3–4.

Ross, R., 1999. Atherosclerosis–an inflammatory disease. N. Engl. J. Med. 340, 115–126.

Rott, D., Zhu, J., Burnett, M.S., Zhou, Y.F., Wasserman, A., Walker, J., Epstein, S.E., 2001. Serum of cytomegalovirus-infected mice induces monocyte chemoattractant protein-1 expression by endothelial cells. J. Infect. Dis. 184, 1109–1113.

Ruan, Y., Takahashi, K., Naito, M., 1995. Immunohistochemical detection of macrophage-derived foam cells and macrophage colony-stimulating factor in pulmonary atherogenesis of cholesterol-fed rabbits. Pathol. Int. 45, 185–195.

Rumsaeng, V., Cruikshank, W.W., Foster, B., Prussin, C., Kirshenbaum, A.S., Davis, T.A., Kornfeld, H., Center, D.M., Metcalfe, D.D., 1997. Human mast cells produce the CD4+ T lymphocyte chemoattractant factor, IL-16. J. Immunol. 159, 2904–2910.

Rus, H.G., Vlaicu, R., Niculescu, F., 1996a. Interleukin-6 and interleukin-8 protein and gene expression in human arterial atherosclerotic wall. Atherosclerosis 127, 263–271.

Rus, H.G., Vlaicu, R., Niculescu, F., 1996b. Interleukin-6 and interleukin-8 protein and gene expression in human arterial atherosclerotic wall. Atherosclerosis 127, 263–271.

Sakai, M., Kobori, S., Miyazaki, A., Horiuchi, S., 2000. Macrophage proliferation in atherosclerosis. Curr. Opin. Lipidol. 11, 503–509.

Schecter, A.D., Calderon, T.M., Berman, A.B., McManus, C.M., Fallon, J.T., Rossikhina, M., Zhao, W., Christ, G., Berman, J.W., Taubman, M.B., 2000. Human vascular smooth muscle cells possess functional CCR5. J. Biol. Chem. 275, 5466–5471.

Schecter, A.D., Rollins, B.J., Zhang, Y.J., Charo, I.F., Fallon, J.T., Rossikhina, M., Giesen, P.L., Nemerson, Y., Taubman, M.B., 1997. Tissue factor is induced by monocyte chemoattractant protein-1 in human aortic smooth muscle and THP-1 cells. J. Biol. Chem. 272, 28568–28573.

Scheinman, R.I., Cogswell, P.C., Lofquist, A.K., Baldwin Jr., A.S., 1995. Role of transcriptional activation of I kappa B alpha in mediation of immunosuppression by glucocorticoids (see comments). Science 270, 283–286.

Schieffer, B., Schieffer, E., Hilfiker-Kleiner, D., Hilfiker, A., Kovanen, P.T., Kaartinen, M., Nussberger, J., Harringer, W., Drexler, H., 2000. Expression of angiotensin II and interleukin 6 in human coronary atherosclerotic plaques: potential implications for inflammation and plaque instability. Circulation 101, 1372–1378.

Schmitz, G., Herr, A.S., Rothe, G., 1998. T-lymphocytes and monocytes in atherogenesis. Herz 23, 168–177.

Sciaky, D., Brazer, W., Center, D.M., Cruikshank, W.W., Smith, T.J., 2000. Cultured human fibroblasts express constitutive IL-16 mRNA: cytokine induction of active IL-16 protein synthesis through a caspase-3-dependent mechanism. J. Immunol. 164, 3806–3814.

Seino, Y., Ikeda, U., Ikeda, M., Yamamoto, K., Misawa, Y., Hasegawa, T., Kano, S., Shimada, K., 1994. Interleukin 6 gene transcripts are expressed in human atherosclerotic lesions. Cytokine 6, 87–91.

Seli, E., Selam, B., Mor, G., Kayisli, U.A., Pehlivan, T., Arici, A., 2001. Estradiol regulates monocyte chemotactic protein-1 in human coronary artery smooth muscle cells: a mechanism for its antiatherogenic effect. Menopause 8, 296–301.

Sellke, F.W., Laham, R.J., Edelman, E.R., Pearlman, J.D., Simons, M., 1998. Therapeutic angiogenesis with basic fibroblast growth factor: technique and early results. Ann. Thorac. Surg. 65, 1540–1544.

Shimizu, S., Gabazza, E.C., Hayashi, T., Ido, M., Adachi, Y., Suzuki, K., 2000. Thrombin stimulates the expression of PDGF in lung epithelial cells. Am. J. Physiol. Lung Cell Mol. Physiol. 279, L503–L510.

Shin, W.S., Szuba, A., Rockson, S.G., 2002. The role of chemokines in human cardiovascular pathology: enhanced biological insights. Atherosclerosis 160, 91–102.

Shu, H.B., Agranoff, A.B., Nabel, E.G., Leung, K., Duckett, C.S., Neish, A.S., Collins, T., Nabel, G.J., 1993. Differential regulation of vascular cell adhesion molecule 1 gene expression by specific NF-kappa B subunits in endothelial and epithelial cells. Mol. Cell. Biol. 13, 6283–6289.

Simonini, A., Moscucci, M., Muller, D.W., Bates, E.R., Pagani, F.D., Burdick, M.D., Strieter, R.M., 2000. IL-8 is an angiogenic factor in human coronary atherectomy tissue. Circulation 101, 1519–1526.

Smith, J.K., Dykes, R., Douglas, J.E., Krishnaswamy, G., Berk, S., 1999. Long-term exercise and atherogenic activity of blood mononuclear cells in persons at risk of developing ischemic heart disease. JAMA 281, 1722–1727.

Stanford, S.J., Pepper, J.R., Mitchell, J.A., 2000. Cyclooxygenase-2 regulates granulocyte-macrophage colony-stimulating factor, but not interleukin-8, production by human vascular cells: role of cAMP. Arterioscler. Thromb. Vasc. Biol. 20, 677–682.

Stary, H.C., 1990. The sequence of cell and matrix changes in atherosclerotic lesions of coronary arteries in the first forty years of life. Eur. Heart J. 11 (Suppl. E), 3–19.

Sugawara I., 2000. Interleukin-18 (IL-18) and infectious diseases, with special emphasis on diseases induced by intracellular pathogens (In Process Citation). Microbes Infect. 2, 1257–1263.

Sumpio, B.E., Du, W., Galagher, G., Wang, X., Khachigian, L.M., Collins, T., Gimbrone Jr., M.A, Resnick, N., 1998. Regulation of PDGF-B in endothelial cells exposed to cyclic strain. Arterioscler. Thromb. Vasc. Biol. 18, 349–355.

Swanson, M.A., Lee, W.T., Sanders, V.M., 2001. IFN-gamma production by Th1 cells generated from naive CD4+ T cells exposed to norepinephrine. J. Immunol. 166, 232–240.

Takeshita, A., Chen, Y., Watanabe, A., Kitano, S., Hanazawa, S., 1995. TGF-beta induces expression of monocyte chemoattractant JE/monocyte chemoattractant protein 1 via transcriptional factor AP-1 induced by protein kinase in osteoblastic cells. J. Immunol. 155, 419–426.

Taki, H., Sakai, T., Sugiyama, E., Mino, T., Kuroda, A., Taki, K., Hamazaki, T., Koizumi, H., Kobayashi, M., 1999. Monokine stimulation of interleukin-11 production by human vascular smooth muscle cells in vitro. Atherosclerosis 144, 375–380.

Tedgui, A., Mallat, Z., 2001. Interleukin-10: an anti-atherogenic cytokine? Eur. J. Clin. Invest. 31, 1–2.

Temaru, R., Urakaze, M., Satou, A., Yamazaki, K., Nakamura, N., Kobayashi, M., 1997. High glucose enhances the gene expression of interleukin-8 in human endothelial cells, but not in smooth muscle cells: possible role of interleukin-8 in diabetic macroangiopathy. Diabetologia 40, 610–613.

Tenaglia, A.N., Buda, A.J., Wilkins, R.G., Barron, M.K., Jeffords, P.R., Vo, K., Jordan, M.O., Kusnick, B.A., Lefer, D.J., 1997. Levels of expression of P-selectin, E-selectin, and intercellular adhesion molecule-1 in coronary atherectomy specimens from patients with stable and unstable angina pectoris. Am. J. Cardiol. 79, 742–747.

Thorlacius, H., Lindbom, L., Raud, J., 1997. Cytokine-induced leukocyte rolling in mouse cremaster muscle arterioles in P-selectin dependent. Am. J. Physiol. 272, H1725–H1729.

Thorne, S.A., Abbot, S.E., Stevens, C.R., Winyard, P.G., Mills, P.G., Blake, D.R., 1996. Modified low density lipoprotein and cytokines mediate monocyte adhesion to smooth muscle cells. Atherosclerosis 127, 167–176.

Tipping, P.G., Hancock, W.W., 1993. Production of tumor necrosis factor and interleukin-1 by macrophages from human atheromatous plaques. Am. J. Pathol. 142, 1721–1728.

Toborek, M., Barger, S.W., Mattson, M.P., Barve, S., McClain, C.J., Hennig, B., 1996. Linoleic acid and TNF-alpha cross-amplify oxidative injury and dysfunction of endothelial cells. J. Lipid Res. 37, 123–135.

Toborek, M., Blanc, E.M., Kaiser, S., Mattson, M.P., Hennig, B., 1997. Linoleic acid potentiates TNF-mediated oxidative stress, disruption of calcium homeostasis, and apoptosis of cultured vascular endothelial cells. J. Lipid Res. 38, 2155–2167.

Tojo, N., Asakura, E., Koyama, M., Tanabe, T., Nakamura, N., 1999. Effects of macrophage colony-stimulating factor (M-CSF) on protease production from monocyte, macrophage and foam cell in vitro: a possible mechanism for anti-atherosclerotic effect of M-CSF. Biochim. Biophys. Acta 1452, 275–284.

Uyemura, K., Demer, L.L., Castle, S.C., Jullien, D., Berliner, J.A., Gately, M.K., Warrier, R.R., Pham, N., Fogelman, A.M., Modlin, R.L., 1996. Cross-regulatory roles of interleukin (IL)-12 and IL-10 in atherosclerosis. J. Clin. Invest. 97, 2130–2138.

Vasse, M., Paysant, I., Soria, J., Mirshahi, S.S., Vannier, J.P., Soria, C., 1996. Down-regulation of fibrinogen biosynthesis by IL-4, IL-10 and IL-13. Br. J. Haematol. 93, 955–961.

von Hundelshausen, P., Weber, K.S., Huo, Y., Proudfoot, A.E., Nelson, P.J., Ley, K., Weber, C., 2001. RANTES deposition by platelets triggers monocyte arrest on inflamed and atherosclerotic endothelium. Circulation 103, 1772–1777.

Wang, C.Y., Mayo, M.W., Korneluk, R.G., Goeddel, D.V., Baldwin Jr., A.S, 1998. NF-kappaB antiapoptosis: induction of TRAF1 and TRAF2 and c-IAP1 and c-IAP2 to suppress caspase-8 activation (In Process Citation). Science 281, 1680–1683 (MEDLINE record in).

Wang, N., Tabas, I., Winchester, R., Ravalli, S., Rabbani, L.E., Tall, A., 1996a. Interleukin 8 is induced by cholesterol loading of macrophages and expressed by macrophage foam cells in human atheroma. J. Biol. Chem. 271, 8837–8842.

Wang, N., Tabas, I., Winchester, R., Ravalli, S., Rabbani, L.E., Tall, A., 1996b. Interleukin 8 is induced by cholesterol loading of macrophages and expressed by macrophage foam cells in human atheroma. J. Biol. Chem. 271, 8837–8842.

Wang, X., Feuerstein, G.Z., Clark, R.K., Yue, T.L., 1994. Enhanced leukocyte adhesion to interleukin-1 beta stimulated vascular smooth muscle cells is mainly through intercellular adhesion molecule-1. Cardiovasc. Res. 28, 1808–1814.

Ward, M.R., Pasterkamp, G., Yeung, A.C., Borst, C., 2000. Arterial remodeling. Mechanisms and clinical implications. Circulation 102, 1186–1191.

Wasowska, B., Hancock, W.W., Onodera, K., Korom, S., Stadlbauer, T.H., Zheng, X.X., Strom, T.B., Kupiec-Weglinski, J.W., 1997. Rapamycin and cyclosporine A treatment: a novel regimen to prevent chronic allograft rejection in sensitized hosts. Transplant Proc. 29, 333.

Watanabe, Y., Inaba, T., Shimano, H., Gotoda, T., Yamamoto, K., Mokuno, H., Sato, H., Yazaki, Y., Yamada, N., 1994. Induction of LDL receptor-related protein during the differentiation of monocyte-macrophages. Possible involvement in the atherosclerotic process. Arterioscler. Thromb. 14, 1000–1006.

Weeks, B.S., 1998. The role of HIV-1 activated leukocyte adhesion mechanisms and matrix metalloproteinase secretion in AIDS pathogenesis. Int. J. Mol. Med. 1, 361–366.

Wilcox, J.N., Nelken, N.A., Coughlin, S.R., Gordon, D., Schall, T.J., 1994. Local expression of inflammatory cytokines in human atherosclerotic plaques. J. Atheroscler. Thromb. 1 (Suppl. 1), S10 S13.

Woenckhaus, C., Kaufmann, A., Bussfeld, D., Gemsa, D., Sprenger, H., Grone, H.J., 1998. Hypochlorite-modified LDL: chemotactic potential and chemokine induction in human monocytes. Clin. Immunol. Immunopathol. 86, 27–33.

Wong, M.L., Xie, B., Beatini, N., Phu, P., Marathe, S., Johns, A., Gold, P.W., Hirsch, E., Williams, K.J., Licinio, J., Tabas, I., 2000. Acute systemic inflammation up-regulates secretory sphingomyelinase in vivo: a possible link between inflammatory cytokines and atherogenesis. Proc. Natl. Acad. Sci. USA 97, 8681–8686.

Wuttge, D.M., Eriksson, P., Sirsjo, A., Hansson, G.K., Stemme, S., 2001. Expression of interleukin-15 in mouse and human atherosclerotic lesions. Am. J. Pathol. 159, 417–423.

Yamashita, N., Koizumi, H., Murata, M., Mano, K., Ohta, K., 1999. Nuclear factor kappa B mediates interleukin-8 production in eosinophils. Int. Arch. Allergy Immunol. 120, 230–236.

Yazdani, S., Simon, A.D., Vidhun, R., Gulotta, C., Schwartz, A., Rabbani, L.E., 1998. Inflammatory profile in unstable angina versus stable angina in patients undergoing percutaneous interventions. Am. Heart J. 136, 357–361.

Yudkin, J.S., Kumari, M., Humphries, S.E., Mohamed-Ali, V., 2000. Inflammation, obesity, stress and coronary heart disease: is interleukin-6 the link? Atherosclerosis 148, 209–214.

G. Krishnaswamy et al.

Yue, T.L., Mckenna, P.J., Gu, J.L., Feuerstein, G.Z., 1993. Interleukin-8 is chemotactic for vascular smooth muscle cells. Eur. J. Pharmacol. 240, 81–84.

Zidovetzki, R., Wang, J.L., Chen, P., Jeyaseelan, R., Hofman, F., 1998. Human immunodeficiency virus Tat protein induces interleukin 6 mRNA expression in human brain endothelial cells via protein kinase C- and cAMP-dependent protein kinase pathways. AIDS Res. Hum. Retroviruses 14, 825–833.

**Advances in
Cell Aging and
Gerontology**

Endothelium-mediated signaling and vascular aging

Bernd van der Loo and Thomas F. Lüscher*

*Division of Cardiology, Cardiovascular Center, University Hospital, Raemistrasse 100,
CH-8091 Zurich, Switzerland*

Contents

Abbreviations

NO	nitric oxide
ROS	reactive oxygen species
$O_2^{\bullet-}$	superoxide
$ONOO^-$	peroxynitrite
EC	endothelial cell
eNOS (=NOS III)	endothelial nitric oxide synthase
PG	prostaglandin

*Corresponding author. Tel.: +41-1-255-2121; fax: +41-1-255-4251.
E-mail address: cardiotfl@gmx.ch (T.F. Lüscher).

Advances in Cell Aging and Gerontology, vol. 11, 127–144

VSMC	vascular smooth muscle cell
cGMP	cyclic guanylmonophosphate
nNOS (=NOS I)	neuronal nitric oxide synthase
iNOS (=NOS II)	inducible nitric oxide synthase
H_4B	tetrahydrobiopterin
SHR	spontaneously hypertensive rats
ET	endothelin
SOD	superoxide dismutase
ECE	endothelin-converting enzyme
DPI	diphenyleniodonium
MnSOD	manganese superoxide dismutase
GSH	glutathione
Cu/ZnSOD	copper/zinc superoxide dismutase
EC-SOD	extracellular superoxide dismutase
HUVECs	human umbilical vein endothelial cells

1. Introduction

In this chapter, we will review the molecular and cellular mechanisms involved in endothelial aging. The endothelium is located in a strategic position between the blood stream and the vascular smooth muscle cells (VSMCs). Under physiological conditions, it is an important modulator of vascular function (Lüscher and Vanhoutte, 1991). The endothelium and its signaling processes are known to be altered by a variety of pathophysiological conditions, among them aging. Aging, in general, and endothelial aging, in particular, as one of the most important biological features of age-related vascular dysfunction, has gained remarkable interest as it may be considered as an independent risk factor for the development of cardiovascular disease. Understanding of the underlying mechanisms of endothelial aging might eventually lead to the design of specific therapies to delay this process and thereby many forms of cardiovascular disease. Therefore, a large amount of research has been dedicated to understand these mechanisms during the past several years. This has led to new and important insights which we will discuss. These experimental observations relate to:

(a) alterations of the endothelial cell L-arginine/nitric oxide (NO) synthase system including potential changes in the availability of cofactors;

(b) enhanced formation of reactive oxygen species (ROS), namely, superoxide (O_2^-) and peroxynitrite ($ONOO^-$) which are likely to be central regulators of endothelial aging;

(c) the characterization of the enzymatic and/or non-enzymatic sources of enhanced ROS production;

(d) changes of the antioxidant capacity with increasing age; and

(e) loss of the balance between vasodilatory and vasoconstrictive elements.

At last, based upon the current experimental evidence, we will propose a model how changes in the endothelial signaling network, normally controlling vascular function, eventually lead to an imbalance between vasoprotective elements and increasing vascular damage, so that the physiological modulatory role of the endothelium cannot be preserved any more in the aged vasculature.

2. Endothelial dysfunction

Vascular aging is mainly characterized by endothelial dysfunction. The endothelium exerts a multimodal regulation of vascular smooth muscle tone and structure by the release of NO and other vasoactive substances such as endothelium-derived hyperpolarizing factor, endothelin (ET) and prostacyclin (Lüscher and Noll, 1995). Endothelial dysfunction is closely associated with a decline of endothelium-dependent relaxation with increasing age (Tschudi et al., 1996; Küng and Lüscher, 1995; Dohi et al., 1990). Relaxation to both receptor-dependent (acetylcholine) and-independent (calcium ionophore) agonists has been shown to be dramatically reduced (up to 60%) in aortas obtained from old normotensive rats as compared with aortas from young rats (Tschudi et al., 1996). Most studies of vascular aging have been performed in rats as their life span is reasonably short, background knowledge is extensive, and genetic and environmental conditions as well as nutrition can easily be controlled. Furthermore, they do not develop atherosclerosis which often hampers studies of human cardiovascular aging (Folkow and Svanborg, 1993). However, Zeiher et al. (1993) were the first to show that the close association between endothelial dysfunction and vascular aging may also be applicable to humans. They demonstrated a strong reduction of acetylcholine-mediated dilator capacity of the coronary microvasculature with increasing age. In the same patients, a strong dilator response to acetylcholine of angiographically normal epicardial arteries ruled out the presence of atherosclerotic lesions. Therefore, the authors concluded that endothelial dysfunction (as assessed by the reduced acetylcholine-dependent dilator capacity) of the human coronary microvasculature was a direct function of age.

Pulse pressure may also increase with age (Tschudi et al., 1996). The notion that mechanical factors might be involved in vascular aging is supported by the fact that aging occurs in the aorta which is exposed to high pressure and pulsatility but not in the pulmonary artery where pressure and pulsatility are low (Tschudi et al., 1996). Pulsatile stretch in normal aortic endothelial cells has been shown to stimulate not only NO, but also $O_2^{\bullet-}$ production from endothelial cells (ECs) (Hishikawa and Lüscher, 1997; Hishikawa et al., 1997). Simultaneous upregulation of endothelial nitric oxide synthase (=eNOS, NOS III) found in these studies may either be a scavenger mechanism of $O_2^{\bullet-}$ or a source of $O_2^{\bullet-}$ itself. Interestingly, shear-stress induced upregulation of eNOS expression is impaired in aged ECs (Hoffmann et al., 2001). Upregulation of production by increased mechanical forces may, therefore, play a key role in age-related endothelial dysfunction as a very early step of atherosclerosis.

Most commonly, the aorta has been investigated in aging studies, and little is known about other vascular beds. However, the mechanisms responsible for endothelial dysfunction might be different from one vessel to the other. An anatomic heterogeneity of vascular aging has been shown by Barton (Barton et al., 1997) who found an age-dependent impaired relaxation in the aorta, but not in the femoral artery of the rat. It has been suggested that the equilibrium between endothelial vasoconstrictor products from the cyclooxygenase pathway, such as thromboxan A_2 and prostaglandin H_2 (PGH_2) on one hand and endothelial NO may be differently altered with age due to vascular bed heterogeneity (Matz et al., 2000). Indeed, PGH_2 synthase-, unlike PGH_1 synthase-, dependent vasoconstriction is increased with aging (Stewart et al., 2000). To date, many aspects of the differential regulation of vascular aging remain unclear.

Finally, the possibility of environmental influences has been brought up by a study in which age-associated endothelial dysfunction was not found in a group of Chinese subjects but in aged white individuals (Woo et al., 1997).

3. Nitric oxide

NO is synthesized from L-arginine by the nitric oxide synthases through the L-arginine–NO pathway (Moncada and Higgs, 1993; Moncada, 1992; Vanhoutte, 1989; Palmer et al., 1988). It is released from ECs after stimulation of muscarinic receptors by acetylcholine or other agonists, and crosses the subendothelial space. NO reacts with the ferrous iron in the heme group of the soluble guanylate cyclase in VSMCs. It thereby increases the concentration of cyclic guanylmonophosphate (cGMP), leading to vascular relaxation (Waldman and Murad, 1988). The NO-producing enzymes consist of three isoforms: (1) neuronal nitric oxide synthase (nNOS=NOS I), (2) inducible nitric oxide synthase (iNOS=NOS II), and (3) eNOS=NOS III. eNOS and nNOS are constitutively expressed, generally calcium-dependent enzymes. Activity of iNOS is independent of an increase in calcium (Andrew and Mayer, 1999).

The short half-life of NO had made it difficult to directly measure NO in biological samples. However, since the introduction of highly sensitive electrochemical methods (Malinski and Taha, 1992), in situ monitoring of NO release on the endothelial surface of blood vessels has become possible. Furthermore, when a receptor-independent agonist such as the calcium ionophore A23187 is used for stimulation of eNOS, the resulting NO release will reflect NOS activity rather than possible age-related changes in receptor-operated signal transduction. Using this technique originally developed by Malinski (Malinski and Taha, 1992), Tschudi et al. (1996) have investigated the kinetics of endothelial NO release as a function of prolonged vascular aging. Fig. 1 shows that NO peak concentrations are significantly reduced in the aorta of 32–33-month-old normotensive female rats. Furthermore, it was shown that aging had no significant effect on endothelial NO release in the pulmonary circulation (Fig. 1). In contrast, in pulmonary arteries, NO concentration even slightly increased with age. This was the first study to clearly demonstrate directly that a reduced bioavailability of NO is causally at the origin of an impaired vasorelaxation in the aged blood vessel. Furthermore, this study supported the notion that age differently alters NO release in the vasculature and is, therefore, fully in line with the hypothesis of an anatomic heterogeneity of vascular aging (Barton et al., 1997). The anatomic heterogeneity might be due to chronic exposure to higher pulse pressure and higher mean flow velocity, parameters which importantly

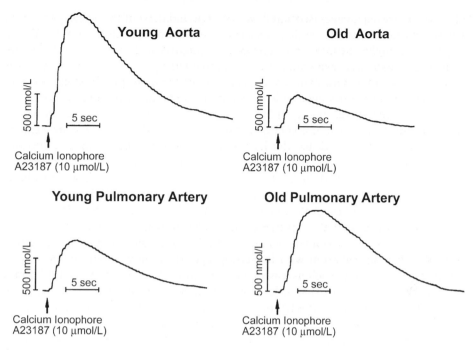

Fig. 1.   Representative amperograms of NO release from isolated aortas and pulmonary arteries of young (8–9-month-old) and old (32–33-month-old) normotensive female rats. NO release was stimulated by the calcium ionophore A23187 (10 µmol/L) and measured on the endothelial surface using a prophyrinic microsensor. With age, there was a significant decrease of NO release in the aorta, whereas a non-signifi-cant, mild increase could be observed in the pulmonary artery. Reproduced from Tschudi et al. (1996) (J. Clin. Invest. 1996; 98: 899–905) by permission of the American Society for Clinical Investigation.

contribute to structural and functional changes eventually leading to a derangement of endothelial function (Lüscher et al., 1995).

3.1. *eNOS*

The main source of endothelial NO is eNOS (Vanhoutte, 1997). eNOS is generally considered to be localized within the plasmalemmal caveolae, chief components of which are the caveolins. eNOS in caveolae is mostly inactive; however, it is still controversial in which fraction eNOS eventually becomes active (Fleming and Busse, 1999). eNOS may well be the most crucial enzyme to determine the state of the vasculature (Fleming and Busse, 1999). There are conflicting data in the literature regarding the regulation of eNOS with increasing age. Both upregulation of eNOS and reduced levels of enzyme expression have been observed. Challah et al. (1997) observed reduced levels of eNOS mRNA in the aorta of 30-month-old normotensive rats compared with 10-month-old animals. Barton (Barton et al., 1997) also demonstrated a reduction of eNOS mRNA expression in aortic endothelial cells. However, other authors have demonstrated an age-related increase of eNOS enzyme expression, both on the transcriptional and on the protein level. Goettsch (Goettsch et al., 2001) reported an age-associated twofold upregulation of the eNOS gene in the aortic vasculature. Cernadas et al. (1998) found in the aorta of 18-month-old Wistar rats a twofold higher expression of eNOS as compared with 6-month-old animals. However, this increased expression was accompanied by a significant reduction in eNOS enzyme activity. Our own recent data support the concept of eNOS becoming a part of a compensatory mechanism to counter-regulate the decreased bioavailability of NO with increasing age (van der Loo et al., 2000). As Fig. 2 shows, we found a sevenfold increase of eNOS expression in the aged rat aorta. Furthermore, subcellular analysis revealed that this increased expression was exclusively associated with the membrane fraction containing the biological activity of the enzyme (Sessa et al., 1993; Busconi and Michel, 1993). This overexpression was exactly paralleled by a significantly higher activity, suggesting that fully active eNOS is upregulated with increasing age, although the intended product, NO, is diminished. However, to date, it is not yet clear if this upregulation of eNOS, which, at first glance, seems paradoxical, solely is a counter-regulatory mechanism against impaired endothelium-mediated vasorelaxation with increasing age. It is known that eNOS, in particular, under conditions such as absence of cofactors (Cosentino et al., 1998), may exhibit oxidase activity. In that case, it may well be possible that eNOS might be involved in increased O_2^- production with aging. Full NOS activity can only be carried out after assembly of the reductase and oxygenase domain to a homodimer. Only at very high concentrations of one of the most important cofactors, tetrahydrobiopterin (H_4B), NOS functions solely as an NO synthase (Andrew and Mayer, 1999). Low levels of H_4B lead to the formation of an NO synthase that catalyzes production of both NO and O_2^-. O_2^- production by eNOS has been shown in the context of endothelial dysfunction seen in spontaneously hypertensive rats (SHR) (Cosentino et al., 1998). The fact that O_2^- production by eNOS is inhibited

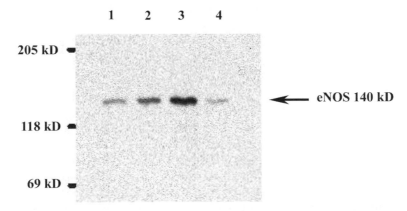

Fig. 2. Aortic protein expression as a function of age. Homogenates of aortic endothelium from 4–6-month-old (1), 19-month-old (2), and 32–35-month-old (3) male normotensive F1 rats were analyzed by western blotting for eNOS expression. Molecular mass markers are indicated and expressed in kD. Human umbilical vein endothelial cells (HUVECs) were used as a positive control (4). Reproduced from van der Loo et al. (2000) (J. Exp. Med. 2000; 192: 1731–1743) by permission of the Rockefeller University Press.

by H_4B (Xia et al., 1998a; Vasquez-Vivar et al., 1998) points to a decisive role for H_4B. Although never shown to date, age-associated changes in H_4B might partly be responsible for which end product results.

As suitable animal models and/or selective inhibitors of the reductase or oxidase activity of eNOS are not yet available, the exact role of eNOS in the setting of vascular aging remains to be determined.

Aging of ECs is furthermore associated with an increased sensitivity to apoptosis (Hoffmann et al., 2001) which is prevented by eNOS overexpression. This work done in cultured ECs was further supported by experiments in a primate model, in which vascular endothelial dysfunction was found to be associated with endothelial apoptosis (Asai et al., 2000).

3.2. *iNOS*

Expression of iNOS has been documented in most vascular cells, in particular, VSMCs (Papapetropoulos et al., 1999). iNOS is capable of catalyzing O_2^- production (Xia et al., 1998b) and may, therefore, be important for the development of age-related endothelial dysfunction. However, as is the case for eNOS, there are also conflicting data for vascular iNOS (NOS II) in the literature regarding its expression and activity with increasing age. In the work done by Cernadas (Cernadas et al., 1998), iNOS was virtually absent in the aortic segments of young rats. In contrast, a marked expression of the iNOS protein was observed in segments of aging rats. In parallel, a marked calcium-independent (=iNOS) activity was detected in aortic extracts of aging animals. Goettsch et al. (2001) also found an upregulated NOS II gene in the aorta of aged rats. Unlike these authors, Challah et al. (1997) found a significant decrease of iNOS mRNA expression levels in the aorta of old rats. In our own work (van der Loo et al., 2000), iNOS was low in aortic vessels of young rats and remained virtually unchanged with increasing age, suggesting that iNOS does not contribute to the compensatory mechanism of age-associated NOS upregulation, at least not in chronic situations such as vascular aging.

The considerably different age of the old age cohorts, the use of different strains and (macroscopically) undetected accompanying diseases might all serve as further explanations for these discrepancies.

3.3. *nNOS*

Expression of nNOS has been shown in endothelial (Papapetropoulos et al., 1997) and in VSMCs (Boulanger et al., 1998). In the later study, increased production of NO from nNOS was seen in carotid arteries of old, but not young SHR. However, although nNOS expression could be detected both in normotensive and SHR, enzyme activity was only demonstrated in SHR (Boulanger et al., 1998). Furthermore, Wilcox et al. (1997) only demonstrated nNOS mRNA in atherosclerotic lesions, but not in normal human blood vessels. This group observed a shift from eNOS expression in normal arteries to increased expression of the other isoforms in atherosclerosis. Therefore, one may assume that, based upon the current literature, nNOS may only be expressed *and* active under distinct pathophysiological conditions, aging is possibly not a part of Clearly, more work will be necessary to establish the role of nNOS for impaired endothelium-dependent relaxation in the context of vascular aging.

4. Endothelin

ETs, synthesized, among others, by endothelial and VSMCs, are converted by ET-converting enzymes (ECE) originating from preproendothelin peptides (Spieker et al., 2001). The major isoform in the cardiovascular system is ET-1 which exerts its vascular effects through activation of specific receptors (ET_A and ET_B) on VSMCs.

The pathogenetic role of ET in hypertension, atherosclerosis and heart failure (Spieker et al., 2001) is extensively documented. An increase in ET production might also contribute to the age-related reduction of endothelium-dependent relaxation. Plasma levels of ET-1, released abluminally from ECs, increase with age and are inversely correlated to plasma superoxide dismutase (SOD) activity (Barton et al., 1997). Furthermore, functional ECE activity, expressing the ratio of contraction of big ET-1 to ET-1, was found to be increased in old aortas compared with young ones (Barton et al., 1997). This was caused by increased contractions of aortic vessels to big ET-1, but decreased contractions to ET-1 in aged aortas (Marin and Rodriguez-Martinez, 1999). Selective downregulation of ET_A receptors (Lüscher et al., 1992) and/or possibly ET_B receptors (d'Uscio et al., 2000) (which contribute to mediation of NO formation) may explain these findings. Alternatively, increased ET-1 plasma levels and increased ECE activity, reflecting impaired endothelial function in the old aorta, could explain a downregulation of the response to ET-1. Consistent with increased ET-1 plasma levels, vascular ET-1 protein expression as well as pre-proendothelin-1 mRNA expression increased with age (Goettsch et al., 2001). Reduced bioavailability of NO (Boulanger and Lüscher, 1990) and increased levels of ROS (Gwinner et al., 1998) known to stimulate the release of ET-1 peptide are likely to contribute to the age-dependent upregulation of ET-1.

Taken together, alterations of the balance between NO and ET-1 of the endothelium are well known key events in the initiation of atherosclerosis (Kunz, 2000) and might also be involved in the early steps of vascular aging (Vanhoutte, 2000).

5. Reactive oxygen species

ROS are important modulators of NO availability under various conditions (Harrison, 1997) and are also thought be involved in the aging process (Stadtman, 1992). The oxygen free radical theory of aging in general has become widely accepted. Increased breakdown of NO due to an augmented production of O_2^- has directly been shown in vitro (Gryglewski et al., 1986), and there is increasing evidence that augmented release of O_2^-, and subsequent inactivation of NO may also be an important key mechanism leading to the decline of endothelium-dependent vasorelaxation with increasing age. The interaction of these two free radicals will result in subsequent formation of $ONOO^-$, a powerful oxidant which can easily penetrate cells to initiate oxidative modifications of proteins and which can thereby exhibit new messenger functions.

5.1. *Superoxide*

$O_2^{\bullet-}$ is the main oxidant for NO (Dinerman et al., 1993). The decrease in endothelial NO bioavailability with aging (Dohi et al., 1990, 1995) occurs concurrent with an increase in $O_2^{\bullet-}$ production (van der Loo et al., 2000; Hamilton et al., 2001). Hamilton et al. (2001) have demonstrated an increased production of $O_2^{\bullet-}$ both in the aorta and in the carotid artery of 12-month-old Wistar-Kyoto rats. Our own data (van der Loo et al., 2000) in the aorta of 32–35-month-old rats showed a threefold increase in basal and a twofold increase in calcium ionophore A23167-stimulated $O_2^{\bullet-}$ generation as compared to 4–6-month-old animals. Interestingly, when aortic rings of old animals were denuded, $O_2^{\bullet-}$ fell to levels comparable to those obtained in young animals. This strongly suggests that the age-associated increase in $O_2^{\bullet-}$ generation primarily occurs within the endothelium.

However, the source of this age-associated $O_2^{\bullet-}$ increase still remains unknown. Once the oxidase activity which is ultimately responsible for the age-associated increased one-electron transfer to molecular oxygen will have been identified, it will become an attractive novel target for the design and development of drugs to alleviate vascular aging. Potential sources are discussed in this chapter. They include eNOS (Cosentino et al., 1998), NAD(P)H oxidase (Griendling et al., 2000), xanthin oxidase (Marczin et al., 1996) and enzymes of the mitochondrial respiratory chain (Beckman and Ames, 1998). Studies to identify the enzymatic source of $O_2^{\bullet-}$ have been hampered so far by the fact that specific inhibitors are not available to date. Although diphenyleniodonium (DPI) and apocynin have been shown to attenuate $O_2^{\bullet-}$ production in blood vessels from old rats (Hamilton et al., 2001), thus apparently indicating an inhibition of the vascular NAD(P)H oxidase, it has to be pointed out that these compounds also have an inhibitory effect on NOS. L-NMMA would inhibit NOS as a whole (reductase and oxidase activity) and, therefore, not be suitable to reveal the role of eNOS. If, in accordance with the "oxidative stress hypothesis" of vascular aging (Finkel and Holbrook, 2000), increased $O_2^{\bullet-}$ formation is the primary cause of age-associated endothelial dysfunction, studies with genetically modified animals showing a prolonged or reduced life span will help in the future to further shed new light on the role of oxidative stress.

5.2. *Peroxynitrite*

Strong experimental evidence has recently been presented for a close association between the formation of $ONOO^-$ and age-associated vascular endothelial dysfunction (van der Loo et al., 2000). The link between increased $O_2^{\bullet-}$ production and decreased NO bioavailability to form $ONOO^-$ is obvious in view of the known chemistry, kinetics, and diffusion properties of both free radicals. Unlike $O_2^{\bullet-}$, $ONOO^-$ in its protonated form can easily cross cell membranes because of its high diffusibility (pK of 6.8) (Marla et al., 1997). The formation of ONOO$^-$, in turn, exhibits new messenger functions, including tyrosine nitration (Goldstein et al., 2000; Reiter et al., 2000). By initiation of the oxidative modification of proteins, in particular, nitration of aromatic rings (Beckman et al., 1992), ONOO$^-$ renders inactive certain functionally important regulatory proteins. As it is not possible to directly measure ONOO$^-$ formation in vivo, the detection of typical end products of its reaction with biological compounds is the current gold standard to prove that ONOO$^-$ is indeed formed after capture of NO by O_2^-.

To this end, we have recently demonstrated (van der Loo et al., 2000) an increased deposition of 3-nitrotyrosinated proteins in the vasculature, in particular, within the endothelium of old rats. Fig. 3A shows a significant accumulation of nitrotyrosine in the endothelium of old aortas compared with young ones (Fig. 3B). A particularly high amount of nitrotyrosine was found in the mitochondria of endothelial cells, a fact which strongly supports that the most significant generation of O_2^- and ONOO$^-$, occurs within the mitochondria, and in particular, in those within the endothelium.

6. Mitochondria

The importance of mitochondria, in particular, of those within the endothelium, for the process of age-related endothelial dysfunction is underlined by the fact that increased nitrotyrosination with age has been shown to be dominant in these organelles (van der Loo et al., 2000). This supports their importance in the cascade of events involved in the vascular aging process. Although not yet proven directly, mitochondria themselves may be a major source of O_2^- and ONOO$^-$ in the aging vasculature (Beckman and Ames, 1998). Under physiological conditions, approximately 1% of O_2 consumed by mitochondria is reduced by enzymes of the mitochondrial electron transport chain to O_2^-. Under particular conditions such as aging, this percentage may increase by misdirection of electrons from the respiratory chain into ROS production. This may be due to an age-related decline of mitochondrial function, affecting enzyme function, as it has been shown for aconitase (Yan et al., 1997). Such a decline could recently be demonstrated in an enzyme knockout model of heterozygous mice with a partial deficiency in manganese superoxide dismutase (MnSOD) (Kokoszka et al., 2001). A role for mitochondrial ROS production in the aging process has recently been suggested (Kokoszka et al., 2001). Additional evidence for mitochondria and an increased oxidation of respiratory chain components being involved in the initial reactions leading to endothelial dysfunction comes from findings regarding MnSOD. This enzyme is solely expressed in mitochondria, and age-related changes in its expression and activity can, therefore, well serve as a molecular footprint of mitochondrial oxidative stress in the aged vasculature. It has recently been shown that although expression levels of this enzyme did not change with age, a significantly increased nitration of tyrosine residues within MnSOD could be observed in aortas from 3-year-old rats as compared with young adult animals (van der Loo et al., 2000). Nitration of an essential tyrosine residue in MnSOD has

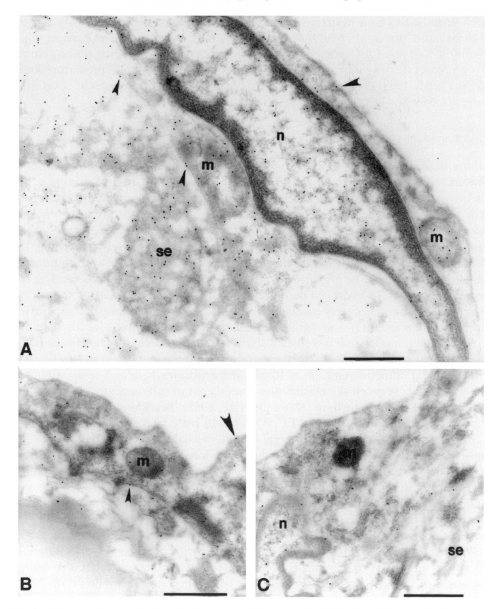

Fig. 3. Electron micrographs showing the pattern of immunogold labeling for 3-nitrotyrosine in sections of the intima of old (A) and young (B) aortas. Primary antibody binding sites were visualized with a secondary antibody conjugated to 10 nm gold particles. (A) Label is densest over endothelial cell mitochondria (m) and strong over nucleoplasm (n). Strong labeling is also seen in the subendothelial space (se). (B) In the intima of the aorta from a young rat, label is lower over mitochondria and cytoplasm. (C) Intima of an old rat. The primary antibody against nitrotyrosine was preincubated with nitrotyrosine before labeling as in (A) and (B). Label density is reduced to levels lower than those seen in the young rats. Reproduced from van der Loo et al. (2000) (J. Exp. Med. 2000; 192: 1731–1743) by permission of the Rockefeller University Press.

been proposed to be a mechanism leading to a significant reduction of its activity (MacMillan-Crow et al., 1999). MnSOD is the major antioxidant enzyme in mitochondria, and proof for an important role of this enzyme in the aging process comes from a report showing that genetic inactivation of MnSOD results in premature death (Melov et al., 1998). This also suggests that MnSOD may be a potential novel drug target to combat vascular aging.

7. Antioxidant systems

Apart from MnSOD, other enzyme systems, which, under physiological conditions, ensure the direct detoxification of the vasculature from ROS exist, but their role, and in particular, their changes with age, are less well studied. However, it is generally accepted that a gradual loss of antioxidant capacity as a whole is involved in age-related endothelial dysfunction (Azhar et al., 1995). As a counter-regulation, glutathione (GSH) and SOD will react with O_2^-, thereby preventing the formation of $ONOO^-$. Evidence for detrimental effects of O_2^- on endothelial function in age would be provided by protective effects of SOD. SODs catalyze the conversion of O_2^- to hydrogen peroxide. All three SOD isoenzymes are thought to function in a complementary manner. From these isoforms, copper/zinc superoxide dismutase (Cu/ZnSOD) and MnSOD are intracellular enzymes, localized in the cytoplasm and mitochondria, respectively, whereas extracellular SOD (EC-SOD) is the principal scavenger of O_2^- in the extracellular space (Stralin et al., 1995). It is either present in the interstitium of tissues, in particular, the blood vessel wall, and the plasma, i.e. between the plasma phase and heparan sulfate proteoglycans in the glycocalyx of the endothelium (Karlsson et al., 1988). Marklund et al. (1997) have demonstrated increased plasma EC-SOD levels with increasing age in Swedish subjects aged 25–74 years. This might be interpreted as a protective adaptation against enhanced oxidative stress. Furthermore, low levels were associated with an increased risk for cardiovascular disease. These findings were supported by a more recent study done by Adachi et al. (2000) who found that plasma levels of EC-SOD changed in an age-dependent manner. Total SOD activity in this study also increased with age. Therefore, one may conclude that the protective effect provided by EC-SOD, which normally forms an equilibrium between the outer endothelial cell surface and the plasma, cannot be maintained with increasing age, leading to a decreased antioxidant potential. However, in contrast to these studies, age-related decreases of SOD plasma activity have also been reported (Guemouri et al., 1991). Transgenic animals, overexpressing isoforms of SODs, are an excellent tool to study the effects of those enzymes on aging, in particular, if overexpression had a positive effect on life span, this would be a direct proof of causality. However, transgenic mice overexpressing Cu/ZnSOD had no extended life span compared with non-transgenic littermate controls (Huang et al., 2000) suggesting that CuZnSOD, at least alone, is not sufficient for a prolongation of life span. Genetic inactivation of EC-SOD had also no significant effect on longevity (Carlsson et al., 1995). In contrast, lack of the MnSOD gene resulted in premature death (Melov et al., 1998).

8. NAD(P)H oxidase

The endothelium contains membrane-bound oxidases that use NADH and NADPH as substrates for the electron transfer to molecular oxygen (Harrison, 1997; Mohazzab et al., 1994). NAD(P)H oxidase consists of membrane-bound cytochrome b_{558} (containing p22^{phox} and gp91^{phox}) and cytosolic components (p40^{phox}, p47^{phox}, p67^{phox}). To become active, the cytosolic components have to be transferred to the membrane in order to assemble there with the membrane-bound components. In the setting of other cardiovascular risk factors, such as diabetes (Hink et al., 2001), hypertension (Rajagopalan et al., 1996) and hypercholesterolemia (Ohara et al., 1993), the NAD(P)H oxidase, to a significant extent, appears to be responsible for oxidative stress and hence endothelial dysfunction. In the pathophysiological setting of age-related endothelial dysfunction, NAD(P)H oxidase as a potential source for enhanced O_2^- production has been less well investigated to date (Griendling et al., 2000). Recent immunohistochemical (semiquantitative) data suggested that p22^{phox} levels were higher in the endothelium of aortas from old rats compared with young ones (Hamilton et al., 2001). When using DPI and apocynin to inhibit the NAD(P)H oxidase pathway, O_2^- production in aortas from old animals was indeed significantly attenuated, being consistent with a role for NAD(P)H oxidase as one potential source of age-associated O_2^- production, in particular, within the endothelium. However, more work, especially investigation of all subunits of the endothelial NAD(P)H oxidase and their changes in terms of expression and activity with increasing age, will be necessary in order to definitely establish a causal role for the NAD(P)H oxidase in the cascade of events eventually leading to age-related endothelial dysfunction.

9. Summary

As depicted in Fig. 4, we propose a mechanistic model of vascular aging, in which increased O_2^- production, mainly derived from the endothelium, is the centerpiece. The source of this increased O_2^- formation remains obscure, but might involve the endothelial NAD(P)H oxidase system, mitochondrial respiratory chain components and/or eNOS. Current evidence suggests a particularly intriguing role for eNOS. There is a steep upregulation of the eNOS enzyme system, exactly paralleled by an increase in enzyme activity. As the bioavailability of its intended product, NO, is diminished, this upregulation may be interpreted as a feedback mechanism to counter-regulate the loss of NO and hence reduced vasodilation. However, under certain conditions, eNOS may well exhibit oxidase activities and further enhance O_2^- production. These conditions, which have not yet been thoroughly investigated to date, would include the absence of cofactors (H_4B) or insufficient substrate supply (L-arginine). The development of genetically altered animals expressing only specific eNOS domains should help in the future to elucidate this double-faced role.

Increased O_2^- production leads to an inactivation of equimolar amounts of NO by the formation of $ONOO^-$. $ONOO^-$ exhibits new messenger functions by oxidative modification of proteins after production of 3-nitrotyrosine residues. Interestingly,

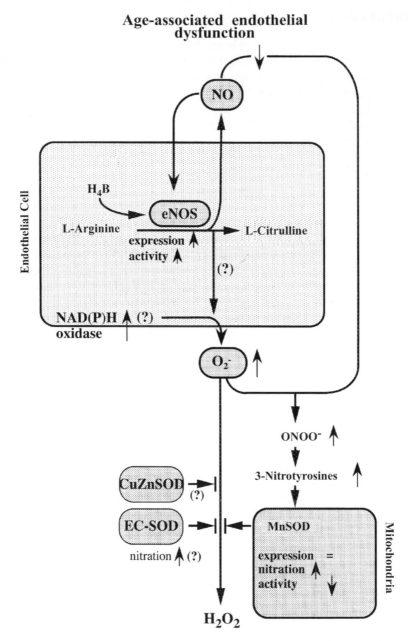

Fig. 4. A proposed mechanism for the development of age-associated endothelial dysfunction. For further explanation, see text under Section 9. Signaling pathways drawn outside the endothelial cell may primarily take place within the endothelium, but also in other cells or compartments of the vasculature.

the most significant generation of oxidants occurs within the endothelial mito-chondria, a finding which supports their central role in endothelial aging. Similar to eNOS, mitochondria may also have a double-faced role. On one hand, they may themselves be a major source of ROS in the aging vascular system. On the other hand, mitochondrial enzymes are a part of the counter-balance to prevent endo-thelial dysfunction. However, selective nitration of an essential tyrosine residue in MnSOD by $ONOO^-$, subsequently leading to inactivation of MnSOD, suggests that this counter-balance, normally a key element of the antioxidant defense, cannot be maintained with increasing age. To date, less is known about the two other isoforms of SOD, in particular, it is not known if nitration and dityrosine formation within these enzymes are mediated by $ONOO^-$, in the same way as in MnSOD.

New data elucidating the molecular pathways of age-associated endothelial dys-function will lead to a better understanding of vascular aging and to the development of therapeutic strategies to delay this process.

Acknowledgements

Original research of the authors reported in this chapter has been supported by grants from the Swiss National Research Foundation (grants no. 32-51069.97 and 32-49126.96), the Swiss Heart Foundation, the Roche Research Foundation, Aetas, Foundation for Research into Ageing, and the European Society of Cardiology.

References

Adachi, T., Wang, J., Wang, X.L., 2000. Age-related change of plasma extracellular-superoxide dismutase. Clin. Chim. Acta 290, 169–178.

Andrew, P.J., Mayer, B., 1999. Enzymatic function of nitric oxide synthases. Cardiovasc. Res. 43, 521–531.

Asai, K., Kudej, R.K., Shen, Y.T., Yang, G.P., Takagi, G., Kudej, A.B., Geng, Y.J., Sato, N., Nazareno, J.B., Vatner, D.E., Natividad, F., Bishop, S.P., Vatner, S.F., 2000. Peripheral vascular endothelial dys-function and apoptosis in old monkeys. Arterioscler. Thromb. Vasc. Biol. 20, 1493–1499.

Azhar, S., Cao, L., Reaven, E., 1995. Alteration of the adrenal antioxidant defense system during aging in rats. J. Clin. Invest. 95, 1414–1424.

Barton, M., Cosentino, F., Brandes, R.P., Moreau, P., Shaw, S., Lüscher, T.F., 1997. Anatomic hetero-geneity of vascular aging: role of nitric oxide and endothelin. Hypertension 30, 817–824.

Beckman, K.B., Ames, B.N., 1998. Mitochondrial aging: open questions. Ann. NY Acad. Sci. 854, 118–127.

Beckman, J.S., Ischiropoulos, H., Zhu, L., van der Woerd, M., Smith, C., Chen, J., Harrison, J., Martin, J.C., Tsai, M., 1992. Kinetics of superoxide dismutase- and iron-catalyzed nitration of phenolics by peroxynitrite. Arch. Biochem. Biophys. 298, 438–445.

Boulanger, C., Heymes, C., Benessiano, J., Geske, R.S., Levy, B.I., Vanhoutte, P.M., 1998. Neuronal nitric oxide synthase is expressed in rat vascular smooth muscle cells: activation by angiotensin II in hypertension. Circ. Res. 83, 1271–1278.

Boulanger, C., Lüscher, T.F., 1990. Release of endothelin from the porcine aorta. Inhibition by endothe-lium-derived nitric oxide. J. Clin. Invest. 85, 587–590.

Busconi, L., Michel, T., 1993. Endothelial nitric oxide synthase. N-terminal myristoylation determines subcellular localization. J. Biol. Chem. 268, 8410–8413.

Carlsson, L.M., Jonsson, J., Edlund, T., Marklund, S.L., 1995. Mice lacking extracellular superoxide dis-mutase are more sensitive to hyperoxia. Proc. Natl. Acad. Sci. USA 92, 6264–6268.

Cernadas, M.R., Sanchez de Miguel, L., Garcia-Duran, M., Gonzalez-Fernandez, F., Millas, I., Monton, M., Rodrigo, J., Rico, L., Fernandez, P., de Frutos, T., Rodriguez-Feo, J.A., Guerra, J., Caramelo, C., Casado, S., Lopez-Farre, A., 1998. Expression of constitutive and inducible nitric oxide synthases in the vascular wall of young and aging rats. Circ. Res. 83, 279–286.

Challah, M., Nadaud, S., Philippe, M., Battle, T., Soubrier, F., Corman, B., Michel, J.B., 1997. Circulating and cellular markers of endothelial dysfunction with aging in rats. Am. J. Physiol. 273, H1941–H1948.

Cosentino, F., Patton, S., d'Uscio, L.V., Werner, E.R., Werner-Felmayer, G., Moreau, P., Malinski, T., Lüscher, T.F., 1998. Tetrahydrobiopterin alters superoxide and nitric oxide release in prehypertensive rats. J. Clin. Invest. 101, 1530–1537.

Dinerman, J., Lowenstein, C.J., Snyder, S.H., 1993. Molecular mechanisms of nitric oxide regulation. Potential relevance to cardiovascular disease. Circ. Res. 73, 217–222.

Dohi, Y., Kojima, M., Sato, K., Lüscher, T.F., 1995. Age-related changes in vascular smooth muscle and endothelium. Drugs Aging 7, 278–291.

Dohi, Y., Thiel, M.A., Bühler, F.R., Lüscher, T.F., 1990. Activation of endothelial L-arginine pathway in resistance arteries. Effect of age and hypertension. Hypertension 15, 170–179.

d'Uscio, L.V., Barton, M., Shaw, S., Lüscher, T.F., 2000. Endothelin in atherosclerosis: importance of risk factors and therapeutic implications. J. Cardiovasc. Pharmacol. 35 (Suppl. 2), S55–S59.

Finkel, T., Holbrook, N.J., 2000. Oxidants, oxidative stress and the biology of ageing. Nature 408, 239–247.

Fleming, I., Busse, R., 1999. Signal transduction of eNOS activation. Cardiovasc. Res. 43, 532–541.

Folkow, B., Svanborg, A., 1993. Physiology of cardiovascular aging. Physiol. Rev. 73, 725–764.

Goettsch, W., Lattmann, T., Amann, K., Szibor, M., Morawietz, H., Munter, K., Muller, S.P., Shaw, S., Barton, M., 2001. Increased expression of endothelin-1 and inducible nitric oxide synthase isoform II in aging arteries in vivo: implications for atherosclerosis. Biochem. Biophys. Res. Comm. 280, 908–913.

Goldstein, S., Czapski, G., Lind, J., Merenyi, G., 2000. Tyrosine nitration by simultaneous generation of NO and O_2^- under physiological conditions. How the radicals do the job. J. Biol. Chem. 275, 3031–3036.

Griendling, K.K., Sorescu, D., Ushio-Fukai, M., 2000. NAD(P)H oxidase: role in cardiovascular biology and disease. Circ. Res. 86, 494–501.

Gryglewski, R.J., Palmer, R.M., Moncada, S., 1986. Superoxide anion is involved in the breakdown of endothelium-derived vascular relaxing factor. Nature 320, 454–456.

Guemouri, L., Artur, Y., Herbeth, B., Jeandel, C., Cuny, G., Siest, G., 1991. Biological variability of superoxide dismutase, glutathione peroxidase, and catalase in blood. Clin. Chem. 37, 1932–1937.

Gwinner, W., Deters-Evers, U., Brandes, R.P., Kubat, B., Koch, K.M., Pape, M., Olbricht, C.J., 1998. Antioxidant–oxidant balance in the glomerulus and proximal tubule of the rat kidney. J. Physiol. 509, 599–606.

Hamilton, C.A., Brosnan, M.J., McIntyre, M., Graham, D., Dominiczak, A.F., 2001. Superoxide excess in hypertension and aging: a common cause of endothelial dysfunction. Hypertension 37 (part 2), 529–534.

Harrison, D.G., 1997. Cellular and molecular mechanisms of endothelial cell dysfunction. J. Clin. Invest. 100, 2153–2156.

Hink, U., Li, H., Mollnau, H., Oelze, M., Matheis, E., Hartmann, M., Skatchkov, M., Thaiss, F., Stahl, R.A., Warnholtz, A., Meinertz, T., Griendling, K., Harrison, D.G., Forstermann, U., Munzel, T., 2001. Mechanisms underlying endothelial dysfunction in diabetes mellitus. Circ. Res. 88, e14–e22.

Hishikawa, K., Lüscher, T.F., 1997. Pulsatile stretch stimulates superoxide production in human aortic endothelial cells. Circulation 96, 3610–3616.

Hishikawa, K., Oemar, B.S., Yang, Z., Lüscher, T.F., 1997. Pulsatile stretch stimulates superoxide production and activates nuclear factor-kappa B in human coronary smooth muscle. Circ. Res. 81, 797–803.

Hoffmann, J., Haendeler, J., Aicher, A., Rossig, L., Vasa, M., Zeiher, A.M., Dimmeler, S., 2001. Aging enhances the sensitivity of endothelial cells toward apoptotic stimuli: important role of nitric oxide. Circ. Res. 89, 709–715.

Huang, T.T., Carlson, E.J., Gillespie, A.M., Shi, Y., Epstein, C.J., 2000. Ubiquitous overexpression of CuZn superoxide dismutase does not extend life span in mice. J. Gerontol. A Biol. Sci. Med. Sci. 55, B5–B9.

Karlsson, K., Lindahl, U., Marklund, S.L., 1988. Binding of human extracellular superoxide dismutase C to sulphated glycosaminoglycans. Biochem. J. 256, 29–33.

Kokoszka, J.E., Coskun, P., Esposito, L., Wallace, D.C., 2001. Increased mitochondrial oxidative stress in the Sod2 (+/−) mouse results in the age-related decline of mitochondrial function culminating in increased apoptosis. Proc. Natl. Acad. Sci. USA 98, 2278–2283.

Küng, C.F., Lüscher, T.F., 1995. Different mechanisms of endothelial dysfunction with aging and hypertension in rat aorta. Hypertension 25, 194–200.

Kunz, J., 2000. Initial lesions of vascular aging disease. Gerontology 46, 295–299.

Lüscher, T.F., Boulanger, C.M., Dohi, Y., Yang, Z.H., 1992. Endothelium-derived contracting factors. Hypertension 19, 117–130.

Lüscher, T.F., Noll, G., 1995. The endothelium in coronary vascular control. Heart Dis. 3, 1–10.

Lüscher, T.F., Noll, G., Wenzel, R.R., 1995. Systemic hypertension and related vascular diseases. Vasc. Pathol. 553–569.

Lüscher, T.F., Vanhoutte, P.M., 1991. The Endothelium: Modulator of Cardiovascular Function. CRC Press, Boca Raton, FL, USA.

MacMillan-Crow, L.A., Crow, J.P., Thompson, J.A., 1999. Peroxynitrite-mediated inactivation of manganese superoxide dismutase involves nitration and oxidation of critical tyrosine residues. Biochemistry 37, 1613–1622.

Malinski, T., Taha, Z., 1992. Nitric oxide release from a single cell measured in situ by a porphyrinic-based microsensor. Nature 358, 676–678.

Marczin, N., Antonov, A., Papapetropoulos, A., Munn, D.H., Virmani, R., Kolodgie, F.D., Gerrity, R., Catravas, J.D., 1996. Monocyte-induced downregulation of nitric oxide synthase in cultured aortic endothelial cells. Arterioscler. Thromb. Vasc. Biol. 16, 1095–1103.

Marin, J., Rodriguez-Martinez, M.A., 1999. Age-related changes in vascular responses. Exp. Gerontol. 34, 503–512.

Marklund, S., Nilsson, P., Israelsson, K., Schampi, I., Peltonen, M., Asplund, K., 1997. Two variants of extracellular-superoxide dismutase: relationship to cardiovascular risk factors in an unselected middle-aged population. J. Intern. Med. 242, 5–14.

Marla, S.S., Lee, J., Groves, J.T., 1997. Peroxynitrite rapidly permeates phospholipid membranes. Proc. Natl. Acad. Sci. USA 94, 14243–14248.

Matz, R.L., de Sotomayor, M.A., Schott, C., Stoclet, J.C., Andriantsitohaina, R., 2000. Vascular bed heterogeneity in age-related endothelial dysfunction with respect to NO and eicosanoids. Br. J. Pharmacol. 131, 303–311.

Melov, S., Schneider, J.A., Day, B.J., Hinerfeld, D., Coskun, P., Mirra, S.S., Crapo, J.D., Wallace, D.C., 1998. A novel neurological phenotype in mice lacking mitochondrial manganese superoxide dismutase. Nat. Genet. 18, 159–163.

Mohazzab, K.M., Kaminski, P.M., Wolin, M.S., 1994. NADH oxidoreductase is a major source of superoxide anion in bovine coronary artery endothelium. Am. J. Physiol. 266, H2568–H2572.

Moncada, S., 1992. The 1991 Ulf von Euler Lecture. The L-arginine: nitric oxide pathway. Acta Physiol. Scand. 145, 201–227.

Moncada, S., Higgs, A., 1993. The L-arginine-nitric oxide pathway. New Engl. J. Med. 329, 2002–2012.

Ohara, Y., Peterson, T.E., Harrison, D.G., 1993. Hypercholesterolemia increases endothelial superoxide anion production. J. Clin. Invest. 91, 2546–2551.

Palmer, R.M.J., Ashton, D.S., Moncada, S., 1988. Vascular endothelial cells synthesize nitric oxide from L-arginine. Nature 333, 664–666.

Papapetropoulos, A., Desai, K.M., Rudic, R.D., Mayer, B., Zhang, R., Ruiz-Torres, M.P., Garcia-Cardena, G., Madri, J.A., Sessa, W.C., 1997. Nitric oxide synthase inhibitors attenuate transforming-growth-factor-beta 1-stimulated capillary organization in vitro. Am. J. Pathol. 150, 1835–1844.

Papapetropoulos, A., Rudic, R.D., Sessa, W.C., 1999. Molecular control of nitric oxide synthases in the cardiovascular system. Cardiovasc. Res. 43, 509–520.

Rajagopalan, S., Kurz, S., Munzel, T., Tarpey, M., Freeman, B.A., Griendling, K.K., Harrison, D.G., 1996. Angiotensin II-mediated hypertension in the rat increases vascular superoxide production via membrane NADH/NADPH oxidase activation. Contribution to alterations of vasomotor tone. J. Clin. Invest. 97, 1916–1923.

Reiter, C.D., Teng, R.J., Beckman, J.S., 2000. Superoxide reacts with nitric oxide to nitrate tyrosine at physiological pH via peroxynitrite. J. Biol. Chem. 275, 32460–32466.

Sessa, W.C., Barber, C.M., Lynch, K.R., 1993. Mutation of N-myristoylation site converts endothelial cell nitric oxide synthase from a membrane to a cytosolic protein. Circ. Res. 72, 921–924.

Spieker, L.E., Noll, G., Ruschitzka, F.T., Lüscher, T.F., 2001. Endothelin receptor antagonists in congestive heart failure: a new therapeutic principle for the future? J. Am. Coll. Cardiol. 37, 1493–1505.

Stadtman, E.R., 1992. Protein oxidation and aging. Science 257, 1220–1224.

Stewart, K.G., Zhang, Y., Davidge, S.T., 2000. Aging increases PGHS-2-dependent vasoconstriction in rat mesenteric arteries. Hypertension 35, 1242–1247.

Stralin, P., Karlsson, K., Johansson, B.O., Marklund, S.L., 1995. The interstitium of the human arterial wall contains very large amounts of extracellular superoxide dismutase. Arterioscler. Thromb. Vasc. Biol. 15, 2032–2036.

Tschudi, M., Barton, M., Bersinger, N.A., Moreau, P., Cosentino, F., Noll, G., Malinski, T., Lüscher, T.F., 1996. Effect of age on kinetics of nitric oxide release in rat aorta and pulmonary artery. J. Clin. Invest. 98, 899–905.

van der Loo, B., Labugger, R., Skepper, J.N., Bachschmid, M., Kilo, J., Powell, J.M., Palacios-Callender, M., Erusalimsky, J.D., Quaschning, T., Malinski, T., Gygi, D., Ullrich, V., Lüscher, T.F., 2000. Enhanced peroxynitrite formation is associated with vascular aging. J. Exp. Med. 192, 1731–1743.

Vanhoutte, P.M., 1989. Endothelium and control of vascular function. State of the Art lecture. Hypertension 13, 658–667.

Vanhoutte, P.M., 1997. Endothelial dysfunction and atherosclerosis. Eur. Heart J. 18 (Suppl. E), E19–E29.

Vanhoutte, P.M., 2000. Say NO to ET. J. Autonom. Nerv. Syst. 81, 271–277.

Vasquez-Vivar, J., Kalyanaraman, B., Martasek, P., Hogg, N., Masters, B.S., Karoui, H., Tordo, P., Pritchard Jr., K.A., 1998. Superoxide generation by endothelial nitric oxide synthase: the influence of cofactors. Proc. Natl. Acad. Sci. USA 95, 9220–9225.

Waldman, S.A., Murad, F., 1988. Biochemical mechanisms underlying vascular smooth muscle relaxation: the guanylate cyclase-cyclic GMP system. J. Cardiovasc. Pharmacol. 12 (Suppl. 5), S115–S118.

Wilcox, J.N., Subramanian, R.R., Sundell, C.L., Tracey, W.R., Pollock, J.S., Harrison, D.G., Marsden, P.A., 1997. Expression of multiple isoforms of nitric oxide synthase in normal and atherosclerotic vessels. Arterioscler. Thromb. Vasc. Biol. 17, 2479–2488.

Woo, K.S., McCrohon, J.A., Chook, P., Adams, M.R., Robinson, J.T., McCredie, R.J., Lam, C.W., Feng, J.Z., Celermajer, D.S., 1997. Chinese adults are less susceptible than whites to age-related endothelial dysfunction. J. Am. Coll. Cardiol. 30, 113–118.

Xia, Y., Tsai, A.L., Berka, V., Zweier, J.L., 1998a. Superoxide generation from endothelial nitric-oxide synthase. A Ca^{2+}/calmodulin-dependent and tetrahydrobiopterin regulatory process. J. Biol. Chem. 273, 25804–25808.

Xia, Y., Roman, L.J., Masters, B.S., Zweier, J.L., 1998b. Inducible nitric-oxide synthase generates superoxide from the reductase domain. J. Biol. Chem. 273, 22635–22639.

Yan, L.J., Levine, R.L., Sohal, R.S., 1997. Oxidative damage during aging targets mitochondrial aconitase. Proc. Natl. Acad. Sci. USA 94, 11168–11172.

Zeiher, A.M., Drexler, H., Saurbier, B., Just, H., 1993. Endothelium-mediated coronary blood flow modulation in humans. Effects of age, atherosclerosis, hypercholesterolemia, and hypertension. J. Clin. Invest. 92, 652–662.

Nitric oxide, gender and hypertension in humans

Stefano Taddei*, Agostino Virdis, Lorenzo Ghiadoni, Guido Salvetti, Daniele Versari and Antonio Salvetti

Department of Internal Medicine, University of Pisa, Via Roma 67, 56100 Pisa, Italy

Contents

Abbreviations

EDRF	endothelium-derived relaxing factor
NO	nitric oxide
NOS	nitric oxide synthase
EDHF	endothelium-derived hyperpolarizing factor
ET-1	endothelin-1

*Corresponding author. Tel.: +39-050-551110; fax: +39-050-553407.
E-mail address: s.taddei@med.unipi.it (S. Taddei).

Advances in Cell Aging and Gerontology, vol. 11, 145–163

L-NMMA   L-*N*(G)-monomethyl-arginine
EDCFs   endothelium-dependent contracting factors
FMD   flow-mediated dilation
FBF   forearm blood flow

1. Introduction

Endothelial cells play an important local regulatory role by secreting substances that control both vascular tone and structure (Lüscher and Vanhoutte, 1990). The best characterized endothelium-derived relaxing factor (EDRF) is nitric oxide (NO) (Furchgott and Zawadzky, 1980; Palmer et al., 1987), which is derived from the metabolism of L-arginine (Palmer et al., 1998) by NO-synthase (NOS) (Bredt et al., 1991), a constitutive enzyme present in endothelial cells. NO is produced and released both tonically and under the influence of endothelial agonists, such as acetylcholine, bradykinin, substance P, serotonin and others acting on specific receptors (Lüscher and Vanhoutte, 1990), and by mechanical forces, such as shear stress (Rubanyi et al., 1986). Endothelial cells can also induce relaxation by causing hyperpolarization (Cohen and Vanhoutte, 1995). However, at the present time, arguments for the existence of an endothelium-derived hyperpolarizing factor (EDHF) in humans are plausible only on the basis that endothelium-dependent relaxation cannot be abolished by NO-synthase antagonists, thus ruling out NO as responsible for this activity (Cohen and Vanhoutte, 1995).

Endothelial cells can also produce and release endothelium-derived contracting factors. Such substances include cyclooxygenase derivatives, at this time partially identified with prostanoids (TXA2 and PGH2) (Miller and Vanhoutte, 1985; Altiere et al., 1986), and oxygen free radicals (Katusic and Vanhoutte, 1989), which can impair endothelial function by directly evoking contractions or causing NO break-down (Gryglewski et al., 1986). Finally, endothelial cells can also produce endo-thelin-1 (ET-1), a peptide characterized by sustained and potent vasoconstrictor action (Yanagisawa et al., 1988; Inoue et al., 1989) and mitogenic activity. ET-1 acts through specific receptors named ETA and ETB (Arai et al., 1990). ETA receptors are represented only on smooth muscle cells and have the function of promoting growth and mediating contractions (Seo et al., 1990). In contrast, ETB receptors are located on both endothelial and smooth muscle cells, with different effects. Smooth muscle cell ETB receptors evoke contractions (Seo et al., 1990; Haynes et al., 1995), whereas endothelial ETB receptors induce relaxation by production of EDRFs, including NO (Tsukahara et al., 1994) and prostacyclin (De Nucci et al., 1988).

NO and endothelium-derived contracting factors not only exert an opposite effect on vascular tone but also, respectively, inhibit and activate those mechanisms such as platelet aggregation (Radomski et al., 1987), vascular smooth cell proliferation (Garg and Hassid, 1989) and migration (Dubey and Lüscher, 1993), monocyte adhesion (Kubes et al., 1991) and adhesion molecule expression (De Caterina et al., 1995) that exert an important role in the genesis of thrombosis and atherosclerotic plaque. Thus, endothelial dysfunction, caused by an impairment of the L-arginine-NO pathway (Panza et al., 1993) and production of endothelium-derived contracting factors (Taddei et al., 1993), can be considered a relevant mechanism causing atherosclerosis and thrombosis.

This hypothesis is in agreement with the finding that endothelial dysfunction is detectable in the presence of various cardiovascular risk factors, such as hypertension (Linder et al., 1990; Panza et al., 1990), hypercholesterolemia (Creager et al., 1990; Casino et al., 1993), diabetes mellitus (Williams et al., 1996; Ting et al., 1996) and smoking (Celermajer et al., 1996; Heitzer et al., 1996), and that the association of several risk factors further impairs endothelial function (Vita et al., 1990). In the present paper, we will examine the influence of aging on endothelial function both in normotensive subjects and in hypertensive patients, the mechanism(s) through which aging can modify endothelial function, the relationship between aging, gender and endothelial function and finally the possibility of therapeutic intervention which can prevent age-related endothelial dysfunction.

2. Aging and endothelium-dependent vasodilation in healthy subjects

Experimental data indicate that aging alters endothelium-dependent relaxation in large and small resistance arteries of rat (Moritoki et al., 1986; Soltis, 1987; Hongo et al., 1988; Mayhan et al., 1990; Dohi et al., 1990).

2.1. *Studies in the coronary circulation*

In humans, the first findings demonstrating the association between advancing age and impaired endothelium-dependent vasodilation have been obtained in the coronary circulation. Yasue et al. (1990) compared the epicardial vasomotor response to intracoronary injection of acetylcholine in 74 patients with angiographically normal coronary arteries. Patients were divided into a younger and older subgroup (9–29 and 31–68 yr, respectively). While in younger subjects, acetylcholine caused coronary vasodilation, in older patients, the muscarinic agonist determined a paradoxical vasoconstriction, an established marker of endothelial dysfunction. It must, however, be noted that older subjects were also characterized by a greater prevalence of cardiovascular risk factors, which at least partially could contribute to the endothelial dysfunction observed in this study subgroup. Similar results were obtained by Vita et al. (1990). In 34 patients with a difference in prevalence of cardiovascular risk factors, but angiographically smooth coronary arteries, the authors tested the vasomotor response to intracoronary injection of acetylcholine. The acetylcholine response ranged from +37% (dilation) to –53% (constriction) and by multiple stepwise regression analysis, age, but also other risk factors, was independently associated with the acetylcholine response. However, in these preliminary reports, the impaired response to acetylcholine associated with increased age was explained by the presence in older individuals of early atherosclerosis not detectable by angiography.

A few years later, Egashira et al. (1993) addressed the impact of advancing age on endothelium-dependent vasodilation induced by acetylcholine in the coronary microcirculation. They studied a small number of subjects ($n = 18$; age range from 23 to 70 yr) with atypical chest pain but angiographically normal coronary arteries and no cardiovascular risk factor. In these subjects, the authors demonstrated that the acetylcholine-induced increase in coronary blood flow showed a highly significant inverse correlation with age ($r = -0.86$; $P < 0.001$) whereas the vascular effect of the endothelium-independent vasodilator adenosine was slightly affected by aging ($r = -0.44$, $P = 0.7$). However, again in aged individuals, these authors observed a paradoxical vasoconstrictor response to acetylcholine in epicardial coronary arteries. Thus, the blunted increase in coronary blood flow in these patients, especially at the highest dose of acetylcholine, might be explained by the constriction of epicardial arteries, leading to reduced vascular conductivity and thereby limiting the increases in blood flow, especially during high-flow states. Therefore, as in the previous studies, the possible presence of early atherosclerosis may represent a confounding factor to establish whether aging has a clear negative impact on endothelial function in humans.

Interestingly, Zeiher et al. (1993) addressed the effect of aging on endothelium-dependent vasodilation in a mixed population including normal subjects, patients with hypercholesterolemia, essential hypertension and coronary artery disease. Endothelial function was assessed as the response of epicardial diameter and coronary blood flow to injection of acetylcholine. Multivariate analysis using the stepwise multiple-regression technique revealed a significant negative correlation of acetylcholine-induced coronary blood flow responses with total cholesterol levels ($r = -0.70$; $P < 0.0001$) and with age ($r = -0.62$; $P < 0.0001$), whereas other risk factors were not independently related to the vasodilating effect of acetylcholine. It is worth noting that in this study the strongest relation between age and acetylcholine-mediated dilator capacity of the coronary microvasculature was observed in those patients who exhibited a dilator response of their epicardial conductance vessels to acetylcholine. Thus, these results first strongly suggested that aging per se contributes to the impaired acetylcholine-induced vasodilation of the human coronary microcirculation.

2.2. Studies in the peripheral circulation

However, the definitive conclusion that aging is associated with impaired endothelium-dependent vasodilation derives from studies in the peripheral circulation. Assessment of endothelial function in the peripheral vascular beds can be safely performed in large samples of population, including healthy subjects.

By injecting acetylcholine or metacholine into the brachial artery and measuring forearm blood flow (FBF) modifications by strain-gauge venous plethysmography, it was clearly demonstrated that advancing age can progressively alter endothelial function in humans (Taddei et al., 1995; Gerhard et al., 1996). In 53 healthy subjects (age range from 19 to 79 yr), with no cardiovascular risk factors, the maximum forearm vasodilating response to acetylcholine, as well as the slope of the FBF

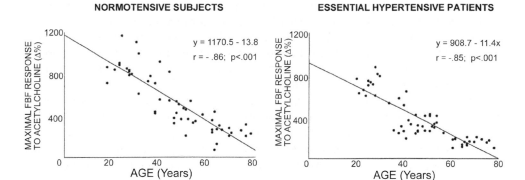

Fig. 1.   Scatterplot of relation between age (*x*-axis) and maximum of the FBF to acetylcholine (*y*-axis) in normotensive control subjects (left) and essential hypertensive patients (right). The maximum effect is calculated as percent increase above basal level (Taddei et al., 1995).

response to acetylcholine, showed a significant inverse correlation with increasing age (maximum FBF response: $r = -0.86$, $P < 0.001$; slope of the FBF response: $r = -0.83$, $P < 0.001$) (Fig. 1) (Taddei et al., 1995). On the other hand, vasodilation to sodium nitroprusside, an endothelium-independent vasodilator, was minimally affected by aging (maximum FBF response: $r = -0.37$, $P < 0.01$; slope of the FBF response: $r = -0.37$, $P < 0.01$). It is also important to observe that in this study older individuals were selected in order to have clinical characteristics (including blood pressure values, lipid and glucidic profile) comparable to those observed in the younger study population. This is an important issue in order to distinguish the direct impact of age on endothelial function from the confounding effect of the usual greater prevalence of cardiovascular risk factors that is generally observed in aged individuals.

These data were confirmed using metacholine as an endothelial agonist. In a very large study population of healthy subjects ($n = 119$; age range from 19 to 69 yr), Gerhard et al. (1996) observed an evident inverse correlation between advancing age and the response to metacholine ($r = -081$; $P < 0.001$), while no correlation was observed with the vasodilating effect of sodium nitroprusside ($r = -0.10$; $P = NS$).

Taken together, these results indicate that aging per se impairs endothelium-dependent vasodilation in healthy subjects, raising the possibility that this alteration could be one of the main mechanisms through which advancing age increases cardiovascular risk in humans.

3. Aging and endothelium-dependent vasodilation in patients with essential hypertension

The possibility that aging could have a negative impact on endothelial function in patients with essential hypertension is of extreme interest, since, as compared to normotensive subjects, hypertensive patients show impaired endothelial-dependent vasodilation (Linder et al., 1990; Panza et al., 1990; Taddei et al., 1993). Therefore, advancing age should have a negative additive effect in respect of a vascular endothelium which is already characterized by an altered function.

In line with this hypothesis, in 57 patients with essential hypertension (age range from 20 to 78 yr), increasing age showed an inverse correlation with the maximum FBF response to acetylcholine ($r = -0.85$; $P < 0.001$) as well as with the slope of the forearm blood response to acetylcholine ($r = -0.83$; $P < 0.001$) (Fig. 1) (Taddei et al., 1995). In contrast, forearm vasodilation to sodium nitroprusside showed a poor inverse correlation with patient age (maximum FBF response: $r = -0.36$, $P < 0.01$; slope of the FBF response: $r = -0.30$, $P < 0.05$). It is relevant that aging causes a similar degree of alteration in endothelium-dependent vasodilation in both normotensive subjects and essential hypertensive patients. This finding is of particular interest since it indicates that advancing age is such a powerful inductor of endothelial dysfunction that it is possible to detect its negative effect even in the presence of hypertension, which itself is a clinical condition able to cause impaired endothelium-dependent vasodilation.

4. Mechanisms responsible for age-induced endothelial dysfunction

4.1. *Alteration in the NO-pathway*

The mechanisms through which aging impairs endothelium-dependent vasodilation may involve various different alterations. In humans, it is possible to assess the integrity of the L-arginine NO pathway by evaluating the effect of L-arginine, the substrate for NO-synthase, or L-N(G)-monomethyl-arginine (L-NMMA), a selective inhibitor of NO-synthase, on vasodilation of acetylcholine (Lüscher and Noll, 1996). In normotensive subjects younger than 30 yr, L-arginine did not affect the vasodilation induced by acetylcholine (Taddei et al., 1997a), while L-NMMA clearly inhibited the relaxing effect of the muscarinic agonist (Taddei et al., 2001) (Fig. 2). Thus, at this age, endothelial function is preserved and sustained by NO-mediated bioactivity. In normotensive subjects aged between 31 and 60 yr, L-arginine was able to increase the blunted response to acetylcholine up to the level observed in the youngest subgroup. On the other hand, in the same age range, the degree of inhibition exerted by L-NMMA progressively declined (Fig. 2). Finally, in normotensive individuals older than 60 yr, L-arginine still exerted a potentiating effect on the response to acetylcholine, which, however, remained impaired as compared to the youngest subgroup (Taddei et al., 1997a). Moreover, L-NMMA no longer showed inhibitory ability on acetylcholine-induced vasodilation (Fig. 2) (Taddei et al., 2001). These results seem to indicate that in normotensive subjects age-related endothelial dysfunction is characterized by a progressive derangement in the L-arginine-NO pathway, which can be reversed by L-arginine administration, at least up to the age of 60. Beyond this age, NO availability seems to be totally compromised, since the response to acetylcholine is completely resistant to L-NMMA and can only minimally be improved by L-arginine administration.

It is interesting that in essential hypertensive patients a more serious derangement in the L-arginine NO pathway can be observed (Taddei et al., 1997a, 2001).

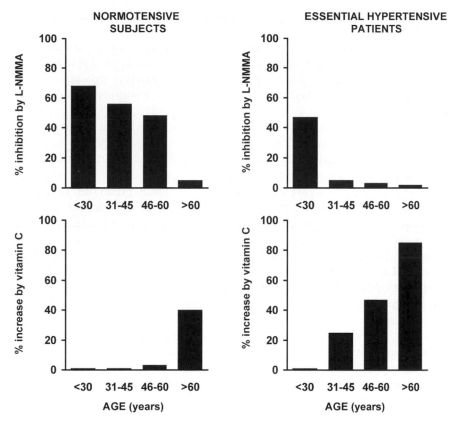

Fig. 2. Bars show the degree of inhibition and potentiation induced by L-NMMA and vitamin C, respectively, on FBF increase above basal induced by acetylcholine in four groups of normotensive subjects (left) and essential hypertensive patients (right) characterized by a different age profile (Taddei et al., 2001).

In young (< 30 yr) essential hypertensive patients, the blunted response to acetylcholine was restored by intrabrachial administration of L-arginine, while L-NMMA exerted a marked inhibitory effect (Fig. 2). In older hypertensive patients (between 31 and 45 yr), the facilitating effect of L-arginine or the inhibitory activity of L-NMMA was notably reduced (Fig. 2). Finally, in two further groups of older essential hypertensive patients (46–60 and >60 yr, respectively), L-arginine no longer improved vasodilation to acetylcholine (Taddei et al., 1997a) whereas the response to the muscarinic agonist was completely resistant to L-NMMA (Fig. 2) (Taddei et al., 2001). Taken together, and in comparison with evidence from healthy subjects, these results indicate that young hypertensive patients are characterized by an impairment in NO availability, which, however, seems to be reversible by L-arginine supplementation. As the effect of aging starts to be noticeable, the NO-pathway is completely compromised and no longer reversible by L-arginine.

4.2. *Production of endothelium-dependent contracting factors (EDCFs)*

Experimental evidence indicates that endothelial function can be impaired by the production of EDCFs (Miller and Vanhoutte, 1985; Altiere et al., 1986; Katusic and Vanhoutte, 1989). These substances can be cyclooxygenase prostanoids and/or oxygen free radicals. Cyclooxygenase itself can also be a source of oxidative stress (Cosentino et al., 1994).

Therefore, the possible impact of cyclooxygenase activity on age-related endothelial dysfunction was assessed by testing the effect of indomethacin on the vasodilating response to acetylcholine (Taddei et al., 1997a). In normotensive subjects younger than 30 yr, indomethacin did not affect the vasodilation induced by acetylcholine, confirming that at this age endothelial function is preserved. In normotensive subjects aged between 31 and 60 yr, indomethacin was still devoid of any effect on acetylcholine-induced vasodilation, but in normotensive individuals older than 60 yr, the cyclooxygenase inhibitor was able to increase the vascular response to acetylcholine. These results seem to indicate that in normotensive subjects, only after 60 yr does EDCF production participate in causing dysfunction of endothelium-dependent vasodilation. The same mechanism seems to operate in essential hypertensive patients, the only difference being the time of onset (Taddei et al., 1997a). Thus, in young (< 30 yr) essential hypertensive patients, the blunted response to acetylcholine was not affected by indomethacin administration. However, in older hypertensive patients (between 31 and 45 yr), indomethacin began to enhance the response to acetylcholine and the facilitating effect of the cyclooxygenase inhibitor became increasingly evident in the two further groups of older essential hypertensive patients (46–60 and >60 yr, respectively).

Since evidence in essential hypertensive patients seems to suggest that cyclooxygenase could be a source of oxidative stress (Taddei et al., 1997b, 1998), it was natural to propose testing the effect of an antioxidant such as vitamin C on age-related impaired endothelium-dependent vasodilation in both normotensive subjects and essential hypertensive patients.

Interestingly, the results obtained with vitamin C proved to be virtually superimpossible on those observed with indomethacin. Thus, in healthy subjects, vitamin C infusion into the brachial artery improved the impaired vasodilation to acetylcholine in aged (over 60 yr) individuals only, whereas in the younger subgroups, the antioxidant was devoid of any effect on the relaxing ability of the muscarinic agonist (Fig. 2) (Taddei et al., 2001). In essential hypertensive patients, the potentiating effect of vitamin C on acetylcholine-mediated vasodilation started to be evident after the age of 30 and the degree of potentiation progressively increased in parallel with advancing age (Fig. 2). It is important to observe that in essential hypertensive patients, vitamin C completely prevented the age-related reduction of endothelium-dependent vasodilation. Thus, in hypertensive patients aged more than 60 yr, the degree of vasodilation induced by acetylcholine, at the maximum infusion rate, in the simultaneous presence of vitamin C, was no longer different as compared to the vasodilation induced by acetylcholine in the youngest (age less than 30 yr) subgroup of hypertensive patients (Taddei et al., 2001). However, the most significant finding of the vitamin C study is probably related to the restoration of NO availability. Crucially, vitamin C is active only in those sub-groups of individuals (normotensive subjects and hypertensive patients older than 60 and 30 yr, respectively) who are also characterized by an L-NMMA-resistant response to acetylcholine. In these same patients, when L-NMMA was tested again in the presence of vitamin C administration, the ability of the NO-synthase inhibitor to blunt the vasodilating response to acetylcholine was restored (Taddei et al., 2001). Taken together, these results indicate that in healthy individuals oxidative stress, produced after a certain age, leads to a complete compromise of NO availability. This alteration seems to have much earlier onset in essential hypertensive patients.

4.3. *Is cyclooxygenase the source of oxidative stress in aging?*

No direct evidence is available in these patients to support the possibility that cyclooxygenase could be the source of oxidative stress. However, several indirect findings may at least suggest this possibility.

Thus, it has been demonstrated that these substances can curtail endothelium-dependent vasodilation not only by inducing vasoconstriction, but also by impairing the L-arginine-NO pathway. In essential hypertensive patients (aged around 50 yr), cyclooxygenase blockade by indomethacin restores the facilitating and inhibiting effect of L-arginine and L-NMMA on vasodilation to acetylcholine, respectively, indicating that cyclooxygenase-derived EDCFs can impair NO availability (Taddei et al., 1997b). Moreover, in a similar group of essential hypertensive patients, both indomethacin and vitamin C exerted a similar degree of facilitation on acetylcholine-induced vasodilation. However, when in the same patients, acetylcholine was repeated in the presence of the simultaneous infusion of indomethacin and vitamin C, no additive effect was observed (Taddei et al., 2001). Taken together, these results seem to indicate that in essential hypertensive patients cyclooxygenase could be a source of oxidative stress. Whether and to what degree cyclooxygenase-dependent prostanoids also take part in this vascular abnormality is still to be established, since at the present time, selective antagonists for the thromboxane A2/prostaglandin H2 receptor or inhibitors of thromboxane synthase are not available for intraarterial human utilization.

Therefore, the above-described conclusion that in essential hypertensive patients cyclooxygenase activity is a main source of oxidative stress, together with the almost identical effect of indomethacin and vitamin C on the response to acetylcholine in aged healthy subjects and hypertensive patients, allows the interpretation that aging could determine endothelial dysfunction at least partially by a mechanism involving cyclooxygenase as a major source of oxygen free radical production in human endothelial cells.

In conclusion, the relationship between aging and endothelial dysfunction seems to be mediated by different mechanisms depending on which age range is considered. In healthy individuals, the alteration seems to be caused by a primary alteration in the NO-L-arginine pathway, and only in the elderly, is production of oxidative stress a major cause of this alteration. By contrast, among essential hypertensive patients, in subjects younger than 30 yr, endothelial dysfunction seems to be selectively caused by a defect in the L-arginine-NO pathway. In patients older than 30 yr, production of oxidative stress (cyclooxygenase-dependent?) progressively increases in parallel with advancing age, and once oxidative stress production becomes detectable, NO availability appears completely compromised.

The possibility that oxidative stress could be one of the main determinants of age-related endothelial dysfunction is in line with experimental evidence. It is well documented that enhanced peroxynitrite (van der Loo et al., 2000) or superoxide (Hamilton et al., 2001) formation is associated with vascular aging.

A final comment opens up new avenues of research. Given this finding that the mechanisms responsible for aging and hypertension related endothelial dysfunction are the same, and that the only difference consists in time of appearance, a fascinating possibility, in agreement with experimental evidence (Hamilton et al., 2001), is that impaired endothelium-dependent vasodilation in essential hypertension could be just a mere acceleration of changes seen in advancing age.

5. Aging, gender and endothelial function

It is well documented that menopause and consequent estrogen deprivation increase the risk of cardiovascular disease in women (Kannel et al., 1976; Barrett-Connor and Bush, 1991). However, the mechanisms responsible for the cardioprotective effect of estrogen in women are not clear. Although the estrogen-mediated favorable effect on lipid profile can explain around 50% of the beneficial effect of this hormone on cardiovascular risk (Wahl et al., 1983; Lobo, 1990; Walsh et al., 1991; Collins et al., 1993), increasing evidence supports the possibility that estrogens can act directly on the arterial wall by improving endothelial function (Gisclard et al., 1998; Hayashi et al., 1992). Therefore, it is conceivable that the augmented prevalence of cardiovascular disease in post-menopausal women could be related to endothelial dysfunction caused by endogenous estrogen deficiency.

Celermajer et al. (1994) first studied endothelium-dependent vasodilation separately in men and women. They enrolled 238 subjects (103 men, 135 women, age range from 15 to 72 yr) and assessed endothelium-dependent vasodilation as brachial artery diameter increase (measured by vascular ultrasound) induced by reactive hyperemia (flow-mediated dilation, FMD) induced by distal post-ischemic vasodilation (obtained by deflating a pediatric cuff placed around the forearm and inflated up to 300 mm Hg for 4.5 min). In this study population, the authors observed that in men, FMD was preserved in subjects aged less than 40 yr, but declined thereafter at 0.21% per year. In women, FMD was stable until the early 1950s, after which it declined at 0.49% per year. The decline observed in women was significantly ($P = 0.002$) faster compared with men. Endothelium-independent vasodilation was assessed as brachial artery diameter modification induced by sublingual glyceryl trinitrate administration. Results showed no significant change in the vascular response with aging in either gender. The authors thus concluded that although endothelial dysfunction appears earlier in men than in women, the steep decline observed in women around the time of menopause is consistent with a protective effect of estrogen on the arterial wall.

The relationship between gender and endothelial function has been further addressed by evaluating whether the onset of menopause is associated with detectable impairment of endothelium-dependent vasodilation either in healthy women or female patients with essential hypertension (Taddei et al., 1996). To distinguish the possible role of menopause from the age-related decline in endothelial function, endothelium-dependent vasodilation was compared in matched women and men, to ascertain whether females are characterized by an attenuation of age-dependent endothelial dysfunction when still menstruating and by a sharp worsening after menopause compared to males.

In this study population (73 normotensive subjects: 37 women; 36 men; age range: 18–76 yr; 73 essential hypertensive patients: 36 women; 37 men; age range: 20–76 yr), the presence of endothelial dysfunction was confirmed in essential hypertension. In addition, in both normotensive and hypertensive subjects, a highly significant inverse correlation was confirmed between increasing age and response to acetylcholine (normotensive subjects: $r = -0.88$, $P < 0.001$; hypertensive patients: $r = -0.87$, $P < 0.001$) while only a weaker negative correlation was observed between the vasodilating effect of sodium nitroprusside and aging (normotensive subjects: $r = -46$, $P < 0.01$; hypertensive patients: $r = -48$, $P < 0.01$). These findings are in line with the above-commented evidence that aging is associated with endothelial dysfunction.

However, the main finding of this study was that menopause affects endothelium-dependent, but not endothelium-independent vasodilation both in normotensive subjects and essential hypertensive patients. Thus, in normotensive males, endothelial responses started to decline after age 30 yr, a derangement which was gradual and progressive until old age. By contrast, in premenopausal normotensive women, advancing age only slightly affected endothelium-dependent vasodilation, while after menopause, endothelium-dependent vasodilation showed a steeper decline as compared to men. But this gender-related difference in endothelium-dependent vasodilation was no longer evident after 60 yr. In male essential hypertensive patients, advancing age was associated with a decrease in endothelium-dependent vasodilation to acetylcholine, which was most evident up to 40 yr after which the rate of decline began to slow. The more rapid decline in endothelium-dependent vasodilation in younger hypertensive men as compared to those aged over 40 yr reinforces the earlier discussed possibility that hypertension anticipates age-related endothelial dysfunction. Moreover, the fact that after a certain age (around 40 yr) the decline seems to slow is probably explainable by the fact that response to acetylcholine cannot be depressed above a certain degree. In hypertensive women, at variance with these results observed in hypertensive males, endothelial dysfunction seems to exhibit the opposite pattern. Thus, the rate of age-related dysfunction in vasodilation induced by acetylcholine was evident but slower up to 44 yr, while a steeper decline commenced at around the age of menopause. In older groups (>60 yr), no difference was observed in the age-related decrease in endothelial function in women as compared to men. In both normotensive subjects and essential hypertensive patients, we observed no gender difference in the response to sodium nitroprusside.

Taken together, these results seem to indicate that while in normotensive males endothelial dysfunction associated with increasing age is a constant and homogenous event, in normotensive females menopause is a crucial moment characterized by a remarkable deterioration of endothelial function. Particularly noteworthy is the finding that in both male and female essential hypertensive patients impairment in endothelium-dependent vasodilation is already detectable in early age. However, in early maturity age-related endothelial dysfunction is more accentuated in male than in female hypertensive patients, while after age 60, the extent of impairment of endothelium-dependent vasodilation is lower in men than in post-menopausal women. These findings indicate that endogenous estrogen can protect endothelial function against the negative influence of aging both in normotensive and hypertensive women.

In conclusion, the present study indicates that both in normotensive and essential hypertensive females, menopause is associated with onset or worsening of aging-associated endothelial dysfunction, respectively, a finding which suggests that loss of endogenous estrogen could be a possible mechanism responsible for the acceleration of cardiovascular risk in post-menopausal women.

6. Clinical relevance of endothelial dysfunction in aging

Aging and hypertension are well documented cardiovascular risk factors (Roberts, 1980; Kannel et al., 1971). Moreover, it is well documented that endothelium plays a primary role in the control of vascular tone and structure (Lüscher and Vanhoutte, 1990). Therefore, the clinical relevance of the presence of endothelial dysfunction in aging is attributable to the fact that NO and EDCFs not only exert an opposite effect on vascular tone but also, respectively, inhibit and activate mechanisms such as platelet aggregation (Radomski et al., 1987), vascular smooth muscle cell proliferation (Garg and Hassid, 1989) and migration (Dubey and Lüscher, 1993), monocyte adhesion (Kubes et al., 1991) and adhesion molecule expression (De Caterina et al., 1995), which exerts an important role in the genesis of thrombosis and atherosclerotic plaque. Endothelial dysfunction is thus a mechanism promoting atherosclerosis and thrombosis or altering vasomotricity and thereby contributing to cardiovascular events. This concept is reinforced by the evidence that endothelial dysfunction is not specific to aging, gender and essential hypertension. Rather, it is a common alteration of the major cardiovascular risk factors, including hypercholesterolemia (Creager et al., 1990; Casino et al., 1993), diabetes mellitus (Williams et al., 1996; Ting et al., 1996), smoking (Celermajer et al., 1996; Heitzer et al., 1996), and hyperhomocysteinemia (Tawakol et al., 1997; Virdis et al., 2001). It is conceivable that such an alteration may be a common pathogenetic mechanism determining cardiovascular events in patients with cardiovascular risk factors.

6.1. *Association of endothelial dysfunction with markers of vascular damage and with cardiovascular events*

Evidence is mounting that the presence of endothelial dysfunction is associated with markers of vascular damage and with cardiovascular events. In essential hypertensive patients, impaired forearm response to acetylcholine is correlated with intima-media thickening of carotid arteries, an index of atherosclerosis (Ghiadoni et al., 1998). Moreover, in epicardial coronary arteries of normotensive subjects, the response to acetylcholine shows an inverse correlation with intramural plaque as detected by intravascular ultrasounds (Zeiher et al., 1994). Finally, in epicardial coronary arteries of patients with cardiac transplantation, endothelial dysfunction is a predictor of the subsequent development of arteriolosclerosis (Davis et al., 1996).

It should be kept in mind that the presence of endothelial dysfunction has been associated with the occurrence of cardiovascular events in longitudinal studies. Suwaidi et al. (2000) evaluated the outcome of patients with mild coronary artery disease on the basis of endothelial function. Only patients with severe endothelial dysfunction (assessed as coronary microcirculatory response to acetylcholine) had cardiovascular events in a mean follow-up period of 28 months (range, 11–52 months). Similar results were obtained by Schachinger et al. (2000), who demonstrated that cardiovascular events (in a median follow-up period of 7.7 yr) had a significantly greater association with coronary endothelial dysfunction, assessed as response to intracoronary acetylcholine, sympathetic activation by the cold pressure test and FMD induced by distal infusion of papaverine. Furthermore, the presence of endothelial dysfunction in the peripheral large arteries (FMD in the brachial artery) has also been associated with increased coronary events (Neunteufl et al., 2000). Finally, Heitzer et al. (2001) showed that in the forearm macrocirculation of 281 patients with coronary artery disease, during a follow-up period of 4.5 yr, the degree of vasodilation to acetylcholine and the facilitating effect of vitamin C coinfusion were independent predictors of cardiovascular events.

Although these studies may be biased by low numerosity in the study population, concordant evidence is accumulating which demonstrates that endothelial dysfunction acts as a pathogenetic mechanism causing cardiovascular disease.

7. Is aging-related endothelial dysfunction reversible?

If endothelial dysfunction could be shown to be one of the main pathogenetic mechanisms through which advancing age acts as a promoter of atherosclerosis and cardiovascular events, it would be clinically relevant to prevent this vascular alteration.

At the present time, available evidence indicates that the only intervention which proves to be effective in preventing age-related impaired endothelium-dependent vasodilation is dynamic physical activity.

Endothelial function was assessed as forearm vasodilator response to acetylcholine and sodium nitroprusside in 12 young and elderly (age 26.9 ± 2.3 and

62.9 ± 5.8 yr, respectively) healthy subjects and 11 young and 14 matched endurance athletes (age 27.5 ± 1.9 and 66.4 ± 6.1 yr) (Taddei et al., 2000). In young sedentary individuals and athletes, the vasodilating response to acetylcholine was not different. In both elderly sedentary subjects and athletes, vasodilation to acetylcholine was found to be reduced as compared to younger subgroups. However, in elderly endurance exercise trained men, the vasodilating effect was significantly increased as compared to healthy, but sedentary individuals of the same age. Since the response to sodium nitroprusside was similar between trained and nontrained groups, these results indicate that in healthy individual dynamic physical activity can partially prevent age-related endothelial dysfunction.

As regards the mechanism responsible for the beneficial effect of exercise, available evidence seems to indicate that physical activity can prevent age-related onset of oxidative stress. In young sedentary and trained subjects, vasodilation to acetylcholine was inhibited by L-NMMA and remained unchanged by vitamin C. In elderly athletes, the response to acetylcholine, albeit reduced, was still sensitive to L-NMMA and not modified by vitamin C administration (Fig. 3). By contrast, in elderly healthy sedentary subjects, the vasodilating effect induced by the endothelial agonist proved not only to be decreased as compared to trained individuals, but also resistant to L-NMMA (Fig. 3). Moreover, in this sedentary subgroup, vitamin C administration was able to increase the response to acetylcholine and restore the inhibiting activity of L-NMMA up to values observed in elderly trained individuals (Fig. 3) (Taddei et al., 2000).

Taken together, these results indicate that in young healthy individuals, when endothelial function is normal, physical activity has no additive beneficial effect. In contrast, dynamic exercise can partially prevent age-related endothelial dysfunction by a mechanism probably involving antioxidant activity and the consequent preservation of NO availability.

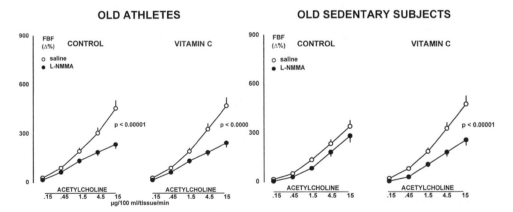

Fig. 3.   Line graphs show the forearm vasodilation induced by intrabrachial administration of acetylcholine during saline L-NMMA, in the absence and presence of vitamin C, in old (>60 yr) athletes and sedentary subjects. Results are represented as percent FBF changes as compared to baseline (Taddei et al., 2000).

Finally, the question of the amount of exercise and training required in order for sedentary individuals to obtain an improvement of endothelium-dependent vasodilation has also been addressed. In a cross-sectional study, DeSouza et al. (2000) confirmed that regular aerobic exercise prevents the age-related decline in forearm endothelium-dependent vasodilation to acetylcholine in healthy men. Furthermore, the novel finding of this study is the demonstration of a beneficial effect of an intervention trial. Thirteen sedentary middle aged and elderly healthy men (age 56 ± 2 yr) underwent a 3-month exercise training program, consisting of 30 min of walking per day, 3–4 days per week, at an intensity of around 60% of their individually determined maximal heart rate. This training program did not change the clinical characteristics of the study subjects, including body weight, blood pressure or lipid and glucidic profile, but significantly increased the forearm vasodilation induced by intrabrachial infusion of acetylcholine, without modification in the response to sodium nitroprusside. After the training program, endothelium-dependent vasodilation was no longer different from that observed in endurance trained individuals of the same age. Therefore, this study demonstrates that the negative effect of aging on endothelium-dependent vasodilation can be prevented by a home-based aerobic exercise training and with a mode (walking) and intensity (moderate) of exercise that can safely be performed by most if not all sedentary healthy older men.

Data indicating whether other types of therapeutic intervention, such as L-arginine or antioxidant supplementation, could be effective in preventing age-related endothelial dysfunction would be of extreme interest, but remain to be determined.

8. Conclusions

Aging is associated with the development of cardiovascular structural and functional alterations, which can explain the age-related increase in cardiovascular risk. Available data indicate that aging causes endothelial dysfunction both in normotensive subjects and in essential hypertensive patients. This alteration is caused by a progressive impairment of the L-arginine-NO pathway and production of cyclooxygenase-dependent EDCFs and oxygen free radicals. Once EDCF production becomes detectable, NO availability proves to be completely compromised.

Essential hypertension seems to anticipate and amplify the negative impact of aging on endothelial function. In contrast, endogenous estrogen probably protects premenopausal women from the negative effect of aging on endothelium-dependent vasodilation.

Since endothelial dysfunction is a strong predictor of cardiovascular events, the possibility exists that impairment in endothelium-dependent vasodilation could represent one of the main mechanisms through which advancing age leads to the development of atherosclerotic lesions and, therefore, of cardiovascular events. If this hypothesis is well founded, the correction of endothelial dysfunction could be a rational therapeutic target. In this regard, results are available indicating that dynamic exercise trained individuals are characterized by preserved endothelium-dependent vasodilation while a moderate training program can improve endothelial function in aged healthy individuals. It may thus be suggested that any therapeutic intervention which prevents or reverses endothelial dysfunction associated with advancing age could reduce age-related vascular alterations and consequently also the age-related increase in cardiovascular risk.

References

Altiere, R.J., Kiritsy-Roy, J.A., Catravas, J.D., 1986. Acetylcholine-induced contractions in isolated rabbit pulmonary arteries: role of thromboxane A2. J. Pharmacol. Exp. Ther. 236, 535–541.

Arai, H., Hori, S., Aramori, I., Ohkubo, H., Nakanishi, S., 1990. Cloning and expression of a cDNA encoding an endothelin receptor. Nature 348, 730–732.

Barrett-Connor, E., Bush, T.L., 1991. Estrogen and coronary heart disease in women. JAMA 265, 1861–1867.

Bredt, D.S., Hwang, P.M., Glatt, C.E., Lowenstein, C., Reed, R.R., Snyder, S.H., 1991. Cloned and expressed nitric oxide synthase structurally resembles cytochrome P-450 reductase. Nature 351, 714.

Casino, P.R., Kilcoyne, C.M., Quyyumi, A.A., Hoeg, J.M., Panza, J.A., 1993. The role of nitric-oxide in endothelium-dependent vasodilation of hypercholesterolemic patients. Circulation 88, 2541–2547.

Celermajer, D.S., Sorensen, K.E., Spiegelhalter, D.J., Georgakopoulos, D., Robinson, J., Deanfield, J.E., 1994. Aging is associated with endothelial dysfunction in healthy men years before the age-related decline in women. J. Am. Coll. Cardiol. 24, 471–476.

Celermajer, D.S., Adams, M.R., Clarkson, P., Robinson, J., McCredie, R., Donald, A., Deanfield, J.E., 1996. Passive smoking and impaired endothelium-dependent arterial dilatation in healthy young adults. N. Engl. J. Med. 334, 150–154.

Cohen, R.A., Vanhoutte, P.M., 1995. Endothelium-dependent hyperpolarization-beyond nitric oxide and cyclic GMP. Circulation 92, 3337–3349.

Collins, P., Rosano, G.M.C., Jiang, C., Lindsay, D., Sarrel, P.M., Poole-Wilson, P.A., 1993. Hypothesis: cardiovascular protection by oestrogen – a calcium antagonist effect? Lancet 341, 1264–1265.

Cosentino, F., Sill, J.C., Katusic, Z.S., 1994. Role of superoxide anions in the mediation of endothelium-dependent contractions. Hypertension 23, 229–235.

Creager, M.A., Cooke, J.P., Mendelsohn, M.E., Gallagher, S.J., Coleman, S.M., Loscalzo, J., Dzau, V.J., 1990. Impaired vasodilation of forearm resistance vessels in hypercholesterolemic humans. J. Clin. Invest. 86, 228–234.

Davis, S.F., Yeung, A.C., Meredith, I.T., Charbonneau, F., Ganz, P., Selwyn, A.P., Anderson, T.J., 1996. Early endothelial dysfunction predicts the development of transplant coronary artery disease at 1 year posttransplant. Circulation 93, 457–462.

De Caterina, R., Libby, P., Peng, H.B., Thannickal, V.J., Rajavashisth, T.B., Gimbrone, M.A., Shin, W.S., Liao, J.K., 1995. Nitric oxide decreases cytokine-induced endothelial activation. J. Clin. Invest. 96, 60–68.

De Nucci, G., Thomas, R., D'Orleans Juste, P., Antunes, E., Walder, C., Warner, T.D., Vane, J.R., 1988. Pressor effects of circulating endothelin are limited by its removal in the pulmonary circulation and by the release of prostacyclin and endothelium-derived relaxing factor. Proc. Natl. Acad. Sci. USA 85, 9797–9800.

DeSouza, C.A., Shapiro, L.F., Clevenger, C.M., Dinenno, F.A., Monahan, K.D., Tanaka, H., Seals, D.R., 2000. Regular aerobic exercise prevents and restores age-related declines in endothelium-dependent vasodilation in healthy men. Circulation 102, 1351–1357.

Dohi, Y., Thiel, M.A., Bühler, F.R., Lüscher, T.F., 1990. Activation of endothelial L-arginine pathway in pressurized mesenteric resistance arteries: effect of age and hypertension. Hypertension 15, 170–175.

Dubey, O.B., Lüscher, T.F., 1993. Nitric oxide inhibits angiotensin II induced migration of vascular smooth muscle cells. Hypertension 22, 412–416.

Egashira, K., Inou, T., Hirooka, Y., Kai, H., Sugimachi, M., Suzuki, S., Kuga, T., Urabe, Y., Takeshita, A., 1993. Effects of age on endothelium-dependent vasodilation of resistance coronary artery by acetylcholine in humans. Circulation 88, 77–81.

Furchgott, R.F., Zawadzky, J.V., 1980. The obligatory role of endothelial cells in the relaxation of arterial smooth muscle by acetylcholine. Nature 288, 373–376.

Garg, U.C., Hassid, A., 1989. Nitric oxide-generating vasodilators and 8-bromo-cyclic guanosine monophosphate inhibit mitogenesis and proliferation of cultured rat vascular smooth muscle cells. J. Clin. Invest. 83, 1774–1777.

Gerhard, M., Roddy, M.A., Creager, S.J., Creager, M.A., 1996. Aging progressively impairs endothelium-dependent vasodilation in forearm resistance vessels of humans. Hypertension 27, 849–853.

Ghiadoni, L., Taddei, S., Virdis, A., Sudano, I., Di Legge, V., Meola, M., Di Venanzio, L., Salvetti, A., 1998. Endothelial function and common carotid wall thickening in essential hypertensive patients. Hypertension 32, 25–32.

Gisclard, V., Miller, V.M., Vanhoutte, P.M., 1988. Effect of 17beta-estradiol on endothelium-dependent responses in the rabbit. J. Pharmacol. Exp. Ther. 244, 19–22.

Gryglewski, R.J., Palmer, R.M.J., Moncada, S., 1986. Superoxide anion is involved in the breakdown of endothelium-derived vascular relaxing factor. Nature 320, 454–456.

Hamilton, C.A., Brosnan, M.J., McIntyre, M., Graham, D., Dominiczak, A.F., 2001. Superoxide excess in hypertension and aging: a common cause of endothelial dysfunction. Hypertension 37 (2; Part 2), 529–534.

Hayashi, T., Fukuto, J.M., Ignarro, L.J., Chaudhuri, G., 1992. Basal release of nitric oxide from aortic rings is greater in female rabbits than in male rabbits: implications for atherosclerosis. Proc. Natl. Acad. Sci. USA 89, 11259–11263.

Haynes, W.G., Strachan, F.E., Webb, D.J., 1995. Endothelin ETA and ETB receptors cause vasoconstriction of human resistance and capacitance vessels in vivo. Circulation 92, 357–363.

Heitzer, T., Ylä-Herttauala, S., Luoma, J., Kurz, S., Münzel, T., Just, H., Olschewski, M., Drexeler, H., 1996. Cigarette smoking potentiates endothelial dysfunction of forearm resistance vessels in patients with hypercholesterolemia. Role of oxidized LDL. Circulation 93, 1346–1353.

Heitzer, T., Schlinzig, T., Krohn, K., Meinertz, T., Munzel, T., 2001. Endothelial dysfunction, oxidative stress, and risk of cardiovascular events in patients with coronary artery disease. Circulation 104, 2673–2678.

Hongo, K., Nakagomi, T., Kassel, N.F., Sasaki, T., Lehmann, M., Vollmer, D.G., Tsukahara, T., Ogawa, H., Torner, J., 1988. Effects of aging and hypertension on endothelium-dependent vascular relaxation in rat carotid artery. Stroke 19, 892–897.

Inoue, A., Yanagisawa, M., Kimura, S., Kasuya, Y., Miyauchi, T., 1989. The human endothelin family: 3 structurally and pharmacologically distinct isopeptides predicted by 3 separate genes. Proc. Natl. Acad. Sci. USA 86, 2863–2867.

Kannel, W.B., Gordon, T., Schwartz, M.J., 1971. Systolic versus diastolic blood pressure and risk of coronary artery disease: the Framingham Study. Am. J. Cardiol. 27, 335–346.

Kannel, W.B., Hjortland, M.C., McNamara, P.M., 1976. Menopause and the risk of cardiovascular disease: the Framingham Study. Ann. Intern. Med. 8 S, 447–456.

Katusic, Z.S., Vanhoutte, P.M., 1989. Superoxide anion is an endothelium-derived contracting factor. Am. J. Physiol. 257, H33–H37.

Kubes, P., Suzuki, M., Granger, D.N., 1991. Nitric oxide: an endogenous modulator of leucocyte adhesion. Proc. Natl. Acad. Sci. USA 88, 4651–4655.

Linder, L., Kiowski, W., Buhler, F.R., Luscher, T.F., 1990. Indirect evidence for the release of endothelium-derived relaxing factor in the human forearm circulation in vivo: blunted response in essential hypertension. Circulation 81, 1762–1767.

Lobo, R.A., 1990. Estrogen and cardiovascular disease. Ann. NY Acad. Sci. 592, 286–294.

Lüscher, T.F., Vanhoutte, P.M., 1990. The Endothelium: Modulator of Cardiovascular Function. CRC Press, Boca Raton, FL.

Lüscher, T.F., Noll, G., 1996. Endothelial function as an end-point in intervention trials: concepts, methods and current data. J. Hypertens. 14 (Suppl. 2), S111–S121.

Mayhan, W.G., Faraci, F.M., Baumbach, G.L., Heistad, D.D., 1990. Effects of aging on responses of cerebral arterioles. Am. J. Physiol. 258, H1138–H1143.

Miller, V.M., Vanhoutte, P.M., 1985. Endothelium-dependent contractions to arachidonic acid are mediated by products of cyclooxygenase. Am. J. Physiol. 248, H432–H437.

Moritoki, H., Hosoki, E., Ishida, Y., 1986. Age-related decrease in endothelium-dependent dilator response to histamine in rat mesenteric artery. Eur. J. Pharmacol. 126, 61–67.

Neunteufl, T., Heher, S., Katzenschlager, R., Wolfl, G., Kostner, K., Maurer, G., Weidinger, F., 2000. Late prognostic value of flow-mediated dilation in the brachial artery of patients with chest pain. Am. J. Cardiol. 86 (2), 207–210.

Palmer, R.M.J., Ferrige, A.G., Moncada, S., 1987. Nitric oxide release accounts for the biological activity of endothelium-derived relaxing factor. Nature 327, 524–526.

Palmer, R.M.J., Ashton, D.S., Moncada, S., 1998. Vascular endothelial cells synthesize nitric oxide from L-arginine. Nature 333, 664–666.

Panza, J.A., Quyyumi, A.A., Brush Jr., J.E., Epstein, S.E., 1990. Abnormal endothelium dependent vascular relaxation in patients with essential hypertension. N. Engl. J. Med. 323, 22–27.

Panza, J.A., Casino, P.R., Kilcoyne, C.M., Quyyumi, A.A., 1993. Role of endothelium-derived nitric oxide in the abnormal endothelium-dependent vascular relaxation of patients with essential hypertension. Circulation 87, 1468–1474.

Radomski, M.W., Palmer, R.M.J., Moncada, S., 1987. Endogenous nitric oxide inhibits human platelet adhesion to vascular endothelium. Lancet 2, 1057–1068.

Roberts, W.C., 1980. The hypertensive diseases. In: Laragh, J.H. (Ed.), Topics in Hypertension, vol. 17. York Medical Books, New York, NY, pp. 368–388.

Rubanyi, G.M., Romero, J.C., Vanhoutte, P.M., 1986. Flow-induced release of endothelium-derived relaxing factor. Am. J. Physiol. 250, H1145–H1149.

Schachinger, V., Britten, M.B., Zeiher, A.M., 2000. Prognostic impact of coronary vasodilator dysfunction on adverse long-term outcome of coronary heart disease. Circulation 101, 1899–1906.

Seo, B., Oemar, B.S., Siebermann, R., Segesser, L., Luscher, T., 1994. Both ETA and ETB receptors mediate contraction to endothelin-1 in human blood vessels. Circulation 89, 1203–1208.

Soltis, E.E., 1987. Effect of age on blood pressure and membrane-dependent vascular responses in the rat. Circ. Res. 61, 889–897.

Suwaidi, J.A., Hamasaki, S., Higano, S.T., Nishimura, R.A., Holmes Jr., D.R., Lerman, A., 2000. Long-term follow-up of patients with mild coronary artery disease and endothelial dysfunction. Circulation 101, 948–954.

Taddei, S., Virdis, A., Mattei, P., Salvetti, A., 1993. Vasodilation to acetylcholine in primary and secondary forms of human hypertension. Hypertension 21, 929–933.

Taddei, S., Virdis, A., Mattei, P., Ghiadoni, L., Gennari, A., Basile-Fasolo, C., Sudano, I., Salvetti, A., 1995. Aging and endothelial function in normotensive subjects and essential hypertensive patients. Circulation 91, 1981–1987.

Taddei, S., Virdis, A., Ghiadoni, L., Mattei, P., Sudano, I., Bernini, G.P., Pinto, S., Salvetti, A., 1996. Menopause is associated with endothelial dysfunction in women. Hypertension 28, 576–582.

Taddei, S., Virdis, A., Mattei, P., Ghiadoni, L., Basile-Fasolo, C., Sudano, I., Salvetti, A., 1997a. Hypertension causes premature aging of endothelial function in humans. Hypertension 29, 736–743.

Taddei, S., Virdis, A., Ghiadoni, L., Magagna, A., Salvetti, A., 1997b. Cyclooxygenase inhibition restores nitric oxide activity in essential hypertension. Hypertension 29 (Part 2), 274–279.

Taddei, S., Virdis, A., Ghiadoni, L., Magagna, A., Salvetti, A., 1998. Vitamin C improves endothelium-dependent vasodilation by restoring nitric oxide activity in essential hypertension. Circulation 97, 2222–2229.

Taddei, S., Galetta, F., Virdis, A., Ghiadoni, L., Solvetti, G., Franzoni, F., Giusti, C., Salvetti, A., 2000. Physical activity prevents age-related impairment in nitric oxide availability in elderly athletes. Circulation 101, 2896–2901.

Taddei, S., Virdis, A., Ghiadoni, L., Salvetti, G., Bernini, G., Magagna, A., Salvetti, A., 2001. Age-related reduction of NO availability and oxidative stress in humans. Hypertension 38, 274–279.

Tawakol, A., Omland, T., Gerhard, M., Wu, J.T., Creager, M.A., 1997. Hyperhomocyst(e)inemia is associated with impaired endothelium-dependent vasodilation in humans. Circulation 95, 1119–1121.

Ting, H.H., Timini, F.K., Boles, K.S., Creager, S.J., Ganz, P., Creager, M.A., 1996. Vitamin C improves endothelium-dependent vasodilation in patients with non-insulin-dependent diabetes mellitus. J. Clin. Invest. 97, 22–28.

Tsukahara, H., Ende, H., Magazine, H.I., Bahou, W.F., Gologorsky, M.S., 1994. Molecular and functional characterization of the non-isopeptide-selective ETB receptor in endothelial cells: receptor coupling to nitric oxide synthase. J. Biol. Chem. 269, 21778–21785.

van der Loo, B., Labugger, R., Skepper, J.N., Bachschmid, M., Kilo, J., Powell, J.M., Palacios-Callender, M., Erusalimsky, J.D., Quaschning, T., Malinski, T., Gygi, D., Ullrich, V., Luscher, T.F., 2000. Enhanced peroxynitrite formation is associated with vascular aging. J. Exp. Med. 192, 1731–1744.

Virdis, A., Ghiadoni, L., Cardinal, H., Favilla, S., Duranti, P., Birindelli, R., Magagna, A., Solvetti, G., Taddei, A., Solvetti, A., 2001. Mechanisms responsible for endothelial dysfunction induced by fasting hyperhomocyst(e)inemia in humans. J. Am. Coll. Cardiol. 38, 1106–1115.

Vita, J.A., Treasure, C.B., Nabel, E.G., McLenachan, J.M., Fish, R.D., Yeung, A.C., Vekshtein, V.I., Selwyn, A.P., Ganz, P., 1990. Coronary vasomotor response to acetylcholine relates to risk factors for coronary artery disease. Circulation 81, 491–497.

Wahl, P., Walden, C., Knopp, R., Hoover, J., Wallace, R., Heiss, G., Rifkind, B., 1983. Effect of estrogen/progestin potency on lipid/lipoprotein cholesterol. N. Engl. J. Med. 308, 862–867.

Walsh, B.W., Schiff, I., Rosner, B., Greenberg, L., Ravnikar, V., Sacks, F.M., 1991. Effects of postmenopausal estrogen replacement therapy on the concentrations and metabolism of plasma lipoproteins. N. Engl. J. Med. 325, 1196–1204.

Williams, S.B., Cusco, J.A., Roddy, M.-A., Johnstone, M.T., Creager, M.A., 1996. Impaired nitric oxide mediated vasodilation in patients with non insulin-dependent diabetes mellitus. J. Am. Coll. Cardiol. 27, 567–574.

Yanagisawa, M., Kurihawa, H., Kimura, S., Tomobe, Y., Koboyashi, M., Mitsui, Y., Yazaki, Y., Goto, K., Masaki, T., 1988. A novel potent vasoconstrictor peptide produced by vascular endothelial cells. Nature 332, 411–415.

Yasue, H., Matsuyama, K., Matsuyama, K., Okumura, K., Morikami, Y., Ogawa, H., 1990. Responses of angiographically normal human coronary arteries to intracoronary injection of acetylcholine by age and segment. Possible role of early coronary atherosclerosis. Circulation 81, 482–490.

Zeiher, A.M., Drexter, H., Saurbier, B., Just, H., 1993. Endothelium-mediated coronary blood flow modulation in humans. Effects of age, atherosclerosis, hypercholesterolemia, and hypertension. J. Clin. Invest. 92, 652–662.

Zeiher, A.M., Schachlinger, V., Hohnloser, S.H., Saurbier, B., Just, H., 1994. Coronary atherosclerotic wall thickening and vascular reactivity in humans. Elevated high-density lipoprotein levels ameliorate abnormal vasoconstriction in early atherosclerosis. Circulation 89, 2525–2532.

Advances in
Cell Aging and
Gerontology

Alterations of ion channels in vascular muscle cells and endothelial cells during hypertension and aging

Yusuke Ohya* and Masatoshi Fujishima

*Department of Medicine and Clinical Science, Graduate School of Medical Sciences,
Kyushu University, Maidashi 3-1-1, Higashi-ku, Fukuoka 812-8582, Japan*

Contents

* Corresponding author. Present address. Third Department of Internal Medicine, School of Medicine, University of Ryukyus, 207 Uehara, Nishihara-cho, Okinawa 903-0215, Japan Tel.: +81-98-895-1150; fax: +81-98-895-1416.

E-mail address: ohya@med.u-ryukyu.ac.jp (Y. Ohya).

Advances in Cell Aging and Gerontology, vol. 11, 165–182

Abbreviations

Ca^{2+}	calcium
SHRs	spontaneously hypertensive rats
WKY	Wistar Kyoto rats
K^+	potassium
K_{Ca} channel	Ca^{2+}-activated K^+ channel
K_V channel	delayed voltage-dependent K^+ channel
K_{ATP}	ATP-sensitive K^+ channel
K_{IR}	inwardly rectifying K^+ channel
$[Ca^{2+}]$	intracellular concentration of Ca^{2+}
BK_{Ca}	large-conductance K_{Ca} channel
MRNA	messenger ribonucleic acid
ACE	angiotensin-converting enzyme
4-AP	4-aminopyridine
DOCA	deoxycorticosterone acetate
GDP	guanosine diphosphate
UDP	uridine diphosphate
Camp	cyclic adenosine monophosphate
NO	nitric oxide
Cl^-	chloride
PGH_2	prostaglandin H_2
EDHF	endothelium-derived hyperpolarizing factor(s)
NAD(P)H	nicotinamide adenosine dinucleotide (phosphate)

1. Introduction

Growing evidence suggests that properties of ion channels in vascular cells, including smooth muscle cells and endothelial cells, are altered during various disease states including hypertension and during aging. A patch-clamp technique enables us to record macroscopic currents (whole-cell currents) and unit currents (single-channel currents), and evaluate the functional alteration of ion channels. In addition, recent progress in the molecular biology also facilitates qualitative and quantitative evaluation of ion channels, although only a few studies have examined vascular tissues. In this review, we attempt to summarize information regarding the alteration of ion channels in vascular muscle cells and endothelial cells during hypertension and aging. Due to the limited space available, we do not review the basic characteristics of ion channels and their regulation by various vasoactive substances. For such information, several good reviews are available (Hughe, 1995; Beech, 1997; Quayle et al., 1997; Jackson, 2000; Hill et al., 2001; Nilius and Droogmans, 2001; Sobey, 2001).

2. Smooth muscle cells

2.1. *Alteration during hypertension*

2.1.1. *Voltage-operated calcium (Ca^{2+}) channels*
In vascular muscle cells, Ca^{2+} influx through voltage-operated Ca^{2+} channels, receptor-operated channels (including store-operated channels), and mechano-sensitive channels, as well as Ca^{2+} release from intracellular store sites is an important trigger of muscle contraction (Fig. 1). Several types of voltage-operated Ca^{2+} channels exist in vascular smooth muscles. The L-type Ca^{2+} channel, which is sensitive to dihydropyridine derivatives, appears to be dominant in most vascular muscle cells (Hughe, 1995); however, fast-inactivating, dihydropyridine-insensitive channels also exist in some vessels (Hughe, 1995; Ohya and Sperelakis, 1989; Morita et al., 1999).

2.1.1.1. Alteration in spontaneously hypertensive rats (SHRs) In arterial muscle cells, membrane potentials are more depolarized in hypertensive rats than in their nor-motensive controls (Chung, 1984; Fujii et al., 1992; Wellman et al., 2001). Thus, depolarization stimulates opening of voltage-operated Ca^{2+} channels in vascular muscles. In addition, accumulating evidence suggests that the activity of L-type Ca^{2+} channels is enhanced in hypertensive rats, regardless of membrane potential levels. Patch-clamp experiments show that the amplitudes of macroscopic current through L-type Ca^{2+} channels are increased in arterial muscle cells from SHR compared to those from Wistar Kyoto rats (WKY). This was firstly reported in cultured venous cells (Rusch and Hermsmeyer, 1988), and then in freshly isolated muscle cells from the mesenteric artery (Ohya et al., 1993; Cox and Lozinskaya, 1995), cerebral artery (Wilde et al., 1994), and renal resistance artery (Gelband et al., 1999).

Amplitudes of the L-type Ca^{2+} channel currents (current densities) are greater in SHR than in WKY at all membrane potential levels. In addition, no apparent changes are observed in the voltage-dependent kinetics (both activation and inacti-vation) of L-type Ca^{2+} channels in arterial muscle cells between SHR and WKY (Ohya et al., 1993; Cox and Lozinskaya, 1995; Wilde et al., 1994; Gelband et al., 1999). However, one study has shown that both activation and inactivation curves of L-type Ca^{2+} channels are negatively shifted in arterial muscle cells from SHR-SP (Self et al., 1994). Thus, the voltage-dependent kinetics of the L-type Ca^{2+} channels are not altered in arterial muscle cells from hypertensive rats, although some dis-crepancy exists.

The alteration of L-type Ca^{2+} channels is also demonstrated by single-channel recording with the cell-attached patch-clamp recording. The channel opening is more frequent in mesenteric arterial muscle cells from SHR than in those from WKY (Ohya et al., 1998). This observation suggests that the channel availability (the product of open probability of the channel and the number of functional channels) is increased in SHR membrane. In contrast, other parameters, such as the single-channel conductance (amplitude of the single-channel current) and the mean open time of unit currents, do not differ between SHR and WKY.

Amounts of the channels distributed in the cell membrane, could be estimated by the numbers of dihydropyridine binding sites and expression levels of L-type Ca^{2+} channel protein. The numbers of dihydropyridine (PN200-110) binding sites to the aortic membrane do not differ between SHR and WKY (Ikeda et al., 1994). In contrast, one preliminary report has shown that the dihydropyridine (PN200-110) binding is greater in the tail artery from SHR rather than in WKY (Galletti et al., 1991). In another report, an increased number of dihydropyridine (nicardipine) binding sites have been noted in the pulmonary artery and vein from SHR, as compared with WKY (Ricci et al., 2000). On the contrary, only one study has examined the expression of L-type Ca^{2+} channel protein in arterial tissues from hypertensive animals. Western blot analysis has shown that levels of α subunit of the L-type Ca^{2+} channel in small renal arteries do not differ between SHR and WKY (Gelband et al., 1999). An accumulation of data is needed to know whether the number of the functional channels is increased.

One study has shown that the amplitude of Ca^{2+} currents in arterial muscle cells is larger in SHR than in WKY at all ages examined from 5 to 23 weeks of age (Lozinskaya and Cox, 1997). These authors have also shown that the increased Ca^{2+} channel activity parallels blood pressure levels among all ages. In contrast, another study has shown that the difference in the current amplitude of L-type Ca^{2+} channel currents decreases after hypertension is established in adult SHR (Ohya et al., 1993). Further information is necessary to understand the contribution of altered L-type Ca^{2+} channel activity to the development and maintenance of hypertension.

The alteration of L-type Ca^{2+} channels appears in cultured venous muscle cells (Rusch and Hermsmeyer, 1988), which are not exposed to pressure stress, and in muscle cells from arteries of young SHR (5 weeks old) (Ohya et al., 1993), in which blood pressure is not apparently different from WKY, this alteration results from the genetic background of this model. Systemic administration of antisense to angiotensin II type 1 receptor gene or to angiotensin-converting enzyme (ACE) gene normalizes the blood pressure of SHR (Gelband et al., 1999, 2000). This therapy also normalizes the alteration of L-type Ca^{2+} channel currents in renal artery muscle cells of SHR. Thus, the rennin–angiotensin system likely has a profound contribution to the alteration of L-type Ca^{2+} channels in vascular muscle cells. However, controversy still exists; it has been reported that treatment with an ACE inhibitor to SHR from 5 to 12 weeks of age decreases the blood pressure, but does not normalize the alteration of Ca^{2+} channels (Ohya et al., 1996b).

Ca^{2+} channel blockers effectively and safely decrease blood pressure in hypertensive animals and humans. The decrease in blood pressure in response to Ca^{2+} channel blockers is more evident in hypertension than in normotension (Herpin et al., 1992). It has therefore been hypothesized that the sensitivity of Ca^{2+} channel blockers to vascular L-type Ca^{2+} channels is higher in hypertension than in normotension. From dihydropyridine binding studies (Ikeda et al., 1994; Galletti et al., 1991; Ricci et al., 2000), the dissociation constant of dihydropyridines to vascular tissues does not differ between SHR and WKY, suggesting that dihydropyridine sensitivity is not altered in SHR. In whole-cell recording, the actions of dihydropyridine Ca^{2+} channel antagonist (nicardipine) and agonist (Bay K 8644) on macroscopic L-type Ca^{2+} channel currents do not apparently differ between SHR and WKY cells (Ohya et al., 1993; Matsuda et al., 1997). However, in single-channel recording, sensitivity to both dihydropyridine Ca^{2+} channel antagonist and agonist is higher in SHR than in WKY cells (Kubo et al., 1998). Accordingly, alteration of the dihydropyridine sensitivity of L-type Ca^{2+} channels in hypertension is still controversial.

Alteration of Ca^{2+} channels other than L-type Ca^{2+} channels has not been fully evaluated. One study has shown that the amplitude of the T-type Ca^{2+} channel current is larger in SHR-SP cells than in WKY cells (Self et al., 1994). In contrast, others have shown that T-type Ca^{2+} channel current in cerebral artery muscle cells and a fast-inactivating Ca^{2+} channel current (possibly non-L non-T type) in mesenteric artery muscle cells are not altered in SHR compared to WKY (Ohya et al., 1993; Wilde et al., 1994).

2.1.1.2. Alteration in other hypertensive rat models In renal hypertension rats (2-kidney 1-clip model, 2–11 weeks after the surgery), the amplitude of Ca^{2+} channel currents in muscle cells from the basilar artery is larger than that in normotensive controls (Simard et al., 1998). The amplitude of Ca^{2+} channel currents correlates with the duration of hypertension and systolic blood pressure levels. In addition, the sensitivity to dihydropyridine Ca^{2+} channel agonist (Bay K 8644) is not altered in renal hypertensive rats. In single-channel recordings, opening of the L-type Ca^{2+} channels is increased in hypertensive rats; in contrast, other parameters, including single-channel conductance, open times, and the distribution of two open states do not differ between hypertensive and normotensive rats. As this alteration appears after the blood pressure elevation in this model, factors related to mechanism of renal hypertension may secondarily affect the channel property.

Dahl salt-sensitive rats develop hypertension when fed a high-salt diet. The amplitude of the L-type Ca^{2+} channel current is larger in muscle cells from small mesenteric arteries of Dahl salt-sensitive rats fed a high-salt diet compared to those fed a low-salt diet (Ohya et al., 2000). The increase in current amplitude is most evident at potentials near resting potentials. The voltage-dependent kinetics are altered after salt loading; the voltage-dependent activation is negatively shifted, while voltage-dependent inactivation kinetics remain the same. This result suggests that a window component of Ca^{2+} channels (non-inactivating component) is increased after salt loading. These observations are in good accord with the observation that salt loading facilitates the spontaneous electrical activity in the mesenteric artery of Dahl salt-sensitive rats (Fujii et al., 1997). Since this alteration appears after salt loading, factors related to salt loading and/or hypertension would affect the channel characteristics.

2.1.2. Potassium (K$^+$) channels

K$^+$ channels play an important role in the regulation of membrane potential in smooth muscle cells (Beech, 1997; Quayle et al., 1997; Jackson, 2000; Sobey, 2001) (Fig. 1). The opening of K$^+$ channels hyperpolarizes the membrane, closes voltage-operated Ca^{2+} channels, and thus induces vasodilation. In contrast, closing of K$^+$ channels depolarizes the membrane, activates voltage-operated Ca^{2+} channels, and increases vascular tone. In vascular muscle cells, at least four types of K$^+$ channels exist: Ca^{2+}-activated K$^+$ (K$_{Ca}$) channels, delayed voltage-dependent K$^+$ (K$_V$) channels, ATP-sensitive K$^+$ (K$_{ATP}$) channels, and inwardly rectifying K$^+$ (K$_{IR}$) channels.

2.1.2.1. Ca^{2+}-activated K$^+$ channels

Large-conductance Ca^{2+}-activated K$^+$ (BK$_{Ca}$) channels are abundantly distributed in membrane of vascular muscle cells. These channels are activated by increases in intracellular Ca^{2+} concentrations ([Ca^{2+}]$_i$) and membrane depolarization. Evidence suggests that activity of the BK$_{Ca}$ channel is enhanced in arterial muscle cells of hypertension model rats. For example, the amplitude of the macroscopic BK$_{Ca}$ current is greater in muscle cells from the aorta, renal small artery, and cerebral artery of SHR and the aorta of aldosterone–salt hypertensive rats (Rusch et al., 1992; Martens and Gelband, 1996; Liu et al., 1997, 1998). In single-channel recording, the channel opening occurs more frequently in muscle cells of the cerebral artery from SHR than those from WKY; however, the amplitude of the unit current, the Ca^{2+} sensitivity, and the voltage-dependency do not differ between SHR and WKY (Liu et al., 1998). Thus, the major mechanism for the increased BK$_{Ca}$ channel activity appears to be an increase in the channel availability (the product of number of the functional channel and open probability of the channel). In contrast to this observation, in aortic muscle cells, the Ca^{2+} sensitivity of the BK$_{Ca}$ channel from SHR is increased compared to WKY (England et al., 1993).

Western blot analysis has shown that levels of the α subunit of BK$_{Ca}$ channels increased in the aorta and cerebral arteries of hypertensive rats (Liu et al., 1997, 1998). Thus, the increase in the number of functional channels is at least one relevant mechanism for the enhancement of BK$_{Ca}$ current. However, mRNA levels as evaluated by ribonuclease protection assays are not altered in SHR (Liu et al., 1997). It is, thus, possible that an alteration exists in the posttranscriptional rather than in the transcriptional process.

The enhanced activity of BK$_{Ca}$ channels is a secondary change due to the increase in blood pressure, as antihypertensive treatment of SHR with an ACE inhibitor normalizes this alteration (Rusch and Runnells, 1994). This conclusion is also supported by several reports that the increase in BK$_{Ca}$ channel activity is similarly observed in different hypertensive rat models and at the proximal segment of the coarcted aorta that is exposed to high blood pressure (Rusch et al., 1992).

In addition to this increased availability of BK$_{Ca}$ channels, the increased [Ca^{2+}]$_i$ and more depolarized membrane potential of arterial muscle cells in hypertension further stimulate the channel activity. The opening of BK$_{Ca}$ channels counteracts the increased [Ca^{2+}]$_i$ and membrane depolarization. Thus, BK$_{Ca}$ channel function is enhanced as a protective mechanism against increases in vascular tone. Indeed, inhibition of

BK_{Ca} channels by blockers depolarizes the membrane and increases vascular tone (Liu et al., 1998; Rusch and Runnells, 1994). In addition, the BK_{Ca} channel knock-out mouse (knock-out of β1 subunit) exhibits hypertension as well as increased vascular tone and decreased BK_{Ca} currents in vascular muscle cells (Pluger et al., 2000).

Little information is available regarding the alteration of other K_{Ca} channels in hypertension. One study has shown that apamin, which inhibits small-conductance K_{Ca} channels, induces a larger contraction of the aorta in SHR than in WKY (Silva et al., 1994). This finding suggests that the activity of small-conductance K_{Ca} channels is stimulated more in SHR than in WKY.

Small-conductance and intermediate-conductance K_{Ca} channels as well as BK_{Ca} channels are activated during endothelium-dependent hyperpolarization of vascular muscle cells (Feletou and Vanhoutte, 2000). Since endothelium-dependent hyper-polarization is decreased in hypertension (Fujii et al., 1992; Sunano et al., 1999; Van de Voorde et al., 2000), it is hypothesized that function of small-conductance and intermediate-conductance K_{Ca} channels is impaired, however, no direct evidence of such alteration has been demonstrated.

2.1.2.2. K_V channels K_V channels are distributed in most arterial smooth muscle cells and are sensitive to 4-aminopyridine (4-AP). Molecular biological studies have shown that various K_V proteins are responsible for the channel formation. In renal interlobar arteries of SHR and deoxycorticosterone acetate (DOCA) rats, the am-plitude of the K_V current is smaller than that of their normotensive controls (Martens and Gelband, 1996). The K_V current is also decreased in aortic muscle cells from SHR compared to WKY (Cox, 1996). It is suggested that the decreased K_V current is one mechanism for the cell depolarization in hypertension (Martens and Gelband, 1996; Cox, 1996).

An intracardiac injection of ACE antisense or that of angiotensin II type 1 receptor antisense prevents the alteration of K_V channel currents as well as the development of hypertension in SHR (Martens et al., 1998; Gelband et al., 2000). Thus, the rennin–angiotensin system and/or hypertension is considered to play an important role to cause this alteration of K_V currents.

The mechanism for the decreased amplitude of K_V current has not been fully determined. One possible mechanism is that the higher $[Ca^{2+}]_i$ in hypertension suppresses K_V currents to a greater extent (Gelband and Hume, 1994). Another is that expression of K_V channel proteins is decreased in hypertension. However, a recent study has shown that levels of the K_V protein are rather increased in arteries from SHR ($K_V1.2$, $K_V1.5$, and $K_Vβ$) (Cox et al., 2001). In addition, same authors have shown that the amplitude of the K_V current is greater in muscle cells from SHR arteries than those from WKY arteries, when K_V currents are recorded at low $[Ca^{2+}]_i$.

2.1.2.3. K_{ATP} channels Opening of K_{ATP} channels in vascular muscle cells is in-hibited by intracellular ATP and stimulated by intracellular nucleotide diphosphates such as guanosine diphosphate (GDP) and uridine diphosphate (UDP). In addition, stimulations, that increase cyclic adenosine monophosphate (cAMP) concentration, and synthetic K^+ channel openers stimulate the opening of K_{ATP} channels, and then cause vasodilation.

K^+ channel openers induce a less potent vasodilating action in the basilar artery and renal small arteries from SHR, and in mesenteric artery from nitric oxide (NO)-deficient hypertensive rats (Kitazono et al., 1993; Mimuro et al., 1998; Kalliovalkama et al., 1999). However, relaxation is not impaired by other stimulations of K_{ATP} channels, stimulations that increase cAMP levels (forskolin and norepinephrine) in the basilar artery from SHR (Kitazono et al., 1993). Thus, the mechanism by which K^+ channel openers activate K_{ATP} is impaired in chronic hypertension. In contrast, vasodilation induced by K^+ channel openers is exaggerated in carotid arteries from SHR (Miyata et al., 1990), and is not altered in mesenteric arteries from SHR (Fujii et al., 1992). A possible explanation of this discrepancy is that the increased oxidative stress under hypertension may stimulate K_{ATP} channel opening (Wei et al., 1996; Kinoshita et al., 2001). Another possible explanation is that alterations of K_{ATP} channels occur differently in different vessels.

Macroscopic K_{ATP} current, which is activated by a K^+ channel opener (levocromakalim), is smaller in muscle cells from mesenteric arteries of SHR than in those of WKY (Ohya et al., 1996a). In contrast, the opening of K_{ATP} channels in single-channel recording in response to dizoxide is increased in the membrane of tail arteries from SHR, compared to WKY (Furspan and Webb, 1993). In addition, the ATP concentrations required for K_{ATP} channel inhibition are greater in SHR-SP than in WKY. Different results may be due to the use of different arteries and/or different K^+ channel openers.

2.1.2.4. K_{IR} channels K_{IR} channels exist and contribute to the regulation of vascular tone in some arteries (Quayle et al., 1997; Jackson, 2000). The application of Ba^{2+}, which possibly inhibits K_{IR}, induces a smaller vasodilation of arteries in SHR-SP and in DOCA hypertensive pigs than in their normotensive controls (Webb, 1982; McCarron and Halpern, 1990). It is, thus, postulated that the function of K_{IR} channels in these arteries is impaired. However, no direct evidence exists to demonstrate the alteration of K_{IR} channels in arteries from hypertensive animals.

2.1.3. *Mechanosensitive channels*

The myogenic mechanical responses of small arteries (renal microvessels, skeletal muscle arterioles, and small mesenteric arteries) are enhanced in hypertensive rats, as compared to normotensive rats (Hayashi et al., 1989; Falcone et al., 1993; Izzard et al., 1996). In addition, depolarization of arterial muscle in response to increases in transmural pressure is greater in cerebral arteries from SHR than that from WKY (Harder et al., 1985). Thus, enhanced depolarization by mechanical stimuli is a possible mechanism for the enhanced myogenic tone of these arteries.

Mechanical stimuli to the cell membrane activate mechanosensitive channels (Hill et al., 2001). For example, membrane stretch activates non-selective cation channels and depolarizes the cell, as well as allowing Ca^{2+} and Na^+ to enter the cell (Davis et al., 1992; Setoguchi et al., 1997). Stretch-activated non-selective cation channels in arterial muscle cells from SHR and WKY have been compared by the use of whole-

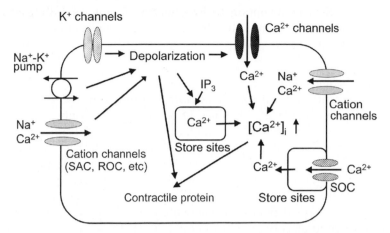

Fig. 1.   Membrane potential, ion channels and Ca^{2+} influx in vascular muscle cells. Membrane potential has a pivotal role in the regulation of Ca^{2+} mobilization and then muscle contraction. In hypertension, membrane potential of vascular muscle cells is more depolarized than in normotension. Limited opening of K^+ channels, altered function of $Na^+–K^+$ pump, and increased Na^+ influx through non-selective cation channels are possible mechanisms for the depolarization. Membrane depolarization activates voltage-operated Ca^{2+} channels, which enhances Ca^{2+} influx. Depolarization also stimulates inositol-triphosphate (IP_3)-induced Ca^{2+} release from intracellular Ca^{2+} store sites and enhances Ca^{2+} sensitivity of contractile protein. Ca^{2+} enters cell-inside also through various cation channels including stretch-activated cation channels (SAC), receptor-operated channels (ROC), and store-operated Ca^{2+} channels (SOC).

cell and single-channel recordings (Ohya et al., 1998). The amplitude of the macroscopic stretch-activated current is larger in muscle cells from SHR than in those from WKY. In single-channel recording, the channel opening, in response to the same degree of stretch-stimulation, is more frequent in SHR cells than in WKY cells. However, single-channel conductance does not differ between SHR and WKY. This enhanced activation of stretch-activated channels would explain the exaggerated myogenic responses observed in small arteries of hypertensive animals by inducing more depolarization and greater Ca^{2+} influx in vascular muscle cells (Fig. 1).

2.1.4. *Store-operated channels*

Store-operated channel is another kind of Ca^{2+} entry channels, that is activated when intracellular calcium stores are empty (Gibson et al., 1998). Electro-physiological characterization of this channel is insufficient in vascular muscle cells; this channel is, however, considered to play an important role in the regulation of vascular tone. The alteration of store-operated channels in vascular muscle cells and its contribution to hypertension has not yet been determined.

2.1.5. *Chloride (Cl^-) channels*

Cl^- channels (Ca^{2+}-activated Cl^- channel and voltage-activated Cl^- channel) also contribute to the control of vascular tone (Jackson, 2000; Kitamura and Yamazaki,

2001). However, their contribution to hypertension is not yet fully evaluated. In addition, no study has examined the alteration of Cl^- currents in vascular muscle cells in hypertension.

2.1.6. *Membrane potentials*

Membrane potential activates and inactivates various voltage-dependent channels including voltage-operated Ca^{2+} channels. Depolarization not only activates voltage-operated Ca^{2+} channels, but also stimulates inositol 1,4,5-triphosphate-induced release of Ca^{2+} from intracellular store sites, and increases the Ca^{2+} sensitivity of the contractile apparatus in vascular muscle cells (Yamagishi et al., 1992; Ganitkevich and Isenberg, 1993) (Fig. 1). Thus, the membrane potential of arterial muscle cells plays an important role in the regulation of vascular tone. In SHR, the membrane potentials of vascular muscle are more depolarized in mesenteric arteries (Chung, 1984; Fujii et al., 1992) and in cerebral arteries (Wellman et al., 2001). Depolarization of membrane potentials is also observed in vascular muscle cells from salt-loaded Dahl salt-sensitive rats (Fujii et al., 1997), 2-kidney, 1-clip renal hypertensive rats (Shoemaker and Overbeck, 1986; Callera et al., 2001), and DOCA salt-hypertensive rats (Friedman and Tanaka, 1987). The mechanism of this depolarization has not been fully clarified; however, the increased Na^+ influx through cation channels, decreased K^+ channel activity (BK_{Ca} channels, K_V channels), and altered function of Na^+–K^+ pump have been suggested (Shoemaker and Overbeck, 1986; Hermsmeyer and Harder, 1986; Friedman and Tanaka, 1987; Callera et al., 2001). In addition, prostaglandin H_2 (PGH_2) is considered to contribute to this depolarization, as the expression of prostaglandin H_2 synthase is increased in hypertension (Davidge, 2001) and an inhibitor of PGH_2 hyperpolarizes the membrane in hypertensive rats (Fujii et al., 1997).

2.1.7. *β receptor-mediated hyperpolarization*

β stimulation activates K_{ATP} channels and hyperpolarizes the membrane potential of vascular smooth muscle cells. This β receptor-mediated hyperpolarization is impaired in small arteries in the cremaster muscle from reduced renal mass hypertensive rats and in mesenteric arteries from young, prehypertensive SHR, compared to their controls (Stekiel et al., 1993; Goto et al., 2001). Direct Gs protein activation by cholera toxin fails to induce hyperpolarization, but direct adenylate cyclase stimulation by forskolin induces comparable hyperpolarization in hypertensive and prehypertensive rats, compared to their controls. Accordingly, Gs protein–adenylate cyclase coupling is likely to be altered in hypertensive and prehypertensive rats. It is likely that such alteration occurs during the development of hypertension secondarily in reduced renal mass hypertensive rats, but the alteration also occurs primarily in young SHR due to the genetic background of this model.

2.1.8. *Endothelium-dependent hyperpolarization*

Various factors released from endothelium, including nitric oxide, endothelium-derived hyperpolarizing factor (EDHF), and prostacyclin relax vascular tissue (Lüscher, 1990; Feletou and Vanhoutte, 2000). Evidence suggests that the contribution of EDHF to endothelium-dependent relaxation is reduced in genetic and non-genetic hypertension rats (Fujii et al., 1992; Sunano et al., 1999; Van de Voorde et al., 2000). Endothelium-dependent hyperpolarization is decreased in the mesenteric artery of SHR and SHR-SP, as well as in the aorta of renal hypertensive rats (Fujii et al., 1992; Sunano et al., 1999; Van de Voorde et al., 2000). Although consensus regarding nature of EDHF has not been obtained (Feletou and Vanhoutte, 2000), a release of EDHF or the mechanism of hyperpolarization by EDHF may be impaired in chronic hypertension. Antihypertensive treatments restore this impairment (Onaka et al., 1998), suggesting that the chronic hypertension primarily impairs the EDHF action. An ACE inhibitor more efficiently improves this impairment than does a combination of hydrochlorothiazide and hydralazine. It is, thus, considered that the renin–angiotensin system also has a contribution to the impairment of EDHF action in hypertension.

2.2. *Alteration during aging*

In vascular tissues from aged animals, endothelium-dependent and endothelium-independent relaxations are impaired, although anatomical heterogeneity does exist (Barton et al., 1997). Several mechanisms of this alteration, have been suggested. For example, it has been postulated that superoxide production is increased, antioxidant systems are suppressed, and endothelial nitric oxide-dependent relaxation is impaired with aging (Barton et al., 1997; Azhar et al., 1995; Sohal et al., 1994; Shigenaga et al., 1994; Reckelhoff et al., 1994). Alterations in vascular muscle responsiveness to catecholamines, endothelin, and endothelium-derived contracting factors have also been reported in arteries from aged animal (Duckles, 1983; Moritoki et al., 1986; Koga et al., 1989; Dohi and Lüscher, 1990). However, little is known regarding the alterations in ion channels in vascular tissues.

2.2.1. *Voltage-operated Ca^{2+} channels*
With increases in age, the amplitude of Ca^{2+} channel current is increased until adulthood in WKY (Ohya et al., 1993; Lozinskaya and Cox, 1997). In addition, a voltage-dependent activation kinetics are shifted negatively with maturation. These alterations increase Ca^{2+} influx. However, no study has examined alterations in Ca^{2+} channels of arterial muscle cells in aged animals including human.

2.2.2. *K^+ channels*
Patch-clamp experiments have shown that the amplitude of BK_{Ca} current in rat aortic muscle cells increases with maturation from 4 to 12 weeks of age; however, that of 4-AP-sensitive K_V currents does not change (Gomez et al., 2000). In coronary muscle cells from rats (F344 rats), the BK_{Ca} current density decreases with increasing age from 3 to 25–30 months (Marijic et al., 2001). Western blot analysis has also shown that levels of the α subunit of BK_{Ca} channels in this tissue decrease with aging. This decrease in channel protein has also been noted in coronary arteries from humans (61–70 yr old vs. 3–18 yr old) (Marijic et al., 2001). Consistently with the decrease in BK_{Ca} channels in aged rats, the inhibition of BK_{Ca} channels by

iberiotoxin induces smaller contractions in aged rats than in young rats. However, western blot analysis has shown that BK_{Ca} channel expression in corporal smooth muscle in aged rats (>9 months old) is decreased (Christ et al., 1998), and that in pulmonary artery from aged rats (25–30 months old) is not altered (Marijic et al., 2001), as compared to the young rats. These observations, thus, suggest that changes in protein expression of BK_{Ca} channels in various vascular tissues are not uniform.

Vasodilation in response to K^+ channel openers (levocromakalim and Y-26763) is impaired in the small basilar artery of aged rats (24–26 months old), compared to that of adult rats (4–6 months old); however the vasodilation in the large branch and main trunk of the basilar artery is not impaired (Toyoda et al., 1997). Vasodilation of the aorta in response to K^+ channel opener (cromakalim) is also impaired in aged rabbit (3 yr old), as compared to young rabbit (3–5 months old) (Ferrer et al., 1998). In contrast to these reports, hyperpolarization and relaxation in response to K^+ channel opener (cromakalim) in smooth muscle of mesenteric arteries does not differ between young (6–8 months old) and old (>24 months old) rats (Fujii et al., 1993, 1999b). The alteration of K_{ATP} channel activation in response to K^+ channel openers may not be uniform in various arteries of aged animals.

2.2.3. *Membrane potentials*

In aged rats, membrane potential in smooth muscle cells of mesenteric arteries from aged rats (20–26 months old) is more depolarized than that from young and adult rats (<20 months old) (Fujii et al., 1993, 1999a,b). In addition, smooth muscle cells in mesenteric arteries from aged SHR exhibit spontaneous electrical activity that is absent in young WKY and SHR and aged WKY (Fujii et al., 1999a). The coexistence of aging and hypertension likely promotes the appearance of spontaneous electrical activity. PGH_2 synthase inhibitor corrects both depolarization and spontaneous electrical activity in arteries from aged SHR. Thus, increased production of PGH_2 contributes to the increased electrical activity in aged SHR artery. It has been reported that expression of PGH_2 synthase 2 is increased in arteries from aged rats (Stewart et al., 2000).

2.2.4. *β receptor-mediated hyperpolarization*

β receptor-mediated hyperpolarization in muscle cells of mesenteric arteries from aged WKY (>24 months old) is decreased compared to adult WKY (12–20 weeks old) (Fujii et al., 1999b). Decreased β receptor-mediated hyperpolarization is likely to be associated with the impaired vasodilation in response to β stimulation. The same authors suggest that in addition to the decreased activity of adenylate cyclase, the cAMP-dependent pathway to stimulate K_{ATP} channels is impaired in arteries from aged rats, as a direct Gs protein activation by a cholera toxin fails to induce hyperpolarization and direct adenylate cyclase stimulation by forskolin induces less hyperpolarization in aged rats than in young rats.

2.2.5. *Endothelium-dependent hyperpolarization*

In aged rats, endothelium-dependent hyperpolarization due to EDHF is impaired in aged rats (20–26 months old) compared to young rats (6–8 months) (Fujii et al.,

1993). This alteration parallels the impaired endothelium-dependent relaxation occurring with aging. ACE inhibitor treatment for 3 months restores the hyperpolarization in mesenteric arteries from aged WKY, whereas a combination of hydrochlorothiazide and hydralazine exerts less effect (Goto et al., 2000). Thus, the rennin–angiotensin system contributes to the age-related impairment of EDHF action.

3. Endothelial cells

Various functional alterations occur in endothelial cells during hypertension and aging. For example, endothelial-dependent vasodilation (NO and EDHF) is impaired and production of vasoconstricting factors and superoxide is increased during hypertension and aging (Moritoki et al., 1986; Koga et al., 1989; Dohi and Lüscher, 1990; Lüscher, 1990). However, only a few studies are available regarding the alteration of ion channels in endothelial cells during hypertension. Furthermore, no information regarding age-related alterations in ion channels is available at the present.

Patch-clamp studies have shown that agonist-operated (non-selective) cation channels, store-operated Ca^{2+} channels, several types of K^+ channels, amiloride-sensitive Na^+ channels, at least two types of Cl^- channels (Ca^{2+}-activated Cl^- channels and voltage-dependent Cl^-), and several types of mechanosensitive channels are present in endothelial cells (Nilius and Droogmans, 2001) (Fig. 2).

3.1. *Alterations during hypertension*

3.1.1. *Mechanosensitive channels*

Endothelial cells are continuously exposed to mechanical stimuli, including shear stress and transmural pressure (Fisher et al., 2001). Endothelial cells translate mechanical stimuli to cellular responses via various mechanisms including mechanosensitive channels. In general, the opening of mechanosensitive non-selective cation channels in endothclial cells increases $[Ca^{2+}]_i$ by permeating Ca^{2+}.

Two types of macroscopic stretch-activated cation currents have been recorded in intact and freshly isolated endothelial cells from rat aorta (Hoyer et al., 1997). One is stretch-activated non-selective cation channel current, which is permeable to Na, K^+, and Ca^{2+}. Another type is stretch-activated K^+ selective channel current. The amplitudes of both non-selective cation current and K^+-selective current are larger in cells from adult SHR than those from age-matched WKY. However, this alteration is not evident in young SHR. Thus, chronic hypertension may change the distribution and/or properties of these stretch-activated cation channels. Since opening of non-selective cation channels allows Ca^{2+} to enter the cell, and opening of K^+-selective channels hyperpolarizes the cell and increases the driving force of Ca^{2+}, enhanced openings of both non-selective and K^+-selective channels stimulate increase in $[Ca^{2+}]_i$ (Fig. 2).

Pressure-activated channels are another type of mechanosensitive cation channels; these channels are activated by exposure to pressure. The opening of

Y. Ohya and M. Fujishima

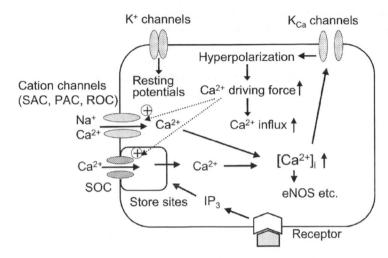

Fig. 2. Membrane potential, ion channels and Ca^{2+} influx in endothelial cells. Various K^+ channels exist in endothelial cells and primarily control membrane potential. However, voltage-operated Ca^{2+} channels are absent. Ca^{2+} enters cell-inside mainly through various cation channels including SOC, ROC, SAC, and pressure-activated cation channels (PAC). In addition to direct activation of cation channels by receptor activation, release of intracellular Ca^{2+}, and mechanical stimulation, hyperpolarization of the cell enhances the Ca^{2+} influx through cation channels by increasing the Ca^{2+} driving force. Receptor stimulation increases intracellular Ca^{2+} concentration by releasing Ca^{2+} from intracellular store sites. Increase in the intracellular Ca^{2+} concentration activates Ca^{2+}-activated K^+ (K_{Ca}) channels and hyperpolarizes the cell. This hyperpolarization facilitates the Ca^{2+} influx through cation channels.

pressure-activated channels in endothelial cells of the aorta and mesenteric arteries is more frequent in SHR-SP than in WKY (Köhler et al., 2001b). Single-channel conductance and the pressure sensitivity of pressure-activate channels are not altered in SHR-SP. Antihypertensive treatment by an ACE inhibitor normalizes this alteration, suggesting that chronic hypertension and/or rennin–angiotensin system alter this channel in this model. In contrast, the activity of PA channels is decreased in endothelial cells from salt-sensitive hypertensive rats (DOCA loaded Sabra salt-sensitive rats), as compared to non-treated Sabra salt-sensitive rats and Sabra salt-resistant rats (Köhler et al., 2001a). The opposite alterations observed in SHR and salt-induced hypertension are probably due to differences in the pathophysiology of these models.

Luminar shear stress for 4 hours to cultured human umbilical venous endothelial cells increases the densities of stretch-activated cation channels and their sensitivity to mechanical stimulation (Brakemeier et al., 2002). Inhibition of tyrosine kinase and protein kinase C prevents this channel alteration, suggesting that activation of these protein kinases contributes to this alteration. In addition, the density of stretch-activated channels in endothelial cells of umbilical vein from mothers with preeclampsia is increased compared to those from mothers with normotensive pregnancy (Köhler et al., 1998). Other properties of channels including single-channel conductance and ion selectivity do not differ between normal pregnancy and preeclampsia. The condition that is related with preeclampsia may modify the properties of stretch-activated channels in human endothelial cells.

3.1.2. K^+ channels

Several types of K^+ channels exist in endothelial cells: K_{IR} channels, BK_{Ca} channels, intermediate-conductance K_{Ca} channels, small-conductance K_{Ca} channels, and K_V channels (Nilius and Droogmans, 2001). The K_{IR} channel contributes significantly to the control of resting membrane potential. Large-conductance, intermediate-conductance, and small-conductance Ca^{2+}-dependent K^+ channels also play some role in the regulation of membrane potentials. Openings of K_{Ca} channels are especially important in the agonist-induced hyperpolarization of endothelial cells, since membrane hyperpolarization is known to increase Ca^{2+} influx. However, alteration of K_{IR} channels and K_{Ca} channels in endothelial cells during hypertension has not yet been evaluated by voltage-clamp methods so far.

Delayed K^+ current is recorded in freshly isolated or intact endothelial cells from some arteries (Nilius and Droogmans, 2001). The amplitude of 4-AP sensitive delayed K^+ current is smaller in endothelial cells from SHR-SP aorta than in those from WKY aorta (Sadanaga et al., 2002). Immunostaining of endothelia cells by anti-$K_V1.5$ antibody is less evident in SHR-SP compared to WKY. It is possible that decreased expression of the $K_V1.5$ channel might be associated with this alteration. In contrast, mechanical stretch for 24 hours under culture conditions increased the amplitude of charybdotoxin-sensitive delayed K^+ currents in endothelial cells from rat cardiac microvasculature (Fan and Walsh, 1999). Continuous mechanical stretch under culture conditions and chronic hypertension in vitro may not induce the same alteration in delayed K^+ currents in endothelial cells. In addition, responses to mechanical stress may differ among different arteries.

3.1.3. Membrane potentials

The membrane potential of endothelial cells plays an important role in the production of vasoactive substances. Hyperpolarization increases driving force of Ca^{2+} and then increases Ca^{2+} influx (Fig. 2). In contrast, depolarization decreases Ca^{2+} influx. Depolarization also increases superoxide production by stimulating NAD(P)H oxidase (Sohn et al., 2000).

Membrane potential in endothelial cells of coronary arteries from 1-kidney, 1-clip renal hypertensive rats is slightly depolarized (by 3 mV compared to those from normotensive controls (Gauthier and Rusch, 2001). However, degrees of hyperpolarization induced by acetylcholine, substance P, and bradykinin do not differ between renal hypertensive rats and normotensive rats. These observations, thus, suggest that altered endothelial function may result from a mechanism other than the decreased agonist-induced hyperpolarization of endothelial cells in this model. The resting membrane potential of freshly isolated aortic endothelial cells from SHR-SP is more depolarized (by 8 mV than that of cells from WKY (Sadanaga et al., 2002). Application of 4-AP abolishes the difference in membrane potential between the two strains, suggesting that impaired activation of 4-AP sensitive delayed K^+ channels might contribute to the depolarized membrane potentials. This is in good accord with the observation that 4-AP sensitive K^+ current is decreased in endothelial cells from SHR-SP (Sadanaga et al., 2002).

4. Conclusion

This brief review summarizes available evidence for the alteration of ion channels in vascular muscle cells and endothelial cells during hypertension and aging. In vascular muscle cells, L-type Ca^{2+} channels, BK_{Ca} channels, and K_V channels are altered with hypertension and aging; however alteration of K_{ATP} channels is controversial. The activity of stretch-activated channels in smooth muscle cells is enhanced in hypertension. In addition, membrane potential is depolarized and hyperpolarization to EDHF or β-stimulation is impaired with hypertension and aging. In endothelial cells, alterations occur in mechanosensitive channels and K_V channels during hypertension. Although hypertension and aging induce similar alterations in ion channels, it has not been clarified whether the mechanisms responsible for these alterations are the same with hypertension and aging. In addition, altered expression of protein and mRNA has been evaluated in some channels, though no clear evidence exists indicating that such an alteration is genetic in origin. Further accumulation of evidence in cellular, molecular, and genetic levels is needed. Such information could provide a key to a novel strategy for preventing and treating vascular diseases induced by hypertension and aging.

References

Azhar, S., Cao, L., Reaven, E., 1995. J. Clin. Invest. 96, 1414–1424.
Barton, M., Cosentino, C., Brandes, R.P., Moreau, R., Shaw, S., Lüscher, T.F., 1997. Hypertension 30, 817–824.
Beech, D.J., 1997. Pharmacol. Ther. 73, 91–119.
Brakemeier, S., Eichler, I., Hopp, H., Köhler, R., Hoyer, J., 2002. Cardiovasc. Res. 53, 209–218.
Callera, G.E., Varanda, W.A., Bendhack, L.M., 2001. Hypertension 38, 592–596.
Christ, G.J., Rehman, J., Day, N., Salkoff, L., Valcic, M., Melman, A., Geliebter, J., 1998. Am. J. Physiol. 275, H600–H608.
Chung, D.W., 1984. Can. J. Physiol. Pharmacol. 62, 957–960.
Cox, R.H., 1996. Am. J. Hypertens. 9, 884–894.
Cox, R.H., Folander, K., Swanson, R., 2001. Hypertension 37, 1315–1322.
Cox, R.H., Lozinskaya, I.M., 1995. Hypertension 26, 1060–1064.
Davidge, S.T., 2001. Circ. Res. 89, 650–660.
Davis, M.J., Donovitz, J.A., Hood, J.D., 1992. Am. J. Physiol. 262, C1083–C1088.
Dohi, Y., Lüscher, T.F., 1990. Br. J. Pharmacol. 100, 889–893.
Duckles, S.P., 1983. Neurobiol. Aging 4, 151–156.
England, S.K., Wooldridge, T.A., Stekiel, W.J., Rusch, N.J., 1993. Am. J. Physiol. 264, H1337–H1345.
Falcone, J.C., Granger, H.J., Meininger, G.A., 1993. Am. J. Physiol. 265, H1847–H1855.
Fan, J., Walsh, K.B., 1999. Circ. Res. 84, 451–457.
Feletou, M., Vanhoutte, P.M., 2000. Acta Pharmacol. Si. 21, 1–18.
Ferrer, M., Tejera, N., Marin, J., Balfagon, G., 1998. Life Sci. 63, 2071–2078.
Fisher, A.B., Chien, S., Barakat, A.I., Nerem, R.M., 2001. Am. J. Physiol. 281, L529–L533.
Friedman, S.M., Tanaka, M., 1987. J. Hypertens. 5, 341–345.
Fujii, K., Ohmori, S., Tominaga, M., Abe, I., Takata, Y., Ohya, Y., Kobayashi, K., Fujishima, M., 1993. Am. J. Physiol. 265, H509–H516.

Fujii, K., Onaka, U., Abe, I., Fujishima, M., 1999a. J. Hypertens. 17, 75–80.

Fujii, K., Onaka, U., Goto, K., Abe, I., Fujishima, M., 1999b. Hypertension 34, 222–228.

Fujii, K., Onaka, U., Ohya, Y., Ohmori, S., Tominaga, M., Abe, I., Takata, Y., Fujishima, M., 1997. Br. J. Pharmacol 120, 1207–1214.

Fujii, K., Tominaga, M., Ohmori, S., Kobayashi, K., Koga, T., Takata, Y., Fujishima, M., 1992. Circ. Res. 70, 660–669.

Furspan, P.B., Webb, R.C., 1993. J. Hypertens. 11, 1067–1072.

Galletti, F., Rutledge, A., Krogh, V., Triggle, D.J., 1991. Gen. Pharmacol. 22, 173–176.

Ganitkevich, V.Y., Isenberg, G., 1993. J. Physiol. (Lond.) 470, 35–44.

Gauthier, K.M., Rusch, N.J., 2001. Hypertension 37, 66–71.

Gelband, C.H., Hume, J.R., 1994. Circ. Res. 77, 121–130.

Gelband, C.H., Reaves, P.Y., Evans, J., Wang, H., Katovich, M.J., Raizada, M.K., 1999. Hypertension 33, 360–365.

Gelband, C.H., Wang, H., Gardon, M.L., Keene, K., Goldberg, D.S., Reaves, P.Y., Katovich, M.J., Raizada, M.K., 2000. Hypertension 35, 209–213.

Gibson, A., McFadzean, I., Wallace, P., Wayman, C.P., 1998. Trends Pharmacol. Sci. 19, 266–269.

Gomez, J.P., Ghisdal, P., Morel, N., 2000. Pflügers Arch. 441, 388–397.

Goto, K., Fujii, K., Abe, I., 2001. Hypertension 37, 609–613.

Goto, K., Fujii, K., Onaka, U., Abe, I., Fujishima, M., 2000. Hypertension 36, 581–587.

Harder, D.R., Smeda, J., Lombard, J., 1985. Circ. Res. 57, 319–322.

Hayashi, K.M., Epstein, M., Loutzenhiser, R., 1989. Circ. Res. 65, 1475–1484.

Hermsmeyer, K., Harder, D.R., 1986. Am. J. Physiol. 250, C557–C562.

Herpin, D., Vaisse, B., Pitiot, M., de Gaudemaris, R., Mallion, J.M., Poggi, L., Demange, J., 1992. Am. J. Cardiol. 69, 923–926.

Hill, M.A., Zou, H., Potocnik, S.J., Meininger, G.A., Davis, M.J., 2001. J Appl. Physiol. 91, 973–983.

Hoyer, J., Köhler, R., Distler, A., 1997. Hypertension 30, 112–119.

Hughe, A.D., 1995. J. Vasc. Res. 32, 353–370.

Ikeda, S., Amano, Y., Adachi-Akahane, S., Nagao, T., 1994. Eur. J. Pharmacol. 264, 223–226.

Izzard, A.S., Bund, S.J., Heagerty, A.M., 1996. Am. J. Physiol. 270, H1–H6.

Jackson, W.F., 2000. Hypertension 35, 173–178.

Kalliovalkama, J., Jolma, P., Tolvanen, J.-P., Kahonen, M., Hutri-Kahonen, N., Wu, X., Holm, P., Porsti, I., 1999. Cardiovasc. Res. 42, 773–782.

Kinoshita, H., Kakutani, T., Iranami, H., Hatano, Y., 2001. Jpn. J. Pharmacol. 85, 29–33.

Kitamura, K., Yamazaki, J., 2001. Jpn. J. Pharmacol. 85, 351–357.

Kitazono, T., Heistad, D.D., Faraci, F.M., 1993. Hypertension 22, 677–681.

Koga, T., Takata, Y., Kobayashi, K., Takishita, S., Yamashita, Y., Fujishima, M., 1989. Hypertension 14, 542–548.

Köhler, R., Kreutz, R., Grundig, A., Rothermund, L., Yagil, C., Yagil, Y., Pries, A.R., Hoyer, J., 2001a. J. Am. Soc. Nephrol. 12, 1624–1629.

Köhler, R., Grundig, A., Brakemeier, S., Rothermund, L., Distler, A., Kreutz, R., Hoyer, J., 2001b. Am. J. Hypertens. 14, 716–721.

Köhler, R., Schonfelder, G., Hopp, H., Distler, A., Hoyer, J., 1998. J. Hypertens. 16, 1149–1156.

Kubo, T., Taguchi, K., Ueda, M., 1998. Hypertens. Res. 21, 33–37.

Liu, Y., Hudetz, A.G., Knaus, H.G., Rusch, N.J., 1998. Circ. Res. 82, 729–737.

Liu, Y., Pleyte, K., Knaus, H.G., Rusch, N.J., 1997. Hypertension 30, 1403–1409.

Lozinskaya, I.M., Cox, R.H., 1997. Hypertension 29, 1329–1336.

Lüscher, T.F., 1990. Hypertension 15, 482–485.

Marijic, J., Li, Q., Song, M., Nishimaru, K., Stefani, E., Toro, L., 2001. Circ. Res. 88, 210–216.

Martens, J.R., Gelband, C.H., 1996. Circ. Res. 79, 295–301.

Martens, J.R. Reaves, P.Y., Lu, D., Katovich, M.J., Berecek, K.H., Bishop, S.P., Raizada, M.K., Gelband, C.H., 1998. Proc. Natl. Acad. Sci. USA 95, 2664–2669.

Matsuda, K., Lozinskaya, I., Cox, R.H., 1997. Am. J. Hypertens. 10, 1231–1239.

McCarron, J.G., Halpern, W., 1990. Circ. Res. 67, 609–619.

Mimuro, T., Kawata, T., Onuki, T., Hashimoto, S., Tsuchiya, K., Nihei, H., Koike, T., 1998. Eur. J. Pharmacol. 358, 153–160.

Miyata, N., Tsuschida, K., Otomo, S., 1990. Eur. J. Pharmacol. 182, 209–210.

Morita, H., Cousins, H., Onoue, H., Ito, Y., Inoue, R., 1999. Circ. Res. 85, 596–605.

Moritoki, H., Hosoki, E., Ishida, Y., 1986. Eur. J. Pharmacol. 126, 61–67.

Nilius, B., Droogmans, G., 2001. Physiol. Rev. 81, 1415–1459.

Ohya, Y., Sperelakis, N., 1989. Circ. Res. 64, 145–154.

Ohya, Y., Abe, I., Fujii, K., Takata, Y., Fujishima, M., 1993. Circ. Res. 73, 1090–1099.

Ohya, Y., Adachi, N., Nakamura, Y., Setoguchi, M., Abe, I., Fujishima, M., 1998. Hypertension 31, 254–258.

Ohya, Y., Fujii, K., Eto, K., Abe, I., Fujishima, M., 2000. Hypertens. Res. 23, 701–707.

Ohya, Y., Setoguchi, M., Fujii, K., Nagao, T., Abe, I., Fujishima, M., 1996a. Hypertension 27, 1234–1239.

Ohya, Y., Tsuchihashi, T., Kagiyama, S., Abe, I., Fujishima, M., 1998. Hypertension 31, 1125–1129.

Ohya, Y., Tsuchihashi, T., Kagiyama, S., Abe, I., Fujishima, M., 1996b. Hypertension 28, 530 (Abst.).

Onaka, U., Fujii, K., Abe, I., Fujishima, M., 1998. Circulation 98, 175–182.

Pluger, S., Faulhaber, J., Furstenau, M., Lohn, M., Waldschutz, R., Gollasch, M., Haller, H., Luft, F.C., Ehmke, H., Pongs, O., 2000. Circ. Res. 87, E53–E60.

Quayle, L.M., Nelson, M.T., Standen, N.B., 1997. Physiol. Rev. 77, 1165–1232.

Reckelhoff, J.F., Kellum, J.A., Blanchard, E.J., Bacon, E.E., Wesley, A.J., Kruckeberg, W.C., 1994. Life Sci. 55, 1895–1902.

Ricci, A., Bronzetti, E., El-Assouad, D., Felici, L., Greco, S., Mariotta, S., Sabbatini, M., Amenta, F., 2000. Mech. Ageing Dev. 120, 33–44.

Rusch, N.J., De Lucena, R.G., Wooldridge, T.A., England, S.K., Cowley, A.W., 1992. Hypertension 19, 301–307.

Rusch, N.J., Hermsmeyer, K., 1998. Circ. Res. 63, 997–1002.

Rusch, N.J., Runnells, A.M., 1994. Hypertension 23, 941–945.

Sadanaga, T., Ohya, Y., Goto, K., Fujii, K., Abe, I., 2002. Hypertens. Res. 25, 589–596.

Self, D.A., Bian, K., Mishra, S.K., Hermsmeyer, K., 1994. J. Vasc. Res. 31, 359–366.

Setoguchi, M., Ohya, Y., Abe, I., Fujishima, M., 1997. J. Physiol. (Lond.) 501, 343–353.

Shigenaga, M.K., Hagen, T.M., Ames, B.N., 1994. Proc. Natl. Acad. Sci. USA 91, 10771–10778.

Shoemaker, R.L., Overbeck, H.W., 1986. Proc. Soc. Exp. Biol. Med. 181, 529–534.

Silva, E.G., Frediani-Neo, E., Ferreira, A.T., Paiva, A.C.M., Paiva, T.B., 1994. Br. J. Pharmacol. 113, 1022–1028.

Simard, J.M., Li, X., Tewari, K., 1998. Circ. Res. 82, 1330–1337.

Sobey, C.G., 2001. Arterioscler. Thromb. Vasc. Biol. 21, 28–38.

Sohal, R.S., Ku, H.H., Agarwal, S., Forster, M.J., Lal, H., 1994. Mech. Ageing Dev. 74, 121–133.

Sohn, H.-Y., Keller, M., Gloe, T., Morawietz, H., Rueckschloss, U., Pohl, U., 2000. J. Biol. Chem. 275, 18745–18750.

Stekiel, W.J., Contney, S.J., Rusch, N.J., 1993. Hypertension 21, 1005–1009.

Stewart, L.G., Ahang, Y., Davidge, S.T., 2000. Hypertension 35, 1242–1247.

Sunano, S., Watanabe, H., Tanaka, S., Sekiguchi, F., Shimamura, K., 1999. Br. J. Phamacol. 126, 709–116.

Toyoda, K., Fujii, K., Takata, Y., Ibayashi, S., Kitazono, T., Nagao, T., Fujikawa, M., Fujishima, M., 1997. Stroke 28, 171–175.

Van de Voorde, J., Vanheel, B., Leusen, I., 2000. Circ. Res. 87, 112–117.

Webb, R.C., 1982. Hypertension 67, 609–619.

Wei, E.P., Kontos, H.A., Beckman, J.S., 1996. Am. J. Physiol. 271, H1262–H1266.

Wellman, G.C., Cartin, L., Eckman, D.M., Stevenson, A.S., Saundry, C.M., Lederer, W.J., Nelson, M.T., 2001. Am. J. Physiol. 281, H2559–H2567.

Wilde, D.W., Furspan, P.B., Szocik, J.F., 1994. Hypertension 24, 739–746.

Yamagishi, T., Yanagisawa, T., Taira, N., 1992. Naunyn. Schmiedebergs Arch. Pharmacol. 346, 691–700.

**Advances in
Cell Aging and
Gerontology**

Extracellular matrix changes and vascular smooth muscle signaling

Emily Wilson* and Gerald A. Meininger

*Department of Medical Physiology and Cardiovascular Research Institute,
College of Medicine, Texas A&M University System Health Science Center,
College Station, TX, USA*

Contents

Abbreviations

AGE	advanced glycation endproduct
ALT-711	3-phenacyl-4,5-dimethylthiazolium chloride
ECM	extracellular matrix
ecNOS	endothelial nitric oxide synthase
GAGs	glycosaminoglycans
LDL	low-density lipoprotein
LDV	leucine–aspartic acid–valine
MMP	matrix metalloprotease
NO	nitric oxide
PDGF	platelet-derived growth factor
PDGF-BB	platelet-derived growth factor-BB
PPE	porcine pancreatic elastase

* Corresponding author. Tel.: +1-979-862-8673; fax: +1-979-847-8635.
  E-mail address: emilyw@tamu.edu (E. Wilson).

Advances in Cell Aging and Gerontology, vol. 11, 183–199

RGD   arginine–glycine–aspartic acid
ROS   reactive oxygen species
SPARC   secreted protein acidic and rich in cysteine/osteonectin/BM-40
TGF-β   transforming growth factor-β
TIMPs   tissue inhibitors of metalloproteases

1. Introduction

Changes within the vasculature with aging contribute to the risk of developing cardiovascular diseases, including atherosclerosis and hypertension, that may lead to stroke and heart failure (Benetos et al., 1993; Hariri et al., 1986; Kannel and Gordon, 1980). Biomechanical studies of both humans and rats show an increase in stiffness and a reduction in elasticity with aging (Kalth et al., 1986; Kawasaki et al., 1987; Sonesson et al., 1993; Spina et al., 1983; Vogel, 1978). More recent studies have focused on changes in expression, post-translational modification, crosslinking, and glycation of extracellular matrix (ECM) proteins with aging. These alterations in connective tissue expression and properties are likely to contribute to both the mechanical alterations and functional changes in contractile properties of the vasculature with age-related remodeling. In addition, alterations in extracellular matrix proteins have been implicated in regulation of smooth muscle phenotype, gene expression, and reactivity in vascular disease and in cultured cells. In this review, we will focus on enumerating changes in extracellular matrix proteins, alterations in smooth muscle responsiveness with aging, and potential therapeutics that may aid in prevention of cardiovascular diseases that accompany aging.

2. Alterations in biomechanical properties of arteries with aging

Vascular aging is associated with structural and functional changes that include intimal–medial thickening (Howard et al., 1993), arterial dilation (Crouse et al., 1994), and deterioration of elastic wall properties with vascular stiffening (Hansen et al., 1995; Kelly et al., 1989; Van Merode et al., 1988). The gross changes in mechanical properties of arteries with aging have been assessed by a number of groups, using both human subjects and animal models to assess changes. Crucial to these studies is the ability to separate the changes that occur with aging from other cardiovascular risk factors that correlate with age, such as hypertension, diabetes, and atherosclerosis. Generalized changes in the vasculature with aging included a 15–20% increase in the diameter of large vessels (aorta, carotid, and coronary arteries) in human and animal models. The length of vessels was found to increase with age, contributing to the tortuosity of vessels, as observed in angiography of older patients. Many of these changes appear to be independent of increases in blood pressure as chronic blockade of the angiotensin system did not alter age-related changes in diameter (Belmin, 1999). For example, Schmidt-Trucksass and coworkers utilized a cohort of 69 males between the ages of 16 and 75, who were screened for the absence of major atherosclerotic risk factors and evaluated for multiparametric changes in common carotid artery function, structure, and hemodynamics (Schmidt-Trucksass et al., 1999). Their findings showed a nearly linear increase in media thickness (0.052 mm/10 years) and diastolic diameter (0.17 mm/10 years) with age. Additionally, diastolic/systolic diameter change diminished by 0.10 mm/10 years and peak expansion velocity dropped by 0.12 cm/s per 10 years. Peak blood flow velocity decreased continuously with age by 9.3 cm/s per 10 years. Groenink et al. (1999) studied the relationship between aging and aortic stiffness as related to the extent of irreversible deformation and breaking stress of the human thoracic aorta. Aortic segments derived from human heart valve donors without aortic disease were subjected to increasing hydrostatic loads while radius and all thicknesses were monitored echocardiographically. Mean breaking stress was found to be 2.7×10^6 N/m^2. Breaking stress correlated negatively with age and positively with distensibility and collagen recruitment pressure. In contrast, the number of vessels that survived a pressure load of 800 mmHg, the extent of irreversible dilation, was positively correlated with age and negatively correlated with distensibility and collagen recruitment pressure. Bulpitt et al. (1999) reviewed 22 studies relating aortic compliance to age in order to determine the relationship between vascular compliance and age. Their findings showed that alterations in compliance of the aorta and carotid arteries closely related to age. However, peripheral artery compliance is less closely related to age. These authors concluded that the compliance of aorta and carotid arteries is more closely related to chronological age than other indices of aging such as skin elasticity and graying of the hair, and therefore, deviations of vascular compliance from age predicted norms may be indicators of cardiovascular pathologies. Thus, there is a strong interrelationship between mechanical and structural changes within the vasculature with aging. The mechanical changes within the vasculature closely correlated with changes in expression and modification of the major connective tissue protein present in the vessel wall.

3. Alterations in vascular collagens and elastin with aging

Collagens and elastin serve as the major structural proteins of the arterial wall, providing tensile strength and elasticity, respectively. In addition to the amount of connective tissue proteins present in arteries, the specific isoforms that are present and post-translational modifications, such as crosslinking, play important roles in connective tissue function(s) of arteries. Approximately 80–90% of the collagens found in the aorta are type I and type III. Minor amounts of types IV, V, VI, and VII are also present. Types I, II, and VI are present throughout the intimal, medial, and adventitial layers. Type IV is a component of the subendothelial basement membrane and the basement membranes surrounding smooth muscle cells. Less is known about the localization and functions of collagen types V and VIII. The types of collagen present in vessels vary depending on the size and function of blood vessels (Barnes, 1988). For example, Marshall et al. (1990) utilized ultrastructural immunogold labeling techniques to identify collagen types found in large arteries, small arteries, and capillaries of the retina. Collagen types I, III, IV, V, and VI were found in large arteries; collagen types I, IV, and V (with a smaller amount of III and VI) were found in small arteries, while types I, IV, and V were present in capillaries. How these proportions and collagen types change with age and other diseases associated with age is still an area of active investigation.

Cattell et al. (1996) have systematically studied changes in collagen and elastin in aortic walls from post mortem analysis or aorta taken from normotensive subjects ranging in age from 14 to 90 years. The concentrations of both collagen and elastin increased significantly—72% and 90%, respectively, over the age range studied, with the most substantial increases occurring after the age of 45 years. However, when expressed as absolute amounts (milligrams per sample or lipid dry weight milligrams per sample), there is significant decrease in both collagen (92%) and elastin (62%) between the ages of 14 and 90. These data suggest that there is a parallel loss of other aortic components at a rate that outstrips both collagen and elastin with age. Bruel and Oxlund (1996) utilized three age groups of rats—young (4.5 months), adult (14 months), and old (27 months)—to compare biomechanical properties, composition of elastins, collagen, and advanced glycation endproducts (AGEs) of the aorta with age. Aorta from old rats showed an increase in diameter and stiffness in comparison to adult rat aorta. The total hydroxyproline, a measure of collagen content, and elastin content per sample were not changed. However, hydroxyproline content per square millimeter of the aortic wall was reduced by 20% and the elastin content of the wall was reduced by 19% in old rats when compared to adult rats. These investigators observed marked increases in collagen (42%) and elastin (17%) AGEs in old rats as compared to adult animals. The increase in AGEs correlated with increased stiffness of the aorta in old rats.

Age-dependent expression of collagen-, elastin-, and fibrosis-related genes has been studied by a number of investigators. Elastin protein is produced early in life and has a turnover rate that approaches the life span of the animal (Shapiro et al., 1991). Hsuwong et al. (1994) utilized a transgenic mouse line expressing an elastin promoter–reporter construct and found that promoter activity peaked at 3 months of age and decreased at older ages. However, the promoter may be reactivated during wound healing or during pathological processes. Numerous studies have shown that growth factors, including insulin-like growth factor I and transforming growth factor-β (TGF-β), may modulate elastin expression. In addition, dietary factors, hypoxia, and cell density may modulate elastin mRNA expression levels. Tumor necrosis factor, interleukin 1β, 1,25-dihydroxyvitamin D3 and glucocorticoids have been shown to reduce expression in various tissues (Robert et al., 1998). Thus, elastin expression may be influenced both positively and negatively throughout life. In addition to effects of quantitative changes in elastin expression with aging, Hanon et al. (2001) have identified a polymorphism in the elastin gene that results in a serine to glycine mutation that may contribute to increased age-associated alterations in carotid artery distensibility.

Annoni et al. (1998) followed mRNA expression and protein deposition of four genes: procollagen α2 (I) and α1 (III), transforming growth factors β1 and β3—associated with cardiac fibrosis during maturational growth and early aging. An age-related decrease in procollagen I mRNA expression was seen in the left ventricle but not in the right ventricle. Procollagen type III expression decreased during maturational growth in both ventricles. Collagen deposition increased during this time period and at a higher rate during early aging. There were no major changes in mRNA levels for TGF-β—a growth factor that regulates connective tissue synthesis—during this time.

Other components of the vascular extracellular matrix have been reported to change with age and development of vascular diseases that correlate with age such as hypertension, diabetes, and atherosclerosis. Fibronectin expression has been investigated during development and its expression correlated with smooth muscle cell phenotype and expression of smooth muscle specific contractile proteins. High levels of fibronectin are expressed in human aorta during fetal development. Smooth muscle cells during this time express a low level of smooth muscle specific contractile proteins. Adult differentiated smooth muscle cells express low levels of fibronectin, whereas intimal smooth muscle cells from atherosclerotic plaques re-expressed many of the fetal characteristics, including increased fibronectin (Glukhova et al., 1991). Takasaki et al. (1994) investigated fibronectin expression in aorta of male Dahl salt-sensitive rats in response to age and hypertension. They found that mRNA levels were dramatically increased at 37 weeks of age in salt-loaded Dahl-S rats that corresponded to severe hypertension and high mortality. In contrast, no change in blood pressure or aortic expression of fibronectin was seen in Dahl-R rats in response to salt loading. Aging in the absence of hypertension did not affect fibronectin expression. However, Li et al. (1999) show that fibronectin expression in aorta of old Fischer 344XBN rats (30 months) was fivefold higher than in adult controls (6 months) as determined by western blot analysis. Thus, although fibronectin expression is closely correlated with diseases that have increased incidence with age, such as atherosclerosis and hypertension, it remains an area of active research to determine if fibronectin expression correlates with aging in the absence of other vascular diseases.

Laminin and collagen IV are the major ECM proteins that make up both the subendothelial basement membrane and the basement membrane surrounding individual medial smooth muscle cells. Gavazzi et al. (1995) studied laminin immunoreactivity using densitometric application of confocal microscopy. A 50% decrease in laminin reactivity at the medial–adventitial border of 24-month-old rats was observed. A parallel decrease in innervation of the basilar artery was also evident. However, no change in laminin staining was seen in the endothelial basilar lamina or in the adventitia. These studies support the hypothesis that changes in connective tissue and extracellular matrix proteins may be very localized during the aging process and that generalized conclusions from "bulk" analysis may yield conflicting results. Similarly, Bleys and Cowen (2001) investigated the effects of innervation of cerebral blood vessels with plasticity and age-related and Alzheimer's disease-related neurodegeneration. These investigators conclude that focal expression of target-associated factors such as neurotrophins and extracellular matrix factors such as laminin is important in these processes.

Glycosaminoglycans (GAGs) and proteoglycans are important components of the extracellular matrix. GAGs bind low-density lipoprotein (LDL) and may contribute to the progression of atherosclerosis. Tovar et al. (1998) investigated GAGs in intimal and media layers of normal human thoracic aortas from donors of different ages. Total GAG content increases during the first 40 years of life. Chondroitin sulfate increased most remarkably, whereas changes in hyaluronic acid, heparin sulfate, and dermatan sulfate were less noticeable. LDL-binding GAGs do not appear to increase in disease-free areas of the aorta with age, suggesting that the changes in GAG concentration do not contribute to increased susceptibility to atherosclerosis. Proteoglycan distribution in the intima and media of aorta of young and aging rabbits was studied using ultrastructural analysis (Richardson et al., 1988). These studies concluded that the thickened intimal area of aging rabbit aorta contained more proteoglycan than that of younger animals and a higher concentration than that found in the media of the same vessel. The increase in intimal proteoglycan was not associated with increased lipid deposition. The amount of proteoglycan in the endothelial basement membrane decreased with age. Clearly, more precise quantification, localization, and correlation of functional changes in expression of these complicated extracellular matrix components during the aging process are required.

4. Age-related changes in connective tissue post-translational modifications

Covalent crosslinks in collagen and elastin are necessary to provide stability and tensile strength to the proteins. Collagen crosslinks are essential for binding collagen molecules into higher-ordered fibers and fibrils. Lysyl oxidase catalyzes the oxidative deamination of specific lysyl or hydroxylysyl residues, the first step in the cross-linking process, generating lysyl and hydroxylysyl aldehydes. The divalent crosslinks dehydro-hydroxylysinonorleucine and dihydro-dihydroxylysinonorleucine can then spontaneously be formed by a condensation reaction between these aldehydes and the ε-amino group of lysyl or hydroxylysyl residues of a neighboring collagen molecule. These divalent crosslinks then react with a third lysyl or hydroxylysyl residue to form a mature trivalent crosslink that is detected as either pyridinoline or deoxy-pyridinoline (Eyre et al., 1984; Robins, 1982). Inhibition of collagen crosslinks by β-aminoproprionitrile changes the biomechanical properties, including reduced maximum load and stiffness of the thoracic aorta of young rats (Bruel et al., 1998).

Similarly, crosslinks are associated with the functional maturation of elastin. Elastin crosslinks are referred to as desmosines, and their formation is initiated by oxidative deamination of lysyl residues to lysyl aldehydes. Tetrafunctional desmosines occur through a series of spontaneous condensation reactions of three reactive lysyl aldehydes with a fourth lysyl residue (Resier, 1992). Watanabe et al. (1996) investigated age-related changes in elastin crosslinking in human aorta. Elastin crosslinks were rapidly formed in childhood and decreased with age. Increased formation of crosslinks in older individuals is associated with age-related weakening and/or damage to elastin.

The relationship between collagen and elastin crosslinking, lysyl oxidase activity, and increased stiffening in aging arteries has been investigated. Reiser (1991) and coworkers examined collagen crosslinking in skin and lungs from rats, monkeys, and humans ranging in age from fetal to old. Biological aging was found to regulate changes during the first part of life. These changes included a decrease in difunctional crosslinks and a gradual rise in hydroxypyridium and lysyl pyridinium content (the mature forms of the crosslinks). Changes during the second half of life were less predictable, with there being species-related discrepancies, and suggest that drawing too many conclusions from short-lived animal studies regarding effects of collagen crosslinking changes with aging may not be advisable. Overall, these studies concluded that there are fewer collagen crosslinks in skin and lung of older animals, suggesting that increased tissue stiffness with aging is not directly related to lysyl oxidase-mediated crosslinks and is more complicated (Reiser et al., 1987). Reiser also investigated the effects of long-term dietary restriction and age on enzymatically mediated crosslinks and nonenzymatic glycation of collagen. Difunctional crosslinks were found to decrease with age, with no change in mature crosslinks being found. However, AGEs increased in skin and tail tendon and a specific AGE, pentosidine, increased in the aorta of aging mice. Diet-restricted mice showed a decrease in stiffness that is not explained by alterations in lysyl oxidase-mediated crosslinking and is more likely caused by decreased AGE formation with dietary restriction. These studies suggest that lysyl oxidase-mediated crosslinking and nonenzymatic glycation of collagen are independently regulated by diet and aging. Nonenzymatic glycation of collagen (AGE) formation is increased both with aging (Reiser, 1994) and as a consequence of diabetes (Reiser, 1994).

The effect of AGE on vascular stiffening and function has recently come under study. Aminoguanidine, an inhibitor of AGE production, prevents age-related arterial stiffening and cardiac hypertrophy. Corman et al. utilized normotensive WAG/Rij rats treated from ages 24 to 30 months with aminoguanidine to study the effects of inhibition of AGE formation on a number of cardiovascular functions. Treatment with aminoguanidine did not alter body and kidney weights as compared to untreated control animals. However, age-related cardiac hypertrophy was prevented in the aminoguanidine-treated animals and mesangial surface area was decreased by 30%. Aminoguanidine did not affect age-related increase in collagen content of the aorta between 24 and 30 months and did not alter elastin content, media thickness, and smooth muscle cell number as compared to the untreated control animals. Age-related increase in aortic impedance and decrease in carotid distensibility were inhibited by blocking AGE formation. Vaitkevicius et al. (2001) tested the effects of 3-phenacyl-4,5 dimethylthiazolium chloride (ALT-711), a novel nonenzymatic breaker of AGE crosslinks, on arterial and ventricular properties in older rhesus monkey. ALT-711 improved both arterial and ventricular function and optimized ventriculo-vascular coupling in healthy, older primates without diabetes. Similarly, ALT-711 was shown to improve arterial compliance and lower pulse pressure in older humans with vascular stiffening (Kass et al., 2001). These studies strongly suggest that formation of AGEs with age and diabetes contributes to the striking changes seen in increased arterial stiffness and reduced compliance seen with age.

5. Age-related changes in matrix degradation

Increased matrix degradation has been associated with vascular remodeling associated with aging, hypertension, and atherosclerosis (Galis and Khatri, 2002). Matrix metalloproteases (MMPs) are a large family of endopeptidases that are involved in degrading extracellular matrix proteins. MMPs have been implicated in both physiological and pathophysiological remodeling of the vasculature and other tissues (Sternlicht and Werb, 2001). Protease activity is regulated at multiple levels including gene transcription, synthesis of inactive zymogens, activation of zymogens, and interaction with tissue inhibitors of metalloproteases (TIMPs). Nondiseased human arteries and experimental animal models express MMP-2, TIMP-1, and TIMP-2 evenly across the arterial wall; no enzymatic activity is observed, suggesting tight control. However, in vascular diseases such as atherosclerosis and restenosis, focal increases in expression and activity of several MMPs has been detected and implicated in arterial morphological changes associated with these diseases.

Expression and activity of MMPs and TIMPs in the vasculature are regulated by a number of factors that are known to contribute to vascular remodeling, including hemodynamics and mechanical forces, injury, inflammatory mediators, and oxidative stress. Nitric oxide (NO) has been implicated as a modulator of MMP production and activity in flow-induced remodeling (Tronc et al., 2000), and in vitro endothelial nitric oxide synthase (ecNOS) transfer into smooth muscle cells was shown to reduce the expression of MMP-2 and MMP-9. Thus, reduced NO expression associated with aging may contribute to some of the alterations in the extracellular matrix. Reactive oxygen species (ROS) (Rajagopalan et al., 1996) and oxidative stress have also been implicated in regulating expression and activation of MMPs in pathologic conditions in the vasculature and are potentially responsible for alterations in MMP activity during normal aging processes.

Morphological analysis of arteries obtained from old Fischer 344XBN rats (30 months) shows an increased number of breaks in the internal elastic lamina as compared with young adult rats (6 months) (Li et al., 1999). These and other findings suggest that increases in matrix degrading activity may contribute to the alterations seen in arteries with aging. Li et al. found that activity and expression of MMP-2, a normal constituent of the vascular wall, increased in the intima of aged rats. MMP-2 mRNA expression was found to be threefold higher in aortic wall of old rats (30 month) than young rats (6 months). Both latent and activated forms of MMP-2 protein were at least twofold higher in old vs. young rats and increased presence coincided with breaks in the internal elastic lamina and in areas of thickened intima. Wang and Lakatta (2002) followed up these studies and concluded that in addition to an increase in MMP-2 expression between 2 and 30 months of age, there is a corresponding increase in a number of factors that regulate activity of MMP-2 including an increase in plasminogen and plasminogen receptors. Imai et al. (1997) propose that one of the mechanisms for altered regulation of collagenases is an age-related decrease in one of the transcription factors (Oct-1) responsible for down-regulating expression of several proteolytic enzymes. Yamada et al. (1986) also showed an increase in collagenase activity with increasing age of spontaneously hypertensive rats and normotensive rats, and cathepsin D also shows age dependence of expression in normotensive rats. Elastase expression has been shown to increase with passage number in cultured vascular smooth muscle cells (Robert et al., 1986). Interestingly, porcine pancreatic elastase (PPE) has been used since 1981 to treat elderly Japanese patients for the prevention of arterial aging. Patients receiving elastase treatment show decreased age-related increases in pulse wave velocity as compared to untreated control subjects. The mechanisms by which elastase treatment improves vascular function with age are still under investigation.

6. Connective tissue- and extracellular matrix-associated changes in smooth muscle and vascular function with aging

The studies presented above clearly show that there are numerous alterations in the composition and organization of connective tissue and extracellular matrix environment in blood vessels with aging. Which of these changes are most important in contributing to the functional changes that occur during the aging process is still an area of active investigation. In the second half of this chapter we will focus on changes in vascular function and changes in smooth muscle phenotype and function in response to alterations in extracellular matrix and try to relate these. While there are not many studies that have been performed on vessels from old animals, some analogies will be drawn from studies on vessels from normal and hypertensive animals.

Evidence from animal models and humans suggests that skeletal muscle blood flow is reduced in old age. Recently, Muller-Delp et al. (2002) have systematically studied the function of soleus and gastrocnemius skeletal muscle arterioles from young (4-month-old) and old (24-month-old) Fischer 344 rats. The authors of this study hypothesized that there would be increased vasoconstriction in the arterioles from the older animals. The response to norepinephrine and KCl was similar in both soleus and gastrocnemius vessels from old and young animals. Additionally, measuring passive diameter responses to pressure and mechanical stiffness assessed alterations in mechanical properties. No change in either of these parameters was seen with age in either type of arteriole. However, in contrast to the authors' original hypothesis that arterioles from old animals would show increased myogenic vasoconstriction, they found reduced rather than increased myogenic response in both soleus and gastrocnemius arterioles. The mechanical distensibility of arterioles from old animals was also increased over that of young animals. Lack of change in mechanical and material properties of vessels from old animals suggests that gross change in the structure of these skeletal muscle arterioles is not responsible for blunting of the myogenic response. One mechanism that has been proposed for blunting of the myogenic response is an increase in release of endothelium-derived relaxing factors such as NO. However, other studies have shown that there is decreased endothelial responsiveness and endothelial NO production with age. The authors suggest that the difference in responsiveness is most likely due to impairment of pressure-sensitive signaling mechanisms that are linked to change in the composition of the vessel wall with the aging process.

The findings of Muller-Delp suggest that the differences seen between old and young skeletal muscle arterioles may be related to changes in composition in the vessel wall that are involved in mediating pressure-induced responses. One of the mechanisms by which mechanical stimuli are transduced into biological responses is thought to be through the interaction of ECM and their integrin receptor (Alenghat and Ingber, 2002). In this regard, recent studies from Meininger's laboratory have implicated extracellular matrix–integrin-mediated signals in regulating vascular tone. Integrin-binding peptides containing the arginine–glycine–aspartic acid (RGD) sequence can elicit arteriolar vasodilation or vasoconstriction when applied to the abluminal surface of cannulated, cremaster skeletal muscle arterioles by interacting with $\alpha v \beta 3$ and $\alpha 5 \beta 1$ integrins, respectively (Mogford et al., 1996, 1997). One mechanism by which these integrins influence vascular tone is through modulation of L-type calcium channel activity. Ligation of $\alpha v \beta 3$ integrin leads to reduced current through the calcium channel; whereas ligation of $\alpha 5 \beta 1$ integrin causes increased calcium entry, leading to vasoconstriction (Wu et al., 1998). Src tyrosine kinase has been implicated in this signal transduction cascade (Wu et al., 2001).

Further studies have investigated the role of other integrin-binding extracellular matrix motifs. Leucine–aspartic acid–valine (LDV), an amino acid found in the CS-1 region of alternatively spliced fibronectin, has previously been shown to bind to and activate $\alpha 4 \beta 1$ integrin. LDV peptides cause sustained vasoconstriction of cremaster muscle arterioles and increased intracellular calcium concentrations (Waitkus-Edwards et al., 2002). These and other studies provide support to the hypothesis that in addition to structural and mechanical properties provided by extracellular matrix proteins to blood vessels, these proteins have profound influence on the function of arteries and arterioles and may contribute to the pathogenesis of vascular disease (Intengan and Schiffrin, 2000). Although similar studies have not been performed on arteries or arterioles from aging models, given the changes in connective tissue expression, crosslinking, and degradation seen in many models of aging, it is likely that the extracellular matrix–integrin signaling system will be important in understanding the aging process and changes in vascular tone and responsiveness in the cardiovascular system with increased age.

The role of extracellular matrix proteins in providing signals that regulate adhesion, migration, proliferation, differentiation, and gene expression is now widely accepted. Davis et al. (2000) have recently proposed that within the extracellular matrix are biologically cryptic sites that are exposed upon structural or conformational changes in extracellular matrix proteins. For example, collagen contains multiple RGD sites that do not appear to play an important role in integrin ligation of native collagen. However, cell attachment to denatured collagen was found to be mediated through these RGD motifs, suggesting that the denaturation process reveals "new" biologically active sites. Additionally, it is now evident that degradation of collagen by MMP-1 reveals functional RGD sites. These "matricryptic" sites are now thought to be revealed by a number of stimuli, including enzymatic breakdown of the ECM, multimerization, mechanical stimuli, and denaturation or modification of the ECM (such as enzymatic crosslinking or formation of AGEs). Such modifications have been proposed to occur at sites of injury or inflammation and are hypothesized to play important regulatory roles in the wound healing process. In addition to the role of newly revealed matricryptic sites in wound healing and the related vascular remodeling, new synthesis and deposition of matrix molecules from plasma may also regulate cellular functions in the wound healing process. Increased vascular permeability results in recruitment of plasma proteins, including vitronectin, fibronectin, and fibrinogen, that permeate into the vascular wall. Cells within the injury site increase synthesis and deposition of ECM components, such as osteopontin, secreted protein acidic and rich in cysteine/osteonectin/BM-40 (SPARC), thrombospondins, tenascins, and alternatively spliced fibronectins, that are involved in coordinating the wound healing process. We would propose that alterations seen in localized expression patterns, organization, and degradation of matrix proteins that have been observed during vascular aging are important in orchestrating the remodeling process seen in aging, contributing to alterations in the mechanical properties of blood vessels, influencing changes in vascular tone, and regulating cellular responsiveness and phenotype of vascular smooth muscle.

7. Alterations in smooth muscle cell proliferation, phenotype, responsiveness, and gene expression with aging

Several pivotal studies established that neointimal formation and related smooth muscle cell growth in response to arterial injury was greater in aged animals than in younger animals. Stemerman et al. (1982) investigated the kinetics of proliferation of vascular smooth muscle cells from denuded aortas of old (21–24 months) and young (3–4 months) rats by measuring [^{3}H]thymidine incorporation. Old animals had greater incorporation at day 2 that peaked at day 4, whereas young animals showed peak incorporation at day 2 and sharp decrease thereafter. Increased uptake of [^{3}H]thymidine represented increased smooth muscle cell intimal growth as determined by morphometric analysis. Similarly, Hariri et al. (1986) utilized two models of arterial injury to investigate smooth muscle cell growth in response to arterial trauma in old and young animals. In the first model, vessels underwent severe mechanical damage caused by repeated overinflation of a balloon catheter resulting in endothelial denudation, platelet binding and activation, and mechanical damage to the medial layer with breaks of the elastic lamina and medial cell death. In this model, vessels from both young and old animals developed large neointimas at the site of injury. In a less traumatic injury model in which a fine wire coil was used to gently denude the endothelial layer, the injury resulted in platelet binding and activation at the injury site, but minimal damage to the medial layer was observed. In contrast to the model where there was more extensive damage to the vessel, fundamentally different responses were seen in old and young animals. Vessels in young animals did not develop a neointima, whereas vessels from old animals developed an injury response similar to that seen with the more extensive trauma of the balloon catheter. In addition to the increase in intimal size with injury or localized trauma, there is also an increase in the thickness of the intima as part of the normal aging process. Again, smooth muscle cells are the most prevalent cell type in age-associated thickened media (Guyton et al., 1983). These and other studies provide evidence that the growth properties of smooth muscle cells from old and young animals are quantitatively different and may contribute to the increased susceptibility of older animals to the development of atherosclerosis.

To further investigate the mechanisms regulating increased cellular proliferation of smooth muscle cells from old rats as compared to young rats, a number of laboratories have utilized primary smooth muscle cell cultures derived from aortas of young and old animals. Dysregulation of the cell cycle is one mechanism by which smooth muscle cells from old animals may differ from cells from young animals. Rivard et al. (2002) utilized primary aortic smooth muscle cell cultures isolated from young (6–8 months) or old (4–5 years) New Zealand rabbits and compared pro-liferation rates, expression of cell cycle proteins, and growth-related transcription factors. Vascular smooth muscle cells from old animals show a shortened cycle and increased expression of cyclin A and cyclin-dependent kinase II with no change in expression of cyclin E as compared to cells from young animals. Furthermore, an increase in c-fos expression and activity was seen in cells from the old rabbits. Increased expression of c-fos is proposed to drive the increased expression of cyclin A and shortened cell cycle in this model. However, Moon et al. (2001) have shown that isolated smooth muscle cells from aortas of young (4 months) and old (16 months) mice differ in a number of proliferation related measurements. Cells from old mice showed decreased proliferative response to thrombin, increased generation of ROS, and constitutively increased mitogen activated protein (MAP) kinase activity as compared to cells from young mice. These authors also suggest that aging is asso-ciated with dysregulation of cell cycle regulatory proteins and that increased gen-eration of ROS in cells from old animals is associated with increased lipid peroxidation and mitochondrial DNA damage. The authors propose that decreased cell proliferation and increased oxidant-induced damage may be associated with plaque instability in human atherosclerosis. Clearly, one of the important issues yet to be resolved is the identification of fundamental alterations in signal transduction pathways that determine whether there is an increase or decrease in smooth muscle cell proliferation with age.

Changes in responsiveness to serum growth factors with age or with phenotypic modulation of smooth muscle cells from a contractile status (as seen in normal medial cells) to a proliferative status (as in intimal smooth muscle cells) have been proposed to be an important regulatory factor in the injury response of smooth muscle cells. In this regard, McCaffrey and Falcone (1993) investigated whether increased proliferation of aged smooth muscle cells was due to a loss in respon-siveness to such antiproliferative signals as TGF-β1. Equivalent mRNA and latent and active protein for TGF-β1 was found in smooth muscle cultures from young (3–4 months) or old (>19 months) rat aortas. However, smooth muscle cells from old rats did not exhibit the marked inhibition of proliferation (80%) of cells from young rats upon exposure to low levels of TGF-β. Decreased TGF-β binding to smooth muscle cells from old rats was observed. Additionally, Bilato et al. (1997) have shown that smooth muscle cells from young rats (3–4 months) require signals from both platelet-derived growth factor (PDGF) and fibroblast growth factor

(FGF) for PDGF-induced migratory responses. Smooth muscle cells from old animals (18–20 months) did not require FGF-mediated activation of calmodulin kinase II. Thus, smooth muscle cells from older animals were able to bypass some signals that were required for the smooth muscle cells from younger animals. These results may explain differences in response to injury seen in vivo.

Additionally, the localized extracellular matrix environment surrounding smooth muscle cells is important in regulating signal transduction pathways, gene expression, phenotype, and proliferation rates. For example, primary smooth muscle cells seeded on fibronectin have increased transition to a synthetic, proliferative phenotype, whereas cells seeded on the basement membrane protein, laminin, are retained in a contractile phenotype longer in culture (Thyberg et al., 1990). The transition to a more proliferative phenotype of cells on fibronectin is mediated by interaction of RGD domain binding to $\alpha5\beta1$ integrin of the smooth muscle cells. This interaction results in reorganization of the actin cytoskeleton into stress fibers, decreased expression of smooth muscle specific contractile proteins, increased abundance of biosynthetic organelles, increased synthesis and secretion of extracellular matrix proteins, and increased ability to respond to exogenous mitogens (Hedin et al., 1990). Similarly, Wilson et al. (1995) showed that neonatal rat aortic smooth muscle cells exposed to cyclic mechanical strain in vitro showed increased proliferation when the cells adhered to fibronectin, but not when the smooth muscle cells adhered to laminin. Reusch et al. (1996) showed that rat aortic smooth muscle cells that adhered to laminin or collagen I increased expression of the differentiation marker smooth muscle myosin heavy chain in response to cyclic mechanical strain, whereas cells that adhered to pronectin, a synthetic poly-RGD substrate, did not. These studies indicate that the types of extracellular matrix with which smooth muscle cells are in contact greatly affect the response of the cells.

Further studies suggest that it is not just the type of matrix protein that smooth muscle cells are in contact with that influences growth and differentiation properties but also the organization and presentation of specific matrix components. Koyama et al. (1996) showed that smooth muscle cells adhering to native fibrillar collagen did not undergo mitogenesis when stimulated with PDGF-BB. However, smooth muscle cells adhering to denatured collagen responded to PDGF-BB and underwent cell division. Cells adhering to fibrillar collagen showed increased expression of cell cycle inhibitor proteins. Carragher et al. (1999) followed up these studies and showed that degraded collagen fragments caused smooth muscle cells to lose their focal adhesion and to round up. The authors hypothesize that in vivo cryptic sites that are revealed in collagen and other matrix proteins after degradation with MMPs may be important in modulating smooth muscle cell behavior in response to injury and may play a role in the progression of atherosclerosis.

As discussed earlier in this chapter, matrix protease expression and activity are modulated with age and influence the remodeling processes associated with the aged artery. It is likely that changes in the matrix seen during aging contribute to changes in smooth muscle phenotype and responsiveness. This hypothesis is supported by several studies. Lovdahl et al. (2000) showed that batimastat, a synthetic metalloproteinase inhibitor, suppresses injury-induced phosphorylation of mitogen-activated protein kinase ERK1/ERK2 and phenotypic modification of arterial smooth muscle cells in vitro. Antisense oligonucleotides to stromelysin mRNA inhibit injury-induced proliferation of arterial smooth muscle cells in a balloon injury model in rat carotid arteries. While these studies do not directly address the effect of MMP inhibition on aging, they do suggest that targeting these enzymes may inhibit intimal thickening associated with aging (Lovdahl et al., 1999).

8. Conclusions

Hopefully, this chapter will aid in the appreciation of the complexity of changes in the connective tissue and extracellular matrix proteins of the arterial wall with aging and how these changes affect the mechanical and functional properties of arteries and will contribute to stimulating new research in this area. The approaches that have been taken in the past have been to study individual target molecules and how their expression of activity changes at any given moment in time. This type of investigation has clearly strengthened our understanding of the aging process but does not give a good indication of how interacting molecules, such as matrix molecules, integrins, and MMPs, are coordinately regulated or what the temporal patterns of regulation are. With the expansion of gene array analysis, some of this information should be available soon. Furthermore, future studies should be aimed not just at identifying changes, but at aiding in the understanding of the interactions of the many factors (extracellular matrix, growth factors, cell–cell interaction, and mechanical change) that contribute to normal remodeling with aging and how this process contributes to increased susceptibility to other vascular diseases.

References

Alenghat, F.J., Ingber, D.E., 2002. Mechanotransduction: all signals point to cytoskeleton, matrix and integrins. Sci. STKE 1, PE6.

Annoni, G., Luvara, G., Arosio, B., Gagliano, N., Fiordaliso, F., Santambrogio, D., Jeremic, G., Mircoli, L., Latini, R., Vergani, C., Masson, S., 1998. Age-dependent expression of fibrosis-related genes and collagen deposition in the rat myocardium. Mech. Ageing Dev. 101, 57–72.

Barnes, M.J., 1988. Collagens of normal and diseased blood vessel wall. In: Nimni, M.E. (Ed.), Biochemistry, Collagens, vol. I. CRC Press, Inc, Boca Raton, pp. 275–290.

Belmin, J., 1999. Vascular aging. In: Levy, B.I., Tedgui, A. (Eds.), Biology of the Arterial Wall. Kluwer Academic Publishers, Boston, pp. 129–147.

Benetos, A., Laurent, S., Hoeks, A.P., Boutouyrie, P.H., Safar, M.E., 1993. Arterial alterations with aging and high blood pressure. A noninvasive study of carotid and femoral arteries. Arterioscler. Thromb. 13, 90–97.

Bilato, C., Curto, K.A., Monticone, R.E., Pauly, R.R., White, A.J., Crow, M.T., 1997. The inhibition of vascular smooth muscle cells migration by peptide and antibody antagonists of the $\alpha v \beta 3$ integrin complex is reversed by activated calcium/calmodulin kinase II. J. Clin. Invest. 100, 693–704.

Bleys, R.L.A.W., Cowen, T., 2001. Innervation of cerebral blood vessels: morphology, plasticity, age-related, and Alzheimer's disease-related neurodegeneration. Microsc. Res. Tech. 53, 106–118.

Bruel, A., Oxlund, H., 1996. Changes in biomechanical properties, composition of collagen and elastin, and advanced glycation endproducts of rat aorta in relation to age. Atherosclerosis 127, 155–165.

Bruel, A., Ortoft, G., Oxlund, H., 1998. Inhibition of cross-link in collagen is associated with reduced stiffness of the aorta in young rats. Atherosclerosis 140, 135–145.

Bulpitt, C.J., Rajkumar, C., Caeron, J.D., 1999. Vascular compliance as a measure of biological age. J. Am. Geriatr. Soc. 47, 657–663.

Carragher, N.O., Levkau, B., Ross, R., Raines, E.W., 1999. Degraded collagen fragments promote rapid disassembly of smooth muscle focal adhesions that correlates with cleavage of pp125FAK, paxillin and tallin. J. Cell Biol. 147, 619–629.

Cattell, M.A., Anderson, J.C., Hasleton, P.S., 1996. Age-related changes in amounts and concentrations of collagen and elastin in normotensive human thoracic aorta. Clin. Chim. Acta 245, 73–84.

Crouse, J.R., Goldbourt, U., Evans, G., Pinsky, J., Sharrett, A.R., Sorlie, P., Riley, W., Heiss, G., 1994. Arterial enlargement in the Atherosclerosis Risk in Communities (ARIC) cohort. In vivo quantification of carotid arterial enlargement. The ARIC investigators. Stroke 25, 1354–1359.

Davis, G.E., Bayless, K.J., Davis, M.J., Meininger, G.A., 2000. Regulation of tissue injury responses by the exposure of matricryptic sites within extracellular matrix molecules. Am. J. Pathol. 156, 1489–1498.

Eyre, D.R., Paz, M.A., Gallop, P.M., 1984. Crosslinking in collagen and elastin. Annu. Rev. Biochem. 53, 717–748.

Galis, Z.S., Khatri, J.J., 2002. Matrix metalloproteinases in vascular remodeling and atherogenesis. Circ. Res. 90, 251–262.

Gavazzi, I., Boyle, K.S., Edgar, D., Cowen, T., 1995. Reduced laminin immunoreactivity in the blood vessels wall of ageing rats correlates with reduced innervation in vivo and following transplantation. Cell Tissue Res. 281, 23–32.

Glukhova, M.A., Frid, M.G., Koteliansky, V.E., 1991. Phenotypic changes of human aortic smooth muscle cells during development and in the adult vessel. Am. J. Physiol. 26, 78–80.

Groenink, M., Langerak, S.E., Vanbavel, E., van der Wall, E.E., Mulder, B.J.M., van der Wal, A., Spaan, J.A.E., 1999. The influence of aging and aortic stiffness on permanent dilation and breaking stress of the thoracic descending aorta. Cardiovasc. Res. 43, 471–480.

Guyton, J.R., Lindsay, K.L., Dao, D.T., 1983. Comparison of aortic intima and inner media in young adult versus aging rats. Am. J. Pathol. 111, 234–246.

Hanon, O., Luong, V., Mourad, J.J., Bortolotto, L.A., Jeunemaitre, X., Girerd, X., 2001. Aging, carotid artery distensibility and Ser422Gly elastin gene polymorphism in humans. Hypertension 38, 1185–1189.

Hansen, F., Mangell, P., Sonesson, B., Lanne, T., 1995. Diameter and compliance in the human common carotid artery—variation with age and sex. Ultrasound Med. Biol. 21, 1–9.

Hariri, R.J., Alonso, D.R., Hajjar, D.P., Coletti, D., Weksler, M.E., 1986. Aging and arteriosclerosis. I. Development of myointimal hyperplasia after endothelial injury. J. Exp. Med. 164, 1171–1178.

Hedin, U., Sjolund, M., Hultgard-Nilsson, A., Thyberg, J., 1990. Changes in expression and organization of smooth-muscle-specific α-actin during fibronectin-mediated modulation of arterial smooth muscle cell phenotype. Differentiation 44, 222–232.

Howard, G., Sharrett, A.R., Heiss, G., Evans, G.W., Chambless, L.E., Riley, W.A., Burke, G.L., 1993. Carotid artery intimal–medial thickness distribution in general populations as evaluated by B-mode ultrasound. ARIC investigators. Stroke 24, 1297–1304.

Hsuwong, S., Katchman, S.D., Ledo, I., Wu, M., Khillan, J., Bashir, M.M., Rosenbloom, J., Uitto, J., 1994. Tissue-specific and developmentally regulated expression of human elastin promoter activity in transgenic mice. J. Biol. Chem. 269, 18072–18075.

Imai, S.I., Nishibayashi, S., Tako, K., Tomifuji, M., Fujino, T., Hasegawa, M., Takano, T., 1997. Dissociation of oct-1 from the nuclear peripheral structure induces the cellular aging-associated collagenase gene expression. Mol. Biol. Cell 8, 2407–2419.

Intengan, H.D., Schiffrin, E.L., 2000. Structure and mechanical properties of resistance arteries in hypertension: role of adhesion molecules and extracellular matrix determinants. Hypertension 36, 312–318.

Kalth, S., Tsipouras, P., Silver, F.H., 1986. Non-invasive assessment of aortic mechanical properties. Ann. Biomed. Eng. 14, 513–524.

Kannel, W.B., Gordon, T., 1980. Cardiovascular risk factors in the aged: the Framingham Study. In: Haynes, S.G., Feinlieb, M. (Eds.), Epidemiology of Aging. NIH Publication 80-969, Bethesda, MD, pp. 65–98.

Kass, D.A., Shapiro, E.P., Kawaguchi, M., Capriotti, A.R., Scuteri, A., deGroof, R.C., Lakatta, E.G., 2001. Improved arterial compliance by a novel advanced glycation end-product crosslink breaker. Circulation 104, 1464–1470.

Kawasaki, T., Sasayama, S., Yagi, S., Asakawa, T., Hirai, T., 1987. Non-invasive assessment of the age related changes in stiffness of major branches of the human arteries. Cardiovasc. Res. 21, 678–687.

Kelly, R., Hayward, C., Avolio, A., O'Rourke, M., 1989. Noninvasive determination of age-related changes in the human arterial pulse. Circulation 80, 1652–1659.

Koyama, H., Raines, E.W., Bornfeldt, K.E., Roberts, J.M., Ross, R., 1996. Fibrillar collagen inhibits arterial smooth muscle proliferation through regulation of Cdk2 inhibitors. Cell 87, 1069–1078.

Li, Z., Froehilich, J., Galis, Z.S., Lakatta, E.G., 1999. Increased expression of matrix metalloproteinase-2 in the thickened intima of aged rats. Hypertension 33, 116–123.

Lovdahl, C., Thyber, J., Cercek, B., Bomgren, K., Dimayuga, P., Kallin, B., Hultgardh-Nilsson, A., 1999. Antisense oligonucleotides to stromelysin mRNA inhibit injury-induced proliferation of arterial smooth muscle cells. Histol. Histopathol. 14, 1101–1112.

Lovdahl, C., Thyberg, J., Hultgardh-Nilsson, A., 2000. The synthetic metalloproteinase inhibitor batimastat suppresses injury-induced phosphorylation of MAP kinase ERK1/ERK2 and phenotypic modification of arterial smooth muscle cells in vitro. J. Vasc. Res. 37, 345–354.

Marshall, G.E., Konstas, A.G., Lee, W.R., 1990. Ultrastructural distribution of collagen types I–VI in aging human retinal vessels. Br. J. Ophthalmol. 74, 228–232.

McCaffrey, T.A., Falcone, D.J., 1993. Evidence for an age-related dysfunction in the antiproliferative response to transforming growth factor-beta in vascular smooth muscle cells. Mol. Biol. Cell 4, 315–322.

Mogford, J.E., Platts, S.H., Davis, G.E., Meininger, G.A., 1996. Vascular smooth muscle $\alpha v \beta 3$ integrin mediates arteriolar vasodilation in response to RGD peptides. Circ. Res. 79, 821–826.

Mogford, J.E., Davis, G.E., Meininger, G.A., 1997. RGDN peptide interaction with endothelial $\alpha 5 \beta 1$ integrin causes sustained endothelin-dependent vasoconstriction of rat skeletal muscle arterioles. J. Clin. Invest. 100, 1647–1653.

Moon, S.-K., Thompson, L.F., Madamanchi, N., Ballinger, S., Papconstantinou, J., Horaist, C., Runge, M.S., Patterson, C., 2001. Aging, oxidative responses, and proliferative capacity in cultured mouse aortic smooth muscle cells. Am. J. Physiol. Heart Circ. Physiol. 280, H2779–H2788.

Muller-Delp, J., Spier, S.A., Ramsey, M.W., Lesniewski, L.A., Papadopoulos, A., Humphrey, J.S., Delp, M.D., 2002. Effects of aging on vasoconstrictor and mechanical properties of rat skeletal muscle arterioles. Am. J. Physiol. Heart Circ. Physiol. 282, H1843–H1845.

Rajagopalan, S., Meng, X.P., Ramasamy, S., Harrison, D.G., Galis, Z.S., 1996. Reactive oxygen species produced by macrophage-derived foam cells regulate the activity of vascular matrix metalloproteinases in vitro. J. Clin. Invest. 98, 2572–2579.

Reiser, K.M., 1991. Nonenzymatic glycation of collagen in aging and diabetes. Proc. Soc. Exp. Biol. Med. 196, 17–29.

Reiser, K.M., 1994. Influence of age and long-term dietary restriction on enzymatically mediated crosslinks and nonenzymatic glycation of collagen in mice. J. Gerontol. 49, B71–B79.

Reiser, K.M., Hennessy, S.M., Last, J.A., 1987. Analysis of age-associated changes in collagen crosslinking in the skin and lung in monkeys and rats. Biochim. Biophys. Acta 926, 339–348.

Resier, K.M., 1992. Enzymatic and non-enzymatic crosslinking of collagen and elastin. FASEB J. 6, 2439–2449.

Reusch, P., Wagdy, H., Reusch, R., Wilson, E., Ives, H.E., 1996. Mechanical strain increases smooth muscle and decreases nonmuscle myosin expression in rat vascular smooth muscle cells. Circ. Res. 79, 1046–1053.

Richardson, M., Hatton, M.W., Moore, S., 1988. Proteoglycan distribution in the intima and media of the aortas of young and aging rabbits: an ultrastructural analysis. Atherosclerosis 71.

Rivard, A., Principe, N., Andres, V., 2000. Age-dependent increase in c-fos activity and cyclin A expression in vascular smooth muscle cells. A potential link between aging, smooth muscle cell proliferation and atherosclerosis. Cardiovasc. Res. 45, 1026–1034.

Robert, L., Labat-Robert, J., Hornebeck, W., 1986. Aging and atherosclerosis. In: Gotto, A.M., Paoletti, R., (Eds.), Atherosclerosis Reviews. Raven Press, New York, pp. 143–170.

Robert, L., Robert, A.M., Jacotot, B., 1998. Elastin–elastase—atherosclerosis revisited. Atherosclerosis 140, 281–295.

Robins, S., 1982. Analysis of crosslinking components in collagen and elastin. Meth. Biochem. Anal. 28, 329–379.

Schmidt-Trucksass, A., Grathwohl, D., Schmid, A., Boragk, R., Upmeier, C., Keul, J., Huonker, M., 1999. Structural, functional, and hemodynamic changes in the common carotid artery with ageing in male subjects. Arterioscler. Thromb. Vasc. Biol. 19, 1091–1097.

Shapiro, S.D., Endicott, S.K., Province, M.A., Pierce, J.A., Campbell, E.J., 1991. Marked longevity of human lung parenchyma elastic fiber from prevalence of D-aspartate and nuclear weapons related radiocarbon. J. Clin. Invest. 87, 1828–1834.

Sonesson, B., Hansen, F., Stale, H., Lanne, T., 1993. Compliance and diameter in the human abdominal aorta—the influence of age and sex. Eur. J. Vasc. Surg. 7, 690–697.

Spina, M., Garbisa, S., Hinnie, J., Hunter, J.C., Serafini-Fracassini, A., 1983. Age-related changes in composition and mechanical properties of the tunica media of the upper thoracic human aorta. Arteriosclerosis 3, 64–76.

Stemerman, M.B., Weinstein, R., Rowe, J.W., Maciag, T., Fuhro, R., Gardner, R., 1982. Vascular smooth muscle cell growth kinetics in vivo in aged rats. Proc. Natl. Acad. Sci. U. S. A. 79, 3863–3866.

Sternlicht, M.D., Werb, Z., 2001. How matrix metalloproteinases regulate cell behavior. Annu. Rev. Cell Dev. Biol. 17, 463–516.

Takasaki, I., Takizawa, T., Sugimoto, K., Gotoh, E., Shionoiri, H., Ishii, M., 1994. Effects of hypertension and aging on fibronectin expression in aorta of Dahl salt-sensitive rats. Am. J. Physiol. 267, H1523–H1529.

Thyberg, J., Hedin, U., Sjolund, M., Palmberg, L., Bottger, B.A., 1990. Regulation of differentiated properties and proliferation of arterial smooth muscle cells. Atherosclerosis 10, 966–990.

Tovar, A.M.F., Cesar, D.C.F., Leta, G.C., Mourao, P.A.S., 1998. Age-related changes in populations of aortic glycosaminoglycans. Species with low affinity for plasma low-density lipoproteins, and not species with high affinity, are preferentially affected. Arterioscler. Thromb. Vasc. Biol. 18, 604–614.

Tronc, F., Mallat, Z., Lehoux, S., Wassef, M., Espositio, B., Tedgui, A., 2000. Role of matrix metalloproteinases in blood flow-induced arterial enlargement: Interaction with NO. Arterioscler. Thromb. Vasc. Biol. 20, e120–e126.

Vaitkevicius, P.V., Lane, M., Spurgeion, H., Ingram, D.K., Roth, G.S., Egan, J.J., Vasan, S., Wagle, D.R., Ulrich, P., Brines, M., Wuerth, J.P., Cerami, A., Lakatta, E.G., 2001. A cross-link breaker has sustained effects on arterial and ventricular properties in older rhesus monkeys. Proc. Natl. Acad. Sci. 98, 1171–1175.

Van Merode, T., Hick, P.J., Hoeks, A.P., Rahn, K.H., Reneman, R.S., 1988. Carotid artery wall properties of in normotensive and borderline hypertensive subjects of various ages. Ultrasound Med. Biol. 14, 563–569.

Vogel, H.G., 1978. Influence of maturation and age on mechanical and biochemical parameters of connective tissue of various organs in the rat. Connect. Tissue Res. 6, 161–166.

Waitkus-Edwards, K.R., Martinez-Lemus, L.A., Wu, X., Trzeciakowski, J.P., Davis, M.J., Davis, G.E., Meininger, G.A., 2002. α4β1 integrin activation of L-type calcium channels in vascular smooth muscle causes arteriole vasoconstriction. Circ. Res. 90, 473–480.

Wang, M., Lakatta, E.G., 2002. Altered regulation of matrix metalloproteinases-2 in aortic remodeling during aging. Hypertension 39, 865–873.

Watanabe, M., Sawai, T., Hagura, H., Suyama, K., 1996. Age-related alteration of cross-linking amino acids of elastin in human aorta. Tohoku J. Exp. Med. 180, 115–130.

Wilson, E., Sudhir, K., Ives, H.E., 1995. Mechanical strain of rat vascular smooth muscle cells is sensed by specific extracellular matrix/integrin interactions. J. Clin. Invest. 96, 2364–2372.

Wu, X., Mogford, J.E., Platts, S.H., Davis, G.E., Davis, M.J., 1998. Modulations of calcium current in arteriolar smooth muscle by αvβ3 and α5β1 integrin receptor ligands. J. Cell Biol. 143, 241–252.

Wu, X., Davis, G.E., Meininger, G.A., Wilson, E., Davis, M.J., 2001. Integrin-dependent L-type calcium channel by α5β1 integrin requires signaling between focal adhesion proteins. J. Biol. Chem. 276, 30285–30292.

Yamada, E., Hazama, F., Amano, S., Sasahara, M., Kataoka, H., 1986. Elastase, collagenase and cathepsin D activities in the aortas of spontaneously hypertensive and renal hypertensive rats. Exp. Mol. Pathol. 44, 147–156.

**Advances in
Cell Aging and
Gerontology**

Mitochondrial electron transport and aging in the heart

Edward J. Lesnefsky[a,d], Bernard Tandler[d], Shadi Moghaddas[a],
Medhat O. Hassan[d] and Charles L. Hoppel[b,c,d,*]

[a]*Division of Cardiology, Department of Medicine, Case Western Reserve University
and Medical Services and Geriatric Research, Education and Clinical Center, 10701 East Boulevard,
Cleveland, OH 44106, USA*
[b]*Division of Clinical Pharmacology, Department of Medicine, Case Western Reserve University and Medical
Services and Geriatric Research, Education and Clinical Center, 10701 East Boulevard,
Cleveland, OH 44106, USA*
[c]*Departments of Medicine and Pharmacology, Case Western Reserve University
and Medical Services and Geriatric Research, Education and Clinical Center, 10701 East Boulevard,
Cleveland, OH 44106, USA*
[d]*Department of Medicine, Case Western Reserve University and Medical Services
and Geriatric Research, Education and Clinical Center, Louis Stokes Veterans Affairs Medical Center,
10701 East Boulevard, Cleveland, OH 44106, USA*

Contents

* Corresponding author. Tel.: +1-216-791-3800x5657; fax: +1-216-707-0254.
E-mail address: clh5@po.cwru.edu (C.L. Hoppel).

Advances in Cell Aging and Gerontology, vol. 11, 201–232

Abbreviations

SSM	subsarcolemmal mitochondria
IFM	interfibrillar mitochondria
CL	cardiolipin
PC	phosphatidylcholine
PE	phosphatidylethanolamine
PI	phosphatidylinositol
ISP	Iron–sulfur protein
BNPAGE	blue native polyacrylamide electrophoresis
DHQ	durohydroquinone
EPR	electron paramagnetic resonance
Q	coenzyme Q
mtDNA	mitochondrial DNA

1. Introduction

This chapter addresses the role of mitochondrial defects in the aging heart from the structural and biochemical perspectives. First, the insights into the alterations in mitochondria during aging that are gained from the study of myocardial histology and histochemistry are reviewed. The preservation of mitochondrial morphology during aging is then addressed. In the second part of the chapter, the biochemistry of aging defects in mitochondrial metabolism is examined. The review of mitochondrial metabolism during aging begins with the procedure used to isolate mitochondrial subpopulations, with a focus on mitochondrial recovery as determined by the balance study of mitochondrial marker enzymes. Next, aging defects in interfibrillar mitochondria (IFM) are reviewed, especially the localization of aging damage to specific molecular sites within electron transport chain complexes III and IV. Finally, the mechanisms whereby aging defects contribute to myocyte dysfunction and potential cell death in the aging heart in the baseline state and during the metabolic stress of ischemia are discussed.

2. Structure

Each cardiac muscle fiber consists of a series of cardiomyocytes joined end-to-end by intercalated disks. The latter are made up of attachment devices and gap junctions arranged in stepwise fashion. The gap junctions are low impedance structures, so that an action potential passes uninterruptedly from myocyte to myocyte, in effect producing a functional syncitium. Aside from the myofilaments that constitute the contractile apparatus, the cardinal cytoplasmic organelles in the myocytes are the mitochondria, which, in young hearts, make up 24–43% of the fractional volume of the cytoplasm, according to species (Schaper et al., 1985). The mitochondria are ovoid to ellipsoid and have numerous, transversely oriented cristae. Based on both morphological and biochemical criteria (Palmer et al., 1977), there are two distinct populations of mitochondria, one beneath the sarcolemma (subsarcolemmal mitochondria, SSM), the other interspersed among the myofilaments (interfibrillar mitochondria, IFM) (Fig. 1); it should be noted that this functional difference is not reflected at the morphological level: mitochondria at both sites are structurally identical based on transmission electron microscopic examination.

There have been relatively few morphological studies of the aging heart. In Fischer rats, interstitial fibrosis occurs at 6–12 months of age and increases in frequency and degree with advancing age (Coleman et al., 1977). These changes were not considered to be of vascular origin, but rather due to degenerative and inflammatory changes. In a histometric analysis of cardiac papillary muscle in these rats, Anversa et al. (1989) found significant replacement fibrosis in aged animals, especially in the left papillary muscle. Because this study was based entirely on transverse sections of the cardiac fibers, it was not possible to determine the linear extent of these lesions. In other words, were cardiac fibers affected for their entire length or were the defects segmental, i.e., in sporadic cardiomyocytes?

The matter of ventricular fibrosis in aging is unsettled. Most studies of this phenomenon are based on study of human hearts. Some reports aver that there is little or no fibrosis in elderly hearts (Lakatta et al., 1987; Olivetti et al., 1991). Other studies claim that fibrosis occurs only in scattered foci or in specific restricted regions (Olivetti et al., 1991; Wanagat et al., 2002), and that extensive regions of the ventricles remain unaffected (Olivetti et al., 1991; Wanagat et al., 2002). In review on aging hearts, Wei (1992) concludes that there is a slight increase in the amount of elastic tissue, fat, and collagen, as well as in the number of fibrotic foci. In our unpublished study of aged rat hearts examined in semithin epoxy sections, we found several hearts wherein the connective tissue spaces between cardiac fibers were exaggerated and contained a homogeneous matrix in which collagen fiber bundles were not discernible, and, in agreement with the electron microscope observations of Tomanek and Karlsson (1973), various types of connective tissue cells were present. However, many of the aged hearts in our study were indistinguishable from those in 6-month adults.

Another feature of aging hearts, in general, is the presence, usually at the poles of the nuclei, of deposits of lipofuscin (wear-and-tear pigment). This material represents, at the light microscopic level, lysosomes, autophagic vacuoles, and residual bodies (Travis and Travis, 1972). These structures, which increase progressively in number with aging, appear to be of no physiological significance (Lakatta et al., 1987).

An ultracytochemical study of aging human heart by Müller-Höcker (1989) found that scattered individual cardiomyocytes to varying degrees lack cytochrome c oxidase activity and that such cells show degenerative changes. All of the mitochondria in a given cell are affected; the lesion ends at the intercalated disks. Similar defects were noted in the hearts of aged monkeys (Müller-Höcker, 1989; Müller-Höcker et al., 1996). In a histochemical study of hearts from aged hybrid rats, Wanagat et al. (2002) observed occasional myocytes that lacked activities of cytochrome c oxidase and of succinic dehydrogenase. Staining with hematoxylin and eosin did not show

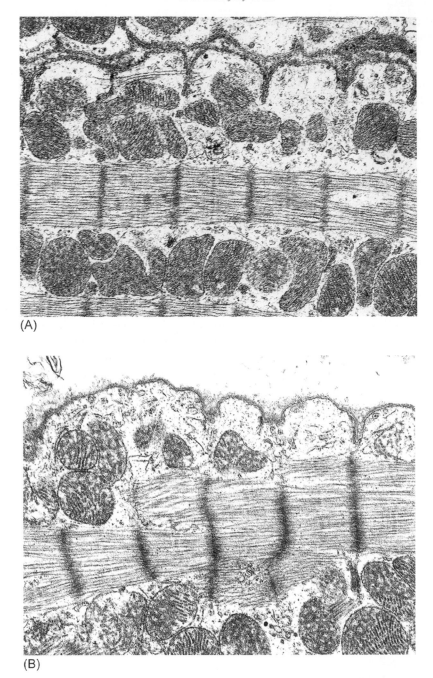

(A)

(B)

Fig. 1.   Electron micrographs of myocardium from adult (6 months) (panel A) and aged (28 months) (panel B) Fischer 344 rat hearts. Subsarcolemmal mitochondria (SSM) are located beneath the plasma membrane whilst IFM are ensconced among the myofibrils. The appearance of myocardium from adult and aged rat hearts is, in general, similar. See text for details. A and B: $18,000 \times$.

morphologically defective myocytes. It seems probable that cardiac fibers with altered mitochondria are indistinguishable from normal ones using conventional histological staining.

We have examined in semithin sections the microscopic structure of the left ventricle of hearts from a large number of rats aged 6, 24, and 28 months. By and large, the hearts were identical across the board. Some of the 28-month rats showed a relatively minor increase in fibrosis. We encountered no evidence of degenerating or degenerated cells. Several, but not all, of the 24-month rats had numerous, small droplets of neutral lipids scattered throughout their cytosol. Although we did not perform a strict cytometric analysis, our subjective impression was that there was no obvious change in either mitochondrial population. Frenzel and Feiman (1984) found that in aged Wistar rats, there was a reduction in mitochondrial volume that was offset by an increase in mitochondrial number.

The discrepancy between our findings and that of others probably is due to differences in technique. We customarily employ a triple aldehyde-DMSO mixture (Kalt and Tandler, 1971), which, because of its rapid penetration into solid tissues, yields optimal fixation. For example, in a previous ultrastructural study, we (Lesnefsky et al., 1997) found that, with this fixative, even cardiomyocytes subjected to 15–45 min of ischemia almost matched those fixed immediately upon extirpation from rabbits. We believe that when cardiomyocytes are subjected to stress (in the present case, aging), they become progressively more fragile and that less-than-optimal fixation results in cytological disruption. When, however, appropriate fixatives are applied, the native structure of these cells is preserved.

Through the use of balance studies, we are able to account for the total mito-chondrial activity present in the intact heart and all mitochondrial and supernatant fractions obtained from these organs from animals subjected to ischemia or not, whether adult or aged. Our recovery of mitochondria was 60–70%. We found virtually no morphological differences among cardiac mitochondrial pellets prepared from control or aged rats, whether or not the animals had been subjected to ischemia (Fannin et al., 1999; Lesnefsky et al., 2001a). There were relatively few structurally damaged mitochondria in our pellets, regardless of their source.

It should be noted that if intact mitochondrial pellets are fixed, they may show a gradient of structural preservation based on centrifugal stratification and that it becomes possible to obtain non-representative images that show a high level of structural preservation. To guard against such a possibility, we fix all of our fractions in suspension, so that any given view is representative of the fraction as a whole.

3. Physiology

3.1. *Isolation of two populations of cardiac mitochondria*

The two mitochondrial populations, SSM and IFM, are fundamentally different (Fannin et al., 1999; Hoppel et al., 1982; Lesnefsky et al., 1997; Palmer et al., 1977; Palmer et al., 1985; Piper et al., 1985; Shin et al., 1989). In the adult heart, state 3 respiratory rates are greater in IFM than in SSM; the coupling of respiration is

Isolation of Two Population of Cardiac Mitochondria

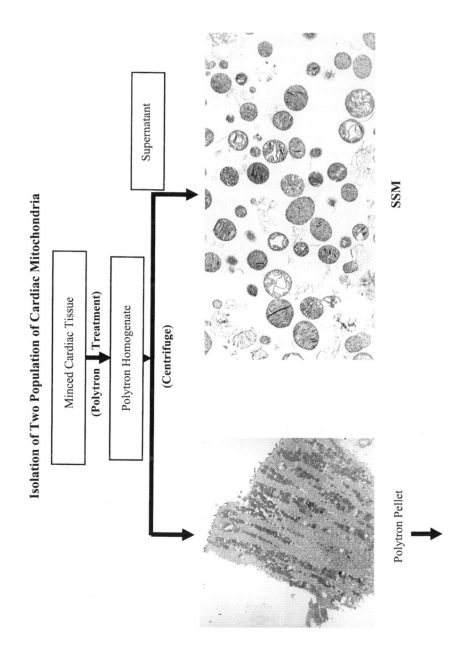

Minced Cardiac Tissue

(Polytron Treatment)

Polytron Homogenate

(Centrifuge)

Supernatant

SSM

Polytron Pellet

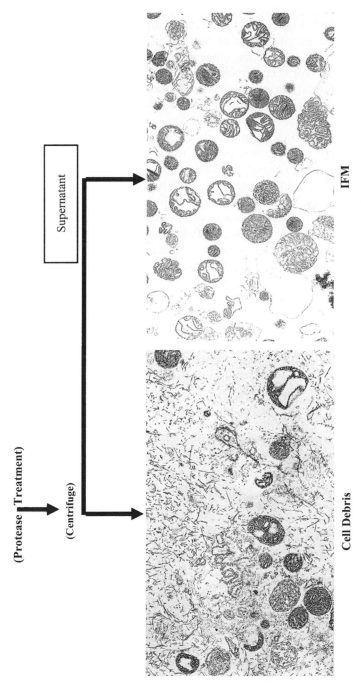

Fig. 2.   Schematic diagram displaying the method used to isolate subsarcolemmal and interfibrillar populations of mitochondria. Cardiac tissue is finely minced, placed in Chappell-Perry buffer (100 mM KCl, 50 mM MOPS, 1 mM EDTA, 5 mM MgSO$_4$ 7 H$_2$O, 1 mM ATP, pH 7.4) containing 0.2% BSA and homogenized with a polytron tissue processor for 2.5 s at a rheostat setting of 6.0. The resulting polytron homogenate was centrifuged at 500 g, the supernatant saved for isolation of SSM, and the pellet washed. The combined supernatants are centrifuged at 3000 g to sediment SSM, which were washed twice, then suspended in KME (100 mM KCl, 50 mM MOPS, 0.5 mM EGTA). The final SSM pellet is shown (6200 ×). The polytron pellet consisting of skinned myofibers (1200 ×) is resuspended in Chappell-Perry buffer; nagarse added to a final concentration of 5 mg/g wet weight of tissue, the suspension immediately homogenized with a Potter–Elvejhem homogenizer, then diluted with Chappell–Perry buffer containing 0.2% BSA, and centrifuged at 5000 g to rapidly separate mitochondria from the protease-containing supernatant. The pellet was resuspended in Chappell–Perry buffer containing 0.2% BSA and centrifuged at low speed (500 g) to sediment cell debris (7700 ×). The pellet was washed, the mitochondrial-containing supernatants combined, and IFM isolated by centrifugation at 3000 g. IFM were washed twice and suspended in KME (6200 ×).

similar in both populations (Lesnefsky et al., 1997; Palmer et al., 1977). IFM have an increased content of respiratory cytochromes and activity of electron transport chain complexes (Hoppel et al., 1982; Lesnefsky et al., 1997; Palmer et al., 1977). Differences in respiratory rates and enzyme contents persist following exposure of each population to the methods used to isolate the other population (Palmer et al., 1985). A distinctive structural marker for each population is yet to be identified. The two populations are affected differently in pathologic states, including calcium overload (Palmer et al., 1986), cardiomyopathy (Hoppel et al., 1982), and ischemia (Lesnefsky et al., 2001a; Lesnefsky et al., 1997; Piper et al., 1985; Shin et al., 1989). The study of the response of each population to the aging process may identify novel, regionally specific mitochondrial defects that are not evident when a combined population composed of potentially affected and unaffected mitochondria is used.

We considered that aging might affect only one of the two populations of cardiac mitochondria. SSM are released by the initial tissue homogenization, whereas the liberation of IFM from the resulting skinned myocytes requires additional disruption of the myofilaments by brief exposure to protease (Palmer et al., 1977; Fannin et al., 1999). Two populations of cardiac mitochondria were isolated from the aging heart using the procedure of Palmer et al. (1977) (Fig. 2), except that a modified Chappell–Perry buffer (myofibril relaxing buffer including magnesium and ATP) was used for mitochondrial isolation (Fannin et al., 1999). Briefly, cardiac tissue was finely minced, placed in Chappell–Perry buffer containing bovine serum albumin (BSA) and homogenized with a polytron tissue processor (Fannin et al., 1999). The polytron homogenate was centrifuged at low speed (500 g), the polytron supernatant saved for isolation of SSM, and the polytron pellet washed. The combined supernatants were centrifuged to sediment SSM (3000 g), washed twice, and suspended in KCl–MOPS–EGTA buffer for study. The polytron pellet was resuspended in Chappell–Perry buffer, the protease nagarse added, and the suspension immediately homogenized. The mixture was diluted with Chappell–Perry buffer containing albumin, and centrifuged to rapidly sediment IFM away from the nagarse (5000 g). The IFM pellet was resuspended in Chappell–Perry containing albumin and centrifuged at low speed (500 g) to sediment myofibrillar debris. The pellet was washed, the mitochondria-containing supernatants combined, and IFM isolated by centrifugation (3000 g). IFM were washed twice and suspended in KCl–MOPS–EGTA buffer for study.

The protein yield of SSM and IFM was similar in 6-month old adult Fischer 344 rat hearts. In hearts obtained from either 24 or 28-month old elderly groups, the yield of IFM was decreased by 20–30% compared to the yield of IFM from the adult heart, whereas the yield of SSM remained unaltered (Fannin et al., 1999).

The enzyme cytology approach of DeDuve (1967) was used in order to address whether the relative recovery of SSM and IFM was similar in adult and elderly hearts. Citrate synthase, present in the mitochondrial matrix, was employed as a mitochondrial marker enzyme. The specific activity of citrate synthase enrichment relative to the specific activity in the initial myocardial homogenate was measured in the cellular fractions obtained during the isolation of SSM and IFM (Fannin et al., 1999). The enrichment of citrate synthase in each fraction, the protein yield, and thus the percentage recovery of total citrate synthase in each fraction was similar in adult and elderly hearts (Fannin et al., 1999). Succinate dehydrogenase, present in the inner mitochondrial membrane, was used as a second marker enzyme and yielded results similar to those observed with citrate synthase. Based on the recovery of marker enzyme activity, the relative recovery of both SSM and IFM populations of mitochondria was similar in the adult and aging heart. Morphologic analysis of the nagarse pellets did not suggest greater entrapment of IFM in this fraction in the aging heart. Thus, the aging-related decrease in protein yield and oxidative phosphorylation in aging IFM does not occur as a result of the isolation process.

Trypsin also has been used as the protease to release IFM (Fannin et al., 1999; Moghaddas et al., 2002c). The protein yield and the rate of oxidative phosphorylation in IFM were similar to results obtained using nagarse. Enzyme cytology studies were performed when trypsin was used as the protease to isolate IFM. Again, a similar relative recovery of SSM and IFM was obtained in adult and aging hearts (unpublished data). With the use of trypsin, a decrease in the protein yield of IFM from aging hearts was again observed (Moghaddas et al., 2002c). Thus, irrespective of the protease used, a decreased yield of IFM is obtained in the aging heart. Enzyme cytology studies support a similar recovery of mitochondria from adult and aging hearts regardless of the protease used to isolate IFM. Thus, the decreased protein yield of IFM is intrinsic to the aging heart and is not a consequence of the procedure used to isolate the mitochondria.

3.2. *Mitochondrial oxidative physiology*

The study of oxidative phosphorylation in isolated mitochondria identifies defects in the electron transport chain and characterizes damage to the phosphorylation apparatus that leads to diminished coupling of respiration. Substrates that donate electrons to specific sites in the electron transport chain are used to localize the site of defects within the sequence of electron transport (Fig. 3). Measurement of uncoupled respiration tests if damage to the phosphorylation apparatus is the mechanism of decreased rate of oxygen consumption. Exposure of mitochondria to freezing-thawing and hypotonic conditions permeabilizes the inner mitochondrial membrane, removing transport barriers. Measurement of oxygen consumption in permeabilized mitochondria bypasses defects in substrate carriers or dehydrogenases and confirms the localization of defects to the electron transport chain itself. The measurement of the enzyme activities of individual electron transport chain complexes directly localizes defects within the chain that are predicted from studies of intact and permeabilized mitochondria.

In many tissues, mitochondrial oxidative metabolism declines with age. However, the presence and severity of aging-induced decreases in the rate of oxidative phosphorylation of cardiac mitochondria had remained problematic (Chen et al., 1972; Chiu and Richardson, 1980; Hansford, 1978; Manzelmann and Harmon, 1987; Takasawa et al., 1993). Some investigators observed a decreased rate of oxidative phosphorylation in mitochondria isolated from the hearts of aging animals (Chen et al., 1972; Chiu and Richardson, 1980), whereas others did not (Hansford, 1978;

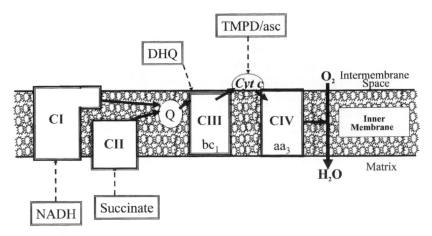

Fig. 3.   Schematic diagram of electron transport chain. The entry of reducing equivalents from NADH, succinate, durohydroquinone (DHQ), and TMPD-ascorbate (TMPD-asc) into the electron transport chain is shown. Glutamate generates NADH via glutamate dehydrogenase, which is oxidized by complex I with electron flow via coenzyme Q (Q), complex III, cytochrome c, and complex IV (cytochrome oxidase). Succinate is oxidized by complex II. DHQ is oxidized by complex III. TMPD-ascorbate reduces cytochrome c, which is oxidized by complex IV. Complex III contains cytochromes b and c_1. Complex IV contains cytochrome aa_3.

Manzelmann and Harmon, 1987; Takasawa et al., 1993). The study of cardiac mitochondria isolated by tissue homogenization alone (Takasawa et al., 1993), yielding SSM, observed similar rates of oxidative phosphorylation in mitochondria from adult and aging hearts. Mitochondria isolated following homogenization in the presence of protease (Chen et al., 1972; Hansford, 1978; Manzelmann and Harmon, 1987) yielded a mixed population of SSM and IFM. Findings in the aging heart using a mixed population of cardiac mitochondria yielded inconsistent results. Some workers observed a decrease in the rate of oxidative phosphorylation (Chen et al., 1972) with age, while others did not (Hansford, 1978; Manzelmann and Harmon, 1987). These conflicting observations suggest that previous work utilized a mixed population of cardiac mitochondria with a variable enrichment of IFM. Based upon the findings of the prior studies, we proposed that aging-induced decreases in mitochondrial oxidative phosphorylation would involve only IFM.

    We tested the hypothesis that aging-related decreases in oxidative function selectively involve IFM. Oxidative phosphorylation was studied in SSM and IFM isolated from adult and elderly hearts using the Fischer 344 rat heart model of aging with a median animal survival of 29 months (Fannin et al., 1999; Lesnefsky et al., 2001b). Glutamate, an electron donor to complex I via glutamate dehydrogenase and NADH, was the substrate (Fig. 3). The maximal rate of oxidative phosphorylation, measured in the presence of 2 mM ADP, was decreased in IFM from 24- and 28-month elderly hearts compared to IFM from 6-month old adults (Fannin et al., 1999). In contrast, the rate of oxidative phosphorylation in SSM remained unaltered by aging. The rate of oxidative phosphorylation in IFM did not decrease with age between 24 and 28 months.

The rate of oxidative phosphorylation stimulated by durohydroquinone, an electron donor to complex III, was decreased by aging in IFM, but not in SSM (Fannin et al., 1999; Lesnefsky et al., 2001b). This observation localized aging defects to a site distal to complex I (Fig. 3). The rate of uncoupled respiration was decreased, localizing the aging defect to the electron transport chain rather than to the phosphorylation apparatus. In IFM from the aging heart, respiratory rates were decreased for TMPD-ascorbate, an electron donor to complex IV via cytochrome c. Since the content of cytochrome c was unaltered by aging in IFM (Fannin et al., 1999), this observation localizes a site of aging-induced damage at least to cytochrome oxidase in IFM.

The aging-related decrease in cytochrome oxidase was previously described using a mixed population of cardiac mitochondria (Paradies et al., 1993; Paradies et al., 1997). The decrease in oxidation through cytochrome oxidase in IFM was observed at oxidation rates that represent only 30% of the maximal rate of oxidative phosphorylation and under conditions that result in maximally expressed rates of respiration (Fannin et al., 1999). The mechanism of the aging-induced defect in cytochrome oxidase is discussed below.

Aging decreased the activity of electron transport complexes III (Lesnefsky et al., 2001b) and IV (Fannin et al., 1999) in IFM (see below). The specific activities of NADH-cytochrome c oxidoreductase (complexes I and III) and succinate-cytochrome c oxidoreductase (complexes II and III) (Fig. 3) were unchanged by aging in both SSM and IFM from elderly compared to adult hearts (Fannin et al., 1999). Thus, aging does not decrease the activity of either complex I or II (the rate limiting activity for the NADH and succinate oxidoreductase assays). One laboratory found a decrease in complex I activity with aging in a mitochondrial population prepared solely by homogenization (Takasawa, 1993) (probably consisting of SSM) whereas Davies et al. (2001) did not observe a decrease. Aging decreased the activity of complex V ATPase in heart mitochondria (Davies et al., 2001; Guerrieri et al., 1993).

The rate of oxidative phosphorylation stimulated by carbohydrate as well as by fatty-acid substrates was decreased in IFM from the aging heart. The oxidation of pyruvate, a complex I substrate derived from carbohydrate metabolism, was decreased in IFM from aging hearts (Fannin et al., 1999). The oxidation of palmitoylcarnitine, a long chain fatty-acid substrate for beta oxidation, also was decreased in IFM with aging (Fannin et al., 1999).

Although aging decreased the maximal rate of oxidation in IFM, respiration remained tightly coupled in both SSM and IFM during aging (Fannin et al., 1999). State 4 respiration, respiratory control ratio, and the ADP:O ratio were unaltered by aging in both SSM and IFM. Thus, the inner mitochondrial membrane in both SSM and IFM retains functional integrity with aging.

In summary, aging-related decreases in fatty-acid oxidation (Hansford, 1978) and cytochrome oxidase activity (Paradies et al., 1993; Paradies et al., 1994; Paradies et al., 1997) previously described in mixed populations of cardiac mitochondria were localized to IFM (Fannin et al., 1999). In previous work in other laboratories, heart mitochondria isolated by tissue homogenization alone (Takasawa et al., 1993) that were expected to yield a population consisting of SSM did not exhibit aging-related decreases in mitochondrial respiration. Thus, previous results are reconciled by the finding that aging-induced decreases in oxidative phosphorylation occur only in IFM.

3.3. *Aging defect in complex IV*

Aging decreased the rate of oxidative phosphorylation stimulated by TMPD-ascorbate, an electron donor to cytochrome oxidase via cytochrome c in IFM (Fannin et al., 1999). The rate of uncoupled respiration was decreased, localizing the aging defect to the electron transport chain (Fannin et al., 1999). Cytochrome oxidase enzyme activity was measured in freshly isolated, permeabilized mitochondria in the presence of exogenous cytochrome c (Fannin et al., 1999). Polarographic cytochrome oxidase activity decreased with aging in IFM, localizing the aging defect to complex IV rather than to cytochrome c. The decrease in cytochrome oxidase activity with aging was reversed by the addition of phospholipid liposomes (Fannin et al., 1999). In a mixed population of cardiac mitochondria, aging-related decreases in cytochrome oxidase activity were ameliorated by the addition of the mitochondrial phospholipid, cardiolipin (Paradies et al., 1994).

In contrast to the above results obtained with freshly isolated mitochondria, deoxycholate detergent-expressed cytochrome oxidase activity measured in frozen-thawed IFM was unaltered by aging (Fannin et al., 1999). Interventions that alter the membrane environment of cytochrome oxidase, such as the addition of phospholipid liposomes (Fannin et al., 1999; Paradies et al., 1994), detergents (Fannin et al., 1999), or freezing and thawing (Fannin et al., 1999), augmented cytochrome oxidase activity. Cytochrome oxidase is composed of 13 peptide subunits, including three catalytic subunits, with one cytochrome aa_3 per complex (Cooper and Nicholls, 1990). Aging did not alter the content of cytochrome aa_3 in IFM from aging hearts, indicative of a preserved content of cytochrome oxidase in IFM from aging heart (Fannin et al., 1999). These findings suggest the role of an altered inner membrane environment, rather than a reduced content of cytochrome oxidase subunits, in the decrease of cytochrome oxidase activity in IFM from aging hearts.

3.4. *Aging does not alter the cardiolipin composition or content in IFM in the aging heart*

Cytochrome oxidase and complex III requires an inner membrane lipid microenvironment enriched in cardiolipin for optimal activity (Abramovitch et al., 1990; Robinson et al., 1980; Vik and Capaldi, 1977). Cardiolipin is an oxidatively sensitive phospholipid located in the inner mitochondrial membrane (Hoch, 1992). Tightly bound cardiolipin residues are an integral component of complexes III (Fry and Green, 1981; Gomez and Robinson, 1999; Hunte et al., 2000a) and IV (Fry et al., 1980; Fry and Green, 1980; Robinson et al., 1980). A decrease in the content of cardiolipin has been reported to occur during aging in heart (Hansford et al., 1999) and liver (Hagen et al., 1998). The functional studies of cytochrome oxidase in aging IFM discussed above suggest that an aging-induced cardiolipin defect would be a plausible mechanism for the complex IV defect. Thus, we asked if a decreased content or altered composition of cardiolipin occurs in IFM as a potential mechanism for the observed aging-related defects in complexes III and IV.

The content of cardiolipin was quantified by the measurement of lipid phosphate (Lesnefsky et al., 2000) in SSM and IFM obtained from adult and aging hearts (Moghaddas et al., 2002c). Mitochondrial phospholipids from adult and elderly IFM were extracted, phospholipids isolated as a fraction using silica gel columns, and individual phospholipids separated via normal phase HPLC (Moghaddas et al., 2002c). Phospholipids are quantified by measurement of organic phosphate in serial fractions to generate a "phosphate chromatogram" from the normal phase HPLC (Lesnefsky et al., 2000).

The chromatographic separation pattern of phospholipids is similar in adult and elderly hearts. Mitochondria contain phosphatidylcholine (PC), phosphatidylethanol-amine (PE), phosphatidylinositol (PI), and cardiolipin (CL). The content of the cardiolipin was unaltered by aging in both SSM and IFM (Moghaddas et al., 2002c). The content of the remaining phospholipids also was unchanged with age in SSM and IFM (Moghaddas et al., 2002c). Thus, in the population that contains aging-induced defects in mitochondrial oxidative physiology (IFM), cardiolipin content was unaltered by aging.

Total phospholipid phosphate was independently measured in the phospholipid fraction obtained from the silica gel columns (Lesnefsky et al., 2000). The recovery of total phospholipid phosphate as the sum of individual phospholipids was excellent in both adult and aging hearts (Moghaddas et al., 2002c). The excellent recovery of phospholipids does not support the presence of additional lipid phosphorus contain-ing compounds such as lysophospholipids (Lesnefsky et al., 2000) in the aging heart.

Paradies and coworkers estimated cardiolipin content by UV absorbance at 206 nm (a function of acyl-group composition) relative to the other phospholipids and described a decrease in the cardiolipin content in a mixed population of mito-chondria from the aged heart (Paradies et al., 1993, 1997). We also used this approach to estimate the ratio of cardiolipin to other phospholipids; additionally, bovine cardiolipin was used to generate a standard curve and cardiolipin content quantified by peak area of 206 nm absorbance using the standard curve. Cardiolipin content measured in this manner also was similar in IFM from adult and aging hearts (Moghaddas et al., 2002c). Thus, when quantified either by UV absorbance or by phosphate content, cardiolipin content is unchanged in IFM from aging hearts, as well as in the unaffected SSM.

While the content of cardiolipin was unaffected by age, an altered composition of cardiolipin is also a potential mechanism of decreased cytochrome oxidase activity in IFM. The acyl-group composition of cardiolipin was measured following alkaline hydrolysis, derivitization to form fatty-acid methyl esters, and separation and quantitation by gas chromatography (Ingalls et al., 1995). Cardiolipin was composed predominantly of linoleic acid (C18:2) with minor amounts of oleic acid (C18:1) and stearic acid (C18:0). The fraction of total measured acyl-groups represented by linoleic acid was similar in SSM and IFM from both adult and aging hearts, representing approximately 90% of the total acyl residues, and did not support an alteration in acyl-group composition of cardiolipin in IFM from aging hearts (Moghaddas et al., 2002c).

An additional approach was used to study if aging altered the composition of cardiolipin in IFM. The composition of cardiolipin based upon individual molecular species was examined using reverse phase HPLC followed by electrospray ionization mass spectrometry (Lesnefsky et al., 2000, 2001c). The major and minor molecular species of cardiolipin were determined in IFM from 6-month adult and 24-month aged hearts. The composition of cardiolipin as indicated by the molecular species of cardiolipin was similar in IFM from adult and senescent hearts (Fig. 4). The composition of the molecular species of cardiolipin was determined using collision-induced dissociation of the parent ion to generate daughter ions for analysis via MS/MS and MS^3 (Lesnefsky et al., 2000). Consistent with the acyl-group analysis of total cardiolipin, the major molecular species of cardiolipin (m/z 1448) corresponds to cardiolipin containing four C18:2 acyl residues (Lesnefsky et al., 2000, 2001c; Moghaddas et al., 2002c). The composition of cardiolipin molecular species was unaltered by aging in both SSM and IFM (Moghaddas et al., 2002c).

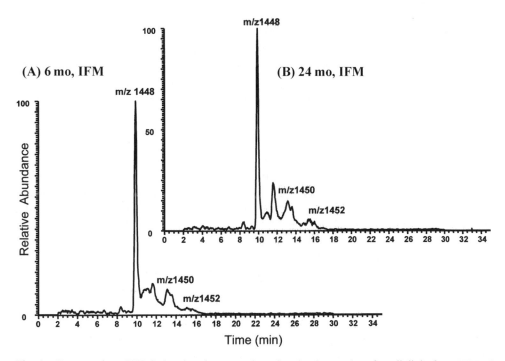

Fig. 4.   Reverse phase HPLC showing the separation of molecular species of cardiolipin from IFM of adult (chromatogram A; total ion current 3.7×10^7 arbitrary units) and elderly (chromatogram B; total ion current 3.5×10^7 arbitrary units) hearts. The major molecular species (m/z 1448) eluted at a retention time of 9.9 min and the minor species at 12 (m/z 1450) and 13 (m/z 1452) min for m/z range of 1445–1452. The molecular species were similar in IFM from adult and aging hearts.

Aging does not alter the content or composition of cardiolipin in IFM. Cardiolipin content is preserved in IFM that manifest aging-related decreases in the rate of oxidative phosphorylation and the activities of complex III (Fannin et al., 1999; Lesnefsky et al., 2001b) (see below) and cytochrome oxidase (Fannin et al., 1999; Lesnefsky et al., 2001b). Hence, damage to cardiolipin is not the mechanism for the aging-induced decrement in complexes III or IV in IFM in the aging Fischer 344 heart.

The finding of preserved cardiolipin content and composition, as well as preserved content of other phospholipids, with aging in IFM raises new questions regarding the mechanism of the aging-induced decrease in cytochrome oxidase activity. The results obtained in the study of cytochrome oxidase activity, namely, that the addition of liposomes containing cardiolipin (Paradies et al., 1994, 1996), the addition of asolectin-containing liposomes (Fannin et al., 1999), detergents (Fannin et al., 1999), or freezing-thawing (Fannin et al., 1999) enhances cytochrome oxidase activity in the aged heart points to the presence of an inner mitochondrial membrane defect that decreases cytochrome oxidase activity. This defect is not reflected in the content of inner membrane phospholipids, including cardiolipin. A further characterization of the alterations in the inner mitochondrial membrane that lead to the decrease in fluidity of the inner mitochondrial membrane described in the aging heart (Paradies et al., 1993, 1994) might provide insight into the membrane alterations that also impair the activity of cytochrome oxidase. Potential causes of the inner membrane defect may include oxidative damage to phospholipids (Paradies et al., 2000) or the depletion of n-3 acyl-groups in the inner membrane (Hansford et al., 1999; Pepe, 2000). The nature of this aging-induced defect in the inner mitochondrial membrane is a key area for understanding the aging-induced changes in cardiac mitochondria.

3.5. *Aging defect in complex III*

Duroquinol-supported state 3 respiration (Fig. 3) was decreased in IFM but was unchanged in SSM (Fannin et al., 1999; Lesnefsky et al., 2001b) during aging. Uncoupled respiration supported by duroquinol was also decreased in IFM from the aging heart, localizing the defect to the electron transport chain (Fannin et al., 1999; Lesnefsky et al., 2001b). Since duroquinol-supported respiration requires electron flow via complex III, cytochrome c, and cytochrome oxidase, assessment of potential aging defects in complex III requires the direct measurement of activity of the complex.

Complex III spans the central part of the respiratory chain, catalyzing electron transfer from ubiquinol to cytochrome c that is coupled to proton translocation (Trumpower, 1990) (Figs. 3 and 5). Mammalian complex III consists of two monomers, each containing 11 subunits. Three of the subunits, cytochrome b, cytochrome c_1, and the iron–sulfur protein (ISP), participate in electron transfer (Hunte et al., 2000; Iwata et al., 1998; Xia et al., 1997; Zhang et al., 1998a). The three-dimensional crystal structure of complex III provides insight into the structure–function relationship of electron flow within the complex (Hunte et al.,

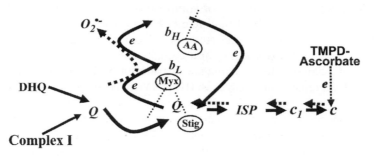

Fig. 5.   Schematic representation of the electron flow within complex III designed to illustrate the partial reactions used to localize the aging defect at the Q_o binding site. Reductants enter complex III in the forward direction either via exogenous donors to complex III (durohydroquinone-DHQ) or via the endogenous quinol pool (Q) from complex I. Quinol is oxidized by heme b_L of cytochrome b and the iron–sulfur protein (ISP). The electron on cytochrome b then equilibrates between hemes b_L and b_H. Reversed electron transport from cytochrome c (c) reduced by TMPD-ascorbate occurs sequentially to cytochrome c_1 (c_1) to ISP and finally to endogenous quinol (Q). The sites of inhibition of antimycin A (AA), myxothiazol (myx), and stigmatellin (stig) are shown.

2000; Iwata et al., 1998; Xia et al., 1997; Zhang et al., 1998a). Electron transfer within complex III occurs in a bifurcated fashion to cytochromes b and c_1 due to movement of the ISP during the redox cycle. ISP begins a redox cycle in proximity to cytochrome b ("b orientation" of ISP) in Fig. 6. When quinol is located within the binding "pocket" of cytochrome b (the Q_o site), a concerted oxidation of quinol by ISP and cytochrome b occurs (Crofts et al., 1999a,b; Snyder et al., 2000). The Q_o binding site is a bifurcated space, with "distal" (closer to ISP) and "proximal" (closer to heme b_L) segments (Crofts et al. 1999b) as shown in Fig. 6. The concerted oxidation of quinol by ISP and heme b_L of cytochrome b is favored by the quinol/ semiquinone species at the proximal location of the binding pocket in proximity to cytochrome b (Snyder et al., 2000). Alternatively, the Q_o site may contain two quinones, with "motion" of the semiquinone species occurring via electron transfer between the two quinone species (Bartoschek et al., 2001). Reduced ISP then moves toward cytochrome c_1 ("c_1 orientation"), as shown by the dashed arrow in Fig. 6, and transfers the electron to cytochrome c_1. The electron on ISP sequentially reduces cytochrome c_1, then cytochrome c via a docking interaction facilitated by subunits VIII and X (Kim et al., 1987; Nakai et al., 1993; Schmitt and Trumpower, 1991). Oxidation releases ISP to return to the "b orientation" for the next cycle.

Complex III (ubiquinol:ferricytochrome c oxidoreductase) activity was measured by the method of Krahenbuhl et al. modified to express maximal enzyme activity in heart mitochondria (Krahenbuhl et al., 1994; Lesnefsky et al., 2001b). Complex III activity was decreased by aging in IFM, but remained unchanged in SSM (Lesnefsky et al., 2001b). Complex III activity also was found to be unaltered by aging in mitochondria isolated by homogenization alone (probably representing SSM) (Davies et al., 2001; Takasawa et al., 1993). The decrease in complex III activity was observed under both maximal and submaximal conditions (Lesnefsky et al., 2001b).

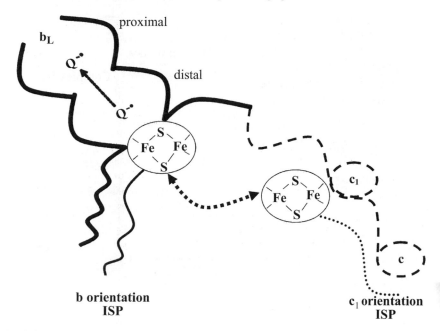

Fig. 6. Schematic representation of the ubiquinol oxidation site (Q_o) binding pocket showing proximal and distal portions of the binding pocket for ubiquinol. Myxothiazol binds in the proximal portion of the pocket near heme b_L of cytochrome b, while stigmatellin binds in the distal portion of the pocket and interacts with iron–sulfur protein. The iron–sulfur protein moves between the "b" and "c_1" orientations as indicated by the dashed arrow and described in the text.

The content of cytochromes b and c_1 in complex III measured by the difference spectrum of reduced minus oxidized states was unaltered by aging in both SSM and IFM (Lesnefsky et al., 2001b). Next, the content of the ISP was measured using the EPR spectra of the iron–sulfur cluster in submitochondrial particles obtained from pools of SSM and IFM obtained from adult or elderly hearts. EPR spectra were obtained following reduction of complex III in the presence of stigmatellin (Ohnishi and Trumpower, 1980). The EPR spectrum of the iron–sulfur cluster in complex III is characterized by g_y and g_x values of 1.89 and 1.79, respectively (Ohnishi and Trumpower, 1980; von Jagow and Ohnishi, 1985). The content of the iron–sulfur protein estimated using the amplitude of the g_y signal at 1.89 was unaltered by aging in IFM (Lesnefsky et al., 2001a).

The contents of cytochrome c_1 and the iron–sulfur peptide in complex III also were estimated using two-dimensional blue native polyacrylamide gel electrophoresis (BNPAGE) (Schagger, 1995). BNPAGE separates intact electron transport complexes under non-denaturing conditions (Schagger, 1996). Electron transport complexes were separated using BNPAGE in the first dimension (Fig. 7) and complex III isolated and subunits separated in a second dimension via denaturing tricine-SDS-PAGE (Fig. 7). Subunits were identified using silver stain. The five highest molecular weight subunits (core 1, core 2, cytochrome b, cytochrome c_1,

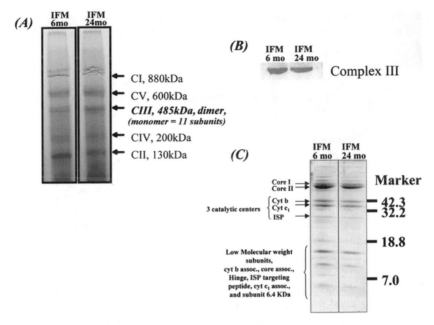

Fig. 7. Panel A: electron transport complexes obtained from IFM from adult and aged hearts were separated using blue native polyacrylamide gel electrophoresis (BNPAGE) (I-complex I; III-complex III; V-complex V ATPase; IV-cytochrome oxidase (complex IV); II-complex II). Panel B: immunoblots of complex III obtained from IFM from adult and aged hearts separated using BNPAGE, transferred to PVDF membrane, and decorated utilizing a polyclonal rabbit antibody raised to bovine complex III. Panel C: the subunit peptides composing complex III were separated using 16.5% tricine-SDS-PAGE in the second dimension. Individual subunits are identified (c_1-cyt c_1, ISP-iron–sulfur protein, molecular weight markers are indicated).

iron–sulfur peptide) were identified along with three of the five detectable lower molecular weight subunits (Schagger, 1995) (Fig. 7). The content of the iron–sulfur protein and cytochrome c_1 was estimated by the intensity of the silver-stained bands, and expressed relative to the intensity of cytochrome b. The ratio of the iron–sulfur peptide to cytochrome b as well as the ratio of cytochrome c_1/b was similar in IFM from adult and elderly hearts (Lesnefsky et al., 2001a). Thus, the aging defect in complex III did not alter the content of catalytic subunits.

Subunits VIII and X enhance the binding of the electron-acceptor cytochrome c to cytochrome c_1 and enhance electron transfer from cytochrome c_1 to c (Kim et al., 1987; Nakai et al., 1993; Schmitt and Trumpower, 1991). A loss of subunits VIII or X predicts a decrease in the maximal activity of complex III (Kim et al., 1987; Nakai et al., 1993; Schmitt and Trumpower, 1991). We asked if aging led to the loss of these subunits in complex III from IFM from elderly hearts. Using BNPAGE to isolate complex III and tricine-SDS-PAGE to separate individual subunits, a band at approximately 9 kDa (subunit VIII) was present in IFM from aging hearts, with identity confirmed using an antibody generated against a partial peptide sequence of subunit VIII. Subunit X (7.4 kDa) was identified using an antibody generated against a partial amino acid sequence of subunit X (Lesnefsky et al., 2001a). The aging defect in complex III in IFM was not due to the absence of either subunit VIII or subunit X, both of which bind cytochrome *c* (Lesnefsky et al., 2001a).

We utilized partial reactions of electron flow within complex III in order to further characterize the nature of the aging defect in the complex. The rate of reduction of cytochrome *b* was measured during either forward or reversed electron transport reactions within complex III. Substrates and inhibitors were chosen to select for studying specific parts of the reaction sequence of complex III (Fig. 5). The reduction of cytochrome *b* in the presence of the inhibitor antimycin A also was rapid in both adult and aging hearts. Antimycin A was included in subsequent experiments to prevent reoxidation of cytochrome *b* (Matsuno-Yagi and Hatefi, 1996; Matsuno-Yagi and Hatefi, 1997; Trumpower, 1990). When the quinol oxidation site inhibitors, myxothiazol or stigmatellin, were used, there was a marked slowing in the reduction of cytochrome *b* in submitochondrial particles from adult hearts.

In the presence of myxothiazol and stigmatellin as inhibitors of quinol oxidation of complex III, the reduction of cytochrome *b* in submitochondrial particles of IFM from aging hearts was increased compared to particles from IFM of adult hearts (Fig. 8). Aging did not alter the rate of reduction of cytochrome *b* in particles derived from SSM. The rate of cytochrome *b* reduction was increased by aging when myxothiazol alone was the quinol oxidation site inhibitor, but not when stigmatellin was the inhibitor (Hoppel et al., 2002; Moghaddas et al., 2001, 2002a,b). Thus, in IFM

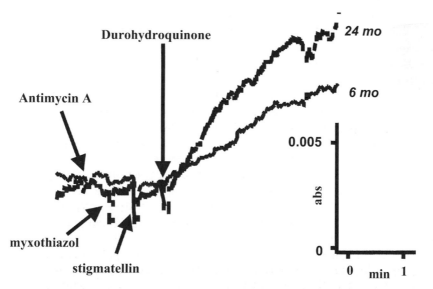

Fig. 8.   Aging increased the rate of reduction of cytochrome *b* (562–575 nm, 30 °C) by durohydroquinone in submitochondrial particles obtained from IFM from senescent hearts (dashed line) compared to adult hearts (solid line). All reactions were performed in the presence of myxothiazol, stigmatellin, and antimycin A as indicated (Moghaddas et al., 2001, 2002a,b).

from aging hearts, there is an increased leak of electrons through myxothiazol blockade to reduce cytochrome b, while stigmatellin inhibition is unaffected (Hoppel et al., 2002; Moghaddas et al., 2001, 2002a,b). The aging leak through myxothiazol blockade was observed when complex III was reduced by the endogenous quinol pool via complex I, using NADH as the substrate.

The aging-induced leak observed during the reduction of cytochrome b in the forward direction also was evident when complex III was reduced in the reversed electron transport from reduced cytochrome c (Hoppel et al., 2002; Moghaddas et al., 2001, 2002a,b). The rate of reduction of cytochrome b in the presence of myxothiazol in the reverse direction remained greater in submitochondrial particles from IFM from aging hearts than in particles from adult hearts. In the reverse direction, an age difference was not observed when stigmatellin was present either alone or in combination with myxothiazol. The aging leak at the myxothiazol site occurs regardless of whether electrons enter cytochrome b in the reverse direction via cytochrome c and ISP functions as the electron donor to the Q_o site, or when electrons enter in the forward direction from quinol and ISP acts as electron acceptor (Moghaddas et al., 2002b) (Fig. 6). Stigmatellin blocks the aging leak when electrons enter in the reverse direction but not when electrons enter via quinol.

Myxothiazol and stigmatellin bind to distinct amino acids within the quinol oxidation (Q_o) site (Fig. 6) (Crofts et al., 1999a,b). Stigmatellin interacts with ISP and binds to the distal domain of Q_o, whereas myxothiazol binds near heme b_L in the proximal domain (Crofts et al., 1999a). The selectivity of the aging-induced leak for myxothiazol, and not for stigmatellin, provides additional localization of the aging defect within the Q_o site.

Mutants of the bacterium *Rhodobacter spheroides* have provided further insight into possible structural defects that lead to aging complex III phenotype present in IFM. Aging decreases complex III activity with a preserved EPR signal (Lesnefsky et al., 2001a) in the setting of increased leak through myxothiazol blockade to reduce cytochrome b with preservation of inhibition by stigmatellin (Moghaddas et al., 2001, 2002a,b). Amino acids in the Q_o site are highly conserved from *R. spheroides* to mammalian cytochrome b (Crofts et al., 1999a,b). *R. spheroides* point mutations with resistance to myxothiazol but not to stigmatellin (A126, Y132, V133, M139, G143, F275) (Crofts et al., 1999a) are potential sites of aging damage (Fig. 6). In addition to myxothiazol resistance, Y132 is a site that decreases complex III activity in the presence of a preserved EPR signal (Crofts et al., 1999a). Thus, Y132 is a potential site for modification of cytochrome b that could match the aging phenotype of complex III in IFM. Localization of the defect at the Q_o site has focused our ongoing studies of the structural nature of the aging defect on functionally relevant portions of cytochrome b.

In summary, aging decreased the rate of oxidative phosphorylation and the activity of complex III in IFM (Lesnefsky et al., 2001b). Aging increased the leak of electrons through myxothiazol blockade within the Q_o site, while inhibition by stigmatellin was unaffected. These functional studies localize the site of aging defect to the proximal domain of the Q_o site in proximity to heme b_L of cytochrome b. The aging-induced alteration of the quinol oxidation site of complex III is a likely site for the increased production of reactive oxygen species that contributes to aging in the heart.

3.6. *Aging increases the production of reactive oxygen species from mitochondria*

Aging defects in mitochondrial electron transport are probable sources of the increase in chronic oxidative injury that occurs in aging tissues (Barja, 1998; Kwong and Sohal, 2000). Mitochondria isolated from senescent animals exhibit higher rates of production of reactive oxygen species compared to younger animals. The production of reactive oxygen species by mitochondria has been inversely correlated with mean lifespan (Barja, 1998). The production of reactive oxygen species is greater in cardiac mitochondria isolated from the senescent mouse heart (Kwong and Sohal, 2000). The enhanced production of reactive oxygen species generally occurs during state 4 respiration, when redox centers in the electron transport chain are relatively reduced (Kwong and Sohal, 2000). Mitochondria from aging hearts also appear to have an increased sensitivity to oxidative damage (Cusack et al., 1991). Consistent with this observation, mitochondria from aging tissues display increased oxidative stress in the baseline state in most (Corral-Debrinski et al., 1992; Nagley et al., 1992; Richter et al., 1988), including an increased content of 8-hydroxydeoxyguanosine, a marker of oxidative damage to mtDNA (Wallace, 2000), but not all studies (Davies et al., 2001).

The defects in complex III and cytochrome oxidase that occur in IFM in the aging heart are sources of enhanced oxidative damage in the aging heart. Complex III directly reduces molecular oxygen to form superoxide ($\bullet O_2^-$), providing a major site for the production of reactive oxygen species (Demin et al., 1998a,b; Turrens et al., 1985). Electron leak to molecular oxygen from the Q_o site is energetically feasible at inner mitochondrial membrane potentials observed during cellular respiration in vivo. The Q_o site directs superoxide release into the intermembrane space (Gille and Nohl, 2001). Electron leak to molecular oxygen is minimized by the concerted oxidation of quinol by ISP and cytochrome b (Snyder et al., 2000). The aging defect likely decreases binding interactions in the proximal portion of the Q_o site and may impair concerted oxidation, leading to the formation of a highly reactive semiquinone at the Q_o site. Semiquinone formation increases the probability of reaction with molecular oxygen to form superoxide, rather than electron transfer to heme b_L (Snyder et al., 2000). Aging increased the production of superoxide in submitochondrial particles from IFM, whereas superoxide production was not increased in particles from SSM (Moghaddas et al., 2001, 2002a,b). Furthermore, aging increased the production of superoxide measured as H_2O_2 in particles from IFM in the presence of myxothiazol and antimycin, consistent with increased leak through myxothiazol blockade leading to increased production of reactive oxygen species (unpublished data). Thus, the Q_o site defect provides a probable mechanism for the increased oxidative damage from complex III in IFM during aging.

The aging defect in cytochrome oxidase is likely to further augment the production of reactive oxygen species from the Q_o site of complex III. Cytochrome oxidase is not a site of production of reactive oxygen species even though the active site of complex IV contains reactive oxygen intermediates including $\bullet O_2^-$, H_2O_2, and hydroxyl radical (Varotsis et al., 1993). These intermediates are chemically bound to prevent release from cytochrome oxidase (Varotsis et al., 1993). Cytochrome oxidase nonetheless has a key antioxidant role due to the modulation of local O_2 content and the redox status of complex III. Electron flow through cytochrome oxidase is under respiratory control by coupling to the inner membrane potential, as well as independent of respiratory control (Kadenbach et al., 2000; Papa et al., 1997). Independent electron flow occurs via a proton leakage current within cytochrome oxidase (Kadenbach et al., 2000; Papa et al., 1997), allowing flux through cytochrome oxidase independent of the membrane potential. During state 4 conditions resulting in a high membrane potential and decreased flux through the electron transport chain, cytochrome oxidase allows for continued electron flow, decreasing the relative reduction of cytochrome b, minimizing the probability of electron leak to molecular oxygen from the Q_o site (Kadenbach et al., 2000; Papa et al., 1997). Conversely, inhibition of cytochrome oxidase increases cell death from oxidative damage generated by the electron transport chain (Qian et al., 1997). Senescence-related decreases in cytochrome oxidase activity in IFM predisposes to the increased reduction of cytochrome b in complex III that contains the Q_o site aging defect discussed above. Thus, the aging-induced decrease in cytochrome oxidase is likely to facilitate the upstream production of reactive oxygen species from the Q_o site from complex III in IFM in the aging heart.

3.7. Significance of complex III defect

Aging decreases the rate of oxidative phosphorylation and the activity of complex III in IFM (Lesnefsky et al., 2001b). Aging increases electron leak through myxothiazol blockade within the Q_o site, whereas inhibition by stigmatellin was unaffected. Using structure–function insights obtained from the three-dimensional crystal structure of complex III (Iwata et al., 1998; Xia et al., 1997; Zhang et al., 1998b), and from the functional responses of complex III containing mutant cytochrome b (Crofts et al., 1999a), the aging defect resides within the myxothiazol-binding domain in proximity to heme b_L of cytochrome b. The aging defect in complex III augments the production of superoxide. Defects within the quinol oxidation site of complex III provide a locus for greater production of reactive oxygen species that contributes to cardiac aging and may enhance oxidative damage during ischemia and reperfusion in the senescent heart.

3.8. Predisposition to cytochrome c release during aging

The release of cytochrome c from mitochondria is a key step leading to apoptosis (Green and Reed, 1998; Yang et al., 1997), but activation of cellular programs resulting in apoptosis can occur in the absence of cytochrome c release (Li et al., 1997). However, the release of cytochrome c from mitochondria is probably the predominant pathway leading to activation of apoptotic programs in cardiac myocytes during cellular stress. Following release of cytochrome c from mitochondria, a complex (apoptosome) consisting of cytochrome c, APAF-1, deoxyATP, and caspase-9 forms in the cytosol. Downstream effectors of the apoptotic pathway including caspase-3 are directly activated by this complex.

In view of the dire consequences of cytochrome *c* release for the cardiac myocyte, it is not surprising that cytochrome *c* release is highly regulated. Release of cytochrome *c* from mitochondria can occur via the onset of mitochondrial permeability transition, the formation of an inner membrane pore permeable to solutes of less than 1200 Da (Crompton, 1999) that leads to loss of mitochondrial membrane potential, swelling of the matrix space, and eventual disruption of mitochondrial membranes (Crompton, 1999; Green and Reed, 1998). However, cytochrome *c* release probably occurs in situations other than the catastrophic mitochondrial damage that is observed when permeability transition is induced in experimental studies. Permeability transition probably is a transient and reversibly regulated phenomenon in vivo (Hatano et al., 2000; Lemasters et al., 1999). Proteins located in the mitochondrial membrane also modulate the predisposition toward cytochrome *c* release independent of the onset of permeability transition (Hatano et al., 2000; Lemasters et al., 1999). The Bax and Bcl-X families exert countervailing influences on cytochrome *c* release, favoring and inhibiting release, respectively (Green and Reed, 1998).

A predisposition to myocyte apoptosis might contribute to the loss of myocytes observed during aging in the heart (Wei, 1992). Release of cytochrome *c* from mitochondria in the aging heart would predispose the myocyte toward activation of apoptotic programs (Green and Reed, 1998; Hatano et al., 2000; Lemasters et al., 1999). The content of cytochrome *c*, measured using spectrophotometric technique, is preserved during aging in both SSM and IFM (Fannin et al., 1999). In a separate study, the content of cytochrome *c* in the cytosol fraction obtained from myocardium was increased in 16- and 24-month Fischer 344 rats compared to 6-month adult controls (Phaneuf and Leeuwenburgh, 2002). Bcl-2 tended to decrease with age (Phaneuf and Leeuwenburgh, 2002), also observed in mice (Liu et al., 1998). Thus, there may be a tendency toward apoptosis in the aged heart.

3.9. *Ischemia*

The elderly heart sustains greater injury during ischemia and reperfusion compared to the adult heart in both patients (Lesnefsky et al., 1996) and in experimental models (Frolkis et al., 1991; Lesnefsky et al., 1994; Lucas and Szweda, 1998). The aging heart displays greater oxidative damage (Frolkis et al., 1991; Lucas and Szweda, 1998) including oxidative protein modification (Frolkis et al., 1991; Lucas and Szweda, 1998), as well as calcium-mediated damage (Ataka et al., 1992), compared to the adult heart. The enhanced calcium-mediated and oxidative damage in the aged heart suggests mitochondria-driven mechanisms of injury. The addition of ischemic mitochondrial damage to aging-related mitochondrial defects can augment mitochondrial-derived injury in the aging heart (Lesnefsky et al., 2001a).

Ischemia damages complex III by functional inactivation of the iron–sulfur protein (ISP) subunit (Lesnefsky et al., 2001a). The ISP is a 22 kDa protein that contains a 2 Fe–2 S redox-active iron–sulfur cluster. Ischemic damage to the ISP results in loss of the EPR signal of the iron–sulfur cluster without loss of the ISP peptide, suggesting that ischemia results in disruption of the cluster without degradation of the ISP subunit (Lesnefsky et al., 2001a). Conserved cysteine and histidine residues are ligands for the Fe atoms in the cluster (Xia et al., 1997). In vitro oxidative damage to the histidine residues leads to loss of complex III activity (Miki et al., 1991). In addition to the ligands of the Fe atoms, the integrity of the cluster requires that the native conformation of ISP be preserved. An intramolecular disulfide bond between two highly conserved cysteine residues remote from the cluster itself is required to preserve the integrity of the cluster (Denke et al., 1998). These sites provide likely targets for ischemia to disrupt the 2 Fe–2 S cluster without loss of the peptide.

Complex III, implicated as a source of reactive oxygen species during reperfusion in the adult heart, is a probable source of enhanced oxidative damage during reperfusion in the aging heart (Lesnefsky et al., 2001a). The addition of ischemia-induced defects in complex III to the preexisting aging-related defects can enhance mitochondrial-derived injury during reperfusion. Ischemia damages the iron–sulfur subunit of complex III (Lesnefsky et al., 2001a). Aging causes a defect at the quinol oxidation site (Moghaddas et al., 2001, 2002a,b). Thus, during ischemia and at the onset of reperfusion in the aging heart, complex III in IFM contains sequential defects in the path of electron flow. The two partial blocks in sequence are likely to act in concert to further slow electron flow within complex III, increase the reduction of cytochrome b, and enhance production of reactive oxygen species compared to either defect alone. An increase in intracellular oxidative injury leads to cell death by necrosis or apoptosis, processes that are increased in the aged heart during reperfusion.

3.10. *Role of mitochondria in myocardial protection mediated by ischemic preconditioning in aged heart*

Brief antecedent periods of ischemia blunt the myocardial damage that results from a subsequent period of ischemia (Murry et al., 1990). Myocardial protection derived from preconditioning results in part from the generation of adenosine that activates G-protein-coupled adenosine (A-1) receptors (Grover and Garlid, 2000). Ischemia also leads to the generation of free radicals. Both of these processes activate intracellular signaling pathways including protein kinase C and tyrosine kinase that open mitochondrial potassium-ATP channels with subsequent cardiac protection (Grover and Garlid, 2000; Pain et al., 2000). The mechanism by which protein kinase C activates mitochondrial potassium-ATP channels remains uncertain. Activation of mitochondrial potassium-ATP channels induces partial depolarization of the inner mitochondrial membrane (Liu et al., 1998) and partial uncoupling of respiration with increased oxygen consumption and decreased ATP synthesis (Holmuhamedov et al., 1998). Membrane depolarization mediated by opening of mitochondrial K-ATP channels may protect the myocyte via reduction of mitochondrial calcium overload (Murata et al., 2001). The partial uncoupling of respiration may also decrease the production of reactive oxygen species by mitochondria.

Although the aging heart sustains greater damage than the adult heart during ischemia and reperfusion (Lesnefsky et al., 1994, 1996), the myocardial protection derived from ischemic preconditioning is blunted in elderly patients (Ishihara et al., 2000; Lee et al., 2002) and in experimental models, including the Fischer 344 rat (Tani et al., 2001). The blunted preconditioning protection observed in the Fischer 344 rat occurs in part because of a decreased activation of protein kinase C (Tani et al., 2001). Activation was reduced following both ischemic preconditioning as well as following the administration of direct pharmacological agonists of protein kinase C, suggestive of defects in protein kinase C itself. However, the preconditioning protection afforded by direct administration of pharmacological activators of mitochondrial potassium-ATP channels also was decreased, suggesting that a defective mitochondrial response also might contribute (Tani et al., 2001).

Nevertheless, isolated mitochondria from senescent Fischer 344 rats retain the ability to respond to diazoxide, a pharmacological agonist of mitochondrial potassium-ATP channels (Jahangir et al., 2001). Jahangir et al. (2001) studied a mixed population of cardiac mitochondria from senescent Fischer 344 rats and observed that mitochondria from senescent hearts had a decreased capacity for calcium uptake and an enhanced susceptibility to calcium-mediated damage. In the adult heart, SSM are more susceptible to calcium-mediated damage than IFM (Palmer et al., 1986). These findings raise the possibility that aging alters IFM such that their response to calcium-loading becomes similar to that of SSM. Diazoxide enhanced the calcium tolerance of the mixed population of cardiac mitochondria obtained from senescent hearts (Jahangir et al., 2001). Since ischemic injury in the aging heart is accompanied by an increased calcium accumulation (Ataka et al., 1992), and ischemic preconditioning production is blunted in the aging heart (Lee et al., 2002; Tani et al., 2001), direct pharmacological activation of potassium-ATP channels is a potentially attractive therapeutic approach to blunt mitochondrial-derived injury in the aging heart during ischemia.

3.11. *Significance of IFM in the aged heart*

An appreciation of the selective effect of aging on IFM is critical to the study of aging-related cardiac dysfunction and damage. Ironically, the use of tissue homogenization alone to isolate cardiac mitochondria targets for study SSM, which are devoid of aging defects. Two studies of the production of reactive oxygen species (Muscari et al., 1990) and protein import (Craig and Hood, 1997) in the aging heart did not find alterations in these processes with age. However, the approach to mitochondrial isolation utilized in those two studies probably yielded only SSM. The study of IFM, the population of mitochondria altered by aging, without contamination by unaltered SSM, will add specificity and selectivity to the study of the contributions of mitochondria to aging-related dysfunction in the heart.

Aging decreases the yield of IFM and reduces their rate of oxidative phosphorylation. In the heart, oxygen extraction across the myocardium is near maximal even at rest. The 25–30% decrease in the rate of oxidative phosphorylation combined with a 25–30% decrease in the protein content of IFM leads to an approximately 50%

decrease in oxidative capacity in the interfibrillar region of the myocyte. Thus, in the highly aerobic myocardium, even modest decreases in oxygen utilization related to tissue stress in the aging heart are likely to have a physiologic impact. IFM, situated among the myofibrils, undoubtedly, are the primary energy source for the contractile apparatus. Decreased rates of oxidative phosphorylation in IFM persist even at non-maximal rates of oxygen consumption through complexes III and IV, and thus may contribute to altered myocardial physiology. Furthermore, the aging-related mito-chondrial defects appear to segregate in a mosaic fashion, with more profound defects occurring in sporadic myocytes (Muller-Hocker, 1989). Thus, aging defects in IFM are even more likely to impact the physiology of the aging heart. IFM, but not SSM, from aging hearts generate an increased flux of reactive oxygen species that are likely to contribute to the increased oxidative injury in the aging heart in the baseline state (Ide et al., 1999; Van Remmen and Richardson, 2001). Defects in IFM are likely to increase the susceptibility of the aging heart to damage during ischemia and reperfusion as well.

4. Conclusions

Aging decreases the protein yield and the rate of oxidative phosphorylation in IFM, whereas the yield of mitochondria and the rate of oxidative phosphorylation in SSM are unchanged during aging. Aging decreases the activity of electron transport complexes III and IV in IFM, but not in SSM. Aging-related decreases in oxidative mitochondrial metabolism previously described in mixed populations of cardiac mitochondria occur only in IFM.

An appreciation of the selective effect of aging on IFM is critical to the study of aging-related alterations in the heart. The study of IFM, the population that contains the aging-related mitochondrial defects, without the confounding effects of unaltered SSM, will facilitate the study of mitochondrial-related mechanisms of dysfunction in the aging heart.

Complex III activity is decreased by aging in IFM. A defect in the ubiquinol binding site (Q_o) exists within cytochrome b in complex III in IFM during aging. The aging defect in complex III is localized in the myxothiazol-binding locus within the proximal segment of the Q_o binding pocket of cytochrome b. The defect is associated with an increased production of superoxide radical. Alteration of the quinol oxi-dation site of complex III in IFM increases the production of reactive oxygen species that contributes to cardiac aging.

The elderly heart sustains greater injury during ischemia and reperfusion com-pared to the adult heart in both patients and animal models. The addition of ischemic mitochondrial damage to preexisting aging-related mitochondrial defects is a probable mechanism of enhanced mitochondrial-derived injury during ischemia and reperfusion in the aging heart. Excess mitochondrial-mediated injury leads to cell death by necrosis or apoptosis, processes that are increased in the aging heart during reperfusion.

Acknowledgements

This work was supported by Grants 2RO1AG12447 and 1POAG15885 from the National Institutes of Health, and by the Office of Research and Development, Medical Research Service, Department of Veterans Affairs and the Geriatric Research, Education, and Clinical Center, Louis Stokes VAMC, Cleveland, OH.

References

Abramovitch, D.A., Marsh, D., Powell, G.L., 1990. Activation of beef-heart cytochrome *c* oxidase by cardiolipin and analogues of cardiolipin. Biochim. Biophys. Acta 1020, 34–42.

Anversa, P., Puntillo, E., Nikitin, P., Olivetti, G., Capasso, J.M., Sonnenblick, E.H. 1989. Effects of age on mechanical and structural properties of myocardium of Fischer 344 rats. Am. J. Physiol. 256, H1440–H1449.

Ataka, K., Chen, D., Levitsky, S., Jimenez, E., Feinberg, H., 1992. Effect of aging on intracellular Ca2+, pHi, and contractility during ischemia and reperfusion. Circulation 86, II371–II376.

Barja, G., 1998. Mitochondrial free radical production and aging in mammals and birds. Ann. NY Acad. Sci. 854, 224–238.

Bartoschek, S., Johansson, M., Geierstanger, B.H., Okun, J.G., Lancaster, C.R., Humpfer, E., Yu, L., Yu, C.A., Griesinger, C., Brandt, U., 2001. Three molecules of ubiquinone bind specifically to mitochondrial cytochrome *bc*1 complex. J. Biol. Chem. 276, 35231–35234.

Chen, J.C., Warshaw, J.B., Sanadi, D.R., 1972. Regulation of mitochondrial respiration in senescence. J. Cell Physiol. 80, 141–148.

Chiu, Y.J., Richardson, A., 1980. Effect of age on the function of mitochondria isolated from brain and heart tissue. Exp. Gerontol. 15, 511–517.

Coleman, G.L., Barthold, W., Osbaldiston, G.W., Foster, S.J., Jonas, A.M., 1977. Pathological changes during aging in barrier-reared Fischer 344 male rats. J. Gerontol. 32, 258–278.

Cooper, C.E., Nicholls, P., 1990. Structure and vectorial properties of proteoliposomes containing cytochrome oxidase in the submitochondrial orientation. Biochemistry 29, 3865–3871.

Corral-Debrinski, M., Shoffner, J.M., Lott, M.T., Wallace, D.C., 1992. Association of mitochondrial DNA damage with aging and coronary atherosclerotic heart disease. Mutat. Res. 275, 169–180.

Craig, E.E., Hood, D.A., 1997. Influence of aging on protein import into cardiac mitochondria. Am. J. Physiol. 272, H2983–H2988.

Crofts, A.R., Barquera, B., Gennis, R.B., Kuras, R., Guergova-Kuras, M., Berry, E.A., 1999a. Mechanism of ubiquinol oxidation by the bc(1) complex: different domains of the quinol binding pocket and their role in the mechanism and binding of inhibitors. Biochemistry 38, 15807–15826.

Crofts, A.R., Guergova-Kuras, M., Huang, L., Kuras, R., Zhang, Z., Berry, E.A., 1999b. Mechanism of ubiquinol oxidation by the bc(1) complex: role of the iron sulfur protein and its mobility. Biochemistry 38, 15791–15806.

Crompton, M., 1999. The mitochondrial permeability transition pore and its role in cell death. Biochem. J. 341, 233–249.

Cusack, B.J., Mushlin, P.S., Andrejuk, T., Voulelis, L.D., Olson, R.D., 1991. Aging alters the force-frequency relationship and toxicity of oxidative stress in rabbit heart. Life Sci. 48, 1769–1777.

Davies, S.M., Poljak, A., Duncan, M.W., Smythe, G.A., Murphy, M.P., 2001. Measurements of protein carbonyls, ortho- and meta-tyrosine and oxidative phosphorylation complex activity in mitochondria from young and old rats. Free Radic. Biol. Med. 31, 181–190.

DeDuve, C., 1967. In: Roodyn, D.B. (Ed.), Enzyme Cytology, Academic Press, New York, pp. 1–26.

Demin, O.V., Kholodenko, B.N., Skulachev, V.P., 1998a. A model of O2-generation in the complex III of the electron transport chain. Mol. Cell Biochem. 184, 21–33.

Demin, O.V., Westerhoff, H.V., Kholodenko, B.N., 1998b. Mathematical modelling of superoxide generation with the *bc*1 complex of mitochondria. Biochemistry (Mosc.) 63, 634–649.

Denke, E., Merbitz-Zahradnik, T., Hatzfeld, O.M., Snyder, C.H., Link, T.A., Trumpower, B.L., 1998. Alteration of the midpoint potential and catalytic activity of the rieske iron–sulfur protein by changes of amino acids forming hydrogen bonds to the iron–sulfur cluster. J. Biol. Chem. 273, 9085–9093.

Fannin, S.W., Lesnefsky, E.J., Slabe, T.J., Hassan, M.O., Hoppel, C.L., 1999. Aging selectively decreases oxidative capacity in rat heart interfibrillar mitochondria. Arch Biochem. Biophys. 372, 399–407.

Frenzel, H., Feimann, J., 1984. Age-dependent structural changes in the myocardium of rats. A quantitative light- and electron-microscopic study on the right and left chamber wall. Mech. Ageing Dev. 27, 29–41.

Frolkis, V.V., Frolkis, R.A., Mkhitarian, L.S., Fraifeld, V.E., 1991. Age-dependent effects of ischemia and reperfusion on cardiac function and Ca2+ transport in myocardium. Gerontology 37, 233–239.

Fry, M., Blondin, G.A., Green, D.E., 1980. The localization of tightly bound cardiolipin in cytochrome oxidase. J. Biol. Chem. 255, 9967–9970.

Fry, M., Green, D.E., 1980. Cardiolipin requirement by cytochrome oxidase and the catalytic role of phospholipid. Biochem. Biophys. Res. Commun. 93, 1238–1246.

Fry, M., Green, D.E., 1981. Cardiolipin requirement for electron transfer in complex I and III of the mitochondrial respiratory chain. J. Biol. Chem. 256, 1874–1880.

Gille, L., Nohl, H., 2001. The ubiquinol/bc1 redox couple regulates mitochondrial oxygen radical formation. Arch Biochem. Biophys. 388, 34–38.

Gomez Jr., B., Robinson, N.C., 1999. Phospholipase digestion of bound cardiolipin reversibly inactivates bovine cytochrome bc1. Biochem 38, 9031–9038.

Green, D.R., Reed, J.C., 1998. Mitochondria and apoptosis. Science 281, 1309–1312.

Grover, G.J., Garlid, K.D., 2000. ATP-Sensitive potassium channels: a review of their cardioprotective pharmacology. J. Mol. Cell Cardiol. 32, 677–695.

Guerrieri, F., Capozza, G., Fratello, A., Zanotti, F., Papa, S., 1993. Functional and molecular changes in FoF1 ATP-synthase of cardiac muscle during aging. Cardioscience 4, 93–98.

Hagen, T.M., Ingersoll, R.T., Wehr, C.M., Lykkesfeldt, J., Vinarsky, V., Bartholomew, J.C., Song, M.H., Ames, B.N., 1998. Acetyl-L-carnitine fed to old rats partially restores mitochondrial function and ambulatory activity. Proc. Natl. Acad. Sci. USA 95, 9562–9566.

Hansford, R.G., 1978. Lipid oxidation by heart mitochondria from young adult and senescent rats. Biochem. J. 170, 285–295.

Hansford, R.G., Tsuchiya, N., Pepe, S., 1999. Mitochondria in heart ischaemia and aging. Biochem. Soc. Symp. 66, 141–147.

Hatano, E., Bradham, C.A., Stark, A., Iimuro, Y., Lemasters, J.J., Brenner, D.A., 2000. The mitochondrial permeability transition augments Fas-induced apoptosis in mouse hepatocytes. J. Biol. Chem. 275, 11814–11823.

Hoch, F.L., 1992. Cardiolipins and biomembrane function. Biochim. Biophys. Acta 1113, 71–133.

Holmuhamedov, E.L., Jovanovic, S., Dzeja, P.P., Jovanovic, A., Terzic, A., 1998. Mitochondrial ATP-sensitive K+ channels modulate cardiac mitochondrial function. Am. J. Physiol. 275, H1567–H1576.

Hoppel, C.L., Moghaddas, S., Lesnefsky, E.J., 2002. Interfibrillar cardiac mitochondrial complex III defects in the aging rat heart. Biogerontology 3, 41–44.

Hoppel, C.L., Tandler, B., Parland, W., Turkaly, J.S., Albers, L.D., 1982. Hamster cardiomyopathy. A defect in oxidative phosphorylation in the cardiac interfibrillar mitochondria. J. Biol. Chem. 257, 1540–1548.

Hunte, C., Koepke, J., Lange, C., Rossmanith, T., Michel, H., 2000. Structure at 2.3 A resolution of the cytochrome bc(1) complex from the yeast *Saccharomyces cerevisiae* co-crystallized with an antibody Fv fragment. Structure Fold Des. 8, 669–684.

Ide, T., Tsutsui, H., Kinugawa, S., Utsumi, H., Kang, D., Hattori, N., Uchida, K., Arimura, K.i., Egashira, K., Takeshita, A., 1999. Mitochondrial electron transport complex I is a potential source of oxygen free radicals in the failing myocardium. Circ. Res. 85, 357–363.

Ingalls, S.T., Xu, Y., Hoppel, C.L., 1995. Determination of plasma non-esterified fatty acids and triglyceride fatty acids by gas chromatography of their methyl esters after isolation by column chromatography on silica gel. J. Chromatogr. B Biomed. Appl. 666, 1–12.

Ishihara, M., Sato, H., Tateishi, H., Kawagoe, T., Shimatani, Y., Ueda, K., Noma, K., Yumoto, A., Nishioka, K., 2000. Beneficial effect of prodromal angina pectoris is lost in elderly patients with acute myocardial infarction. Am. Heart J. 139, 881–888.

Iwata, S., Lee, J.W., Okada, K., Lee, J.K., Iwata, M., Rasmussen, B., Link, T.A., Ramaswamy, S., Jap, B.K., 1998. Complete structure of the 11-subunit bovine mitochondrial cytochrome *bc*1 complex. Science 281, 64–71.

Jahangir, A., Ozcan, C., Holmuhamedov, E.L., Terzic, A., 2001. Increased calcium vulnerability of senescent cardiac mitochondria: protective role for a mitochondrial potassium channel opener. Mech. Ageing Dev. 122, 1073–1086.

Kadenbach, B., Huttemann, M., Arnold, S., Lee, I., Bender, E., 2000. Mitochondrial energy metabolism is regulated via nuclear-coded subunits of cytochrome *c* oxidase. Free Radic. Biol. Med. 29, 211–221.

Kalt, M.R., Tandler, B., 1971. A study of fixation of early amphibian embryos for electron microscopy. J. Ultrastruct. Res. 36, 633–645.

Kim, C.H., Balny, C., King, T.E., 1987. Role of the hinge protein in the electron transfer between cardiac cytochrome *c*1 and *c*. Equilibrium constants and kinetic probes. J. Biol. Chem. 262, 8103–8108.

Krahenbuhl, S., Talos, C., Wiesmann, U., Hoppel, C.L., 1994. Development and evaluation of a spectrophotometric assay for complex III in isolated mitochondria, tissues and fibroblasts from rats and humans. Clin. Chim. Acta 230, 177–187.

Kwong, L.K., Sohal, R.S., 2000. Age-related changes in activities of mitochondrial electron transport complexes in various tissues of the mouse. Arch Biochem. Biophys. 373, 16–22.

Lakatta, E.G., Mitchell, J.H., Pomerance, A., Rowe, G.G., 1987. Human aging: changes in structure and function. J. Am. Coll. Cardiol. 10, 42A–47A.

Lee, T.M., Su, S.F., Chou, T.F., Lee, Y.T., Tsai, C.H., 2002. Loss of preconditioning by attenuated activation of myocardial ATP-sensitive potassium channels in elderly patients undergoing coronary angioplasty. Circulation 105, 334–340.

Lemasters, J.J., Qian, T., Trost, L.C., Herman, B., Cascio, W.E., Bradham, C.A., Brenner, D.A., Nieminen, A.L., 1999. Confocal microscopy of the mitochondrial permeability transition in necrotic and apoptotic cell death. Biochem. Soc. Symp. 66, 205–222.

Lesnefsky, E.J., Gallo, D.S., Ye, J., Whittingham, T.S., Lust, W.D., 1994. Aging increases ischemia-reperfusion injury in the isolated, buffer-perfused heart. J. Lab. Clin. Med. 124, 843–851.

Lesnefsky, E.J., Gudz, T.I., Migita, C.T., Ikeda-Saito, M., Hassan, M.O., Turkaly, P.J., Hoppel, C.L., 2001a. Ischemic injury to mitochondrial electron transport in the aging heart: damage to the iron–sulfur protein subunit of electron transport complex III. Arch. Biochem. Biophys. 385, 117–128.

Lesnefsky, E.J., Gudz, T.I., Moghaddas, S., Migita, C.T., Ikeda-Saito, M., Turkaly, P.J., Hoppel, C.L., 2001b. Aging decreases electron transport complex III activity in heart interfibrillar mitochondria by alteration of the cytochrome *c* binding site. J. Mol. Cell Cardiol. 33, 37–47.

Lesnefsky, E.J., Lundergan, C.F., Hodgson, J.M., Nair, R., Reiner, J.S., Greenhouse, S.W., Califf, R.M., Ross, A.M., 1996. Increased left ventricular dysfunction in elderly patients despite successful thrombolysis: the GUSTO-I angiographic experience. J. Am. Coll. Cardiol. 28, 331–337.

Lesnefsky, E.J., Slabe, T.J., Stoll, M.S., Minkler, P.E., Hoppel, C.L., 2001c. Myocardial ischemia selectively depletes cardiolipin in rabbit heart subsarcolemmal mitochondria. Am. J. Physiol. Heart Circ. Physiol. 280, H2770–H2778.

Lesnefsky, E.J., Stoll, M.S., Minkler, P.E., Hoppel, C.L., 2000. Separation and quantitation of phospholipids and lysophospholipids by high-performance liquid chromatography. Anal. Biochem. 285, 246–254.

Lesnefsky, E.J., Tandler, B., Ye, J., Slabe, T.J., Turkaly, J., Hoppel, C.L., 1997. Myocardial ischemia decreases oxidative phosphorylation through cytochrome oxidase in subsarcolemmal mitochondria. Am. J. Physiol. 273, H1544–H1554.

Li, F., Srinivasan, A., Wang, Y., Armstrong, R.C., Tomaselli, K.J., Fritz, L.C., 1997. Cell-specific induction of apoptosis by microinjection of cytochrome *c*. Bcl-xL has activity independent of cytochrome *c* release. J. Biol. Chem. 272, 30299–30305.

Liu, L., Azhar, G., Gao, W., Zhang, X., Wei, J.Y., 1998. Bcl-2 and Bax expression in adult rat hearts after coronary occlusion: age-associated differences. Am. J. Physiol. 275, R315–R322.

Lucas, D.T., Szweda, L.I., 1998. Cardiac reperfusion injury: aging, lipid peroxidation, and mitochondrial dysfunction. Proc. Natl. Acad. Sci. USA 95, 510–514.

Manzelmann, M.S., Harmon, H.J., 1987. Lack of age-dependent changes in rat heart mitochondria. Mech. Ageing Dev. 39, 281–288.

Matsuno-Yagi, A., Hatefi, Y., 1996. Ubiquinol-cytochrome c oxidoreductase. The redox reactions of the bis-heme cytochrome b in ubiquinone-sufficient and ubiquinone-deficient systems. J. Biol. Chem. 271, 6164–6171.

Matsuno-Yagi, A., Hatefi, Y., 1997. Ubiquinol:cytochrome c oxidoreductase. The redox reactions of the bis-heme cytochrome b in unenergized and energized submitochondrial particles. J. Biol. Chem. 272, 16928–16933.

Miki, T., Yu, L., Yu, C.A., 1991. Hematoporphyrin-promoted photoinactivation of mitochondrial ubiquinol-cytochrome c reductase: selective destruction of the histidine ligands of the iron–sulfur cluster and protective effect of ubiquinone. Biochemistry 30, 230–238.

Moghaddas, S., Hoppel, C.L., Lesnefsky, E.J., 2001. Defect in cytochrome b reduction in the mitochondrial $bc1$ complex (complex III) in the aging heart. J. Inves. Med. 49, 271A.

Moghaddas, S., Hoppel, C.L., Lesnefsky, E.J., 2002a. Aging leads to a defect at the quinol oxidation site of complex III in rat heart interfibrillar mitochondria (submitted for publication).

Moghaddas, S., Hoppel, C.L., Lesnefsky, E.J., 2002b. Myxothiazol-resistant reduction of Cytochrome b in complex III in aging interfibrillar heart mitochondria. FASEB J. 16, A490.

Moghaddas, S., Stoll, M.S., Minkler, P.E., Salomon, R.G., Hoppel, C.L., Lesnefsky, E.J., 2002c. Preservation of cardiolipin content during aging in rat heart interfibrillar mitochondria. J. Gerontol. A Biol. Sci. Med. Sci. 57, B22–B28.

Moseley, M.A., Deterding, L.J., Tomer, K.B., Jorgenson, J.W., 1991. Nanoscale packed-capillary liquid chromatography coupled with mass spectrometry using a coaxial continuous-flow fast atom bombardment interface. Anal. Chem. 63, 1467–1473.

Müller-Höcker, J., 1989. Cytochrome-c-oxidase deficient cardiomyocytes in the human heart–an age-related phenomenon. A histochemical ultracytochemical study. Am. J. Pathol. 134, 1167–1173.

Müller-Höcker, J., Schafer, S., Link, T.A., Possekel, S., Hammer, C., 1996. Defects of the respiratory chain in various tissues of old monkeys: a cytochemical-immunocytochemical study. Mech. Ageing Dev. 86, 197–213.

Murata, M., Akao, M., O'Rourke, B., Marban, E., 2001. Mitochondrial ATP-sensitive potassium channels attenuate matrix Ca(2+) overload during simulated ischemia and reperfusion: possible mechanism of cardioprotection. Circ. Res. 89, 891–898.

Murry, C.E., Richard, V.J., Reimer, K.A., Jennings, R.B., 1990. Ischemic preconditioning slows energy metabolism and delays ultrastructural damage during a sustained ischemic episode. Circ. Res. 66, 913–931.

Muscari, C., Frascaro, M., Guarnieri, C., Caldarera, C.M., 1990. Mitochondrial function and superoxide generation from submitochondrial particles of aged rat hearts. Biochim. Biophys. Acta 1015, 200–204.

Nagley, P., Mackay, I.R., Baumer, A., Maxwell, R.J., Vaillant, F., Wang, Z.X., Zhang, C., Linnane, A.W., 1992. Mitochondrial DNA mutation associated with aging and degenerative disease. Ann. NY Acad. Sci. 673, 92–102.

Nakai, M., Endo, T., Hase, T., Tanaka, Y., Trumpower, B.L., Ishiwatari, H., Asada, A., Bogaki, M., Matsubara, H., 1993. Acidic regions of cytochrome $c1$ are essential for ubiquinol-cytochrome c reductase activity in yeast cells lacking the acidic QCR6 protein. J. Biochem. (Tokyo) 114, 919–925.

Ohnishi, T., Trumpower, B.L., 1980. Differential effects of antimycin on ubisemiquinone bound in different environments in isolated succinate cytochrome c reductase complex. J. Biol. Chem. 255, 3278–3284.

Olivetti, G., Melissari, M., Capasso, J.M., Anversa, P., 1991. Cardiomyopathy of the aging human heart. Myocyte loss and reactive cellular hypertrophy. Circ. Res. 68, 1560–1568.

Pain, T., Yang, X.M., Critz, S.D., Yue, Y., Nakano, A., Liu, G.S., Heusch, G., Cohen, M.V., Downey, J.M., 2000. Opening of mitochondrial K(ATP) channels triggers the preconditioned state by generating free radicals. Circ. Res. 87, 460–466.

Palmer, J.W., Tandler, B., Hoppel, C.L., 1977. Biochemical properties of subsarcolemmal and interfibrillar mitochondria isolated from rat cardiac muscle. J. Biol. Chem. 252, 8731–8739.

Palmer, J.W., Tandler, B., Hoppel, C.L., 1985. Biochemical differences between subsarcolemmal and interfibrillar mitochondria from rat cardiac muscle: effects of procedural manipulations. Arch Biochem. Biophys. 236, 691–702.

Palmer, J.W., Tandler, B., Hoppel, C.L., 1986. Heterogeneous response of subsarcolemmal heart mitochondria to calcium. Am. J. Physiol. 250, H741–H748.

Papa, S., Guerrieri, F., Capitanio, N., 1997. A possible role of slips in cytochrome C oxidase in the antioxygen defense system of the cell. Biosci. Rep. 17, 23–31.

Paradies, G., Petrosillo, G., Pistolese, M., Ruggiero, F.M., 2000. The effect of reactive oxygen species generated from the mitochondrial electron transport chain on the cytochrome *c* oxidase activity and on the cardiolipin content in bovine heart submitochondrial particles. FEBS Lett. 466, 323–326.

Paradies, G., Ruggiero, F.M., Dinoi, P., Petrosillo, G., Quagliariello, E., 1993. Decreased cytochrome oxidase activity and changes in phospholipids in heart mitochondria from hypothyroid rats. Arch Biochem. Biophys. 307, 91–95.

Paradies, G., Ruggiero, F.M., Petrosillo, G., Quagliariello, E., 1994. Enhanced cytochrome oxidase activity and modification of lipids in heart mitochondria from hyperthyroid rats. Biochim. Biophys. Acta 1225, 165–170.

Paradies, G., Ruggiero, F.M., Petrosillo, G., Quagliariello, E., 1996. Age-dependent impairment of mitochondrial function in rat heart tissue. Effect of pharmacological agents. Ann. NY Acad. Sci. 786, 252–263.

Paradies, G., Ruggiero, F.M., Petrosillo, G., Quagliariello, E., 1997. Age-dependent decline in the cytochrome *c* oxidase activity in rat heart mitochondria: role of cardiolipin. FEBS Lett. 406, 136–138.

Pepe, S., 2000. Mitochondrial function in ischaemia and reperfusion of the ageing heart. Clin. Exp. Pharmacol. Physiol. 27, 745–750.

Phaneuf, S., Leeuwenburgh, C., 2002. Cytochrome *c* release from mitochondria in the aging heart: a possible mechanism for apoptosis with age. Am. J. Physiol. 282, R423–R430.

Piper, H.M., Sezer, O., Schleyer, M., Schwartz, P., Hutter, J.F., Spieckermann, P.G., 1985. Development of ischemia-induced damage in defined mitochondrial subpopulations. J. Mol. Cell. Cardiol. 17, 885–896.

Qian, T., Nieminen, A.L., Herman, B., Lemasters, J.J., 1997. Mitochondrial permeability transition in pH-dependent reperfusion injury to rat hepatocytes. Am. J. Physiol. 273, C1783–C1792.

Richter, C., Park, J.W., Ames, B.N., 1988. Normal oxidative damage to mitochondrial and nuclear DNA is extensive. Proc. Natl. Acad. Sci. USA 85, 6465–6467.

Robinson, N.C., Strey, F., Talbert, L., 1980. Investigation of the essential boundary layer phospholipids of cytochrome *c* oxidase using Triton X-100 delipidation. Biochemistry 19, 3656–3661.

Schagger, H., 1995. Native electrophoresis for isolation of mitochondrial oxidative phosphorylation protein complexes. Meth. Enzymol. 260, 190–202.

Schagger, H., 1996. Electrophoretic techniques for isolation and quantification of oxidative phosphorylation complexes from human tissues. Meth. Enzymol. 264, 555–566.

Schaper, J., Meiser, E., Stammler, G., 1985. Ultrastructural morphometric analysis of myocardium from dogs, rats, hamsters, mice, and from human hearts. Circ. Res. 56, 377–391.

Schmitt, M.E., Trumpower, B.L., 1991. The petite phenotype resulting from a truncated copy of subunit 6 results from loss of assembly of the cytochrome *bc*1 complex and can be suppressed by overexpression of subunit 9. J. Biol. Chem. 266, 14958–14963.

Shin, G., Sugiyama, M., Shoji, T., Kagiyama, A., Sato, H., Ogura, R., 1989. Detection of mitochondrial membrane damages in myocardial ischemia with ESR spin labeling technique. J. Mol. Cell Cardiol. 21, 1029–1036.

Snyder, C.H., Gutierrez-Cirlos, E.B., Trumpower, B.L., 2000. Evidence for a concerted mechanism of ubiquinol oxidation by the cytochrome *bc*1 complex. J. Biol. Chem. 275, 13535–13541.

Takasawa, M., Hayakawa, M., Sugiyama, S., Hattori, K., Ito, T., Ozawa, T., 1993. Age-associated damage in mitochondrial function in rat hearts. Exp. Gerontol. 28, 269–280.

Tani, M., Honma, Y., Hasegawa, H., Tamaki, K., 2001. Direct activation of mitochondrial K(ATP) channels mimics preconditioning but protein kinase C activation is less effective in middle-aged rat hearts. Cardiovasc. Res. 49, 56–68.

Tomanek, R.J., Karlsson, U.L., 1973. Myocardial ultrastructure of young and senescent rats. J. Ultra-struct. Res. 42, 201–220.

Travis, D.F., Travis, A., 1972. Ultrastructural changes in the left ventricular rat myocardial cells with age. J. Ultrastruct. Res. 39, 124–148.

Trumpower, B.L., 1990. The protonmotive Q cycle. Energy transduction by coupling of proton transloca-tion to electron transfer by the cytochrome bc1 complex. J. Biol. Chem. 265, 11409–11412.

Turrens, J.F., Alexandre, A., Lehninger, A.L., 1985. Ubisemiquinone is the electron donor for superoxide formation by complex III of heart mitochondria. Arch Biochem. Biophys. 237, 408–414.

Van Remmen, H., Richardson, A., 2001. Oxidative damage to mitochondria and aging. Exp. Gerontol. 36, 957–968.

Varotsis, C., Zhang, Y., Appelman, E.H., Babcock, G.T., 1993. Resolution of the reaction sequence during the reduction of O2 by cytochrome oxidase. Proc. Natl. Acad. Sci. USA 90, 237–241.

Vik, S.B., Capaldi, R.A., 1977. Lipid requirements for cytochrome c oxidase activity. Biochemistry 16, 5755–5759.

von Jagow, G., Ohnishi, T., 1985. The chromone inhibitor stigmatellin-binding to the ubiquinol oxidation center at the C-side of the mitochondrial membrane. FEBS Lett. 185, 311–315.

Wallace, D.C., 2000. Mitochondrial defects in cardiomyopathy and neuromuscular disease. Am. Heart J. 139, S70–S85.

Wanagat, J., Wolff, M.R., Aiken, J.M., 2002. Age-associated changes in function, structure and mitochon-drial genetic and enzymatic abnormalities in the Fischer 344 x Brown Norway F(1) hybrid rat heart. J. Mol. Cell Cardiol. 34, 17–28.

Wei, J.Y., 1992. Age and the cardiovascular system. N. Eng. J. Med. 327, 1735–1739.

Xia, D., Yu, C.A., Kim, H., Xia, J.Z., Kachurin, A.M., Zhang, L., Yu, L., Deisenhofer, J., 1997. Crystal structure of the cytochrome bc1 complex from bovine heart mitochondria. Science 277, 60–66.

Yang, J., Liu, X., Bhalla, K., Kim, C.N., Ibrado, A.M., Cai, J., Peng, T.I., Jones, D.P., Wang, X., 1997. Prevention of apoptosis by Bcl-2: release of cytochrome c from mitochondria blocked. Science 275, 1129–1132.

Zhang, L., Yu, L., Yu, C.A., 1998a. Generation of superoxide anion by succinate-cytochrome c reductase from bovine heart mitochondria. J. Biol. Chem. 273, 33972–33976.

Zhang, Z., Huang, L., Shulmeister, V.M., Chi, Y.I., Kim, K.K., Hung, L.W., Crofts, A.R., Berry, E.A., Kim, S.H., 1998b. Electron transfer by domain movement in cytochrome bc1. Nature 392, 677–684.

**Advances in
Cell Aging and
Gerontology**

Superoxide, superoxide dismutases,
and cardiovascular dysfunction

Marsha P. Cole[a], Luksana Chaiswing[b,*], Terry D. Oberley[b],
Kelley K. Kiningham[c] and Daret K. St. Clair[c,*]

[a]*Graduate Center for Nutritional Sciences, University of Kentucky, Lexington, KY 40536, USA*
[b]*Department of Pathology, V.A. Medical Center, University of Wisconsin, Madison, WI 53705, USA*
[c]*Graduate Center for Toxicology, 363 Health Science Research Building, University of Kentucky,
Lexington, KY 40536-0305, USA*
Faculty of Medical Technology, Mahidol University, Bangkok, Thailand 10700

Contents

---

* Corresponding author. Tel.: +1-859-257-3956; fax: +1-859-257-3955.
  E-mail address: dstcl00@pop.uky.edu (D.K. St. Clair).

Advances in Cell Aging and Gerontology, vol. 11, 233–281

Abbreviations

ROS	reactive oxygen species
RNS	reactive nitrogen species
SOD	superoxide dismutase
CuZnSOD	copper,zinc superoxide dismutase
MnSOD	manganese superoxide dismutase
ECSOD	extracellular superoxide dismutase
TNFα	tumor necrosis factor α
BH$_4$	tetrahydrobiopterin
eNOS	endothelial nitric oxide dismutase
iNOS	inducible nitric oxide dismutase
IRP-1	iron responsive protein-1
CPK	creatine phosphokinase
MB-CPK	myofibrillar-bound creatine phosphokinase
NF-κB	nuclear factor-kappa B
AP-1	activator protein-1
EPR	electron paramagnetic resonance spectroscopy
GSHPx	glutathione peroxidase
GSH	glutathione
GSSG	glutathione disulfide
FALS	familial amyotrophic lateral sclerosis
DS	Down's Syndrome
IL-1-β	interleukin-1-β
IL-2	interleukin-2
PMA	phorbol-12-myristate-13-acetate
ADR	adriamycin
IRI	ischemia-reperfusion injury
4-HNE	4-hydroxynonenal
IHD	ischemic heart disease
TIA	transient ischemic attacks
MDA	malondialdehyde
AIF	apoptosis-inducing factor
IFN-γ	interferon-γ
STAT	signal transducer and activator of transcription
MT	metallothionein
MPG	mercaptoproprionyl glycine
8OHdG	8-hydroxy-2' -deoxyguanosine
DOXol	doxorubicinol
SERCA	sarcoendoplasmic reticulum calcium ATPase
ICRF-187	dexrazone

1. Introduction

All aerobic organisms must cope with reactive oxygen species (ROS), e.g. superoxide radicals ($O_2^{\bullet-}$), hydrogen peroxide (H_2O_2), and hydroxyl radicals ($OH^\bullet$), that are formed as incomplete reduction products of molecular oxygen in metabolizing cells. These ROS can serve as signal mediators regulating gene expression, or they can inactivate certain target macromolecules such as proteins, lipid, and DNA.

Under physiological conditions, superoxide radicals are detoxified by superoxide dismutase (SOD). However, under oxidative stress, the level of superoxide radicals may overwhelm the basal level of this enzyme defense system, leading to an adaptive response or toxicity. Generation of $O_2^{\bullet-}$ radicals is likely to play a major role in cardiac dysfunction because cardiomyocytes contain a large number of mitochondria required for energy production. Ironically, mitochondria are particularly prone to free radical-induced changes because most oxygen utilization by mammalian cells occurs in this organelle. Some components of the electron transport chain such as the NADH–coenzyme Q reductase complex and the reduced form of coenzyme Q leak electrons onto oxygen, which produces a univalent reduction to give rise to super-oxide radicals. Mitochondrial DNA is highly susceptible to mutation because mitochondrial DNA is not protected by histones. Mutations in any of the genes encoding for cytochrome oxidase, cytochrome b-c_1, NADH dehydrogenase, or ATPase complexes may lead to defective function of these enzymes. Additionally, $O_2^{\bullet-}$ can directly inactivate mitochondrial enzymes leading to mitochondrial dys-function and increased ROS generation. It has been demonstrated that Fe–S-containing enzymes, which include several components of the electron transport chain, are highly sensitive to redox-induced inactivation. Thus, if the level of SOD is insufficient to remove excess superoxide radicals, mitochondrial respiration will cause increased oxidative stress in the mitochondria, leading to mitochondrial injury and subsequent cardiac dysfunction.

This review provides background information on ROS and their defense systems in the heart. Special emphases are given to the chemistry of superoxide radicals, the biochemical and molecular biology properties of SODs, and the role of oxidative stress in cardiovascular diseases.

2. Prooxidants and antioxidants in the heart

2.1. Prooxidants

2.1.1. Free radicals

2.1.1.1. Oxygen radicals   Since the appearance of oxygen in the Earth's atmosphere 2–3 billion years ago, we, as multicellular organisms, were forced to develop anti-oxidant defenses against prooxidant formation as a consequence of normal cellular metabolism and aerobic respiration (Halliwell, 1999). Gerschman et al. (1956) first suggested the toxicity of oxygen due to its potential to generate molecules with unpaired electrons or free radicals. Oxygen, a di-radical, participates in numerous one-electron reduction reactions involving both enzymatic and non-enzymatic mechanisms that result in the production of superoxide and other ROS. Reactive oxygen species are derivatives of molecular oxygen that can abstract electrons from other molecules. Reactive oxygen species are classified into two categories: free radicals and non-radicals. Free radicals are highly reactive molecules or atoms that contain one or more unpaired electrons in their valence shells. Examples include the superoxide radical ($O_2^{\bullet-}$) and hydroxyl radical ($OH^{\bullet}$). A molecule can become a free radical by either losing or gaining an electron. Free radicals can act as oxidizing or reducing agents, depending on their substrate. Due to their high reactivity and short half-life, most free radical species react in the proximity of their production sites. Non-radical ROS are molecules that promote or accelerate oxidation of other biomolecules. An example is H_2O_2. These non-radical ROS can also have deleterious biological effects at their production sites. Reactive oxygen species are generated in mitochondria of normal mammalian cells as byproducts of normal respiration and in other subcellular locations as a result of biochemical reactions utilizing oxygen.

2.1.1.2. Superoxide radical Oxygen has two unpaired electrons in the outer orbitals. Reduction of oxygen produces superoxide radicals. The superoxide radical is the first intermediate in the sequential univalent reduction of oxygen that eventually leads to formation of H_2O. Superoxide radical can lead to the formation of other ROS, including $OH^{\bullet}$ and H_2O_2. Protonation of superoxide leads to the formation of peroxyl radical, which is more reactive than $O_2^{\bullet-}$. The superoxide radical is produced by macrophages, neutrophils, fibroblasts, and vascular endothelial cells (Kuhn and Brash, 1990). It is an important intracellular signaling molecule, which participates in growth regulation and in host defense mechanisms. Excessive amounts of superoxide radicals have been implicated in many diseases.

2.1.1.3. Hydroxyl radical The hydroxyl radical is one of the most potent oxidants encountered in biological systems and has a very short half-life. It is very reactive and therefore does not pass through cell membranes. The biological importance of $OH^{\bullet}$ was first suggested in studies of X-ray irradiation. The hydroxyl radical can be generated by two major biological reactions: the Fenton reaction and the Haber–Weiss reaction. In the Fenton reaction, H_2O_2 decomposes by accepting an electron from a reduced metal ion (Basaga, 1990):

$$Fe^{2+} + H_2O_2 \rightarrow Fe^{3+} + OH^{\bullet} + OH^-$$

In the Haber–Weiss reaction, $OH^{\bullet}$ is generated by the interaction of $O_2^{\bullet-}$ and H_2O_2:

$$O_2^{\bullet-} + H_2O_2 \rightarrow O_2 + H_2O + OH^{\bullet}$$

When generated, $OH^{\bullet}$ can induce significant damage in cells through reaction with proteins, lipids, carbohydrates, and DNA. The hydroxyl radical is capable of initiating free radical chain reactions, an example being initiation of lipid peroxidation.

2.1.1.4. Nitric oxide Nitric oxide ($^{\bullet}NO$) has an unpaired electron and is therefore a free radical. It is an important neurotransmitter, has a role in vasodilation (endothelium-derived relaxing factor), and is an effective antimicrobial agent. It is synthesized from the amino acid L-arginine by vascular endothelial cells, phagocytes, and certain cells in the brain (Moncada and Higgs, 1993). Nitric oxide at high concentrations is a potentially toxic compound. Superoxide participates in a near diffusion-limited reaction with $^\bullet$NO to form the reactive nitrogen species (RNS) peroxynitrite ($ONOO^-$). Peroxynitrite is a compound that has been implicated in the vasoconstriction of vascular smooth muscle cells. Steady state levels of both $O_2^{\bullet-}$ and $^\bullet$NO have been reported in the literature to exist in vivo (Beckman et al., 1990; Pfeiffer et al., 1999). When there are equimolar concentrations of $O_2^{\bullet-}$ and $^\bullet$NO, the rate constant for the formation of peroxynitrite is 4.3×10^9 to $6.7 \times 10^9 \, M^{-1} s^{-1}$ (Pfeiffer et al., 1999). Peroxynitrite is a very potent oxidant with a reduction potential of 1.6 V at pH 7.0 (Pfeiffer et al., 1999). Once generated, peroxynitrite can cause enzyme inactivation, lipid peroxidation, DNA damage, and inhibition of mitochondrial respiration (Muijsers et al., 1997). Peroxynitrite, other RNS, and ROS have been implicated in cardiac injury and aging.

2.2. Non-free radical oxidants

2.2.1. Hydrogen peroxide

Hydrogen peroxide is the two-electron reduction product of molecular oxygen in biological systems. It is generated from a radical compound such as $O_2^{\bullet-}$, with an example of its generation being the dismutation of superoxide radical by SOD to H_2O_2. The enzymes xanthine oxidase, NADPH oxidase, amino acid oxidase, and flavoprotein dehydrogenase are capable of producing H_2O_2. Hydrogen peroxide has been implicated in many pathologic states. Recent studies show that H_2O_2 plays an important role in the regulation of several genes by activation of NF-κB transcription factor (Dhalla et al., 2000a,b). Hydrogen peroxide can freely diffuse within and between cells. In the presence of superoxide radical and metal catalysts, H_2O_2 can form hydroxyl radical. In the presence of myeloperoxidase and chloride ion, H_2O_2 forms hypochlorous acid (HOCl) both inside and outside phagocytes, followed by the formation of other non-radical oxidants (Dhalla et al., 2000a).

2.3. Role of metal chelators in oxidative stress

Several of the essential trace elements, including iron (Fe), copper (Cu), and manganese (Mn), exist in multiple oxidation states and are able to catalyze some or all of the reactions that result in oxidative stress. Transition metals are remarkably good promoters of free radical reactions. The redox potentials of these metals, particularly Fe^{3+} and Cu^{2+}, are profoundly influenced by their ligand environment. These metals are soluble only when they are bound to a variety of low molecular weight ligands, including endogenous amino acids, organic acids, and carbohydrates, or to high molecular weight proteins and nucleic acids.

Bound metals have several important and different functions, including the role of cofactor in many antioxidant enzymes such as SOD and catalase. Bound metals can act both as reactants, an example being Fe^{2+} in the Fenton reaction, and electron transfer agents, examples being Mn, Cu, and Zn in the active sites of SOD in the dismutase reaction.

2.4. *Sources of ROS in mammalian cells*

There are many subcellular sources of ROS (Table 1). Reactive oxygen species are generated in the mitochondria of mammalian cells as a byproduct of respiration. Enzymes and transport molecules also generate free radicals as a normal consequence of their catalytic functions. Kojda and Harrison (1999) reviewed the numerous enzymatic sources of ROS in mammalian cells, including mitochondrial electron transport chain, xanthine oxidase, cyclooxygenase, lipoxygenase, NO synthase, heme oxygenases, peroxidases, hemoproteins such as heme and hematin, and NADH oxidases. Non-enzymatic sources of ROS generation include Fe^{2+} and other redox-active metals.

Examples of two enzymes that have been extensively studied in biological systems are xanthine oxidase and aldehyde oxidase. Both of these enzymes generate superoxide anion radical by adding a single electron to molecular oxygen. Other enzymes may also use $O_2^{\bullet-}$ for their normal catalytic activity.

Autoxidation reactions produce free radicals from the spontaneous oxidation of biological molecules involved in non-enzymatic electron transfers. Although these reactions are a normal part of cellular metabolism, free radicals generated may, under certain adverse conditions, have serious clinical significance. Examples of compounds that may be autoxidized in the body include thiols, hydroquinones, catecholamines, flavins, ferredoxins, and hemoglobin. In all of these autoxidation reactions, $O_2^{\bullet-}$ is the main free radical species that is produced initially. The processes involved in oxidation–reduction reactions are of immense biochemical importance since the transfer of electrons is the means by which the body derives most of its free energy.

A variety of factors influence the cellular capacity to produce free radicals, including cell type, subcellular microenvironment, and physiological state of the cell. In addition, exogenous sources of free radicals include exposure to certain chemicals such as toxins (e.g. carbon tetrachloride, paraquat, toluene), drugs (e.g. adriamycin,

Table 1
Cellular sources of free radicals

Subcellular localization	Source
Plasma membrane	Lipoxygenase, prostaglandin synthetase, NADPH oxidase
Mitochondrial electron transport	NADH dehydrogenase, dihydroorotate dehydrogenase
Peroxisomes	Oxidases
Endoplasmic reticulum	Cytochrome P_{450}, Cytochrome b_5
Cytosol	
Soluble enzymes and protein	Hemoglobin, tryptophan dioxygenase, xanthine oxidase
Small molecules	Reduced flavins, thiols, divalent metals, epinephrine

bleomycin, mitomycin C), air pollutants (e.g. carbon monoxide), ingested substances (e.g. smoked and barbecued food, alcohol), radiation, and sunlight.

Among these endogenous sources of ROS, mitochondria remain a major site of ROS production. Within the mitochondria exists a very strong reducing environment with many single electrons, polyunsaturated fatty acids, and transition metals, therefore providing a potential site for generation of ROS. During normal respiration, approximately 1–2% of the electron flow in the electron transport chain is diverted and results in partial reduction of oxygen, and thus generation of $O_2^{\bullet-}$ (Raha et al., 2000).

The mitochondrial electron transport chain is composed of four electron transporting complexes (I–IV) and one proton translocator known as an ATPase (complex V) for ATP synthesis. Two of these complexes have been shown to produce $O_2^{\bullet-}$. Through affinity labeling with rotenone analogs, NADH–ubiquinone oxidoreductase or complex I was found to be a possible site for semiquinone generation (Earley et al., 1987). Through a one-electron reduction reaction, semiquinone is able to donate an electron to molecular oxygen, thus producing $O_2^{\bullet-}$. Also, ubiquinol production occurring at complex I or II is oxidized by complex III. Hence, complex III is an additional site for superoxide generation from the generation of ubisemiquinone (Raha and Robinson, 2001).

2.4.1. Sources of ROS/RNS in myocardial, vascular, and endothelial tissues during cardiovascular diseases

2.4.1.1. Mitochondrial electron transport
In biological systems, oxygen is essential for mitochondrial oxidative phosphorylation and for production of ATP. Electrons leaking from the electron transport chain can convert oxygen molecules into superoxide, which can be further reduced to H_2O_2. Thus, ROS are formed during mitochondrial electron transport and are controlled by intracellular antioxidant defenses such as SOD. Lack of oxygen supply because of hypoxia or ischemia disrupts the mitochondrial electron transport chain, resulting in an accumulation of toxic metabolites, acidosis, ATP depletion, intracellular Ca^{2+} overload, mitochondrial membrane depolarization, mitochondrial matrix swelling, and cell death. Several experiments have shown that injury in myocardium is caused by superoxide radicals derived from respiratory electron transport (Wattanapitayakul and Bauer, 2001).

2.4.2. Reactions of oxidative enzymes
Many enzymes generate free radicals during catalytic reactions, including xanthine oxidase, NADH/NADPH oxidase, and nitric oxide synthase (NOS).

2.4.2.1. Xanthine oxidase
Xanthine oxidoreductase is a molybdo-enzyme capable of catalyzing the oxidation of hypoxanthine and xanthine during the process of purine metabolism. Xanthine oxidoreductase can exist in two interconvertible forms,

as either xanthine dehydrogenase or xanthine oxidase. The reaction of xanthine oxidase occurs as follows (Cai and Harrison, 2000):

$$\text{hypoxanthine} + H_2O + O_2 \xrightarrow{\text{xanthine oxidase}} \text{xanthine} + O_2^{\bullet-}$$

$$\text{xanthine} + H_2O + O_2 \xrightarrow{\text{xanthine oxidase}} \text{uric acid} + O_2^{\bullet-}$$

Xanthine oxidase is widely distributed in the lung, intestine, and liver. In endothelial cells, the activity and expression of xanthine oxidase is enhanced by interferon. The production of $O_2^{\bullet-}$ by xanthine oxidase is widely studied in ischemia reperfusion injury (IRI). Hypoxia and the presence of inflammatory cytokines have been shown to elevate xanthine oxidase activities.

2.4.2.2. NADH/NADPH oxidase   In several studies, investigators have attempted to define the source of ROS using homogenates of either vascular cells or tissues. When homogenates of endothelial and vascular smooth muscle cells have been studied, NADH is the predominant substrate capable of driving $O_2^{\bullet-}$ production. NADPH oxidase generally is found in phagocytic cells. It acts as a non-specific host defense during infection. NADH/NADPH oxidase contributes to $O_2^{\bullet-}$ production in the vasculature. Its activity is regulated by cytokines, hormones, and mechanical forces that are known to be involved in the pathogenesis of vascular diseases. Stimulation of vascular smooth muscle cells with angiotensin II, thrombin, platelet-derived growth factor, and tumor necrosis factor (TNF) increases vascular ROS formation and NADH/NADPH oxidase activity (Griendling et al., 2000).

There is evidence supporting the hypothesis that activation of NADH/NADPH oxidase can lead to endothelial dysfunction by reducing $^{\bullet}$NO bioavailability. This mechanism is postulated to play an important role in several vascular diseases.

2.4.2.3. Nitric oxide synthase   A third source of vascular ROS production is endothelial NOS (eNOS). Endothelial NOS is a cytochrome P_{450} reductase-like enzyme that catalyzes flavin-mediated electron transport from the electron donor NADPH to a prosthetic heme group. The enzyme requires tetrahydrobiopterin (BH_4) bound near this heme group to transfer electrons to a guanidino nitrogen of L-arginine to form nitric oxide. There has also been evidence presented that eNOS can potentiate injury in pathophysiological conditions. In addition, proinflammatory conditions stimulate expression of an inducible isoform of NO synthase (iNOS), resulting in $^{\bullet}$NO production. Not only is inducible NOS expressed by tissue macrophages, but cardiac myocytes can also express iNOS. These observations may help to explain the progression of inflammatory myocardial diseases and eventual heart failure (Michel and Feron, 1997). Both eNOS and iNOS are NADPH-dependent enzymes. However, eNOS is calmodulin dependent, whereas iNOS is calmodulin independent. Activation of eNOS requires high levels of intracellular Ca^{2+} for calmodulin binding. In contrast, calmodulin remains tightly bound to iNOS, allowing for activation even at low concentrations of Ca^{2+}. Almost every intracellular organelle has been proposed as a possible site of NOS, including the nucleus, endoplasmic reticulum, mitochondria, cytoskeleton, and plasma membrane. Endothelial NOS in endothelial cells is activated in many ways, including by shear stress and agonists such as bradykinin (O'Donnell and Freeman, 2001).

2.4.3. Activation of inflammatory cells

It is well documented that inflammatory cells can produce free radicals as a means of host defense with resultant pathogen killing. Activated neutrophils produce superoxide, hydrogen peroxide, and hydroxyl radicals in order to kill pathogens. Infiltration of activated phagocyte cells into cardiac muscle is a potential mechanism of cardiac oxidant production. In addition, phagocytes present in the blood can be rapidly recruited into the tissues when they are required during the inflammatory process. Activated white blood cells may cause additional damage to tissues by the secretion of several mediators, including proteolytic enzymes and proinflammatory cytokines (Mims et al., 1993). As inflammatory cell infiltration during cardiovascular disease will be reviewed in a different chapter, we will not address this topic.

2.5. Role of ROS in the cell

Reactive oxygen species have both physiologic functions and pathologic effects within cells. Physiologic functions include regulation of signal transduction pathways, transcription factor activities, mitochondrial function, and cytoskeleton assembly. The molecular targets in disease are probably the same molecules involved in physiologic function.

2.5.1. ROS and biomolecules

Reactive oxygen species can react with many biomolecules, including lipids, proteins, and DNA, leading to their oxidation and a decrease in their half-life.

2.5.1.1. ROS and proteins   Free radicals induce damage to proteins by modification of primary, secondary, and tertiary structures, resulting in fragmentation, cross-linking, and aggregation of proteins. These changes are usually manifested by a change in the biological activity of enzymes. Activation of some enzymes by ROS may also occur. For example, $O_2^{\bullet-}$ is capable of oxidizing and inactivating aconitase, a key enzyme in the citric acid cycle and a regulator of iron transport and storage (Gardner et al., 1994, 1995). In order for aconitase to have full enzyme activity, the [4Fe–4S] complex at the active site must be intact. Upon enzyme inactivation by $O_2^{\bullet-}$, ferrous iron (Fe^{2+}) is released. The resulting apoenzyme acquires RNA-binding activity through an increase in the transcription of iron responsive protein one (IRP-1) (Minotti et al., 1999). When IRP-1 binds to the iron responsive element in the $3'$ region of transferrin mRNA, the transferrin receptor is stabilized. However, when bound to the iron responsive element in the $5'$ region of ferritin mRNA, the translation of ferritin is suppressed. Ferritin is a protein that facilitates the binding and storage of iron. The free Fe^{2+} can initiate and react with $O_2^{\bullet-}$ and/or H_2O_2 through Fenton-type chemistry to generate a more damaging species, the hydroxyl radical. The hydroxyl radical is the most potent oxidizing species, having a reduction potential of 2.3 V (Buettner, 1993). Therefore, in an increased oxidative state, stabilization of transferrin and suppression of ferritin increases availability of ferrous iron, thereby promoting the Haber–Weiss reaction. The propagation of the hydroxyl radical in this iron-catalyzed reaction can cause lipid peroxidation, protein oxidation, enzyme inactivation, and DNA damage (Halliwell and Gutteridge, 1989).

Creatine phosphokinase (CPK) is another enzyme that is sensitive to oxidative inactivation (McCord and Russell, 1988). CPK is a component of the myofibrils and participates in the regulation of energy transduction in muscle cells (i.e. cardiomyocytes). Enzymatically, CPK facilitates the transfer of high energy phosphates in cross-bridge signaling. Upon cardiac injury, myofibrillar-bound CPK (MB-CPK) is released into the serum and often measured as an indicative marker of myocardial injury.

Other key enzymes have been reported to be sensitive to inactivation by reaction with $O_2^{\bullet-}$, including 3-α-3-phosphate dehydrogenase (Armstrong and Buchana, 1978), glyceraldehyde-3-phosphate dehydrogenase (Armstrong and Buchana, 1978), papain (Armstrong and Buchana, 1978), ornithine decarboxylase (Guarnieri et al., 1982), catalase (Kono and Fridovich, 1982), glutathione peroxidase (Blum and Fridovich, 1985), 3-alpha-hydroxysteroid dehydrogenase (Kim et al., 1986) and α,β-dihydroxyisovalerate dehydratase (Kuo et al., 1987). Glutathione peroxidase and catalase along with SOD comprise the primary antioxidant defense system in the heart. Therefore, increases in superoxide may cause the activities of catalase and/or glutathione peroxidase to be inactivated, thereby compromising the ability of the defense system.

2.5.1.2. ROS and lipids   Unsaturated fatty acids play an important role in cellular metabolism and cellular structure. Polyunsaturated fatty acids are particularly vulnerable to free radical attack. This oxidative damage is termed lipid peroxidation and causes a reduction in membrane fluidity and permeability. Peroxidation is initiated by any species that can attack and abstract a hydrogen atom from a methylene group to leave unpaired electrons on the carbon. This abstraction is easier on a methyl group adjacent to a double bond. In polyunsaturated fatty acids, a molecular rearrangement follows at the carbon radicals to form peroxyl radicals, which, in turn, abstract a hydrogen atom from another lipid molecule (RH) to give a lipid hydroperoxide, thus initiating a chain reaction. Cyclic peroxides may also form, with subsequent rearrangement to lipoperoxides, which upon further oxidation yields aldehyde (Kuhn and Brash, 1990). The reactions are:

$$RH + OH^{\bullet} \rightarrow R^{\bullet} + H_2O$$

$$R^{\bullet} + O_2 \rightarrow ROO^{\bullet}$$

$$ROO^{\bullet} + RH \rightarrow ROOH + R^{\bullet}$$

and these chain termination reactions follow:

$$R^{\bullet} + R^{\bullet} \rightarrow RR$$

$$ROO^{\bullet} + ROO^{\bullet} \rightarrow O_2 + ROOR$$

$$ROO^{\bullet} + R^{\bullet} \rightarrow ROOR$$

2.5.1.3. ROS and DNA   Interaction of free radicals and DNA can result in DNA base modification, strand breakage, and deoxyribose fragmentation. The presence of modified bases in template DNA can induce miscoding in the transcripted DNA strand (Allen and Tresini, 2000). This results in cytotoxicity, mutation, and potential for malignant change as a result of induced chromosomal aberrations. The hydroxyl radical is the most common ROS that causes DNA damage. Sources of ROS that can cause damage to DNA include ionizing radiation, photooxidation, and effects due to chemical production of ROS.

2.5.1.4. ROS and carbohydrates   At physiological pH and temperature, autoxidation of monosaccharides such as glucose can produce H_2O_2, peroxide, and oxaldehydes. Linkage of carbohydrates to proteins (glycation) seems to increase the susceptibility of proteins to free radical attack (Erenel et al., 1993).

2.5.2. *ROS, signal transduction, and gene expression*

Recent studies have demonstrated that ROS may indeed act as signal transduction molecules. For example, cellular H_2O_2 was transiently increased upon activation of platelet-derived growth factor. Several signaling pathways are affected by the platelet-derived growth factor-induced increase in H_2O_2 concentration. Additionally, H_2O_2 activates hypertrophic and apoptotic signaling pathways in cardiac myocytes. Reactive oxygen species activate a wide variety of cellular signaling molecules, including Ca^{2+} levels, protein tyrosine kinases, serine threonine kinases, and phospholipases (Allen and Tresini, 2000).

It has become increasingly evident that ROS are more than cellular toxicants and that they may be important modulators of cellular gene expression patterns. For example, redox cycling of cysteine residues is one of the important mechanisms of ROS regulated activity of transcription factors and signaling molecules. Disruption (reduction) or formation (oxidation) of disulfide bonds plays a central role in determining protein conformation. Conformation is critical for proper protein–protein and protein–DNA interactions, which, in turn, drive specific signal transduction pathways. Many studies show that at least two important transcription factors, NF-κB and AP-1, are controlled by the intracellular redox state (reviewed in Allen and Tresini, 2000). These redox regulated transcription factors bind to several promoter regions of genes that are involved in the pathogenesis of several diseases.

2.6. *Identification of oxidative damage*

Methods for identification of oxidative damage include direct measurement of ROS and indirect measurement of levels of antioxidant enzymes and oxidative damage products. The identification of antioxidant enzymes proved the existence of ROS, while the presence of DNA repair enzymes specific for oxidative DNA damage documented the inherent toxicity of ROS for cellular DNA. In general, ROS have a short half-life because of their high reactivity and are therefore difficult to detect with standard biochemical methods. Advanced physical–chemical techniques such as electron paramagnetic resonance spectroscopy (EPR) with spin traps allow detection and identification of free radicals. However, these techniques require expensive instrumentation and quantification of the amount of oxygen free radicals in tissues is difficult. Reactive oxygen species can be detected by methods allowing detection of fluorescence signals, e.g. luciferase assays with a fluorometer or use of redox-sensitive dyes with flow cytometry or confocal microscopy. These fluorescent techniques suffer from a lack of specificity, but have high sensitivity.

Because of the disadvantage of direct techniques, investigators have turned to analyzing the footprints of oxidative damage, e.g. analysis of oxidative damage products, including products of lipid, protein, and DNA oxidation. Oxidative damage products can be measured with biochemical assays. Antibodies to oxidative damage products have been developed and may be used in either biochemical or morphologic studies (Oberley, 2002).

2.7. *Antioxidant defense systems in the heart*

Superoxide production is ongoing, both intentionally, for processes such as phagocytosis and cell signaling, and as an unwanted byproduct of physiological processes (Halliwell, 1999). Aerobic organisms have developed antioxidant defenses as an adaptive process to maintain a state of redox balance. "A disturbance in the prooxidant–antioxidant balance in the favor of the former" has been used to define oxidative stress (Sies, 1991). Antioxidant activity may be accomplished by many different mechanisms, including the inhibition of the generation of ROS or their precursors, by directly scavenging free radicals by means of antiradical enzymes such as SOD or catalase, and by enhancing endogenous antioxidant generation. The antioxidant defense system has both non-enzymatic and enzymatic components. The enzymatic components are usually classified as primary antioxidant enzymes (manganese and copper, zinc superoxide dismutases, catalase, glutathione peroxidase), secondary antioxidant enzymes such as glutathione reductase, glucose-6-phosphate dehydrogenase, and the glutathione, glutaredoxin, and thioredoxin systems. Protein and DNA repair enzymes may also be considered part of the antioxidant system.

There are three primary antioxidant enzymes located in the heart, with different sites of action in cardiomyocytes. Superoxide dismutase catalyzes the reaction of $O_2^{\bullet -}$ to form H_2O_2 and molecular oxygen. Catalase is another primary antioxidant enzyme found mainly in peroxisomes. Catalase catalyzes the breakdown of H_2O_2 to molecular oxygen and water. In addition, another antioxidant enzyme that targets the breakdown of H_2O_2 is glutathione peroxidase (GSHPx). Glutathione peroxidase is found in the cytoplasm, membrane, and plasma, and its antioxidant action depends upon the availability of reduced glutathione. Hydrogen peroxide is converted to water via GSHPx through oxidation of glutathione (GSH) to glutathione disulfide (GSSG). The enzyme responsible for recycling the glutathione disulfide back to reduced glutathione is known as glutathione reductase. These antioxidant enzymes are briefly discussed below, except for SOD, which is detailed in Section 3.

2.7.1. Catalase

Catalase is a heme-dependent enzyme. It scavenges H_2O_2 as follows (Halliwell and Gutteridge, 1989):

$$H_2O_2 + \text{catalase} - Fe^{3+} \xrightarrow{k_1} \text{compound I}$$

$$\text{compound I} + H_2O_2 \xrightarrow{k_2} \text{catalase} - Fe^{3+} + O_2 + H_2O$$

Compound I is generated as an intermediate depending upon the concentration of catalase and H_2O_2, as well as the values of rate constants k_1 and k_2. The Michaelis constant (K_m) for the catalase reaction is relatively higher than that of GSHPx (Yu, 1994). Catalase is not present in all cellular compartments where H_2O_2 is generated, and the distribution of catalase is primarily in the peroxisome.

2.7.2. Glutathione and glutathione-dependent enzymes

Glutathione peroxidase enzymes exist in both selenium-dependent and selenium-independent forms. Glutathione peroxidase catalyzes the decomposition of H_2O_2 to water and simultaneously oxidizes GSH. High concentrations of reduced GSH and low levels of the oxidized form (GSSG) are necessary for the survival of mammalian cells. Maintenance of high GSH and low GSSG levels is important because higher GSSG levels can react with protein sulfhydryls to form mixed glutathione protein disulfides that can inactivate proteins. The necessary GSH–GSSG ratios are maintained by the enzymes glutathione reductase and glucose-6-phosphate dehydrogenase (G6PD) in the following reactions (Erenel et al., 1993):

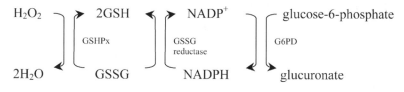

Glutathione peroxidases play an important role in the inhibition of lipid peroxidation of intracellular membranes.

2.8. Non-enzymatic defense systems

Several vitamins and other non-enzymatic defense systems are also critical in maintaining redox balance in the heart. Vitamin C, vitamin E, carotenoids, uric acid, and selenium are discussed below.

2.8.1. Ascorbic acid (vitamin C)

Vitamin C is water-soluble and an essential dietary vitamin, which humans and most mammals cannot synthesize due to absence of the enzyme L-gulono-lactone oxidase. Vitamin C deficiency results in scurvy and dysfunctions in collagen formation and iron absorption. Ascorbic acid is an important cofactor for both proline hydroxylase and dopamine-beta-hydroxylase, the latter enzyme catalyzing the conversion of dopamine to noradrenaline. Vitamin C is a powerful reducing agent and antioxidant, which reacts with superoxide, hydrogen peroxide, and hydroxyl radicals to form the metabolite dehydroascorbic acid (DHA) via a semidehydroascorbate intermediate (Yu, 1994). Under certain physiological conditions, ascorbate can promote lipid peroxidation by the reduction of ferric iron (Fe^{3+}) to ferrous ion (Fe^{2+}). The Fe^{2+} ion can subsequently participate in the Fenton reaction. Vitamin C is regenerated by glutathione in a reaction catalyzed by dehydroascorbate reductase. Vitamin C and vitamin E work synergistically, with vitamin E acting as the primary antioxidant (Erenel et al., 1993).

2.8.2. *Vitamin E (α-tocopherol)*

Vitamin E is a hydrophobic molecule. It has a higher activity toward the membrane surface than the membrane interior. Studies have found that vitamin E is a powerful scavenger of singlet oxygen and can react with superoxide and lipid peroxyl radicals. The mechanism by which vitamin E can block the propagation of lipid peroxyl radicals is thought to be via the intercalation of the hydrocarbon chain into the lipid bilayer. The reaction between α-tocopherol and the lipid peroxyl radical is one in which the peroxyl radical abstracts a hydrogen from the hydroxyl group located on the aromatic moiety of the vitamin. This reaction yields a weak radical known as the α-tocopherol radical as shown below (Erenel et al., 1993):

$$ROO^\bullet + \alpha\text{-tocopherol} \rightarrow ROOH + \alpha\text{-tocopherol}^\bullet$$

α-tocopherol$^\bullet$ can either be oxidized by reacting with a second lipid radical:

$$ROO^\bullet + \alpha\text{-tocopherol}^\bullet \rightarrow ROO\text{-}\alpha\text{-tocopherol}^\bullet$$

or converted back to vitamin E by ascorbate:

$$\text{vitamin E}^\bullet + \text{vitamin C} \rightarrow \text{vitamin E} + \text{ascorbyl}^\bullet$$

The conversion of ascorbyl$^\bullet$ back to vitamin C requires NADH.

2.8.3. *Carotenoids*

Beta-carotene, an efficient biological antioxidant, is considered to be the most efficient scavenger of singlet oxygen. Beta-carotene is the major carotenoid precursor of vitamin A. Vitamin A, however, does not quench singlet oxygen and has a very small capability of scavenging free radicals (Yu, 1994). Carotenoids protect lipids against peroxidation by quenching free radicals and other reactive species.

Beta-carotene, like vitamin C, seems to function as both an antioxidant and a prooxidant. Under low oxygen partial pressures, beta-carotene exhibits excellent radical-scavenging activity. At higher oxygen partial pressures, its capacity to trap free radicals shows autocatalytic prooxidant effects, with simultaneous loss of its antioxidant activity (Yu, 1994). Beta-carotene traps free radicals through its inhibition of lipid peroxidation.

2.8.4. *Uric acid*

Uric acid is an end product of purine metabolism. More recently, uric acid has become recognized as an important biological antioxidant. Studies have demonstrated that uric acid is a potent physiological antioxidant, playing a major role in both extracellular and intracellular defense mechanisms. The one-electron oxidation of uric acid generates the relatively stable urate radical. Urate can react with peroxyl radicals and other oxidizing species very rapidly. In contrast, the rate of reaction for urate radicals with oxygen is very slow. Furthermore, uric acid may serve as an important component of the overall antioxidant defense systems, thus helping to increase the life span of the individual (Yu, 1994).

2.8.5. *Selenium*

The antioxidant ability of GSHPx is dependent upon the selenium residing in the active site of the enzyme. Selenium has unique chemical properties and appears on the periodic table of the elements in a position between the metals and non-metals. The protective actions of selenium seem to operate at several levels. Selenium inhibits microsomal enzymes responsible for the generation of some forms of carcinogens. It may also act at the cellular level to prevent the enzymatic conversion of precarcinogens to carcinogens. Evidence suggests that selenium enhances the detoxification process of carcinogenic substances and protects against carcinogen-induced chromosomal damage. Most carcinogens are thought to be activated through a free radical-mediated interaction with DNA. Selenium may interfere with the DNA–free radical interaction processes. This hypothesis is further supported by the distribution of selenium within the cell since the highest concentration is in the nucleus, followed by the cytosol, mitochondria, and the microsomes. The precise mechanism of the protective action of selenium against cancer has not been fully defined. It is believed that selenium's protective action against cancer is probably linked to its role in maintaining the cell's optimum level of selenium-dependent GSHPx (Lawrence and Burk, 1976).

2.9. *Summary*

Table 2 summarizes the enzymatic and non-enzymatic endogenous antioxidants found in cardiomyocytes (modified from Dhalla et al., 2000b).

Table 2
Endogenous antioxidants and antioxidant enzyme defenses found in cardiomyocytes

Antioxidant	Cellular location	Action
MnSOD	Mitochondria	$2O_2^{\bullet-}+2H^+{\rightarrow}H_2O_2+O_2$
CuZnSOD	Cytoplasm, peroxisomes, mitochondria, and nucleus	
Catalase	Peroxisomes and membrane	$H_2O_2{\rightarrow}2H_2O+O_2$
Glutathione peroxidase	Cytoplasm	$H_2O_2+2GSH{\rightarrow}2H_2O+GSSG$
Vitamin C (ascorbic acid)	Cytoplasm, mitochondria, and plasma	Block propagation of radicals and/or as a cofactor for vitamin E
Vitamin E (α-tocopherol)	Cytoplasm and plasma	Block propagation of lipid peroxyl radicals
Carotenoids	Plasma	Scavenges ROS
Selenium	Nucleus, cytosol, mitochondria, and microsomes	Component of glutathione peroxidase and may interfere with formation of DNA-free radical processes

3. Superoxide dismutase

3.1. *Brief history of SODs*

Beginning in the late 1930s and for approximately the two decades that followed, the Cu-containing proteins erythrocuprein, hepatocuprein, cerebrocuprein, and cytocuprein were discovered and studied (reviewed in Beyer et al., 1991). Mann and Keilin (1939) first assigned the name hemocuprein to a protein whose function was thought to be copper storage. In independent studies, McCord and Fridovich (1969) observed enzymatic functions of this same Cu-containing protein, which led to the isolation and discovery of SOD from bovine erythrocytes.

The development of both a spectrophotometric assay and activity gel, partly based upon the cyanide sensitivity of CuZnSOD, allowed for measurement of SOD activity (Beauchamp and Fridovich, 1971). McCord and Keele soon after isolated a Mn-containing SOD (MnSOD) from *Escherichia coli* (*E. coli*), while Weisiger discovered a similar, but organelle specific, SOD in the mitochondria of chicken liver (Keele et al., 1970; Weisiger and Fridovich, 1973). In addition, Yost and Fridovich (1973) reported isolation of a different SOD from *E. coli*, one that contained iron at its active site. Iron SOD expression in *E. coli* was found to be constitutive, being present in both anaerobic and aerobic cultures (Fridovich, 2001), whereas in *E. coli*, MnSOD was regulated in part by the soxRS regulon and shown only to be expressed in aerobic cultures (Yost and Fridovich, 1973; Amabile-Cuevas and Demple, 1991).

3.2. *Family of SODs*

The family of SODs catalyze the dismutation of $O_2^{\bullet-}$, as shown below, at near diffusion-limited rates:

$$O_2^{\bullet-} + O_2^{\bullet-} + 2H^+ \xrightarrow{\text{SOD}} H_2O_2 + O_2$$

These metalloenzymes contain Cu and Zn, Mn, Fe, or Ni at their active sites (Fridovich, 2001). The highest levels of SOD are found in the liver, adrenal gland, kidney, and spleen. Three different types of SOD have been discovered in humans, including MnSOD, CuZnSOD, and extracellular or ECSOD.

3.3. *CuZnSOD (SOD1)*

The gene coding for SOD containing Cu and Zn in the active site, *SOD1*, is located on chromosome 21 in humans and chromosome 16 in mice (Tippett and Kaplan, 1986). Copper–zinc SOD is homodimeric and is the most abundant SOD of this metalloenzyme family. Copper–zinc SOD exerts its defense in the cytosols of eukaryotes, periplasms of gram negative bacteria, and extracellular space of mammals (Fridovich, 1998). The existence of CuZnSOD in mitochondria has previously been noticed, but only recently has been conclusively determined (Okado-Matsumoto and Fridovich, 2001). Tainer et al. (1982) determined the structure of CuZnSOD by X-ray crystallography.

The subunit molecular weight of CuZnSOD ranges from 14 to 16 kDa and contains approximately 2 g each of Cu and Zn atoms per mole. The Cu and Zn in the active site are thought to play different roles in the activity of the enzyme. The Zn atom may play a structural role, whereas the Cu atom changes valence during catalytic activity (Fridovich, 1998). Sequencing of *SOD1* has been completed for humans (Sherman et al., 1983), rats (Hallewell et al., 1985), and mice (Delabar et al., 1987). There is 97% homology between the mouse and rat *SOD1* genes (Bewley, 1988). Human and mouse *SOD1* genes are 84% homologous (Ho and Crapo, 1987a,b), and the human and rat genes have 83% homology (Bewley, 1988). Transcription of *SOD1* yields more than one polyadenylated mRNA (Sherman et al., 1984). The resultant mRNAs differ in size by 200 nucleotides, the longest being 0.9 kb (Sherman et al., 1984). It has been shown that the longer mRNA produces three times more enzyme than the shorter form (Kilk et al., 1995). The two forms of mRNA differ in their polyadenylation sites.

The familial form of amyotrophic lateral sclerosis (FALS) has been associated with mutations in the cytosolic CuZnSOD (Brown, 1995; Price et al., 1996). Upon investigation, the CuZnSOD gene seems to gain a toxic function as opposed to a loss in activity (Fridovich, 1998). Fifty or more mutations in the CuZnSOD of FALS patients have been reported. However, the activity of the mutated genes varied.

Transgenic mice overexpressing CuZnSOD were generated first by Epstein et al. in 1987 and later by both Ceballos-Picot in 1991 and Mirochnitchenko et al. in 1996 (Epstein et al., 1987; Ceballos-Picot et al., 1991; Mirochnitchenko and Inouye, 1996). These transgenic mouse models were used to study Down's syndrome (DS). Down's syndrome patients have three copies of chromosome 21. Numerous studies have been published and extensively reviewed using CuZnSOD transgenic mice (Yen and St. Clair, 1997). Despite several findings linking overexpression of CuZnSOD to DS, studies using CuZnSOD transgenic mice overall demonstrated protection against oxidative brain and pulmonary injury (reviewed in Yen and St. Clair, 1997). Alterations in other antioxidant enzymes have been demonstrated in some studies with overexpression of CuZnSOD (Yen and St. Clair, 1997).

CuZnSOD knockout mice were generated through gene-targeting techniques (Shefner et al., 1999; Café et al., 2000). These mice were normal, viable, and showed no obvious motor deficiencies up to 6 months of age. However, female *SOD1* knockout mice demonstrated an increase in embryonic postimplantation lethality (Ho et al., 1998). One may conclude from studies using CuZnSOD knockout mice that CuZnSOD is not essential for normal development, but is protective when challenged oxidatively.

3.4. MnSOD (SOD2)

The human gene encoding *SOD2* is located on chromosome 6 (Cregan et al., 1973). Church et al. (1992) reported that the human *SOD2* gene locates to 6q25. In mice, the *SOD2* gene locates on chromosome 8 (Church et al., 1992). Rat (Ho et al., 1991), human (Wan et al., 1994), bovine (Meyrick and Magnuson, 1994), and mouse (DiSilvestre et al., 1995) *SOD2* genes have been completely sequenced. The *SOD2* gene is highly conserved between species. Mouse and rat are 96% homologous (Hallewell et al., 1986), mouse and man are 94% homologous (Ho and Crapo, 1987a,b), and rat and man have 93% homology (Ho and Crapo, 1988). Manganese superoxide dismutase may be either dimeric or tetrameric and contains one Mn(III) per subunit. The *SOD2* gene found in *E. coli* is expressed only under aerobic conditions and is dimeric. In eukaryotes, MnSOD is homotetrameric with a molecular weight of 88 kDa, and located exclusively in the mitochondrial matrix of eukaryotes (Weisiger and Fridovich, 1973). The structure of the protein has been determined by X-ray crystallography (Wagner et al., 1993).

Transcription of *SOD2* in mammalian species results in multiple copies of mRNA processed by alternate polyadenylation (Church, 1990; Hurt et al., 1992). Each mRNA species has high probability to be translated and express the MnSOD protein. The mRNA is translated in the cytosol and contains a leader sequence allowing for transportation to the mitochondria (reviewed in St. Clair, 2001). The peptide sequence responsible for the movement into the mitochondrial matrix is then cleaved by a protease specific to the matrix (Schatz and Butow, 1983; Eilers and Schatz, 1988).

The human *SOD2* gene consists of five exons interrupted by four introns. The promoter region of the gene is GC rich and lacks the typical TATA or CAAT sequence near the start site. The *SOD2* gene contains multiple SP-1 and AP-2 binding sites within the basal promoter region. Yeh et al. (1998) showed that SP-1 is a key regulator for transcription of the human *SOD2* gene through co-transfection studies using insect cells. The human *SOD2* gene contains an intronic enhancer region responsible for the induction of the gene by cytokines such as tumor necrosis factor alpha (TNF-α) and interleukin-1-beta (IL-1-β) (Xu et al., 1999). True to definition, this enhancer region of the gene functions in both an orientation- and position-independent manner. Binding sites within this enhancer region include C/EBP-1, C/EBPX, C/EBP-2, NF-κB, and NF-1. The *SOD2* gene is inducible in response to a variety of agents that alter cellular redox status such as cytokines (Wong and Goeddel, 1988; Masuda et al., 1988), dinitrophenol (Dryer et al., 1988), paraquat (Krall et al., 1988), and phorbol-12-myristate-13-acetate (PMA) (Fujii and Taniguchi, 1991; Kiningham et al., 2001). Induction of the human *SOD2* gene by TNF-α and IL-1-β requires the NF-κB site in the intronic enhancer. In addition, it has been shown that the C/EBP sites are important for synergistic induction of the *SOD2* by cytokine and PMA treatment (Kiningham et al., 2001).

Overexpression of MnSOD has been shown to provide protection against oxidative stress. Transgenic mice overexpressing MnSOD were first generated by Wispe et al. (1992). The expression of the *SOD2* gene was linked to a segment of the human growth hormone, and mRNA was predominately expressed in the lung. When challenged with hyperoxic conditions, MnSOD transgenic mice demonstrated prolonged survival compared to non-transgenic mice. In 1996, Yen et al. produced three lines of MnSOD transgenic mice, low, medium, and high expressors (Yen et al., 1996). The use of the human β-actin promoter targeted MnSOD mRNA expression to be predominantly in the heart. The high MnSOD expressors (Tg-SOD-H) demonstrated protection against adriamycin (ADR)-induced cardiac injury compared to non-transgenic mice (Yen et al., 1996). In addition, MnSOD transgenic mice have been shown to be more resistant to IRI (Chen et al., 1998). In both studies, MnSOD transgenic mice did not exhibit changes in other antioxidant enzymes or heat shock proteins (Yen et al., 1996; Chen et al., 1998).

In addition to the protective role of MnSOD, it is well established that MnSOD is essential for survival of aerobic life. Two different lines of MnSOD knockout mice have been generated through homologous recombination (Li et al., 1995; Lebovitz et al., 1996). The mice produced appeared healthy at birth, but demonstrated poor growth and died within 1–18 d. Depending upon genetic background, MnSOD homozygous knockout mice suffered from either neurodegeneration or dilated cardiomyopathy (Li et al., 1995; Lebovitz et al., 1996). Around day 7, MnSOD null mice exhibited extensive mitochondrial damage within both neurons and cardiomyocytes.

Through studies using MnSOD heterozygous knockout mice, Van Remmen et al. (2001) reported that there was increased induction of the permeability transition in heart mitochondria associated with increased cytochrome *c* release and increased DNA fragmentation. These data support the hypothesis that MnSOD may play a critical role in the mitochondrial activation of apoptosis *in vivo*.

3.5. *ECSOD (SOD3)*

Extracellular SOD (*SOD3*) is located on chromosome 4 in humans and chromosome 5 in mice (Oury et al., 1996; Hendrickson et al., 1990). Human ECSOD is a homotetrameric glycoprotein and has a subunit molecular weight of 30 kDa. Human (Hjalmarsson et al., 1987; Folz and Crapo, 1994), rat (Willems et al., 1993; Perry et al., 1993; Carlsson et al., 1996), and mouse (Folz et al., 1997) ECSOD sequences are known. Homology between species remains the lowest compared to *SOD1* and *SOD2*. Mouse and rat *SOD3* are 79% homologous, and both are only 60% homologous to human *SOD3* (Folz et al., 1997). The primary function of ECSOD is thought to be the scavenging of superoxide released from the surface of cells (Fridovich, 1998). Cytokine induction of ECSOD has been reported (Marklund, 1992).

Extracellular SOD transgenic mice were produced by Oury et al. (1992). Studies showed that the CNS of ECSOD transgenic mice was more susceptible to hyperbaric oxygen than the wild type mice. This finding was conflicting to what was found with the generation of ECSOD knockout mice (Carlsson et al., 1995). The ECSOD knockout mice demonstrated a greater sensitivity to hyperoxia conditions. Folz et al. (1997) showed ECSOD expression to be greatest in the lung and kidney. In addition, when investigated further, increased expression of ECSOD in type II alveolar cells was found. This finding was interesting, considering that a large amount of NO is released under oxidative injury in this area; thus the expression of ECSOD may reduce the formation of peroxynitrite. Thus, ECSOD is not essential to the development of mice under physiological conditions, although it provides protection under oxidative injury.

4. Role of myocardial antioxidants

Cellular defense against free radicals in myocytes includes previously discussed endogenous antioxidant enzymes such as SOD, catalase, and GSHPx. Other endogenous antioxidants, including GSH, vitamin E, vitamin C, and vitamin A, are also present in the myocardium. Many *in vivo* studies have demonstrated that activities of antioxidant enzymes in heart muscle were less than activities in other organs. In both mice and rats, the activities of catalase and CuZnSOD in heart were less than those in liver about 50 fold and 15 fold, respectively (Chen et al., 1994; Doroshow et al., 1980). In rat, it has also been shown that GSHPx activity was lower in heart when compared with liver (Chen et al., 1994). However, in mice, there was no difference in GSHPx activity between heart and liver (Chen et al., 1994). In addition, the activity of glutathione reductase in mouse heart was four times lower than in liver (Doroshow et al., 1980). Based on this information, it appears that ROS generated under physiological conditions were sufficiently neutralized by cardiac antioxidant capacity, but under pathological conditions, including oxidative stress, the capacity of antioxidant systems was not sufficient to neutralize generated ROS, resulting in oxidative injury.

4.1. *Cardiomyocyte dysfunction induced by oxidative stress*

Abnormalities in myocyte function due to oxidative stress are considered in association with effects of ROS on subcellular organelles. Effects on subcellular organelles may be a consequence of either increased formation of ROS and/or a decrease of antioxidant reserve. Many studies have shown that sarcoplasmic reticulum, mitochondria, myofibrils, and nucleus were injured by oxidative stress in myocytes. Exposure of sarcoplasmic membranes to xanthine plus xanthine oxidase and H_2O_2 caused inhibition of the sarcoplasmic reticulum Na^+–K^+ ATPase activity, which was partially prevented by treatment with antioxidants such as catalase and mannitol (Shao et al., 1995). Hydroxyl radicals have been reported to suppress the cardiac sarcoplasmic reticulum-Ca^{2+} pump ATPase activity (Shao et al., 1995) by oxidation of the ATP binding site. In additional studies, $OH^{•-}$, $O_2^{•-}$, and $^•NO$ have all been demonstrated to enhance sarcoplasmic reticulum-Ca^{2+} release by their interactions with sulfhydryl groups of the cardiac and skeletal muscle ryanodine receptor (Xu et al., 1997). Nitric oxide was shown to inhibit cytochrome *c* oxidase activity, and eventually affected the electron transport chain in isolated mitochondria (Cassina and Radi, 1996). Superoxide radicals and H_2O_2 have been reported to inhibit myofibrillar creatine kinase and myofibrillar Ca^{2+} ATPase activities (Kaneko et al., 1993). The accumulation of 4-hydroxynonenal (4-HNE) in mitochondria caused a rapid decrease in NADH linked state 3 respiration and resulted in uncoupling of respiration (Anzai et al., 1998; Favero et al., 1995). Defects in these enzymes result in Ca^{2+} handling abnormalities, decrease in sensitivity to Ca^{2+}, and decrease in energy stores, all leading to myocyte dysfunction. It has been demonstrated that $O_2^{•-}$ can induce apoptosis in cardiomyocytes (Von Harsdorf et al., 1999). In cardiofibroblasts, ROS can induce proliferation and expression of transforming growth factor β-1, and stimulate the synthesis of extracellular matrix components such as collagen, fibronectin, and proteoglycans (Li et al., 1999). On the other hand, Siwik et al. (2001) showed that increased oxidative stress activates matrix metalloproteinase activity and decreased fibrillar collagen synthesis in cardiac fibroblasts. In view of these observations, it appears that oxidative stress may alter the activities of different subcellular structures, proteins, and enzymes in both cardiomyocytes and cardiofibroblasts. These changes may play an important role in many cardiovascular diseases.

4.2. *Role of oxidative stress in specific cardiovascular diseases*

Oxidative stress results from an imbalance between the intracellular production of ROS/RNS and the cellular antioxidant defense mechanisms. If oxidative stress persists, oxidative damage to critical biomolecules can occur, eventually resulting in cell injury and death.

Oxidative stress is known to be involved in several types of cardiovascular disease as a direct cause and/or consequence of the disease. In this chapter, we will focus on only IRI and adriamycin-induced cardiac toxicity, since these diseases have particular relevance to ROS-induced pathology.

5. Ischemia reperfusion injury

5.1. *Pathophysiology of IRI*

Ischemic heart disease (IHD) is due to an imbalance between the supply and demand of the heart for oxygenated blood. This, in turn, leads to tissue hypoxia (reduced oxygen) or anoxia (absence of oxygen). Myocardial ischemia is caused not only by insufficiency of oxygen (hypoxia, anoxia), but also by reduced availability of nutrient substrates and inadequate removal of metabolites (Cotran et al., 1994). The most common causes of ischemia are acute arterial thrombus formation, chronic narrowing (stenosis) of an artery that is often caused by atherosclerotic disease, and arterial vasospasm.

Ischemia can be silent or symptomatic. Symptomatic ischemia is characterized by chest pain (angina pectoris) (Cotran et al., 1994). People with angina are at risk of having a heart attack. Stable angina occurs during exertion and can be quickly relieved by resting. Unstable angina, which increases the risk of a heart attack, occurs more frequently, lasts longer, is more severe, and causes discomfort during rest or light exertion. Angina is usually caused by increased oxygen demand when the heart is working harder than usual, for example, during exercise or mental or physical stress.

Short, repeated episodes of ischemia, transient ischemic attacks (TIAs), do not result in cumulative damage, but rather protect the heart from subsequent damage caused by a larger ischemic insult. This adaptive response by the heart is termed preconditioning and may be a significant protective mechanism in angina patients (Cotran et al., 1994).

Hypoxia resulting from coronary occlusion is a major factor in cardiac stunning (prolonged ischemic vascular dysfunction) and infarct development. However, there is a second major component that can contribute to impaired function, electrical disturbances, and infarct size. This component is associated with coronary reperfusion and is termed reperfusion injury, which occurs when the ischemic myocardium is reperfused and oxygen is reintroduced. Reperfusion of the ischemic myocardium is essential to prevent cardiac damage. Reperfusion of the ischemic heart after a certain critical period has been shown to have effects due to the generation of ROS. Ischemia reperfusion injury is known to occur during several different procedures, including angioplasty, coronary bypass surgery, and thrombolytic therapy, and also after a prolonged period of ischemia (Dhalla et al., 1999). Reperfusion injury also results in upregulation of endothelial and leukocyte adhesion molecules, causing leukocyte adhesion to the vascular endothelium, leukocyte activation, and leukocyte accumulation within tissues. Inflammatory mediators released by activated leukocytes result in further tissue damage and functional impairment. Studies have shown that inhibiting leukocyte adhesion or scavenging oxygen free radicals will reduce reperfusion-associated ventricular dysfunction, arrhythmias, and infarct size. Ischemia reperfused hearts may demonstrate many alterations, including depression in contractile function, arrhythmias, changes in gene expression, and loss of adrenergic pathways. It has been demonstrated that global ischemia (30 min) followed by reperfusion (60 min) in isolated rat hearts was associated with depressed contractile function, as indicated by decreased left ventricular developed pressure and increased left ventricular end diastolic pressure (Zweier et al., 1989).

5.2. *Role of oxidative stress in IRI*

The cellular mechanisms of myocardial IRI are multifactorial. In addition to cardiomyocytes, endothelial cells and inflammatory cells may be involved. Most of these cells are capable of ROS generation. In this section, we will focus only on cardiac myocytes and endothelial cells.

Several studies implicated ROS in the pathogenesis of myocardial reperfusion injury: ROS can be detected in postischemic and reperfused myocardium, overexpression of antioxidant enzymes can protect against IRI, and treatment of myocardium with exogenous ROS sources results in myocyte dysfunction that mimics IRI.

Superoxide production during ischemia has been demonstrated by EPR and chemiluminescence studies (Zweier et al., 1989). Reperfusion of the ischemic myocardium can result in a burst of $O_2^{\bullet-}$ production with maximal oxidant production at 10 to 30 s after reperfusion. In experiments performed by Wang and Zweier (1996), maximal levels of oxidant production was observed at 40 s of reperfusion and gradually decreased to preischemia levels after 5 min of reperfusion. This study was confirmed by McCord (1985); subsequent direct and spin trapping EPR measurements demonstrated that a burst of $O_2^{\bullet-}$ and superoxide-derived radical generation occurs during the early period of reperfusion. The enzyme xanthine oxidase was shown to be an important source of this radical generation. Electron paramagnetic resonance spectroscopy has also been used to demonstrate enhanced ROS production in experimental models of stunning, representing the reversible ventricular dysfunction that often accompanies reperfusion of the ischemic myocardium (Bolli, 1990). The $O_2^{\bullet-}$ produced as a result of reperfusion of ischemic tissue has been proposed to be a mediator of reperfusion injury to the myocardium in many studies. It has been suggested that the increase of ROS production during ischemia reperfusion leads to lipid peroxidation and sulfhydryl group oxidation. Increases in levels of malondialdehyde (MDA) also have been reported in heart exposed to 30 min of ischemia (Ceconi et al., 1991). Hill and Singal (1996) showed that increased oxidative stress and lipid peroxidation were associated with heart failure following myocardial infarction.

Although increases in ROS production have been implicated in heart failure and chemotherapeutic drug-induced heart injury, there is still the question as to the contribution of superoxide, hydrogen peroxide, or the hydroxyl radical, or all three. Growing evidence implicates oxidative stress in myocardial failure and disease progression (Sawyer and Colucci, 2000). Recently, Ide et al. (2000) obtained direct evidence of $OH^{\bullet}$ formation from $O_2^{\bullet-}$ generation in myocardial heart failure using EPR. In an earlier observation, Ide et al. (1999) showed an increase in ROS production in failing versus non-failing myocardium.

Due to the high numbers of mitochondria in cardiac tissue, it is believed that mitochondria are the major intracellular sites of free radical production during ischemia reperfusion. However, it is well known that other cytosolic sites also generate free radicals. The membrane components of mitochondria may represent the most important target of ROS-mediated myocardial dysfunction. During ischemia, the mitochondrial carriers are in a reduced state due to the degradation of the adenine nucleotide pool (Freeman and Crapo, 1982). Increased electron leakage leads to increase in the formation of $O_2^{\bullet-}$ due to interaction with molecular oxygen trapped within the inner membranes of the mitochondria. During reperfusion, there will be further leakage of electrons due to the lack of ADP, resulting in increased production of $O_2^{\bullet-}$. Increased production of ROS precedes mitochondrial permeability transition (MPT) pore opening and is the result of the permeability change of the mitochondrial membranes (Kantrow and Piantadosi, 1997). At low levels of ROS, the MPT pore opening is reversible and does not enhance large amplitude swelling of the mitochondrial matrix. At high levels of ROS, the MPT pore opening is irreversible and leads to large amplitude swelling of the mitochondrial matrix. During this event, cytochrome c and the apoptosis inducing factor (AIF) are released from mitochondria, which may be one reason for injury in ischemia reperfusion (Kantrow and Piantadosi, 1997). Ide et al. (2001) have reported that an increase in $OH^{\bullet}$ and lipid peroxidation can result in mitochondrial DNA damage, which may contribute to defects in mitochondrial DNA encoding the genes expressing subunits of complexes I and III [cytochrome b] and IV [cytochrome c oxidase]. These defects may result in left ventricular remodeling failure.

Several investigations have demonstrated that eNOS expression and activity are reduced during ischemia reperfusion (Mehta et al., 2000). There are some reports suggesting that iNOS expression and activity may be increased during myocardial ischemia reperfusion (Wang et al., 1999). Experimental studies demonstrated that ROS are released during the early phase of myocardial reperfusion. Reactive oxygen species can also cause breakdown of $^\bullet$NO, thereby setting the stage for intense vasoconstriction and a reduction in coronary flow reserve (Mehta et al., 1989). Endothelial dysfunction may be induced by reduction in endothelial-dependent relaxation due to the inactivation of $^\bullet$NO by ROS formed upon reperfusion (Lefer et al., 1991; Hearse et al., 1993).

A number of studies have shown that $^\bullet$NO formation also increased during the early period of ischemia and reperfusion. Nitric oxide formation is markedly increased during ischemia in isolated rat heart (Wang et al., 1996). During the early period of postischemia reperfusion, $^\bullet$NO is greatly increased above normal control values. Immediately upon reflow, $^\bullet$NO levels increased 30-fold higher than preischemia levels and remained at levels 10-fold above preischemia throughout the ischemia reperfusion after 5 min of reflow. However, a gradual decrease was seen over the next 15 min, but the level was still higher when compared to the preischemia value (Wang et al., 1996). Markedly increased $^\bullet$NO levels occurred concurrent with the reperfusion-associated burst of $O_2^{\bullet-}$ generation, leading to the formation of the potent oxidant $ONOO^-$ with a magnitude and time course parallel to the generation of $O_2^{\bullet-}$. This peroxynitrite generation caused protein nitration and cellular injury. Blockade or scavenging of either $^\bullet$NO or $O_2^{\bullet-}$ was sufficient to prevent reperfusion injury and greatly enhanced the recovery of contractile function (Wang et al., 1996). However, $ONOO^-$ at low concentrations has been found to exert beneficial effects on ischemia reperfusion-induced arrhythmias in isolated rat heart mediated by induction of cAMP (Altug et al., 1999).

Endothelial cells, leukocytes, myocytes, mast cells, and macrophages are all capable of producing the ROS detected after reperfusion of the ischemic myocardium. *In vitro* models of IRI using monolayers of cultured endothelial cells suggested that vascular endothelial cells not only can generate the significant fluxes of ROS detected in postischemia tissues, but also can adapt an inflammatory phenotype that promotes the recruitment and activation of leukocytes into postischemia tissue, amplifying ROS production (Granger, 1999).

Another group of investigators postulated that injury caused by ischemia reperfusion is related to Ca^{2+} overload caused by oxidative stress. Oxidative stress may result in a depression in sarcolemmal Ca^{2+} pump ATPase and Na^+–K^+ ATPase activities. These changes lead to decreased Ca^{2+} efflux and increased Ca^{2+} influx, respectively (Dixon et al., 1990, 1992). Oxidative stress has also been reported to depress the sarcoplasmic reticulum Ca^{2+} pump ATPase, thus inhibiting Ca^{2+} sequestration from the cytoplasm in cardiomyocytes (Netticadan et al., 1999). The increase in Ca^{2+} during ischemia reperfusion is proposed to induce the conversion of xanthine dehydrogenase to xanthine oxidase, resulting in generation of $O_2^{\bullet-}$.

Furthermore, exposure of the normal myocardium to ROS generating systems alters myocardial function in a way that mimics reperfusion injury, including persistent cellular loss of K^+, depletion of high energy phosphates, elevated intracellular calcium concentration, loss of systolic force, development of a progressive increase in diastolic tension, depressed metabolic function, and arrhythmias (Bolli, 1990).

5.2.1. *Role of cytokine induction in IRI and heart failure*

Neurohormones have been identified as important biomolecules in the progression of myocardial failure. However, most recently, cytokines have been implicated as an equally important class of biologically active molecules that participate in both the development and progression of cardiac failure. While less is known about circulating levels of the cytokines IL-1, interleukin-2 (IL-2), and interferon-γ (IFN-γ), TNF was found to be elevated in all but two clinical studies of heart failure reviewed by Baumgarten et al. (2000). Both Munger et al. and Pritchett et al. were unable to detect increased levels of TNF, perhaps due to a lack of sensitivity in the assay used (Munger et al., 1996 and Pritchett et al., 1995). Interleukin-6 (IL-6) was also elevated in clinical cardiac failure (Torre-Amione et al., 1996; MacGowan et al., 1997). The roles of these cytokines have not been entirely elucidated, but the signaling cytokine cascade may play a role in the beneficial homeostatic response of myocardial failure. For example, Kurrelmeyer et al. (2000) demonstrated that TNF receptor double knockout mice exhibit a 40% larger infarct size as compared to wild type mice or either single receptor knockout genotype. TNF-α has been shown to induce both the 1 and 4 kb MnSOD mRNAs (Wong and Goeddel, 1988). Thus, Kurrelmeyer's findings suggest that TNF signaling is a cytoprotective response to ischemic injury. Using a mouse model that overexpressed MnSOD, Chen et al. (1998) showed a limited infarct size *in vivo*, suggesting that the protection seen with TNF from Kurrelmeyer's work to be due to an increase in MnSOD. In other studies, it was shown that TNF can protect brain neurons in cell culture and *in vivo* against oxidative and ischemic insults in models of stroke by a mechanism involving increased production of MnSOD (Bruce et al., 1996; Mattson et al., 1997). Moreover, ischemic brain injury was significantly decreased in transgenic mice overexpressing MnSOD (Keller et al., 1998).

5.3. *Role of antioxidants in ischemia reperfusion*

Myocardial antioxidants are defined as substances that inhibit or delay oxidative stress. Various studies have reported the beneficial effects of antioxidants in IRI. A recent investigation has reported a depletion of endogenous antioxidants in the ischemic heart upon reperfusion. Moreover, several studies have demonstrated an imbalance of antioxidant defense enzymes to ROS in myocardial failure. Dhalla and Singal (1994) showed that in addition to an increase in the formation of ROS, decreases in endogenous antioxidant enzymes such as SOD, GSHPx, and catalase could exacerbate the injury seen in IRI. Hill and Singal (1996) have shown that SOD activity was unchanged in mild and moderate cardiac failure, but significantly depressed at 16 weeks after severe cardiac failure due to infarction. An *in vitro* study used diethyl dithiocarbamic acid to inhibit CuZnSOD and ECSOD and subsequently cause a dose-dependent increase in superoxide concentration (Siwik et al., 1999). This model of hypertrophy caused by an increase in $O_2^{\bullet-}$ due to the inhibition of SOD induced activation of apoptosis in cardiomyocytes. The phenotype was verified using a xanthine and xanthine oxidase system to generate $O_2^{\bullet-}$ in the same model. Prasad et al. (1992) showed a decrease in SOD and catalase activities in heart exposed to 30 min of ischemia. Catalase activities also progressively decreased through mild, moderate, and severe cardiac failure stages after myocardial infarction (Hill and Singal, 1996). Ascorbate and GSH levels were decreased during 40 min of reperfusion, but not after ischemia reperfusion. Levels of oxidized compounds, including dehydroascorbate and glutathione disulfide, were markedly increased during reperfusion in the isolated rat heart (Dhalla et al., 1999). Regional differences were observed in GSHPx levels (normal in the left ventricle of the ischemia and reperfused heart but increased in the right ventricle) (Prasad et al., 1992). Dhalla et al. (1999) showed no change in vitamin E levels during ischemia reperfusion, whereas Hill and Singal (1996) demonstrated that vitamin E levels were depressed at moderate and severe cardiac failure stages.

Ischemia reperfusion injury may therefore be associated with antioxidant changes as well as increased myocardial oxidative stress.

5.4. *Therapeutic implications of antioxidant treatment*

Much of the evidence implicating ROS in the pathogenesis of myocardial IRI is based on experiments that examine the ability of free radical scavengers to alter the injury response both *in vivo* and *in vitro*. Superoxide dismutase and catalase have received the most attention in this regard. Although the activity of catalase in the myocardium has been reported to be low (Chen et al., 1994), many studies have suggested its important role in ischemia reperfusion. A number of studies have shown that intravenous administration of antioxidant enzymes such as SOD and/or catalase can reduce infarct size (Bolli, 1991). Inducing ischemia reperfusion in the presence of combined SOD and catalase for 20 min resulted in a decrease in infarct size, an improvement in cardiac function, and sarcoplasmic reticulum regulatory function associated with Ca^{2+}/calmodulin protein kinase (Temsah et al., 1999).

Vitamin E has also been studied and shown to cause a decrease in mortality and infarct size secondary to coronary occlusion by inhibition of the deposition of atherogenic oxidized LDL in rats (Sethi et al., 2000). Vitamin E also prevented the depression of left ventricular function and the elevation of MDA content and conjugated diene formation in the infarcted rat heart (Sethi et al., 2000). These results indicated reduction of oxidative stress by vitamin E.

However, other studies have failed to demonstrate a protective effect of antioxidants. Many investigators hypothesized that differences reported were due to variation in experimental conditions and the inability of high molecular weight antioxidant enzymes such as GSHPx, SOD, and catalase to penetrate cells. These limitations can potentially be overcome by using gene therapy to increase intracellular antioxidant enzymes. More informative data can also be produced by using mutant mice in which a gene encoding a specific antioxidant protein has been deleted to study the role of the protein in ischemia reperfusion. Woo et al. (1998) showed, using recombinant adenovirus-mediated cardiac gene transfer of SOD and catalase, attenuation of postischemia contractile dysfunction after ischemia reperfusion in isolated reperfused neonatal mouse heart. Chen et al. (1998) have shown that overexpression of mitochondrial MnSOD in transgenic mice significantly protected against IRI. Recently, Negoro et al. (2001) have shown that overexpression of STAT 3 (signal transducer and activator of transcription) protected cardiomyocytes against increased ROS following IRI by activation of the *SOD2* gene and its enzyme activity.

Other recent studies demonstrated prevention of postischemic injury by over-expression of CuZnSOD. Chen et al. (2000) demonstrated that overexpression of CuZnSOD in the cytoplasm of the coronary vasculature of both endothelial and smooth muscle cells rendered the heart more resistant to IRI, as demonstrated by improved heart rate and reduction in lactate dehydrogenase release. The role of CuZnSOD in cardioprotection has been confirmed by Yoshida et al. (2000); $SOD1^{-/-}$ mouse hearts were more susceptible to IRI compared with corresponding wild type mouse hearts as demonstrated by increased infarct size. Li et al. (2001) showed that directed gene transfer of cDNA encoding membrane EC-SOD, which binds to heparan sulfate proteoglycans on cellular surfaces, afforded more powerful cardioprotection than freely soluble forms of SOD, as demonstrated by reduced infarct size. These SOD studies demonstrated that all SOD isoforms affected myo-cardial cells.

Glutathione peroxidase is an important enzyme that performs several vital functions. Transgenic mice that overexpress GSHPx appeared to be resistant to myocardial IRI (Yoshida et al., 1996), whereas GSHPx knockout mice are more susceptible to myocardial reperfusion injury compared with wild type mice (Yoshida et al., 1997).

Metallothionein (MT) is a highly conserved, low molecular weight, thiol rich protein. Metallothionein can bind to and be induced by heavy metal ions. Studies using a cell-free system have demonstrated the ability of MT to act as a free radical scavenger (Kang, 1999). Kang et al. (1999) have applied a Langendorff perfusion model to examine directly the effects of MT on ischemia reperfusion-induced derangements of contractile activity of the heart, myocyte injury as estimated by creatine phosphokinase release, and cell death as measured by the size of infarct zone. They showed that there was no significant difference in the contractile force between transgenic and control hearts during a 30 min equilibration period. Trans-genic hearts, however, showed significantly better postischemia recovery of sup-pressed contractile force. Creatine phosphokinase activity in the collected perfusion effluent samples was measured, and high activity was detected in the effluent col-lected from non-transgenic mouse hearts. This observation suggested that the MT overexpressing transgenic hearts were highly resistant to myocardial infarction induced by ischemia reperfusion. It is speculated that MT can only be effective as a free radical scavenger in vivo if it is located sufficiently close to the site of production of the radicals before interaction with other cellular components.

A frequently studied antioxidant agent is the sulfhydryl-containing amino acid derivative mercaptoproprionyl glycine (MPG), a safe and well-tolerated drug that is used clinically to reduce radiation-induced tissue injury. MPG reacts with free radical species, promoting the resynthesis of glutathione, thereby limiting the cyto-toxic effects of H_2O_2 and subsequent lipid peroxidation. This compound has been shown to significantly reduce myocardial infarct size both in the early moments and for as long as 48 h after reperfusion (Uma Devi, 1983). In addition to antioxidant agents, other agents have been shown to exert some cardioprotective action in IRI models, such as deferoxamine (an iron chelator), which resulted in improvement of functional and metabolic recovery of myocardium during the ischemia reperfusion period (Williams et al., 1991). Also, administration of L-arginine, the substrate for NOS, has been shown to limit reperfusion injury. Allopurinol, an inhibitor of xanthine oxidase, has been shown to improve functional recovery of the stunned myocardium and reduce infarct size in dog heart (Bolli, 1990).

Therapeutic intervention with antioxidants in IRI is an area that requires additional investigation.

5.5. *Summary*

Many studies support the role of oxidative stress in IRI due to generation of free radicals in both postischemic and reperfusion myocardium. Reactive oxygen species and RNS can contribute to impaired contractile function, electric disturbances, abnormal gene expression, increased infarct size, myocardial cell damage, and cardiac dysfunction. Mitochondria have been suggested to be the major intracellular site of radical production. Elevation of free radicals was observed with decreasing endogenous antioxidant enzymes levels during the ischemia reperfusion period. Exposure of the normal myocardium to ROS generating systems alters myocardial function in a way that mimics IRI. The actions of antioxidants resulted in improvement in cardiac function in both experimental and clinical studies. Whether the critical factor of cardiac injury lies primarily within the increase in production of ROS or the decrease in antioxidant enzyme defense response, numerous studies have shown protection against the oxidative injury associated with both cardiac failure and IRI through genetic and recombinant technologies by which MnSOD activity is increased.

6. Adriamycin-induced cardiotoxicity

6.1. *Features and structural characteristics of ADR*

The anthracycline antibiotic adriamycin, or doxorubicin (DOX), is one of the most effective antitumor agents against human malignancies, including leukemias, lymphomas, and many solid tumors (Young et al., 1981). Adriamycin was originally isolated from a mutant fungus *Streptomyces peucetius* var *caesius* obtained 30 years ago. The ADR molecule contains an amino sugar, daunosamine, linked through a glycosidic bond to adriamycinone, a red-pigmented naphthacenequinone nucleus, as shown in Fig. 1. Because of its unique structure, the drug is highly lipophilic and has a relatively long half-life in the body. The major antitumor effect of this drug involves DNA intercalation and interference with the catalytic cycle of DNA topoisomerase II (Cummings et al., 1991). The drug inserts non-specifically between adjacent base pairs and binds to the sugar phosphate backbone of DNA, causing local uncoiling, resulting in a block of DNA and RNA synthesis and inhibition of DNA repair. Intercalation can interfere with topoisomerase II-catalyzed breakage reunion reaction of DNA strands to cause an unrepairable break. However, further

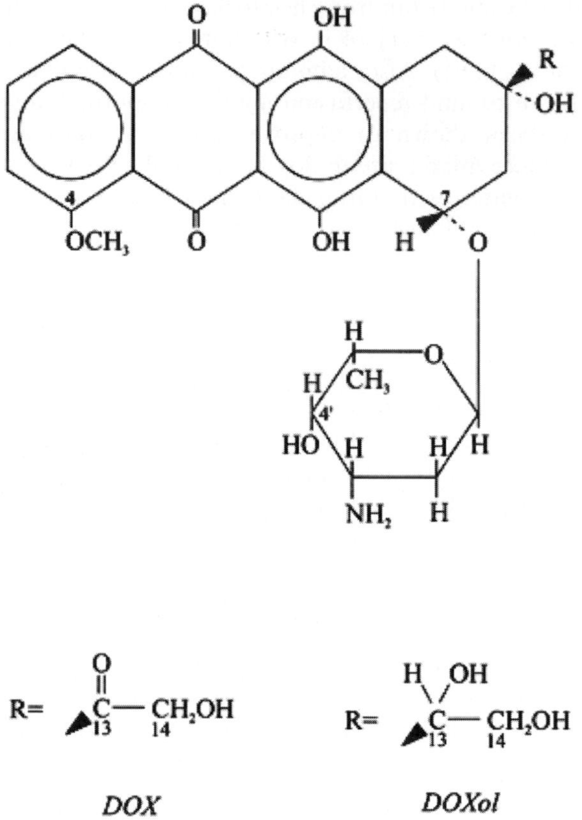

Fig. 1.	Structure of adriamycin (DOX) and its metabolite (DOXol).

studies have shown additional antitumor effects of ADR, including binding of negatively charged phospholipids, e.g. cardiolipin of mitochondrial membranes, resulting in defects of mitochondrial membrane functions (Cummings et al., 1991).

6.2. Mechanism of ADR-induced cardiotoxicity

Adriamycin is an anthracycline antibiotic with broad spectrum antitumor activity. However, ADR administration can also result in toxic side effects. Long term treatment with ADR and other extracted or pharmaceutically engineered anthracyclines is limited by acute and chronic cardiotoxicity. The total dose limit of ADR treatment is 500–550 mg per square meter of body surface area in patients with no underlying heart disease (Young et al., 1981). Acute toxicity manifests as transient and clinically treatable arrhythmias and hypotension (Singal, 2000). However, the acute effects of ADR are not of major concern because these are generally reversible and/or clinically manageable. Chronic treatment can lead to cardiotoxicity and heart failure (Cummings et al., 1991), which are serious side effects of this drug.

Typical clinical characteristics of ADR cardiotoxicity are a profound decrease in blood pressure and ventricular dilation with subsequent cardiac failure (Cummings et al., 1991). Papadopoulou et al. (1999) have shown that ADR caused cardiovascular arrhythmias characterized by bradycardia, extension of ventricular depolarization time (tQRS), and failure of QRS at high concentrations (10–14 mg per kilogram body weight). ADR caused significant left ventricle dysfunction as measured by echocardiography (Weinstein et al., 2000) and reduced reflex control of circulation by causing both systolic and diastolic dysfunction without changes in cardiac output or baroreflex control of heart rate (Rabelo et al., 2001). Many studies have suggested that mitochondria are the site of ADR-induced cardiotoxicity (Kang et al., 1996; Yen et al., 1996, 1999). Disruption of mitochondrial cristae, mitochondrial swelling, the presence of myelin figures, swelling of sarcoplasmic reticulum, and myofibrillar degeneration were ultrastructural pathologic changes observed following treatment with ADR for 5 d (Yen et al., 1996). Adriamycin has been shown to cause mitochondrial functional impairment by inhibition of respiratory control and stimulation of ATPase activity, which is associated with decreased ATP production in cardiomyocytes (Jeyaseelan et al., 1997a). Yen et al. (1999) showed a significant decrease in state 3 respiration and respiratory control ratio in mitochondrial complexes I and II after treatment with ADR. In addition to effects on mitochondria, ADR has been also shown to inhibit mRNA levels of sarcomeric genes such as alpha actin, troponin I, and myosin light chain (Ito et al., 1990). These changes were supported by ultrastructural analysis showing changes in myofibril and sarcoplasmic reticulum structures. Recent studies have reported that ADR also can induce apoptosis or necrosis in cardiomyocytes (Arola et al., 2000). Studies have suggested that ADR may have at least two mechanisms of action that cause cellular damage. One of the major theories of ADR-induced cardiotoxicity is that it is due to the production of free radicals, with subsequent damage being inhibited by free radical scavengers. The other major hypothesis is that ADR injury is mediated by alternative mechanisms in which free radicals are not produced, an example being altered calcium metabolism, which is unaffected by antioxidants.

6.2.1. *Production of free radicals*

The ability of ADR to trigger formation of free radicals was first reported by Sato et al. (1977). They demonstrated that microsomal enzyme P-450 reductase was able to catalyze the reduction of anthracycline to semiquinone free radicals. In the presence of oxygen, redox cycling of ADR from quinones to semiquinones results in the production of $O_2^{\bullet-}$. This observation has been confirmed by other investigators. Other flavo-reductase enzymes such as mitochondrial NADH dehydrogenase (Doroshow, 1983), the hypoxanthine–xanthine oxidase system, and cytochrome b_5 reductase (Marcillat et al., 1989) were shown to produce similar reduction of ADR to semiquinone free radicals. A current study has demonstrated that eNOS also mediates reduction of ADR to semiquinone (Weinstein et al., 2000).

The mitochondrial electron transport chain is postulated to be an important site of ADR-induced ROS generation. Mitochondria are abundant in cardiomyocytes. Thus, it is possible that heart mitochondria represent a particularly rich source of

ADR stimulated generation of $O_2^{\bullet-}$ and H_2O_2. Increased free radical levels generated by ADR have been measured directly by EPR (Bachur et al., 1977) and indirectly via increased levels of oxidative damage product formation in cardiomyocytes, endothelial cells, and cardiofibroblasts. Doroshow (1983) has shown free radical formation induced by ADR in heart homogenates, sarcoplasmic reticulum, mitochondria, and cytosol by biochemical assay of $O_2^{\bullet-}$. Several studies have demonstrated that ADR treatment results in lipid peroxide formation. Praet and Ruysschaert (1993) demonstrated that ADR induced damage to the mitochondrial membrane and the mitochondrial respiratory chain, affected mitochondrial membrane fluidity, and increased lipid peroxidation both *in vivo* and *in vitro*. These results indicated that impairment of mitochondrial structure and function were induced by generation of ROS following ADR treatment. Another recent study demonstrated that ADR caused preferential accumulation of 8-hydroxy-2'-deoxyguanosine (8OHdG) in heart mitochondrial DNA (Palmeira et al., 1997). Mitochondrial damage resulted in decreased levels of overall mitochondrial gene transcription and decreased expression of several mitochondrial genes, including genes encoding cytochrome *c* oxidase and the adenine nucleotide translocator (Zhou et al., 2001a). These observations provide an explanation for mitochondrial injury following ADR treatment. The accumulation and persistence of oxidized mitochondrial DNA also resulted in long-lasting stimulation of ROS generation by ADR. This persistent generation of ROS may contribute to the cumulative and irreversible nature of cardiotoxicity (Zhou et al., 2001a).

Recently, the role of $^{\bullet}NO$ in cardiotoxicity has been considered, since the combination of ADR and NOS could lead to $O_2^{\bullet-}$ generation (Fig. 2). Vásquez-Vivar et al. (1997) demonstrated that eNOS reduced ADR to the semiquinone radical. As a consequence, superoxide formation is enhanced and nitric oxide levels are decreased. The disruption of the balance between $^{\bullet}NO$ and $O_2^{\bullet-}$ levels may lead to the generation of $ONOO^-$, H_2O_2, and other potent oxidants implicated in the pathogenesis of ADR toxicity. Increased production of either $^{\bullet}NO$ or $O_2^{\bullet-}$ may be sufficient to drive the formation of $ONOO^-$. The consequent formation of peroxynitrite may play a key role in the cardiotoxicity of ADR.

It is possible that the cardiovascular toxicity of ADR is linked to the transformation of eNOS from a nitric oxide synthase to an NADPH oxidase. Cardiac dysfunction has been shown to be associated with severe loss of nitric oxide control by increasing tissue levels of eNOS and extensive myocyte protein nitration by $ONOO^-$ (Weinstein et al., 2000). Nitric oxide can alter myocyte energetics by inhibition of activity of MCK (the monomeric myofibrillar isoform of CK) in vitro (Andreu et al., 1998). Several studies have shown that ADR can activate signal transduction pathways that result in disruption of the cardiac gene expression programs. Adriamycin has been demonstrated to decrease intracardiac levels of mRNA for several important proteins and enzymes by suppression of transcription (Jeyaseelan et al., 1997a; Ito et al., 1990; Zhou et al., 2001b). Adriamycin has been shown to suppress transcription of α-actin, myosin light chain, and troponin I genes, resulting in myofibrillar degeneration, and also to inhibit transcription of Rieske iron sulfur protein, ADP/ATP translocase, phosphofructokinase, and creatine kinase

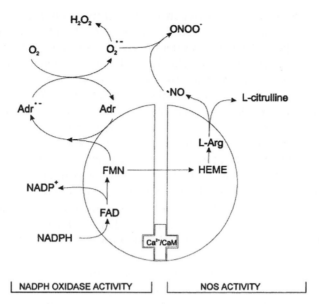

Fig. 2. eNOS-dependent superoxide formation from redox cycling of ADR semiquinone. ADR, at low concentrations, increases superoxide production from eNOS by binding the reductase domain of eNOS and concomitantly inhibits formation of nitric oxide. The resultant shift in the balance between superoxide and nitric oxide could lead to formation of peroxynitrite. Peroxynitrite ($ONOO^-$) production is biomolecular, and increased production of either nitric oxide or superoxide may be sufficient to drive the formation of peroxynitrite. From Vásquez-Vivar et al. (1997), with permission.

(M isoform, the muscle specific enzyme in skeletal muscle), resulting in energy impairment (Jeyaseelan et al., 1997a). Adriamycin treatment also resulted in suppression of cytochrome *c* oxidase II gene expression, resulting in structural and functional impairment of mitochondria (Kang et al., 1996). Recently, one study reported that mRNA of cardiac ADR responsive protein, a transcriptional regulatory protein expressed selectively in myocytes, was also sensitive to ADR (Jeyaseelan et al., 1997b).

The effects of ADR on these mRNA levels are not clearly independent of free radicals. Many studies attempt to prove that one of the roles of ROS induced by ADR is to regulate signal transduction, which leads to abnormal gene expression. However, the molecular mechanisms of ADR-induced cardiotoxicity remain unclear.

6.2.2. *Alternative mechanism not involving free radicals*

Alternative mechanisms of cardiotoxicity other than generation of free radicals have been proposed, including toxicity of an adriamycin metabolite (DOXol) or Ca^{2+} or iron overload.

6.2.2.1. *ADR metabolite (DOXol)* An alternative mechanism of proposed cardiotoxicity has implicated an ADR metabolite other than semiquinone free radical.

Doxorubicinol (DOXol) is a hydroxy metabolite formed upon two-electron reduction of the C-13 carbonyl group in the side chain of ADR (Fig. 1). Doxorubicinol is formed by cytosolic NADPH-dependent enzymes sharing similarities with the multigene family of carbonyl and aldoketoreductases. From a pharmacokinetic standpoint, it has been demonstrated that DOXol accumulates in the heart of rats receiving multiple ADR injections. Experiments utilizing transgenic mice overexpressing carbonyl or aldehyde reductases resulted in increased DOXol and enhanced the development of ADR-induced cardiotoxicity in vivo (Forrest et al., 2000). Doxorubicinol also causes cardiotoxicity by inducing oxidative stress subsequent to perturbation of iron homeostasis (Licata et al., 2000). Doxorubicinol can potently and directly inhibit the Ca^{2+}–Mg^{2+} ATPase of sarcoplasmic reticulum, the f_0–f_1 proton pump of mito-chondria (Boucek et al., 1987), and the Na^+–K^+ ATPase and Na^+–Ca^{2+} exchanger of sarcolemma (Olson et al., 1988). DOXol can therefore affect myocardial energy metabolism, ionic gradients, and Ca^{2+} movements, ultimately impairing cardiac contraction and relaxation.

6.2.2.2. Ca^{2+} and iron overload Interference with Ca^{2+} regulation has been proposed to be one of the causative events in the mechanism of ADR-induced cardiotoxicity. Solem et al. (1994) reported that ADR treatment *in vivo* causes a dose-dependent and irreversible decrease in mitochondrial Ca^{2+} loading capacity by suppression of adenine nucleotide translocase and alteration of the calcium-dependent regulation of the MPT pore, which is related to the persistent decrease in mitochondrial Ca^{2+} loading capacity. Sarcoendoplasmic reticulum Ca^{2+}-ATPase2 (SERCA2) is a major transport protein in sarcoplasmic reticulum that regulates intracellular Ca^{2+} concentration. Studies in neonatal cardiac myocytes have shown that SERCA2 is decreased in ADR-treated heart (Arai et al., 2000).

There are at least two pathways in which iron may be involved in ADR-induced cardiotoxicity. The first mechanism acts by reduction of ADR–Fe^{3+}(III) complex to ADR–Fe^{2+}, resulting in production of superoxide mediated by NADH dehydrogenase (Zweier, 1984). The ADR–Fe^{3+}(III) complex also acts as a potential mutagen (Kostoryz and Yourtee, 2001). Secondly, ADR may induce cardiotoxicity by disturbing iron homeostasis. Intramyocardial formation of DOXol disturbs the homeostatic process associated with cluster assembly or disassembly and the reversible switch between aconitase enzyme and IRP-1 (iron regulatory protein, which controls the balance between ferritin and transferrin) by delocalizing low molecular weight Fe^{2+} from the [4Fe-4s] cluster of the cytoplasmic aconitase enzyme (Minotti et al., 1999). In addition to aconitase enzyme and IRP-1, IRP-2 was inactivated also (Minotti et al., 2001). However, Minotti et al. (2001) have suggested that inactivation of IRP-2 occurs by ROS generation rather than by DOXol accumulation.

An additional study has been reported by Link et al. (1998). Treatment of myocytes with iron resulted in loss of mitochondrial respiratory enzyme activities, which resulted in a decrease in ATP levels. This observation was more dramatically affected when myocytes were treated with combined iron and ADR. These studies have proposed that iron loading impaired cardiac mitochondrial respiratory enzymes. In conclusion, disruption of iron homeostasis leads to posttranscriptional dysfunction in selected cardiac genes, and dysfunction of several enzymes and proteins such as cytochromes, catalase, lipoxygenases, and respiratory protein complexes. Due to imbalance of iron homeostasis, several oxidant reactions are disturbed by accumulation of iron, resulting in elevation of ROS generation.

The above studies have demonstrated that the mechanisms of ADR-induced cardiotoxicity are multifactorial and complex.

6.3. *Role of antioxidants in ADR-induced cardiotoxicity*

Several studies have shown that the heart is generally low in SOD levels (Chen et al., 1994; Doroshow et al., 1980). In addition, cardiac tissues also have low catalase levels and thus are unable to detoxify H_2O_2 (Chen et al., 1994). Three enzymes, SOD, GSHPx, and catalase, are important in mitigating free radical-induced cell injury. Analysis of these three antioxidant enzymes has been reported in different animal species treated with different doses and over different times following ADR treatment. Li and Singal (2000) demonstrated that activities and protein levels of GSHPx and MnSOD were significantly decreased from 2 to 24 h and 1 to 2 h, respectively, after treatment with ADR. However, MnSOD activity was recovered by 4 h and unchanged after both 24 h and 3 weeks following treatment with ADR (Li et al., 2000). Catalase activity also decreased from 2 to 24 h but protein levels were not changed (Li and Singal, 2000). CuZnSOD activity was not changed at any time (Li and Singal, 2000). Further studies suggested that MDA, a byproduct of lipid peroxidation, might diminish GSHPx activity by oxidizing the active site or by forming protein cross-links. Early and persistent decreased MnSOD and GSHPx activities may play an important role in the pathogenesis of ADR-induced cardiotoxicity. It is concluded from these studies that depression of the antioxidant system is due to the global inhibitory effect of ADR on DNA, RNA, and protein synthesis.

6.4. *Prevention of ADR-induced cardiotoxicity*

Many studies have been attempted to prevent the cardiotoxic side effects of ADR. Strategies for the prevention of ADR-induced cardiotoxicity have focused on combination therapies.

6.4.1. *Combination therapy with antioxidants*

Cardiotoxic effects of ADR have been demonstrated by free radical overproduction and/or reduction in endogenous antioxidant sources. Combinations of ADR and antioxidants have been tried in both *in vivo* and *in vitro* studies. Transgenic mouse models provide powerful tools to study mechanisms of ADR-induced cardiotoxicity *in vivo*. The rat model is also considered suitable because ADR injury in rat seems to resemble human injury as judged by several features (Jones et al., 1990). Since mitochondria may be a critical site of ADR-induced cardiotoxicity, overexpression of MnSOD in heart has been a focus of study. One of the most interesting observations was that of Yen et al. (1996), who noted that overexpression of MnSOD in mice protects against cardiotoxicity from ADR treatment by reducing mitochondrial damage. This reduced damage was correlated with reduction of LDH and CK levels, protection of mitochondria complex I activity, and inhibition of peroxynitrite formation (Yen et al., 1999). Recently, the protective property of signaling molecules has been proposed. Transgenic mice with cardiac specific over-expression of the STAT 3 gene (signal transducer and activator of transcription) have shown protective activity against ADR-induced cardiotoxicity by inhibiting reduction of cardiac contractile genes and inducing cardiac protective factor (Kunisada et al., 2000). Reduced glutathione was also reported to decrease acute myocardial toxicity of ADR (Yoda et al., 1986).

Catalase is the other antioxidant enzyme whose role in ADR toxicity has been the subject of study. Kang et al. demonstrated that overexpression of catalase activity in a transgenic mouse model by 60- or 100-fold resulted in significant resistance to ADR-induced cardiac lipid peroxidation, elevation of serum CPK, and functional changes in the isolated atrium. Interestingly, 200-fold or greater elevation of catalase activity did not provide protection (Kang et al., 1996). The results provide direct evidence for the role of catalase in the ADR cardiotoxic response. However, tissue culture models studying transfection of catalase cDNA have shown that catalase-enriched cells were actually more sensitive to the cytotoxicity of ADR than the untransfected cells from which they were derived (Speranza et al., 1993). It was speculated that overexpression of catalase may cause imbalance between SOD and catalase (Orr and Sohal, 1994), which may lead to an accumulation of $O_2^{\bullet-}$ due to regeneration of molecular oxygen from H_2O_2 and continued redox cycling of ADR. In addition, catalase is an iron-dependent enzyme, so iron released from degradation of catalase may form a complex with ADR. It has been shown that an iron–ADR complex is toxic.

Metallothionein, the highly conserved, low molecular weight, thiol rich protein, can bind to and be induced by heavy metal ions and detoxify transition metals. Recent studies show that overexpression of metallothionein *in vivo* resulted in significant resistance to cardiac injury and a reduction in serum CPK (Sun et al., 2001).

Probucol is a lipid-lowering drug. The structure of probucol resembles that of vitamin E, a well-known antioxidant that has one phenolic group. Since probucol has two phenolic groups in its molecular structure, it has been reported to be a strong antioxidant. Effects of probucol on ADR-induced cardiotoxicity have been examined in detail in the rat model, and it has been reported that probucol completely prevented cardiotoxicity without interfering with the antitumor properties of ADR by preventing both myocardial lipid peroxidation and ADR-induced decrease in antioxidant activity. Probucol also increased GSHPx activity (Li et al., 2000).

Melatonin, a pineal hormone, has recently been shown to be equally effective as probucol. Melatonin preserved both cardiac function and myocardial ultrastructural changes by preventing lipid peroxidation formation following ADR treatment in the rat (Morishima et al., 1998).

These studies clearly indicate that a stable increase in the intramyocardial levels of antioxidants may effectively protect the heart from ADR toxicity. However, some studies have reported failure of antioxidant protection against ADR cardiotoxicity.

The protective effects of diets rich in antioxidant compounds have also been demonstrated. Vitamin E has been shown to prevent cardiotoxicity and delay the toxic effects of ADR. Vitamin E does not completely protect against ADR cardiotoxicity (Singal and Tong, 1988). The administration of ascorbic acid and ADR to mice significantly prolonged the life of animals and decreased ultrastructural alterations due to ADR-induced cardiotoxicity (Shimpo et al., 1991). Flavonoids and synthetic flavonoids have also been reported to reduce the redox toxicity induced by ADR in left atrium (Van Acker et al., 2001). Moreover, dietary supplementation of *N*-acetylcysteine, a glutathione precursor, has also been shown to offer some protection against ADR-induced cardiotoxicity in mice (Doroshow et al., 1981).

6.4.2. *Combination therapy with iron chelators*

Iron chelators have been analyzed in many studies. EDTA and dexrazoxane (ICRF-187) were shown to prevent cardiac lesions and dysfunction induced by anthracyclines in both isolated and whole heart (Hasinoff et al., 1986). Abnormalities associated with ADR were reduced in the heart of dog pretreated with dexrazoxane (Herman and Ferrans, 1981). The cardioprotective action of ICRF-187 is to inhibit the conversion of Fe^{3+} to Fe^{2+}, which also inhibits the formation of hydroxyl radical. Unfortunately, combination therapy with dexrazoxane and ADR was shown to be associated with an increase in hematological toxicity, thus limiting the clinical application of dexrazoxane (Von Hoff et al., 1981).

6.4.3. *Inhibition of the production of DOXol*

One last cardiac protective strategy might be to decrease the formation of DOXol. Drug inhibition of aldoketoreductase or anthracyclines forming fewer C-13 metabolites could prove useful in prevention of cardiotoxicity. Decreasing the formation of this metabolite should delay the process of cardiotoxicity. Tamoxifen, an antiestrogen drug, has demonstrated cardioprotective properties by reducing the formation of DOXol in the cytosol of myocytes in vitro (Vaidyanathan and Boroujerdi, 2000).

It is important to note that the combination of antioxidant approaches and the inhibition of DOXol may be synergistic in therapies for ADR-induced cardiotoxicity.

Another option of therapy proposed was the use of myocet (liposome encapsulated ADR), which reduced cardiotoxicity while preserving its antitumor property. Myocet reduced the distribution of ADR to the heart and delivered ADR effectively to tumor cells. This experiment has been tried with 297 patients with metastatic breast cancer. Variables such as lipid composition, liposome size, and drug to lipid ratio need to be investigated to determine the best therapeutic result (Batist et al., 2001).

6.5. *Summary*

Chronic ADR treatment may induce cardiotoxicity through several mechanistic pathways. Oxidative stress seems to correlate with ADR-induced cardiotoxicity due to production of free radicals as well as a decrease in endogenous antioxidant enzymes levels and activities. Free radical production occurs by both enzymatic and non-enzymatic redox cycling of ADR. The generated free radicals are considered to be associated with the disruption of mitochondrial function and structure. In addition to mitochondrial disruption, production of free radicals is also responsible for damage of myofibrils and modulation of intracellular Ca^{2+} concentration and cardiac gene expression. Moreover, interactions of oxidative stress effects with other mechanisms such as iron overload or accumulation of DOXol should be considered in designing therapeutic strategies against ADR-induced cardiotoxicity.

7. Oxidative cardiac injury in aging

Cardiac dysfunction as a consequence of aging includes chronic heart failure, IRI, and myocardial infarction. These conditions, just to name a few, cause a disturbance in the redox balance of the heart, and thus an overproduction of free radical species. Several studies have reported increases in mitochondrial $O_2^{\bullet-}$ and H_2O_2 production in aged vs. young rats (Nohl and Hegner, 1978; Sawada and Carlson, 1987; Sohal et al., 1994). The "free radical theory" of aging, postulated by Denham Harman (1957), supports the hypothesis that the endogenous generation of oxygen-derived radicals results in cumulative damage to cells.

Suh et al. (2001), using cardiomyocyte cultures from aged (24–28 months) and young (2–5 months) rats, found that levels of ascorbic acid were decreased as a function of increasing age, whereas α-tocopherol levels were unchanged. In addition, there is a correlative increase in the levels of oxidative mitochondrial DNA damage reported as a measure of increasing 8OHdG levels; however, F_2-isoprostanes did not change (Suh et al., 2001). The authors speculate that there was no increase in iso-prostanes as a function of age due to their cellular location (Suh et al., 2001). In addition, Suh et al. (2001) reported that supplementation with lipoic acid for 2 weeks attenuated mitochondrial-induced oxidative stress and restored ascorbic acid levels.

Hamilton et al. (2001) also reported increasing levels of 8OHdG as a function of an age-related sensitivity to oxidative stress in rats. The age-related increases in 8OHdG ranged from 21% in the kidneys to 225% in the hearts of male B6D2F1 mice as compared to 40% in the kidneys to 78% in the hearts of male C57BL/6 mice (Hamilton et al., 2001). Age-related increases in 8OHdG were also observed in female C57BL/6 mice. The 8OHdG levels were 107% for the kidneys and 143% in the hearts. Dietary restriction was found to significantly reduce levels of 8OHdG in male B6D2F1 mice (Hamilton et al., 2001). Through subsequent testing, activities of antioxidant enzymes, including catalase, GSHPx, MnSOD, and CuZnSOD, were found to be the same in both young (6–7 months) and old (26–28 months) C57BL/6 female mice (Hamilton et al., 2001). The authors conclude that there is an age-related increase in 8OHdG; however, the increases do not appear to be due to a change in the antioxidant defense systems of the aged animals.

Overall, evidence suggests that ROS are involved in the aging processes and in cardiac disease progression. Studies have shown a correlation between increases in

8OHdG with increasing age. In addition, primary antioxidant enzymes have been reported to remain unchanged between young and old animals. These findings suggest that the older animals are unable to adapt to increasing oxidative stress as a function of increasing age. It is possible that intervention to increase endogenous levels of antioxidant enzymes would be protective against increasing oxidative stress in older animals.

8. Future directions

Many investigators have suggested that mitochondria are the source of ROS production in age-associated cardiac dysfunction. Measurement and localization of oxidative damage products is one way to address this hypothesis. Immunogold labeling for detection of oxidative damage products at the ultrastructural level is a technique available to correlate sites of oxidant production with sites of oxidant damage.

If the oxidative stress hypothesis is correct, the optimal therapy for ROS-induced cardiotoxicity should be antioxidant interventions. However, the overexpression of a single antioxidant enzyme such as MnSOD may cause an imbalance between MnSOD and catalase/GSHPx levels, which may lead to an imbalance of ROS. Also, the ability of a single antioxidant enzyme to protect against ROS-induced cardiotoxicity may not be sufficient. The techniques that combine two antioxidant enzymes such as MnSOD and catalase/GSHPx in ADR-treated patients should be investigated in the future.

Iron is an important element that may play a role in ROS generation and ROS-induced cardiotoxicity. However, it is still unclear whether iron is a cause or consequence of ROS-induced cardiotoxicity. For example, the ADR–Fe^{3+} complex may play a central role in free radical generation. Future experiments should analyze the degree of myocardium damage in heart treated with ADR–Fe^{3+} complex. For maximal therapeutic results, antioxidant therapy combined with an iron chelator should be considered for future study.

References

Allen, R.G., Tresini, M., 2000. Oxidative stress and gene regulation. Free Rad. Biol. Med. 28, 463–499.

Altug, S., Demiryurek, A.T., Cakici, I., Kanzik, I., 1999. The beneficial effects of peroxynitrite on ischaemia-reperfusion arrhythmias in rat isolated hearts. Eur. J. Pharmacol. 384, 157–162.

Amabile-Cuevas, C.F., Demple, B., 1991. Molecular characterization of the *soxRS* genes of *Escherichia coli*. Two genes control a superoxide stress regulon. Nucl. Acids Res. 19, 4479–4484.

Andreu, A.L., Arbos, M.A., Perez-Martos, A., Lopez-Perez, M.J., Asin, J., Lopez, N., Montoya, J., Schwartz, S., 1998. Reduced mitochondrial DNA transcription in senescent rat heart. Biochem. Biophys. Res. Commun. 252, 577–581.

Anzai, K., Ogawa, K., Kuniyasu, A., Ozawa, T., Yamamoto, H., Nakayama, H., 1998. Effects of hydroxyl radical and sulfhydryl reagents on the open probability of the purified cardiac ryanodine receptor channel incorporated into planar lipid bilayers. Biochem. Biophys. Res. Commun. 249, 938–942.

Arai, M., Yoguchi, A., Takizawa, T., Yokoyama, T., Kanda, T., Kurabayashi, M., Nagai, R., 2000. Mechanism of doxorubicin-induced inhibition of sarcoplasmic reticulum Ca(2+)-ATPase gene transcription. Circ. Res. 86, 8–14.

Armstrong, D.A., Buchana, J.D., 1978. Reactions of $O_2^{\bullet-}$, H_2O_2 and other oxidants with sulfhydryl enzymes. Photochem. Photobiol. 28, 743–755.

Arola, O.J., Saraste, A., Pulkki, K., Kallajoki, M., Parvinen, M., Voipio-Pulkki, L.M., 2000. Acute doxorubicin cardiotoxicity involves cardiomyocyte apoptosis. Cancer Res. 60, 1789–1792.

Bachur, N.R., Gordon, S.L., Gee, M.V., 1977. Anthracycline antibiotic augmentation of microsomal electron transport and free radical formation. Mol. Pharmacol. 13, 901–910.

Basaga, H.S., 1990. Biochemical aspects of free radicals. Biochem. Cell Biol. 68, 989–998.

Batist, G., Ramakrishnan, G., Rao, C.S., Chandrasekharan, A., Gutheil, J., Guthrie, T., Shah, P., Khojasteh, A., Nair, M.K., Hoelzer, K., Tkaczuk, K., Park, Y.C., Lee, L.W., 2001. Reduced cardiotoxicity and preserved antitumor efficacy of liposome-encapsulated doxorubicin and cyclophosphamide compared with conventional doxorubicin and cyclophosphamide in a randomized, multicenter trial of metastatic breast cancer. J. Clin. Oncol. 19, 1444–1454.

Baumgarten, G., Knuefermann, P., Mann, D.L., 2000. Cytokines as emerging targets in the treatment of heart failure. Trends Cardiovasc. Med. 10, 216–223.

Beauchamp, C., Fridovich, I., 1971. Superoxide dismutase. Improved assays and an assay applicable to acrylamide gels. Anal. Biochem. 44, 276–287.

Beckman, J.S., Beckman, T.W., Chen, J., Marshall, P.A., Freeman, B.A., 1990. Apparent hydroxyl radical production by peroxynitrite: implications for endothelial injury from nitric oxide and superoxide. Proc. Natl. Acad. Sci. U. S. A. 87, 1620–1624.

Bewley, G.C., 1988. cDNA and deduced amino acid sequence of murine Cu–Zn superoxide dismutase. Nucl. Acids Res. 16, 2728.

Beyer, W., Imlay, J., Fridovich, I., 1991. Superoxide dismutases. Prog. Nucl. Acid Res. Mol. Biol. 40, 221–253.

Blum, J., Fridovich, I., 1985. Inactivation of glutathione peroxidase by superoxide radical. Arch. Biochem. Biophys. 240, 500–508.

Bolli, R., 1990. Mechanism of myocardial "stunning". Circulation 82, 723–738.

Bolli, R., 1991. Oxygen-derived free radicals and myocardial reperfusion injury: an overview. Cardiovasc. Drugs Ther. 5, 249–268.

Boucek Jr., R.J., Olson, R.D., Brenner, D.E., Ogunbunmi, E.M., Inui, M., Fleischer, S., 1987. The major metabolite of doxorubicin is a potent inhibitor of membrane-associated ion pumps. A correlative study of cardiac muscle with isolated membrane fractions. J. Biol. Chem. 262, 15851–15856.

Brown Jr., R.H., 1995. Amyotrophic lateral sclerosis: recent insights from genetics and transgenic mice. Cell 80, 687–692.

Bruce, A.J., Boling, W., Kindy, M.S., Peshon, J., Kraemer, P.J., Carpenter, M.K., Holtsberg, F.W., Mattson, M.P., 1996. Altered neuronal and microglial responses to excitotoxic and ischemic brain injury in mice lacking TNF receptors. Nat. Med. 2, 788–794.

Buettner, G.R., 1993. The pecking order of free radicals and antioxidants: lipid peroxidation, α-tocopherol, and ascorbate. Arch. Biochem. Biophys. 300, 535–543.

Café, C., Testa, M.P., Sheldon, P.J., French, W.P., Ellerby, L.M., Bredesen, D.E., 2000. Loss of oxidation-reduction specificity in amyotrophic lateral sclerosis-associated CuZnSOD mutants. J. Mol. Neurosci. 15, 71–83.

Cai, H., Harrison, D.G., 2000. Endothelial dysfunction in cardiovascular diseases: the role of oxidant stress. Circ. Res. 87, 840–844.

Carlsson, L.M., Jonsson, J., Edlund, T., Marklund, S.L., 1995. Mice lacking extracellular superoxide dismutase are more sensitive to hyperoxia. Proc. Natl. Acad. Sci. U. S. A. 92, 6264–6268.

Carlsson, L.M., Marklund, S.L., Edlund, T., 1996. The rat extracellular superoxide dismutase dimer is converted to a tetramer by the exchange of a single amino acid. Proc. Natl. Acad. Sci. U. S. A. 93, 5219–5222.

Cassina, A., Radi, R., 1996. Differential inhibitory action of nitric oxide and peroxynitrite on mitochondrial electron transport. Arch. Biochem. Biophys. 328, 309–316.

Ceballos-Picot, I., Nicole, A., Briand, P., Grimber, G., Delacourt, A., Defossez, A., Javoy-Agid, F., Lafon, M., Blouin, J.L., Sinet, P.M., 1991. Neuronal-specific expression of human copper–zinc superoxide dismutase gene in transgenic mice carrying the human CuZn superoxide dismutase gene than in brains of their non-transgenic littermates. Brain Res. 552, 198–214.

Ceconi, C., Cargnoni, A., Pasini, E., Condorelli, E., Curello, S., Ferrari, R., 1991. Evaluation of phospholipid peroxidation as malondialdehyde during myocardial ischemia and reperfusion injury. Am. J. Physiol. 260, H1057–H1061.

Chen, Y., Saari, J.T., Kang, Y.J., 1994. Weak antioxidant defenses make the heart a target for damage in copper-deficient rats. Free Rad. Biol. Med. 17, 529–536.

Chen, Z., Siu, B., Ho, Y.-S., Vincent, R., Chua, C.C., Hamdy, R.C., Chua, B.H.L., 1998. Overexpression of MnSOD protects against myocardial ischemia/reperfusion injury in transgenic mice. J. Mol. Cell Cardiol. 30, 2281–2289.

Chen, Z., Oberley, T.D., Ho, Y., Chua, C.C., Siu, B., Hamdy, R.C., Epstein, C.J., Chua, B.H., 2000. Overexpression of CuZnSOD in coronary vascular cells attenuates myocardial ischemia/reperfusion injury. Free Rad. Biol. Med. 29, 589–596.

Church, S.L., 1990. Manganese superoxide dismutase: nucleotide and deduced amino acid sequence of a cDNA encoding a new human transcript. Biochim. Biophys. Acta 1087, 250–252.

Church, S.L., Grant, J.W., Meese, E.U., Trent, J.M., 1992. Sublocalization of the gene encoding manganese superoxide dismutase (MnSOD/*SOD2*) to 6q25 by fluorescence in situ hybridization and somatic cell hybrid mapping. Genomics 14, 823–825.

Cotran, R.S., Kumar, V., Robbins, S.L., 1994. The heart. In: Schoen, F.J. (Ed.), Pathologic Basis of Disease, fifth edition. W.B. Saunders, Philadelphia, pp. 517–539.

Cregan, R., Tischfield, J., Ricciuti, F., Ruddle, F.H., 1973. Chromosome assignment of genes in man using mouse–human somatic cell hybrids: mitochondrial superoxide dismutase (indophenol oxidase B, tetrameric) to chromosome 6. Humangenetik 20, 203–209.

Cummings, J., Anderson, L., Willmott, N., Smyth, J.F., 1991. The molecular pharmacology of doxorubicin in vivo. Eur. J. Cancer 27, 532–535.

Delabar, J.-M., Nicole, A., D'Auriol, L., Jacob, Y., Meunier-Rotival, M., Galibert, F., Sinet, P.-M., Jerome, H., 1987. Cloning and sequencing of a rat CuZn superoxide dismutase cDNA. Correlation between CuZn superoxide dismutase mRNA level and enzyme activity in rat and mouse tissues. Eur. J. Biochem. 166, 181–187.

Dhalla, A.K., Singal, P.K., 1994. Antioxidant changes in hypertrophied and failing guinea pig hearts. Am. J. Physiol. 266, H1280–H1285.

Dhalla, N.S., Golfman, L., Takeda, S., Takeda, N., Nagano, M., 1999. Evidence for the role of oxidative stress in acute ischemic heart disease: a brief review. Can. J. Cardiol. 15, 587–593.

Dhalla, N.S., Temsah, R.M., Netticadan, T., 2000a. Role of oxidative stress in cardiovascular diseases. J. Hypertens. 18, 655–673.

Dhalla, J.S., Elmoselhi, A.B., Hata, T., Makino, N., 2000b. Status of myocardial antioxidants in ischemia-reperfusion injury. Cardiovasc. Res. 47, 446–456.

DiSilvestre, D., Kleeberger, S.R., Johns, J., Levitt, R.C., 1995. Structure and DNA sequence of the mouse MnSOD gene. Mamm. Genome 6, 281–284.

Dixon, I.M., Kaneko, M., Hata, T., Panagia, V., Dhalla, N.S., 1990. Alterations in cardiac membrane Ca^{2+} transport during oxidative stress. Mol. Cell. Biochem. 99, 125–133.

Dixon, I.M., Hata, T., Dhalla, N.S., 1992. Sarcolemmal Na(+)–K(+)-ATPase activity in congestive heart failure due to myocardial infarction. Am. J. Physiol. 262, C664–C671.

Doroshow, J.H., 1983. Effect of anthracycline antibiotics on oxygen radical formation in rat heart. Cancer Res. 43, 460–472.

Doroshow, J.H., Locker, G.Y., Myers, C.E., 1980. Enzymatic defenses of the mouse heart against reactive oxygen metabolites: alterations produced by doxorubicin. J. Clin. Invest. 65, 128–135.

Doroshow, J.H., Locker, G.Y., Ifrim, I., Myers, C.E., 1981. Prevention of doxorubicin cardiac toxicity in the mouse by *N*-acetylcysteine. J. Clin. Invest. 68, 1053–1064.

Dryer, S.E., Dryer, R.L., Autor, A.P., 1980. Enhancement of mitochondrial, cyanide-resistant superoxide dismutase in the livers of rats treated with 2,4-dinitrophenol. J. Biol. Chem. 255, 1054–1057.

Earley, F.G., Patel, S.D., Ragan, I., Attardi, G., 1987. Photolabelling of a mitochondrially encoded subunit of NADH dehydrogenase with [^{3}H]dihydrorotenone. FEBS Lett. 219, 108–112.

M. P. Cole et al.

Eilers, M., Schatz, G., 1988. Protein unfolding and the energetics of protein translocation across biological membrane. Cell 52, 481–483.

Epstein, C.J., Avraham, K.B., Lovett, M., Smith, S., Elroy-Stein, O., Rotman, G., Bry, C., Groner, Y., 1987. Transgenic mice with increased Cu/Zn-superoxide dismutase activity: animal model of dosage effects in Down's syndrome. Proc. Natl. Acad. Sci. U. S. A. 84, 8044–8048.

Erenel, G., Erbas, D., Aricioglu, A., 1993. Free radicals and antioxidant systems. Mater. Med. Pol. 25, 37–43.

Favero, T.G., Zable, A.C., Abramson, J.J., 1995. Hydrogen peroxide stimulates the Ca^{2+} release channel from skeletal muscle sarcoplasmic reticulum. J. Biol. Chem. 270, 25557–25563.

Folz, R.J., Crapo, J.D., 1994. Extracellular superoxide dismutase (*Sod3*): tissue-specific expression, genomic characterization, and computer-assisted sequence analysis of the human EC-SOD gene. Genomics 22, 162–171.

Folz, R.J., Guan, J., Seldin, M.F., Oury, T.D., Enghild, J.J., Crapo, J.D., 1997. Mouse extracellular superoxide dismutase: primary structure, tissue-specific gene expression, chromosomal localization, and lung in situ hybridization. Am. J. Respir. Cell Mol. Biol. 17, 393–403.

Forrest, G.L., Gonzalez, B., Tseng, W., Li, X., Mann, J., 2000. Human carbonyl reductase overexpression in the heart advances the development of doxorubicin-induced cardiotoxicity in transgenic mice. Cancer Res. 60, 5158–5164.

Freeman, B.A., Crapo, J.D., 1982. Biology of disease: free radicals and tissue injury. Lab. Invest. 47, 412–426.

Fridovich, I., 1998. Oxygen toxicity: a radical explanation. J. Exp. Biol. 201, 1203–1209.

Fridovich, I., 2001. Reflections of a fortunate biochemist. J. Biol. Chem. 276, 28629–28636.

Fujii, J., Taniguchi, N., 1991. Phorbol ester induces manganese superoxide dismutase in tumor necrosis factor-resistant cells. J. Biol. Chem. 266, 23142–23146.

Gardner, P.R., Nguyen, D.D., White, C.W., 1994. Aconitase is a sensitive and critical target of oxygen poisoning in cultured mammalian cells and in rat lungs. Proc. Natl. Acad. Sci. U. S. A. 91, 12248–12252.

Gardner, P.R., Raineri, I., Epstein, L.B., White, C.W., 1995. Superoxide radical and iron modulate aconitase activity in mammalian cells. J. Biol. Chem. 270, 13399–13405.

Gerschman, R., Gilbert, D.L., Nye, S.W., Dwyer, P., Fenn, W.O., 1956. Oxygen poisoning and X-irradiation: a mechanism in common. Science 119, 623–626.

Granger, D.N., 1999. Ischemia-reperfusion: mechanisms of microvascular dysfunction and the influence of risk factors for cardiovascular disease. Microcirculation 6, 167–178.

Griendling, K.K., Sorescu, D., Ushio-Fukai, M., 2000. NAD(P)H oxidase: role in cardiovascular biology and disease. Circ. Res. 86, 494–501.

Guarnieri, C., Lugaresi, A., Flamigni, F., Muscari, C., Caldarera, C.M., 1982. Effect of oxygen radicals and hyperoxia on rat heart ornithine decarboxylase activity. Biochim. Biophys. Acta 718, 157–164.

Hallewell, R.A., Masiarz, F.R., Najarian, R.C., Puma, J.P., Quiroga, M.R., Randolph, A., Sanchez-Pescador, R., Scandella, C.J., Smith, B., Steimer, K.S., Mullenback, G.T., 1985. Human Cu/Zn superoxide dismutase cDNA: isolation of clones synthesizing high levels of active or inactive enzyme from an expression library. Nucl. Acids Res. 13, 2017–2034.

Hallewell, R.A., Mullenbach, G.T., Stempien, M.M., Bell, G.I., 1986. Sequence of a cDNA coding for mouse manganese superoxide dismutase. Nucl. Acids Res. 14, 9539.

Halliwell, B., 1999. Antioxidant defence mechanisms: from the beginning to the end (of the beginning). Free Rad. Res. 31, 261–272.

Halliwell, B., Gutteridge, J.M.C., 1989. Free Radicals in Biology and Medicine, 2nd ed. Oxford University Press, New York.

Hamilton, M.L., Van Remmen, H., Drake, J.A., Yang, H., Guo, Z.M., Kewitt, K., Walter, C.A., Richardson, A., 2001. Does oxidative damage to DNA increase with age? Proc. Natl. Acad. Sci. U. S. A. 98, 10469–10474.

Harman, D., 1957. Aging: a theory based on free radical and radiation chemistry. J. Gerontol. 2, 298–300.

Hasinoff, B.B., Yalowich, J.C., Ling, Y., Buss, J.L., 1986. The effect of dexrazoxane (ICRF-187) on doxorubicin- and daunorubicin-mediated growth inhibition of Chinese hamster ovary cells. Anticancer Drugs 7, 558–567.

Hearse, D.J., Maxwell, L., Saldanha, C., Gavin, J.B., 1993. The myocardial vasculature during ischemia and reperfusion: a target for injury and protection. J. Mol. Cell. Cardiol. 25, 759–800.

Hendrickson, D.J., Fisher, J.H., Jones, C., Ho, Y.-S., 1990. Regional localization of human extracellular superoxide dismutase gene to 4pter–q21. Genomic 8, 736–738.

Herman, E.H., Ferrans, V.J., 1981. Reduction of chronic doxorubicin cardiotoxicity in dogs by pretreatment with $(+/-)$-1,2-bis-(3,5-dioxopiperazinyl-1-yl) propane (ICRF-187). Cancer Res. 41, 3436–3440.

Hill, M.F., Singal, P.K., 1996. Antioxidant and oxidative stress changes during heart failure subsequent to myocardial infarction in rats. Am. J. Pathol. 148, 291–300.

Hjalmarsson, K., Mardlund, S.L., Engstrom, A., Edlund, T., 1987. Isolation and sequence of complementary DNA encoding human extracellular superoxide dismutase. Proc. Natl. Acad. Sci. U. S. A. 84, 6340–6344.

Ho, Y.-S., Crapo, J.D., 1987a. Nucleotide sequences of cDNAs coding for rat manganese-containing superoxide dismutase. Nucl. Acids Res. 15, 10070.

Ho, Y.-S., Crapo, J.D., 1987b. cDNA and deduced amino acid sequences of rat copper-zinc containing superoxide dismutase. Nucl. Acids Res. 15, 6746.

Ho, Y.-S., Crapo, J.D., 1988. Isolation and characterization of complementary DNAs encoding human manganese-containing superoxide dismutase. FEBS Lett. 229, 256–260.

Ho, Y.-S., Howard, A.I., Crapo, J.D., 1991. Molecular structure of a functional rat gene for manganese-containing superoxide dismutase. Am. J. Respir. Cell Mol. Biol. 4, 278–286.

Ho, Y.-S., Magnenat, J.L., Gargano, M., Cao, J., 1998. The nature of antioxidant defense mechanisms: a lesson from transgenic studies. Environ. Health Perspect. 106 (Suppl.), 1219–1228.

Hurt, J., Hsu, J.L., Dougall, W.C., Visner, G.A., Burr, I.M., Nick, H.S., 1992. Multiple mRNA species generated by alternative polyadenylation from the rat manganese superoxide dismutase gene. Nucl. Acids Res. 12, 2985–2990.

Ide, T., Tsutsui, H., Kinugawa, S., Utsumi, H., Kang, D., Hattori, N., Uchida, K., Arimura, K., Egashira, K., Takeshita, A., 1999. Mitochondrial electron transport complex I is a potential source of oxygen free radicals in the failing myocardium. Circ. Res. 85, 357–363.

Ide, T., Tsutsui, H., Kinugawa, S., Suematsu, N., Hayashidani, S., Ichikawa, K., Utsumi, H., Machida, Y., Egashira, K., Takeshita, A., 2000. Direct evidence for increased hydroxyl radicals originating from superoxide in the failing myocardium. Circ. Res. 86, 151–157.

Ide, T., Tsutsui, H., Hayashidani, S., Kang, D., Suematsu, N., Nakamura, K., Utsumi, H., Hamasaki, N., Takeshita, A., 2001. Mitochondrial DNA damage and dysfunction associated with oxidative stress in failing hearts after myocardial infarction. Circ. Res. 88, 529–535.

Ito, H., Miller, S.C., Billingham, M.E., Akimoto, H., Torti, S.V., Wade, R., Gahlmann, R., Lyons, G., Kedes, L., Torti, F.M., 1990. Doxorubicin selectively inhibits muscle gene expression in cardiac muscle cells in vivo and in vitro. Proc. Natl. Acad. Sci. U. S. A. 87, 4275–4279.

Jeyaseelan, R., Poizat, C., Wu, H.Y., Kedes, L., 1997a. Molecular mechanisms of doxorubicin-induced cardiomyopathy. Selective suppression of Reiske iron-sulfur protein, ADP/ATP translocase, and phosphofructokinase genes is associated with ATP depletion in rat cardiomyocytes. J. Biol. Chem. 272, 5828–5832.

Jeyaseelan, R., Poizat, C., Baker, R.K., Abdishoo, S., Isterabadi, L.B., Lyons, G.E., Kedes, L., 1997b. A novel cardiac-restricted target for doxorubicin. CARP, a nuclear modulator of gene expression in cardiac progenitor cells and cardiomyocytes. J. Biol. Chem. 272, 22800–22808.

Jones, S.M., Kirby, M.S., Harding, S.E., Vescova, G., Wanless, R.B., Dalla Libera, L.D., Poole-Wilson, P.A., 1990. Adriamycin cardiomyopathy in the rabbit: alterations in contractile proteins and myocyte function. Cardiovasc. Res. 24, 834–842.

Kaneko, M., Masuda, H., Suzuki, H., Matsumoto, Y., Kobayashi, A., Yamazaki, N., 1993. Modification of contractile proteins by oxygen free radicals in rat heart. Mol. Cell. Biochem. 125, 163–169.

Kang, Y.J., 1999. The antioxidant function of metallothionein in the heart. Proc. Soc. Exp. Biol. Med. 222, 263–273.

Kang, Y.J., Chen, Y., Epstein, P.N., 1996. Suppression of doxorubicin cardiotoxicity by overexpression of catalase in the heart of transgenic mice. J. Biol. Chem. 271, 12610–12616.

Kang, Y.J., Li, G., Saari, J.T., 1999. Metallothionein inhibits ischemia-reperfusion injury in mouse heart. Am. J. Physiol. 276, H993–H997.

Kantrow, S.P., Piantadosi, C.A., 1997. Release of cytochrome *c* from liver mitochondria during permeability transition. Biochem. Biophys. Res. Commun. 232, 669–671.

Keele Jr., B.B., McCord, J.M., Fridovich, I., 1970. Superoxide dismutase from *Escherichia coli* B. A new manganese-containing enzyme. J. Biol. Chem. 245, 6176–6181.

Keller, J.N., Kindy, M.S., Holtsberg, F.W., St. Clair, D.K., Yen, H.C., Germeyer, A., Steiner, S.M., Bruce-Keller, A.J., Hutchins, J.B., Mattson, M.P., 1998. Mitochondrial manganese superoxide dismutase prevents neural apoptosis and reduces ischemic brain injury: suppression of peroxynitrite production, lipid peroxidation, and mitochondrial dysfunction. J. Neurosci. 18, 687–697.

Kilk, A., Laan, M., Torp, A., 1995. Human CuZn superoxide dismutase enzymatic activity in cells is regulated by the length of the mRNA. FEBS Lett. 362, 323–327.

Kim, H.S., Minard, P., Legoy, M.D., Thomas, D., 1986. Inactivation of 3-alpha-hydroxysteroid dehydrogenase by superoxide radicals. Modification of histidine and cysteine residues causes the conformational change. Biochem. J. 233, 493–497.

Kiningham, K.K., Xu, Y., Daosukho, C., Popova, B., St. Clair, D.K., 2001. Nuclear factor κB-dependent mechanisms coordinate the synergistic effect of PMA and cytokines on the induction of superoxide dismutase 2. Biochem. J. 353, 147–156.

Kojda, G., Harrison, D., 1999. Interactions between NO and reactive oxygen species: pathophysiological importance in atherosclerosis, hypertension, diabetes and heart failure. Cardiovasc. Res. 43, 562–571.

Kono, Y., Fridovich, I., 1982. Superoxide radical inhibits catalase. J. Biol. Chem. 257, 5751–5754.

Kostoryz, E.L., Yourtee, D.M., 2001. Oxidative mutagenesis of doxorubicin-Fe(III) complex. Mutat. Res. 490, 131–139.

Krall, J., Bagley, A.C., Mullenback, G.T., Hallewell, R.A., Lynch, R.E., 1988. Superoxide mediates the toxicity of paraquat for cultured mammalian cells. J. Biol. Chem. 263, 1910–1914.

Kuhn, H., Brash, A.R., 1990. Occurrence of lipoxygenase products in membranes of rabbit reticulocytes. Evidence for a role of the reticulocyte lipoxygenase in the maturation of red cells. J. Biol. Chem. 265, 1454–1458.

Kunisada, K., Negoro, S., Tone, E., Funamoto, M., Osugi, T., Yamada, S., Okabe, M., Kishimoto, T., Yamauchi-Takihara, K., 2000. Signal transducer and activator of transcription 3 in the heart transduces not only a hypertrophic signal but a protective signal against doxorubicin-induced cardiomyopathy. Proc. Natl. Acad. Sci. U. S. A. 97, 315–319.

Kuo, C.F., Mashino, T., Fridovich, I., 1987. Alpha, beta-dihydroxyisovalerate dehydratase: a superoxide-sensitive enzyme. J. Biol. Chem. 262, 4724–4727.

Kurrelmeyer, K.M., Michael, L.H., Baumgarten, G., Taffet, G.E., Peschon, J.J., Sivasubramanian, N., Entman, M.L., Mann, D.L., 2000. Endogenous tumor necrosis factor protects the adult cardiac myocyte against ischemic-induced apoptosis in a murine model of acute myocardial infarction. Proc. Natl. Acad. Sci. U. S. A. 97, 5456–5461.

Lawrence, R.A., Burk, R.F., 1976. Glutathione peroxidase activity in selenium-deficient rat liver. Biochem. Biophys. Res. Commun. 71, 952–958.

Lebovitz, R.M., Zhang, H., Vogel, H., Cartwright Jr., J., Dionne, L., Lu, N., Huang, S., Matzuk, M.M., 1996. Neurodegeneration, myocardial injury, and perinatal death in mitochondrial superoxide dismutase-deficient mice. Proc. Natl. Acad. Sci. U. S. A. 93, 9782–9787.

Lefer, A.M., Tsao, P.S., Lefer, D.J., Ma, X.L., 1991. Role of endothelial dysfunction in the pathogenesis of reperfusion injury after myocardial ischemia. FASEB J. 5, 2029–2034.

Li, P.F., Dietz, R., Von Harsdorf, R., 1999. Superoxide induces apoptosis in cardiomyocytes, but proliferation and expression of transforming growth factor-beta1 in cardiac fibroblasts. FEBS Lett. 448, 206–210.

Li, Q., Bolli, R., Qiu, Y., Tang, X.L., Guo, Y., French, B.A., 2001. Gene therapy with extracellular superoxide dismutase protects conscious rabbits against myocardial infarction. Circulation 103, 1893–1898.

Li, T., Singal, P.K., 2000. Adriamycin-induced early changes in myocardial antioxidant enzymes and their modulation by probucol. Circulation 102, 2105–2110.

Li, T., Danelisen, I., Bello-Klein, A., Singal, P.K., 2000. Effects of probucol on changes of antioxidant enzymes in adriamycin-induced cardiomyopathy in rats. Cardiovasc. Res. 46, 523–530.

Li, Y., Huang, T.T., Carlson, E.J., Melov, S., Ursell, P.C., Olson, J.L., Noble, L.J., Yoshimura, M.P., Berger, C., Chan, P.H., Wallace, D.C., Epstein, C.J., 1995. Dilated cardiomyopathy and neonatal lethality in mutant mice lacking manganese superoxide dismutase. Nat. Genet. 11, 376–381.

Licata, S., Saponiero, A., Mordente, A., Minotti, G., 2000. Doxorubicin metabolism and toxicity in human myocardium: role of cytoplasmic deglycosidation and carbonyl reduction. Chem. Res. Toxicol. 13, 414–420.

Link, G., Saada, A., Pinson, A., Konijn, A.M., Hershko, C., 1998. Mitochondrial respiratory enzymes are a major target of iron toxicity in rat heart cells. J. Lab. Clin. Med. 131, 466–474.

MacGowan, G.A., Mann, D.L., Kormas, R.L., Feldman, A.M., Murali, S., 1997. Circulating interleukin-6 in severe heart failure. Am. J. Cardiol. 79, 1128–1131.

Mann, T., Keilin, D., 1939. Haemocuprein and hepatocuprein, copper-protein compounds of blood and liver in mammals. Proc. R. Soc. London 126, 303–315.

Marcillat, O., Zhang, Y., Davies, K.J., 1989. Oxidative and non-oxidative mechanisms in the inactivation of cardiac mitochondrial electron transport chain components by doxorubicin. Biochem. J. 259, 181–189.

Marklund, S.L., 1992. Regulation by cytokines of extracellular superoxide dismutase and other superoxide dismutase isoenzymes in fibroblasts. J. Biol. Chem. 267, 6696–6701.

Masuda, A., Longo, D.L., Kobayashi, Y., Appella, E., Oppenheim, J.J., Matsushima, K., 1988. Induction of mitochondrial manganese superoxide dismutase by interleukin 1. FASEB J. 15, 3087–3091.

Mattson, M.P., Goodman, Y., Luo, H., Fu, W., Furukawa, K., 1997. Activation of NF-kappaB protects hippocampal neurons against oxidative stress-induced apoptosis: evidence for induction of manganese superoxide dismutase and suppression of peroxynitrite production and protein tyrosine nitration. J. Neuorsci. Res. 49, 681–697.

McCord, J.M., 1985. Oxygen-derived free radicals in postischemic tissue injury. N. Engl. J. Med. 312, 159–163.

McCord, J.M., Fridovich, I., 1969. Superoxide dismutase: an enzymatic function for erythrocuprein (hemocuprein). J. Biol. Chem. 244, 6049–6055.

McCord, J.M., Russell, W.J., 1988. Inactivation of creatine phosphokinase by superoxide during reperfusion injury. Basic Life Sci. 49, 869–873.

Mehta, J.L., Nichols, W.W., Donnelly, W.H., Lawson, D.L., Thompson, L., ter Riet, M., Saldeen, T.G., 1989. Protection by superoxide dismutase from myocardial dysfunction and attenuation of vasodilator reserve after coronary occlusion and reperfusion in dog. Circ. Res. 65, 1283–1295.

Mehta, J.L., Chen, H., Li, D., Phillips, I.M., 2000. Modulation of myocardial SOD and iNOS during ischemia-reperfusion by antisense directed at ACE mRNA. J. Mol. Cell. Cardiol. 32, 2259–2268.

Meyrick, B., Magnuson, M.A., 1994. Identification and functional characterization of the bovine manganous superoxide dismutase promoter. Am. J. Respir. Cell Mol. Biol. 10, 113–121.

Michel, T., Feron, O., 1997. Nitric oxide synthases: which, where, how, and why? J. Clin. Invest. 100, 2146–2152.

Mims, C.A., Playfair, J.H.L., Roitt, I.M., Wakelin, D., Williams, R., 1993. In: Anderson, R.M. (Ed.), Medical Microbiology. Mosby Europ Limited, London, pp. 4.5–4.8 (Chapter 4).

Minotti, G., Cairo, G., Monti, E., 1999. Role of iron in anthracycline cardiotoxicity: new tunes for an old song? FASEB J. 13, 199–212.

Minotti, G., Ronchi, R., Salvatorelli, E., Menna, P., Cairo, G., 2001. Doxorubicin irreversibly inactivates iron regulatory proteins 1 and 2 in cardiomyocytes: evidence for distinct metabolic pathways and implications for iron-mediated cardiotoxicity of antitumor therapy. Cancer Res. 61, 8422–8428.

Mirochnitchenko, O., Inouye, M., 1996. Effect of overexpression of human Cu, Zn superoxide dismutase in transgenic mice on macrophage functions. Biochim. Biophys. Acta 949, 58–64.

Moncada, S., Higgs, A., 1993. The L-arginine–nitric oxide pathway. N. Engl. J. Med. 329, 2002–2012.

Morishima, I., Matsui, H., Mukawa, H., Hayashi, K., Toki, Y., Okumura, K., Ito, T., Hayakawa, T., 1998. Melatonin, a pineal hormone with antioxidant property, protects against adriamycin cardiomyopathy in rats. Life Sci. 63, 511–521.

Muijsers, R.B.R., Folkerts, G., Henricks, P.A.J., Sadeghi-Hashjin, G., Nijkamp, F.P., 1997. Minireview: peroxynitrite: a two-faced metabolite of nitric oxide. Life Sci. 60, 1833–1845.

Munger, M.A., Johnson, B., Amber, I.J., Callahan, K.S., Gibert, E.M., 1996. Circulating concentrations of proinflammatory cytokines in mild or moderate heart failure secondary to ischemic or idiopathic dilated cardiomyopathy. Am. J. Cardiol. 77, 723–727.

Negoro, S., Kunisada, K., Fujio, Y., Funamoto, M., Darville, M.I., Eizirik, D.L., Osugi, T., Izumi, M., Oshima, Y., Nakaoka, Y., Hirota, H., Kishimoto, T., Yamauchi-Takihara, K., 2001. Activation of signal transducer and activator of transcription 3 protects cardiomyocytes from hypoxia/reoxygenation-induced oxidative stress through the upregulation of manganese superoxide dismutase. Circulation 104, 979–981.

Netticadan, T., Temsah, R., Osada, M., Dhalla, N.S., 1999. Status of Ca^{2+}/calmodulin protein kinase phosphorylation of cardiac SR proteins in ischemia-reperfusion. Am. J. Physiol. 277, C384–C391.

Nohl, H., Hegner, D., 1978. Do mitochondria produce oxygen radicals in vivo? Eur. J. Biochem. 82, 563–567.

Oberley, T.D., 2002. Oxidative damage and cancer. Am. J. Pathol. 160, 1–6.

O'Donnell, V.B., Freeman, B.A., 2001. Interactions between nitric oxide and lipid oxidation pathways: implications for vascular disease. Circ. Res. 88, 12–21.

Okado-Matsumoto, A., Fridovich, I., 2001. Subcellular distribution of superoxide dismutases (SOD) in rat liver. J. Biol. Chem. 276, 38388–38393.

Olson, R.D., Mushlin, P.S., Brenner, D.E., Fleischer, S., Cusack, B.J. Chang, B.K., Boucek Jr., R.J., 1988. Doxorubicin cardiotoxicity may be caused by its metabolite, doxorubicinol. Proc. Natl. Acad. Sci. U. S. A. 85, 3585–3589.

Orr, W.C., Sohal, R.S., 1994. Extension of life-span by overexpression of superoxide dismutase and catalase in *Drosophila melanogaster*. Science 263, 1128–1130.

Oury, T.D., Ho, Y.-S., Piantadosi, C.A., Crapo, J.D., 1992. Extracellular superoxide dismutase, nitric oxide, and central nervous system O_2 toxicity. Proc. Natl. Acad. Sci. U. S. A. 89, 9715–9719.

Oury, T.D., Day, B.J., Crapo, J.D., 1996. Extracellular superoxide dismutase: a regulator of nitric oxide bioavailability. Lab. Invest. 75, 617–636.

Palmeira, C.M., Serrano, J., Kuehl, D.W., Wallace, K.B., 1997. Preferential oxidation of cardiac mitochondrial DNA following acute intoxication with doxorubicin. Biochim. Biophys. Acta 1321, 101–106.

Papadopoulou, L.C., Theophilidis, G., Thomopoulos, G.N., Tsiftsoglou, A.S., 1999. Structural and functional impairment of mitochondria in adriamycin-induced cardiomyopathy in mice: suppression of cytochrome *c* oxidase II gene expression. Biochem. Pharmacol. 57, 481–489.

Perry, A.C.F., Jones, R., Hall, L., 1993. Isolation and characterization of a rat cDNA clone encoding a secreted superoxide dismutase reveals the epididymis to be a major site of its expression. J. Biochem. 293, 21–25.

Pfeiffer, S., Mayer, B., Hemmens, B., 1999. Nitric oxide: chemical puzzles posed by a biological messenger. Angew. Chem. Int. Ed. Engl. 38, 1714–1731.

Praet, M., Ruysschaert, J.M., 1993. In-vivo and in-vitro mitochondrial membrane damages induced in mice by adriamycin and derivatives. Biochim. Biophys. Acta 1149, 79–85.

Prasad, K., Lee, P., Mantha, S.V., Kalra, J., Prasad, M., Gupta, J.B., 1992. Detection of ischemia-reperfusion cardiac injury by cardiac muscle chemiluminescence. Mol. Cell. Biochem. 115, 49–58.

Price, D.L., Becher, M.W., Wong, P.C., Borchelt, R., Lee, M.K., Sisidia, S.S., 1996. Inherited neurodegenerative diseases and transgenic models. Brain Pathol. 6, 467–480.

Pritchett, G., Cohen, H.J., Rao, K.M.K., Cobb, F., Sullivan, M., Currie, M.S., 1995. Tumor necrosis factor, natural killer activity and other measures of immune function and inflammation in elderly men with heart failure. Gerontology 41, 45–56.

Rabelo, E., De Angelis, K., Bock, P., Gatelli Fernandes, T., Cervo, F., Bello Klein, A., Clausell, N., Claudia Irigoyen, M., 2001. Baroreflex sensitivity and oxidative stress in adriamycin-induced heart failure. Hypertension 38, 576–580.

Raha, S., Robinson, B.H., 2001. Mitochondria, oxygen free radicals, and apoptosis. Am. J. Med. Genet. 106, 62–70.

Raha, S., McEachern, G.E., Myint, A.T., Robinson, B.H., 2000. Superoxides from mitochondrial complex III: the role of manganese superoxide dismutase. Free Radic. Biol. Med. 29, 170–180.

Sato, S., Iwaizumi, M., Handa, K., Tamura, Y., 1977. Electron spin resonance study on the mode of generation of free radicals of daunomycin, adriamycin, and carboquone in NAD(P)H–microsome system. Gann 68, 603–608.

Sawada, M., Carlson, J.C., 1987. Changes in superoxide radical and lipid peroxide formation in the brain, heart and liver during the lifetime of the rat. Mech. Ageing Dev. 41, 125–137.

Sawyer, D.B., Colucci, W.S., 2000. Mitochondrial oxidative stress in heart failure. "Oxygen wastage" revisited. Circ. Res. 86, 119–120.

Schatz, G., Butow, R.A., 1983. How are proteins imported into mitochondria? Cell 32, 316–318.

Sethi, R., Takeda, N., Nagano, M., Dhalla, N.S., 2000. Beneficial effects of vitamin E treatment in acute myocardial infarction. J. Cardiovasc. Pharmacol. Ther. 5, 51–58.

Shao, Q., Matsubara, T., Bhatt, S.K., Dhalla, N.S., 1995. Inhibition of cardiac sarcolemma Na(+)−K+ ATPase by oxyradical generating systems. Mol. Cell. Biochem. 147, 139–144.

Shefner, J.M., Reaume, A.G., Flood, D.G., Scott, R.W., Kowall, N.W., Ferrante, R.J., Siwek, D.F., Upton-Rice, M., Brown Jr., R.H., 1999. Mice lacking cytosolic copper/zinc superoxide dismutase display a distinctive motor axonopathy. Neurology 53, 1239–1246.

Sherman, L., Dafni, N., Lieman-Hurwitz, J., Groner, Y., 1983. Nucleotide sequence and expression of human chromosome 21-encoded superoxide dismutase mRNA. Proc. Natl. Acad. Sci. U. S. A. 80, 5465–5469.

Sherman, L., Levanon, D., Lieman-Hurwitz, J., Dafni, N., Groner, Y., 1984. Human Cu/Zn superoxide dismutase gene: molecular characterization of its two mRNA species. Nucl. Acids Res. 12, 9349–9365.

Shimpo, K., Nagatsu, T., Yamada, K., Sato, T., Niimi, H., Shamoto, M., Takeuchi, T., Umezawa, H., Fujita, K., 1991. Ascorbic acid and adriamycin toxicity. Am. J. Clin. Nutr. 54, 1298S–1301S.

Sies, H., 1991. Oxidative Stress, Oxidants and Antioxidants. Academic Press, San Diego, CA, pp. XV–XXII.

Singal, P.K., 2000. Adriamycin-induced heart failure: mechanism and modulation. Mol. Cell. Biochem. 207, 77–85.

Singal, P.K., Tong, J.G., 1988. Vitamin E deficiency accentuates adriamycin-induced cardiomyopathy and cell surface changes. Mol. Cell. Biochem. 84, 163–171.

Siwik, D.A., Tzortzis, J.D., Pimental, D.R., Chang, D.L.-F., Pagano, P.J., Singh, K., Sawyer, D.B., Colucci, W.S., 1999. Inhibition of copper–zinc superoxide dismutase induces cell growth, hypertrophic phenotype, and apoptosis in neonatal rat cardiac myocytes in vitro. Circ. Res. 85, 147–153.

Siwik, D.A., Pagano, P.J., Colucci, W.S., 2001. Oxidative stress regulates collagen synthesis and matrix metalloproteinase activity in cardiac fibroblasts. Am. J. Physiol. Cell Physiol. 280, C53–C60.

Sohal, R.S., Ku, H.H., Agarwal, S., Forster, M.J., Lal, H., 1994. Oxidative damage, mitochondrial oxidant generation and antioxidant defenses during aging and in response to food restriction in the mouse. Mech. Ageing Dev. 74, 121–133.

Solem, L.E., Henry, T.R., Wallace, K.B., 1994. Disruption of mitochondrial calcium homeostasis following chronic doxorubicin administration. Toxicol. Appl. Pharmacol. 129, 214–222.

Speranza, M.J., Bagley, A.C., Lynch, R.E., 1993. Cells enriched for catalase are sensitized to the toxicities of bleomycin, adriamycin, and paraquat. J. Biol. Chem. 268, 19039–19043.

St. Clair, D.K., 2001. Antioxidants and Free Radicals in Health and Disease. Prominent Press, Arizona.

Suh, J.H., Shigeno, E.T., Morrow, J.D., Cox, B., Rocha, A.E., Frei, B., Hagen, T.M., 2001. Oxidative stress in the ageing rat heart is reversed by dietary supplementation with (*R*)-α-lipoic acid. FASEB J. 15, 700–706.

Sun, X., Zhou, Z., Kang, Y.J., 2001. Attenuation of doxorubicin chronic toxicity in metallothionein-overexpressing transgenic mouse heart. Cancer Res. 61, 3382–3387.

Tainer, J.A., Getzoff, E.D., Beem, K.M., Richardson, J.S., Richardson, D.C., 1982. Determination and analysis of the 2 angstrom structure of copper, zinc superoxide dismutase. J. Mol. Biol. 160, 181–217.

Temsah, R.M., Netticadan, T., Chapman, D., Takeda, S., Mochizuki, S., Dhalla, N.S., 1999. Alterations in sarcoplasmic reticulum function and gene expression in ischemic-reperfused rat heart. Am. J. Physiol. 277, H584–H594.

Tippett, P., Kaplan, J.C., 1986. Report of the committee on the genetic constitution of chromosomes 20, 21, and 22. Cytogenet. Cell Genet. 40, 268–295.

Torre-Amione, G., Kapadia, S., Benedict, C.R., Oral, H., Young, J.B., Mann, D.L., 1996. Proinflammatory cytokine levels in patients with depressed left ventricular ejection fraction: a report from the studies of left ventricular dysfunction (SOLVD) J. Am. Coll. Cardiol. 27, 1201–1206.

Uma Devi, P., 1983. Chemical radiation protection by alpha-mercaptopropionylglycine. J. Nucl. Med. Allied Sci. 27, 327–336.

Vaidyanathan, S., Boroujerdi, M., 2000. Effect of tamoxifen pretreatment on the pharmacokinetics, metabolism and cardiotoxicity of doxorubicin in female rats. Cancer Chemother. Pharmacol. 46, 185–192.

Van Acker, F.A., Hulshof, J.W., Haenen, G.R., Menge, W.M., Van der Vijgh, W.J., Bast, A., 2001. New synthetic flavonoids as potent protectors against doxorubicin-induced cardiotoxicity. Free Radic. Biol. Med. 31, 31–37.

Van Remmen, H., Williams, M.D., Guo, Z., Estlack, L., Yang, H., Carlson, E.J., Epstein, C.J., Huang, T.T., Richardson, A., 2001. Knockout mice heterozygous for $Sod2$ show alterations in cardiac mitochondrial function and apoptosis. Am. J. Physiol. Heart Circ. Physiol. 281, H1422–H1432.

Vásquez-Vivar, J., Martasek, P., Hogg, N., Masters, B.A., Pritchard, K.A., Kalyanaraman, B., 1997. Endothelial nitric oxide synthase-dependent superoxide generation from adriamycin. Biochemistry 36, 11293–11297.

Von Harsdorf, R., Li, P.F., Dietz, R., 1999. Signaling pathways in reactive oxygen species-induced cardiomyocyte apoptosis. Circulation 99, 2934–2941.

Von Hoff, D.D., Howser, D., Lewis, B.J., Holcenberg, J., Weiss, R.B., Young, R.C., 1981. Phase I study of ICRF-187 using a daily for 3 days schedule. Cancer Treat. Rep. 65, 249–252.

Wagner, U.G., Pattridge, K.A., Judwig, M.L., Stallings, W.C., Werber, M.W., Oefner, C., Frolow, F., Sussman, J.L., 1993. Comparison of the crystal structures of genetically engineered human manganese superoxide dismutase and manganese superoxide dismutase from the $Thermus$ $thermophilus$: differences in dimer–dimer interaction. Protein Sci. 2, 814–825.

Wan, X.S., Devalaraja, M.N., St. Clair, D.K., 1994. Molecular structure and organization of the human manganese superoxide dismutase gene. DNA Cell Biol. 13, 1127–1136.

Wang, D., Yang, X.P., Liu, Y.H., Carretero, O.A., LaPointe, M.C., 1999. Reduction of myocardial infarct size by inhibition of inducible nitric oxide synthase. Am. J. Hypertens. 12, 174–182.

Wang, P., Zweier, J.L., 1996. Measurement of nitric oxide and peroxynitrite generation in the postischemic heart. Evidence for peroxynitrite-mediated reperfusion injury. J. Biol. Chem. 271, 29223–29230.

Wattanapitayakul, S.K., Bauer, J.A., 2001. Oxidative pathways in cardiovascular disease: roles, mechanisms, and therapeutic implications. Pharmacol. Ther. 89, 187–206.

Weinstein, D.M., Mihm, M.J., Bauer, J.A., 2000. Cardiac peroxynitrite formation and left ventricular dysfunction following doxorubicin treatment in mice. J. Pharmacol. Exp. Ther. 294, 396–401.

Weisiger, R.A., Fridovich, I., 1973. Superoxide dismutase. Organelle specificity. J. Biol. Chem. 248, 3582–3592.

Willems, J.A., Zwijsen, H., Slegers, S., Nicolai, J., Bettadpura, J., Raymackers, J., Scarcez, T., 1993. Purification and sequence of rat extracellular superoxide dismutase B secreted by C_6 glioma. J. Biol. Chem. 268, 24614–24621.

Williams, R.E., Zweier, J.L., Flaherty, J.T., 1991. Treatment with deferoxamine during ischemia improves functional and metabolic recovery and reduces reperfusion-induced oxygen radical generation in rabbit hearts. Circulation 83, 1006–1014.

Wispe, J.R., Warner, B.B., Clark, J.C., Dey, C.R., Neuman, J., Glasser, S.W., Crapo, J.D., Chang, L.Y., Whitsett, J.A., 1992. Human Mn-superoxide dismutase in pulmonary epithelial cells of transgenic mice confers protection from oxygen injury. J. Biol. Chem. 267, 23937–23941.

Wong, G.H.W., Goeddel, D.V., 1988. Induction of manganous superoxide dismutase by tumor necrosis factor: possible protective mechanism. Science 242, 941–944.

Woo, Y.J., Zhang, J.C., Vijayasarathy, C., Zwacka, R.M., Englehardt, J.F., Gardner, T.J., Sweeney, H.L., 1998. Recombinant adenovirus-mediated cardiac gene transfer of superoxide dismutase and catalase attenuates postischemic contractile dysfunction. Circulation 98, II255–II260.

Xu, K.Y., Zweier, J.L., Becker, L.C., 1997. Hydroxyl radical inhibits sarcoplasmic reticulum Ca(2+)-ATPase function by direct attack on the ATP binding site. Circ. Res. 80, 76–81.

Xu, Y., Kiningham, K.K., Devalaraja, M.N., Yeh, C.C., Majima, H., Kasarskis, E.J., St. Clair, D.K., 1999. An intronic NFκB element is essential for induction of the human manganese superoxide dismutase gene by tumor necrosis factor alpha and interleukin-1β. DNA Cell Biol. 18, 709–722.

Yeh, C.C., Wan, X.S., St. Clair, D.K., 1998. Transcriptional regulation of the 5′ proximal promoter of the human manganese superoxide dismutase gene. DNA Cell Biol. 17, 921–930.

Yen, H.-C., St. Clair, D.K., 1997. Transgenic and knockout mice in the study of superoxide dismutases. J. Biomed. Lab. Sci. 9, 40–54.

Yen, H.-C., Oberley, T.D., Vichitbandha, S., Ho, Y.-S., St. Clair, D.K., 1996. The protective role of manganese superoxide dismutase against adriamycin-induced acute cardiac toxicity in transgenic mice. J. Clin. Invest. 98, 1253–1260.

Yen, H.C., Oberley, T.D., Gairola, C.G., Szweda, L.I., St. Clair, D.K., 1999. Manganese superoxide dismutase protects mitochondrial complex I against adriamycin-induced cardiomyopathy in transgenic mice. Arch. Biochem. Biophys. 362, 59–66.

Yoda, Y., Nakazawa, M., Abe, T., Kawakami, Z., 1986. Prevention of doxorubicin myocardial toxicity in mice by reduced glutathione. Cancer Res. 46, 2551–2556.

Yoshida, T., Watanabe, M., Engelman, D.T., Engelman, R.M., Schley, J.A., Maulik, N., Ho, Y.S., Oberley, T.D., Das, D.K., 1996. Transgenic mice overexpressing glutathione peroxidase are resistant to myocardial ischemia reperfusion injury. J. Mol. Cell. Cardiol. 28, 1759–1767.

Yoshida, T., Maulik, N., Engelman, R.M., Ho, Y.S., Magnenat, J.L., Rousou, J.A., Flack, J.E., Deaton, D., Das, D.K., 1997. Glutathione peroxidase knockout mice are susceptible to myocardial ischemia reperfusion injury. Circulation 96, II216–II220.

Yoshida, T., Maulik, N., Engelman, R.M., Ho, Y.S., Das, D.K., 2000. Targeted disruption of the mouse Sod I gene makes the hearts vulnerable to ischemic reperfusion injury. Circ. Res. 86, 264–269.

Yost Jr., F.J., Fridovich, I., 1973. An iron-containing superoxide dismutase from *Escherichia coli*. J. Biol. Chem. 248, 4905–4908.

Young, R.C., Ozols, R.F., Myers, C.E., 1981. The anthracycline antineoplastic drugs. N. Engl. J. Med. 305, 139–153.

Yu, B.P., 1994. Cellular defenses against damage from reactive oxygen species. Physiol. Rev. 74, 139–162.

Zhou, S., Palmeira, C.M., Wallace, K.B., 2001a. Doxorubicin-induced persistent oxidative stress to cardiac myocytes. Toxicol. Lett. 121, 151–157.

Zhou, S., Starkov, A., Froberg, M.K., Leino, R.L., Wallace, K.B., 2001b. Cumulative and irreversible cardiac mitochondrial dysfunction induced by doxorubicin. Cancer Res. 61, 771–777.

Zweier, J.L., 1984. Reduction of O_2 by iron-adriamycin. J. Biol. Chem. 259, 6056–6058.

Zweier, J.L., Kuppusamy, P., Williams, R., Rayburn, B.K., Smith, D., Weisfeldt, M.L., Flaherty, J.T., 1989. Measurement and characterization of postischemic free radical generation in the isolated perfused heart. J. Biol. Chem. 264, 18890–18895.

**Advances in
Cell Aging and
Gerontology**

Aging and the Red Cell

Joseph M. Rifkind*, O.O. Abugo, Enika Nagababu, Somasundaram Ramasamy, Andrew Demehin and Rajadas Jayakumar

*Molecular Dynamics Section, National Institute on Aging, National Institutes of Health,
5600 Nathan Shock Drive, Baltimore, MD 21224, USA*

Contents

Abbreviations

ESI	excess surface area index
GSH	glutathione
NADH	nicotinamide adenine dinucleotide (reduced form)

* Corresponding author.
E-mail address: rifkindj@grc.nia.nih.gov (J.M. Rifkind).

Advances in Cell Aging and Gerontology, vol. 11, 283–307

NADPH	nicotinamide adenine dinucleotide phosphate (reduced form)
SOD	superoxide dismutase
IgG	immunoglobulin G
ROS	reactive oxygen species
βAP	amyloid beta protein

1. Introduction

Red cells are essential for the transport of oxygen from the lungs to the tissues. In the lungs, the red cell hemoglobin becomes fully oxygenated picking up four oxygen molecules. The oxygenated blood goes back to the heart and is pumped through the circulatory system releasing oxygen to the tissues as it passes through the micro-circulation at a lower partial pressure of oxygen. In the circulation, the red cell undergoes environmental stress. It undergoes extreme fluctuations in oxygen pressure and attack by oxygen radicals from inside the cell and outside the cell. In order to pass through the narrow capillaries with pore sizes less than the diameter of the red cell, it undergoes drastic shear forces and shape changes (deformability) necessary to traverse these pores. It is, therefore, not surprising that in order to maintain functional red cells, the cells have a relatively short life span (120 d in humans) and are continuously being replenished by new cells.

In this article, we will discuss the relationship of the red cell to the deleterious changes, which take place as individuals age. Because of the short life span of red cells, a distribution of cells with different cellular ages is always present. Chronological aging and the red cell cannot be discussed without taking into consideration the aging of the red cell and possible changes in the cellular aging process.

The role of the red cell on aging involves two factors. (1) Possible age induced changes in the erythropoietic system responsible for the formation of red cells. Are the cells in older individuals, therefore, less efficient in performing the crucial roles of the red cell? These may involve functional decrements in the newly formed cells and/or changes in these cells, which affect the ability of the cell to deal with stress. (2) Does the red cell released into circulation in older individuals undergo more rapid changes, which affect red cell function? These changes can result from alterations in the red cell, vascular changes that influence pore sizes and shear stresses as well as extracellular changes, which influence the composition of the plasma and the oxidative stress experienced by the red cell.

There is extensive literature on cellular aging of the red cell (Clark, 1988; Danon and Marikovsky, 1988). A number of properties of the red cell have been reported to change during cellular aging including enzyme activities (Brok et al., 1996; Shimizu and Susuki, 1991), membrane structure (Bartosz, 1991; Suzuki and Dale, 1989; Low et al., 1985; Rifkind et al., 1985), anion and cation transport (Romero and Romero, 1999; Aiken et al., 1992; Park et al., 1999), cell volume (Waugh et al., 1997), surface charge (Danon et al., 1983), deformability (Waugh et al., 1992; Sutera et al., 1985; Nash and Wyard, 1981; Bartosz et al., 1982), fragility (Bartosz, 1982; Rifkind et al., 1983), membrane potential (Grzelinska and Bartosz, 1988) and exposure of antigenic sites (Kay, 1990; Graldi et al., 1999).

In the study of cellular aging, the focus has been on the changes that are responsible for the removal of the cell from circulation, and not necessarily on changes that affect the ability of the circulating red cells to adequately deliver oxygen. Metabolic changes, which influence transport, and thereby, the size of the cell and cell deformability and fragility, can influence the removal of cells by the reticuloendothelial system. Changes in surface charge, rearrangements of red cell proteins as well as oxidative damage to membrane proteins may lead to the exposure of new antigenic sites on the red cell membrane, which bind IgG (Kay, 1978; Rettig et al., 1999) and result in the eventual removal of senescent red cells by macrophages. While the cells removed from circulation generally exhibit impaired function, the processes, which trigger the removal of the cell from circulation, are not directly related to a loss in cell function.

In evaluating the contribution of red cells to individual aging, the emphasis is on changes that impair the function of the red cells still retained in circulation. The more rapid removal of cells from circulation, as long as the supply of red cells can be replenished, results in a younger distribution of cells, which may actually have improved functional capabilities.

2. Hematopoietic changes

2.1. *Alterations in hematopoiesis during aging*

Hemopoiesis involves pluripotential cells that produce multipotential stem cells that differentiate into progenitor-committed cells and finally red cells, white cells and platelets (Chatta and Dale, 1996; Baldwin, 1988). Proliferation and differentiation (Kaushansky and Karplus, 1993) requires intimate contact between stem cells, stromal cells and the extracellular matrix and is mediated by a number of growth factors and cytokines. Basal hematological parameters generally show no change with age (Globerson, 1999) indicating that the hematopoietic system is able to maintain the necessary level of blood cells even during aging. However, there is evidence, both in animals and humans, that the reserve capacity under conditions requiring extensive hematopoietic function is compromised in the aged (Lipschitz, 1995). This phenomenon is seen as a decrease in the erythropoietic response to iron deficiency anemia in the elderly (Matsuo et al., 1995) and a blunted erythropoietic response to hemorrhage in aged mice (Boggs and Patrene, 1985).

Although the specific changes responsible for the decrease in reserve capacity have not been established, age dependent decrements have been reported at every stage of the hemopoiesis process (Balducci et al., 2001). Thus, a decrease in progenitor cells (Hirota et al., 1988) and their proliferative ability (Marley et al., 1999) have been reported. In addition, there are changes in the marrow microenvironment (Boggs et al., 1984; Lee et al., 1989) and decreases in regulatory growth factors (Buchanan et al., 1996).

2.2. *Changes in red cell life span during aging*

The lower reserve capacity in older subjects is coupled with a greater demand on the hemopoietic system. This is indicated by a shorter red cell life span in mice, rats, rabbits and humans. [59]Fe labeling of WF rats (Glass et al., 1983) indicates that the life span decreases from 40 d for 6-month-old rats to 25 d in 27–31-month-old rats. [59]Fe labeling of C57/BL6J mice indicates that the 50% survival time decreases from 52 d for 10-month-old mice to 20 d for 37-month-old mice (Abraham et al., 1978). [51]Cr labeling, which does not have the same problem of reutilization as ^{59}Fe labeling, has been used to determine the effect of aging on the red cell life span in BALB/c mice (Magnani et al., 1988) and SPF line "white Russian" rabbits (Vomel and Platt, 1981). For the mice, the half-life decreased from 12 to 8 d and in rabbits, it was found that the Cr labeled red cells from a young animal remained in the circulation three times longer. In these chromium-labeling studies, the investigators injected labeled cells from young and old donors into young and old animals. In this way, the effect of aging on both the red cells and the reticuloendothelial system could be delineated. In the mouse study, the age of the recipient had no effect, while in the rabbit study the red cells were removed more rapidly in the older animals.

Labeling studies have not been performed on humans. However, evidence for a shorter life span is indicated by increased levels of reticulocytes (Glass et al., 1985), an increase, in the less dense, presumably younger cells and decreased activity of aspartate amino transferase (Shperling and Danon, 1990) which decreases linearly with age of the cell (Brok et al., 1996).

2.3. *Stress erythropoiesis*

The attempt to maintain an adequate blood supply in the older organism places stress on the hemopoietic system, which is already impaired (see above). Although the hematocrit is generally maintained in older individuals, the higher incidence of non-explained anemia in the elderly (Carmel, 2001; Baldwin, 1988; Timiras and Brownstein, 1987; Hershko et al., 1979) has been attributed to the impaired reserve capacity, which is stressed by the greater demand to resupply the short-lived red cells in older subjects.

However, it is also necessary to consider the changes in the red cells produced under stress in older subjects (Rifkind et al., 1999). Red cell changes including larger cells, which were less deformable and had a shorter life span, have been reported to take place when the hemopoietic system is stressed. This phenomenon was found following hemorrhage (Brecher et al., 1975), after phenylhydrazine-induced anemia (Stohlman, 1961) and after treatment with erythropoietin (Norton, 1990; Rifkind, 1999). In older individuals, the decreased reserve capacity coupled with a higher demand for red cell production would be expected to exacerbate the red cell changes attributed to stress erythropoiesis. The finding that the stress of chronic erythropoietin treatment is more pronounced in older rats than in younger rats (Rifkind et al., 1999) supports this contention.

2.4. *Altered properties of cells released into the circulation during aging*

On the basis of differences in the properties of cells separated by both Percoll gradients and Stractan gradients (Glass et al., 1983; Glass and Gershon, 1984; Glass et al., 1985; Gershon and Gershon, 1988), it has been proposed that the red cells entering the circulation in older subjects are impaired. Thus, an appreciable decrease in the activity of enzymes has been found in the least dense (youngest) fraction of red cells from old subjects when compared with the same fraction of cells from young subjects. In fact, the levels of enzyme activities in the youngest fraction of cells from old subjects are frequently comparable to that of the densest (oldest) fraction of cells from young subjects. In old rats, the decreased activity in the youngest cells includes the activity of glucose-6-phosphate dehydrogenase, catalase, glutathione reductase, glutathione peroxidase and superoxide dismutase. In humans, the least dense fraction in old subjects has decreased activity of superoxide dismutase, aldolase, pyruvate kinase, 5′-pyrimidine nucleotidase, Na–K ATPase and acetylcholine esterase. Most of the decreased enzyme activities reported by Gershon and collaborators involve enzymes that are necessary to protect the red cell from oxidative stress. They have, therefore, proposed (Gershon and Gershon, 1988) that the red cells entering the circulation in old subjects are impaired and less able to deal with the oxidative stress experienced as the cells pass through the circulation.

We have expanded on these studies by comparing the red cell volumes of the 1% least dense cells of rats. In the earlier studies, the fraction of cells included in the least dense fraction corresponded to the entire lowest density band obtained using Percoll gradients. This band, which contains a range of cell densities, contains more cells in the old subjects than in the young subjects because of the shorter life span in old subjects (see above). In humans this fraction contains 25% of the cells and in rats as much as 50% of the cells. In order to study the actual least dense, and presumably the youngest cells, we have limited our measurements to the 1% least dense cells, which contained no detectable reticulocytes. We obtained a significant increase in the mean cell volume of this fraction in F344 Fischer rats from 47.1 ± 1.1 in 6–7 months rats to 51.6 ± 1.7 in 23–26 months rats (Table 1). In addition, the total surface area increased and the cells were found to have a lower excess surface area index (ESI) indicating that the cells are more spherical in old rats than in young rats. We also confirmed these measurements using biotin labeling to separate the youngest cells instead of density. The cells of the rat were first fully labeled with biotin. Two days later, the new cells entering into the circulation, which were not labeled with biotin, were separated using streptavidin magnetic beads (Rettig et al., 1999) and again the youngest cells in old rats were found to be larger and more spherical than those in the young rat.

This increase in mean cell volume and sphericity mimics the larger less deformable cells formed during stressed erythropoiesis, and is consistent with the hypothesis that the changes in the cells entering the circulation in old subjects are at least in part due to stressed erythropoiesis. While the decreased enzyme activities in the youngest fraction of cells in old subjects impair the ability of the cell to deal with oxidative stress, the increased cell volume, increased sphericity and associated decreased

Table 1
Red cell shape factors for young and old rats[a] separated by density

Age (months)	Young (6–7)	Old (23–26)
Mean cell volume (YF)[b,d] (fl)	47.1 ± 1.1^{g}	51.6 ± 1.7
Mean cell volume (OF)[c,d] (fl)	45.2 ± 1.0	49.6 ± 1.6
Surface area (YF)[b] (μm^2)	87.9 ± 1.7	90.0 ± 3.9
Surface area (OF)[c] (μm^2)	79.1 ± 3.0	80.1 ± 3.8
ESI[e] (YF)	1.40 ± 0.01	1.35 ± 0.08
ESI[e] (OF)[f]	1.29 ± 0.04	1.23 ± 0.05

[a] Fischer 344 rats.
[b] YF is the 1% least dense cells separated by Percoll gradient.
[c] OF is the 1% most dense cells separated by Percoll gradient.
[d] The cells from young and old rats were significantly different by a two tailed t-test, $P < 0.001$.
[e] ESI is the excess surface area index, which is the ratio of the surface area to the surface area of a sphere with a volume equal to the mean cell volume.
[f] The cells from young and old rats were significantly different by a two tailed t-test, $P < 0.05$.
[g] Values given are means $\pm$ standard deviation.

deformability is expected to actually increase the oxidative stress experienced by the cells. The decreased deformability of these larger more spherical cells slows down the passage of cells through the microcirculation resulting in increased deoxygenation of hemoglobin in these cells. Since increased deoxygenation of hemoglobin increases the rate of hemoglobin autoxidation and the associated production of superoxide (Fig. 1),

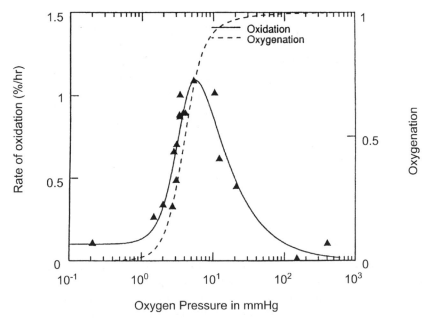

Fig. 1.   Autoxidation of hemoglobin as a function of the oxygen pressure.

this hypoxic stress resulting from larger less deformable cells produces oxidative stress. This coupled with the decreased activity of the antioxidant enzymes in these cells makes the red cells in older subjects more susceptible to oxidative damage.

3. Changes in red cells during aging

3.1. *Methodological problems associated with aging results*

A number of changes have been reported to take place when comparing young and old subjects. It is important to recognize that for many of the measurements there are conflicting results in the literature. While some of these differences may depend on the methods used by various investigators, there are a number of other non-trivial factors that contribute to variability in aging results.

Aging can affect red cells differently in males and females as well as in different species. Thus, in mice, the mean cell volume decreases (Magnani et al., 1988) and in humans (Araki and Rifkind, 1980a), the mean cell volume increases. Many parameters are affected by diseases, and, particularly in an older population, results can depend on how rigorously diseased subjects were eliminated. Finally changes reported are not necessarily linear with respect to age. Therefore, different results can be obtained depending on the range of ages studied.

One important example of this factor is with regard to red cell glutathione (GSH). A number of studies have been performed both on humans and animals and a decrease in red cell glutathione has usually been reported (Al-Turk et al., 1987; Hazelton and Lang, 1985; Farooqui et al., 1987; Matsubara and Machado, 1991). A recent paper by Kasapoglu and Ozben (2001), however, did not report a change in GSH. This study was, however, limited to subjects ranging in age from 20 to 69. The limited age range can possibly explain the absence of a drop in glutathione during aging in this study. In a study (Lang et al., 1992), where the changes in glutathione during aging were analyzed with respect to different age groups, the highest prevalence of low glutathione levels was found in the age group 60–79 years old, with much smaller differences in the other age groups. Similar findings were found in mice (Abraham et al., 1978), for which glutathione levels increase between 10 and 20 months of age and decrease later, with the most dramatic decrease after 30 months of age.

These various factors frequently make it difficult to analyze age dependent changes. Although these questions are important in evaluating the significance of age dependent differences, it is beyond the scope of this review to critically evaluate every study referred to.

3.2. *Younger age distribution*

Many of the reported changes with subject age can be attributed to a younger distribution of cellular ages. This includes density distribution (Shperling and Danon, 1990; Pinkofsky, 1997), changes in enzyme activities such as aspartate amino transferase, hexokinase, glucose-6-phosphate dehydrogenase, pyruvate kinase and glutamate-oxaloacetate transaminase (Glass and Gershon, 1984; Gershon and

Gershon, 1988; Shperling and Danon, 1990; Magnani et al., 1988), increased charge density (Abe et al., 1984) and the associated agglutination (Shperling and Danon, 1990). In a comparison of 6- and 24-month Fischer 344 rats, we found a number of changes, which reflect a younger distribution of cells. We confirmed the previously reported age dependent decrease in density and increase in aspartate amino transferase (Shperling and Danon, 1990), and also found an increase in glycosylated hemoglobin reflecting a longer exposure of the hemoglobin to glucose (Krzisnik and Lukac-Bajalo, 1993; Elseweidy et al., 1983).

3.3. *Oxidative stress*

Most of the reported changes in the red cell as a function of subject age that are not attributed to a younger distribution of cellular ages are indicative of oxidative stress. A decrease in the reductive capacity of red cells has been reported (Al-Turk et al., 1987; Hazelton and Lang, 1985; Farooqui et al., 1987; Matsubara and Machado, 1991; Berr et al., 1993) as indicated by a decrease in GSH, total thiols, NADH, NADPH and selenium. In a recent report (Demehin et al., 2001), it has been shown that the red cell membrane antioxidant capacity, which protects the cell from oxidative damage decreases during aging. The activities of a number of enzymes, including a number of antioxidant enzymes, decrease during aging resulting in cells being more susceptible to oxidative damage. The enzymes, which decrease in activity, include superoxide dismutase, glutathione reductase, glutathione peroxidase, catalase and glucose-6-phosphate dehydrogenase (Glass and Gershon, 1984; Gershon and Gershon, 1988; Perrin et al., 1990).

In a study of superoxide dismutase in rat erythrocytes (Glass and Gershon, 1981), it was found that in addition to the decreased activity, there was evidence of damaged enzyme. This was indicated by a decrease in catalytic activity per unit enzyme antigen determined by the use of monospecific rabbit anti-rat superoxide dismutase (SOD) IgG. These studies suggest that old animals contain significant amounts of catalytically altered molecules, implying that the decrease in enzyme activities found in old animals represents oxidative damage of these enzymes. Oxidative damage to red cell proteins is also implied by the decrease in hemoglobin content of red cells in older subjects.

Evidence for increased susceptibility to oxidative stress of red cells from older subjects has been shown in experiments where the red cells were stressed. Thus, Tyan (1982) has shown that when blood from old mice is subjected to oxidative stress by adding sodium ascorbate, the red cells accumulate more methemoglobin and undergo increased lysis. Glass and Gershon (1984) found a decrease in the inability of red cells from old rats to exclude trypan blue when treated with xanthine/xanthine oxidase.

Increased oxidative damage during aging is indicated by increased lipid peroxidation, red cell rigidity and lysis (Glass and Gershon, 1984; Rifkind et al., 1997; Ajmani et al., 2000; Detraglia et al., 1974) as well as increased binding of IgG associated with exposure of a senescent antigen on the red cell (Danon and Marikovsky, 1988; Glass et al., 1985; Gershon and Gershon, 1988). We have confirmed a link between IgG binding and oxidative stress by showing that cells treated with hydrogen peroxide or phenylhydrazine bind more IgG. The possible involvement of heme degradation products is suggested by the finding that oxidation of the hemoglobin, which prevents the formation of heme degradation products, decreases the effect of hydrogen peroxide.

Lipid peroxidation is a direct measure of oxidative damage to the bilayer. Red cell rigidity depends on both the rigidity of the lipid bilayer as well as on the protein matrix. A change in deformability as a measure of rigidity has been related to hydrogen peroxide induced crosslinking of membrane proteins (Snyder et al., 1985). Rigidity associated with the lipid bilayer will be affected by lipid peroxidation as well as by changes in the composition of the bilayer. In addition to increased lipid peroxidation, the age dependent increase in red cell cholesterol (Araki and Rifkind, 1980b) can increase red cell rigidity (Peddada et al., 1997). Red cell cholesterol is thought to be determined by an increase in the level of plasma cholesterol (Araki and Rifkind, 1980b). It has, however, been suggested that the accumulation of cholesterol is also associated with oxidative stress (Gesquiere et al., 1999). The exposure of the senescent antigen has been attributed to oxidative damage to band 3 of the red cell membrane (Kay et al., 1986; Beppu et al., 1990).

Decreases in red cell deformability during aging have been reported (Avellone et al., 1993; Tozzi-Ciancarelli et al., 1989; Franzini et al., 1988; Abe et al., 1984; Ajmani and Rifkind, 1998). These changes are in part related to an increase in membrane rigidity (Rifkind et al., 1997) and an increase in the shear modulus of elasticity of the bilayer (Rifkind et al., 1999). The increased deformability also depends on the change in the size and shape of the cell, which limit the ability of the cell to deform as the cell passes through narrow pores.

We have recently completed a study on rats in order to determine the factors, which contribute to the decreased deformability during aging. Table 2 shows a decrease in deformability as indicated by the time necessary to pass through a 5-μ pore. In addition, it is found that there is an appreciably larger fraction of cells with a particularly long transit time. In attempting to evaluate the factors contributing to

Table 2
Effect of age on red cell deformability in rats[a]

Age (months)	Young (4–7)	Old (23–26)
Mean cell transit time (ms)[c]	1.941 ± 0.028[b]	2.033 ± 0.045
Percent slow cells (>2.3 ms)[e]	9.0 ± 1.1	13.2 ± 4.0
Shear modulus (dynes/cm $\times 10^3$)[c]	4.8 ± 0.3	14.8 ± 1.8
Mean cell volume (fl)[c]	46.4 ± 1.1	50.7 ± 3.3
Maximum swollen volume (fl)	75.4 ± 2.4	76.9 ± 5.1
Surface area (μm^2)	86.3 ± 1.9	87.4 ± 4.0
ESI[c,d]	1.39 ± 0.02	1.32 ± 0.06

[a] Fischer 344 rats.

[b] Values given are mean ± standard deviation.

[c] The difference between young and old rats is significantly different by a two tailed *t*-test, $P < 0.0001$.

[d] ESI is the excess surface area index, which is the ratio of the surface area to the surface area of a sphere with a volume equal to the mean cell volume.

[e] The difference between young and old rats is significantly different by a two tailed *t*-test, $P < 0.02$.

this decrease in deformability, we find that the shear modulus decreases by a factor of three indicating increased rigidity of the bilayer. The cells are also larger and more spherical with less excess surface area (a lower ESI) necessary to pass through narrow pores. The increased shear modulus reflects oxidative damage to the red cell membrane (see above); the increased size of the cell is related to the observation that in older subjects the cells entering the circulation are larger (Table 1). The increased sphericity is in part due to the properties of the cells entering the circulation (Table 1), but is further exacerbated by changes taking place while the cells are in circulation (see below). The change in shape is also responsible for reported changes in osmatic fragility (Rifkind et al., 1983; Detraglia et al., 1974).

3.4. *Origin of increased red cell oxidative stress during aging*

The oxidative changes in the red cell are in part related to impairment of the cells entering the circulation. These cells are larger and have lower activities of the anti-oxidant enzymes. However, this greater susceptibility to oxidative stress should be compensated for by the shorter life span in old subjects resulting in a younger distribution of cells, which should be less oxidatively damaged.

However, a careful examination of the data indicates that red cells in old subjects undergo greater oxidative damage in the circulation and that many of the red cells still in circulation are more oxidatively damaged than the cells in young subjects. Comparing the densest fraction of red cells, which contains a greater proportion of old cells, in young and old subjects perhaps best indicates this phenomenon. It has, thus, been reported that 50% more malondialdehyde and 30% more of the fluorescent byproducts of lipid peroxidation are found in old rats than in young rats (Gershon et al., 1988). We have compared the size and shape of the cells in the densest fraction of cells for young and old rats (Table 1). Although the young cells are also more spherical having a lower ESI in the old rats, this difference only becomes significant in the older cell fraction suggesting that the increased sphericity is in part generated while the cells are in circulation. The increased sphericity for cells in circulation longer in old rats can be attributed to altered cation homeostasis associated with a decrease in the activity of the Mg-Na-K and Mg-Na ATPases (Platt and Rieck, 1988).

Additional evidence that the cells in old subjects undergo greater damage before being removed from circulation is indicated by the density distribution of the cells. We, thus, find that in old rats there is an appreciably larger fraction of cells with a density >1.110 g/ml with as much as 10% of the cells having a density of 1.18 g/ml (Fig. 2). In addition, we find that cells removed from circulation of old subjects are lyzed appreciably faster than cells removed from young subjects.

The data are consistent with studies (Van Remmen and Richardson, 2001; Roberts and Reckelhoff, 2001, Beckman and Ames, 1998) that there is an increase in oxidative stress in older subjects. There is, thus, evidence for increased leakage of free radicals by mitochondria in old subjects (Van Remmen and Richardson, 2001). Increased inflammation in old subjects releases free radicals in the circulation and is in part responsible for increased fibrinogen (Ajmani and Rifkind, 1998). Fibrinogen increases

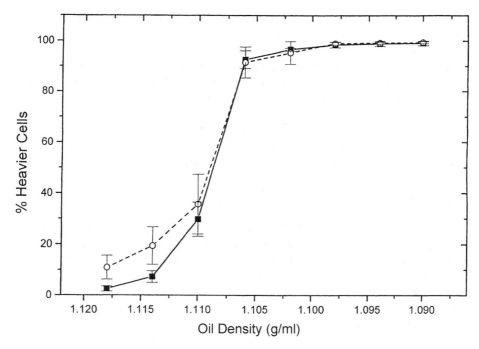

Fig. 2.   Density distribution of red cells from Fischer 344 rats: (■) young rats; (○) old rats.

red cell aggregation and leads to the formation of fibrin degradation products associated with coagulation. Plasma generated oxidants, known to increase in older subjects, contribute to red cell lipid peroxidation and red cell rigidity. In addition, these oxidants can react with hemoglobin, an excellent sink for plasma oxidants.

4. Red cell oxidative stress

4.1. *Autoxidation*

An understanding of red cell oxidative stress needs to consider the unique role of hemoglobin, which accounts for almost all of the red cell protein. The function of hemoglobin involves the reversible binding of oxygen to reduced Fe(II) hemoglobin, which is responsible for the transport of oxygen from the lungs to the tissues. Hemoglobin is, however, susceptible to oxidation both by exogenous oxidants originating from plasma and tissues as well as by autoxidation:

$$HbO_2 \rightarrow Hb^+ + \dot{O}_2^- \tag{1}$$

It has been estimated that in a 24 h period 3% of hemoglobin undergoes oxidation. The Fe(III) hemoglobin formed no longer binds oxygen and for an average human subject this reaction generates ~0.05 mol of potentially detrimental superoxide molecules. Cellular enzymes (methemoglobin reductase and diphorase) reduce almost all the oxidized hemoglobin and the cellular antioxidant enzymes (superoxide dismutase, catalase and glutathione peroxidase) convert most of the superoxide into oxygen and water.

The significance of the hemoglobin autoxidation reaction, however, hinges on unique properties of hemoglobin. We have shown (Levy et al., 1988; Abugo and Rifkind, 1994) that the rate for hemoglobin autoxidation, unlike most other oxidative reactions involving oxygen, increases several orders of magnitude when hemoglobin is partially oxygenated (Fig. 1). This phenomenon has been attributed to an altered configuration around the heme for partially oxygenated hemoglobin, which increases the susceptibility of the Fe(II) heme to oxidation (Levy et al., 1992; Rifkind et al., 1991). Therefore, most of the autoxidation and superoxide production takes place as the blood passes through the microcirculation and delivers oxygen to the tissues. This contention has recently been confirmed by the observation that red cell hemoglobin is more oxidized in venous blood right after passing through the capillary bed than in arterial blood (Fig. 3). The production of most of the superoxide in the microcirculation where the red blood cells are in intimate contact with the tissue suggests that these free radicals are a potential source for free radical induced tissue damage.

The red cell, dependent on the partial pressure of oxygen, can either act as a sink for tissue generated reactive oxygen species (ROS) or be a source for oxidants, which can damage tissue. We have demonstrated that under hypoxic conditions superoxide is able to leak out of the red cell (Rifkind et al., 1989). The ROS which leak out of the red cell were also shown to be able to damage low-density lipoproteins (Balagopalakrishna et al., 1997) and fibroblasts (Rifkind et al., 1993).

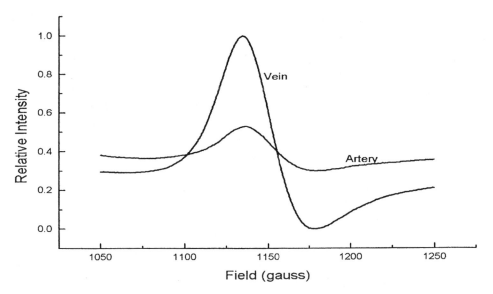

Fig. 3.   Electron paramagnetic resonance spectrum of arterial and venous blood showing the intensity of the signal due to oxidized hemoglobin.

4.2. *Reactions with hydrogen peroxide*

The production of superoxide during hemoglobin autoxidation is, however, only the beginning of a cascade of reactions, which can generate oxidative damage. Superoxide by the reaction with superoxide dismutase as well as through spontaneous dismutation forms hydrogen peroxide:

$$\dot{O}_2^{\;-} + \dot{O}_2^{\;-} + 2H^+ \rightarrow H_2O_2 + O_2 \tag{2}$$

Hydrogen peroxide and superoxide in the presence of metal ions can generate hydroxyl radicals through the Haber-Weiss reaction and Fenton chemistry:

$$\dot{O}_2^{\;-} + H_2O_2 + H^+ \rightarrow H\dot{O} + H_2O + O_2 \tag{3}$$

This reaction is accelerated in the presence of metal ion contaminants:

$$\dot{O}_2^{\;-} + Fe(III) \rightarrow Fe(II) + O_2 \tag{4}$$

resulting in the Fenton reaction:

$$H_2O_2 + Fe(II) \rightarrow H\dot{O} + HO^- + Fe(III) \tag{5}$$

Hydrogen peroxide also reacts with hemoglobin to produce ferrylhemoglobin:

$$HbO_2 + H_2O_2 \rightarrow FerrylHb \tag{6}$$

Ferrylhemoglobin is a strong oxidizing agent and is considered a putative source for cellular and tissue damage (Comair et al., 1993; Everse and Hsia, 1997; Goldman et al., 1998; Gorbunov et al., 1995; Svistunenko et al., 1997). We have also shown (Nagababu and Rifkind, 2000) that in the absence of other substrates ferryl hemoglobin reacts with an additional molecule of hydrogen peroxide to produce methemoglobin and superoxide:

$$FerrylHb + H_2O_2 \rightarrow Hb^+ + \dot{O}_2^{\;-} \tag{7}$$

We have detected this superoxide by electron paramagnetic resonance and shown that this superoxide generated from ferrylHb is properly located in the heme pocket to attack the heme resulting in a damaged heme that eventually leads to heme degradation (Nagababu and Rifkind, 1998, 2000).

The first damaged heme product detected is a rhombic heme (Fig. 4). The high-spin rhombic heme not normally observed with hemoglobin, which favors a tetragonal geometry, is formed as a result of cleaving the porphyrin backbone, thereby, stabilizing this altered heme geometry. This signal appears in a region of the spectrum where no other hemoglobin signals are observed and can, therefore, be quantitated in whole blood. The fact that these reactions take place in vivo is indicated by the observation that we have been able to detect rhombic heme in fresh blood samples (Fig. 4). We also find that the level of rhombic heme increases after the subject underwent an ischemia–reperfusion procedure known to produce oxidative stress. The finding of rhombic heme in blood is an indication that the antioxidant systems to scavenge hydrogen peroxide are not able to handle all the hydrogen peroxide produced.

These damaged hemes further react producing two fluorescent degradation products and free iron. Flow cytometry has been used to determine the levels of these

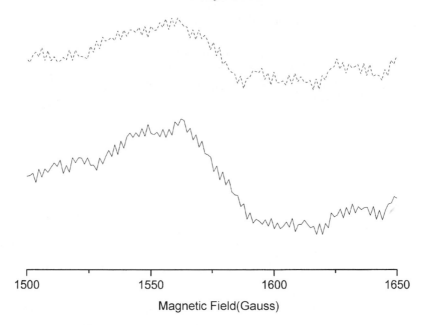

Fig. 4.   Electron paramagnetic resonance spectrum in the region from 1500–1650 gauss. This region of the spectrum measures exclusively the high-spin Fe(II) rhombic heme. A venous blood sample from a cardiac patient prior to (- - -) and after (—) an ischemic-reperfusion procedure.

fluorescent products produced while the red cells are in circulation. The increased autofluorescence in the denser cells (Table 3) in circulation for a longer period of time confirms that fluorescent heme degradation products are produced in vivo. These products are a potential source for red cell damage, which cannot be neutralized by the available red cell antioxidant systems.

4.3. *Role of hemoglobin-membrane interactions*

The red cell contains large amounts of superoxide dismutase, catalase and glutathione peroxidase to neutralize the superoxide and hydrogen peroxide formed within the red cell. These enzymes together with the low molecular weight anti-

Table 3
Fluorescence levels in human red cells separated by density centrifugation

Type of cells	Fluorescence intensity[a]
Least dense	6.423 ± 0.023
Medium density	6.715 ± 0.016[b]
Most dense	7.172 ± 0.026[b]

[a] Fluorescence intensity is measured by flow cytometry and is in arbitrary units.

[b] Values are significantly different from those of the least dense fraction, $P < 0.0001$.

oxidants like tocopherol, uric acid, ascorbic acid and glutathione would be expected to eliminate all ROS including superoxide and hydrogen peroxide, which are responsible for the propagation of red cell damage. We have, however, observed that at least under hypoxic conditions superoxide can leak out of the red cell (Rifkind et al., 1989); red cell damage indicated by crosslinking of hemoglobin with band 3 increased red cell rigidity, decreased deformability of the red cell and increased lysis is also observed (Rifkind and Abugo, 1994).

In order to explain this phenomenon, we have proposed (Rifkind et al., 1993) that oxidative reactions involving the small fraction of hemoglobin bound to the red cell membrane are responsible. Since hemoglobin bound to the red cell generates free radicals in close proximity to the membrane, it is both less available to react with the predominantly cytoplasmic antioxidants and is at the same time located near the membrane, which is the site for damage by ROS. Because of the enhanced binding of hemoglobin to the membrane when hemoglobin is deoxygenated (Tsuneshige et al., 1987), hypoxia not only increases the production of ROS, but makes it more difficult for the cell's antioxidant enzymes to protect the cell from the production of super-oxide and hydrogen peroxide.

The role of hemoglobin-membrane interactions on the propagation of red cell oxidative stress was recently demonstrated by comparing the effects of catalase inhibition by azide and glutathione peroxidase inhibition by iodoacetamide on the increased fluorescence observed during incubation of intact cells (Rifkind et al., 2001). Red cells begin to form fluorescent products after a lag phase. The elimination of this lag phase when glutathione peroxidase is inhibited, but not when catalase is inhibited, was explained by the ability of glutathione peroxidase, but not catalase to react with membrane associated peroxides as well as with hydrogen peroxide generated in close proximity to the membrane during the oxidation of membrane bound hemoglobin. The relationship between glutathione levels and glutathione peroxidase activity and the ability to protect the cell from oxidative damage implicates hemoglobin-membrane interactions.

These membrane interactions are thought to be involved in the production of fluorescent products while the cells are in circulation (Table 3). It has, thus, been found that the increased fluorescence is associated with a decrease in glutathione, which would limit the ability of glutathione peroxidase to react with hydrogen peroxide generated in the region of the membrane.

It was reported that amyloid beta-peptide 1–42 induces oxidative stress and membrane lipid peroxidation in red blood cells, and that levels of lipid peroxidation were increased in red blood cells from patients with Alzheimer's disease (Mattson et al., 1997).

We have also shown that the association of amyloid fibrils with red cells, which damages the membrane cytoskeleton, enhances the time dependent increase in the production of autofluorescence (Fig. 5). These changes are also thought to be associated with increased hemoglobin interactions with the cytoskeleton and are exacerbated when glutathione peroxidase is inhibited (Fig. 5).

The putative linkage between hemoglobin-membrane interactions and red cell oxidative processes provides a unique way to specifically turn off red cell induced

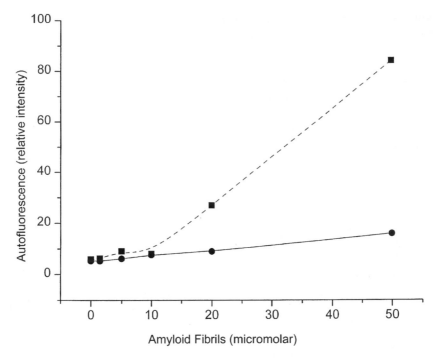

Fig. 5.   Autofluorescence detected by flow cytometry after a 16 h incubation at 37°C. Red cells treated with different concentrations of beta amyloid fibrils without the addition of any inhibitor of antioxidant enzymes (—) and with iodoacetamide added to inhibit glutathione peroxidase (- - -).

oxidative stress. Instead of requiring large concentrations of antioxidants to neutralize the ROS formed, blocking the interaction of hemoglobin with the membrane will make it possible for the large supply of red cell antioxidants and antioxidant enzymes to eliminate the hemoglobin generated oxidants, and thereby, prevent red cell oxidative stress.

We are currently exploring various hemoglobin and/or membrane modifications designed to see if it is possible to inhibit hemoglobin-membrane interactions. Our initial studies involve the reaction of cyanate with the hemoglobin alpha-amino groups. This reaction blocks the binding of the cytoplasmic end of band 3 to the cavity between the beta chains (Walder et al., 1984). We have shown that this reaction inhibits hemoglobin binding (Rifkind et al., 2001) and at the same time inhibits red cell oxidative damage generated by hydrogen peroxide and cumene hydroperoxide (Fig. 6).

We have also investigated the effect of crosslinking on the hemoglobin by bis(3,5dibromosalicyl)fumarate between the lysine 99 residues on two of the alpha subunits. This crosslink extends through the central cavity. While it results in low affinity hemoglobin, which binds oxygen cooperatively, binding to the membrane is inhibited. Use of this hemoglobin as a cell free blood substitute actually increases the formation of heme degradation products (Nagababu et al., 2002). However, in a cell

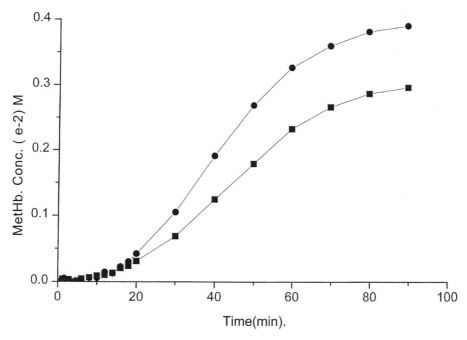

Fig. 6. Oxidation of human red cell hemoglobin by cumene hydroperoxide: (●) normal red cells; (■) hemoglobin in the red cells was reacted with cyanate before adding cumene hydroperoxide.

with the full repertoire of red cell antioxidants, these oxidative reactions may be better neutralized. Since it does not bind to the membrane, leakage of oxidants from the cell and damage to the membrane will be prevented. Hemoglobin-induced reduction of nitroblue tetrazolium (Abugo and Rifkind, 1994; Demehin et al., 2001) has been used as a measure of red cell oxidative membrane interactions. Enhanced oxidative interactions resulting in a more rapid reduction of nitroblue tetrazolium in the presence of membranes is suggested as shown in Table 4. The much smaller enhancement for crosslinked hemoglobin implies much less binding to the membrane resulting in reduced oxidative stress.

Table 4
Oxidative reaction[a] between human hemoglobin and nitroblue tetrazolium in the absence of oxygen

	Normal hemoglobin	Crosslinked hemoglobin
No added membrane	0.0314[b]	0.0047[b]
Plus membrane	0.2879[b]	0.0827[b]

[a] The reaction of hemoglobin with nitroblue tetrazolium results in the oxidation of hemoglobin and the reduction of nitroblue tetrazolium. The reduction of the tetrazolium was followed spectroscopically.

[b] The values of reduced nitroblue tetrazolium 2 min after the reaction began are given.

5. Red cell oxidative stress during aging

This cascade of oxidative processes takes place continuously in red cells. We have in fact shown by measuring hemoglobin oxidation in arterial and venous blood (Fig. 3) that increased autoxidation and the associated release of superoxide and hydrogen peroxide occurs every time the blood passes through the microcirculation. The extent of this reaction is further dramatized by the fact that the cellular reducing enzymes (methemoglobin reductase and diaphorase) are not able to keep up with the production of oxidants.

During aging, these processes are expected to be exacerbated. The increased size and sphericity, increased rigidity, decreased deformability and increased shear modulus of elasticity (Table 2) are expected to impair the flow of blood through the microcirculation in older subjects. Vascular changes known to occur in older subjects (Tanaka et al., 1998) are expected to further impair blood flow. All of these changes result in a greater hypoxic stress and increased oxidative stress during aging in the red cell. In vivo these changes in the normal healthy circulation can be partially compensated for by the release of nitric oxide (NO), which causes vasodilation. A pool of available nitric oxide has been postulated to be stored in the red cell (Jia et al., 1996). This nitric oxide would be preferentially released under hypoxic conditions and be available to compensate for the hypoxic stress in the microcirculation. It has, however, been shown that in older subjects less nitric oxide is synthesized (Matsushita et al., 2001; Amrani et al., 1996) and the response to nitric oxide is blunted (Okamoto et al., 2001; Matz et al., 2000) resulting in the inability to maintain optimal blood flow and to, thereby, limit oxidative stress.

The proposed decrement in blood flow as a result of increased oxidative stress in the aged is consistent with studies of the carotid arteries and middle cerebral arteries responsible for cerebral blood flow (Ajmani et al., 2000). An age dependent decrease in CBF is found in the left and right common carotid arteries. In addition, age dependent decreases in flow velocities and increases in peripheral vascular resistance were found for the common carotid, anterior carotid and middle cerebral arteries. The relationship between these age dependent changes in flow properties and oxidative stress was indicated by partial correlation analysis of the age dependent changes corrected for lipid peroxidation fluorescent products.

6. Functional impairment and altered red cell properties

The relationship between age associated red cell changes and the flow properties of blood suggests that the red cell may contribute to an aging induced decrement in the ability to deliver oxygen to the tissues. The tissues expected to be most affected are the brain and the heart, which have the greatest demand for oxygen.

The role of red cell impairment on cardiovascular function is indicated by the independent risk factors for cardiovascular disease (Lowe et al., 2000) involving whole blood viscosity and fibrinogen. Red cell rigidity, which contributes to red cell viscosity, has been shown to be associated with oxidative stress (Rifkind et al., 1997).

Fibrinogen, which is involved in red cell aggregation and increases whole blood viscosity, is synthesized in response to stress (Mansoor et al., 1997).

We have recently initiated a controlled study designed to test the effect of oxidative stress on the flow properties of the red cell and how it impacts on aging and cardiovascular impairment. In this study, maximal treadmill exercise is used to initiate stress. Our preliminary studies indicate increased oxidative stress during exercise, but have not yet been able to investigate the effect of age and cardiovascular impairment.

A relationship between red cell flow properties and cognitive function in rats was indicated (Rifkind et al., 1999) by a negative correlation between the errors made in a maze and the shear modulus of elasticity, a measure of deformability. This correlation was only observed in old rats (24-month Fischer 344 rats) and not in young rats indicating that the young rats are able to compensate for changes in red cell deformability and still deliver the necessary oxygen to the brain.

Amyloid beta protein (βAP) is associated with plaques, which develop during Alzheimer's disease. Previous studies have shown that βAPs can induce oxidative stress and lysis of red blood cells (Mattson et al., 1997). We have found that amyloid fibrils are taken up by red cells causing a swelling of the cells and a decrease in red cell deformability (Table 5). These results were obtained with relatively small amyloid fibrils produced by a 4 h incubation of beta amyloid. The larger fibrils present after a 72-h incubation produced a much greater swelling of the cells with the mean cell volume increasing to 106.27 ± 2.07 femtoliters at $20 \mu M$ amyloid. These perturbations would impair oxygen delivery to the tissues and be a potential source for oxidative stress. The increased time dependent increase in autofluorescence with amyloid treated red cells (Fig. 5) supports the contention that amyloids induce greater red cell oxidative stress.

Cells in the nervous systems as well as in peripheral tissues continuously produce amyloids and low levels of these proteins are found in blood (Mehta et al., 2000). The production of these amyloids increases under pathological conditions and may also be increased during normal aging (Thomas et al., 2000; Kuo et al., 1999; Kalaria, 1992). We are currently investigating APP transgenic mice, which produce

Table 5
Alterations in human red cells by beta amyloid fibrils[a]

Amyloid concentration (μM)	MCV[b] (fl)	MCTT[c] (ms)	CS[d]	Percentage of slow cells (>6.4 ms)
0	81.56	3.73	11.67	2.64
5	84.19	3.58	8.62	1.64
15	85.14	4.08	5.79	4.29
20	85.98	4.13	4.86	5.53

[a] Fibrils produced by incubation for 4 h.

[b] MCV is the mean cell volume.

[c] MCTT is the mean transit time for the red cells to pass through a 5 μ pore.

[d] CS is the cells per second that pass through the pores. With the same concentration of cells, this parameter reflects the ability of the cells to successfully pass through the pores.

more βAP, to determine whether amyloid associated with red cells can be detected in vivo. We have, thus far, not been able to confirm the presence of increased red cell amyloid in these mice. Some of our preliminary results suggest that red cells in these APP mice may be removed from circulation more rapidly. While this will not produce cells with elevated amyloids, it places an increased hemopoietic stress on the mice and may, thereby, further impair the red cell properties.

7. Conclusion

The red cell plays a crucial role being instrumental in supplying oxygen to the tissues. However, because of the short life span of 120 d (in humans), the contribution of red cells to aging is frequently neglected. In this review, we have indicated how the red cell may, nevertheless, contribute to the pathophysiological changes, which occur during aging. In old subjects, the red cell life span decreases, placing a stress on the hemopoietic system, which has a reduced reserve capacity. This results in a form of stress erythropoiesis producing larger less deformable cells. These larger less deformable cells are also shown to be more susceptible to oxidative stress.

It is generally considered that oxidative stress in the organism involves mitochondria, neutrophils, etc. However, any potential contribution from the red cell is neglected. The red cell, however, contains the largest pool of oxygen. In the red cell, the bulk of this molecular oxygen is transported to the tissues without the generation of partially reduced ROS. However, ROSs are continuously produced by red cells with a dramatic enhancement at low oxygen pressures where the rates of autoxidation increase and the cellular antioxidant systems are bypassed because of hemoglobin interactions with the membrane.

The red cell changes during aging exacerbate red cell oxidative stress and provide the bases for potential functional decrements that occur during aging.

Acknowledgement

The help of Catherine Smertycha in preparing the bibliography for this review is greatly appreciated.

References

Abe, A., Orita, M., Arichi, S., 1984. Erythrocyte deformality in aging. Mech. Ageing Dev. 27, 383–390.

Abraham, E.C., Taylor, J.F., Lang, C.A., 1978. Influence of mouse age and erythrocyte age on glutathione metabolism. Biochem. J. 174, 819–825.

Abugo, O.O., Rifkind, J.M., 1994. Oxidation of hemoglobin and the enhancement produced by nitroblue tetrazolium. J. Biol. Chem. 269, 24845–24853.

Aiken, N.R., Satterlee, J.D., Galey, W.R., 1992. Measurement of intracellular Ca2+ in young and old human erythrocytes using 19F-NMR spectroscopy. Biochim. Biophys. Acta 1136, 155–160.

Ajmani, R.S., Rifkind, J.M., 1998. Hemorheological changes during human aging. Gerontology 44, 111–120.

Ajmani, R.S., Metter, E.J., Jaykumar, R., Ingram, D.K., Spangler, E.L., Abugo, O.O., Rifkind, J.M., 2000. Hemodynamic changes during aging associated with cerebral blood flow and impaired cognitive functions. Neurobiol. Aging 21, 257–269.

Al-Turk, W.A., Stohs, S.J., el-Rashidy, F.H., Othman, S., 1987. Changed in glutathione and its metabolizing enzymes in human erythrocytes and lymphocytes with age. J. Pharm. Pharmacol. 39, 13–16.

Amrani, M., Goodwin, A.T., Gray, C.C., Yacoub, M.H., 1996. Ageing is associated with reduced basal and stimulated release of nitric oxide by the coronary endothelium. Acta Physiol. Scand. 157, 79–84.

Araki, K., Rifkind, J.M., 1980a. Age dependent changes in osmotic hemolysis of human erythrocytes. J. Gerontol. 35, 499–505.

Araki, K., Rifkind, J.M., 1980b. Erythrocyte membrane cholesterol: an explanation of the aging effect on the rate of hemolysis. Life Sci. 26, 2223–2230.

Avellone, G., Di Garbo, V., Panno, A.V., Cordova, R., Alletto, G., Raneli, G., DeSimone, R., Strano, A., Bompiani, G.D., 1993. Haemorheological components in the pre-geriatric and geriatric age range in a randomly selected western Sicily population sample (Casteldaccia Study). Clin. Hemorheol. 13, 83–92.

Balagopalakrishna, C., Nirmala, R., Rifkind, J.M., Chatterjee, S., 1997. Modification of low density lipoproteins by erythrocytes and hemoglobin under hypoxic conditions. Adv. Exp. Med. Biol. 411, 337–345.

Balducci, L., Hardy, C.L., Lyman, G.H., 2001. Hematopoietic growth factors in the older cancer patient. Curr. Opin. Hematol. 8, 170–187.

Baldwin Jr., J.G., 1988. Hematopoietic function in the elderly. Arch Intern. Med. 148, 2544-2546.

Bartosz, G., 1982. Aging of the erythrocyte, XV. Isoosmotic lysis times. Experientia 38, 1484–1485.

Bartosz, G., 1991. Erythrocyte aging: physical and chemical membrane changes. Gerontology 37, 33–67.

Bartosz, G., Niewiarowska, J., Jurkiewicz, L., 1982. Decreased deformability in aging erythrocytes. Biochim. Biophys. Acta 693, 262–264.

Beckman, K.B., Ames, B.N., 1998. The free radical theory of aging matures. Physiol. Rev. 78, 547–581.

Beppu, M., Mizukami, A., Nagoya, M., Kikugawa, K., 1990. Binding of anti-band 3 autoantibody to oxidatively damaged erythrocytes. J. Biol. Chem. 265, 3226–3233.

Berr, C., Nicole, A., Godin, J., Ceballos-Picot, I., Thevenin, M., Dartigues, J.-F., Alperovitch, A., 1993. Selenium and oxygen-metabolizing enzymes in elderly community residents: a pilot epidemiological study. JAGS 41, 143–148.

Boggs, D.R., Patrene, K.D., 1985. Hematopoiesis and aging III: anemia and a blunted erythropoietic response to hemorrhage in aged mice. Am. J. Hematol. 4, 327–338.

Boggs, D.R., Saxe, D.F., Boggs, S.S., 1984. Aging and hematopoiesis II. The ability of bone marrow cells from young and aged mice to cure and maintain cure in W/Wv. Transplantation 37, 300–306.

Brecher, G., Prenant, M., Haley, J., Bessis, M., 1975. Origin of stress macroreticulocytes from macronormoblasts. Nouv. Rev. Fr. Hematol. 15, 13–28.

Brok, F., Ramot, B., Zwang, E., Danon, D., 1996. Enzyme activities in human red cells of different age groups. Isr. J. Med. Sci. 2, 291–296.

Buchanan, J.P., Peters, C.A., Rasmussen, C.J., Rothstein, G., 1996. Impaired expression of hematopoietic growth factors: a candidate mechanism for the hematopoietic defect of aging. Exp. Gerontol. 31, 135–144.

Carmel, R., 2001. Anemia and aging: an overview of clinical, diagnostic and biological issues. Blood Rev. 15, 9–18.

Chatta, G.S., Dale, D.C., 1996. Aging and haemopoiesis: implications for treatment with haemopoietic growth factors. Drugs Aging 9, 37–47.

Clark, M.R., 1988. Senescence of red blood cells: progress and problems. Pathol. Rev. 68, 503–554.

Comair, Y.G., Schipper, H.M., Brem, S., 1993. The prevention of oxyhemoglobin-induced endothelial and smooth muscle cytoskeletal injury by deferoxamine. Neurosurgery 32, 58–64.

Danon, D., Marikovsky, Y., 1988. The aging of red blood cell. A multifactor process. Blood Cells 14, 7–15.

Danon, D., Marikovsky, Y., Fischler, H., 1983. Surface charge of old, transformed and experimentally deteriorated erythrocytes. NYAS 149–158.

Demehin, A.A., Abugo, O.O., Rifkind, J.M., 2001. The reduction of nitroblue tertrazolium by red blood cells; a measure of red cell membrane antioxidant capacity and hemoglobin-membrane binding sites. Free Radic. Res. 34, 605–620.

Detraglia, M., Cook, F.B., Stasiw, D.M., 1974. Erythrocyte fragility in aging. Biochim. Biophys. Acta 345, 312–219.

Elseweidy, M.M., Stallings, M., Abraham, E.C., 1983. Changes in glycosylated hemoglobins with red cell aging in normal and diabetic subjects and in newborn infants of normal and diabetic mothers. J. Lab. Clin. Med. 102, 628–636.

Everse, J., Hsia, N., 1997. The toxicities of native and modified hemoglobins. Free Radic. Biol. Med. 22, 1075–1099.

Farooqui, M.Y., Day, W.W., Zamorano, D.M., 1987. Glutathione and lipid peroxidation in the aging rat. Comp. Biochem. Physiol. 88, 177–180.

Franzini, E., Driss, F., Driss, F.R., Darcet, P.H., Thao, C.M., 1988. The role of red cells subpopulations in the determination of erythrocyte deformability. Clin. Hemortheol. 8, 493–499.

Gershon, H., Gershon, D., 1988. Altered enzyme function and premature sequestration of erythrocytes in aged individuals. Blood Cells 14, 93–101.

Gershon, D., Glass, G.A., Gershon, H., 1988. The effect of host and cell age on the rat erythrocyte: biochemical aspects. Blood Cells, Rheol. Aging, 42–50.

Gesquiere, L., Loreau, N., Minnich, A., Davignon, J., Blache, D., 1999. Oxidative stress leads to cholesterol accumulation in vascular smooth muscle cells. Free Radic. Biol. Med. 27, 134–145.

Glass, G.A., Gershon, D., 1981. Enzymatic changes in rat erythrocytes with increasing cell and donor age: loss of superoxide dismutase activity associated with increases in catalytically defective forms. Biochem. Biophys. Res. Commun. 103, 1245–1253.

Glass, G.A., Gershon, D., 1984. Decreased enzymic protection and increased sensitivity to oxidative damage in erythrocytes as a function of cell and donor aging. J. Biochem. 218, 531–537.

Glass, G.A., Gershon, H., Gershon, D., 1983. The effect of donor and cell age on several characteristics of rat erythrocytes. Exp. Hematol. 11, 987–995.

Glass, G.A., Gershon, D., Gershon, H., 1985. Some characteristics of the human erythrocyte as a function of donor and cell age. Exp. Hematol. 13, 1122–1126.

Globerson, A., 1999. Hematopoietic stem cells and aging. Exp. Gerontol. 34, 137–146.

Goldman, D.W., Breyer III, R.J., Yeh, D., Brockner-Ryan, B.A., Alayash, A.I., 1998. Acellular hemoglobin-mediated oxidative stress toward endothelium: a role for ferryl iron. Am. J. Physiol. 275, 1046–1053.

Gorbunov, N.V., Osipov, A.N., Day, B.W., Zayas-Rivera, B., Kagan, V.E., Elsayed, N.M., 1995. Reduction of ferrylmyoglobin and ferrylhemoglobin by nitric oxide: a protective mechanism against ferryl hemoprotein-induced oxidations. Biochemistry 34, 6689–6699.

Graldi, G., Giuliani, A.L., Unis, L., Pora, R., Verenini, M., Lorenzini, F., Melandri, P., Torboli, M., Bergamini, C., Berti, G., 1999. Accelerated elimination from the circulation of homologous aged red blood cells in rats bearing anti-spectrin antibodies. Mech. Ageing Dev. 107, 21–36.

Grzelinska, E., Bartosz, G., 1988. Membrane potential decreases during erythrocyte aging. Cell Biol. Int. Rep. 12, 497–501.

Hazelton, G.A., Lang, C.A., 1985. Glutathione peroxidase and reductase activities in the aging mouse. Mech. Ageing Dev. 29, 71–81.

Hershko, C., Levy, S., Matzner, Y., Grossowicz, N., Izak, G., 1979. Prevalence and causes of anemia in the elderly in Kiryat Shmoneth, Israel. Gerontology 25, 42–48.

Hirota, Y., Okamura, S., Kimura, N., Shibuya, T., Niho, Y., 1988. Haematopoiesis in the aged as studied by in vitro colony assay. Eur. J. Haematol. 40, 83–90.

Kaushansky, K., Karplus, P.A., 1993. Hematopoietic growth factors: understanding functional diversity in structural terms. Blood 82, 3229–3240.

Lowe, G., Rumley, A., Norrie, J., Ford, I., Shepherd, J., Cobbe, S., Macfarlane, P., Packard, C., 2000. Blood rheology, cardiovascular risk factors, and cardiovascular disease: the West of Scotland coronary prevention study. Thromb. Haemost. 84, 553–558.

Jia, L., Bonaventura, C., Stamler, J.S., 1996. *S*-nitrosohaemoglobin: a dynamic activity of blood involved in vascular control. Nature 380, 221–226.

Kalaria, R.N., 1992. Serum amyloid P and related molecules associated with the acute-phase response in Alzheimer's disease. Res. Immunol. 143, 637–641.

Kasapoglu, M., Ozben, T., 2001. Alterations of antioxidant enzymes and oxidative stress markers in aging. Exp. Gerontol. 36, 209–220.

Kay, M.M., 1978. Role of physiologic autoantibody in the removal of senescent human red cells. J. Supramol. Struct. 94, 555–567.

Kay, M.M.B., 1990. Senescent cell antigen, band 3, and band 3 mutations in cellular aging. Biomed. Biochim. Acta 49, 212–217.

Kay, M.M., Bosman, G.J., Shapiro, S.S., Bendich, A., Bassel, P.S., 1986. Oxidation as a possible mechanism of cellular aging: vitamin E deficiency causes premature aging and IgG binding to erythrocytes. Proc. Natl. Acad. Sci. 83, 2463–2467.

Krzisnik, C., Lukac-Bajalo, J., 1993. Glycosylated hemoglobin in fractions of erythrocytes of different ages. J. Endocrinol. Invest. 16, 495–498.

Kuo, Y.M., Emmerling, M.R., Lampert, H.C., Hempelman, S.R., Kokjohn, T.A., Woods, A.S., Cotter, R.J., Roher, A.E., 1999. High levels of circulating Abeta42 are sequestered by plasma proteins in Alzheimer's disease. Biochem. Biophys. Res. Commun. 257, 787–791.

Lang, C.A., Naryshikin, S., Schneider, D.L., Mills, B.J., Lindeman, R.D., 1992. Low blood glutathione levels in healthy aging adults. J. Lab. Clin. Med. 120, 720–725.

Lee, M.A., Segal, G.M., Bagby, G.C., 1989. The hematopoietic microenvironment in the elderly: defects in IL-1-induced CSF expression in vitro. Exp. Hematol. 17, 952–956.

Levy, A., Zhang, L., Rifkind, J.M., 1988. Hemoglobin: a source of superoxide radical under hypoxic conditions. Hemoglobin 11–25.

Levy, A., Sharma, V.S., Zhang, L., Rifkind, J.M., 1992. A new mode for heme–heme interactions in hemoglobin associated with distal perturbations. Biophys. J. 61, 750–755.

Lipschitz, D.A., 1995. Age-related declines in hematopoietic reserve capacity. Seminars Oncol. 22, 3–5.

Low, P.S., Waugh, S.M., Zinke, K., Drenckhahn, D., 1985. The role of hemoglobin denaturation and based 3 clustering in red blood cell aging. Science 227, 531–533.

Magnani, M., Rossi, L., Stocchi, V., Cucchiarini, L., Piacentini, G., Fornaini, G., 1988. Effect of age on some properties of mice erythrocytes. Mech. Ageing Dev. 42, 37–47.

Mansoor, O., Cayol, M., Gachon, P., Boirie, Y., Schoeffler, P., Obled, C., Beaufrere, B., 1997. Albumin and fibrinogen syntheses increase while muscle protein synthesis decreases in head-injured patients. Am. J. Physiol. 273, 898–902.

Marley, S.B., Lewis, J.L., Davidson, R.J., Roberts, I.A., Dokal, I., Goldman, J.M., Gordon, M.Y., 1999. Evidence for a continuous decline in haemopoietic cell function from birth: application to evaluating bone marrow failure in children. Br. J. Haematol. 106, 162–166.

Matsubara, L.S., Machado, P.E.A., 1991. Age-related changes of glutathione content, glutathione reductase and glutathione peroxidase activity of human erythrocytes. Brazilian J. Med. Biol. Res. 24, 449–454.

Matsuo, T., Kario, K., Kodoma, K., Asada, R., 1995. An inappropriate erythropoietic response to iron deficiency anaemia in the elderly. Clin. Lab. Haem. 17, 317–321.

Matsushita, H., Chang, E., Glassford, A.J., Cooke, J.P., Chiu, C.P., Tsao, P.S., 2001. eNOS activity is reduced in senescent human endothelial cells: preservation by hTERT immoralization. Circ. Res. 89, 793–798.

Mattson, M.P., Begley, J.G., Mark, R.J., Furukawa, K., 1997. Abeta 25–35 induces rapid lysis of red blood cells: contrast with Abeta1-42 and examination of underlying mechanisms. Brain Res. 771, 147–153.

Matz, R.L., de Sotomayor, M.A., Schott, C., Stoclet, J.C., Andriantsitohaina, R., 2000. Vascular bed heterogenecity in age-related endothelial dysfunction with respect to NO and eicosanoids. Br. J. Pharmacol. 131, 303–311.

Mehta, P.D., Pirttila, T., Mehta, S.P., Sersen, E.A., Aisen, P.S., Wisniewski, H.M., 2000. Plasma and cerebrospinal fluid levels of amyloid beta proteins 1–40 and 1–42 in Alzheimer disease. Arch Neurol. 57, 100–105.

Nagababu, E., Rifkind, J.M., 1998. Formation of fluorescent heme degradation products during the oxidation of hemoglobin by hydrogen peroxide. Biochem. Biophys. Res. Commun. 247, 592–596.

Nagababu, E., Rifkind, J.M., 2000. Reaction of hydrogen peroxide with ferrylhemoglobin: superoxide production and heme degradation. Biochemistry 39, 12503–12511.

Nagababu, E., Ramasamy, S., Rifkind, J.M., Jia, Y., Alayash, A.I., 2002. Site-specific cross-linking of human and bovine hemoglobins differentially alters oxygen binding and redox side reactions producing rhombic heme and heme degradation. Biochemistry 41, 7407–7415.

Nash, G.B., Wyard, S.J., 1981. Erythrocyte membrane elasticity during in vivo ageing. Biochim. Biophys. Acta 643, 269–275.

Norton, J.M., 1990. The effect of macrocytosis on rat erythrocyte deformability during recovery from phenylhydrazine-induced anemia. Biorheology 27, 21–37.

Okamoto, M., Etani, H., Yagita, Y., Kinoshita, N., Nukada, T., 2001. Diminished reserve for cerebral vasomotor response to l-arginine in the elderly: evaluation by transcranial Doppler sonography. Gerontology 47, 131–135.

Park, S.C., Yeo, E.J., Han, J.A., Hwang, Y.C., Choi, J.Y., Park, J.D., Park, Y.H., Kim, K.O., Kim, I.G., Seong, S.C., Kwak, S.J., 1999. Aging process is accomplished by increase of transglutaminase C. J. Gerontol. A Biol. Sci. Med. Sci. 54, 78–83.

Peddada, R.R., Abugo, O.O., Kelly, J.F., Roth, G.S., Rifkind, J.M., 1997. Effect of cholesterol content in diet on capillary flow of rat erythrocytes. Part II: mechanical properties. Clin. Hemorheol. Microcirc. 17, 445–457.

Perrin, R., Briancon, S., Jeandel, C., Artur, Y., Minn, A., Penin, F., Siest, G., 1990. Blood activity of Cu/Zn superoxide dismutase, glutathione peroxidase and catalase in Alzheimer's disease: a case control study. Gerontology 36, 306–313.

Pinkofsky, H.B., 1997. The effect of donor age on human erythrocyte density distribution. Mech. Ageing Dev. 97, 73–79.

Platt, D., Rieck, W., 1988. Red cell membrane proteins, glycoproteins, and aging. Blood Cells, Rheology, Aging, 29–41.

Rettig, M.P., Low, P.S., Gimm, J.A., Mohandas, N., Wang, J., Christian, J.A., 1999. Evaluation of biochemical changes during in vivo erythrocyte senescence in the dog. Blood 93, 376–384.

Rifkind, J.M., Abugo, O.O., 1994. Alterations in erythrocyte deformability under hypoxia: implications for impaired oxygen transport. Adv. Exp. Med. Biol. 361, 345–351.

Rifkind, J.M., Araki, K., Hadley, E.C., 1983. The relationship between the osmotic fragility of human erythrocytes and cell age. Arch Biochem. Biophys. 222, 582–589.

Rifkind, J.M., Araki, K., Mohanty, J.G., Suda, T., 1985. Age dependent changes in erythrocyte membrane function. Prog. Clin. Biol. Res. 195, 159–172.

Rifkind, J.M., Zhang, L., Heim, J.M., Levy, A., 1989. The role of hemoglobin in generating oxyradicals. Oxygen radicals in biology and medicine, 157–162.

Rifkind, J.M., Zhang, L., Levy, A., Manoharan, P.T., 1991. The hypoxic stress on erythrocytes associated with superoxide formation. Free Radic. Res. Commun. 2, 645–652.

Rifkind, J.M., Abugo, O., Levy, A., Monticone, R., Heim, J., 1993. Formation of free radicals under hypoxia. In: Hochachka, P.W., Lutz, P.L., Sick, T., Rosenthal, M., van den Thillart, G. (Eds.), Surviving Hypoxia: Mechanisms of Control and Adaptation, pp. 509–525.

Rifkind, J.M., Ajmani, R.S., Heim, J., 1997. Impaired hemorheology in the aged associated with oxidative stress. Adv. Exp. Med. Biol. 428, 7–13.

Rifkind, J.M., Abugo, O.O., Peddada, R.R., Patel, N., Speer, D., Balagopalakrishna, C., Danon, D., Ingram, D.K., Spangler, E.L., 1999. Maze learning impairment is associated with stress hemopoiesis recombinant erythropoietin. Life Sci. 64, 237–247.

Rifkind, J.M., Abugo, O.O., Nagababu, E., Ajmani, R.S., Metter, E.J., Demehin, A., Manoharan, P.T., Balagopalakrishna C., Chrest, F.J., 2001. Role of altered blood properties in the propagation of ischemic blood flow: contribution of aging and oxidative stress. In: Fukuuchi, Y., Tomita, M. (Eds.), Ischemic Blood Flow in the Brain, pp. 369–380.

Roberts II, L.J., Reckelhoff, J.F., 2001. Measurement of F(2)-isoprostanes unveils profound oxidative stress in aged rats. Biochem. Biophys. Res. Commun. 287, 254–256.

Romero, P.J., Romero, E.A., 1999. Effect of cell ageing and Ca2+ influx into human red cells. Cell Calcium 26, 131–137.

Shimizu, Y., Suzuki, M., 1991. The relationship between red cell aging and enzyme activities in experimental animals. Comp. Biochem. Physiol. 99, 313–316.

Shperling, T., Danon, D., 1990. Age population distribution of erythrocytes in young and old healthy donors. Exp. Gerontol. 25, 413–422.

Snyder, L.M., Fortier, N.L., Trainor, J., Jacobs, J., Leb, L., Lubin, B., Chiu, D., Shohet., S., Mohandas, N., 1985. Effect of hydrogen peroxide exposure on normal human erythrocyte deformability, morphology, surface characteristics, and spectrin-hemoglobin cross-linking. J. Clin. Invest. 76, 1971–1977.

Stohlman, F., 1961. Humoral regulation of erythropoiesis VII. Shortened survival of erythrocytes produced by erythropoietine or severe anemia. Proc. Soc. Exp. Biol. Med. 107, 884–886.

Sutera, S.P., Gardner, R.A., Boylan, C. W., Carroll, G.L., Chang, K.C., Marvel, J.S., Kilo, C., Gonen, B., Williamson, J.R., 1985. Age-related changes in deformability of human erythrocytes. Blood 65, 275–282.

Suzuki, T., Gale, G.L., 1989. Membrane proteins in senescent erythrocytes. Biochem. J. 257, 37–41.

Svistunenko, D.A., Patel, R.P., Voloshchenko, S.V., Wilson, M.T., 1997. The globin-based free radical of ferryl hemoglobin is detected in normal human blood. J. Biol. Chem. 272, 7114–7121.

Tanaka, J., Dinenno, F.A., Hunt, B.E., Jones, P.P., DeSouza, C.A., Seals, D.R., 1998. Hemodynamic sequelae of age-related increases in arterial stiffness in healthy women. Am. J. Cardiol. 82, 1151–1155.

Thomas, A.J., Morris, C.M., Ferrier, I.N., Kalaria, R.N., 2000. Distribution of amyloid beta 42 in relation to the cerebral microvasculature in an elderly cohort with Alzheimer's disease. Ann. NY Acad. Sci. 903, 83–88.

Timiras, M.L., Brownstein, H., 1987. Prevalence of anemia and correlation of hemoglobin with age in a geriatric screening clinic population. J. Am. Geriatr. Soc. 35, 639–643.

Tozzi-Ciancarelli, M.G., Fedele, F., Tozzi, E., Massimo, D.C., Oratore, A., De-Matteis, G., et al., 1989. Age dependent changes in human erythrocyte properties. Clin. Hemorheol. 9, 999–1007.

Tsumeshige, A., Imai, K., Tyuma, I., 1987. The binding of hemoglobin to red cell membrane lowers its oxygen affinity. J. Biochem. 101, 695–704.

Tyan, M.L., 1982. Age-related increase in erythrocyte oxidant sensitivity. Mech. Ageing Dev. 20, 25–32.

Van Remmen, H., Richardson, A., 2001. Oxidative damage to mitochondria and aging. Exp. Gerontol. 36, 957–968.

Vomel, Th., Platt, D., 1981. Lifespan of rabbit erythrocytes and activity of the reticulohistiocyte system. Mech. Ageing Dev. 17, 261–266.

Walder, J.A., Chatterjee, R., Steck, T.L., Low, P.S., Musso, G.F., Kaiser, E.T., Rogers, P.H., Arnone, A., 1984. The interaction of hemoglobin with the cytoplasmic domain of band 3 of the human erythrocyte membrane. J. Biol. Chem. 259, 10238–10246.

Waugh, R.E., Narla, M., Jackson, C.W., Mueller, T.J., Suzuki, T., Dale, G.L., 1992. Blood 79, 1351–1358.

Waugh, R.E., McKenney, J.B., Bauserman, R.G., Brooks, D.M., Valeri, C.R., Snyder, L.M., 1997. Surface area and volume changes during maturation of reticulocytes in the circulation of the baboon. J. Lab. Clin. Med. 527–535.

Hyperhomocysteinemia and cardiovascular aging

Marco Cattaneo* and Federico Lussana

*Hematology and Thrombosis Unit, Department of Medicine, Surgery and Dentistry,
Ospedale San Paolo, University of Milano, Via di Rudinì, 8, 20142 Milano, Italy*

Contents

---

* Corresponding author. Tel.: +39-2-5503-5404; fax: +39-2-5516-093.
  E-mail address: marco.cattaneo@unimi.it (M. Cattaneo).

Advances in Cell Aging and Gerontology, vol. 11, 309–335

Abbreviations

Hcy	homocysteine
tHcy	total homocysteine
PML	post-methionine loading
MTHFR	methylenetetrahydrofolate reductase.
LDL	low density lipoprotein

1. Introduction

Homocysteine (Hcy) is a sulfhydryl amino acid derived from the metabolic conversion of methionine, its removal is dependent on vitamins (folic acid, B12 and B6) as cofactors or cosubstrates. Its plasma levels increase with age and are higher in post-menopausal than in fertile women. In the past few decades, a growing amount of interest has focused on moderate hyperhomocysteinemia as a risk factor for cardiovascular disease. Several case-control, cross-sectional and prospective studies showed that elevated plasma levels of Hcy are associated with a heightened risk for coronary artery disease, cerebrovascular disease, peripheral artery disease and venous thromboembolism. In addition, the observation that subjects with cardiovascular risk factors and a history of stroke have an increased risk of both dementia and Alzheimer's disease led to the hypothesis that elevated plasma Hcy may be a risk factor for dementia and Alzheimer's disease, which has recently been supported by the results of case-control and prospective studies. These observations suggest that plasma homocysteine has an important role in cardiovascular aging. This review summarizes the metabolism of homocysteine, the genetic and environmental determinants of plasma homocysteine levels, the clinical studies that have evaluated its association with cardiovascular diseases and dementia, the mechanisms by which hyperhomocysteinemia might predispose to vascular disease, and the efficacy of vitamin supplementation in reducing plasma homocysteine levels.

1.1. *Metabolism of homocysteine*

Homocysteine exists both in free and protein-bound forms and is oxidized in plasma to the disulfides homocysteine–homocysteine (homocysteine) and homocysteine–cysteine (mixed disulfide). Free and protein-bound Hcy and its disulfides are globally referred to as total homocysteine (tHcy) (Mudd et al., 2000). The intracellular metabolism of Hcy occurs through two pathways of remethylation to methionine and one pathway of trans-sulfuration to cysteine (Fig. 1). In the

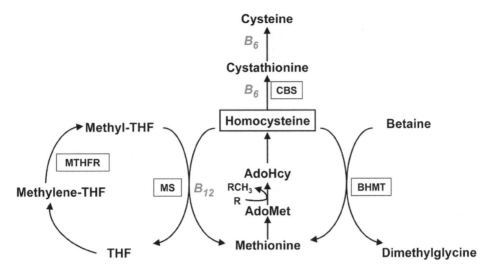

Fig. 1. Schematic representation of homocysteine metabolism. THF, tetrahydrofolate; MTHFR, methylenetetrahydrofolate reductase; MS, methionine synthase; AdoMet, *S*-adenosylmethionine; AdoHcy, *S*-adenosylhomocysteine; BHMT, betaine homocysteine methyltransferase; CBS, cystathionine-β-synthase; B12, vitamin B12; B6, vitamin B6.

remethylation pathway that is catalyzed by methionine synthase, cobalamin acts as a cofactor and the methyl group is donated by 5-methyltetrahydrofolate, while in the other, less important, remethylation pathway, betaine is the methyl donor. In the trans-sulfuration pathway, homocysteine is transformed by cystathionine-β-synthase (CBS) in cystathionine, with pyridoxal-5′-phosphate, a vitamin B-6 derivative, acting as a cofactor. Vitamin B-6 is also necessary for transformation of cystathionine to cysteine and alpha-ketobutyric acid. Under conditions of methionine excess, homocysteine is prevalently metabolized through the trans-sulfuration pathway; in contrast, under conditions of negative methionine balance, homocysteine is mostly transformed in methionine (Finkelstein, 1990; Storch et al., 1990).

1.2. *Determinants of plasma tHcy Levels*

The plasma levels of tHcy increase with age, are lower in fertile women than in men and increase after menopause (Andersson et al., 1992; Nygård et al., 1995; Wouters et al., 1995; Lussier-Cacan et al., 1996; Selhub et al., 1999) (Table 1). Major determinants of plasma tHcy levels include genetic abnormalities, diet (vitamin B12, B6 and folate intake), renal function, cigarette smoking and coffee consumption (Selhub et al., 1993, 1999; Nygård et al., 1995, 1997a, 1998; Cravo et al., 1996; Lussier-Cacan et al., 1996). Strict vegetarians tend to have high tHcy levels, probably due to vitamin B12 depletion (Mann et al., 1999; Mezzano et al., 1999). Other less well-established determinants of tHcy are race (Carmel et al., 1999; Osganian et al., 1999), arterial hypertension, hypercholesterolemia and physical exercise (Cattaneo, 1999a).

Table 1
Factors affecting the plasma levels of tHcy

	Effect on plasma tHcy levels
Age	Increase
Male gender	Increase
Menopause	Increase
Insufficient intake of folate, vitamin B6 and B12	Increase
Cigarette smoking	Increase
Coffee consumption	Increase
Congenital enzymatic defects (see text)	Increase
Renal function	Decrease
Physical exercise	Decrease
Drugs	
Methotrexate	Increase
Trimethoprim	Increase
Anticonvulsants	Increase
Nitrous oxide	Increase
Theophilline	Increase
Fibrates	Increase
Estrogens	Decrease
Tamoxifen	Decrease
Penicillamine	Decrease
Acetylcysteine	Decrease

2. Causes of hyperhomocysteinemia

2.1. *Severe hyperhomocysteinemia (homocystinuria)*

The most frequent cause of severe hyperhomocysteinemia (characterized by fasting levels of tHcy in plasma higher than 100 µmol/l) is the homozygous deficiency of CBS, which has a prevalence in the general population of approximately 1 in 335,000, varying between 1:65,000 (Ireland) and 1:900,000 (Japan) (Naughton et al., 1998). Affected individuals develop the classic syndrome of homocystinuria, characterized by ectopic lens, skeletal abnormalities, premature vascular disease, thromboembolism and mental retardation (Mudd et al., 1995). Approximately 5–10% of cases of severe hyperhomocysteinemia are caused by inherited defects of remethylation (Mudd et al., 1995; Rozen, 1996). Homozygous deficiency of methylene-tetrahydrofolate reductase (MTHFR), which catalyzes the reduction of methylenetetrahydrofolate to methyltetrahydrofolate, is the most common inherited defect of the remethylation pathway and is characterized by neurological dysfunction, psychomotor retardation, seizures, peripheral neuropathy, premature vascular disease and thromboembolism. Rare cases of homocystinuria have been described in subjects with errors of cobalamin metabolism, resulting in decreased activity of methionine synthase (Rosenblatt and Cooper, 1990).

2.2. *Mild-to-moderate hyperhomocysteinemia*

Mild-to-moderate forms of hyperhomocysteinemia (fasting levels of tHcy between 12 and 100 μmol/l) are encountered in phenotypically normal subjects with genetic defects, acquired conditions, or, more frequently, a combination of both. Genetic defects associated with moderate hyperhomocysteinemia cause approximately a 50% reduction in activities of the corresponding enzymes, such as heterozygosity for CBS or MTHFR deficiency, whose cumulative prevalence in the general population is between 0.4% and 1.5% (Rees and Rodgers, 1993). Another genetic defect that is associated with 50% reduction of the enzymatic activity is characterized by the presence of a thermolabile mutant of MTHFR (Kang et al., 1988), which is due to the homozygous C to T substitution at nucleotide 677 of the encoding gene, converting the codon for alanine to that for valine (Frosst et al., 1995). The prevalence of homozygosity for the C677T mutation is between 5% and 20% in subjects of Caucasian descent. Moderate elevations of plasma tHcy levels are not found in all subjects with genetic defects causing a 50% reduction of the corresponding enzyme activities, indicating that their phenotypic expression can be influenced by other factors. For instance, homozygotes for the thermolabile form of MTHFR and heterozygotes for CBS deficiency have high homocysteine levels mainly in the presence of low serum concentrations of folic acid (Kang, 1995; Guttormsen et al., 1996; Ma et al., 1996). Another common mutation in the MTHFR gene, A1298C, is not associated with hyperhomocysteinemia, but might interact with the C677T mutation in raising tHcy levels in plasma (van der Put et al., 1998).

Common causes of acquired hyperhomocysteinemia include deficiencies of folate, cobalamin and pyridoxine, which are essential cosubstrates or cofactors for homocysteine metabolism, and chronic renal insufficiency. Vitamin deficiencies are the most frequent cause of hyperhomocysteinemia (Selhub et al., 1999), especially in elderly people (Joosten et al., 1993; Selhub et al., 1993, 1995). Drugs interfering with the metabolism of folate, such as methotrexate, trimethoprim and anticonvulsants, of cobalamin, such as nitrous oxide, and of vitamin B-6, such as theophylline, can cause moderate hyperhomocysteinemia (McCully, 1996; Ubbink et al., 1996; Rees and Rodgers, 1993; Smulders et al., 1999). The increase in plasma tHcy after therapy with fibrates (De Lorgeril et al., 1999; Dierkes et al., 1999; Landray et al., 1999) may be partly related to an induced functional reduction in renal function (Dierkes et al., 1999; Landray et al., 1999). Estrogens (Van der Mooren et al., 1994; Giltay et al., 1998), tamoxifen (Anker et al., 1995; Cattaneo et al., 1998a), penicillamine (Kang et al., 1986) and acetylcysteine (Wiklund et al., 1996) reduce the plasma tHcy levels.

3. Measurement of tHcy in plasma

Current methods to assay plasma tHcy include gas chromatography–mass spectroscopy and HPLC with fluorometric or electrochemical detection (reviewed in Guba et al., 1996). Recently, manual or fully automated enzyme immunoassays have become commercially available, which should allow tHcy measurements in non-specialized clinical laboratories (Schipchandler and Moore, 1995; Frantzen et al.,

1998). Recent studies, which compared plasma tHcy measurements in different laboratories, pointed to the need to improve analytical precision and to the establishment of an international plasma standard to harmonize tHcy measurement across laboratories (Pfeiffer et al., 1999; Tripodi et al., 2001, 2002).

3.1. *The post-methionine loading (PML) test*

Measurement of plasma homocysteine 4–8 h after a standardized oral methionine loading (3.8 g/m² body surface area or 0.1 g/kg body weight), which was initially developed to detect heterozygosity for CBS deficiency (Fowler et al., 1971; Boers et al., 1985), improves the ability of distinguishing between normal individuals and subjects with mild abnormalities of the homocysteine metabolism (Boers et al., 1985; Falcon et al., 1994; Fermo et al., 1995; Mudd et al., 1995; Cattaneo et al., 1996; Graham et al., 1997). A shortened 2-h protocol has been validated, which may offer advantages of patient acceptability over the 4-h or 8-h protocols (Bostom et al., 1995). However, the equivalence of the 2-h and 4-h protocol has been recently questioned (Cattaneo et al., 1998b). It appears that the PML test is most sensitive to the trans-sulfuration pathway of homocysteine (Selhub and Miller, 1992; Miller et al., 1994). However, it is also abnormal in individuals who are homozygous for the C677T mutation of the MTHFR gene, who have a selective defect of the remethylation pathway of homocysteine (Cattaneo et al., 1997).

3.2. *Normal ranges*

Normal ranges vary widely in different populations, since they are affected by several lifestyle determinants (see above). When determined in a population with adequate vitamin intake (Ubbink et al., 1995; Rasmussen et al., 1996), the upper limit of the normal range may be as low as 12 μmol/l. Reference ranges for the PML *increase* of tHcy above fasting levels (the PML *absolute levels* of tHcy should not be considered, since they are partly affected by the fasting levels) have less extensively been determined.

4. Hyperhomocysteinemia in atherothrombotic disease

In 1969, McCully first reported the presence of severe atherosclerotic lesions in patients with homocystinuria and hypothesized the existence of a pathogenic link between hyperhomocysteinemia and atherogenesis (McCully, 1969). Several epidemiological studies have confirmed the initial hypothesis of McCully, showing that also moderate hyperhomocysteinemia is associated with heightened risk of arterial disease (Refsum et al., 1998; Cattaneo, 1999a).

4.1. *Case-control studies*

In 1976, Wilcken and Wilcken first showed that patients with coronary artery disease have elevated concentrations of plasma cysteine–homocysteine disulfide after an oral methionine load (Wilcken and Wilcken, 1976). Increased plasma levels of homocysteine species before and/or after an oral methionine load were subsequently reported by several other groups on patients with atherothrombosis (coronary artery disease, cerebrovascular disease and peripheral arterial occlusive disease) (Refsum et al., 1998; Cattaneo, 1999a).

A meta-analysis of 27 studies, mostly with a case-control design, published before 1994, revealed that the summary odds ratio as an estimate of the relative risk in subjects with hyperhomocysteinemia was 1.7 (95% CI, 1.5–1.9) for CAD, 2.5 (2.0–3.0) for cerebrovascular disease and 6.8 (2.9–15.8) for peripheral arterial disease (Boushey et al., 1995). For each increase in tHcy concentration of 5 μmol/l, there was an increase of approximately 40% in the relative risk for CAD. The association of hyperhomocysteinemia with arterial occlusive diseases remained statistically significant after adjustment for known risk factors, such as smoking, cholesterol, hypertension and diabetes. Many other case-control studies have been published since then, most of which confirmed the association of hyperhomocysteinemia with cardiovascular diseases. Among them, a multicenter study of 750 patients with vascular disease and 800 controls confirmed that hyperhomocysteinemia conferred a graded risk of vascular disease, which was similar to and independent of that of other risk factors, such as smoking and hypercholesterolemia (Graham et al., 1997). A more recent analysis of the same study revealed that, in addition to plasma homocysteine levels, concentrations of red cell folate below the 10th centile and of vitamin B-6 below the 20th centile for control subjects were also associated with increased risk (Robinson et al., 1998). This risk was independent of conventional risk factors and, for folate, it was explained in part by high levels of tHcy. In contrast, the association between vitamin B-6 and the risk of vascular disease was independent of tHcy levels both before and after methionine loading (Robinson et al., 1998). These results agree with those of those of other studies, which showed that low pyridoxal-5′-phosphate confers an independent risk for coronary artery disease (Folsom et al., 1998; Robinson et al., 1995).

4.2. Cross-sectional studies

Several cross-sectional studies demonstrated the existence of a relationship between homocysteine level and the extent of atherosclerosis in the aorta (Malinow et al., 1993; Selhub et al., 1995; Konecki et al., 1997), coronary (von Eckardstein et al., 1994; Verhoef et al., 1997a) and peripheral arteries (Taylor et al., 1991; van den Berg et al., 1996).

4.3. Prospective studies

4.3.1. Prospective studies of healthy subjects

The results of 13 prospective studies, all with a nested case-control design, of the relationship between tHcy and risk of cardiovascular disease in subjects who were healthy at the time of their enrollment are controversial. Six of them demonstrated that tHcy levels at baseline could predict the risk of future cardiovascular and/or cerebrovascular events, while seven of them failed to demonstrate such an association (Taylor et al., 1991; Stampfer et al., 1992; Malinow et al., 1993; Alfthan et al., 1994;

von Eckardstein et al., 1994; Verhoef et al., 1994; Arnesen et al., 1995; Perry et al., 1995; Chasan-Taber et al., 1996; Stehouwer et al., 1996; van den Berg et al., 1996; Bots et al., 1997; Evans et al., 1997; Konecki et al., 1997; Verhoef et al., 1997a, 1997b; Folsom et al., 1998; Ubbink et al., 1998; Wald et al., 1998; Whincup et al., 1999).

4.3.2. *Prospective studies of elderly healthy subjects*

The results of prospective studies of elderly healthy subjects, one of them including post-menopausal women, showed that high tHcy levels are associated with an increased risk not only for future cardiovascular and cerebrovascular events (Stehouwer et al., 1998; Bots et al., 1999; Bostom et al., 1999a, 1999b; Kark et al., 1999; Ridker et al., 1999; Aronow and Ahn, 2000) but also for all-cause and cardiovascular mortality (Bostom et al., 1999a; Kark et al., 1999).

4.3.3. *Prospective studies of patients with overt coronary artery disease or other conditions at risk*

In 1997, a prospective study of patients with overt coronary artery disease showed that there was a strong, graded and statistically significant relation between tHcy levels and overall mortality, which was independent of other risk factors (Nygård et al., 1997b). When death due to cardiovascular disease was considered as the end point, the relation between tHcy levels and mortality was even stronger. Subgroup analysis revealed that tHcy predicted the risk of death independent of age, gender, serum cholesterol, smoking, blood pressure and serum creatinine. In agreement with these data, more recent studies showed that plasma tHcy levels are independent predictors of long-term survival (Omland et al., 2000; Anderson et al., 2000) and late cardiac events (Stubbs et al., 2000) in patients with acute coronary syndromes or angiographically defined coronary artery disease. In a study of 337 patients with systemic lupus erythematosus, Petri et al. (1996) found that high tHcy concentrations were significantly associated with stroke (odds ratio 2.24; 95% CI, 1.22–4.13) and arterial thrombotic events (3.71; 95% CI, 1.96–7.13). The association remained statistically significant after adjustment for established risk factors.

Patients with chronic renal failure have markedly increased plasma levels of tHcy. In addition to case-controls and cross-sectional studies (Robinson et al., 1996; Bostom and Lathrop, 1997), two prospective studies of maintenance peritoneal dialysis or hemodialysis patients revealed that the adjusted hazard ratios for non-fatal and fatal cardiovascular events were from 3.0 to 4.4 in patients with tHcy levels in the upper quartile, compared to those of patients with tHcy levels in the three lowest quartiles (Bostom et al., 1997) and that the relative risk for cardiovascular events, including death, increased 1% per μmol/l increase in tHcy concentration (RR, 1.01; 95% CI, 1.00–1.01) Moustapha et al. (1998). More recently, hyperhomocysteinemia was shown to be a predictor of mortality in type 2 diabetes (Stehouwer et al., 1999; Hoogeveen et al., 2000).

In conclusion, while case-control studies consistently showed a positive association between hyperhomocysteinemia and atherothrombotic events, prospective cohort studies gave conflicting results. However, a clear distinction should be made between prospective cohort studies of subjects who were healthy at the moment of their enrollment, and prospective cohort studies of patients with overt athero-thrombotic disease or other conditions at risk. While studies of healthy subjects gave conflicting results, studies of patients at risk consistently showed a positive association between baseline tHcy levels and the risk of future atherothrombotic events. This has been demonstrated not only in patients whose high risk was due to the presence of pathological conditions, such as previous cardiovascular disease, diabetes, end-stage renal disease, systemic lupus erythematosus, but also in subjects who were at increased risk due to physiological conditions, such as advanced age and post-menopausal status. Several interpretations of these findings can be given, the simplest one being that hyperhomocysteinemia, a weak risk factor by itself, synergizes with other conditions to increase the risk of future events (Cattaneo, 2001).

In agreement with this interpretation, two recent case-control studies, nested in a population-based cohort study, showed that hyperhomocysteinemia predicts the risk of future CHD events in women (Knekt et al., 2001a) and men (Knekt et al., 2001b) with a positive history of CHD but not in those without previous CHD.

4.4. *Case-control and cross-sectional studies of genetic abnormalities of Hcy Metabolism*

The homozygous C677T mutation of MTHFR was associated with a threefold increase in cardiovascular risk in the initial study by Kluijtmans et al. (1996). After this initial report, several additional studies of the frequency of the C677T MTHFR mutation in cardiovascular patients have been published. A meta-analysis of eight studies revealed that the homozygous genotype for the C677T mutation was present in 299 of 2476 patients (12.1%), and in 257 of 2481 controls (10.4%), resulting in a significant odds ratio of 1.22 (95% CI, 1.01–1.47), relative to the normal genotype (Kluijtmans et al., 1997a). In contrast, a subsequent meta-analysis of 13 studies including a total of 3281 patients with cardiovascular disease and 3218 healthy controls revealed no difference between patients and control subjects neither in the allele frequency (33.7 vs. 35.6, respectively) nor in the frequency of mutant homozygotes (12.2 vs. 13.2, respectively) (Brattsröm et al., 1998). More recent studies suggest that the C677T mutation of MTHFR may be associated with increased risk for early-onset coronary artery disease (Mager et al., 1999) or childhood stroke (Nowak-Gottl et al., 1999).

A common 844ins68 insertion variant in the CBS gene, which was independently described by two groups (Sperandeo et al., 1996; Tsai et al., 1996), is not associated with hyperhomocysteinemia nor with heightened risk of vascular disease (Kluijtmans et al., 1997b).

In line with previous similar studies (see above), two recent cross-sectional studies showed that carotid atherosclerosis was associated with high Hcy levels; however, no such association was found with the C677T mutation (McQuillan et al., 1999; Spence et al., 1999).

The lack of associations between genetic determinants of hyperhomocysteinemia and cardiovascular risk or carotid atherosclerosis is in marked contrast with the results of case-control studies of hyperhomocysteinemia in cardiovascular diseases. Although some explanations have been attempted (Refsum et al., 1998), this paradox questions the hypothesis of the existence of a causal relationship between hyper-homocysteinemia and cardiovascular diseases.

5. Hyperhomocysteinemia in venous thrombosis

5.1. *Case-control studies*

After the publication of two negative studies of a small series of patients (Brattsröm et al., 1991; Bienvenu et al., 1993), the association of moderate hyper-homocysteinemia with venous thrombosis was demonstrated by Falcon et al. in 1994 (Falcon et al., 1994). They showed a high prevalence of moderate hyperhomocys-teinemia in patients with early-onset venous thrombosis, in whom other congenital or acquired causes of thrombophilia had been ruled out (Falcon et al., 1994). In this, as well as in subsequent confirmatory studies (Fermo et al., 1995; Cattaneo et al., 1996), the measurement of tHcy after an oral methionine loading allowed the detection of a greater number of patients with abnormal Hcy metabolism than measurement of fasting levels alone. In 1995, the association between hyperhomo-cysteinemia and venous thrombosis was reported in a study of patients with a history of recurrent venous thrombosis (den Heijer et al., 1995). A high prevalence of hyperhomocysteinemia was later found in patients with first episodes of deep-vein thrombosis of the lower extremities (Amundsen et al., 1995; Cattaneo et al., 1996; den Heijer et al., 1996; Simioni et al., 1996), although the statistical significance was reached in two studies only (den Heijer et al., 1996; Simioni et al., 1996). No asso-ciation was found between hyperhomocysteinemia and the risk of deep-vein thrombosis of the upper extremities (Martinelli et al., 1997).

Two meta-analysis of published case-control studies of hyperhomocysteinemia in venous thrombosis have been published. Both showed that both fasting and post-methionine loading hyperhomocysteinemia associate with a 2- to 3-fold relative risk of venous thrombosis (den Heijer et al., 1998a; Ray, 1998).

Whether hyperhomocysteinemia is associated with increased risk for venous thrombosis by itself or only when combined with other congenital risk factors has been a matter of debate, although the bulk of evidence now suggests that the thrombotic risk associated with hyperhomocysteinemia is independent of the coex-istence of abnormalities of the natural anticoagulant system.

A recent case-control study showed that low plasma levels of vitamin B6 are associated with a heightened risk of deep-vein thrombosis independent of other risk factors, including plasma tHcy levels (Cattaneo et al., 2001).

5.2. *Prospective studies*

5.2.1. *First episodes of venous thromboembolism*
Three prospective studies of tHcy as predictor of the risk for first episodes of venous thromboembolism gave essentially negative results (Petri et al., 1996; Ridker

et al., 1997; Cattaneo et al., 1998c). There was no association of hyperhomocysteinemia and the risk of venous thromboembolism in SLE patients (Petri et al., 1996), nor in patients who underwent elective hip replacement surgery and were screened for post-operative deep-vein thrombosis with bilateral phlebography (Cattaneo et al., 1998c). Ridker et al. (1997), in their nested case-control study of a subset of 22,071 male physicians participating in the Physician Health Study, did find an association between hyperhomocysteinemia and an increased risk to develop future episodes of idiopathic venous thrombosis, but only when hyperhomocysteinemia was associated with factor V Leiden, an established risk factor for venous thromboembolism. The association of hyperhomocysteinemia with idiopathic venous thrombosis in the absence of factor V Leiden only approached statistical significance ($P=0.06$). The inclusion of men only and of patients with cancer in this prospective study is among the possible reasons accounting for the differences with case-control studies, which demonstrated an association between hyperhomocysteinemia and venous thrombosis that was independent of the coexistence of resistance to activated protein C or factor V Leiden (Cattaneo et al., 1998d).

5.2.2. *Recurrent episodes of thromboembolism*

In a prospective, multicenter study of 264 patients with objectively documented single episode of idiopathic venous thromboembolism, Eichinger et al. (1998) recently showed that the risk of recurrent venous thromboemblism is higher (RR 2.7, 95% CI 1.3–5.8) in patients with hyperhomocysteinemia than in patients with normal tHcy levels.

5.3. *Case-control studies of genetic abnormalities of hcy metabolism*

Studies of the prevalence of mutant C677T MTHFR in patients with venous thrombosis gave conflicting results (Arruda et al., 1997; Cattaneo et al., 1997; Tosetto et al., 1997; Kluijtmans et al., 1998; Margaglione et al., 1998; Alhenc-Gelas et al., 1999; Rintelen et al., 1999; Salomon et al., 1999). In three studies, C677T was shown to be a risk factor for venous thrombosis (Arruda et al., 1997; Margaglione et al., 1998; Salomon et al., 1999). The other studies failed to demonstrate an increased prevalence of C677T MTHFR among patients as compared to controls. The coexistence of factor V Leiden or the G20210A mutation of the gene encoding for factor II and mutant C677T MTHFR conferred a particularly high risk for venous thrombosis in some studies (Cattaneo et al., 1997; Salomon et al., 1999; den Heijer et al., 1999), but not in others (Kluijtmans et al., 1998; Alhenc-Gelas et al., 1999; Cattaneo et al., 1999b).

6. Hyperhomocysteinemia as a risk factor for dementia and Alzheimer's disease

It is known that patients with cardiovascular risk factors and previous episodes of stroke are at increased risk for vascular dementia and Alzheimer's disease (Hofman et al., 1997a; Snowdon et al., 1997; Breteler, 2000) and that there is an inverse association between tHcy levels and cognitive function (Bell et al., 1992; Riggs et al.,

1996; Lehmann et al., 1999; Morris et al., 2001). Two case-control studies found higher plasma tHcy levels in patients with Alzheimer's disease than age- and sex-matched healthy controls (McCaddon et al., 1998; Clarke et al., 1998). The association of hyperhomocysteinemia with dementia was confirmed in a prospective study in which plasma tHcy was examined in relation to newly diagnosed dementia and Alzheimer's disease in the elderly, population-based cohort of Framingham Study participants (Seshadri et al., 2002). An increment in the plasma tHcy levels of 5 μmol/l increased the risk of Alzheimer's disease by 40%, and a plasma tHcy level in the upper age-specific quartile doubled the risk of dementia or Alzheimer's disease. The observed association was independent of age, sex, APOE genotype, plasma vitamin levels and other putative risk factors, and could be observed only after a follow-up period of at least 4 yr.

Recent animal studies support a role for elevated homocysteine levels in rendering neurons vulnerable to dysfunction and death in Alzheimer's and Parkinson's diseases, and further suggest that dietary folic acid can be neuroprotective. Transgenic mice expressing a mutant form of amyloid precursor protein that causes familial Alzheimer's disease exhibit age-dependent amyloid deposition in their brains, but no degeneration of neurons under usual animal maintenance conditions. However, when the "Alzheimer's" mice are maintained on a diet with reduced levels of folic acid, homocysteine levels increase and hippocampal pyramidal neurons degenerate (Kruman et al., 2002). In addition, folic acid deprivation and homocysteine rendered cultured neurons vulnerable to being killed by amyloid. In a mouse model of Parkinson's disease, damage to dopamine-producing neurons is increased and motor function is more severely impaired when the mice are maintained on a folic acid deficient diet (Duan et al., 2002). Additional studies suggest that homocysteine promotes neuronal degeneration by impairing DNA repair; this renders neurons vulnerable to oxidative and metabolic stress (Kruman et al., 2000, 2002).

The causal association between hyperhomocysteinemia should be tested in properly designed clinical trials evaluating the effects of tHcy lowering vitamin therapy on the progression and development of dementia and Alzheimer's disease.

7. Hyperhomocysteinemia in other pathologic conditions

In addition to renal failure and cobalamin and folate deficiencies, hyperhomocysteinemia can be found in other pathologic conditions, such as hypothyroidism (Nedrebo et al., 1998), inflammatory bowel disease (Cattaneo et al., 1998e) and rheumatoid arthritis (Roubenoff et al., 1997), suggesting a potential mechanism for the high incidence of thrombotic complications in these patients. Hyperhomocysteinemia was also found in patients with renal or heart transplantation (Sunder-Plassmann et al., 2000) with lymphoproliferative disorders (Refsum et al., 1991), but not in patients with polycytemia (Tonon et al., 1997). It is common in insulin-dependent diabetes mellitus if it is complicated by nephropathy, and may contribute to increased mortality from cardiovascular disease in these patients (Hofman et al.,

1997b); in addition, it is a very strong risk factor for cardiovascular complications in patients with non-insulin-dependent diabetes mellitus (Hoogeveen et al., 1998).

8. Mechanisms by which hyperhomocysteinemia might predispose to vascular disease

The mechanism(s) by which hyperhomocysteinemia might contribute to atherogenesis and thrombogenesis are incompletely understood. In vivo studies in baboons showed that homocysteine causes endothelial cell desquamation, smooth muscle cell proliferation and intimal thickening (Harker et al., 1976). In vitro studies showed that homocysteine-induced endothelial injury requires copper and oxygen and is prevented by catalase but not superoxide dismutase, suggesting that production of hydrogen peroxide is responsible for the toxic effect on endothelial cells (Starkebaum and Harlan, 1986). Other effects of homocysteine include activation of factor V (Rodgers and Kane, 1986) and interference with protein C activation and thrombomodulin expression (Rodgers and Conn, 1990; Lentz and Sadler, 1991; Hayashi et al., 1992); inhibition of the inactivation of factor Va by activated protein C (APC) (Undas et al., 2001); inhibition of tissue plasminogen activator binding (Haijar, 1993) and modulation of tissue plasminogen activator binding to annexin II tail domain (Haijar et al., 1998); impaired generation and decreased bioavailability of endothelium derived relaxing factor/nitric oxide (EDRF/NO) (Haijar, 1993; Stamler et al., 1993; Welch et al., 1997; Haijar et al., 1998) and prostacyclin (Wang et al., 1993), which are potent antiaggregating agents and vasodilators; induction of tissue factor activity (Fryer et al., 1993); suppression of the expression on the vessel wall of the anticoagulant substance heparan sulfate (Nishinaga et al., 1993); inhibition of ecto-ADPase (Broekman et al., 1994); increase of DNA synthesis in aortic smooth muscle cells and inhibition of DNA synthesis in human umbilical vein endothelial cells (HUVEC) (Tsai et al., 1994); enhanced collagen production and accumulation by smooth muscle cells (Majors et al., 1997); endoplasmic reticulum stress and growth arrest in HUVEC (Outinen et al., 1999); acceleration of endothelial cell senescence (Xu et al., 2000); induction of programmed cell death of human vascular endothelial cells (Zhang et al., 2001); induction of monocyte tissue factor expression (Khajuria and Houston, 2000). It must be noted, however, that most in vitro effects of homocysteine on endothelial cells have been demonstrated for very high homocysteine concentrations, usually at least one order of magnitude higher than the plasma concentrations of homocysteine that can be found in patients with homozygous homocystinuria. The lack of control samples in which the effects of other thiols, such as cysteine, were studied, questions the specificity of the observed effects. Therefore, the pathophysiological relevance of most in vitro studies awaits confirmation from in vivo and ex vivo experiments.

The data of an in vivo study of the effects of diet-induced hyperhomocysteinemia on vascular functions in monkeys showed that Hcy decreases vascular relaxation in response to various stimuli and inhibits thrombomodulin-dependent protein C activation in aortic endothelial cells (Lentz et al., 1996). These findings are consistent with the observation that in vitro exposure of endothelial cells to Hcy decreases the activity of nitric oxide and the activation of protein C. However, the finding that circulating plasma levels of activated protein C are not decreased in subjects with hyperhomocysteinemia and are increased in hyperhomocysteinemic patients with previous DVT, questions the pathogenic role of the thrombomodulin-protein C pathway in Hcy-induced thrombosis (Cattaneo et al., 1998f). In agreement with these data, another ex vivo study showed that patients with homocystinuria due to CBS deficiency have high plasma levels of activated protein C (Coppola et al., 1997). These patients also had high plasma levels of markers of thrombin generation, and abnormally high in vivo biosynthesis of thromboxane A_2, as reflected by increased urinary excretion of its metabolite 11-dehydro-thromboxane B_2 (Di Minno et al., 1993; Coppola et al., 1997).

Recent studies of murine models of hyperhomocysteinemia found that Hcy induces endothelial dysfunction (Eberhardt et al., 2000) and vascular inflammation, contributing to the acceleration of the atherogenic process (Hofman et al., 2001).

Compelling evidence indicates that both chronic (Tawakol et al., 1997; Woo et al., 1997) and acute (induced by an oral methionine loading) (Bellamy et al., 1998; Chambers et al., 1998, 1999; Nappo et al., 1999; Kanani et al., 1999; Chao et al., 2000) hyperhomocysteinemia impair the endothelium-dependent flow-mediated dilation of the brachial artery. The inhibitory effects of homocysteine were inhibited by antioxidant vitamins (Chambers et al., 1999; Nappo et al., 1999; Kanani et al., 1999), suggesting that the adverse effects of homocysteiune on vascular endothelial cells are mediated through oxidative stress mechanisms. However, this hypothesis has recently been questioned (Chao et al., 2000).

9. Treatment of hyperhomocysteinemia

Estrogens reduce the plasma tHcy levels in post-menopausal women (Van der Mooren et al., 1994). The estrogen agonist/antagonist tamoxifen, which is the standard endocrine treatment for breast cancer, reduces tHcy levels not only in patients with advanced breast cancer (Anker et al., 1995), but also in healthy women (Cattaneo et al., 1998a), indicating that its lowering effect is not only due to its antitumoral activity, but also to its direct effect on estrogen-regulated targets. This finding may explain the observed reduction in coronary artery disease associated with tamoxifen treatment (McDonald et al., 1995) and bears potentially important implications for the outcome of the ongoing trials of breast cancer prevention.

The mainstay of treatment of hyperhomocysteinemia is folic acid, alone or in combination with cobalamin and vitamin B-6 (Brattsröm, 1996). While the three vitamins were often administered in combination, it appears that folic acid is the most effective agent, since it reduces dramatically the plasma tHcy fasting levels also when given alone (Ubbink et al., 1994; den Heijer et al., 1998b). A meta-analysis of 12 trials of reduction of tHcy by dietary supplementation with folic acid alone, or in combination with vitamin B-6, vitamin B-12 or both, including 1114 individuals, was recently published (Homocysteine Lowering Trialists' Collaboration, 1998). It showed that the proportional and absolute reductions in blood fasting tHcy produced by folic acid supplements were greater at higher pretreatment blood tHcy concentrations and lower pretreatment serum folic acid levels. After standardization to pretreatment tHcy levels of 12 μmol/l and of folate of 12 nmol/l, folic acid, at doses ranging between 0.5 and 5 mg daily, significantly reduced plasma tHcy levels by 25% (95% CI, 23–28%) (Homocysteine Lowering Trialists' Collaboration, 1998). A lower dose of folic acid (0.5 mg every second day) decreased the tHcy levels by only 11% in 50 healthy women (Brouwer et al., 1999). In a recent randomized trial of supplementation of folic acid, a dosage of 0.8 mg/d appeared necessary to achieve the maximum reduction in serum homocysteine level across the range of tHcy levels (Wald et al., 2001). Higher doses of folic acid (2.4 mg) may be necessary to treat hyperhomocysteinemia in renal transplant recipients (Beaulieu et al., 1999). Cereal-grain products in the United States food supply are being fortified with folic acid to prevent neural tube defects. Cereals providing 127 μg of folic acid daily, which approximates the levels of folic acid fortification recommended by the Food and Drug Administration (FDA) (140 μg per 100 g of cereal-grain products), decreased plasma tHcy levels by only 3.7% in a recent controlled trial, which is probably insufficient to prevent cardiovascular disease (Malinow et al., 1998). A subsequent trial showed that a meal providing mean folate intakes of 601 ± 143 μg/d decreased the serum tHcy concentration from 10.8 ± 5.8 to 9.3 ± 4.9 μmol/l, while the normal diet, providing mean folate intakes of 270 ± 107 μg/d had no effects on tHcy levels (Chait et al., 1999). The first published study of the effects of folic acid fortification in the US was done within the frame of the Framingham Offspring Study (Jaques et al., 1999). It showed that folic acid fortification decreased the mean tHcy levels from 10.1 to 9.4 μmol/l and the prevalence of high tHcy concentrations (>13 μmol/l) from 18.7% to 9.8%. The most marked effect of folic acid fortification on tHcy levels was seen in subjects with hyperhomocysteinemia at baseline, whose mean levels decreased from 18.7 to 9.8 μmol/l (Jaques et al., 1999).

Vitamin B-6 should be added to folic acid and vitamin B-12, because it effectively reduces the post-methionine loading tHcy levels (Beaulieu et al., 1999). This finding corroborates the hypothesis that the post-methionine loading test is most sensitive to the trans-sulfuration pathway of Hcy metabolism, in which vitamin B-6 acts as a cofactor (Selhub and Miller, 1992; Miller et al., 1994; Ubbink et al., 1996). In addition to supplementation of vitamins, also dietary interventions can effectively lower the plasma levels of tHcy (Appel et al., 2000).

It is quite clear that the administration of high doses of vitamin B_6, often associated to folic acid and betaine, to patients with homocystinuria due to deficient activity of CBS is associated with considerable reduction of their thrombotic risk, despite the fact that their plasma tHcy levels remain moderately increased (Wilcken and Wilcken, 1997; Yap et al., 2001). The effect of lowering tHcy levels on the risk of thrombosis in individuals with moderate hyperhomocysteinemia is still unknown. In an uncontrolled study, the supplementation of vitamins (folic acid 2.5 mg/d, pyridoxine 25 mg/d and cyanocobalamin 250 μg/d) to 50 patients with vascular disease and hyperhomocysteinemia for about 2 yr decreased the rate of progression of carotid plaque (measured by two-dimensional B-mode ultrasound) from 0.21 ± 0.41 cm^2/yr to -0.049 ± 0.24 cm^2/yr (Jaques et al., 1999). A lower effect of the same vitamin regimen was also seen in 51 vascular disease patients with normal tHcy concentrations (Tucker et al., 1996). A recent controlled trial showed that the combination of folic acid (1 mg), vitamin B12 (400 µg), and pyridoxine (10 mg) administered to 205 patients for six months after successful coronary angioplasty significantly lowered plasma tHcy levels from 11.1 ± 4.3 to 7.2 ± 2.4 µmol/l. At follow-up, the minimal luminal diameter was significantly larger in the group assigned to vitamin treatment (1.72 ± 0.76 vs. 1.45 ± 0.88 mm), and the degree of stenosis was less severe (39.9 ± 20.3 vs. $48.2 \pm 28.3\%$). The rate of restenosis was significantly lower in patients assigned to vitamin treatment (19.6% vs. 37.6%), as was the need for revascularization of the target lesion (10.8% vs. 22.3%) (Schnyder et al., 2001). Vitamin treatment should, therefore, be considered as adjunctive therapy for patients undergoing coronary angioplasty.

To date, the recommended treatment of hyperhomocysteinemia should include folic acid (at least 1 mg/d) and vitamin B-6, with the addition of vitamin B-12 in order to secure full folic acid responsiveness and to avoid the risk of deteriorating cobalamin neuropathy in deficient patients, due to masking by folic acid (Hackam et al., 2000). Ongoing prospective, placebo-controlled clinical trials will tell us whether or not the hypothetical preventive effect of vitamin supplementation on thrombotic diseases is real.

References

Alfthan, G., Pekkanen, J., Jauhiainen, M., Pitkaniemi, J., Karvonen, M., Tuomilehto, T., Salonen, J.T., Ehnholm, C., 1994. Relation of serum homocysteine and lipoprotein (a) concentrations to atherosclerotic disease in a prospective finnish population based study. Atherosclerosis 106, 9–19.

Alhenc-Gelas, M., Arnaud, E., Nicaud, V., Aubry, M.-L., Flessinger, J.-N., Aiach, M., Emmerich, J., 1999. Venous thromboembolic disease and the prothrombin, methylenetetrahydrolfolate reductase and factor V genes. Thromb. Haemost. 81, 506–510.

Amundsen, T., Ueland, P.M., Waage, A., 1995. Plasma homocysteine levels in patients with deep venous thrombosis. Arterioscler. Thromb. Vasc. Biol. 15, 1321–1323.

Andersson, A., Brattsröm, L., Israelsson, B., Isaksson, A., Hamfelt, A., Hultberg, B., 1992. Plasma homocysteine before and after methionine loading with regard to age, gender, and menopausal status. Eur. J. Clin. Invest. 22, 79–87.

Anderson, J.L., Muhlestein, J.B., Horne, B.D., Carlquist, J.F., Bair, T.L., Madsen, T.E., Pearson, R.R., 2000. Plasma homocysteine predicts mortality independently of traditional risk factors and C-reactive protein in patients with angiographically defined coronary artery disease. Circulation Sep. 12 102(11), 1227–1232.

Anker, G., Lonning, P.E., Ueland, P.M., Refsum, H., Lien, E.A., 1995. Plasma levels of the atherogenic amino acid homocysteine in post-menopausal women with breast cancer treated with tamoxifen. Int. J. Cancer 60, 365–368.

Appel, L.J., Miller III, E.R., Jee, S.H., Stolzenberg-Solomon, R., Lin, P.H., Erlinger, T., Nadeau, M.R., Selhub, J., 2000. Effect of dietary patterns on serum homocysteine: results of a randomized, controlled feeding study. Circulation 102, 852–857.

Arnesen, E., Refsum, H., Bonan, K.H., Ueland, P.M., Forde, O.H., Nordrehaug, J.E., 1995. Serum total homocysteine and coronary heart disease. Int. J. Epidemiol. 24, 704–709.

Aronow, W.S., Ahn, C., 2000. Increased plasma homocysteine is an independent predictor of new coronary events in older persons. Am. J. Cardiol. Aug 1 86(3), 346–347.

Arruda, V.R., von Zuben, P.M., Chiaparini, L.C., Annichino-Bizzacchi, J.M., Costa, F.F., 1997. The mutation ALA677→VAL in the methylene-tetrahydrofolate reductase gene: a risk factor for arterial disease and venous thrombosis. Thromb. Haemost. 77, 818–821.

Beaulieu, A.J., Gohh, R.Y., Han, H., Hakas, D., Jaques, P.F., Selhub, J., Bostom, A.G., 1999. Enhanced reduction of fasting total homocysteine levels with supraphysiological versus standard multivitamin dose folic acid supplementation in renal transplant recipients. Arterioscler. Thromb. Vasc. Biol. 19, 2918–2921.

Bell, I.R., Edman, J.S., Selhub, J., Morrow, F.D., Marby, D.W., Kayne, H.L., Cole, J.O., 1992. Plasma homocysteine in vascular disease and in nonvascular dementia of depressed elderly people. Acta Psychiatr. Scand. 86, 386–390.

Bellamy, M.F., McDowell, I.F.W., Ramsey, M.W., Brownlee, M., Bones, C., Newcombe, R.G., Lewis, M.J., 1998. Hyperhomocysteinemia after an oral methionine load acutely impairs endothelial function in healthy adults. Circulation 98, 1848–1852.

Bienvenu, T., Ankri, A., Chadefaux, B., Montalescot, G., Kamoun, P., 1993. Elevated total plasma homocysteine, a risk factor for thrombosis: relation to coagulation and fibrinolytic parameters. Thromb. Res. 70, 123–129.

Boers, G.H.J., Fowler, B., Smals, A.G.H., Trijbels, F.J.M., Leermakers, A.I., Kleijer, W.J., Kloppenborg, P.W.C., 1985. Improved identification of heterozygotes for homocystinuria due to cystathionine synthase deficiency by the combination of methionine loading and enzyme determination in cultured fibroblasts. Hum. Genet. 69, 164–169.

Bostom, A.G., Roubenoff, R., Dellaripa, P., Nadeau, M.R., Sutherland, P., Wilson, P.W.F., Jaques, P.F., Selhub, J., Rosenberg, I.H., 1995. Validation of abbreviated oral methionine-loading test. Clin. Chem. 41, 948–949.

Bostom, A.G., Lathrop, L., 1997. Hyperhomocysteinemia in end-stage renal disease: prevalence, etiology, and potential relationship to arteriosclerotic outcomes. Kidney Internatl. 52, 10–20.

Bostom, A.G., Shemin, D., Verhoef, P., Nadeau, M.R., Jaques, P.F., Selhub, J., Dworkin, L., Rosenberg, I.H., 1997. Elevated fasting total plasma homocysteine levels and cardiovascular disease outcomes in maintenance dialysis patients. A prospective study. Arterioscler. Thromb. Vasc. Biol. 17, 2554–2558.

Bostom, A.G., Silbershatz, H., Rosenberg, I.H., Selhub, J., D'Agostino, R.B., Wolf, P.A., Jaques, P.F., Wilson, P.W.F., 1999a. Nonfasting plasma total homocysteine levels and all-cause and cardiovascular disease mortality in elderly Framingham men and women. Arch. Intern. Med. 159, 1077–1080.

Bostom, A.G., Rosenberg, I.H., Silbershatz, H., Jaques, P.F., Selhub, J., D'Agostino, R.B., Wilson, P.W.F., Wolf, P.A., 1999b. Nonfasting plasma total homocysteine levels and stroke incidence in elderly persons: The Framingham Study. Ann. Intern. Med. 131, 352–355.

Bots, M.L., Launer, L.J., Lindemans, J., Hofman, A., Grobbee, D.E., 1997. Homocysteine, atherosclerosis and prevalent cardiovascular disease in the elderly: The Rotterdam Study. J. Int. Med. 242, 339–347.

Bots, M.L., Launer, L.J., Lindemans, J., Hoes, A.W., Hofman, A., Witteman, J.C.M., Koudstaal, P.J., Grobbee, D.E., 1999. Homocysteine and short-term risk of myocardial infarction and stroke in the elderly. The Rooterdam Study. Arch. Intern. Med. 159, 38–44.

Boushey, C.J., Beresford, S.A.A., Omenn, G.S., Motulsky, A.G., 1995. A quantitative assessment of plasma homocysteine as a risk factor for vascular disease. Probable benefits of increasing folic acid intakes. JAMA 274, 1049–1057.

Brattsröm, L., Tangborn, L., Lagerstedt, C., Israelsson, B., Hultber, B., 1991. Plasma homocysteine in venous thromboembolism. Haemostasis 21, 51–57.

Brattström, L., 1996. Vitamins as homocysteine-lowering agents. J. Nutr. 126, 1276S–1280S.

Brattström, L., Wilcken, D.E.L., Ohrvik, J., Brudin, L., 1998. Common methylenetetrahydrofolate reductase gene mutation leads to hyperhomocysteinemia but not to vascular disease. The results of a meta-analysis. Circulation 98, 2520–2526.

Breteler, M.M., 2000. Vascular risk factors for Alzheimer's disease: an epidemiologic perspective. Neurobiol. Aging 21, 153–160.

Broekman, M.J., Haijar, K.A., Marcus, A.J., Lev, E., Islam, N., Safier, L.B., Fliessbach, J., 1994. Homocysteine inhibits ecto-ADPase activity of human umbilical vein endothelial cells. Blood 84 (Suppl. 1), 77.

Brouwer, I.A., van Dusseldorp, M., Thomas, C.M.G., Duran, M., Hautvast, J.G.A.J., Eskes, T.K.A.B., Steegers-Theunissen, R.P.M., 1999. Low-dose folic acid supplementation decreases plasma homocysteine concentrations: a randomized trial. Am. J. Clin. Nutr. 69, 99–104.

Carmel, R., Green, R., Jacobsen, D.W., Rasmussen, K., Florea, M., Azen, C., 1999. Serum cobalamin, homocysteine, and methylmalonic acid concentrations in a multiethnic elderly population: ethnic and sex differences in cobalamin and metabolite abnormalities. Am. J. Clin. Nutr. 70, 904–910.

Cattaneo, M., Martinelli, I., Mannucci, P.M., 1996. Hyperhomocysteinemia as a risk factor for deep-vein thrombosis. N. Engl. J. Med. 335, 974–975.

Cattaneo, M., Tsai, M.Y., Bucciarelli, P., Taioli, E., Zighetti, M.L., Bignell, M., Mannucci, P.M., 1997. A common mutation in the methylenetetrahydrofolate reductase gene (C677T) increases the risk for deep-vein thrombosis in patients with mutant factor V (factor V:Q506). Arterioscler. Thromb.-Vasc. Biol. 17, 1662–1666.

Cattaneo, M., Baglietto, L., Zighetti, M.L., Bettega, D., Robertson, C., Costa, A., Mannucci, P.M., Decensi, A., 1998a. Tamoxifen reduces plasma homocysteine levels in healthy women. Brit. J. Cancer 77, 2264–2266.

Cattaneo, M., Agati, B., Lecchi, A., Lombardi, R., Zighetti, M.L., Taioli, E., Mannucci, P.M., 1998b. Comparison between the 2-hour and the 4-hour methionine loading test for the identification of subjects with methionine intolerance. Netherlands J. Med. 52 (Suppl.), S37.

Cattaneo, M., Zighetti, M.L., Turner, R.M., Thompson, S.G., Lowe, G.D.O., Haverkate, F., Bertina, R.M., Turpie, A.G.G., Mannucci, P.M., the ECAT DVT Study Group, 1998c. Fasting plasma homocysteine levels do not predict the occurrence of deep-vein thrombosis after elective hip replacement surgery. Netherlands J. Med. 52 (Suppl.), S21.

Cattaneo, M., Monzani, M.L., Martinelli, I., Falcon, C.R., Mannucci, P.M., 1998d. Interrelation of hyperhomocyst(e)inemia, factor V Leiden, and risk of future venous thromboembolism. Circulation 97, 295.

Cattaneo, M., Vecchi, M., Zighetti, M.L., Saibeni, S., Martinelli, I., Omodei, P., Mannucci, P.M., de Franchis, R., 1998e. High prevalence of hyperhomocysteinemia in patients with inflammatory bowel disease: a pathogenic link with thromboembolic complications? Thromb. Haemost. 80, 542–545.

Cattaneo, M., Martinelli, I., Faioni, E., Franchi, F., Zighetti, M.L., Mannucci, P.M., 1998f. Plasma levels of activated protein C in healthy subjects and patients with previous venous thromboembolism. Relationship with plasma homocysteine levels. Arterioscler. Thromb. Vasc. Biol. 18, 1371–1375.

Cattaneo, M., 1999a. Hyperhomocysteinemia, atherosclerosis and thrombosis. Thromb. Haemost. 81, 165–176.

Cattaneo, M., Chantarangkul, V., Taioli, E., Hermida Santos, J., Tagliabue, L., 1999b. The G20210A mutation of the prothrombin gene in patients with previous first episodes of deep-vein thrombosis: prevalence and association with factor V G1691A, methylenetetrahydrofolate reductase C677T and plasma prothrombin levels. Thromb. Res. 93, 1–8.

Cattaneo, M., 2001. Is hyperhomocysteinemia a risk factor or a consequence of coronary heart disease? Arch. Intern. Med. 161, 2628–2629.

Cattaneo, M., Lombardi, R., Lecchi, A., Bucciarelli, P., Mannucci, P.M.., 2001. Low plasma levels of vitamin B(6) are independently associated with a heightened risk of deep-vein thrombosis. Circulation 104 (20), 2442–2446.

Chait, A., Malinow, M.R., Nevin, D.N., Morris, C.D., Eastgard, R.L., Kris-Etherton, P., Pi-Sunyer, F.X., Oparil, S., Resnick, L.M., Stern, J.S., Haynes, R.B., Hatton, D.C., Metz, J.A., Clark, S., McMahon, M., Holcomb, S., Reusser, M.E., Snyder, G.W., McCarron, D.A., 1999. Increased dietary micronutrients decrease serum homocysteine concentrations in patients at high risk of cardiovascular disease. Am. J. Clin. Nutr. 70, 881–887.

Chambers, J.C., McGregor, A., Jean-Marie, J., Kooner, J.S., 1998. Acute hyperhomocysteinaemia and endothelial dysfunction. Lancet 351, 36–37.

Chambers, J.C., McGregor, A., Jean-Marie, J., Obeid, O.A., Kooner, J.S., 1999. Demonstration of rapid onset vascular endothelial dysfunction after hyperhomocysteinemia. An effect reversible with vitamin C therapy. Circulation 99, 1156–1160.

Chao, C.-L., Kuo, T.-L., Lee, Y.-T., 2000. Effects of methionine-induced hyperhomocysteinemia on endothelium-dependent vasodilation and oxidative status in healthy adults. Circulation 101, 485–490.

Chasan-Taber, L., Selhub, J., Rosenberg, I.H., Malinow, M.R., Terry, P., Tishler, P.V., Willett, W., Hennekens, C.H., Stampfer, M.J., 1996. A prospective study of folate and vitamin B6 and risk of myocardial infarction in US physicians. J. Am. Coll. Nutr. 15, 136–143.

Clarke, R., Smith, A.D., Jobst, K.A., Refsum, H., Sutton, L., Ueland, P.M., 1998. Folate, vitamin B12, and serum total homocysteine levels in confirmed Alzheimer's disease. Arch. Neurol. 55, 1449–1455.

Coppola, A., Cerbone, A.M., Guiotto, G., Soriente, L., Piemontino, U., Rugiada, F., Viganò, D'Angelo, S., Della Valle, P., Mancini, F.P., Davì, G., Di Minno, G., Patrono, C., 1997. A hypercoagulable state in homocystinuria due to homozygous cystathionine-β-synthase deficiency. Thromb. Haemost. Suppl., 528.

Cravo, M.L., Gloria, L.M., Selhub, J., Nadeau, M.R., Camilo, M.E., Resende, M.P., Cardoso, J.N., Leitao, C.N., Mira, F.C., 1996. Hyperhomocysteinemia in chronic alcoholism: correlation with folate, vitamin B-12 and vitamin B-6 status. Am. J. Clin. Nutr. 63, 220–224.

De Lorgeril, M., Salen, P., Paillard, F., Lacan, P., Richard, G., 1999. Lipid-lowering drugs and homocysteine. Lancet 353, 209–210.

den Heijer, M., Blom, H.J., Gerrits, W.B.J., Rosendaal, F.R., Haak, H.L., Wijermans, P.W., Bos, G.M.J., 1995. Is hyperhomocysteinaemia a risk factor for recurrent venous thrombosis? Lancet 345, 882–885.

den Heijer, M., Koster, T., Blom, H.J., Bos, G.M.J., Briet, E., Reitsma, P.H., Vanderbroucke, J.P., Rosendaal, F.R., 1996. Hyperhomocysteinemia as a risk factor for deep-vein thrombosis. N. Engl. J. Med. 334, 759–762.

den Heijer, M., Rosendaal, F.R., Blom, H.J., Gerrits, W.B.J., Bos, G.M.J., 1998a. Hyperhomocysteinemia and venous thrombosis: a meta-analysis. Thromb. Haemost. 80, 874–877.

den Heijer, M., Brower, I.A., Bos, G.M., Blom, H.J., van der Put, N.M., Spaans, A.P., Rosendaal, F.R., Thomas, C.M., Haak, H.L., Wijermans, P.W., Gerrits, W.B., 1998b. Vitamin supplementation reduces blood homocysteine levels. A controlled trial in patients with venous thrombosis and healthy volunteers. Arterioscler. Thromb. Vasc. Biol. 18, 356–361.

den Heijer, M., Willems, H.P.J., Bos, G.M.J., Blom, H.J., Gerrits, W.B.J., Rosendaal, F.R., 1999. Homocysteine, serum folate, mutated methylenetetrahydrofolate reductase (MTHFR) and factor V Leiden and the risk of venous thrombosis. Thromb. Haemost. Suppl., 271.

Di Minno, G., Davi, G., Margaglione, M., Cirillo, F., Grandone, E., Ciabattoni, G., Catalano, I., Strisciuglio, P., Andria, G., Patrono, C., Mancini, M., 1993. Abnormally high thromboxane biosynthesis in homozygous homocystinuria. Evidence for platelet involvement and probucol-sensitive mechanism. J. Clin. Invest. 92, 1400–1406.

Dierkes, J., Westphal, S., Luley, C., 1999. Serum homocysteine increases after therapy with fenofibrate or bezafibrate. Lancet 354, 219–220.

Duan, W., Ladenheim, B., Cutler, R.G., Kruman I.I., Cadet, J.L., Mattson MP, 2002. Dietary folate deficiency and elevated homocysteine levels endanger dopaminergic neurons in models of Parkinson's disease. J. Neurochem. 80, 101–110.

Eberhardt, R.T., Forgione, M.A., Cap, A., Leopold, J.A., Rudd, M.A., Trolliet, M., Heydrick, S., Stark, R., Klings, E.S., Moldovan, N.I., Yaghoubi, M., Goldschmidt-Clermont, P.J., Farber, H.W., Cohen, R., Loscalzo, J., 2000. Endothelial dysfunction in a murine model of mild hyperhomocyst(e)inemia. J. Clin. Invest. 106, 483–491.

Eichinger, S., Stümpfen, A., Hirschl, M., Blalonczyk, C., Herkner, K., Stain, M., Schneider, B., Pabinger, I., Lechner, K., Kyrle, P.A., 1998. Hyperhomocysteinemia is a risk factor of recurrent venous thromboembolism. Thromb. Haemost. 80, 566–569.

Evans, R.W., Shaten, B.J., Hempel, J.D., Cutler, J.A., Kuller, L.H., for the MRFIT Research Group, 1997. Homocyst(e)ine and risk of cardiovascular disease in the multiple risk factor intervention trial. Arterioscler. Thromb. Vasc. Biol. 17, 1947–1953.

Falcon, C.R., Cattaneo, M., Panzeri, D., Martinelli, I., Mannucci, P.M., 1994. High prevalence of hyperhomocyst(e)inemia in patients with juvenile venous thrombosis. Arterioscler. Thromb. 14, 1080–1083.

Fermo, I., Viganò-D'Angelo, S., Paroni, R., Mazzola, G., Calori, G., D'Angelo, A., 1995. Prevalence of moderate hyperhomocysteinemia in patients with early-onset venous and arterial occlusive disease. Ann. Intern. Med. 123, 747–753.

Finkelstein, J.D., 1990. Methionine metabolism in mammals. J. Nutr. Biochem. 1, 228–257.

Folsom, A.R., Nieto, F.J., McGovern, P.G., Tsai, M.Y., Malinow, M.R., Eckfeldt, J.H., Hess, D.L., Davi, C.E., 1998. Prospective study of coronary heart disease incidence in relation to fasting total homocysteine, related genetic polymorphisms, and B vitamins. The Atherosclerosis Risk in Communities (ARIC) Study. Circulation 98, 204–210.

Fowler, B., Sardharwalla, I.B., Robins, A.J., 1971. The detection of heterozygotes for homocystinuria by oral loading with L-methionine. Biochem. J. 122, 23–24.

Frantzen, F., Faaren, A.L., Alfheim, I., Nordhei, A.K., 1998. Enzyme conversion immunoassay for determining total homocysteine in plasma or serum. Clin. Chem. 44, 311–316.

Frosst, P., Blom, H.J., Milos, R., Goyette, P., Sheppard, C.A., Matthews, R.G., Boers, G.J.H., den Heijer, M., Kluijtmans, L.A.J., van den Heuvel, L.P., Rozen, R., 1995. A candidate genetic risk factor for vascular disease: a common mutation in methylenetetrahydrofolate reductase. Nature Genet. 10, 111–113.

Fryer, R.H., Wilson, B.D., Gubler, D.B., Fitzgerald, L.A., Rodgers, G.M., 1993. Homocysteine, a risk factor for premature vascular disease and thrombosis, induces tissue factor activity in endothelial cells. Arterioscler. Thromb. 13, 1327–1332.

Giltay, E.J., Hoogeveen, E.K., Elbers, J.M.H., Gooren, L.J.G., Asscheman, H., Stehouwer, C.D.A., 1998. Effects of sex steroids on plasma total homocysteine levels: a study in transsexual males and females. J. Clin. Endocrinol. Metab. 83, 550–553.

Graham, I.M., Daly, L.E., Refsum, H.M., Robinson, K., Brattsröm, L.E., Ueland, P.M., Palma-Reis, R.J., Boers, G.H.J., Sheahan, R.G., Israelsson, B., Uiterwaal, C.S., Meleady, R., McMaster, D., Verhoef, P., Witterman, J., Rubba, P., Bellet, H., Wautrecht, J.C., de Valk, H.W., Sales Luis, A.C., Parrot-Roulaud, F.M., Soon Tan, K., Higgins, I., Garcon, D., Medrano, M.J., Candito, M., Evans, A.E., Andria, G., 1997. Plasma homocysteine as a risk factor for vascular disease. The European Concerted Action Project. JAMA 277, 1775–1781.

Guba, S.C., Fink, L.M., Fonseca, V., 1996. Hyperhomocysteinemia. An emerging and important risk factor for thromboembolic and cardiovascular disease. Am. J. Clin. Pathol. 105, 709–722.

Guttormsen. A.B., Ueland, P.M., Nesthus, I., Nygård, O., Schneede, J., Vollset, S.E., Refsum, H., 1996. Determinants and vitamin responsiveness of intermediate hyperhomocysteinemia (>40 μmol/liter). The Hordaland Homocysteine Study. J. Clin. Invest. 98, 2174–2183.

Hackam, D.G., Peterson, J.C., Spence, J.D., 2000. What levels of plasma homocyst(e)ine should be treated? Effects of vitamin therapy on progression of carotid atherosclerosis in patients with homocyst(e)ine levels above and below 14 μmol/l. Am. J. Hypertens. 13, 105–110.

Haijar, K.A., 1993. Homocysteine-induced modulation of tissue plasminogen activator binding to its endothelial cell membrane receptor. J. Clin. Invest. 91, 2873–2879.

Haijar, K.A., Mauri, L., Jacovina, A.T., Zhong, F., Mirza, U.A., Padovan, J.C., Chait, B.T., 1998. Tissue plasminogen activator binding to annexin II tail domain. Direct modulation by homocysteine. J. Biol. Chem. 273, 9987–9993.

Harker, L.A., Ross, R., Slichter, S.J., Scott, C.R., 1976. Homocysteine-induced arteriosclerosis: the role of endothelial cell injury and platelet response in its genesis. J. Clin. Invest. 58, 731–741.

Hayashi, T., Honda, G., Suzuki, K., 1992. An atherogenic stimulus homocysteine inhibits cofactor activity of thrombomodulin and enhances thrombomodulin expression in human umbilical vein endothelial cells. Blood 79, 2930–2936.

Hofman, A., Ott, A., Breteler, M.M., Bots, M.L., Slooter, A.J., van Harskamp, F., van Duijn, C.N., Van Broeckhoven, C., Grobbee, D.E., 1997a. Atherosclerosis, apolipoprotein E, and prevalence of dementia and Alzheimer's disease in the Rotterdam Study. Lancet 349, 151–154.

Hofman, M.A., Koll, B., Zumbach, M.S., Borces, V., Bierhaus, A., Henkels, M., Amiral, J., Fiehn, W., Ziegler, R., Wahl, P., Nawroth, P.P., 1997b. Hyperhomocyst(e)inemia and endothelial dysfunction in IDDM. Diabetes Care 20, 1880–1886.

Hofman, M.A., Lalla, E., Lu, Y., Gleason, M.R., Wolf, B.M., Tanji, N., Ferran Jr., L.J., Kohl, B., Rao, V., Kisiel, W., Stern, D.M., Schmidt, A.M., 2001. Hyperhomocysteinemia enhances vascular inflammation and accelerates atherosclerosis in a murine model. J. Clin. Invest. 107 (6), 675–683.

Homocysteine Lowering Trialists' Collaboration, 1998. Lowering blood homocysteine with folic acid based supplements: meta-analysis of randomised trials. Br. Med. J. 316, 894–898.

Hoogeveen, E.K., Kostense, P.J., Beks, P.J., Mackaay, A.J., Jakobs, C., Bouter, L.M., Heine, R.J., Stehouwer, C.D., 1998. Hyperhomocysteinemia is associated with an increased risk of cardiovascular disease, especially in non-insulin-dependent diabetes mellitus: a population-based study. Arterioscler. Thromb. Vasc. Biol. 18, 133–138.

Hoogeveen, E.K., Kostense, P.J., Jakobs, C., Dekker, J.M., Nijpels, G., Heine, R.J., Bouter, L.M., Stehouwer, C.D.A., 2000. Hyperhomocysteinemia increases risk of death, especially in type 2 diabetes. 5-year follow-up of the Hoorn Study. Circulation 101, 1506–1511.

Jaques, P.F., Selhub, J., Bostom, A.G., Wilson, P.W.F., Rosenberg, I.H., 1999. The effect of folic acid fortification on plasma folate and total homocysteine concentrations. N. Engl. J. Med. 340, 1449–1454.

Joosten, E., van den Berg, A., Riezler, R., Naurath, H.J., Lindenbaum, J., Stabler, S.P., Allen, R.H., 1993. Metabolic evidence that deficiencies of vitamin B-12 (cobalamin), folate, and vitamin B-6 occur commonly in elderly people. Am. J. Clin. Nutr. 58, 468–476.

Kanani, P.M., Sinkey, C.A., Browning, R.L., Allaman, M., Knapp, H.R., Haynes, W.G., 1999. Role of oxidant stress in endothelial dysfunction produced by experimental hyperhomocyst(e)inemia in humans. Circulation 100, 1161–1168.

Kang, S.-S., Wong, P.W.K., Glickman, P.B., MacLeod, C.M., Jaffe, I.A., 1986. Protein-bound homocyst(e)ine in patients with rheumatoid arthritis undergoing D-penicillamine treatment. J. Clin. Pharmacol. 26, 712–715.

Kang, S.-S., Zhou, J., Wong, P.W.K., Kowalisyn, J., Strokosch, G., 1988. Intermediate homocysteinemia: a termolabile variant of methylenetetrahydrofolate reductase. Am. J. Hum. Genet. 43, 414–421.

Kang, S.-S., 1995. Critical points for determining moderate hyperhomocyst(e)inaemia. Eur. J. Clin. Invest. 25, 806–808.

Kark, J.D., Selhub, J., Adler, B., Gofin, J., Abramson, J.H., Friedman, G., Rosenberg, I.H., 1999. Ann. Intern. Med. 131, 321–330.

Khajuria, A., Houston, D.S., 2000. Induction of monocyte tissue factor expression by homocysteine: a possible mechanism for thrombosis. Blood 96, 966–972.

Kluijtmans, L.A.J., van den Heuvel, L.P.W.J., Boers, G.H.J., Frosst, P., Stevens, E.M.B., van Oost, B.A., den Heijer, M., Trijbels, F.J.M., Rozen, R., Blom, H.J., 1996. Molecular genetic analysis in mild hyperhomocysteinemia: a common mutation in the methylenetetrahydrofolate reductase gene is a genetic risk factor for cardiovascular disease. Am. J. Hum. Genet. 58, 35–41.

Kluijtmans, L.A.J., Kastelein, J.J.P., Lindemans, J., Boers, G.H.J., Heil, S.G., Bruschke, A.V.G., Jukema, J.W., van den Heuvel, L.P.W.J., Trijbels, F.J.M., Boerma, G.J.M., Verheugt, F.W.A., Willems, F., Blom, H.J., 1997a. Thermolabile methylenetetrahydrofolate reductase in coronary artery disease. Circulation 96, 2573–2577.

Kluijtmans, L.A.J., Boers, G.H.J., Trijbels, F.J.M., van Lith-Zanders, H.M.A., van den Heuvel, L.P.W.J., Blom, H.J., 1997b. A common 844ins68 insertion variant in the cystathionine-β-synthase gene. Biochem. Mol. Med. 62, 23–25.

Kluijtmans, L.A.J., den Heijer, M., Reitsma, P.H., Heil, S.G., Blom, H.J., Rosendaal, F.R., 1998. Thermolabile methylenetetrahydrofolate reductase and factor V Leiden in the risk of deep-vein thrombosis. Thromb. Haemost. 79, 254–258.

Knekt, P., Alfthan, G., Aromaa, A., Heliovaara, M., Marniemi, J., Rissanen, H., Reunanen, A., 2001a. Homocysteine and major coronary events: a prospective population study amongst women. J. Intern. Med. 249, 461–465.

Knekt, P., Reunanen, A., Alfthan, G., Heliovaara, M., Rissanen, H., Marniemi, J., Aromaa, A., 2001b. Hyperhomocysteinemia. A risk factor or a consequence of coronary heart disease? Arch. Intern. Med.161, 1589–1594.

Konecki, N., Malinow, R., Tunick, P.A., Freedberg, R.S., Rosenzweig, B.P., Katz, E.S., Hess, D.L., Upson, B., Leung, B., Perez, J., Kronzon, I., 1997. Correlation between plasma homocyst(e)ine and aortic atherosclerosis. Am. Heart J. 133, 534–540.

Kruman, I.I., Culmsee, C., Chan, S.L., Kruman, Y., Guo, Z., Penix, L., Mattson, M.P., 2000. Homocysteine elicits a DNA damage response in neurons that promotes apoptosis and hypersensitivity to excitotoxicity. J. Neurosci. 20, 6920–6926.

Kruman, I.I., Kumaravel, T.S., Lohani, A., Pedersen, W.A., Cutler, R.G., Kruman, Y., Haughey, N., Lee, J., Evans, M., Mattson, M.P., 2002. Folic acid deficiency and homocysteine impair DNA repair in hippocampal neurons and sensitize them to amyloid toxicity in experimental models of Alzheimer's disease. J. Neurosci. 22, 1752–1762.

Landray, M.J., Townend, J.N., Martin, S., Martin, U., Wheeler, D.C., 1999. Lipid-lowering drugs and homocysteine. Lancet 353, 1974–1975.

Lehmann, M., Gottfries, C.G., Regland, B., 1999. Identification of cognitive impairment in the elderly: homocysteine is an early marker. Dement. Geriatr. Cogn. Disord. 10, 12–20.

Lentz, S.R., Sadler, J.E., 1991. Inhibition of thrombomodulin surface expression and protein C activation by the thrombogenic agent homocysteine. J. Clin. Invest. 88, 1906–1914.

Lentz, S.R., Sobey, C.G., Piegors, D.J., Bhopatkar, M.Y., Faraci, F.M., Malinow, M.R., Heistad, D.D., 1996. Vascular dysfunction in monkeys with diet-induced hyperhomocysteinemia. J. Clin. Invest. 98, 24–29.

Lussier-Cacan, S., Xhignesse, M., Piolot, A., Selhub, J., Davignon, J., Genest Jr., J., 1996. Plasma total homocysteine in healthy subjects: sex-specific relation with biological traits. Am. J. Clin. Nutr. 64, 587–593.

Ma, J., Stampfer, M.J., Hennekens, C.H., Frosst, P., Selhub, J., Horsford, J., Malinow, M.R., Willett, W.C., Rozen, R., 1996. Methylenetetrahydrofolate reductase polymorfism, plasma folate, homocysteine, and risk of myocardial infarction in US physicians. Circulation 94, 2410–2416.

Mager, A., Lalezari, S., Shohat, T., Birnbaum, Y., Adler, Y., Magal, N., Shohat, M., 1999. Methylenetetrahydrofolate reductase genotypes and early-onset coronary artery disease. Circulation 100, 2406–2410.

Majors, A., Ehrhart, L.A., Pezacka, E.H., 1997. Homocysteine as a risk factor for vascular disease. Enhanced collagen production and accumulation by smooth muscle cells. Arterioscler. Thromb. Vasc. Biol. 17, 2074–2081.

Malinow, M.R., Nieto, F.J., Szklo, M., Chambless, L.E., Bond, G., 1993. Carotid artery intimal-medial wall thickening and plasma homocyst(e)ine in asymptomatic adults. The Atherosclerosis in Communities (ARIC) Study. Circulation 87, 1107–1113.

Malinow, M.R., Duell, P.B., Hess, D.L., Anderson, P.H., Kruger, W.D., Phillipson, B.E., Gluckman, R.A., Block, P.C., Upson, B.M., 1998. Reduction of plasma homocyst(e)ine levels by breakfast cereal fortified with folic acid in patients with coronary heart disease. N. Engl. J. Med. 338, 1009–1015.

Mann, N.J., Li, D., Sinclair, A.J., Dudman, N.P.B., Guo, X.W., Elsworth, G.R., Wilson, A.K., Kelly, F.D., 1999. The effect of diet on plasma homocysteine concentrations in healthy male subjects. Eur. J. Clin. Nutr. 53, 895–899.

Margaglione, M., D'Andrea, G., d'Addedda, M., Giuliani, N., Cappucci, G., Iannaccone, L., Vecchione, G., Grandone, E., Brancaccio, V., Di Minno, G., 1998. The methylenetetrahydrofolate reductase TT677 genotype is associated with venous thrombosis independently of the coexistence of the FV Leiden and the prothrombin A20210 mutation. Thromb. Haemost. 79, 907–911.

Martinelli, I., Cattaneo, M., Panzeri, D., Taioli, E., Mannucci, P.M., 1997. Risk factors for primary deep vein thrombosis of the upper extremities. Ann. Intern. Med. 126, 707–711.

McCaddon, A., Davies, G., Hudson, P., Tandy, S., Cattell, H., 1998. Total serum homocysteine in senile dementia of Alzheimer type. Int. J. Geriatr. Psychiatry 13, 235–239.

McCully, K.S., 1969. Vascular pathology of homocysteinemia: implications for the pathogenesis of atherosclerosis. Am. J. Pathol. 56, 111–128.

McCully, K.S., 1996. Homocysteine and vascular disease. Nature Med. 2, 386–389.

McDonald, C.C., Alexander, F.E., White, W., Forrest, A.P., Stewart, H.J., 1995. Cardiac and vascular morbidity in women receiving adjuvant tamoxifen for breast cancer in a randomized trial. Br. Med. J. 311, 977–980.

McQuillan, B.M., Beilby, J.P., Nidorf, M., Thompson, P.L., Hung, J., 1999. Hyper-homocysteinemia but not the C677T mutation of methylenetetrahydrofolate reductase is an independent risk determinant of carotid wall thickening. The Perth Carotid Ultrasound Disease Assessment Study (CUDAS). Circulation 99, 2383–2388.

Mezzano, D., Munoz, X., Martinez, C., Cuevas, A., Panes, O., Aranda, E., Guasch, V., Strobel, P., Munoz, B., Rodriguez, S., Pereira, J., Leighton, F., 1999. Vegetarians and cardiovascular risk factors: hemostasis, inflammatory markers and plasma homocysteine. Thromb. Haemost. 81, 913–917.

Miller, J.W., Nadeau, M.R., Smith, D., Selhub, J., 1994.Vitamin B-6 deficiency vs folate deficiency: comparison of responses to methionine loading in rats. Am. J. Clin. Nutr. 59, 1033–1039.

Morris, M.S., Jaques, P.F., Rosenberg, I.H., Selhub, J., 2001. Hyperhomocysteinemia associated with poor recall in the third National Health and Nutrition Examination Survey. Am. J. Clin. Nutr. 73, 927–933.

Moustapha, A., Naso, A., Nahlawi, M., Gupta, A., Arheart, K.L., Jacobsen, D.W., Robinson, K., Dennis, V.W., 1998. Prospective study of hyperhomocysteinemia as an adverse cardiovascular risk factor in end-stage renal disease. Circulation 20, 138–141.

Mudd, S.H., Levy, H.L., Skovby, F., 1995. Disorders of transulfuration. In: Scriver, C.R., Beaudet, A.L., Sly, W.S., Valle, D., Stanbury, J.B., Wyngarden, J.B., Fredrickson, D.S. (Eds.), The Metabolic and Molecular Bases of Inherited Disease. McGraw-Hill, New York, pp. 1279–1327.

Mudd, S.H., Finkelstein, J.D., Refsum, H., Ueland, P.M., Malinow, M.R., Lentz, S.R., Jacobsen, D.W., Brattstrom, L., Wilcken, B., Wilcken, D.E., Blom, H.J., Stabler, S.P., Allen, R.H., Selhub, J., Rosenberg, I.H., 2000. Homocysteine and its disulfide derivatives: a suggested consensus terminology. Arterioscler. Thromb. Vasc. Biol. 20, 1704–1706.

Nappo, F., De Rosa, N., Marfella, R., De Lucia, D., Ingrosso, D., Perna, A.F., Farzati, B., Giugliano, D., 1999. Impairment of endothelial functions by acute hyperhomocysteinemia and reversal by antioxidant vitamins. JAMA 281, 2113–2118.

Naughton, E.R., Yap, S., Mayne, P.D., 1998. Newborn screening for homocystinuria: Irish and world experience. Eur. J. Pediatr. 157 (Suppl. 2), S84–S87.

Nedrebo, B.G., Ericsson, U.B., Nygård, O., Refsum, H., Ueland, P.M., Aakvaag, A., Aanderud, S., Lien, E.A., 1998. Plasma total homocysteine levels in hyperthyroid and hypothyroid patients. Metabolism 47, 89–93.

Nishinaga, M., Ozawa, T., Shimada, K., 1993. Homocysteine, a thrombogenic agent, suppresses anticoagulant heparan sulfate expression in cultured porcine aortic endothelial cells. J. Clin. Invest. 92, 1381–1386.

Nowak-Gottl, U., Strater, R., Heinecke, A., Junker, R., Koch, H.-G., Schierer, G., von Eckardstein, A., for the Childhood Stroke Study Group, 1999. Lipoprotein (a) and genetic polymorphisms of clotting factor V, prothrombin, and methylenetetrahydrofolate reductase are risk factors for spontaneous ischemic stroke in childhood. Blood 94, 3678–3682.

Nygård, O., Vollset, S.E., Refsum, E., Stensvold, I., Tverdal, A., Nordrehaug J.E., Ueland, P.M., KvŒle, G., 1995. Total plasma homocysteine and cardiovascular risk profile. The Hordaland Homocysteine Study. JAMA 274, 1526–1533.

Nygård, O., Refsum, H., Ueland, P.M., Stensvold, I., Nordrehaug, J., Kvale, G., Vollset, S.E., 1997a. Coffee consumption and plasma total homocysteine: The Hordaland Homocysteine Study. Am. J. Clin. Nutr. 65, 136–143.

Nygård, O., Nordrehaug, J.E., Refsum, H., Ueland, P.M., Farstad, M., Vollset, S.E., 1997b. Plasma homocysteine levels and mortality in patients with coronary artery disease. N. Engl. J. Med. 337, 230–236.

Nygård, O., Refsum, H., Ueland, P.M., Vollset, S.E., 1998. Major lifestyle determinants of plasma total homocysteine distribution: the Hordaland Homocysteine Study. Am. J. Clin. Nutr. 67, 263–270.

Omland, T., Samuelsson, A., Hartford, M., Herlitz, J., Karlsson, T., Christensen, B., Caidahl, K., 2000. Serum homocysteine concentration is an indicator of survival in patients with acute coronary syndromes. Arch. Intern. Med. 160, 1834–1840.

Osganian, S.K., Stampfer, M.J., Spiegelman, D., Rimm, E., Cutler, J.A., Feldman, H.A., Montgomery, D.H., Webber, L.S., Lytle, L.A., Bausserman, L., Nader, P.R., 1999. Distribution of and factors associated with serum homocysteine levels in children. Child and adolescent trial for cardiovascular health. JAMA 281, 1189–1196.

Outinen, P.A., Sood, S.K., Pfeifer, S.I., Pamidi, S., Podor, T.J., Li, J., Weitz, J.I., Austin, R.C., 1999. Homocysteine-induced endoplasmic reticulum stress and growth arrest leads to specific changes in gene expression in human vascular endothelial cells. Blood 94, 959–967.

Perry, I.J., Refsum, H., Morris, R.W., Ebrahim, S.B., Ueland, P.M., Shaper, A.G., 1995. Prospective study of serum total homocysteine concentration and risk of stroke in middle-aged British men. Lancet 346, 1395–1398.

Petri, M., Roubenoff, R., Dallal, G.E., Nadeau, M.R., Selhub, J., Rosenberg, I.H., 1996. Plasma homocysteine as a risk factor for atherothrombotic events in systemic lupus erythematosus. Lancet 348, 1120–1124.

Pfeiffer, C.M., Huff, D.L., Smith, S.J., Miller, D.T., Gunter, E.W., 1999. Comparison of plasma total homocysteine measurements in 14 laboratories: an international study. Clin. Chem. 45, 1261–1268.

Rasmussen, K., Möller, J., Lyngbak, M., Pedersen, A.M., Dybkjaer, L., 1996. Age- and gender-specific reference intervals for total homocysteine and methylmalonic acid in plasma before and after vitamin supplementation. Clin. Chem. 42, 630–636.

Ray, J.G., 1998. Meta-analysis of hyperhomocysteinemia as a risk factor for venous thromboembolic disease. Arch. Intern. Med. 158, 2101–2106.

Rees, M.W., Rodgers, G.M., 1993. Homocysteinemia: association of a metabolic disorder with vascular disease and thrombosis. Thromb. Res. 71, 337–359.

Refsum, H., Wesenberg, F., Ueland, P.M., 1991. Plasma homocysteine in children with acute lymphoblastic leukemia. Changes during a chemotherapeutic regimen including methotrexate. Cancer Res. 51, 828–835.

Refsum, H., Ueland, P.M., Nygård, O., Vollset, S.E., 1998. Homocysteine and cardiovascular disease. Ann. Rev. Med. 49, 31–62.

Ridker, P.M., Hennekens, C.H., Selhub, J., Miletich, J.P., Malinow, M.R., Stampfer, M.J., 1997. Interrelation of hyperhomocyst(e)inemia, factor V Leiden, and risk of future venous thromboembolism. Circulation 95, 1777–1782.

Ridker, P.M., Manson, J.E., Buring, J.E., Shih, J., Matias, M., Hennekens, C.H., 1999. Homocysteine and risk of cardiovascular disease among postmenopausal women. JAMA 281, 1817–1821.

Riggs, K.M., Spiro III, A., Tucker, K., Rush, D., 1996. Relations of vitamin B-12, vitamin B-6, folate, and homocysteine to cognitive performance in the Normative Aging Study. Am. J. Clin. Nutr. 63, 306–314 (Abstract).

Rintelen, C., Mannhalter, C., Lechner, K., Eichinger, S., Kyrle, P.A., Papagiannopoulos, M., Schneider, B., Pabinger, I., 1999. No evidence for an increased risk of venous thrombosis in patients with factor V Leiden by the homozygous 677 C to T mutation in the methylenetetrahydrofolate reductase gene. Blood Coag. Fibrinol. 10, 101–105.

Robinson, K., Mayer, E.L., Miller, D.P., Green, R., van Lente, F., Gupta, A., Kattke-Marchant, K., Savon, S.R., Selhub, J., Nissen, S.E., Kutner, M., Topol, E.J., Jacobsen, D.W., 1995. Hyperhomocysteinemia and low pyridoxal phosphate. Common and independent reversible risk factors for coronary artery disease. Circulation 92, 2825–2830.

Robinson, K., Gupta, A., Dennis, V., Arheart, K., Chaudhary, D., Green, R., Vigo, P., Mayer, E.L., Selhub, J., Kutner, M., Jacobsen, D.W., 1996. Hyperhomocysteinemia confers an independent increased risk of atherosclerosis in end-stage renal disease and is closely linked to plasma folate and pyridoxine concentrations. Circulation 94, 2743–2748.

Robinson, K., Arheart, K., Refsum, H., Brattström, L., Boers, G., Ueland, P., Rubba, P., Palma-Reis, R., Meleady, R., Daly, L., Witteman, J., Graham, I., for the European COMAC Group, 1998. Low circulating folate and vitamin B6 concentrations. Risk factors for stroke, peripheral vascular disease, and coronary artery disease. Circulation 97, 437–443.

Rodgers, G.M., Kane, W.H., 1986. Activation of endogenous factor V by a homocysteine-induced vascular endothelial cell activator. J. Clin. Invest. 77, 1909–1916.

Rodgers, G.M., Conn, M.T., 1990. Homocysteine, an atherogenic stimulus, reduces protein C activation by arterial and venous endothelial cells. Blood 75, 895–901.

Rosenblatt, D.S., Cooper, B.A., 1990. Inherited disorders of vitamin-B12 utilization. BioEssays 12, 331–334.

Roubenoff, R., Dellaripa, P., Nadeau, M.R., Abad, L.W., Muldoon, B.A., Selhub, J., Rosenberg, I.H., 1997. Abnormal homocysteine metabolism in rheumatoid arthritis. Arthritis Rheumatism 40, 718–722.

Rozen, R., 1996. Molecular genetics of methylenetetrahydrofolate reductase deficiency. J. Inhertit. Metab. Dis. 19, 589–594.

Salomon, O., Steinberg, D.M., Zivelin, A., Gitel, S., Dardik, R., Rosenberg, N., Berliner, S., Inbal, A., Mani, A., Lubetsky, A., Varon, D., Martinowitz, U., Seligsohn, U., 1999. Single and combined pro-thrombotic factors in patients with idiiopathic venous thromboembolism: prevalence and risk assessment. Arterioscler. Thromb. Vasc. Biol. 19, 511–518.

Schnyder, G., Roffi, M., Pin, R., Flammer, Y., Lange, H., Eberli, F.R., Meier, B., Turi, Z.G., Hess, O.M., 2001. Decreased rate of coronary restenosis after lowering of plasma homocysteine levels. N. Engl. J. Med. 29 345(22), 1593–1600.

Selhub, J., Miller, J.W., 1992. The pathogenesis of homocysteinemia: interruption of the coordinate regulation by *S*-adenosylmethionine of the remethylation and transsulfuration of homocysteine. Am. J. Clin. Nutr. 55, 131–138.

Selhub, J., Jaques, P.F., Wilson, P.W.F., Rush, D., Rosenberg, J.H., 1993. Vitamin status and intake as primary determinants of homocysteinemia in an elderly population. JAMA 270, 2693–2698.

Selhub, J., Jaques, P.F., Bostom, A.G., D'Agostino, R.B., Wilson, P.W.F., Belanger, A.J., O'Leary, D.H., Wolf, P.A., Schaeffer, E.J., Rosenberg, I.H., 1995. Association between plasma homocysteine concentrations and extracranial carotid-artery stenosis. N. Engl. J. Med. 332, 286–291.

Selhub, J., Jaques, P.F., Rosenberg, I.H., Rogers, G., Bowman, B.A., Gunter, E.W., Wright, J.D., Johnson, C.L., 1999. Serum total homocysteine concentrations in the third national health and nutrition examination survey (1991–1994): population reference ranges and contribution of vitamin status to high serum concentrations. Ann. Intern. Med. 131, 331–339.

Seshadri, S., Beiser, A., Selhub, J., Jaques, P.F., Rosenberg, I.H., D'Agostino, R.B., Wilson, P.W., Wolf, P.A., 2002. Plasma homocysteine as a risk factor for dementia and Alzheimer's disease. N. Engl. J. Med. 346, 476–483.

Shipchandler, M.T., Moore, E.G., 1995. Rapid, fully automated measurement of plasma homocyst(e)ine with the Abbott Imx Analyzer. Clin. Chem. 41, 991–994.

Simioni, P., Prandoni, P., Burlina, A., Tormene, D., Sardella, C., Ferrari, V., Beneditti, L., Girolami, A., 1996. Hyperhomocysteinemia and deep-vein thrombosis. A case control study. Thromb. Haemost. 76, 883–886.

Smulders, Y.M., de Man, A.M.E., Stehouwer, C.D.A., Slaats Ed, H., 1999. Trimethoprim and fasting plasma homocysteine. Lancet 352, 1827–1828.

Snowdon, D.A., Greiner, L.H., Mortimer, J.A., Riley, K.P., Greincr, P.A., Markesbery, W.R., 1997. Brain infarction and the clinical expression of Alzheimer disease: the Nun Study. JAMA 277, 813–817.

Spence, J.D., Malinow, M.R., Barnett, P.A., Marian, A.J., Freeman, D., Hegele, R.A., 1999. Plasma homocyst(e)ine concentration but not MTHFR genotype, is associated with variation in carotid plaque area. Stroke 30, 969–973.

Sperandeo, M.P., De Franchis, R., Andria, G., Sebastio, G., 1996. A 68-bp insertion found in a homocystinuric patient is a common variant and is skipped by alternative splicing of the cystathionine β-synthase mRNA. Am. J. Hum. Genet. 59, 1391–1393.

Stamler, J.S., Osborne, J.A., Jaraki, O., Rabbani, L.E., Mullins, M., Singel, D., Loscalzo, J., 1993. Adverse vascular effects of homocysteine are modulated by endothelium-derived relaxing factor and related oxides of nitrogen. J. Clin. Invest. 91, 308–318.

Stampfer, M.J., Malinow, M.R., Willett, W.C., Newcomer, L.M., Upson, D., Tishler, P.V., Hennekens, C.H., 1992. A prospective study of plasma homocyst(e)ine and risk of myocardial infarction in U.S. Physicians. JAMA 268, 877–881.

Starkebaum, G., Harlan, J.M., 1986. Endothelial cell injury due to copper-catalyzed hydrogen peroxide generation from homocysteine. J. Clin. Invest. 77, 1370–1376.

Stehouwer, C.D.A., Weijenberg, M.P., van den Berg, M., 1996. Serum homocysteine and the five year risk of cardiovascular diseases, cancer and cognitive impairment in elderly men. In: Weijenberg, M. (Ed.),

Prospective Studies on Coronary Heart Disease in the Elderly: the Role of Classical and New Risk Factors. Wageningen, The Netherlands: Grafisch Bedrijf Ponsen & Looijen B.V., pp. 83–99.

Stehouwer, C.D.A., Weijenberg, M.P., van den Berg, M., Jakobs, C., Feskens, E.J.M., Kromhout, D., 1998. Serum homocysteine and risk of coronary heart disease and cerebrovascular disease in elderly men. A 10-year follow-up. Arterioscler. Thromb. Vasc. Biol. 18, 1895–1901.

Stehouwer, C.D.A., Gall, A.-A., Hougaard, P., Jakobs, C., Parving, H.-H., 1999. Plasma homocysteine concentration predicts mortality in non-insulin-dependent diabetic patients with and without albuminuria. Kidney Internatl. 55, 308–314.

Storch, K.J., Wagne, D.A., Burke, J.F., Young, V.R., 1990. (1-13C; methyl-2H3) Methionine kinetics in humans: methionine conservation and cysteine sparing. Am. J. Physiol. 258, E790–E798.

Stubbs, P.J., Al-Obaidi, M.K., Conroy, R.M., Mus, B., Collinson, P.O. (MRCPath), Graham, I.M. (Frcpi), Noble, M.I., 2000. Effect of plasma homocysteine concentration on early and late events in patients with acute coronary syndromes. Circulation 102, 605–610.

Sunder-Plassmann, G., Floth, A., Fodinger, M., 2000. Hyperhomocysteinemia in organ transplantation. Curr. Opin. Urol. 10, 87–94.

Tawakol, A., Omland, T., Gerhard, M., Wu, J.T., Creager, M.A., 1997. Hyperhomocyst(e)inemia is associated with impaired endothelium-dependent vasodilation in humans. Circulation 95, 1119–1121.

Taylor, L.M., DeFrang, R.D., Harris, E.J., Porter, J.M., 1991. The association of elevated plasma homocyst(e)ine with progression of symptomatic peripheral arterial disease. J. Vasc. Surg. 13, 128–136.

Tonon, G., Boyd, K., Lecchi, A., Lombardi, R., Porcella, A., Cattaneo, M., 1997. Plasma homocysteine levels in 10 patients with polycythemia. Haematologica 82, 343–344.

Tosetto, A., Missiaglia, E., Frezzato, M., Rodeghiero, F., 1997. The VITA project: C677T mutation in the methylenetetrahydrofolate reductase gene and the risk of venous thromboembolism. Br. J. Haematol. 97, 804–806.

Tripodi, A., Chantarangkul, V., Lombardi, R., Lecchi, A., Mannucci, P.M., Cattaneo, M., 2001. Multicenter study of homocysteine measurement-performance characteristics of different methods, influence of standards on interlaboratory agreement of results. Thromb. Haemost. 85 (2), 291–295.

Tripodi, A., Chantarangkul, V., Tan, Y., Hoffman, R.M., Cattaneo, M., 2002. Evaluation of an enzymatic method to measure total homocysteine in plasma. Thromb. Haemost. 87 (1), 172–173.

Tsai, J.-C., Perrella, M.A., Yoshizumi, M., Hsieh, C.M., Haber, E., Schlegel, R., Lee, M.E., 1994. Promotion of vascular smooth muscle cell growth by homocysteine: a link to atherosclerosis. Proc. Natl. Acad. Sci. USA 91, 6369–6373.

Tsai, M.Y., Bignell, M., Schwichtenberg, K., Hanson, N.Q., 1996. High prevalence of a mutation in the cystathionine β-synthase gene. Am. J. Hum. Genet. 59, 1262–1267.

Tucker, K.L., Mahnken, B., Wilson, P.W.F., Jaques, P., Selhub, J., 1996. Folic acid fortification of the food supply. Potential benefits and risks for the elderly population. JAMA 276, 1879–1885.

Ubbink, J.B., Vermaak, W.J.H., van der Merwe, A., Becker, P.J., Delport, R., Potgeieter, H.C., 1994. Vitamin requirements for the treatment of hyperhomocysteinemia in humans. J. Nutr. 124, 1927–1933.

Ubbink, J.B., Becker, P.J., Vermaak, W.J., Delport, R., 1995. Results of B-vitamin supplementation study used in a prediction model to define a reference range for plasma homocysteine. Clin. Chem. 41, 1033–1037.

Ubbink, J.B., van der Merwe, A., Delport, R., Allen, R.H., Stabler, S.P., Riezler, R., Vermaak, W.J.H., 1996. The effect of a subnormal vitamin B-6 status on homocysteine metabolism. J. Clin. Invest. 98, 177–184.

Ubbink, J.B., Fehily, A.M., Pickering, J., Elwood, P.C., Vermaak, W.J.H., 1998. Homocysteine and ischaemic heart disease in the Caerphilly cohort. Atherosclerosis 140, 349–356.

Undas, A., Williams, E.B., Butenas, S., Orfeo, T., Mann, K.G., 2001. Homocysteine inhibits inactivation of factor Va by activated protein C. J. Biol. Chem. 9 276(6), 4389–4397.

Van den Berg, M., Stehouwer, C.D.A., Bierdrager, E., Rauwerda, J.A., 1996. Plasma homocysteine and severity of atherosclerosis in young patients with lower-limb atherosclerotic disease. Arterioscler. Thromb. Vasc. Biol. 16, 165–171.

Van der Mooren, M.J., Wouters, M.G., Blom, H.J., Schellekens, L.A., Eskes, T.K., Rolland, R., 1994. Hormone replacement therapy may reduce high serum homocysteine in postmenopausal women. Eur. J. Clin. Invest. 24, 733–736.

Van der Put, N.M.J., Gabreels, F., Stevens, E.M.B., Smaitink, J.A.M., Trijbels, F.J.M., Eskes, T.K.A.B., van den Heuvel, L.P., Blom, H.J., 1998. A second mutation in the methylenetetrahydrofolate reductase gene: an additional risk factor for neural-tube defects? Am. J. Hum. Genet. 62, 1044–1051.

Verhoef, P., Hennekens, C.H., Malinow, M.R., Kok, F.J., Willert, W.C., Stampfer, M.J., 1994. A prospective study of plasma homocyst(e)ine and risk of ischemic stroke. Stroke 25, 1924–1930.

Verhoef, P., Kok, F.J., Kruyssen, D.A.C.M., Schouten, E.G., Witteman, J.C., Grobbe, D.E., Ueland, P.M., Refsum, H., 1997a. Plasma total homocysteine, B vitamins and risk of coronary atherosclerosis. Arterioscler. Thromb. Vasc. Biol. 17, 989–995.

Verhoef, P., Hennekens, C.H., Allen, R.H., Stabler, S.P., Willett, W.C., Stampfer, M.J., 1997b. Plasma total homocysteine and risk of angina pectoris with subsequent coronary artery bypass surgery. Am. J. Cardiol. 79, 799–801.

Von Eckardstein, A., Malinow, M.R., Upson, B., Heinrich, T., Schulte, H., Schonfeld, R., Kohler, E., Assmann, G., 1994. Effects of age, lipoproteins, and hemostatic parameters on the role of homocystinemia as a cardiovascular risk factor in men. Arterioscler. Thromb. 14, 460–464.

Wald, D.S., Bishop, L., Wald, N.J., Law, M., Hennessy, E., Weir, D., McPartlin, J., Scott, J., 2001. Randomized trial of folic acid supplementation and serum homocysteine levels. Arch. Intern. Med. Mar 12 161 (5), 695–700.

Wald, N.J., Watt, H.C., Law, M.R., Weir, D.G., McPartlin, J., Scott, J.M., 1998. Homocysteine and ischemic heart disease. Results of a prospective study with implications regarding prevention. Arch. Intern. Med. 158, 862–867.

Wang, J., Dudman, N.P.B., Wilcken, D.E.L., 1993. Effects of homocysteine and related compounds on prostacyclin production by cultured human vascular endothelial cells. Thromb. Haemostas. 70, 1047–1052.

Welch, G.N., Upchurch Jr., G.R., Loscalzo, J., 1997. Hyperhomocyst(e)inemia and atherothrombosis. Ann. NY Acad. Sci. 811, 48–58.

Whincup, P.H., Refsum, H., Perry, I.J., Morris, R., Walker, M., Lennen, L., Thomson, A., Ueland, P.M., Ebrahim, S.B.J., 1999. Serum total homocysteine and coronary heart disease: prospective study in middle aged men. Heart 82, 448–454.

Wiklund, O., Fager, G., Andersson, A., Lundstam, U., Masson, P., Hultberg, B., 1996. *N*-acetylcysteine treatment lowers plasma homocysteine but not serum lipoprotein (a) levels. Atherosclerosis 119, 99–106.

Wilcken, D.E.L., Wilcken, B., 1976. The pathogenesis of coronary artery disease. A possible role for methionine metabolism. J. Clin. Invest. 57, 1079–1082.

Wilcken, D.E.L., Wilcken, B., 1997. The natural history of vascular disease in homocystinuria and the effects of treatment. J. Inherit. Metab. Dis. 20 (2), 295–300.

Woo, K.S., Chook, P., Lolin, Y.I., Cheung, A.S.P., Chan, L.T., Sun, Y.Y., Sanderson, J.E., Metreweli, C., Celermajer, D.S., 1997. Hyperhomocyst(e)inemia is a risk factor for arterial endothelial dysfunction in humans. Circulation 96, 2542–2544.

Wouters, M.G.A.J., Moorrees, M.T.E.C., van der Mooren, M.J., Blom, H.J., Boers, G.H., Schellekens, L.A., Thomas, C.M., Eskes, T.K., 1995. Plasma homocysteine and menopausal status. Eur. J. Clin. Invest. 25, 801–805.

Xu, D., Neville, R., Finkel, T., 2000. Homocysteine accelerates endothelial cell senescence. FEBS Lett. 470, 2024.

Yap, S., Boers, G.H., Wilcken, B., Wilcken, D.E., Brenton, D.P., Lee, P.J., Walter, J.H., Howard, P.M., Naughten, E.R., 2001. Vascular outcome in patients with homocystinuria due to cystathionine beta-synthase deficiency treated chronically: a multicenter observational study. Arterioscler. Thromb. Vasc. Biol. 21 (12), 2080–2085.

Zhang, C., Cai, Y., Adachi, M.T., Oshiro, S., Aso, T., Kaufman, R.J., Kitajima, S., 2001. Homocysteine induces programmed cell death in human vascular endothelial cells through activation of the unfolded protein response. J. Biol. Chem. 21 276(38), 35867–35874.

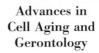

Interactions of selenium, vitamin E, and vitamin C in atherosclerosis

James M. May* and Raymond F. Burk

*Department of Medicine, 715 Preston Research Building, 2220 Pierce Avenue,
Vanderbilt University School of Medicine, Nashville, TN 37232-6303, USA*

Contents

Abbreviations

LDL   low-density lipoprotein
NO   nitric oxide

1. Introduction

Improved health care in the developed countries has resulted in growth of an aging population. Rather than dying from acute illness at a young age, many now live long enough to develop chronic diseases, such as obesity, diabetes, and atherosclerosis (Fries, 1980; Schneider and Brody, 1983). According to American Heart Association statistics, atherosclerosis, whether related to coronary artery disease, stroke, or peripheral vascular disease, remains the leading cause of death in both

---
* Corresponding author. Tel.: +1-615-936-1653; fax: +1-615-936-1667.
  E-mail address: james.may@mcmail.vanderbilt.edu (J.M. May).

Advances in Cell Aging and Gerontology, vol. 11, 337–348

men and women in the US. In addition to standard therapies, such as mechanical intervention, cholesterol lowering, smoking cessation, treatment of hypertension, and weight reduction, attention has focused on alternative therapies, one of which is administration of antioxidants. In this chapter, we review the potential for anti-oxidant interaction of α-tocopherol (vitamin E), ascorbic acid (vitamin C), and selenium and its relevance to atherosclerosis and aging.

2. Role of oxidized low-density lipoprotein in causing atherosclerosis

Evidence accumulated over many years has implicated oxidative modification of low-density lipoprotein (LDL) in the pathogenesis of atherosclerosis (Chisolm and Steinberg, 2000). LDL is the major cholesterol-carrying lipoprotein in human plasma. The bulk of circulating LDL is normally cleared by specific receptors, primarily in liver and muscle. However, oxidative modification of LDL in the sub-endothelial space of arteries results in a particle that is no longer taken up by specific receptors, but rather is cleared by a non-saturable scavenger pathway in monocyte-derived macrophages (Quinn et al., 1987; Steinberg et al., 1989). Moreover, oxidized LDL causes the release of tissue factors that both stimulate the movement of monocytes into the sub-endothelial space and cause differentiation of monocytes into macrophages (Ross, 1999). The latter remain in the sub-intimal space and become the lipid-laden foam cells found in atherosclerotic plaques (Ylä-Herttuala et al., 1989).

The response of the endothelial cells lining the vascular bed is also crucial in the development of atherosclerosis. Oxidized LDL impairs endothelial function (Henriksen et al., 1979; Therond et al., 2000), which manifests as an inability of the endothelium to produce adequate amounts of nitric oxide (NO). Nitric oxide has been shown to inhibit virtually all of the processes that are involved in the pathogenesis of atherosclerosis (Wever et al., 1998). These include monocyte adhesion, platelet aggregation, endothelial permeability, and vascular smooth muscle cell proliferation. Because of these defects associated with endothelial dysfunction, and the fact that it is present before gross changes of atherosclerosis, endothelial dysfunction is considered an early stage in the pathogenesis of atherosclerosis (Ross, 1999). However, not all of the endothelial dysfunction present in early or established atherosclerosis is due to oxidized LDL, since antioxidants also improve endothelial function independent of the toxic effects of oxidized LDL (Diaz et al., 1997).

3. Rationale for use of antioxidant vitamins and selenium to prevent atherosclerosis

3.1. *Atherosclerosis and α-tocopherol*

Both α-tocopherol (Fuller et al., 1996; Steinbrecher et al., 1984) and ascorbic acid (Jialal and Grundy, 1991) have been shown to protect LDL from oxidation by different, but complementary, mechanisms. α-Tocopherol is the major antioxidant in the lipid phase (Niki, 1987). By scavenging hydroperoxyl radicals that form in unsaturated fatty acids, α-tocopherol acts as a chain-breaking antioxidant to halt lipid peroxidation in lipoproteins and in cell membranes (Niki, 1987). As recently reviewed (Diaz et al., 1997; Kaul et al., 2001), numerous ex vivo and in vitro studies have shown that α-tocopherol protects LDL from oxidative modification. However, proving that the ability of α-tocopherol to increase resistance of LDL to oxidative modification translates into clinical benefit in atherosclerosis has been more difficult. Although many animal intervention studies and some epidemiologic studies in humans show benefit from supplemental α-tocopherol in the diet, the results of large, randomized, clinical trials have been contradictory (Kaul et al., 2001). There may be several reasons for this failure to consistently show benefits of α-tocopherol in atherosclerosis. First, most human studies have been done in people with existing atherosclerosis, the progression of which may be dependent on factors that might not respond to α-tocopherol, such as advanced inflammation, calcification, plaque rupture, and local thrombosis (Diaz et al., 1997). Second, administration of α-tocopherol as part of an antioxidant "cocktail," whatever the results obtained, will not help to identify α-tocopherol as the definitive agent. Third, most studies have not had adequate numbers of patients to detect what appears to be a relatively small effect of α-tocopherol. These caveats are exemplified in the recent study by Brown et al. (2001), in which just such an antioxidant mixture (α-tocopherol, vitamin C, β-carotene, and selenium) was administered to 39 subjects with established coronary disease in comparison to similar numbers of subjects who received placebo, simvastatin plus niacin, and antioxidants plus simvastatin and niacin. After 3 years, cholesterol lowering with simvastatin plus niacin decreased both the extent of coronary artery stenosis and the clinical incidence of coronary disease, whereas the antioxidant cocktail mixture showed only a trend towards decreased stenosis and no clinical improvement. It could be argued that this study with 40 patients in each treatment group may not have been adequately powered to detect a small difference due to the antioxidants. However, it seems more likely, given the presumed role of α-tocopherol in preventing endothelial dysfunction and early lesion formation, that much larger studies aimed at primary intervention will be needed.

3.2. *Atherosclerosis and ascorbate*

Ascorbate and uric acid are considered the major water-soluble antioxidants in plasma (Frei et al., 1989). Not only does ascorbate consume oxygen free radicals before they can oxidize α-tocopherol, but it can directly reduce the α-tocopheroxyl free radical in the cell membranes (Leung et al., 1981; Van den Berg et al., 1990). Ascorbate has long been known to recycle α-tocopherol in micelles and biomembranes (Niki, 1987). Ascorbate has also been shown to spare α-tocopherol in intact cells (Stocker et al., 1986; May et al., 1998a). Further, ascorbate is part of the first line of defense against oxidant-induced damage due to lipid and other peroxides that are generated during cellular metabolism (Frei et al., 1989; Halliwell and Gutteridge, 1990; Kaneko et al., 1993). Although ascorbate can act as a prooxidant in the presence of free iron or copper (Halliwell, 1999; Proteggente et al., 2000), given the low free concentrations of such transition metals in vivo, most evidence points to the function of ascorbate as an antioxidant (Carr and Frei, 1999). The antioxidant effects of ascorbic acid could help to explain the observations of Willis almost 50 years ago that acute and chronic scurvy in guinea pigs produced intimal lesions indistinguishable from those of human atherosclerosis (Willis, 1953).

There is increasing evidence that ascorbic acid protects against the deleterious effects of oxidant stress in humans. For example, plasma and tissue concentrations are low in a variety of conditions thought to be associated with chronic excesses of oxygen free radicals, including smoking, diabetes, and atherosclerosis (Levine, 1986). Epidemiologic studies in humans have shown that people who have high intakes of the vitamin have a lower incidence of atherosclerosis (Enstrom et al., 1992), but there are no long-term clinical trials with large numbers of patients. More recently, results from small clinical studies have shown that ascorbate improves or reverses endothelial dysfunction due to lack of NO, and this provides support for a potential effect of the vitamin in early coronary heart disease. These studies strongly suggest a link between ascorbate and endothelial NO generation or metabolism. For example, ascorbate has been shown to reverse endothelial dysfunction due to NO deficiency in coronary or peripheral arteries in smoking (Heitzer et al., 1996), hypercholesterolemia (Wever et al., 1998), hypertension (Solzbach et al., 1997), congestive heart failure (Hornig et al., 1998), and coronary artery disease (Kugiyama et al., 1998; Levine et al., 1996). This effect has been demonstrated with both ascorbate infusion and with oral ascorbate supplements (Gokce et al., 1999; Hornig et al., 1998; Levine et al., 1996). The common mechanism proposed in these studies is that ascorbate preserves the ability of the endothelium to generate NO by diminishing oxidative stress. At the cell level, it appears that ascorbate may stabilize tetrahydrobiopterin, a crucial co-factor required for function of endothelial nitric oxide synthase (Baker et al., 2001; Heller et al., 2001).

3.3. Atherosclerosis and selenium

The postulated role for selenium in preventing atherosclerosis is based on its function as a co-factor in several enzymes that have antioxidant functions. These selenoenzymes include glutathione peroxidase, phospholipid hydroperoxide glutathione peroxidase, and thioredoxin reductase. Each enzyme has been shown to reduce lipid hydroperoxides to alcohols (Björnstedt et al., 1995; Little and O'Brien, 1968; Thomas et al., 1990) and thus detoxify the major end product of oxidant-induced lipid peroxidation. These selenoenzymes also directly reduce H_2O_2, which is a by-product of mitochondrial oxygen metabolism. In addition, the major function of thioredoxin reductase is to maintain intracellular thiols in a reduced state (Arnér and Holmgren, 2000), which will also contribute to the antioxidant defenses of the cell.

An antioxidant role for selenium in protecting endothelial cells has been demonstrated in cultured arterial endothelial cells, which are sensitive to damage from oxidized LDL (Martin and Frei, 1997; Thomas et al., 1993). Culture of cells in medium containing low concentrations of selenium decreases activities of several selenoenzymes, and sensitizes the cells to damage by oxidized LDL and hydroperoxides (Thomas et al., 1993). Further, selenoprotein P, the major selenoprotein in plasma (Read et al., 1990), also binds to endothelial cells (Burk et al., 1997), and its presence correlates with protection of the liver against oxidant damage and damage due to diquat administration (Atkinson et al., 2001).

There is evidence from animal studies that selenium supplements can slow the progression of atherosclerosis due to high-fat diets. In rats (Kang et al., 1998) fed a cholesterol-enriched diet, added selenium above that already present in the diet decreased plasma cholesterol levels as well as the extent of plasma and tissue lipid peroxidation. In fat-feeding studies in rabbits, plasma cholesterol, lipid peroxidation, and aortic atherosclerosis were inhibited by supplements of both α-tocopherol and selenium (Schwenke and Behr, 1998; Wójcicki et al., 1991). In the study by Schwenke and Behr (1998), aortic atherosclerosis was inhibited to a similar extent by selenium and α-tocopherol supplements as it was by an equally hypolipidemic dose of pro-bucol (Schwenke and Behr, 1998), a drug that functions to reduce atherosclerosis at least in part through an antioxidant mechanism (Parthasarathy, 1992). However, a caveat in these studies is that selenium was added in excess of normal dietary amounts. It seems likely that the effects observed were due to pharmacologic, or even toxic, levels of selenium.

In human studies, plasma selenium concentrations (Moore et al., 1984) and ery-throcyte glutathione peroxidase activities (Yegin et al., 1997) were found to vary inversely with the incidence and severity of coronary atherosclerosis. The situation is less clear for carotid intimal thickness and the risk of stoke in that one study showed a negative correlation of plasma selenium concentrations with carotid disease (Salonen et al., 1991), while another did not (Bonithon-Kopp et al., 1997). One large study from China failed to show benefits of selenium supplements on cere-brovascular disease (Blot et al., 1993), although it was designed to test effects of selenium and other antioxidants on cancer. It must be kept in mind that all plasma selenium concentrations above 8 µg/dl indicate nutritional selenium adequacy and that variations in concentration above this value are related to the chemical form of the element ingested and not to its nutritional adequacy (Burk et al., 2001). Thus, the correlations of clinical events with plasma selenium levels that are above 8 µg/dl are not related to nutritional selenium status and must be made with caution.

4. Rationale for antioxidant potentiation by α-tocopherol, ascorbate, and selenium

Because the evidence that ascorbate, α-tocopherol, and selenium individually prevent or ameliorate atherosclerosis is not definitive, it is worth considering whether and how they might interact to enhance antioxidant defenses. Selenium and α-tocopherol have been linked since the 1957 report by Schwarz and Foltz (Schwarz and Foltz, 1957) that addition of selenium to rat diets prevents the vitamin E-responsive condition known as dietary liver necrosis. At the same time, it was shown that selenium also ameliorates the exudative diathesis that develops in chicks made deficient in both vitamin E and selenium (Patterson et al., 1955). After the discovery in 1973 that selenium is an essential constituent of glutathione peroxidase (gluta-thione peroxidase-1) (Rotruck et al., 1973), Hoekstra (1975) presented a scheme that defined the relationship of selenium with vitamin E to enhance antioxidant defenses. He proposed that α-tocopherol and glutathione peroxidase act sequentially to eliminate free radicals and their hydroperoxide metabolites. Thus, α-tocopherol donates a hydrogen atom to a lipid hydroperoxyl free radical to form the hydroperoxide. In turn, glutathione peroxidase reduces the hydroperoxide to a nonreactive alcohol. If either α-tocopherol or glutathione peroxidase (i.e., selenium) is lacking, the other can compensate to some extent. If both are absent, spontaneous lipid peroxidation causes liver necrosis. This hypothesis received support from later studies showing that selenium supplementation in vitamin E-deficient rats prevents both lipid peroxidation and dietary liver necrosis (Awad et al., 1994; Hafeman and Hoekstra, 1977).

However, subsequent studies have questioned whether the classical glutathione peroxidase mediates antioxidant protection through this mechanism. For example, doses of selenium too low to increase glutathione peroxidase reduced mortality in vitamin E-deficient chicks during challenge with the redox cycling agent paraquat (Mercurio and Combs, 1986). Similarly, selenium administration to selenium-deficient rats 10 h prior to treatment with diquat also markedly decreased massive liver necrosis and lipid peroxidation, but before measurable increases in liver glutathione peroxidase activity occurred (Burk et al., 1980). More recently, mice in which the glutathione peroxidase-1 gene was inactivated by targeted gene disruption were found to be viable, fertile, and able to tolerate the oxidative stress of hyperoxia as well as normal mice (Ho et al., 1997). Further, lens epithelial cells (Spector et al., 1996) and other tissues (Ho et al., 1997) from such knockout mice show no impairment in their ability to detoxify H_2O_2 in vitro. However, glutathione peroxidase-1 knockout mice do show defects in mitochondrial sensitivity to oxidant stress (Esposito et al., 2000) as well as the development of cataracts with age (Reddy et al., 2001). The effect of glutathione peroxidase-1 deficiency may not be dramatic, because selenoenzymes other than glutathione peroxidase-1 also help to protect against oxidant stress. One such selenoenzyme is phospholipid hydroperoxide glutathione peroxidase (glutathione peroxidase-4), which reduces phospholipid hydroperoxides in biomembranes (Maiorino et al., 1990), and "spares" α-tocopherol in microsomes (Maiorino et al., 1989).

The discovery that mammalian thioredoxin reductase is also a selenoenzyme (Gladyshev et al., 1996) provides another mechanism by which selenium might spare α-tocopherol. In the mammalian thioredoxin system, thioredoxin reductase uses NADPH as a co-factor to reduce thioredoxin, which, in turn, reduces protein and other disulfides in cells (Holmgren, 1989; Holmgren and Björnstedt, 1995). In this manner, the thioredoxin system is thought to contribute to the maintenance of cellular redox balance (Holmgren and Björnstedt, 1995). Given the failure of glutathione peroxidase-1 to account for protection against selenium-dependent lipid peroxidation, as noted above, Tamura et al. (1996) proposed that the selenium dependency of the thioredoxin system provides the link between selenium and α-tocopherol. They hypothesized the link to involve three steps: (1) reduction of protein disulfide isomerase by the thioredoxin system (Lundström and Holmgren, 1990), (2) reduction of DHA to ascorbate by reduced protein disulfide isomerase

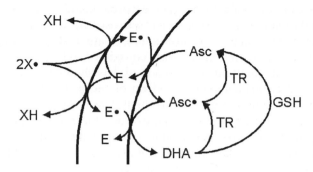

Fig. 1.   Antioxidant interactions of selenium and vitamins C and E in the plasma membrane. A free radical (X•) attacks α-tocopherol in the plasma membrane, generating the α-tocopheroxyl free radical (E•). This is recycled by ascorbate (Asc). The oxidized products of ascorbate, dehydroascorbic acid (DHA), and the ascorbate free radical (Asc•) are then recycled by the selenoenzyme thioredoxin reductase (TR). Reduced glutathione (GSH) can also recycle dehydroascorbic acid to ascorbate.

(Wells et al., 1990), and (3) recycling of α-tocopherol by ascorbate (Liebler et al., 1986; Niki et al., 1995). Since thioredoxin reductase can reduce DHA (May et al., 1997) and the ascorbate free radical (May et al., 1998b) to ascorbate directly, it may be possible to simplify the hypothesis of Tamura et al. In this model, only two steps are required to link selenium to α-tocopherol: reduction of DHA or the AFR by thioredoxin reductase, and recycling of α-tocopherol by ascorbate. The model is diagrammed in Fig. 1.

5. Relevance to atherosclerosis

The caveat in proposing that α-tocopherol, ascorbate, and selenium interact to lessen the oxidant damage that precedes and accompanies atherosclerosis is, of course, that few people in developed countries are likely to be deficient in selenium. However, there is evidence that selenium levels decline with age in humans (Berr et al., 1993; Girodon et al., 1997; Savarino et al., 2001), an effect that may be due to or at least worsened by poor dietary intake in infirm elderly or nursing home inhabitants. Low selenium concentrations have been correlated with decreased activity of plasma and erythrocyte glutathione peroxidase in elderly populations (Berr et al., 1993; Girodon et al., 1997). Illness or poor dietary intake will also decrease α-tocopherol and ascorbate levels, which could result in borderline deficiencies of the three nutrients and bring the hypothesis into play. For example, in one study of 57 hospitalized elderly subjects, there was a substantial incidence of combined selenium, ascorbate, and α-tocopherol deficiency that was reversed by 6 months of replacement therapy (Girodon et al., 1997). Further, the sensitivity of erythrocytes to oxidant damage and hemolysis from a water-soluble free radical initiator in the combined deficiency group was also reversed.

Given the lack of effect of α-tocopherol, ascorbate, and selenium supplements in combination in decreasing established atherosclerosis (Brown et al., 2001), emphasis should be directed towards primary prevention of atherosclerosis in future clinical trials. Although these three antioxidants are considered to be non-toxic individually, a recent study derived from that of Brown et al. has shown that a cocktail of these antioxidants plus β-carotene impairs the effect of statins to raise high-density lipoprotein in patients with decreased levels of high-density lipoprotein (Cheung et al., 2001). These findings reemphasize the need to study the antioxidants individually as well. The rationale that antioxidant vitamins and selenium should help to prevent atherosclerosis is compelling, but the benefit may be limited to certain stages of the disease and to individuals deficient in the nutrients.

References

Arnér, E.S.J., Holmgren, A., 2000. Physiological functions of thioredoxin and thioredoxin reductase. Eur. J. Biochem. 267, 6102–6109.

Atkinson, J.B., Hill, K.E., Burk, R.F., 2001. Centrilobular endothelial cell injury by diquat in the selenium-deficient rat liver. Lab. Invest. 81, 193–200.

Awad, J.A., Morrow, J.D., Hill, K.E., Roberts, L.J., Burk, R.F., 1994. Detection and localization of lipid peroxidation in selenium- and vitamin E-deficient rats using F2-isoprostanes. J. Nutr. 124, 810–816.

Baker, R.A., Milstien, S., Katusic, Z.S., 2001. Effect of vitamin C on the availability of tetrahydrobiopterin in human endothelial cells. J. Cardiovasc. Pharmacol. 37, 333–338.

Berr, C., Nicole, A., Godin, J., Ceballos-Picot, I., Thevenin, M., Dartigues, J.F., Alperovitch, A., 1993. Selenium and oxygen-metabolizing enzymes in elderly community residents: a pilot epidemiological study. J. Am. Geriatr. Soc. 41, 143–148.

Björnstedt, M., Hamberg, M., Kumar, S., Xue, J., Holmgren, A., 1995. Human thioredoxin reductase directly reduces lipid hydroperoxides by NADPH and selenocystine strongly stimulates the reaction via catalytically generated selenols. J. Biol. Chem. 270, 11761–11764.

Blot, W.J., Li, J.-Y., Taylor, P.R., Guo, W., Dawsey, S., Wang, G.-Q., Yang, C.S., Zheng, S.-F., Gail, M., Li, G.-Y., Yu, Y., Liu, B., Tangrea, J., Sun, Y., Liu, F., Fraumeni Jr., J.R., Zhang, Y.-H., Li, B., 1993. Nutrition intervention trials in Linxian, China: supplementation with specific vitamin/mineral combinations, cancer incidence, and disease-specific mortality in the general population. J. Natl. Cancer Inst. 85, 1483–1492.

Bonithon-Kopp, C., Coudray, C., Berr, C., Touboul, P.J., Fève, J.M., Favier, A., Ducimetière, P., 1997. Combined effects of lipid peroxidation and antioxidant status on carotid atherosclerosis in a population aged 59–71 y: the EVA Study. Am. J. Clin. Nutr. 65, 121–127.

Brown, B.G., Zhao, X.-Q., Chait, A., Fisher, L.D., Cheung, M.C., Morse, J.S., Dowdy, A.A., Marino, E.K., Bolson, E.L., Alaupovic, P., Frohlich, J., Albers, J.J., 2001. Simvastatin and niacin, antioxidant vitamins, or the combination for the prevention of coronary disease. N. Engl. J. Med. 345, 1583–1592.

Burk, R.F., Lawrence, R.A., Lane, J.M., 1980. Liver necrosis and lipid peroxidation in the rat as the result of paraquat and diquat administration. Effect of selenium deficiency. J. Clin. Invest. 65, 1024–1031.

Burk, R.F., Hill, K.E., Boeglin, M.E., Ebner, F.F., Chittum, H.S., 1997. Selenoprotein P associates with endothelial cells in rat tissues. Histochem. Cell Biol. 108, 11–15.

Burk, R.F., Hill, K.E., Motley, A.K., 2001. Plasma selenium in specific and non-specific forms. Biofactors 14, 107–114.

Carr, A., Frei, B., 1999. Does vitamin C act as a pro-oxidant under physiological conditions? FASEB J. 13, 1007–1024.

Cheung, M.C., Zhao, X.Q., Chait, A., Albers, J.J., Brown, B.G., 2001. Antioxidant supplements block the response of HDL to simvastatin–niacin therapy in patients with coronary artery disease and low HDL. Arterioscler. Thromb. Vasc. Biol. 21, 1320–1326.

Chisolm, G.M., Steinberg, D., 2000. The oxidative modification hypothesis of atherogenesis: an overview. Free Radic. Biol. Med. 28, 1815–1826.

Diaz, M.N., Frei, B., Vita, J.A., Keaney Jr., J.F., 1997. Mechanisms of disease—antioxidants and atherosclerotic heart disease. N. Engl. J. Med. 337, 408–416.

Enstrom, J.E., Kanim, L.E., Klein, M.A., 1992. Vitamin C intake and mortality among a sample of the United States population. Epidemiology 3, 194–202.

Esposito, L.A., Kokoszka, J.E., Waymire, K.G., Cottrell, B., MacGregor, G.R., Wallace, D.C., 2000. Mitochondrial oxidative stress in mice lacking the glutathione peroxidase-1 gene. Free Radic. Biol. Med. 28, 754–766.

Frei, B., England, L., Ames, B.N., 1989. Ascorbate is an outstanding antioxidant in human blood plasma. Proc. Natl. Acad. Sci. U. S. A. 86, 6377–6381.

Fries, J.F., 1980. Aging, natural death, and the compression of morbidity. N. Engl. J. Med. 303, 130–135.

Fuller, C.J., Chandalia, M., Garg, A., Grundy, S.M., Jialal, I., 1996. *RRR*-α-tocopheryl acetate supplementation at pharmacologic doses decreases low-density-lipoprotein oxidative susceptibility but not protein glycation in patients with diabetes mellitus. Am. J. Clin. Nutr. 63, 753–759.

Girodon, F., Blache, D., Monget, A.L., Lombart, M., Brunet-Lecompte, P., Arnaud, J., Richard, M.J., Galan, P., 1997. Effect of a two-year supplementation with low doses of antioxidant vitamins and/or minerals in elderly subjects on levels of nutrients and antioxidant defense parameters. J. Am. Coll. Nutr. 16, 357–365.

Gladyshev, V.N., Jeang, K.T., Stadtman, T.C., 1996. Selenocysteine, identified as the penultimate C-terminal residue in human T-cell thioredoxin reductase, corresponds to TGA in the human placental gene. Proc. Natl. Acad. Sci. U. S. A. 93, 6146–6151.

Gokce, N., Keaney Jr., J.F., Frei, B., Holbrook, M., Olesiak, M., Zachariah, B.J., Leeuwenburgh, C., Heinecke, J.W., Vita, J.A., 1999. Long-term ascorbic acid administration reverses endothelial vasomotor dysfunction in patients with coronary artery disease. Circulation 99, 3234–3240.

Hafeman, D.G., Hoekstra, W.G., 1977. Lipid peroxidation in vivo during vitamin E and selenium deficiency in the rat as monitored by ethane evolution. J. Nutr. 107, 666–672.

Halliwell, B., 1999. Vitamin C: poison, prophylactic or panacea? Trends Biochem. Sci. 24, 255–259.

Halliwell, B., Gutteridge, J.M.C., 1990. The antioxidants of human extracellular fluids. Arch. Biochem. Biophys. 280, 1–8.

Heitzer, T., Just, H., Münzel, T., 1996. Antioxidant vitamin C improves endothelial dysfunction in chronic smokers. Circulation 94, 6–9.

Heller, R., Unbehaun, A., Schellenberg, B., Mayer, B., Werner-Felmayer, G., Werner, E.R., 2001. L-Ascorbic acid potentiates endothelial nitric oxide synthesis via a chemical stabilization of tetrahydrobiopterin. J. Biol. Chem. 276, 40–47.

Henriksen, T., Evensen, S.A., Carlander, B., 1979. Injury to human endothelial cells in culture induced by low density lipoproteins. Scand. J. Clin. Lab. Invest. 39, 361–368.

Ho, Y.S., Magnenat, J.L., Bronson, R.T., Cao, J., Gargano, M., Sugawara, M., Funk, C.D., 1997. Mice deficient in cellular glutathione peroxidase develop normally and show no increased sensitivity to hyperoxia. J. Biol. Chem. 272, 16644–16651.

Hoekstra, W.G., 1975. Biochemical function of selenium and its relation to vitamin E. Fed. Proc. 34, 2083–2089.

Holmgren, A., 1989. Thioredoxin and glutaredoxin systems. J. Biol. Chem. 264, 13963–13966.

Holmgren, A., Björnstedt, M., 1995. Thioredoxin and thioredoxin reductase. Meth. Enzymol. 252, 199–208.

Hornig, B., Arakawa, N., Kohler, C., Drexler, H., 1998. Vitamin C improves endothelial function of conduit arteries in patients with chronic heart failure. Circulation 97, 363–368.

Jialal, I., Grundy, S.M., 1991. Preservation of the endogenous antioxidants in low density lipoprotein by ascorbate but not probucol during oxidative modification. J. Clin. Invest. 87, 597–601.

Kaneko, T., Kaji, K., Matsuo, M., 1993. Protective effect of lipophilic derivatives of ascorbic acid on lipid peroxide-induced endothelial injury. Arch. Biochem. Biophys. 304, 176–180.

Kang, B.P., Bansal, M.P., Mehta, U., 1998. Selenium supplementation and diet induced hypercholestero-lemia in the rat: changes in lipid levels, malonyldialdehyde production and the nitric oxide synthase activity. Gen. Physiol. Biophys. 17, 71–78.

Kaul, N., Devaraj, S., Jialal, I., 2001. α-Tocopherol and atherosclerosis. Proc. Soc. Exp. Biol. Med. 226, 5–12.

Kugiyama, K., Motoyama, T., Hirashima, O., Ohgushi, M., Soejima, H., Misumi, K., Kawano, H., Miyao, Y., Yoshimura, M., Ogawa, H., Matsumura, T., Sugiyama, S., Yasue, H., 1998. Vitamin C attenuates abnormal vasomotor reactivity in spasm coronary arteries in patients with coronary spastic angina. J. Am. Coll. Cardiol. 32, 103–109.

Leung, H.-W., Vang, M.J., Mavis, R.D., 1981. The cooperative interaction between vitamin E and vitamin C in suppression of peroxidation of membrane phospholipids. Biochim. Biophys. Acta 664, 266–272.

Levine, M., 1986. New concepts in the biology and biochemistry of ascorbic acid. N. Engl. J. Med. 314, 892–902.

Levine, G.N., Frei, B., Koulouris, S.N., Gerhard, M.D., Keaney, J.F., Vita, J.A., 1996. Ascorbic acid reverses endothelial vasomotor dysfunction in patients with coronary artery disease. Circulation 93, 1107–1113.

Liebler, D.C., Kling, D.S., Reed, D.J., 1986. Antioxidant protection of phospholipid bilayers by α-toco-pherol. Control of α-tocopherol status and lipid peroxidation by ascorbic acid and glutathione. J. Biol. Chem. 261, 12114–12119.

Little, C., O'Brien, P.J., 1968. An intracellular GSH-peroxidase with a lipid peroxide substrate. Biochem. Biophys. Res. Commun. 31, 145–150.

Lundström, J., Holmgren, A., 1990. Protein disulfide-isomerase is a substrate for thioredoxin reductase and has thioredoxin-like activity. J. Biol. Chem. 265, 9114–9120.

Maiorino, M., Coassin, M., Roveri, A., Ursini, F., 1989. Microsomal lipid peroxidation: effect of vitamin E and its functional interaction with phospholipid hydroperoxide glutathione peroxidase. Lipids 241, 721–726.

Maiorino, M., Gregolin, C., Ursini, F., 1990. Phospholipid hydroperoxide glutathione peroxidase. Meth. Enzymol. 186, 448–457.

Martin, A., Frei, B., 1997. Both intracellular and extracellular vitamin C inhibit atherogenic modification of LDL by human vascular endothelial cells. Arterioscler. Thromb. Vasc. Biol. 17, 1583–1590.

May, J.M., Mendiratta, S., Hill, K.E., Burk, R.F., 1997. Reduction of dehydroascorbate to ascorbate by the selenoenzyme thioredoxin reductase. J. Biol. Chem. 272, 22607–22610.

May, J.M., Qu, Z.-C., Mendiratta, S., 1998a. Protection and recycling of α-tocopherol in human erythro-cytes by intracellular ascorbic acid. Arch. Biochem. Biophys. 349, 281–289.

May, J.M., Cobb, C.E., Mendiratta, S., Hill, K.E., Burk, R.F., 1998b. Reduction of the ascorbyl free radi-cal to ascorbate by thioredoxin reductase. J. Biol. Chem. 273, 23039–23045.

Mercurio, S.D., Combs, G.F.J., 1986. Selenium-dependent glutathione peroxidase inhibitors increase toxi-city of prooxidant compounds in chicks. J. Nutr. 116, 1726–1734.

Moore, J.A., Noiva, R., Wells, I.C., 1984. Selenium concentrations in plasma of patients with arterio-graphically defined coronary atherosclerosis. Clin. Chem. 30, 1171–1173.

Niki, E., 1987. Antioxidants in relation to lipid peroxidation. Chem. Phys. Lipids 44, 227–253.

Niki, E., Noguchi, N., Tsuchihashi, H., Gotoh, N., 1995. Interaction among vitamin C, vitamin E, and β-carotene. Am. J. Clin. Nutr. 62 (Suppl.), 1322S–1326S.

Parthasarathy, S., 1992. Evidence for an additional intracellular site of action of probucol in the preven-tion of oxidative modification of low density lipoprotein. Use of a new water-soluble probucol deriva-tive. J. Clin. Invest. 89, 1618–1621.

Patterson, E.L., Milstrey, R., Stokstad, E.L.R., 1955. Effect of selenium in preventing exudative diathesis in chicks. Proc. Soc. Exp. Biol. Med. 95, 617–620.

Proteggente, A.R., Rehman, A., Halliwell, B., Rice-Evans, C.A., 2000. Potential problems of ascorbate and iron supplementation: pro-oxidant effect in vivo? Biochem. Biophys. Res. Commun. 277, 535–540.

Quinn, M.T., Parthasarathy, S., Fong, L.G., Steinberg, D., 1987. Oxidatively modified low density lipo-proteins: a potential role in recruitment and retention of monocyte/macrophages during atherogenesis. Proc. Natl. Acad. Sci. U. S. A. 84, 2995–2998.

Read, R., Bellew, T., Yang, J.G., Hill, K.E., Palmer, I.S., Burk, R.F., 1990. Selenium and amino acid composition of selenoprotein P, the major selenoprotein in rat serum. J. Biol. Chem. 265, 17899–17905.

Reddy, V.N., Giblin, F.J., Lin, L.R., Dang, L., Unakar, N.J., Musch, D.C., Boyle, D.L., Takemoto, L.J., Ho, Y.S., Knoernschild, T., Juenemann, A., Lutjen-Drecoll, E., 2001. Glutathione peroxidase-1 deficiency leads to increased nuclear light scattering, membrane damage, and cataract formation in gene-knockout mice. Invest. Ophthalmol. Vis. Sci. 42, 3247–3255.

Ross, R., 1999. Atherosclerosis—an inflammatory disease. N. Engl. J. Med. 340, 115–126.

Rotruck, J.T., Pope, A.L., Ganther, H.E., Swanson, A.B., Hafeman, D.G., Hoekstra, W.G., 1973. Selenium: biochemical role as a component of glutathione peroxidase. Science 179, 588–590.

Salonen, J.T., Salonen, R., Seppanen, K., Kantola, M., Suntioinen, S., Korpela, H., 1991. Interactions of serum copper, selenium, and low density lipoprotein cholesterol in atherogenesis. Br. Med. J. 302, 756–760.

Savarino, L., Granchi, D., Ciapetti, G., Cenni, E., Ravaglia, G., Forti, P., Maioli, F., Mattioli, R., 2001. Serum concentrations of zinc and selenium in elderly people: results in healthy nonagenarians/centenarians. Exp. Gerontol. 36, 327–339.

Schneider, E.L., Brody, J.A., 1983. Aging, natural death, and the compression of morbidity: another view. N. Engl. J. Med. 309, 854–856.

Schwarz, K., Foltz, C.M., 1957. Selenium as an integral part of Factor 3 against dietary necrotic liver degeneration. J. Am. Chem. Soc. 79, 3292–3293.

Schwenke, D.C., Behr, S.R., 1998. Vitamin E combined with selenium inhibits atherosclerosis in hypercholesterolemic rabbits independently of effects on plasma cholesterol concentrations. Circ. Res. 83, 366–377.

Solzbach, U., Hornig, B., Jeserich, M., Just, H., 1997. Vitamin C improves endothelial dysfunction of epicardial coronary arteries in hypertensive patients. Circulation 96, 1513–1519.

Spector, A., Yang, Y., Ho, Y.S., Magnenat, J.-L., Wang, R.-R., Ma, W., Li, W.C., 1996. Variation in cellular glutathione peroxidase activity in lens epithelial cells, transgenics and knockouts does not significantly change the response to H_2O_2 stress. Exp. Eye Res. 62, 521–540.

Steinberg, D., Parthasarathy, S., Carew, T.E., Khoo, J.C., Witztum, J.L., 1989. Modifications of low-density lipoprotein that increase its atherogenicity. N. Engl. J. Med. 320, 915–924.

Steinbrecher, U.P., Parthasarathy, S., Leake, D.S., Witztum, J.L., Steinberg, D., 1984. Modification of low density lipoprotein by endothelial cells involves lipid peroxidation and degradation of low density lipoprotein phospholipids. Proc. Natl. Acad. Sci. U. S. A. 81, 3883–3887.

Stocker, R., Hunt, N.H., Weidemann, M.J., Clark, I.A., 1986. Protection of vitamin E from oxidation by increased ascorbic acid content within *Plasmodium vinckei*-infected erythrocytes. Biochim. Biophys. Acta 876, 294–299.

Tamura, T., Gladyshev, V., Liu, S.-Y., Stadtman, T.C., 1996. The mutual sparing effects of selenium and vitamin E in animal nutrition may be further explained by the discovery that mammalian thioredoxin reductase is a selenoenzyme. Biofactors 5, 99–102.

Therond, P., Abella, A., Laurent, D., Couturier, M., Chalas, J., Legrand, A., Lindenbaum, A., 2000. In vitro study of the cytotoxicity of isolated oxidized lipid low-density lipoproteins fractions in human endothelial cells: relationship with the glutathione status and cell morphology. Free Radic. Biol. Med. 28, 585–596.

Thomas, J.P., Maiorino, M., Ursini, F., Girotti, A.W., 1990. Protective action of phospholipid hydroperoxide glutathione peroxidase against membrane-damaging lipid peroxidation. In situ reduction of phospholipid and cholesterol hydroperoxides. J. Biol. Chem. 265, 454–461.

Thomas, J.P., Geiger, P.G., Girotti, A.W., 1993. Lethal damage to endothelial cells by oxidized low density lipoprotein: role of selenoperoxidases in cytoprotection against lipid hydroperoxide- and iron-mediated reactions. J. Lipid Res. 34, 479–490.

Van den Berg, J.J.M., Kuypers, F.A., Roelofsen, B., Op den Kamp, J.A.F., 1990. The cooperative action of vitamins E and C in the protection against peroxidation of parinaric acid in human erythrocyte membranes. Chem. Phys. Lipids 53, 309–320.

Wells, W.W., Xu, D.P., Yang, Y.F., Rocque, P.A., 1990. Mammalian thioltransferase (glutaredoxin) and protein disulfide isomerase have dehydroascorbate reductase activity. J. Biol. Chem. 265, 15361–15364.

Wever, R., Stroes, E., Rabelink, T.J., 1998. Nitric oxide and hypercholesterolemia: a matter of oxidation and reduction? Atherosclerosis 137, S51–S60.

Willis, G.C., 1953. An experimental study of the intimal ground substance in atherosclerosis. Can. Med. Assoc. J. 69, 17–22.

Wójcicki, J., Rózewicka, L., Barcew-Wiszniewska, B., Samochowiec, L., Juzwiak, S., Kadlubowska, D., Tustanowski, S., Juzyszyn, Z., 1991. Effect of selenium and vitamin E on the development of experimental atherosclerosis in rabbits. Atherosclerosis 87, 9–16.

Yegin, A., Yegin, H., Alicigüzel, Y., Deger, N., Semiz, E., 1997. Erythrocyte selenium-glutathione peroxidase activity is lower in patients with coronary atherosclerosis. Jpn. Heart J. 38, 793–798.

Ylä-Herttuala, S., Palinski, W., Rosenfeld, M.E., Parthasarathy, S., Carew, T.E., Butler, S., Witztum, J.L., Steinberg, D., 1989. Evidence for the presence of oxidatively modified low density lipoprotein in atherosclerotic lesions of rabbit and man. J. Clin. Invest. 84, 1086–1095.

**Advances in
Cell Aging and
Gerontology**

Dietary antioxidants and cardiovascular disease

Brian M. Dixon[1], Swapna V. Shenvi[1] and Tory M. Hagen*

*Department of Biochemistry and Biophysics, Linus Pauling Institute; Oregon State University,
571 Weniger Hall, Corvallis, OR 97331-6512, USA*

Contents

---

* Corresponding author. Tel.: +1-541-737-5083; fax: +1-541-737-5077.
 E-mail address: tory.hagen@orst.edu (T.M. Hagen).
[1] Both authors contributed equally to this manuscript.

Advances in Cell Aging and Gerontology, vol. 11, 349–376

Abbreviations

4-HNE	4-hydroxy-2-nonenal
AA	ascorbic acid (vitamin C)
AGE	advanced glycation endproducts
AHA	American Heart Association
ARIC	atherosclerosis risk in communities
ATBC	α-Tocopherol β-Carotene Cancer Prevention Study
ATP	adenosine triphosphate
BSO	buthionine-S,R-sulfoximine
CLAS	Cholesterol Lowering Atherosclerosis Study
CoQ	coenzyme Q (ubiquinone)
CVD	cardiovascular disease
DHLA	dihydrolipoic acid
DNA	deoxyribonucleic acid
DRI	daily recommended intake
eNOS	endothelial nitric oxide synthase
EU-RAMIC	European Community Multicenter Study on Antioxidants, Myocardial Infarction, and Breast Cancer
γ-GCS	γ-glutamyl cysteine synthetase
GSH	glutathione
GS	glutathione synthetase
GSSG	glutathione disulfide
HOPE	Heart Outcomes Prevention Evaluation
I-κB	inhibitor of nuclear factor-κB
I/R	ischemia-reperfusion
IU	international units (equal to 1 mg α-tocopherol activity)
KGDH	α-ketoglutarate dehydrogenase
LA	lipoic acid
LDL	low density lipoprotein
MI	myocardial infarction
mRNA	messenger ribonucleic acid
NAC	*N*-acetyl cysteine
NADPH	nicotinamide adenine diphosphate
NF-κB	nuclear factor-κB
NO	nitric oxide
RNS	reactive nitrogen species
ROS	reactive oxygen species
THP-1	human acute monocytic leukemia cell line
TNF-α	tumor necrosis factor-α

TBARS   thiobarbituric acid reactive substance
VE   vitamin E (α-tocopherol)

1. Introduction

In 1990, cardiovascular diseases (CVD) of all types were the major cause of hospitalization, disability, and death worldwide (Murray and Lopez, 1997). The leading risk factor for the onset of CVD is age (AHA, 2001). This suggests that the incidence and morbidity associated with CVD will increase enormously in the near future as the worldwide elderly population increases. Recently, much effort has gone into understanding the mechanisms leading to age-related declines in cardiac and vascular function. While the underlying mechanisms leading to heightened onset of CVD with age are not entirely known and are undoubtedly multifactorial, there is growing awareness that oxidative stress may play an important role.

One important aspect of aging appears to be increased cardiovascular oxidative stress and an associated increase in oxidative damage to lipids, proteins, and DNA. This realization has been the impetus to suggest that maintaining or increasing cardiovascular antioxidant status could be an effective means to delay or prevent incidence of CVD, especially in the elderly. Because other chapters present detailed overviews of the underlying pathophysiologies of CVD with age and the effects of other micronutrients and alternative therapies, this chapter will confine discussion to age-related changes in tissue antioxidant status and the available evidence whether dietary antioxidants effectively mitigate onset and/or the progression of CVD.

1.1. *Age-associated increase in myocardial oxidative stress*

According to the free radical theory of aging, reactive oxygen and nitrogen species (ROS/RNS) are constantly produced as byproducts of normal metabolism. A small percentage of these oxidants escape the normal cellular antioxidant defenses and damage lipids, proteins, and DNA. Over one's lifespan, this constant damage can manifest itself as disease pathophysiologies and compromised cardiovascular function. Intracellular sources of ROS/RNS include mixed-function oxidases (P-450 isozymes, xanthine oxidase, NADPH oxidases), nitric oxide synthase, peroxisomes, and oxidants from the mitochondrial electron transport chain. While many sources undoubtedly contribute to overall cellular oxidant production, the mitochondria are the primary producers of ROS/RNS.

Isolated mitochondrial preparations from old versus young hearts produce more ROS, reflecting an age-related decline in electron transport efficiency (Lesnefsky et al., 2001; Fannin et al., 1999). Nohl et al. (1979) showed that the rate of ROS production by heart mitochondria from old rats increased two-fold over that from young rats. Other studies also reported increased superoxide and hydrogen peroxide production (Sohal et al., 1994; Sohal and Dubey, 1994). However, this view has been recently challenged by Hansford et al. (1997), who show that the apparent age-related increase in oxidant production might be an artifact stemming from assay conditions used in earlier studies. If true, this suggests that other ROS/RNS sources and pathologies would be responsible for observed increases in oxidative stress.

To further address this question, Suh et al. (2001) recently examined mitochondrial oxidant production in isolated cardiac myocytes. They found that oxidant production increased by 31% in mitochondria from old compared to young rats. This increase was even more pronounced when normalized to oxygen consumption. Thus, on a whole cell basis, the aging heart muscle experiences a more pro-oxidant environment than that seen in cells from young animals.

Increased oxidative stress causes a number of underlying changes that likely result in a variety of cardiomyopathies. Notably, there is a pronounced myocardial atrophy, mostly of left ventricular myocytes, and a compensatory hypertrophy of the remaining myocytes (Colucci, 1997). Increased oxidants also contribute to myocardial contraction and relaxation pathologies. This is due to an oxidant-induced increase in collagen content (Colucci, 1997; Katz, 1988; Leukjewicz et al., 1972; Yang et al., 1997; Sharov et al., 1997), fragmentation of elastin fibers (Svanborg, 1997), and fibrotic scarring on the endo- and epicardial surfaces (James, 1998). This remodeling may cause a prolongation of both contraction (systolic) and relaxation (diastolic) times, leading to cardiac arrhythmias and, ultimately, heart failure (Katz, 1988; Carré et al., 1993). More specifically, Uchida et al. (1993) showed that α-ketoglutarate dehydrogenase (KGDH) is susceptible to adduction with 4-hydroxy-2-nonenal (4-HNE), a major product of lipid peroxidation. Other in vitro studies showed that 4-HNE adduction lowers KGDH activity (Humphries and Sweda, 1998; Humphries et al., 1998). Thus, oxidative damage to KGDH and, potentially, other important biomolecules may be a significant underlying event during aging.

The heightened increase in oxidant production and attendant oxidative damage may be exacerbated by a decline in certain antioxidants with age. Glutathione (GSH) and vitamin C, two of the most important low molecular weight, water-soluble antioxidants, decline significantly in the aging rat heart (Suh et al., 2001; Hagen et al., 1999, 2000). Antioxidant enzymes may or may not decline, depending on the particular study or antioxidant enzyme examined (Brown-Borg et al., 2002; Kitani et al., 2001). Coenzyme Q (CoQ), which is an electron transport constituent and antioxidant (see below), also declines with age, which would not only affect mitochondrial energy production but also increase oxidant production from the compromised electron transport chain (Genova et al., 2001). Combined, these events lead to a vicious downward spiral of oxidative damage and compromised myocardial functioning.

1.2. *Age-associated increase in vascular endothelial oxidative stress*

As reported in detail elsewhere in this book, aging profoundly affects endothelial function, in both humans and experimental animals. Evidence for the loss of vasomotor function comes from both human and animal studies showing that arteries of aged subjects have a significantly reduced response to vasodilatory agents such as acetylcholine and bradykinin (Hynes and Duckles, 1987; Kung and Luscher, 1995; Dohi et al., 1990; Egashira et al., 1993; Urakami-Harasawa et al., 1997). Interestingly, there is no loss in vessel relaxation response to nitroglycerine or other nitric oxide-donating drugs (Docherty, 1990). Also, there is no decline in guanylate cyclase activity associated with aging in vascular smooth muscle cells (Koga et al., 1989). These results suggest that age-associated impairment in vasodilation is largely centered in vascular endothelial cells. However, vascular endothelial impairment is not universal. Loss of vasomotor function is confined to the major conduit arteries such as the aorta, coronary, and carotid arteries, whereas pulmonary and peripheral arteries show little or no decline in vessel tone (Tschudi et al., 1996). Thus, the age-related loss in vasomotor response is most likely due to endothelial dysfunction and not pathologies associated with the vascular smooth muscle layer.

The mechanism of endothelial cell dysfunction has yet to be fully elucidated. Despite this, there is growing evidence that oxidation alters endothelial nitric oxide synthase (eNOS) activity, nitric oxide release, and/or its bioavailability (Tschudi et al., 1996; Barton et al., 1997). This argument is strengthened by work showing increased oxidative stress in vascular endothelial cells with age. Carrera-Rotlan and Estrada-Garcia (1998) showed that lipid peroxidation, as measured by the thiobarbituric acid reactive substance (TBARS) assay, increased two- to three-fold in endothelial cells from young versus old rats. Other studies demonstrate enhanced oxidative damage in the aging vessel, which may contribute to both arteriosclerosis and atherosclerosis in the aging animal (Basta et al., 2002; Cain and Khalil, 2002). Thus, there is strong evidence that heightened oxidative stress plays a significant role in the age-related loss of arterial compliance and onset of CVD.

1.3. *Antioxidant treatments of cardiovascular disease*

A role for antioxidants in the prevention and treatment of CVD has gained support because of their widespread availability and ease of supplementation. Since oxidative damage appears to be central in cardiovascular aging, antioxidants may provide significant protection. The studies advocating the use of antioxidants suggest that intake should be well above the general levels of consumption (reviewed below). If these results are true, an increase of antioxidant intake in the US population could reduce disease rates, improve treatment, and reduce hospital stays. Thus, it is conceivable that dietary interventions with antioxidants could provide an effective means to improve or maintain myocardial function in the elderly. Despite this strong theoretical rationale, there is currently conflicting evidence to suggest that individual antioxidant supplements actually lessen risk for CVD in the elderly. We now review the available data examining whether certain widely available antioxidants in the diet ameliorate the risk of CVD.

2. Vitamin C

2.1. *Structure and function*

Since its purification and identification in 1933 (Szent-Györgyi, 1933), the effects of ascorbic acid (AA), or vitamin C, have been extensively studied. AA is essential for collagen, carnitine, and neurotransmitter synthesis, and it is also required as a co-substrate for many mono- and dioxygenases (Carr and Frei, 1999). However, AA is probably most known as a potent antioxidant (Frei et al., 1988, 1989) due to its very high redox potential of 280 mV (Buettner, 1993). The redox potential of AA allows it to act as an oxidant scavenger and also to recycle other cellular antioxidants such as α-tocopherol (Buettner, 1993; Nakagawa et al., 1991). Thus, AA plays a profound role as an antioxidant in both aqueous and lipid compartments of the cell.

2.2. *Justification for supplementation in the elderly*

Numerous studies in both experimental animals and humans show that tissue AA levels decline with age (Porrini et al., 1987; Sasaki et al., 1983; Hercberg et al., 1994; Monget et al., 1996; Mezzetti et al., 1996; Vir and Love, 1979). In a meta-analysis of 36 studies, Brubacher et al. (2000) examined age-related changes in AA status. There was a strong correlation between age and plasma AA concentrations relative to the oral dose given. The authors extrapolated that to maintain a plasma concentration of 50 µmol/l, the elderly require double the oral intake. Men also seem more susceptible to AA loss than women (Birlouez-Aragon et al., 2001; Monget et al., 1996; Roine et al., 1974; VanderJagt et al., 1987; Jacob et al., 1988; Garry et al., 1982), which cannot be accounted for by gender-specific differences in renal clearance (Oreopoulos et al., 1993). One explanation for the exacerbated AA loss in men relative to women may be its lower uptake from the diet. When men and women were supplemented with the same dose of vitamin C, women consistently showed approximately two-fold increases in their plasma levels (VanderJagt et al., 1987; Garry et al., 1982). To further explicate this gender-dependent loss in AA levels in elderly men, Heseker and Schneider (1994) compared absorption characteristics in young versus old men. It was found that older male subjects had a decreased capacity for AA absorption compared to their younger counterparts (Heseker and Schneider, 1994). Thus, there appears to be an age-related and gender-specific difference in the absorption of AA from the diet.

Transport characteristics in young and old male rats were recently explored in our laboratory. The rate of radiolabeled AA uptake was 68% lower in hepatocytes from young compared to old male rats (Fig. 1). Increasing exogenous AA concentrations resulted in improved uptake characteristics in cells from old rats (Fig. 1). However, both the rate of uptake and AA accumulation in cells from old rats always remained lower than in cells from young rats (Fig. 1). Since AA uptake is via active transport, these results suggest that defects in AA transporters may explain the observed loss of AA status in the elderly, especially men (Michels et al., submitted).

Many other factors may also contribute to the age-related loss of AA, including poor diet (Roine et al., 1974; Vir and Love, 1979), socio-economic status, and physical disabilities (Mezzetti et al., 1996). For instance, the elderly confined to nursing homes show very low AA plasma concentrations (Monget et al., 1996; Marazzi et al., 1990), with some subjects exhibiting AA levels bordering on scurvy (plasma concentration <5.6 µmol/l) (Birlouez-Aragon et al., 2001). In non-institutionalized subjects, it is less clear whether significant AA loss is observed with age. In a few studies, a decline in plasma AA was not observed in non-institutionalized

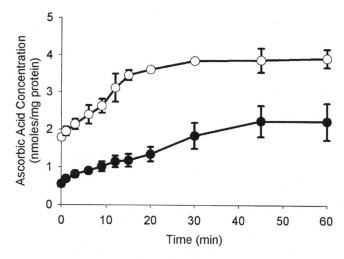

Fig. 1. The rate of hepatocellular AA uptake declines with age. AA (100 μM) was added to hepatocytes (2.0×10^6 cells/ml) freshly isolated from young (open circles) and old (closed circles) rats and incubated at 37°C (N=4). At the times indicated, aliquots were taken and analyzed for intracellular AA concentrations using the method of Frei et al. (1989). Results show an age-related decline in both the rate and steady-state level of AA accumulation in cells isolated from young versus old rats.

subjects (Harrill and Cervone, 1977; Garry et al., 1982; Jacob et al., 1988) but may have been the result of non-representative populations. Conversely, there are other reports that AA concentration does, in fact, decrease in non-institutionalized persons as a function of age, again, especially in men (Hercberg et al., 1994; Heseker and Schneider, 1994) and less frequently in women (Burr et al., 1974).

Further, elderly subjects exhibiting clinical pathologies such as diabetes mellitus (reviewed in Will and Byers, 1996) and Alzheimer's disease (Riviere et al., 1998a,b) tend to have lower plasma AA. These effects can be further magnified by smoking habits, which also adversely affect plasma AA concentration (Heseker and Schneider, 1994; Marangon et al., 1998; Birlouez-Aragon et al., 2001). Therefore, a reduction in AA status occurs in a majority of the elderly population and may be further exacerbated by lifestyle and disease state, with many implications related to CVD risk (discussed below).

2.3. *Epidemiological studies: general population*

Carr and Frei (1999) recently reviewed the available epidemiological data examining the association between vitamin C intake and risk for cardiovascular disease. In seven out of 11 prospective cohort studies, there was a significant inverse correlation between CVD risk and AA status; two other trials also showed correlations between CVD and AA, while only two other studies could not demonstrate an association (Table 1). A more recent study by Yokoyama et al. (2000) also showed a decrease in risk for CVD when high AA status was observed (Table 1). Thus, it appears that AA intake is inversely correlated with risk for CVD.

Table 1
Vitamin C and cardiovascular disease risk

Reference	Population	Duration	Endpoint	Vitamin C	Conclusions
Enstrom et al. (1986)	3119 Men and women	10 years	CVD	>250 compared with <250 mg/d	No decreased risk
Enstrom et al. (1992)	4479 Men	10 years	CVD	>50 mg/d+supplement	Decreased risk by 42%
Enstrom (1993)	6809 Women	10 years	CVD	>50 mg/d+supplement	Decreased risk by 25%
Manson et al. (1992)	87,245 Female nurses	8 years	CAD	>359 compared with <93 mg/d	Decreased risk by 20% (NS)
Manson et al. (1993)	87,245 Female nurses	8 years	Stroke	>359 compared with <93 mg/d	Decreased risk by 24%
Rimm et al. (1993)	39,910 Male health professionals	4 years	CAD	392 compared with 92 mg/d median	No decreased risk
Fehily et al. (1993)	2512 Men	5 years	CVD	>67 compared with <35 mg/d	Decreased risk 37% (NS)
Knekt et al. (1994)	2748 Finnish men	14 years	CAD	>85 compared with <60 mg/d	No decreased risk
Knekt et al. (1994)	2385 Finnish women	14 years	CAD	>91 compared with <61 mg/d	Decreased risk by 51%
Kritchevsky et al. (1995)	4989 Men	3 years	Carotid atherosclerosis	>982 compared with <112 mg/d	Decreased intima thickness
	6318 Women	3 years	Carotid atherosclerosis	>728 compared with <64 mg/d	Decreased intima thickness
Pandey et al. (1995)	1556 Men	24 years	CAD	>113 compared with <82 mg/d	Decreased risk by 25%
Kushi et al. (1996)	34,486 Postmenopausal women	7 years	CAD	>391 compared with <112 mg/d	No decreased risk
				>196 compared with <87 mg/d	No decreased risk
				Supplement versus no supplement	No decreased risk
Yokoyama et al. (2000)	2121 Men and women	20 years	Stroke	Serum vitamin C	Inverse relationship with incidence of stroke
Gale et al. (1995)[a]	730 UK elderly men and women	20 years	Stroke	>45 compared with <28 mg/d	Decreased risk by 50%
Losonczy et al. (1996)[a]	11,178 Elderly men and women	6 years	CAD	>45 compared with <28 mg/d	Decreased risk by 20% (NS)
			CAD	Supplement versus no supplement	No decreased risk
Sahyoun et al. (1996)[a]	725 Elderly men and women	10 years	CVD	>388 compared with <90 mg/d	Decreased risk by 62% (NS)
Wilson et al. (1972)[a]	159 Elderly men and women	4 weeks	Mortality	Buffy coat vitamin C status	Inverse relationship with death (women); inverse relationship with death (men) (NS)
Wilson et al. (1973)[a]	538 Elderly men and women	4 weeks	Mortality	Buffy coat vitamin C status+200 mg/d	Same result as previous study; supplementation did not reverse mortality

[a] Studies in elderly populations.

2.4. *Epidemiological studies: elderly population*

In a 20 year follow-up study in Britain examining the incidences of mortality from stroke and coronary heart disease, Gale et al. (1995) showed that the risk of death from stroke was highest in those with the lowest AA intake (<28 mg/d). Higher AA intake (>45 mg/d) lowered the mortality rate and was independent of social class or other dietary variables. Interestingly, Gale et al. (1995) also showed that AA status was as strong a predictor of death from stroke as was high diastolic blood pressure. Furthermore, while not significant, a reduction in coronary heart disease was also found (Gale et al., 1995). In a study consisting of 725 elderly men and women, Sahyoun et al. (1996) showed that subjects in the upper two quintiles of AA intake (>400 mg/d) had a lower incidence of overall mortality (cancer, injuries, poisoning, and diseases, including: respiratory, endocrine/metabolic, genitourinary, digestive, and nervous systems, and infections) compared to the lowest two quintiles (<90 mg/d). They went on to show that this association was largely due to reduced mortality from heart disease.

In a study examining AA and vitamin E co-supplementation in 11,178 persons, mortality from all causes was reduced, but co-supplementation had a greater effect on mortality from coronary heart disease (Losonczy et al., 1996). The authors could not, however, associate reduced risk for heart disease to vitamin C intake alone. In two older studies, Andrews and co-workers (Wilson et al., 1972, 1973) also showed that plasma AA status was a good predictor of death in men and women (Wilson et al., 1972). However, a subsequent study revealed that this association with mortality could not be reversed by a daily supplementation of 200 mg AA for 4 weeks (Wilson et al., 1973).

Other specific endpoints associated with CVD, although not specifically examined in the elderly, have also been investigated. Increased AA status improved outcomes, including acute myocardial infarction (MI) (Riemersma et al., 2000), endothelial vasomotor relaxation (Gokce et al., 1999), carotid stenosis (Gale et al., 2001), and ambulatory blood pressure (Fotherby et al., 2000). These results further provide a rationale that suggests that AA intake may lower the risk of mortality from CVD in people over the age of 65.

Thus, vitamin C appears to have protective effects in all ages of the population, including the elderly. However, this protection only appears to be afforded to individuals with initially low plasma levels of AA (<50 μmol/l). The optimum dose appears to somewhere between 90 and 100 mg/d, with only slightly improved benefits from higher doses.

3. Vitamin E

3.1. *Structure and function*

The main function of vitamin E (VE) in humans appears to be that of a membrane antioxidant (redox potential 500 mV) (Buettner, 1993). Vitamin E exists naturally in eight different forms: four tocopherols (α, β, γ, δ) and the four corresponding tocotrienols, all of which have relatively potent antioxidant activities in vitro (Li et al., 2001). α-Tocopherol predominates as the major and most biologically active form (Bunyan et al., 1961) of vitamin E in humans and animals and is the only isoform actively maintained in the human body (Traber, 1999). Major sources of VE in the American diet include vegetable oils, nuts, whole grains, green leafy vegetables, and vitamin supplements (Hanninen et al., 2000). The average dietary intake of VE in the US is approximately 9 mg/d for men and 6 mg/d for women, well below the recently revised daily recommended intake (DRI) of 15 mg/d (DRI, 2000).

3.2. *Epidemiological studies: general population*

Oxidative modification of low density lipoprotein (LDL) is considered a key event in the initiation and progression of atherosclerosis (Steinberg et al., 1989). Vitamin E has been postulated as a means to lower risk for atherosclerosis through inhibiting the oxidation of LDL circulating in the plasma (Cherubini et al., 2001). In this regard, LDL isolated from subjects taking vitamin E supplements (>400 IU) was less susceptible to ex vivo oxidation (Devaraj et al., 1997; Jialal et al., 1995). However, epidemiological studies show differing results as to whether VE lowers the risk for atherosclerosis (Table 2). Some studies show an association between high dietary VE intake and/or high serum concentrations and lower rates of CVD (Table 2). Conversely, controlled trials examining VE intake in populations with different risks for CVD reveal differing results (Table 2). The cause for these differences is not clear, and several factors may play a role (Pruthi et al., 2001), including subject compliance, study design, dosage regime, and the isoform of VE used.

3.3. *Epidemiological studies: elderly population*

As described previously, aging increases the likelihood of LDL lipid peroxidation, which suggests a heightened risk for atherogenesis. However, it is not clear whether increased LDL modification even occurs in vivo or whether VE supplementation lowers the susceptibility of LDL oxidation in the elderly. Khalil et al. (1996, 2000) showed that VE was unable to restore the decreased resistance to LDL oxidation from young subjects compared to that from elderly subjects. In contrast, Cherubini et al. (2001) suggested that maintaining VE is important to avoid increased risk for atherosclerosis with advanced age. It is no clearer whether vitamin E supplementation improves other key parameters related to CVD in the elderly. One study with older subjects showed no change in flow-mediated vasodilation following supplementation with 1000 IU/d of VE for 10 weeks (Simons et al., 1999; Celermajer et al., 1994). However, another study that examined VE status and carotid stenosis showed that subjects with low blood concentration of VE were 2.5 times as likely to have a >30% narrowing of the carotid artery (Gale et al., 2001).

Most trials show that the intake of VE derived from food, but not from supplements, is inversely associated with mortality from coronary heart disease. For example, Kushi et al. (1996) and the Finnish trial (Knekt et al., 1994) suggested that modifying dietary habits to increase VE intake may be worthwhile in preventing coronary heart disease. On the other hand, the most recent data on VE utilization suggests that doses of 150 or 300 IU/d replace substantial amounts of circulating plasma VE (Iuliano et al., 2001). Over time, these large doses result in increased total tissue VE concentrations. This increase in tissue vitamin E may explain epidemiological studies that show a decrease in CVD risk in subjects taking supplemental VE in amounts of >100 IU/d for two or more years.

In conclusion, it is unclear whether VE modulates the risk of CVD. The potential role of its antioxidant activity has been called into question because VE accumulates in atherosclerotic lesions in humans (Upston et al., 1999). The dose of VE that is the most effective and safe, as well as the minimum duration of treatment that is required to produce the postulated protective effects of vitamin E, is also unknown. Randomized, placebo-controlled clinical trials are needed before public health recommendations concerning the use of vitamin E supplementation for CVD prevention can be made.

4. Lipoic acid

4.1. *Structure and function*

Lipoic acid (1,2-dithiolane-3-pentanoic acid; LA) is a naturally occurring dithiol compound found in high abundance in green leafy vegetables (spinach, kale, and broccoli) and animal protein (Lodge and Packer, 1999). Though LA is synthesized de novo from octanoic acid in mammals (Bustamante et al., 1998), dietary consumption may also be necessary to maintain adequate cellular levels. Thus, LA is considered a conditionally essential micronutrient.

The chemical reactivity of free LA is mainly conferred by its dithiolane ring. The standard reduction potential for LA is 290 mV making it one of the lowest redox couples in biological systems (Bustamante et al., 1998; Jocelyn, 1972). LA is a potent antioxidant of hydroxyl and peroxyl radicals, singlet oxygen, and hypochlorous acid, as well as a recycler of other antioxidants, including glutathione disulfide (GSSG), CoQ, and vitamins E and C (reviewed in Bustamante et al., 1998). Studies, including those from our laboratory, demonstrate that LA can also act to chelate transition metals, rendering them unable to take part in free radical reactions in vitro (reviewed in Bustamante et al., 1998). This is supported by numerous reports that show LA lowers oxidative stress, both in vitro and in vivo.

In tissues, LA is normally bound to lysine residues in mitochondrial α-ketoacid dehydrogenases (pyruvate dehydrogenase, 2-oxoglutarate dehydrogenase, and the branched chain amino acid oxidase complex), and serves in transfer reactions. Thus, it is critical for cellular bioenergetics. Concentrations of unbound LA are very low in vivo; however, following a meal or dietary supplementation, there is a marked, yet transient, increase in free LA in tissues. LA is normally found in its oxidized form and is readily taken up into cells and reduced either by mitochondrial lipoic acid dehydrogenases or thioredoxin/glutaredoxin reductases to dihydrolipoic acid

Table 2
Vitamin E and cardiovascular disease risk

Reference	Population	Endpoint	Vitamin E	Conclusions
Knekt et al. (1994)	2748 Finnish men, 2385 Finnish women	CVD deaths	>7 mg dietary intake	35% reduction
Boaz et al. (2000)	196 Hemodialysis patients with pre-existing CVD (age 40–75 years)	Non-fatal MI, ischemic stroke, angina	800 IU/d	Lower risk, unstable angina
Rimm et al. (1993)	39,910 Health professionals (age 40–75 years)	CVD risk	60–100 IU/d	Non-significant reduction
Stampfer et al. (1993)	87,245 Female nurses	CVD risk	Supplemental intake	Reduction
CHAOS Study (Stephens et al., 1996; Mitchinson et al., 1999; Ness and Davey-Smith, 1999)	2002 Patients with coronary atherosclerosis	Non-fatal MI, CVD deaths	400–800 IU/d	30–60% decrease in non-fatal MI, no change in CVD deaths
Kushi et al. (1996)	34,486 Post-menopausal women	CVD deaths	Dietary intake, supplemental intake	Lower risk from dietary intake, no change in risk upon supplementation
CLAS (Hodis et al., 1995; Azen et al., 1996)	156 Men with coronary artery bypass surgery (age 40–59 years)	Coronary artery atherosclerosis	≥100 IU/d	Reduced coronary artery atherosclerosis
ARIC Study (Kritchevsky et al., 1995)	6318 Women, 4989 men (age 45–64 years)	Carotid arterial wall thickness	Dietary intake	Reduction in carotid arterial wall thickness
HOPE Study (1996, 2000)	Patients above 55 years with ischemic heart disease, stroke, or peripheral artery disease	400 IU/d	CVD deaths, MI, stroke	No effects
GISSI-Prevenzione Trial (1999)	11,324 Patients with pre-existing CVD	300 mg/d	CVD deaths, non-fatal MI, stroke	No significant reduction
Salonen et al. (1985)	51 Case-control pairs	High serum VE concentration	MI, CVD deaths	No correlation
Kok et al. (1987)	10,532 Patients	High serum VE concentration	CVD deaths	No correlation
Hense et al. (1993)	2023 Men, 1999 Women (age 25–64 years)	High serum VE concentration	CVD development, MI	No association
ATBC Cancer Prevention Study Group (1994)	29,133 Finnish male smokers (age 50–69 years)	50 mg/d	CVD mortality	No effect
Losonczy et al. (1996)	11,178 Subjects (age 67–105 years)	Supplemental intake	CVD mortality	Reduction in risk
DeMaio et al. (1992)	100 Patients with coronary angioplasty	1200 IU/d	Re-stenosis	Non-statistical significant reduction

(DHLA). This reduction occurs at the expense of NAD(P)H, the only known biological compound with sufficient power to reduce oxidized LA (reviewed in Bustamante et al., 1998).

4.2. *Roles of unbound lipoic acid*

Unbound LA/DHLA is only transiently maintained in cells; DHLA appears in culture media only 10 minutes after addition. Feeding studies also show that >80% of a dietary bolus of radiolabeled LA is metabolized and excreted via the urine within 24 hours. Thus, non-protein-bound LA is only transiently available within cells (reviewed in Bustamante et al., 1998).

Lipoic acid supplementation has been reported to increase GSH levels in cell culture, and in vivo, most likely by increasing cysteine and cystine import, the rate-limiting step in GSH synthesis (reviewed in Bustamante et al., 1998). Studies from our laboratory showed that LA reverses the age-related decline in the GSH/GSSG ratio (Fig. 2) and improves resistance to toxins in aged animals (Suh et al., 2001; Hagen et al., 1999, 2000; and preliminary evidence). Thus, LA directly, yet transiently, increases antioxidant capacity, but also indirectly improves antioxidant status by inducing GSH synthesis.

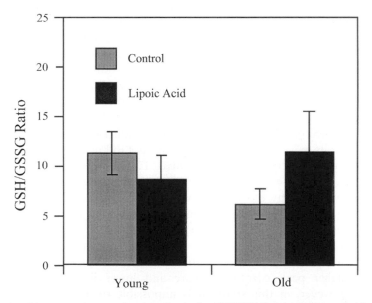

Fig. 2. Lipoic acid reverses the age-related decline in the GSH/GSSG ratio. Young and old rats were fed with or without LA (0.2% [w/w]) for two weeks and the GSH/GSSG ratio determined. Results show that there is a marked decline in the GSH/GSSG ratio in young versus old unsupplemented rats, indicating an overall decline in thiol redox status. LA supplementation reversed the age-related decline in the GSH/GSSG ratio such that it was no longer different from that seen in young rats.

4.3. *Epidemiological studies*

While there have yet to be any large epidemiological studies using LA, it has been clinically used to treat diabetes mellitus, a disease that seems to mirror, in part, the aging condition. It is well established that diabetics experience increased levels of oxidative insult (Baynes, 1991; van Dam et al., 1995; Ruhe and McDonald, 2001) and have a higher likelihood of developing CVD, specifically hypertension and atherosclerosis (DeFronzo et al., 1991; DeFronzo and Ferrannini, 1992; Ruhe and McDonald, 2001). The mechanism potentially responsible for the increased risk of CVD (and organ dysfunction) in diabetic patients is the activation of the polyol pathway and increases in (auto)oxidation of glucose, which can go on to glycate proteins, lipids, and lipoproteins within blood vessels. This ultimately leads to vascular damage both by the accumulation of advanced glycation endproducts (AGE) and by the oxidation of LDL particles. Packer et al. (1995) showed that LA prevents the glycation of proteins (Ruhe and McDonald, 2001), thus leading to a return of normal blood flow to tissues. Furthermore, LA increases sensitivity to insulin treatment, possibly by protecting sulfhydryl groups of glucose transporters (Glut-1 and Glut-4) (Jacob et al., 1996).

The evidence that LA treatment ameliorates certain pathologies associated with diabetes is merely corollary to aging and CVD. However, Suh et al. (2001) showed that the age-related increase in myocardial oxidative stress and steady-state levels of oxidative DNA damage in old rats was reversed by dietary supplementation with LA. These authors also showed that LA supplementation reversed both the age-associated decline in myocardial AA and GSH/GSSG ratio (Figs. 2 and 3). Interestingly, LA had no effect on the antioxidant status or indices of oxidative stress in the myocardium from young rats. This suggests that LA supplementation to old rats reverses loss of normal antioxidant status but does not induce further increases when cellular antioxidant status is normal (Suh et al., 2001) (Fig. 2).

Using an in vitro atherogenesis model, Zhang and Frei (2001) showed that pre-incubation of human aortic endothelial cells with 0.05–1.0 mmol/l LA for 48 hours inhibited tumor necrosis factor (TNF-α)-induced adhesion molecule expression in human THP-1 cells in a dose-dependent manner but did not affect expression of the TNF-α receptor. Furthermore, LA inhibited TNF-α-induced I-κB (inhibitor of nuclear factor-κB,) kinase activation and blocked nuclear translocation of NF-κB. This suggests that LA may block early events in atherogenesis.

Finally, in an animal study that examined whether LA could decrease damage following ischemia-reperfusion (I/R) injury, Coombes et al. (2000) fed a combination of VE and LA to old rats for 14 weeks. Following coronary artery occlusion and reperfusion, the authors demonstrated that rats on the supplemental diet exhibited significantly higher peak carotid pressure and lower lipid oxidation following reperfusion. However, in this study, it is impossible to differentiate between the effects of LA and those of the VE.

While LA has been used for many years to successfully treat diabetes, its roles in the treatment and prevention of other diseases, including CVD, have yet to be fully explored. Early preliminary evidence using LA treatment, predominantly in animal

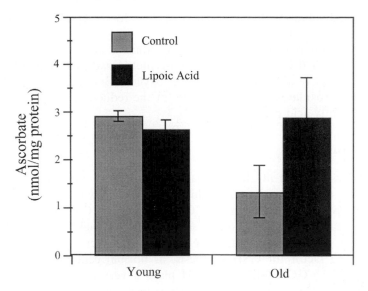

Fig. 3. Lipoic acid supplementation reverses the age-associated decline in myocardial AA status. AA levels in freshly isolated hearts from young and old rats were determined after supplementing the diet for two weeks with and without LA (0.2% [w/w]). Ascorbate levels in old LA-supplemented rats were markedly higher than in old unsupplemented animals. Furthermore, the LA-induced increase was no longer different from that seen in young animals. Interestingly, LA supplementation had no effect on AA status in the young animals.

models, looks promising in ameliorating some indices of CVD. However, much more experimental evidence is needed from both animal studies and clinical trials to fully establish a link between LA supplementation and its therapeutic roles in CVD treatment and prevention in the elderly.

5. Glutathione

5.1. *Structure and function*

Glutathione (γ-glutamyl-cysteinyl-glycine; GSH) is a tripeptide found, with few exceptions, throughout aerobic life. It is composed of glutamate, cysteine, and glycine, where the linkage between glutamate and cysteine is via glutamate's γ carboxyl group. This unusual peptide linkage is not recognized by cellular peptidases and thus confers resistance to proteolysis. GSH must be exported from the cell for turnover to occur. It is broken down by γ-glutamyltransferase, the only known enzyme capable of hydrolyzing the γ-glutamyl bond (Hagen et al., 1991).

GSH is the most abundant low molecular weight thiol in mammalian cells and most plants, ranging in concentration from 1 to 10 mM, which helps maintain intracellular thiol redox balance and many cellular detoxification reactions. Because the concentration of GSH is so high, many foods contain 15 mg or more per 100 g. Asparagus, potatoes, oranges, grapefruit, fresh meats, and fish are particularly high in GSH. For individuals with a high intake of these foods, GSH consumption could be as high as 100–150 mg/d.

GSH has a redox potential of 200–250 mV (Jonas et al., 1999) and therefore can directly scavenge hydroxyl radicals, carbon-centered radicals, hypochlorous acid, peroxynitrite, reactive aldehydes, and singlet oxygen (Buettner, 1993). GSH is also used by GSH peroxidases as a co-substrate for the reduction of hydrogen peroxide and alkyl and fatty acid peroxides.

5.2. *Biosynthesis*

GSH synthesis occurs in all mammalian cells by the concerted action of two ATP-requiring cytosolic enzymes, γ-glutamyl cysteine synthetase (γ-GCS), composed of a heavy and light chain, and GSH synthetase (GS). The heavy chain of γ-GCS is the catalytic subunit, and is sensitive to feedback inhibition from GSH while the light chain controls substrate affinity. However, cysteine availability is the rate-limiting factor for GSH synthesis, as normal cellular cysteine levels are below the K_m of γ-GCS. Although GSH plays a very critical role in detoxification, another function is to serve as a short-term reservoir for cysteine. When cysteine becomes limiting for protein synthesis, GSH pools decrease, and detoxification functions that are dependent on GSH become impaired. Thus, dietary GSH could provide cysteine for both protein and cellular GSH synthesis (Jaeschke and Wendel, 1985).

5.3. *Age-related loss of glutathione*

GSH levels are lower in hepatocytes from old compared to young rats (Hagen et al., 1998, 1999; Liu and Choi, 2000). The GSH/GSSG ratio, an important indicator of oxidative stress, also declines significantly. In addition, Hothersall et al. (1981) reported that the activity of glutathione peroxidase decreases in young compared to old rats. This reduction in the activity of glutathione peroxidase is correlated to the decreased availability of glutathione in aged rats. Thus, age-related loss of cellular detoxification capacity parallels changes in GSH status.

5.4. *Experimental studies*

There is strong evidence that oxidative damage to cellular components of the myocardium is the direct cause of impaired functional performance in the post-ischemic heart (Ambrosio et al., 1991; Brown et al., 1988; Park et al., 1991). It is interesting to note that myocardial I/R injury shares a major etiological mechanism with aging in that both involve increased ROS generation and oxidative stress (Harman, 1956; Lakatta et al., 2001; Beckman and Ames, 1997). Recent literature shows that senescent hearts undergo ultrastructural and biochemical changes that increase their susceptibility to I/R injury (Ataka et al., 1992; Lesnefsky et al., 1994; Tani et al., 1997; Lucas and Szweda, 1998; Abete et al., 1999; Azhar et al., 1999).

Depletion of endogenous GSH by buthionine-*S,R*-sulfoximine (BSO) intensifies the extent of oxidative damage observed in I/R hearts. Conversely, Ramires et al. (2001) showed that GSH supplementation in conjunction with exercise in rats greatly improved myocardial resistance to I/R injury due to an improved antioxidant reserve and GSH homeostasis.

Generation of ROS and RNS produced by several cellular sources like xanthine oxidase, the mitochondrial electron transport chain, and nitric oxide synthase is also an important etiological mechanism for myocardial I/R injury. In isolated perfused rat hearts, GSH supplementation significantly reduced levels of peroxynitrite and enhanced post-ischemic recovery of contractile function (Cheung et al., 2000). One explanation for these results is that GSH spares nitric oxide (NO) and improves coronary vascular tone. These NO-enhancing effects may be of therapeutic benefit in treating acute and chronic manifestations of CVD.

In addition to GSH, *N*-acetyl cysteine (NAC) has also been experimentally administered in an attempt to enhance intracellular GSH concentrations. Supplementation with NAC improves human coronary and peripheral endothelium-dependent vasodilation (Cabassi et al., 2001). Furthermore, addition of NAC to cardioplegic solution protected isolated rat hearts from injury and markedly improved post-arrest recovery following I/R (Menasche et al., 1992). In a more complex model of I/R, Weinbroum et al. (2001) performed dual perfusions of the liver and heart. Isolated livers were first perfused with a Krebs buffer containing 2 mM NAC, and the effluent was collected. They went on to subsequently perfuse isolated rat hearts with the collected liver effluent, presumably enriched in GSH, and showed prevention of remote myocardial injury following cardiac I/R.

Collectively, these findings imply that boosting GSH levels, whether by directly supplementing GSH or NAC, may be an important clinical therapy. However, more data are still needed to establish these supplementation regimes in the intact animal and in clinical practice.

6. Coenzyme Q

6.1. *Structure and function*

CoQ is a lipid-soluble benzoquinone found in all tissues and membranes. The CoQ level is particularly high in the inner mitochondrial membrane, where it functions as an electron carrier in oxidative phosphorylation. CoQ is the only endogenously synthesized lipid-soluble antioxidant (Ernster and Forsmark-Andree, 1993) and protects membrane phospholipids and serum LDL from lipid peroxidation. Two different mechanisms of CoQ antioxidant function have been postulated: (1) it may act independently as a chain-breaking antioxidant, providing hydrogen atoms to reduce peroxyl and/or alkoxyl radicals (Landi et al., 1992), or (2) it may form a redox interaction with other lipid-soluble antioxidants such as VE (Nohl et al., 1999). Regardless of the mechanism, CoQ supplementation has been shown to enhance myocardial antioxidant capacity in rats (Saches et al., 1997).

6.2. *Supplementation studies*

In general, CoQ levels decline in patients with cardiomyopathies (Mortensen, 1993), degenerative diseases, and aging (Pedersen et al., 1999). These age-related changes in CoQ content, along with impaired mitochondrial function, have led to the suggestion that CoQ supplementation may be effective to ameliorate loss of myocardial bioenergetics and improve resistance to I/R injury in the elderly.

However, it is controversial whether CoQ supplementation appreciably increases myocardial levels. Dallner and co-workers (Aberg et al., 1996) showed that CoQ from the diet could be taken up into the blood and incorporated into lipoproteins. The incorporation into the liver was substantial, while little dietary CoQ was found in kidneys, muscle, and the heart (Abete et al., 1996). In contrast, Maulik et al. (2000) demonstrated an $\sim$30% increase in the myocardial content of CoQ after 30 days of feeding. The total antioxidant reserve in the heart was higher and the amount of oxidative stress was lower in the CoQ-fed group compared with controls. They also demonstrated that CoQ feeding resulted in higher post-ischemic ventricular recovery, lower creatine kinase release from hearts, and reduced infarct size, suggesting that CoQ might be instrumental in the reduction of myocardial I/R injury. Further supporting evidence comes from Ferrara et al. (1995), who reported that after 4 weeks of dietary supplementation with CoQ, tissue concentrations rose by 22% and oxidative stress was significantly suppressed.

CoQ supplementation also resulted in greater recovery of aortic and coronary arterial flow, cardiac output, stroke volume, and heart rate in rats in which cardiac function was impaired by repeated episodes of I/R injury (Ali et al., 1993). CoQ supplementation was also effective in reducing myocardial stunning, defined as a reversible decrease in contractility after I/R, and protected the ischemic myocardium in a porcine model (Atar et al., 1993). This protective effect seems to be generated by a humoral rather than an intracellular mechanism. Rowland et al. (1998) also showed that CoQ pre-treatment markedly improved recovery of pump function in old rats after severe aerobic pacing, which otherwise was impaired. Thus, there are numerous reports showing that CoQ supplementation lowers myocardial oxidative stress, lessens the severity of I/R injury, and improves myocardial bioenergetics (Maulik et al., 2000; Genova et al., 1999; Yokoyama et al., 1999). However, there is as yet no consensus on the extent of dietary CoQ incorporation into myocardial tissue.

6.3. *Clinical studies*

Various studies suggest that CoQ treatment may be effective in lowering oxidative stress and/or energy deficits in patients exhibiting CVD (Matsushima et al., 1992). In subjects in which diastolic dysfunction was evident, CoQ administration reduced high blood pressure by 80%, improved diastolic function, and reduced coronary artery thickness by 53% in hypertensive patients (Langsjoen et al., 1993). Matsushima et al. (1992) also showed that pre-treating donated hearts with CoQ resulted in better myocardial recovery, maintenance of ATP, and increased ventricular function.

In clinical studies where patients suffering from dilated cardiomyopathy were treated with CoQ, a marked improvement in echocardiographic parameters was observed (Davini et al., 1992). This suggests that CoQ supplementation may be able to stabilize cardiac function even in patients with advanced disease. However, in a more rigorous placebo-controlled, double-blind cross-over study, chronic treatment with CoQ had no influence on hemodynamic parameters, electrocardiogram, incidence of ventricular arrhythmias, or exercise tolerance (Permanetter et al., 1992). Thus, additional clinical trials will be necessary to determine whether CoQ is an effective therapy for patients suffering from cardiomyopathies. Nonetheless, CoQ treatment appears promising as a means of improving myocardial function in the elderly.

7. Carotenoids

7.1. *Structure and function*

Carotenoids are natural colorants present in various fruits and vegetables. β-Carotene is the most prominent representative of this very lipophilic class of compounds. In addition to β-carotene, other physiologically significant carotenoids include α-carotene, β-cryptoxanthin, lycopene, and leutin+zeaxanthin. Animals and humans are not capable of synthesizing carotenoids but are able to absorb them from the diet.

The basic structure of carotenoids consists of a tetraterpene skeleton, which might be cyclized at one or both ends of the molecule, and an extended system of conjugated double bonds, which confers both color and antioxidant activity to these substances (Britton and Hornero-Mendez, 1997). In general, carotenoids are efficient quenchers of singlet oxygen; this activity depends mainly on the number of conjugated double bonds present in the specific carotenoid molecule. The carotenoids differ in their biological properties, with only some having pro-vitamin A activity. Carotenoids also differ in tissue localization and in their antioxidant properties (Omenn, 1998). Several tissues such as liver, adrenals, and testes are rich in carotenoids, whereas lower amounts are detected in kidney, ovary, and brain.

7.2. *Bioavailability*

Very little is known about the specific distribution of carotenoids in natural sources. Important dietary sources of carotenoids for humans are green, orange, and red vegetables. A study by Tucker et al. (1999) identified and ranked foods that contributed to the majority of intake of each of the carotenoids. Sources of β-carotene included cantaloupe, spinach, and sweet potatoes. β-Cryptoxanthin was found in oranges and peaches. The predominant food source of lycopene was tomatoes, while green leafy vegetables provided leutin+zeaxanthin.

7.3. *Clinical studies*

An increased consumption of a carotenoid-rich diet is associated with a diminished risk for CVD. There are some supporting data from studies within populations that indicate that high levels of carotenoids in the blood (Kristenson et al., 1997; van Poppel, 1996) or adipose tissue (Kohlmeier et al., 1997; Kardinaal et al., 1993) are associated with decreased risk of CVD. On the other hand, low circulating levels of carotenoids are presumed to play a role in atherogenesis (Kontush et al., 1999).

Like many of the other dietary antioxidants, there is conflicting evidence whether diets rich in carotenoids lower risk for CVD in the elderly. To date, most clinical work has examined β-carotene, and few studies specifically examined other carotenoids in relation to cardiovascular health in the elderly. Supplements of β-carotene inhibit lipid peroxidation ex vivo. Jialal et al. (1991) and Gale et al. (2001) showed that elderly men with higher plasma concentrations of β-carotene have less arterial thickening and little or no plaque in their carotid arteries. This suggests that β-carotene is important in lowering the initiation of atherogenesis.

In general, epidemiologic studies find inverse associations between serum or adipose β-carotene levels and CVD outcomes. In contrast to the encouraging, albeit inconsistent, results from epidemiological studies of serum β-carotene, four randomized, placebo-controlled clinical trials found no evidence that supplementation prevents CVD (Table 3). In addition to these, other studies also show inconclusive results regarding the benefits of β-carotene supplementation (Table 3). For instance, two trials studying the protective effects of β-carotene against LDL oxidation could not confirm earlier studies (Princen et al., 1992; Reaven et al., 1993). β-carotene was also ineffective as an antioxidant when added to pre-formed lipid membranes (Liebler et al., 1997).

The concentrations of β-carotene in supplemented diets are much higher than those found normally. The possible toxic effects of high β-carotene are not known but could be severe. For instance, β-carotene is easily incorporated into the atherosclerotic plaque (Prince et al., 1988; Mitchell et al., 1993), and high β-carotene levels could render the plaque more susceptible to rupture. High β-carotene levels may also decrease spontaneous thrombolysis and cause electrical or mechanical instability of the myocardium. Thus, high supplemental intake of β-carotene cannot be presently recommended.

Table 3
Carotenoid intake associated with cardiovascular disease risk

Reference	Conclusions
Gey et al. (1993), Riemersma et al. (1991), Street et al. (1994)	Reduced risk of CVD
Kritchevsky et al. (1998)	Stabilization of arterial plaque
Morris et al. (1994)	Decrease in risk of CVD incidence
Physician's Health Study (Gaziano et al., 1990)	Non-significant increase in cardiovascular deaths
Hennekens et al. (1996), Greenberg et al. (1996)	No evidence of protection against CVD
Omenn et al. (1996), Leppala et al. (2000)	Increase in risk of CVD in long-term smokers
Evans et al. (1998), Sahyoun et al. (1996)	No effect on risk for CVD
The ATBC Cancer Prevention Study Group (1994)	Increase in risk of fatal CVD, non-significant decrease in non-fatal MI

7.4. *Lycopene*

Lycopene is one of the major carotenoids in the diet of Europeans and North Americans. It is an antioxidant carotenoid without pro-vitamin A activity and has been shown to be a more potent antioxidant than α- or β-carotene (DiMascio et al., 1989). Being an open-chain isomer of β-carotene, it exhibits the highest rate of singlet oxygen quenching of all carotenoids. Due to this potent scavenging capability, lycopene has been postulated as a dietary constituent to modulate CVD risk by preventing oxidative modification of LDL (Agarwal and Venkateshwer, 1998). Rissanen et al. (2000) found that in middle-aged men from Eastern Finland, a low concentration of plasma lycopene is associated with early atherosclerosis, as manifested by increased thickness of the carotid artery wall. In the European Community Multicenter Study on Antioxidants, Myocardial Infarction, and Breast Cancer (EU-RAMIC) (Kohlmeier et al., 1997), subjects who previously suffered MI had lower lycopene concentrations in adipose tissue than control subjects. These results suggest that plasma lycopene status may play a role in the early stages of atherogenesis.

Thus, the available epidemiological evidence generally supports the notion that a diet rich in carotenoids is associated with a reduced risk of heart disease. Whether this risk reduction is due to the action of one or several carotenoids or other plant-based substances is unknown.

8. Conclusion

In the last 20 years, there has been a steady rise in the mean age of patients requiring hospitalization. Age has risen in significance as a predictor of mortality for coronary bypass surgery and remains one of the most significant predictors of heart failure following medical intervention. Mortality for elderly patients after MI, post-infarction reperfusion, angioplasty, and cardiac surgery is up to three times greater than for younger patients. Thus, a need for new and alternative intervention therapies to lower progression of CVD, particularly in the elderly, has gained impetus.

Upon reviewing the compendium of literature, there appears to be an association between the use of antioxidants and a reduced risk of CVD in the elderly. However, it is currently very difficult to make definitive conclusions about specific antioxidants and their roles in preventing and/or treating CVD. This is because very few epidemiological studies have addressed these questions in the elderly. Concomitantly, clinical trials involving the general population have given ambiguous results as to antioxidant supplementation and lower morbidity and mortality from heart disease. The reason for these conflicting results may be due to differences in sample size, antioxidant supplementation regimes, study duration, tissues examined, and/or methodologies used. It may also be important to separate cohorts on the basis of lifestyle, diet, genetic predisposition, and disease states to determine which groups may be best aided by antioxidant supplementation.

For example, the results of Kushi et al. (1996) on vitamin E supplementation in post-menopausal women have been hard to extrapolate to the elderly because the population also included middle-aged women. In the case of vitamin C, supplementation proved to be beneficial only in individuals with pre-supplementation plasma levels below 50 µmol/l. Finally, studies using β-carotene have yielded highly controversial and contradictory results.

On the other hand, some antioxidants like LA, GSH, and CoQ convincingly reduce the indices of oxidative stress in animal models, but there are as yet no clinical trials to substantiate their use in humans. Thus, recommendations for the use of these antioxidants to prevent CVD in the elderly may be premature.

In contrast, it is interesting to note that intake of fruits and vegetables is inversely associated with overall morbidity and mortality from CVD. But even here, epidemiological associations pointing to an optimal dietary intake of one type of food or another cannot be presently surmised. For example, fruits and juices high in AA are not associated with changes in mortality, while vegetables are inversely associated with mortality risk (Sahyoun et al., 1996). Thus, independent of their AA concentrations, fruits and vegetables seem to provide added protection against CVD mortality. Similar results have also been shown for fruits and vegetables rich in VE and carotenoids. These results lead to the suggestion that diets rich in many types of antioxidants and chemoprotectants may be more beneficial than any given antioxidant supplement. This suggests that fruits and vegetables may contain other beneficial compounds that also afford protection from CVD other than the antioxidants discussed in this chapter.

Credence to this theory was first lent by Albaugh (1953), who demonstrated that heart disease was responsible for almost three times as many deaths in the US compared to the Greek island of Crete. The people of Crete consume a diet containing large amounts of green leafy vegetables, wild plants, herbs, tomatoes, onions, garlic, fruits, nuts, legumes, wine, and olive oil. What appears to be so special about the Greek diet is the content of bioprotective nutrients, specifically:

(a)   a more balanced intake of essential fatty acids from vegetable, animal, and marine sources;
(b)   a 2:1 ratio of $(n-6)$ to $(n-3)$ fatty acids;
(c)   an abundance of antioxidants, for example: AA, VE, β-carotene, GSH, resveratrol, selenium, folate, phytoestrogens, and other phytochemicals.

The Seven Countries Study that established credible data on CVD prevalence rates in contrasting populations also showed significant differences in CVD incidence (Keys, 1970). There was an overall variance of coronary heart disease of five- to 10-fold, with countries having the highest intake of fruits and vegetables also exhibiting the lowest levels of disease (Keys, 1970). Thus, it must be concluded that diets rich in fruits and vegetables, as compared to supplements alone, appear to correlate better with a decrease in CVD in individuals, including the elderly.

References

Aberg, F., Zhang, Y., Teclebrhan, H., Appelkvist, E.L., Dallner, G., 1996. Chem. Biol. Interact. 99, 205–218.

Abete, P.A.P., Cioppa, A., Calabresa, C., Pascucci, I., Cacciatore, F., Napoli, C., Carnovale, V., Ferrara, N., Rengo, F., 1999. Exp. Gerontol. 34, 875–884.

Agarwal, S., Venkateshwer, R., 1998. Lipids 33, 981–984.

Albaugh, L.G., 1953. Crete: A Case Study of an Underdeveloped Area. Princeton University Press, Princeton, NJ.

Ali, K., Morimoto, M., Fukaya, Y., Furukawa, Y., 1993. Ann. Thorac. Surg. 55, 902–907.

Ambrosio, G., Zweier, J.L., Flaherty, J.T., 1991. J. Mol. Cell. Cardiol. 23, 1359–1374.

American Heart Association (AHA), 2001. Heart and Stroke Statistical Update. www.americanheart.org/statistics/cvd.html.

Ataka, K., Chen, D., Levitsky, S., Jimenez, E., Feinberg, H., 1992. Circulation 86, 1371–1376.

Atar, D., Mortensen, S.A., Flachs, H., Herzog, W.R., 1993. Clin. Invest. 71, S103–S111.

ATBC Cancer Prevention Study Group, The, 1994. N Engl. J. Med. 330, 1029–1035.

Azen, H.P., Mack, W.J., Cashin-Hemphill, L., LaBree, L., Shircore, A.M., Selzer, R.H., Blankenhorn, D.H., Hodis, H.N., 1996. Circulation 93, 34–41.

Azhar, G., Gao, W., Liu, L.Y.W.J., 1999. Exp. Gerontol. 699–714.

Barton, M., Consentino, F., Brandes, R.P., Moreau, P., Shaw, S., Luscher, T.F., 1997. Hypertension 15, 170–179.

Basta, G., Lazzerini, G., Massaro, M., Simoncini, T., Tanganelli, P., Fu, C., Kislinger, T., Stern, D.M., Schmidt, A.M., De Caterina, R., 2002. Circulation 105, 816–822.

Baynes, J.W., Thorpe, S.R., 1999. Diabetes 48, 1–9.

Beckman, K.B., Ames, B.N., 1997. J. Biol. Chem. 272, 19633–19636.

Birlouez-Aragon, I., Delcourt, C., Tessier, F., Papoz, L., POLA Study Group, 2001. Int. J. Vitam. Nutr. Res. 71, 53–59.

Boaz, M., Smetana, S., Weinstein, T., Matas, Z., Gafter, U., Iaina, A., Knecht, A., Weissgarten, Y., Brunner, D., Fainaru, M., et al., 2000. Lancet 356, 1213–1218.

Britton, G. and Hornero-Mendez, D., 1997. Phytochemistry of Fruits and Vegetables, ed. by Tomás-Barberán, F.A. and Robins, R.J. Oxford. Oxford University Press.

Brown, J.M., Terada, L.S., Grosso, M.A., Whitmann, G.J., Velasco, S.E., Patt, A., Harken, A.H., Repine, J.E., 1988. J. Clin. Invest. 81, 297–301.

Brown-Borg, H.M., Rakoczy, S.G., Romanick, M.A., Kennedy, M.A., 2002. Exp. Biol. Med. 227, 94–104.

Brubacher, D., Moser, U., Jordan, P., 2000. Int. J. Vitam. Nutr. Res. 70, 226–237.

Buettner, G.R., 1993. Arch. Biochem. Biophys. 300, 535–543.

Bunyan, J., McHale, D., Green, J., Marcinkiewicz, S., 1961. Br. J. Nutr. 15, 253–257.

Burr, M.L., Elwood, P.C., Hole, D.J., Hurley, R.J., Hughes, R.E., 1974. Am. J. Clin. Nutr. 27, 144–151.

Bustamante, J., Lodge, J.K., Marcocci, L., Tritschler, H.J., Packer, L., Rihn, B.H., 1998. Free Radic. Biol. Med. 24, 1023–1039.

Cabassi, A., Dumont, E.C., Girouard, H., Bouchard, J.F., Le Jossec, M., Lamontagne, D., Besner, J.G., de Champlain, J., 2001. J. Hypertens. 19, 233–244.

Cain, A.E., Khalil, R.A., 2002. Semin. Nephrol. 22, 3–16.

Carr, A.C., Frei, B., 1999. Am. J. Clin. Nutr. 69, 1086–1107.

Carré, F., Rannou, F., et al., 1993. Cardiovasc. Res. 27, 1784–1789.

Carrera-Rotlan, J., Estrada-Garcia, L., 1998. Mech. Ageing Dev. 103, 13–26.

Celermajer, D.S., Sorenson, K.E., Spiegelhalter, D.J., et al., 1994. J. Am. Coll. Cardiol. 24, 471–476.

Cherubini, A., Zuliani, G., Constantini, F., Pierdomenico, S.D., Volpato, S., Mezzetti, A., Mecocci, P., Pezzuto, M., Bregnocchi, M., Fellin, R., Senin, U., The VASA Study Group, 2001. J. Am. Geriatr. Soc. 49, 651–654.

Cheung, P.Y., Wang, W., Schulz, R., 2000. J. Mol. Cell. Cardiol. 32, 1669–1678.

Colucci, W.S., 1997. Am. J. Cardiol. 80, 15L–25L.

Coombes, J.S., Powers, S.K., Hamilton, K.L., Demirel, H.A., Shanely, R.A., Zergeroglu, M.A., Sen, C.K., Packer, L., Ji, L.L., 2000. Am. J. Physiol. Regulat. Integr. Comp. Physiol. 279, R2149–R2155.

Davies, M.B., Austin, J., Partridge, D.A., 1991. The Royal Society of Chemistry, Cambridge.

Davini, A., Cellerini, F., Topi, P.L., 1992. Minerva Cardioangiol. 40, 449–453.

DeFronzo, R.A., Ferrannini, E., 1991. Diabetes Care. 14, 173–194.

DeFronzo, R.A., Bonadonna, R.C., Ferrannini, E., 1992. Diabetes Care. 15, 318–368.

DeMaio, S.J., King III, S.B., Lembo, N.J., Roubin, G.S., Hearn, J.A., Bhagavan, H.N., Sgoutas, D.S., 1992. J. Am. Coll. Nutr. 11, 68–73.

Devaraj, S., Adams-Huet, B., Fuller, C.J., Jialal, I., 1997. Arterioscler. Thromb. Vasc. Biol. 17, 2273–2279.

DiMascio, P., Kaiser, S., Sies, H., 1989. Arch. Biochem. Biophys. 274, 532–538.

Docherty, J.R., 1990. Pharmacol. Rev. 42, 103–125.

Dohi, Y., Thiel, M.A., Buhler, F.R., Luscher, T.F., 1990. Hypertension 15, 170–179.

DRI: Dietary Reference Intakes for Vitamin C, Vitamin E, Selenium, and Carotenoids. Food and Nutrition Board and Institute of Medicine, 2000. National Academy Press, Washington, D.C.

Egashira, K., Inoue, T., Hirooka, Y., Kai, H., Sugimachi, M., Suzuki, S., Kuga, T., Urabe, Y., Takeshita, A., 1993. Circulation 88, 77–81.

Enstrom, J.E., 1993. Nutr. Today 28, 28–32.

Enstrom, J.E., Kanim, L.E., Breslow, L., 1986. Am. J. Public Health 76, 1124–1130.

Enstrom, J.E., Kanim, L.E., Klein, M.A., 1992. Epidemiology 3, 194–202.

Ernster, L., Forsmark-Andree, P., 1993. Clin. Invest. 71, S60–S65.

Evans, R.W., Shaten, B.J., Day, B.W., Kuller, L.H., 1998. Am. J. Epidemiol. 147, 180–186.

Fannin, S.W., Lesnefsky, E.J., Slabe, T.J., Hassan, M.O., Hoppel, C.L., 1999. Arch. Biochem. Biophys. 372, 399–407.

Fehily, A.M., Yarnell, J.W.G., Sweetnam, P.M., Elwood, P.C., 1993. Br. J. Nutr. 69, 303–314.

Ferrara, N., Abete, P., Ambrosio, G., Landino, P., Caccese, P., Cirillo, P., Oradei, A., Littarru, G.P., Chiariello, M., Rengo, F., 1995. J. Pharmacol. Exp. Ther. 274, 858–865.

Fotherby, M.D., Williams, J.C., Forster, L.A., Craner, P., Ferns, G.A., 2000. J. Hypertens. 18, 411–415.

Frei, B., Stocker, R., Ames, B.N., 1988. Proc. Natl. Acad. Sci. U. S. A. 85, 9748–9752.

Frei, B., England, L., Ames, B.N., 1989. Proc. Natl. Acad. Sci. U. S. A. 86, 6377–6381.

Gale, C.R., Martyn, C.N., Winter, P.D., Cooper, C., 1995. Br. Med. J. 310, 1563–1566.

Gale, C.R., Ashurst, H.E., Powers, H.J., Martyn, C.N., 2001. Am. J. Clin. Nutr. 74, 402–408.

Garry, P.J., Goodwin, J.S., Hunt, W.C., Gilbert, B.A., 1982. Am. J. Clin. Nutr. 36, 332–339.

Gaziano, J.M., Manson, J.E., Ridker, P.M., Buring, J.E., Hennekens, C.H., 1990. Circulation 82, 201.

Genova, M.L., Bonacorsi, E., D'Aurelio, M., Formiggini, G., Nardo, B., Cuccomarino, S., Turi, P., Pich, M.M., Lenaz, G., Bovina, C., 1999. Biofactors 9, 345–349.

Genova, M.L., Ventura, B., Giuliano, G., Bovina, C., Formiggini, G., Parenti-Castelli, G., Lenaz, G., 2001. FEBS Lett. 505, 364–368.

Gey, K.F., Stahelin, H.B., Eichholzer, M., 1993. Clin. Invest. 71, 3–6.

GISSI-Prevenzione Trial, 1999. Lancet 354, 447–455.

Gokce, N., Keaney Jr., J.F., Frei, B., Holbrook, M., Olesiak, M., Zachariah, B.J., Leeuwenburgh, C., Heinecke, J.W., Vita, J.A., 1999. Circulation 99, 3234–3240.

Greenberg, R.E., Baron, J.A., Karagas, M.R., Stukel, T.A., Nierenberg, D.W., Stevens, M.M., Mandel, J.S., Haile, R.W., 1996. J. Am. Med. Assoc. 275, 699–703.

Hagen, T.M., Bai, C., Jones, D.P., 1991. FASEB J. 5, 2721–2727.

Hagen, T.M., Ingersoll, R.T., Wehr, C.M., Lykkesfeldt, J., Vinarsky, V., Bartholomew, J.C., Song, M., Ames, B.N., 1998. Proc. Natl. Acad. Sci. U. S. A. 95, 9562–9566.

Hagen, T.M., Ingersoll, R.T., Lykkesfeldt, J., Liu, J., Wehr, C.M., Vinarsky, V., Bartholomew, J.C., Ames, B.N., 1999. FASEB J. 13, 411–418.

Hagen, T.M., Vinarsky, V., Wehr, C.M., Ames, B.N., 2000. Antiox. Redox Signal. 2, 473–483.

Hanninen, Kaartinen, K., Rauma, A.L., Nenonen, M., Torronen, R., Hakkinen, A.S., Adlercreutz, H., Laakso, J., 2000. Toxicology 155, 45–53.

Hansford, R.G., Hogue, B.A., Mildaziene, V., 1997. J. Bioener. Biomem. 29, 89–95.

Harman, D., 1956. J. Gerontol. 11, 298–300.

Harrill, I., Cervone, N., 1977. Am. J. Clin. Nutr. 30, 431–440.

Heart Outcomes Prevention Evaluation (HOPE) Study Investigators, The, 1996. Can. J. Cardiol. 12, 137–147.

Heart Outcomes Prevention Evaluation (HOPE) Study Investigators, The, 2000. N. Engl. J. Med. 342, 154–160.

Hennekens, C.H., Buring, J.E., Manson, J.E., et al., 1996. N. Engl. J. Med. 334, 1145–1149.

Hense, H.W., Stender, M., Bors, W., Keil, U., 1993. Atherosclerosis 103, 21–28.

Hercberg, S., Preziosi, P., Galan, P., Devanlay, M., Keller, H., Bourgeois, C., Potier de Courcy, G., Heseker, H., Schneider, R., 1994. Eur. J. Clin. Nutr. 48, 118–127.

Hodis, H.N., Mack, W.J., LaBree, L., Cashin-Hemphill, L., Sevanian, A., Johnson, R., Azen, S.P., 1995. J. Am. Med. Assoc. 273, 1849–1854.

Hothersall, J.S., El-Hassan, A., McLean, P., Greenbaum, A.L., 1981. Enzyme 26, 271–276.

Humphries, K.M., Szweda, L.I., 1998. Biochemistry 37, 15835–15841.

Humphries, K.M., Yoo, Y., Sweda, L.I., 1998. Biochemistry 37, 552–557.

Hynes, M.R., Duckles, S.P., 1987. J. Pharmacol. Exp. Ther. 241, 387–392.

Iuliano, L., Micheletta, F., Maranghi, M., Frathi, G., Diczfalusy, V., Violi, F., 2001. Arterioscler. Thromb. Vasc. Biol. 21, E34–E37.

Jacob, R.A., Otradovec, C.L., Russel, R.M., Munro, H.N., Hartz, S.C., McGandy, R.B., Morrow, F.D., Sadowski, J.A., 1988. Am. J. Clin. Nutr. 48, 1436–1442.

Jacob, S., Henriksen, E.J., Tritschler, H.J., Augustin, H.J., Dietze, G.J., 1996. Endocrinol. Diabetes 104, 284–288.

Jaeschke, H., Wendel, A., 1985. Biochem. Pharmacol. 34, 1029–1033.

James, T.N., 1998. Ann. Rev. Physiol. 60, 309–325.

Jialal, I., Norkus, E.P., Cristol, L., Grundy, S.M., 1991. Biochim. Biophys. Acta 1086, 134–138.

Jialal, I., Fuller, C.J., Huet, B.A., 1995. Arterioscler. Thromb. Vasc. Biol. 15, 190–198.

Jocelyn, P.C., 1972. Biochemistry of the SH Group. Academic Press, London.

Jonas, C.R., Estivariz, C.F., Jones, D.P., Gu, L.H., Wallace, T.M., Diaz, E.E., Pascal, R.R., Ziegler, T.R., 1999. J. Nutr. 127, 1278–1284.

Kardinaal, A.F.M., Kok, F.J., Ringstad, J., Gomez-Aracena, J., Mazaev, V.P., Kohlmeier, L., Martin, B.C., Aro, A., Kark, J.D., Delgado-Rodriguez, M., et al., 1993. Lancet 342, 1379–1384.

Katz, A.M., 1988. Am. J. Cardiol. 62, 3A–8A.

Keys, A., 1970. Circulation 41, 1–211.

Khalil, A., Wagner, J.R., Lacombe, G., Dangoisse, V., Fulop Jr., T., 1996. FEBS Lett. 392, 45–48.

Khalil, A., Fortin, J., LeHoux, J., Fulop, T., 2000. J. Lipid Res. 41, 1552–1561.

Kitani, K., Minami, C., Yamamoto, T., Maruyama, W., Kanai, S., Ivy, G.O., Carrillo, M.C., 2001. Ann. N. Y. Acad. Sci. 928, 248–260.

Knekt, P., Reunanen, A., Jarvinen, R., Seppanen, R., Heliovaara, M., Aromaa, A., 1994. Am. J. Epidemiol. 139, 1180–1189.

Koga, T., Takata, Y., Kobayashi, K., Takishita, S., Yamashita, Y., Fujishima, M., 1989. Hypertension 14, 542–548.

Kohlmeier, L., Kark, J.D., Gomez-Gracia, E., Martin, B.C., Steck, S.E., Kardinaal, A.F.M., Ringstad, J., Thamm, M., Masaev, V., Riemersma, R., et al., 1997. Am. J. Epidemiol. 146, 618–626.

Kok, F.J., de Bruijn, A.M., Vermeeren, R., et al., 1987. Am. J. Clin. Nutr. 45, 462–468.

Kontush, A., Spranger, T., Reich, A., Baum, K., Beisiegel, V., 1999. Atherosclerosis 144, 117–122.

Kristenson, M., Zieden, B., Kucinskiene, Z., Elinder, L.S., Bergdahl, B., Elwing, B., Abaravicius, A., Razinkoviene, L., Calkauskas, H., Olsson, A.G., 1997. Br. Med. J. 314, 629–633.

Kritchevsky, S.B., Shimakawa, T., Tell, G.S., Dennis, B., Carpenter, M., Eckfeldt, J.H., Peacher-Ryan, H., Heiss, G., 1995. Circulation 92, 2132–2150.

Kritchevsky, S.B., Tell, G.S., Shimakawa, T., Dennis, B., Li, R., Kohlmeier, L., Steere, E., Heiss, G., 1998. Am. J. Clin. Nutr. 68, 726–733.

Kung, C.F., Luscher, T.F., 1995. Hypertension 25, 194–200.

Kushi, L.H., Folsom, A.R., Prineas, R.J., Mink, P.J., Wu, Y., Bostick, R.M., 1996. N. Engl. J. Med. 334, 1156–1162.

Lakatta, E.G., Sollott, S.J., Pepe, S., 2001. Novartis Found. Symp. 235, 172–196; discussion 196–201, 217–220.

Landi, L., Cabrini, L., Fiorentini, D., Stefanelli, C., Pedulli, G.F., 1992. Chem. Phys. Lipids 61, 121–130.

Langsjoen, P.H., Langsjoen, P.H., Folkers, K., 1993. Clin. Invest. 71, S140–S144.

Leppala, J.M., Virtamo, J., Fogelholm, R., et al., 2000. Arterioscler. Thromb. Vasc. Biol. 20, 230–235.

Lesnefsky, E.J., Gallo, D.S., Ye, J., Whittingham, T.S., Lust, W.D., 1994. J. Lab. Clin. Med. 124, 843–851.

Lesnefsky, E.J., Gudz, T.I., Moghaddas, S., et al., 2001. J. Mol. Cell. Cardiol. 33, 37–47.

Leukjewicz, J.E., Davies, M.J., et al., 1972. Cardiovasc. Res. 11, 463–470.

Li, D., Saldeen, T., Romeo, F., Mehta, J.L., 2001. J. Cardiovasc. Pharmacol. Ther. 6, 155–161.

Liebler, D.C., Stratton, S.P., Kaysen, K.L., 1997. Arch. Biochem. Biophys. 338, 244–250.

Liu, R., Choi, J., 2000. Free Radic. Biol. Med. 28, 566–574.

Lodge, J.K., Packer, L., 1999. In: Antioxidant Food Supplements in Human Health. Academic Press, New York, pp. 121–134.

Losonczy, K.G., Harris, T.B., Havlik, R.J., 1996. Am. J. Clin. Nutr. 64, 190–196.

Lucas, D.T., Szweda, L., 1998. Proc. Natl. Acad. Sci. U. S. A. 95, 510–514.

Manson, J.E., Stampfer, M.J., Willett, W.C., Colditz, G.A., Speizer, F.E., Hennekens, C.H., 1992. Circulation 85, 865 (abstract).

Manson, J.E., Stampfer, M.J., Willett, W.C., Colditz, G.A., Speizer, F.E., Hennekens, C.H., 1993. Circulation 87, 678 (abstract).

Marangon, K., Herveth, B., Lecomte, E., Paul-Dauhin, A., Grolier, P., Chancerelle, Y., Arture, Y., Siest, G., 1998. Am. J. Clin. Nutr. 67, 231–239.

Marazzi, M.C., Mancinelli, S., Palombi, L., Martinoli, L., D'Alessandro de Luca, E., Buonomo, E., Riccardi, F., 1990. Int. J. Vitam. Nutr. Res. 60, 351–359.

Matsushima, T., Sueda, T., Matsuura, Y., Kawasaki, T., 1992. J. Thorac. Cardiovasc. Surg. 103, 945–951.

Maulik, N., Yoshida, T., Engelman, R.M., Bagchi, D., Otani, H., Das, D.K., 2000. Am. J. Physiol. Heart Circ. Physiol. 278, H1084–H1090.

Menasche, P., Grousset, C., Gauduel, Y., Mouas, C., Piwnica, A., 1992. J. Thorac. Cardiovasc. Surg. 103, 936–944.

Mezzetti, A., Lapenna, D., Romano, F., et al., 1996. J. Am. Geriatr. Soc. 44, 823–827.

Michels, et al., submitted.

Mitchell, D.C., Prince, M.R., Frisoli, J.K., Smith, R.E., Wood, R.F.M., 1993. Lasers Surg. Med. 13, 149–157.

Mitchinson, M.J., Stephens, N.G., Parsons, A., 1999. Lancet 353, 381.

Monget, A.L., Galan, P., Preziosi, P., Keller, H., Bourgeois, C., Arnaud, J., Favier, A., Hercberg, S., 1996. Int. J. Vitam. Nutr. Res. 66, 71–76.

Morris, D.L., Kritchevsky, S.B., Davis, C.E., 1994. J. Am. Med. Assoc. 272, 1439–1441.

Mortensen, S.A., 1993. Clin. Invest. 71, S116–S123.

Murray, C.J.L., Lopez, A.D., 1997. Lancet 349, 1436–1442.

Nakagawa, Y., Cotgreave, I.A., Moldeus, P., 1991. Biochem. Pharmacol. 42, 883–888.

National Research Council Committee on Diet and Health (DRI), 1989. Food and Nutrition Board, Commission on Life Sciences, National Research Council.

Ness, A., Davey-Smith, G., 1999. Lancet 353, 1017–1018.

Nohl, H., Hegner, D., Summer, K.H., 1979. Mech. Ageing Dev. 11, 145–151.

Nohl, H., Gille, L., Kozlou, A.V., 1999. Biofactors 9, 155–161.

Omenn, G.S., 1998. Annu. Rev. Public Health 19, 73–99.

Omenn, G.S., Goodman, G.E., Thornquist, M.D., et al., 1996. N. Eng. J. Med. 334, 1150–1155.

Oreopoulos, D.G., Lindeman, R.D., VanderJagt, D.J., Tzamaloukas, A.H., Bhagavan, H.N., Garry, P.J., 1993. J Am. Coll. Nutr. 12, 537–542.

Packer, L., Witt, E., Tritschler, H.J., 1995. Free Radic. Biol. Med. 19, 227–250.

Pandey, D.K., Shekelle, R., Selwyn, B.J., Tangney, C., Stamler, J., 1995. Am. J. Epidemiol. 142, 1269–1278.

Park, Y., Kenekal, S., Kehrer, J.P., 1991. Am. J. Physiol. Heart Circ. Physiol. 260, H1395–H1405.

Pedersen, H.S., Martenson, S.A., Rogde, M., Deguchi, Y., Mulvad, G., Bjerregaavid, P., Harsen, J.C., 1999. Biofactors 9, 319–323.

Permanetter, B., Rossy, W., Klein, G., Weingartner, F., Seidl, K.F., Blomer, H., 1992. Eur. Heart J. 13, 1528–1533.

Porrini, M., Simonetti, P., Ciappellano, S., Testolin, G., 1987. Int. J. Vitam. Nutr. Res. 57, 349–355.

Prince, M.R., LaMuraglia, G.M., MacNichol Jr., E.F., 1988. Circulation 78, 338–344.

Princen, H.M., van Poppel, G., Vogelezang, C., Buytenhek, R., Kok, F.J., 1992. Arterioscler. Thromb. Vasc. Biol. 12, 554–562.

Pruthi, S., Allison, T.G., Hensrud, D.D., 2001. Mayo Clin. Proc. 76, 1131–1136.

Ramires, P.R., Ji, L.L., 2001. Am. J. Physiol. Heart Circ. Physiol. 281, H679–H688.

Reaven, P.D., Khouw, A., Beltz, W.F., Parthasarathy, S., Wiztum, J.L., 1993. Arterioscler. Thromb. Vasc. Biol. 13, 590–600.

Riemersma, R.A., Wood, D.A., Macintyre, C.C., Elton, R.A., Gey, K.F., Oliver, M.F., 1991. Lancet 337, 1–5.

Riemersma, R.A., Carruthers, K.F., Elton, R.A., Fox, K.A.A., 2000. Am. J. Clin. Nutr. 71, 1181–1186.

Rimm, E.B., Stampfer, M.J., Ascherio, A., Giovannuci, E., Colditz, G.A., Willett, W.C., 1993. N. Engl. J. Med. 328, 1450–1456.

Rissanen, T., Voutilainen, S., Nyyssonen, K., Salonen, R., Salonen, J.T., 2000. Arterioscler. Thromb. Vasc. Biol. 20, 2677–2681.

Riviere, S., Birlouez-Aragon, I., Narousehmi, S., Velas, B., 1998a. Int. J. Geriat. Psych. 13, 749–754.

Riviere, S., Birlouez-Aragon, I., Vellas, B., 1998b. Glycoconj. J. 5, 1039–1042.

Roine, P., Koivula, L., Pekkarinen, M., Rissanen, A., 1974. Int. J. Vitam. Nutr. Res. 44, 95–106.

Rowland, M.A., Nagley, P., Linnane, A.W., Rosenfeldt, F.L., 1998. Cardiovasc. Res. 40, 165–173.

Ruhe, R.C., McDonald, R.B., 2001. J. Am. Coll. Nutr. 20, 363S–369S; discussion 381S–383S.

Saches, H.L., Saches, M.L., Landau, S.W., Keasten, R., Dooley, F., Sacher, A., Sacher, M., Dietrick, K., Ichkhan, K., 1997. Am. J. Ther. 4, 66–72.

Sahyoun, N.R., Jacques, P.F., Russell, R.M., 1996. Am. J. Epidemiol. 144, 501–511.

Salonen, J.T., Salonen, R., Penttila, I., et al., 1985. Am. J. Cardiol. 56, 226–231.

Sasaki, R., Kurokawa, T., Kobayasi, T., Tero-Kubota, S., 1983. Tohoku J. Exp. Med. 140, 97–104.

Sharov, V.G., Sabbah, H.N., et al., 1997. Int. J. Cardiol. 60, 273–279.

Simons, L.A., von Konigsmark, M., Simons, J., Stocker, R., Celermajer, D.S., 1999. Atherosclerosis 143, 193–199.

Sohal, R.S., Dubey, A., 1994. Free Radic. Biol. Med. 16, 621–626.

Sohal, R.S., Ku, H.H., Agarwal, S., Forster, M.J., Lal, H., 1994. Mech. Ageing Dev. 74, 121–133.

Stampfer, M.J., Hennekens, C.H., Manson, J.E., Colditz, G.A., Rosner, B., Willett, W.C., 1993. N. Engl. J. Med. 328, 1444–1449.

Steinberg, D., Parthasarathy, S., Carew, T.E., Khoo, J.C., Witztum, J.L., 1989. N. Engl. J. Med. 320, 915–924.

Stephens, N.G., Parsons, A., Schofield, P.M., et al., 1996. Lancet 347, 781–786.

Street, D.A., Comstock, G.W., Salkeld, R.M., Schuep, W., Klag, M.J., 1994. Circulation 90, 1154–1161.

Suh, J.H., Shigeno, E.T., Morrow, J.D., Cox, B., Rocha, A.E., Frei, B., Hagen, T.M., 2001. FASEB J. 15, 700–706.

Svanborg, A., 1997. Drugs Aging 10, 463–472.

Szent-Györgyi, A., 1933. Nature 131, 225–226.

Tani, M., Suganuma, Y., Hasegawa, H., Shinmura, K., Ebihara, Y., Hayashi, Y., Guo, X., Takayama, M., 1997. J. Mol. Cell. Cardiol. 29, 3081–3089.

Traber, M.G., 1999. Biofactors 10, 115–120.

Tschudi, M.R., Barton, M., Bersinger, N.A., Moreau, P., Consentino, F., Noll, G., Malinski, T., Luscher, T.F., 1996. J. Clin. Invest. 98, 899–905.

Tucker, K.L. Chen, H., Vogel, S., Wilson, P.W., Schaefer, E.J., Lammi-Keefe, C.J., 1999. J. Nutr. 129, 438–445.

Uchida, K., Szweda, L.I., Chae, H.-Z., Stadman, E.R., 1993. Proc. Natl. Acad. Sci. U. S. A. 90, 8742–8746.

Upston, J.M., Terentis, A.C., Stocker, R., 1999. FASEB J. 13, 977–994.

Urakami-Harasawa, L., Shimokawa, H., Nakashima, M., Egashira, K., Takeshita, A., 1997. J. Clin. Invest. 100, 2793–2799.

van Dam, P.S., van Asbeck, B.S., Erkelens, D.W., Marx, J.J.M., Gispen, W.H., Bravenboer, B., 1995. Diabetes Metab. Rev. 11, 181–192.

VanderJagt, D.V., Garry, P.J., Bhagavan, H.N., 1987. Am. J. Clin. Nutr. 46, 290.

Van Poppel, G., 1996. Eur. J. Clin. Nutr. 50, S57–S61.

Vir, S.C., Love, A.H.G., 1979. Am. J. Clin. Nutr. 32, 1934–1947.

Weinbroum, A.A., Kidron, A., Hochhauser, E., Hochman, A., Rudick, V., Vidne, B.A., 2001. Med. Sci. Monit. 7, 1137–1144.

Will, J.C., Byers, T., 1996. Nutr. Rev. 54, 193–202.

Wilson, T.S., Weeks, M.M., Mukherjee, S.K., Murrell, J.S., Andrews, C.T., 1972. Gerontol. Clin.14, 17–24.

Wilson, T.S., Datta, S.B., Murrell, J.S., Andrews, C.T., 1973. Age Ageing 2, 163–171.

Yang, C.M., Kodaswamy, V., et al., 1997. Cardiovasc. Res. 36, 236–245.

Yokoyama, K., Nakamura, K., Nakamura, K., Kimura, M., Nomoto, K., Itoman, M., 1999. Scand. J. Plast. Reconstr. Surg. Hand. Surg. 33, 1–5.

Yokoyama, T., Date, C., Kokubo, Y., Yoshiike, N., Matsumura, Y., Tanaka, H., 2000. Stroke 31, 2287–2294.

Zhang, W., Frei, B., 2001. FASEB J. 15, 2423–2432.

Advances in
Cell Aging and
Gerontology

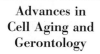

Extension of cardiovascular and cerebrovascular healthspan by dietary restriction: molecular mechanisms

Mark P. Mattson* and Ruiqian Wan

*Laboratory of Neurosciences, National Institute on Aging, Gerontology Research Center,
5600 Nathan Shock Drive, Baltimore, MD 21224, USA*

Contents

Abbreviations

DR	dietary restriction
DHEA	dehydroepiandrosterone sulfate
BMI	body-mass index
BP	blood pressure
HR	heart rate
HDL	high density lipoprotein
LDL	low density lipoprotein
IL-6	interleukin-6
TNF	tumor necrosis factor
BDNF	brain-derived neurotrophic factor

---

* Corresponding author. Tel.: +1-410-558-8463; fax: +1-410-558-8465.
E-mail address: mattsonm@grc.nia.nih.gov (M.P. Mattson).

Advances in Cell Aging and Gerontology, vol. 11, 377–393

Mito-KATP   mitochondrial-derived ATP-sensitive potassium channels
NT-3   neurotrophin-3

1. Introduction: dietary restriction, lifespan and age-related disease

Both the mean and maximum lifespan of many different organisms including yeast, roundworms, rodents and monkeys can be increased by up to 50% simply by reducing their calorie intake (Goodrick et al., 1983; Maeda et al., 1985; Weindruch and Sohal, 1997; Lane et al., 1999; Roth et al., 2001a). Dietary restriction (DR: reduced calorie intake or periodic fasting with maintenance of micronutrients) decreases the incidence of several major age-related diseases including cancers, cardiovascular disease and deficits in immune function in rodents (Weindruch and Sohal, 1997). The disease-reducing and lifespan-extending effects of DR have been observed in every strain of mouse and rat studied, with some variability in the magnitude of the effects among species and strains. DR suppresses many different age-related biochemical and molecular changes in tissues throughout the body including increases in oxidative modification of proteins and DNA, decreases in melatonin and dehydroepiandrosterone sulfate (DHEA), and increases in plasma cholesterol and triglyceride levels (Lane et al., 1997; Roth et al., 2001a,b) (Table 1). One long-standing theory of the mechanism whereby DR increases lifespan and reduces disease is that DR reduces oxyradical production, the majority of which occurs in mitochondria during oxidative phosphorylation, a process in which ATP is produced from glucose (Sohal and Weindruch, 1996). When more calories are consumed, more free radicals are produced and there is more damage to proteins, lipids and nucleic acids in cells. The oxidative damage to cells can impair the function of the cells or can promote cell transformation and cancer. DR suppresses

Table 1

Effects of dietary restriction on physiological parameters relevant to cardiovascular and cerebrovascular aging and disease

Parameter	Effect of DR	References
Blood pressure	Decrease	Taffet et al. (1997), Wan et al. (2002)
Heart rate	Decrease	Nakano et al. (2001), Wan et al. (2002)
Body temperature	Decrease	Lane et al. (1996)
Plasma glucose	Decrease	Weindruch and Sohal (1997)
Plasma insulin	Decrease	Weindruch and Sohal (1997)
Plasma LDL	Decrease	Edwards et al. (1998, 2001)
Plasma HDL	Increase	Verdery et al. (1997)
Plasma triglycerides	Decrease	Roth et al. (2001)
Plasma homocysteine	Decrease	Fig. 4
Plasma melatonin	Increase	Roth et al. (2001b)
Plasma DHEA	Increase	Lane et al. (1997)

oxidative stress and enhances function of the nervous, immune and cardiovascular systems (Duffy et al., 1997).

Data from clinical and epidemiological studies in humans support the striking beneficial effects of DR. Humans with low calorie diets have a decreased risk for many age-related diseases including cardiovascular disease, diabetes and cancers (Lebovitz, 1999; Levi, 1999; Brochu et al., 2000). Recent studies also suggest that low calorie diets can reduce the risk of Parkinson's and Alzheimer's diseases (Logroscino et al., 1996; Mayeux et al., 1999). As in rodents and monkeys, DR improves bio-markers of aging in humans. The most comprehensive data available in humans come from the Biosphere 2 project in which eight people were sealed inside a closed ecological space for 2 yr during which time they consumed a very low calorie, but nutrient rich diet. The participants exhibited marked decreases in blood pressure, blood insulin, glucose and cholesterol levels, and decreased oxidative modification of plasma proteins (Walford et al., 1995).

2. Overeating and obesity: the antithesis of dietary restriction

In industrialized countries in the Western hemisphere overeating and associated obesity is now considered the single most common cause of morbidity and mortality (Aronne, 2001; Visscher and Seidell, 2001). Obesity has an even greater impact on morbidity than on mortality and its monetary impact on society is therefore tremendous. Disability due to obesity-related cardiovascular disease and type 2 diabetes is particularly striking in industrialized countries where patients often survive because of medical interventions. A rapid increase in childhood obesity is particularly worrisome; in the United States childhood obesity has doubled during the past two decades, and it is estimated that 22 million children under the age of 5 are obese worldwide (Deckelbaum and Williams, 2001). Obesity greatly increases the risk of type 2 diabetes, many different types of cancers, and kidney and liver diseases. Overeating has particularly deleterious effects on the cardiovascular and cere-brovascular systems, greatly increasing the risk of hypertension and obstructive coronary artery and cerebrovascular disease (Bronner et al., 1995). Overeating may promote cardiovascular disease by increasing levels of plasma cholesterol, trigly-cerides and glucose (Hecker et al., 1999). These alterations in energy and lipid metabolism result in increased cellular oxidative stress and increased damaging modifications to proteins (e.g., glycation and covalent modification by products of lipid peroxidation such as 4-hydroxynonenal) in cells throughout the body with particularly striking effects on vascular endothelial cells (Ren and Shen, 2000) and postmitotic electrically excitable cells including neurons (Markesbery, 1997) and cardiac myocytes (Horwitz et al., 1996; Ren et al., 1997). The definition of obesity has been quite arbitrary and usually involves determining the individual's body/mass index (BMI), with a BMI of 25 being typically considered as the upper limit of the "normal" range (Seidell and Flegal, 1997). However, two different individuals with the same BMI can differ greatly in their body composition with regard to fat and muscle mass. The individual with a higher level of body fat is at greater risk of cardiovascular disease.

While DR is an obvious and effective treatment for obesity, it is less well recognized that DR can also have striking health benefits for individuals that are not obese. The beneficial effects of DR in non-obese individuals are documented in studies of the effects of long-term DR in rats and mice in which progressive reductions in calorie intake result in progressive extension of lifespan and progressive decreases in tumor incidence (Weindruch and Sohal, 1997). The remainder of this article focuses on the cellular and molecular mechanisms underlying the beneficial effects of DR on the aging cardiovascular and cerebrovascular systems.

3. Dietary restriction and cardiovascular physiology

Previous studies had shown that DR can reduce resting blood pressure and heart rate in humans (Herlihy et al., 1992; Nakano et al., 2001). Mice that were maintained on DR during their adult life exhibited reduced diastolic blood pressure, decreased atrial filling velocity and an increased ratio of early diastolic filling to atrial filling, indicating that DR improves diastolic function during aging (Taffet et al., 1997). The decreased blood pressure and heart rate likely result from changes in the neural and endocrine systems that control blood pressure, including changes in sympathetic and parasympathetic tone, hypothalamic regulation (e.g., changes in leptin, neuropeptide Y and natriuretic peptide signaling) and nitric oxide signaling (Kolta et al., 1989; McShane et al., 1999; VanNess et al., 1999; de Wardener, 2001; Swoap, 2001). Rats maintained on DR throughout their adult life exhibited a highly significant reduction in the development of spontaneous cardiomyopathy compared to rats fed ad libitum (Kemi et al., 2000). Beneficial effects of DR on cardiovascular parameters, including decreased blood pressure and heart rate, were observed within 2–4 weeks of DR in rats (Hilderman et al., 1996). The latter study further showed that levels of epinephrine and norepinephrine in the heart were increased in rats maintained on DR, consistent with an increased sympathetic tone. During 4–5 months of DR (40% calorie reduction diet) rats exhibited decreased body and heart weights, but an increased heart weight to body weight ratio (Kim et al., 1994). Levels of norepinephrine in the synaptosomal fraction from cardiac tissue were increased, and stimulated uptake of norepinephrine was increased, in rats on DR. When taken together with data from numerous studies showing that animals maintained on DR exhibit increased levels of circulating glucocorticoids (Nelson et al., 1995), it seems clear that DR results in a stress-like state. However, unlike other types of chronic stress (psychosocial stress, for example), DR is a unique stressor that improves blood pressure, heart rate and cardiovascular adaptation to physical and psychosocial stress.

The "stress hypothesis" of aging and disease, originally proposed by Selye (for review see Selye, 1976) has received considerable support from studies of animals and humans. An inability to adapt to physiological and psychological stress may contribute to the pathogenesis of cardiovascular disease, cancer and other diseases (Fife et al., 1996; Kawakami and Haratani, 1999; Rozanski et al., 1999; Pedersen et al., 2001). Improved cardiovascular responses to stress can be accomplished by physical exercise (Cox, 1991) and behavioral training programs (Barnes et al., 2001). We have recently shown that cardiovascular stress resistance can also be bolstered by DR (Wan et al., 2002). We used radiotelemetry probes to monitor blood pressure, heart rate and body temperature in adult rats that had been maintained on an every-other-day fasting regimen, and in control rats fed ad libitum daily. The rats on DR had significantly lower basal blood pressure and heart rate which was present on both fasting and non-fasting days; the effects of DR on these cardiovascular parameters became evident only after 2–4 weeks of periodic fasting.

We observed striking reductions in the magnitude of stress-induced increases in HR and BP in rats maintained on the periodic fasting regimen. For example, BP increased to 130–140 mm Hg during a 1 h restraint stress period in control rats, but to only 110–120 mm Hg in periodic fasting rats (Fig. 1). Following release from restraint, BP recovered to pre-stress levels more rapidly in the fasting rats. Periodic fasting also resulted in a significantly reduced HR response to restraint stress, and a more rapid recovery to baseline following release (Wan et al., 2002). There were no differences in body temperature or general activity, during or after restraint stress, in control and fasting rats. Periodic fasting also decreased HR and BP responses in a cold water stress paradigm (data not shown). It should be noted that there is evidence, based on studies of human populations in which calorie intake is low, that DR also benefits cardiovascular function in humans (Alexander et al., 1999).

4. Dietary restriction protects heart and brain cells against ischemic and oxidative injury

Despite the fact that DR can reduce risk of coronary artery and cerebrovascular diseases, surprisingly few studies have been performed to determine whether DR affects the extent of cellular injury and/or functional outcome following a myocardial infarction or stroke. In one study Fisher 344 rats were either fed ad libitum or were maintained on a diet with a 40% reduction in calories beginning at 2 months of age, and when the rats were 12 months old they were subjected to transient occlusion (15 min) of the left anterior descending coronary artery (Chandrasekar et al., 2001). Analyses of heart tissue from the rats revealed increased levels of manganese superoxide dismutase, decreased levels of oxidative damage and decreased production of inflammatory cytokines in the hearts of the calorie-restricted rats. In another study, young adult male Sprague–Dawley rats were maintained on an every-other-day feeding regimen for 3 months; a control group of rats was fed ad libitum. Rats were then subjected to transient occlusion (1 h) of the middle cerebral artery. Twenty four hours later neurological deficits were assessed and then the rats were euthanized and the extent of ischemic damage to their brains was quantified (Yu and Mattson, 1999). The extent of damage to cerebral cortical and striatal neurons was significantly reduced, and functional outcome improved, in the rats that had been

M. P. Mattson and R. Wan

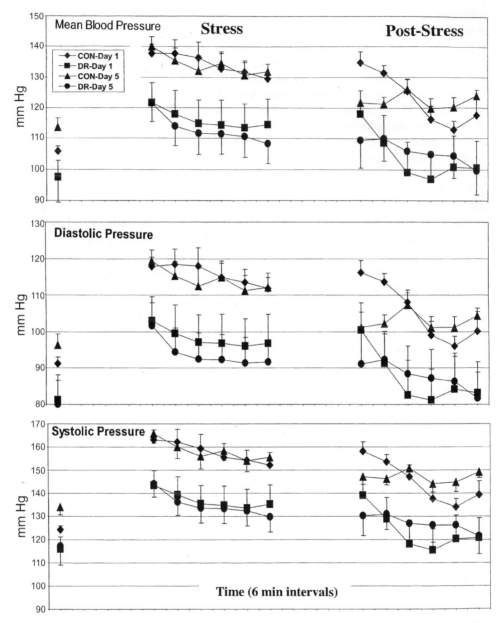

Fig. 1.   Dietary restriction reduces basal blood pressure and attenuates blood pressure responses to stress in rats. Rats were maintained for 3 months on either a control diet in which they were provided continuous access to food, or a DR feeding regimen in which the rats were fed every-other-day. Blood pressure was monitored by telemetry prior to, and for 1 h following exposure of rats to restraint stress. Analyses were performed on two different days (days 1 and 5) separated by a 4-day interval. Values are the mean and SE of measurements made in at least six rats per group. Note that basal diastolic and systolic blood pressures were decreased in DR rats, that blood pressure responses to stress were attenuated in DR rats, and that blood pressure recovered more quickly following stress in the DR rats. Modified from Wan et al. (2002).

maintained on the DR regimen compared to control rats fed ad libitum (Fig. 2). Epidemiological and clinical findings are consistent with reduced heart damage and improved outcome following a myocardial infarction in patients on low calorie diets. For example, Lundergan et al. (2001) reported improved outcome (left ventricular function) in survivors of myocardial infarction with a low body/mass index compared to survivors with a higher body/mass index.

Animal models of stroke involve transient occlusion of the middle cerebral artery which results in degeneration of neurons in the regions of cerebral cortex and striatum supplied by the artery. In these models the reduction in glucose and oxygen availability to neurons results in a depletion of ATP and disruption of cellular ion homeostasis and, upon reperfusion, massive production of oxyradicals (Dirnagl et al., 1999). Rats and mice subjected to such strokes exhibit functional deficits including motor dysfunction. When rats were maintained on a DR feeding regimen for 3 months and then subjected to a stroke, the amount of neuronal damage was significantly decreased and functional outcome was improved (Yu and Mattson, 1999). DR can protect neurons against excitotoxicity a neurodegenerative process in which overactivation of glutamate receptors results in excessive calcium influx and oxyradical production (Bruce-Keller et al., 1999). DR also protects neurons against oxidative injury in animal models of Parkinson's disease (Duan and Mattson, 1999) and Alzheimer's disease (Zhu et al., 1999). It is now believed that, as is the case with cardiovascular disease and type 2 diabetes, DR can also reduce risk of age-related neurodegenerative disorders (Mattson, 2000).

5. Cellular and molecular mechanisms of action of dietary restriction

Many metabolic changes occur in rodents, primates and humans during DR that would be expected to reduce the risk of cardiovascular and cerebrovascular diseases. These include lower plasma insulin levels and greater insulin sensitivity; lower blood pressure and arterial stiffness, lower body temperature; reduced cholesterol and triglyceride levels, elevated HDL levels; and slower age-related decline in levels of DHEA (Table 1). In addition, DR can decrease plasma levels of homocysteine (Fig. 3); elevated levels of homocysteine are associated with increased risk of coronary artery disease and stroke (Mattson et al., 2002). Indeed, recent studies have shown that homocysteine can render neurons vulnerable to dysfunction and death in experimental models relevant to stroke (Fig. 3), Alzheimer's disease (Kruman et al., 2002) and Parkinson's disease (Duan et al., 2002).

One important beneficial effect of DR in the cardiovascular and cerebrovascular systems is inhibition of the process of atherosclerosis. DR may prevent atherosclerosis by multiple mechanisms. By improving plasma lipid profiles (decreased LDL cholesterol, triglycerides and glucose levels) DR reduces oxidative damage to vascular endothelial cells by oxidized LDL and glycated proteins (Kesaniemi et al., 1985; Cefalu et al., 2000; Edwards et al., 1998, 2001). DR may also decrease inflammatory processes resulting from damage to vascular endothelial cells, and may thereby prevent the formation of cholesterol-laden "foam cells" that play a major

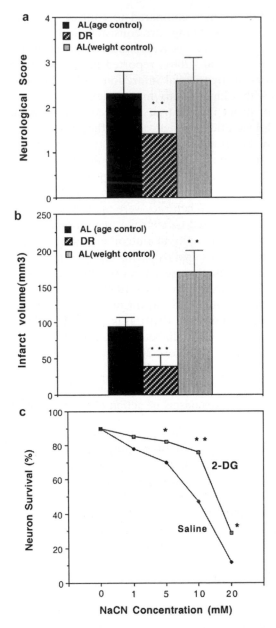

Fig. 2.   Dietary restriction reduces brain cell damage and improves behavioral outcome in a rat model of stroke. Young adult rats were fed ad libitum (AL age control) or were maintained for 3 months on an every-other-day fasting DR regimen. An additional group of younger ad libitum fed rats was matched for body weight with the DR group. Rats were subjected to transient occlusion of the middle cerebral artery. Twenty four hours later the functional deficits of the rats were assessed (a) and then the rats were euthanized and the extent of brain damage (infarct volume) was determined (b). Panel c shows the results of a study in which cultured hippocampal neurons were pretreated with 2-deoxy-D-glucose and then exposed for 24 h to increasing concentrations of sodium cyanide (NaCN) to induce chemical hypoxia. Neuronal survival was quantified. Note that neurons pretreated with 2-deoxy-D-glucose were more resistant to hypoxic injury. Modified from Yu and Mattson (1999).

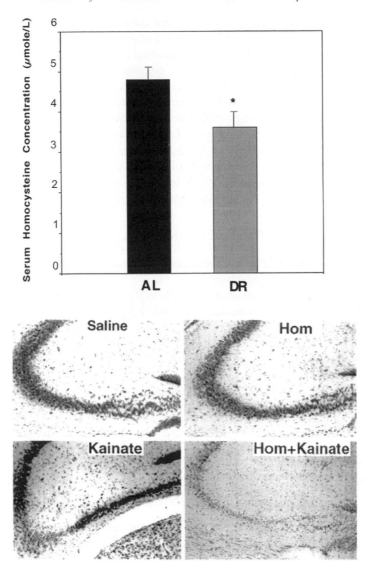

Fig. 3.   Dietary restriction decreases homocysteine levels, and homocysteine renders neurons vulnerable to excitotoxicity. (a) Homocysteine concentrations were measured in serum samples from mice that had been maintained for 3 months on an ad libitum diet (AL; $n = 8$) or an every-other-day DR feeding regimen (DR; $n = 10$). $*P < 0.05$. (b) Micrographs showing neurons in region CA3 of the hippocampus from mice that had received an intrahippocampal injection of either saline, 4.3 ng homocysteine (Hom), 0.2 μg of the excitotoxin kainate or a combination of 4.3 ng homocysteine and 0.2 μg kainate 24 h previously. Note that homocysteine greatly increased the death of CA3 neurons. Modified from Kruman et al. (2000).

role in the progressive occlusion of arteries that occurs during atherosclerosis (Dong et al., 1998; Chung et al., 2001). When a strain of mice (W/BF1) that spontaneously develops coronary vascular disease was maintained on a diet with a 32% reduction in calories, the coronary vascular disease was essentially prevented and lifespan was extended (Mizutani et al., 1994). The vascular disease in the W/BF1 mice is caused by an autoimmune response and DR suppressed the immune response as indicated by decreased levels of circulating anti-cardiolipin antibodies and immune complexes. Inflammatory cytokines such as tumor necrosis factor (TNF) and interleukin-6 (IL-6) play roles in the pathogenesis of cardiovascular and cerebrovascular diseases (Krishnaswamy et al., 2002). Serum levels of TNF and IL-6 increase with age in mice and DR suppresses the age-related increases in these inflammatory cytokines (Spaulding et al., 1997). By suppressing inflammatory processes, DR may prevent atherosclerosis (Fig. 4).

The majority of data concerning the effects of DR on gene expression and cellular physiology have come from recent studies in which levels of gene products (mRNAs and proteins) have been measured in tissues from rats or mice maintained on DR compared with animals fed ad libitum.

Because DR increases the resistance of cells to dysfunction and death in models of myocardial infarction, and stroke and other neurodegenerative disorders, it might be expected that DR modifies a step or steps in the degenerative process that is common to these disorders. Indeed, it has been shown that DR can stabilize mitochondrial function and can reduce oxidative stress in brain cells of rodents (Guo et al., 2000).

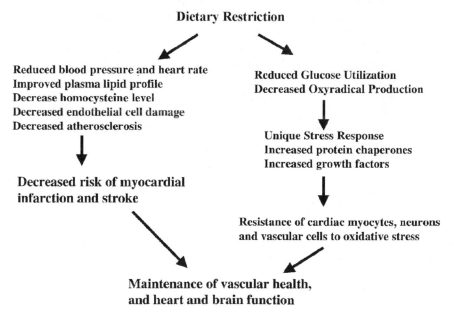

Fig. 4. Model outlining the mechanisms whereby dietary restriction benefits blood vessels and the heart and brain during aging.

DR has also been shown to reduce age-related mitochondrial abnormalities in skeletal muscle cells (Aspnes et al., 1997). Two classes of cytoprotective proteins that are increased by DR are protein chaperones such as heat-shock protein-70 (HSP-70) and glucose-regulated protein-78 (GRP-78), and growth factors such as brain-derived neurotrophic factor (BDNF) (Aly et al., 1994; Duan and Mattson, 1999; Yu and Mattson, 1999; Lee et al., 2000, 2002; Duan et al., 2001). HSP-70 and GRP-78 can protect myocardial cells and neurons against excitotoxic and oxidative injury (Lowenstein et al., 1991; Yu et al., 1999). Similarly, growth factors can protect neurons and cardiac myocytes against ischemic and oxidative injury (Cheng and Mattson, 1994; Cuevas et al., 1997). Growth factors may play particularly important roles in protection of cardiac myocytes and neurons against ischemic injury because infusion of a BDNF blocking antibody into the lateral ventricles of rats and mice significantly attenuated the neuroprotective effect of DR (Duan et al., 2001). It is therefore likely that the increased levels of protein chaperones and growth factors in cells of animals maintained on DR play a major role in the increased resistance of the cells to dysfunction and death (Fig. 4). The transcription factors that mediate the beneficial effects of DR in cells of blood vessels, heart and nervous system have not yet been identified. However, based upon the evidence that DR induces a mild stress response and on the identification of genes upregulated by DR (Prolla and Mattson, 2001), it is likely that NF-kappaB and CREB are two important DR-responsive transcription factors (Mattson and Camandola, 2001).

Interestingly, at least some of the beneficial effects of DR can be mimicked by administering 2-deoxy-D-glucose (a non-metabolizable analog of glucose) to animals fed ad libitum. For example, neurons pretreated with 2-deoxy-D-glucose exhibit increased resistance to chemical hypoxia in an experimental model of stroke (Fig. 2c). Animals given 2-deoxy-D-glucose exhibit increased levels of protein chaperones in their brain cells and increased resistance of neurons to excitotoxic, oxidative and ischemic injury (Duan and Mattson, 1999; Yu and Mattson, 1999; Guo et al., 2000). Presumably by inhibiting glycolysis, 2-deoxy-D-glucose induces increased levels of HSP-70 and GRP-78 in neurons throughout the brain. 2-deoxy-D-glucose can act directly on neurons to increase their resistance to oxidative stress, preserve mitochondrial function, and stabilizes calcium homeostasis; in these ways 2-deoxy-D-glucose protects neurons against excitotoxicity and apoptosis (Lee et al., 1999; Duan and Mattson, 1999; Yu and Mattson, 1999).

When heart or brain cells are subjected to a brief mild ischemia they become resistant to a more severe ischemic insult such as occurs during a myocardial infarction or stroke (Barone et al., 1998; Yellon and Dana, 2000). Studies of cardiac myocytes have provided convincing evidence that mitochondrial ATP-sensitive potassium (Mito-KATP) channels play a central role in such "ischemic preconditioning" (Ghosh et al., 2000). Thus, agents such as diazoxide that selectively open Mito-KATP channels can mimic the cytoprotective effect of preconditioning, whereas drugs such as 5HD that selectively block Mito-KATP channels can abolish ischemic preconditioning (Takashi et al., 1999; Eells et al., 2000). Activation of Mito-KATP channels also protect neurons against ischemic injury in experimental models of stroke (Liu et al., 2002). It has been proposed that mild ischemia activates

Mito-KATP by a mechanism involving oxyradical production and activation of protein kinase-C (Takashi et al., 1999). Other components of the cytoprotective preconditioning response include upregulation of the expression of antioxidant enzymes such as manganese superoxide dismutase (Keller et al., 1998) and anti-apoptotic proteins such as Bcl-2 (Shimizu et al., 2001).

Finally, our hormesis hypothesis for the beneficial effects of dietary restriction in the brain (Mattson et al., 2001) provides a satisfactory explanation for the increased neurogenesis observed in mice and rats maintained on dietary restriction. In situ hybridization analysis showed that the expression of BDNF and neurotrophin-3 (NT-3) are increased in subpopulations of neurons in the hippocampus of mice maintained on dietary restriction; BDNF levels increase in CA3 and CA1 pyramidal neurons and NT-3 levels increase in dentate granule neurons (Lee et al., 2002). Previous findings suggest that the increased levels of BDNF and NT-3 could account for the increased neurogenesis. BDNF promotes the survival and differentiation of hippocampal neural progenitor cells and their newly generated neuronal progeny (Cheng and Mattson, 1994). In addition, stimuli such as seizure activity and enriched environments that increase neurogenesis in the dentate gyrus also increase BDNF expression (Parent et al., 1997; Lowenstein and Arsenault, 1996; Lee et al., 1997; Cameron et al., 1998; Young et al., 1999). NT-3 and BDNF each promote neuronal differentiation of embryonic (Sah et al., 1997) and adult (Takahashi et al., 1999) hippocampal neural progenitor cells. Mice lacking NT-3 exhibit decreased survival of certain populations of neural progenitor cells and their progeny (Kahn et al., 1999). We therefore conclude that the increased expression of BDNF and NT-3 induced by dietary restriction is critical for the enhanced neurogenesis. It will be of considerable interest to determine whether growth factors (e.g., vascular endothelial growth factor or basic fibroblast growth factor) are upregulated in heart or vascular cells in response to DR.

6. Conclusions and future directions

Metabolic and physiological adaptations to DR appear to counteract fundamental mechanisms of aging. For example, DR increases insulin sensitivity, reduces body temperature and blood pressure, and improves blood lipid profiles. In addition, DR induces a number of changes in gene expression in the brain that are associated with protection of cells against age-related diseases including stroke and neurodegenerative disorders. Such beneficial effects of DR may optimize metabolic and physiological functions both in peripheral organs and in the central nervous system. DR enhances cellular resistance to stress and improves the ability of organs and organisms to adapt to stress. The findings described above demonstrate that DR can enhance the ability of the cardiovascular and cerebrovascular systems to adapt to different types of stress.While DR is clearly an effective preventative approach for reducing risk of cardiovascular and cerebrovascular diseases, the extent to which it can be used as a treatment for patients with already severe disease is unclear. However, there is now considerable evidence that the process of atherosclerosis can be reversed by the implementation of stringent DR and exercise programs (Schell and Myers, 1997). DR may therefore be effective in slowing or reversing the disease processes responsible for cardiovascular disease and stroke. Dietary supplements that mimic beneficial effects of DR are being developed (Mattson et al., 2001) with the aim of using them to treat individuals who are unable to comply with DR feeding regimens.

References

Alexander, H., Lockwood, L.P., Harris, M.A., Melby, C.L., 1999. Risk factors for cardiovascular disease and diabetes in two groups of Hispanic Americans with differing dietary habits. J. Am. Coll. Nutr. 18, 127–136.

Aly, K.B., Pipkin, J.L., Hinson, W.G., Feuers, R.J., Duffy, P.H., Lyn-Cook, L., Hart, R.W., 1994. Chronic caloric restriction induces stress proteins in the hypothalamus of rats. Mech. Ageing Dev. 76, 11–23.

Aronne, L.J., 2001. Epidemiology, morbidity, and treatment of overweight and obesity. J. Clin. Psychiatry 23, 13–22.

Aspnes, L.E., Lee, C.M., Weindruch, R., Chung, S.S., Roecker, E.B., Aiken, J.M., 1997. Caloric restriction reduces fiber loss and mitochondrial abnormalities in aged rat muscle. FASEB J. 11, 573–581.

Barnes, V.A., Treiber, F.A., Davis, H., 2001. Impact of transcendental meditation on cardiovascular function at rest and during acute stress in adolescents with high normal blood pressure. J. Psychosom. Res. 51, 597–605.

Barone, F.C., White, R.F., Spera, P.A., Ellison, J., Currie, R.W., Wang, X., Feuerstein, G.Z., 1998. Ischemic preconditioning and brain tolerance: temporal histological and functional outcomes, protein synthesis requirement, and interleukin-1 receptor antagonist and early gene expression. Stroke 29, 1937–1950.

Brochu, M., Poehlman, E.T., Ades, P.A., 2000. Obesity, body fat distribution, and coronary artery disease. J. Cardiopulm. Rehabil. 20, 96–108.

Bronner, L.L., Kanter, D.S., Manson, J.E., 1995. Primary prevention of stroke. N. Engl. J. Med. 333, 1392–1400.

Bruce-Keller, A.J., Umberger, G., McFall, R., Mattson, M.P., 1999. Food restriction reduces brain damage and improves behavioral outcome following excitotoxic and metabolic insults. Ann. Neurol. 45, 8–15.

Cameron, H.A., Hazel, T.G., McKay, R.D., 1998. Regulation of neurogenesis by growth factors and neurotransmitters. J. Neurobiol. 36, 287–306.

Cefalu, W.T., Terry, J.G., Thomas, M.J., Morgan, T.M., Edwards, I.J., Rudel, L.L., Kemnitz, J.W., Weindruch, R., 2000. In vitro oxidation of low-density lipoprotein in two species of nonhuman primates subjected to caloric restriction. J. Gerontol. A Biol. Sci. Med. Sci. 55, B355–B361.

Chandrasekar, B., Nelson, J.F., Colston, J.T., Freeman, G.L., 2001. Calorie restriction attenuates inflammatory responses to myocardial ischemia-reperfusion injury. Am. J. Physiol. Heart Circ. Physiol. 280, H2094–H2102.

Cheng, B., Mattson, M.P., 1994. NT-3 and BDNF protect CNS neurons against metabolic/excitotoxic insults. Brain Res. 640, 56–67.

Chung, H.Y., Kim, H.J., Kim, J.W., Yu, B.P., 2001. The inflammation hypothesis of aging: molecular modulation by calorie restriction. Ann. N.Y. Acad. Sci. 928, 327–335.

Cox, M.H., 1991. Exercise training programs and cardiorespiratory adaptation. Clin. Sports Med. 10, 19–32.

Cuevas, P., Reimers, D., Carceller, F., Martinez-Coso, V., Redondo-Horcajo, M., Saenz de Tejada, I., Gimenez-Gallego, G., 1997. Fibroblast growth factor-1 prevents myocardial apoptosis triggered by ischemia reperfusion injury. Eur. J. Med. Res. 2, 465–468.

Deckelbaum, R.J., Williams, C.L., 2001. Childhood obesity: the health issue. Obes. Res. 9, 239S–243S.

de Wardener, H.E., 2001. The hypothalamus and hypertension. Physiol. Rev. 81, 1599–1658.

Dirnagl, U., Iadecola, C., Moskowitz, M.A., 1999. Pathobiology of ischaemic stroke: an integrated view. Trends Neurosci. 22, 391–397.

Dong, W., Selgrade, M.K., Gilmour, I.M., Lange, R.W., Park, P., Luster, M.I., Kari, F.W., 1998. Altered alveolar macrophage function in calorie-restricted rats. Am. J. Respir. Cell Mol. Biol. 19, 462–469.

Duan, W., Guo, Z., Mattson, M.P., 2001. Brain-derived neurotrophic factor mediates an excitoprotective effect of dietary restriction in mice. J. Neurochem. 76, 619–626.

Duan, W., Ladenheim, B., Cutler, R.G., Kruman, I.I., Cadet, J.L., Mattson, M.P., 2002. Dietary folate deficiency and elevated homocysteine levels endanger dopaminergic neurons in models of Parkinson's disease. J. Neurochem. 80, 101–110.

Duan, W., Mattson, M.P., 1999. Dietary restriction and 2-deoxyglucose administration improve behavioral outcome and reduce degeneration of dopaminergic neurons in models of Parkinson's disease. J. Neurosci. Res. 57, 195–206.

Duffy, P.H., Leakey, J.E., Pipkin, J.L., Turturro, A., Hart, R.W., 1997. The physiologic, neurologic, and behavioral effects of caloric restriction related to aging, disease, and environmental factors. Environ. Res. 73, 242–248.

Edwards, I.J., Rudel, L.L., Terry, J.G., Kemnitz, J.W., Weindruch, R., Cefalu, W.T., 1998. Caloric restriction in rhesus monkeys reduces low density lipoprotein interaction with arterial proteoglycans. J. Gerontol. A Biol. Sci. Med. Sci. 53, B443–B448.

Edwards, I.J., Rudel, L.L., Terry, J.G., Kemnitz, J.W., Weindruch, R., Zaccaro, D.J., Cefalu, W.T., 2001. Caloric restriction lowers plasma lipoprotein (a) in male but not female rhesus monkeys. Exp. Gerontol. 36, 1413–1418.

Eells, J.T., Henry, M.M., Gross, G.J., Baker, J.E., 2000. Increased mitochondrial K(ATP) channel activity during chronic myocardial hypoxia: is cardioprotection mediated by improved bioenergetics? Circ. Res. 87, 915–921.

Fife, A., Beasley, P.J., Fertig, D.L., 1996. Psychoneuroimmunology and cancer: historical perspectives and current research. Adv. Neuroimmunol. 6, 179–190.

Ghosh, S., Standen, N.B., Galinanes, M., 2000. Evidence for mitochondrial K ATP channels as effectors of human myocardial preconditioning. Cardiovasc. Res. 45, 934–940.

Goodrick, C.L., Ingram, D.K., Reynolds, M.A., Freeman, J.R., Cider, N.L., 1983. Differential effects of intermittent feeding and voluntary exercise on body weight and lifespan in adult rats. J. Gerontol. 38, 36–45.

Guo, Z., Ersoz, A., Butterfield, D.A., Mattson, M.P., 2000. Beneficial effects of dietary restriction on cerebral cortical synaptic terminals: preservation of glucose transport and mitochondrial function after exposure to amyloid beta-peptide and oxidative and metabolic insults. J. Neurochem. 75, 314–320.

Hecker, K.D., Kris-Etherton, P.M., Zhao, G., Coval, S., St Jeor, S., 1999. Impact of body weight and weight loss on cardiovascular risk factors. Curr. Atheroscler. Rep. 1, 236–242.

Herlihy, J.T., Stacy, C., Bertrand, H.A., 1992. Long-term calorie restriction enhances baroreflex responsiveness in Fischer 344 rats. Am. J. Physiol. 263, H1021–H1025.

Hilderman, T., McKnight, K., Dhalla, K.S., Rupp, H., Dhalla, N.S., 1996. Effects of long-term dietary restriction on cardiovascular function and plasma catecholamines in the rat. Cardiovasc. Drugs Ther. 10, S247–S250.

Horwitz, L.D., Wallner, J.S., Decker, D.E., Buxser, S.E., 1996. Efficacy of lipid soluble, membrane-protective agents against hydrogen peroxide cytotoxicity in cardiac myocytes. Free Radic. Biol. Med. 21, 743–753.

Kawakami, N., Haratani, T., 1999. Epidemiology of job stress and health in Japan: review of current evidence and future direction. Ind. Health 37, 174–186.

Keller, J.N., Kindy, M.S., Holtsberg, F.W., St Clair, D.K., Yen, H.C., Germeyer, A., Steiner, S.M., Bruce-Keller, A.J., Hutchins, J.B., Mattson, M.P., 1998. Mitochondrial manganese superoxide dismutase prevents neural apoptosis and reduces ischemic brain injury: suppression of peroxynitrite production, lipid peroxidation, and mitochondrial dysfunction. J. Neurosci. 18, 687–697.

Kemi, M., Keenan, K.P., McCoy, C., Hoe, C.M., Soper, K.A., Ballam, G.C., van Zwieten, M.J., 2000. The relative protective effects of moderate dietary restriction versus dietary modification on spontaneous cardiomyopathy in male Sprague–Dawley rats. Toxicol. Pathol. 28, 285–296.

Kesaniemi, Y.A., Beltz, W.F., Grundy, S.M., 1985. Comparison of clofibrate and caloric restriction on kinetics of very low density lipoprotein triglycerides. Arteriosclerosis 5, 153–161.

Kim, S.W., Yu, B.P., Sanderford, M., Herlihy, J.T., 1994. Dietary restriction modulates the norepinephrine content and uptake of the heart and cardiac synaptosomes. Proc. Soc. Exp. Biol. Med. 207, 43–47.

Kolta, M.G., Holson, R., Duffy, P., Hart, R.W., 1989. Effect of long-term caloric restriction on brain monoamines in aging male and female Fischer 344 rats. Mech. Ageing Dev. 48, 191–198.

Krishnaswamy, G., Dube, D., Counts, M., Chi, D.S., 2002. Cytokines and the pathogenesis of atherosclerosis. In: Hagen, T., Mattson, M.P. (Eds.), Mechanisms of Cardiovascular Aging. Elsevier, Amsterdam, 79–126.

Kruman, I.I., Culmsee, C., Chan, S.L., Kruman, Y., Guo, Z., Penix, L., Mattson, M.P., 2000. Homocysteine elicits a DNA damage response in neurons that promotes apoptosis and hypersensitivity to excitotoxicity. J. Neurosci. 20, 6920–6926.

Kruman, I.I., Kumaravel, T.S., Lohani, A., Pedersen, W.A., Cutler, R.G., Kruman, Y., Haughey, N.J., Lee, J., Evans, M., Mattson, M.P., 2002. Folic acid deficiency and homocysteine impair DNA repair in hippocampal neurons and sensitize them to amyloid toxicity in experimental models of Alzheimer's disease. 22, 1752–1762.

Lane, M.A., Baer, D.J., Rumpler, W.V., Weindruch, R., Ingram, D.K., Tilmont, E.M., Cutler, R.G., Roth, G.S., 1996. Calorie restriction lowers body temperature in rhesus monkeys, consistent with a postulated anti-aging mechanism in rodents. Proc. Natl. Acad. Sci. USA 93, 4159–4164.

Lane, M.A., Ingram, D.K., Ball, S.S., Roth, G.S., 1997. Dehydroepiandrosterone sulfate: a biomarker of primate aging slowed by calorie restriction. J. Clin. Endocrinol. Metab. 82, 2093–2096.

Lane, M.A., Ingram, D.K., Roth, G.S., 1999. Nutritional modulation of aging in nonhuman primates. J. Nutr. Health Aging 3, 69–76.

Lebovitz, H.E., 1999. Type 2 diabetes: an overview. Clin. Chem. 45, 1339–1345.

Lee, J., Bruce-Keller, A.J., Kruman, Y., Chan, S., Mattson, M.P., 1999. 2-deoxy-D-glucose protects hippocampal neurons against excitotoxic and oxidative injury: involvement of stress proteins. J. Neurosci. Res. 57, 48–61.

Lee, J., Duan, W., Long, J.M., Ingram, D.K., Mattson, M.P., 2000. Dietary restriction increases survival of newly-generated neural cells and induces BDNF expression in the dentate gyrus of rats. J. Mol. Neurosci. 15, 99–108.

Lee, J., Seroogy, K.B., Mattson, M.P., 2002. Dietary restriction enhances neurotrophin expression and neurogenesis in the hippocampus of adult mice. J. Neurochem. 80.

Levi, F., 1999. Cancer prevention: epidemiology and perspectives. Eur. J. Cancer 35, 1912–1924.

Liu, D., Lu, C., Wan, R., Auyeung, W.W., Mattson, M.P., 2002. Activation of mitochondrial ATP-dependent potassium channels protects neurons against ischemia-induced cell death. J. Cereb. Blood Flow Metab. 22, 431–443.

Logroscino, G., Marder, K., Cote, L., Tang, M.X., Shea, S., Mayeux, R., 1996. Dietary lipids and antioxidants in Parkinson's disease: a population-based, case-control study. Ann. Neurol. 39, 89–94.

Lowenstein, D.H., Chan, P.H., Miles, M.F., 1991. The stress protein response in cultured neurons: characterization and evidence for a protective role in excitotoxicity. Neuron 7, 1053–1060.

Lundergan, C.F., Ross, A.M., McCarthy, W.F., Reiner, J.S., Boyle, D., Fink, C., Califf, R.M., Topol, E.J., Simoons, M.L., Van Den Brand, M., Van de Werf, F., Coyne, K.S., 2001. Predictors of left ventricular function after acute myocardial infarction: effects of time to treatment, patency, and body mass index: the GUSTO-I angiographic experience. Am. Heart J. 142, 43–50.

Maeda, H., Gleiser, C.A., Masoro, E.J., Murata, I., McMahan, C.A., Yu, B.P., 1985. Nutritional influences on aging of Fischer 344 rats: II. Pathology. J. Gerontol. 40, 671–688.

Markesbery, W.R., 1997. Oxidative stress hypothesis in Alzheimer's disease. Free Radic. Biol. Med. 23, 134–147.

Mattson, M.P., Camandola, S., 2001. NF-kappaB in neuronal plasticity and neurodegenerative disorders. J. Clin. Invest. 107, 247–254.

Mattson, M.P., Duan, W., Lee, J., Guo, Z., 2001. Suppression of brain aging and neurodegenerative disorders by dietary restriction and environmental enrichment: molecular mechanisms. Mech. Ageing Dev. 122, 757–778.

Mattson, M.P., Kruman, I.I., Duan, W., 2002. Folic acid and homocysteine in age-related disease. Aging Res. Rev. 1, 95–111.

Mayeux, R., Costa, R., Bell, K., Merchant, C., Tung, M.X., Jacobs, D., 1999. Reduced risk of Alzheimer's disease among individuals with low calorie intake. Neurology 59, S296–S297.

McShane, T.M., Wilson, M.E., Wise, P.M., 1999. Effects of lifelong moderate caloric restriction on levels of neuropeptide Y, proopiomelanocortin, and galanin mRNA. J. Gerontol. A Biol. Sci. Med. Sci. 54, B14–B21.

Mizutani, H., Engelman, R.W., Kinjoh, K., Kurata, Y., Ikehara, S., Matsuzawa, Y., Good, R.A., 1994. Calorie restriction prevents the occlusive coronary vascular disease of autoimmune (NZW × BXSB)F1 mice. Proc. Natl. Acad. Sci. USA 91, 4402–4406.

Nakano, Y., Oshima, T., Sasaki, S., Higashi, Y., Ozono, R., Takenaka, S., Miura, F., Hirao, H., Matsuura, H., Chayama, K., Kambe, M., 2001. Calorie restriction reduced blood pressure in obesity hypertensives by improvement of autonomic nerve activity and insulin sensitivity. J. Cardiovasc. Pharmacol. 38, S69–S74.

Nelson, J.F., Karelus, K., Bergman, M.D., Felicio, L.S., 1995. Neuroendocrine involvement in aging: evidence from studies of reproductive aging and caloric restriction. Neurobiol. Aging 16, 837–843.

Parent, J.M., Yu, T.W., Leibowitz, R.T., Geschwind, D.H., Solviter, R.S., Lowenstein, DH., 1997. Dentate granule cell neurogenesis is increased by seizures and contributes to aberrant network reorganization in the adult rat hippocampus. J. Neurosci. 17, 3727–3738.

Pedersen, W.A., Wan, R., Mattson, M.P., 2001. Impact of aging on stress-responsive neuroendocrine systems. Mech. Ageing Dev. 122, 963–983.

Prolla, T.A., Mattson, M.P., 2001. Molecular mechanisms of brain aging and neurodegenerative disorders: lessons from dietary restriction. Trends Neurosci. 24, S21–31.

Ren, J., Gintant, G.A., Miller, R.E., Davidoff, A.J., 1997. High extracellular glucose impairs cardiac E–C coupling in a glycosylation-dependent manner. Am. J. Physiol. 273, H2876–H2883.

Ren, S., Shen, G.X., 2000. Impact of antioxidants and HDL on glycated LDL-induced generation of fibrinolytic regulators from vascular endothelial cells. Arterioscler. Thromb. Vasc. Biol. 20, 1688–1693.

Roth, G.S., Ingram, D.K., Lane, M.A., 2001a. Caloric restriction in primates and relevance to humans. Ann. N.Y. Acad. Sci. 928, 305–315.

Roth, G.S., Lesnikov, V., Lesnikov, M., Ingram, D.K., Lane, M.A., 2001b. Dietary caloric restriction prevents the age-related decline in plasma melatonin levels of rhesus monkeys. J. Clin. Endocrinol. Metab. 86, 3292–3295.

Rozanski, A., Blumenthal, J.A., Kaplan, J., 1999. Impact of psychological factors on the pathogenesis of cardiovascular disease and implications for therapy. Circulation 99, 2192–2217.

Sah D.W., Ray, J., Gage, F.H., 1997. Regulation of voltage- and ligand-gated currents in rat hippocampal progenitor cells in vitro. J. Neurobiol. 32, 95–110.

Schell, W.D., Myers, J.N., 1997. Regression of atherosclerosis: a review. Prog. Cardiovasc. Dis. 39, 483–496.

Seidell, J.C., Flegal, K.M., 1997. Assessing obesity: classification and epidemiology. Br. Med. Bull. 53, 238–252.

Selye, H., 1976. Forty years of stress research: principal remaining problems and misconceptions. Can. Med. Assoc. J. 115, 53–56.

Shimizu, S., Nagayama, T., Jin, K.L., Zhu, L., Loeffert, J.E., Watkins, S.C., Graham, S.H., Simon, R.P., 2001. bcl-2 Antisense treatment prevents induction of tolerance to focal ischemia in the rat brain. J. Cereb. Blood Flow Metab. 21, 233–243.

Sohal, R.S., Weindruch, R., 1996. Oxidative stress, caloric restriction, and aging. Science 273, 59–63.

Spaulding, C.C., Walford, R.L., Effros, R.B., 1997. Calorie restriction inhibits the age-related dysregulation of the cytokines TNF-alpha and IL-6 in C3B10RF1 mice. Mech. Ageing Dev. 93, 87–94.

Swoap, S.J., 2001. Altered leptin signaling is sufficient, but not required, for hypotension associated with caloric restriction. Am. J. Physiol. Heart Circ. Physiol. 281, H2473–H2479.

Taffet, G.E., Pham, T.T., Hartley, C.J., 1997. The age-associated alterations in late diastolic function in mice are improved by caloric restriction. J. Gerontol. A Biol. Sci. Med. Sci. 52, B285–B290.

Takashi, E., Wang, Y., Ashraf, M., 1999. Activation of mitochondrial K(ATP) channel elicits late preconditioning against myocardial infarction via protein kinase C signaling pathway. Circ. Res. 85, 1113–1114.

VanNess, J.M., DeMaria, J.E., Overton, J.M., 1999. Increased NPY activity in the PVN contributes to food-restriction induced reductions in blood pressure in aortic coarctation hypertensive rats. Brain Res. 821, 263–269.

Verdery, R.B., Ingram, D.K., Roth, G.S., Lane, M.A., 1997. Caloric restriction increases HDL2 levels in rhesus monkeys (*Macaca mulatta*). Am. J. Physiol. 273, E714–E719.

Visscher, T.L., Seidell, J.C., 2001. The public health impact of obesity. Annu. Rev. Public Health. 22, 355–375.

Walford, R.L., Weber, L., Panov, S., 1995. Caloric restriction and aging as viewed from Biosphere 2. Receptor 5, 29–33.

Wan, R., Cutler, R.G., Mattson, M.P., 2002. Periodic fasting enhances cardiovascular and neuroendocrine stress adaptation in rats. FASEB J. submitted.

Weindruch, R., Sohal, R.S., 1997. Seminars in medicine of the Beth Israel Deaconess Medical Center. Caloric intake and aging. N. Engl. J. Med. 337, 986–994.

Yellon, D.M., Dana, A., 2000. The preconditioning phenomenon: a tool for the scientist or a clinical reality? Circ. Res. 87, 543–550.

Young, D., Lawlor, P.A., Leone, P., Dragunow, M., During, M.J., 1999. Environmental enrichment inhibits spontaneous apoptosis, prevents seizures and is neuroprotective. Nat. Med. 5, 448–453.

Yu, Z., Luo, H., Fu, W., Mattson, M.P., 1999. The endoplasmic reticulum stress-responsive protein GRP78 protects neurons against excitotoxicity and apoptosis: suppression of oxidative stress and stabilization of calcium homeostasis. Exp. Neurol. 155, 302–314.

Yu, Z.F., Mattson, M.P., 1999. Dietary restriction and 2-deoxyglucose administration reduce focal ischemic brain damage and improve behavioral outcome: evidence for a preconditioning mechanism. J. Neurosci. Res. 57, 830–839.

Zhu, H., Guo, Q., Mattson, M.P., 1999. Dietary restriction protects hippocampal neurons against the death-promoting action of a presenilin-1 mutation. Brain Res. 842, 224–229.

List of Contributors

Robert Wolk, M.D., Ph.D.

Division of Hypertension
Division of Cardiovascular Diseases
Department of Medicine
Mayo Clinic
St. Mary's Hospital
DO-4-350
1216 Second Street SW
Rochester, MN 55902
Phone: 507-255-1144
Fax: 507-255-7070
Email: wolk.robert@mayo.edu

Virend K. Somers, M.D., Ph.D.

Professor of Medicine
Division of Hypertension
Division of Cardiovascular Diseases
Mayo Clinic and Mayo Foundation
200 First St. SW
DO-4-350
Rochester, MN 55905
Phone: 507-255-1144
Fax: 507-255-7070
Email: somers.virend@mayo.edu

Naohiko Sakai, M.D., Ph.D.

Assistant Professor
Department of Internal Medicine and Molecular
  Science
Osaka University Graduate School of Medicine
2-2 Yamadaoka, Suite, Osaka 565-0871 Japan
Phone: 81-6-6879-3732
Fax: 81-6-6879-3739
Email: naosakai@imed2.med.osaka-u.ac.jp

Makoto Nishida, M.D., Ph.D.

Department of Internal Medicine and Molecular
  Science
Graduate School of Medicine
Osaka University
2-2 B5 Yamadaoka, Suite
Osaka 565-0871, Japan
Email: makoton@imed2.med.osaka-u.ac.jp

Yuji Matsuzawa, M.D., Ph.D.

Professor and Chairman
Department of Internal Medicine and Molecular
  Science

Graduate School of Medicine
Osaka University
2-2 B5 Yamadaoka, Suite
Osaka 565-0871, Japan
Email: yuji@imed2.med.osaka-u.ac.jp

Shizuya Yamashita, M.D., Ph.D.   Associate Professor
Department of Internal
    Medicine and Molecular Science
Graduate School of Medicine
Osaka University
2-2 B5 Yamadaoka, Suite
Osaka 565-0871, Japan
Email: shizu@imed2.med.osaka-u.ac.jp

Guha Krishnaswamy, M.D.   Professor of Medicine and Chief, Clinical
    Immunology Section Chief, Division of
    Allergy and Clinical Immunology
Division of Allergy/Immunology
James H. Quillen, V.A. Medical Center
Department of Medicine
East Tennessee State University
P.O. Box 70622
Johnson City, TN 37614-0622
Phone: 423-439-6282
Fax: 423-439-6387
Email: krishnas@etsu.edu

Daniel Dube, M.D.   Clinical Instructor
Department of Internal Medicine
James H. Quillen College of Medicine
East Tennessee State University
P.O. Box 70622
Johnson City, TN 37614-0622
Phone: 423-439-6283
Fax: 423-439-6387
Email: sijipunda@yahoo.com

Mark Counts, M.D.   Fellow, Division of Cardiology
Department of Internal Medicine
James H. Quillen College of Medicine
East Tennessee State University
P.O. Box 70622
Johnson City, TN 37614-0622
Phone: 423-232-4884
Fax: 423-232-4886
Email: zmdc6@etsu.edu

David S. Chi, Ph.D.

Professor, Medicine/Immunology Chief,
   Division of Biomedical Research
Department of Internal Medicine
James H. Quillen College of Medicine
East Tennessee State University
P.O. Box 70622
Johnson City, TN 37614-0622
Phone: 423-439-6382
Fax: 423-439-6387
Email: chi@mail.etsu.edu

Bernd van der Loo

Division of Cardiology
Cardiovascular Center University Hospital,
   Zurich
Raemistrasse 100 CH-8091
Zurich, Switzerland
Phone: 41-1-255-2121
Fax: 41-1-255-4251
Email: bernd.vanderloo@DIM.usz.ch

Thomas F. Lüscher, FACC,
   FRCP

Professor and Head of Cardiology
Division of Cardiology
Cardiovascular Center University Hospital
Raemistrasse 100
CH-8091
Zurich, Switzerland
Phone: 41-1-255-2121
Fax: 41-1-255-4251
Email: cardiotfl@gmx.ch

Stefano Taddei, M.D.

Department of Internal Medicine
University of Pisa
Via Rome 67
56100
Pisa, Italy
Phone: 39-050-551110
Fax: 39-050-553407
Email: s.taddei@med.unipi.it

Agostino Virdis, M.D.

Department of Internal Medicine
University of Pisa
Via Rome 67
56100 Pisa, Italy
Phone: 39-050-992558
Fax: 39-050-553407
Email: a.virdis@med.unipi.it

Lorenzo Ghiadoni, M.D., Ph.D.   Department of Internal Medicine
University of Pisa
Via Rome 67
56100 Pisa, Italy
Phone: 39-050-992914
Fax: 39-050-553407
Email: l.ghiadoni@med.unipi.it

Guido Salvetti, M.D.   Department of Internal Medicine
University of Pisa
Via Rome 67
56100
Pisa, Italy
Phone: 39-050-992558
Fax: 39-050-553407

Daniele Versari, M.D.   Department of Internal Medicine
University of Pisa
Via Rome 67
56100
Pisa, Italy
Phone: 39-050-992558
Fax: 39-050-553407
Email: dversari@supereva.it

Antonio Salvetti, M.D.   Department of Internal Medicine
University of Pisa
Via Rome 67
56100
Pisa, Italy
Phone: 39-050-992558
Fax: 39-050-553407
Email: a.salvetti@med.unipi.it

Yusuke Ohya, M.D., Ph.D.   Department of Medicine and Clinical Science
Graduate School of Medical Sciences
Kyushu University
Maidashi 3-1-1, Higashi-ku
Fukuoka, 812-8582 Japan
Phone: 81-92-642-5256
Fax: 81-92-642-5271
Email: ohya@intmed2.med.kyushu-u.ac.jp

Masatoshi Fujishima   Department of Medicine and Clinical Science
Graduate School of Medical Sciences
Kyushu University

Maidashi 3-1-1, Higashi-ku
Fukuoka, 812-8582 Japan

Emily Wilson, Ph.D.

Department of Medical Physiology and
   Cardiovascular Research Institute
College of Medicine
Texas A&M University System Health Science
   Center
336 Reynolds Medical Building
College Station, TX 77843-1114
Phone: 979-862-8673
Fax: 979-847-8635
Email: emilyw@tamu.edu

Gerald A. Meininger, Ph.D.

Department of Medical Physiology and
   Cardiovascular Research Institute
College of Medicine
Texas A&M University
   System Health Science Center
336 Reynolds Medical Building
College Station, TX 77843-1114
Phone: 979-845-7491
Email: gam@tamu.edu

Edward J. Lesnefsky

Division of Cardiology, Department of Medicine
Department of Medicine
Case Western Reserve University
Medical Services and Geriatric Research
Education and Clinical Center
10701 East Boulevard
Cleveland, OH 44106

Bernard Tandler

Department of Medicine
Case Western Reserve University
Medical Services and Geriatric Research
Education and Clinical Center
Louis Stokes Veterans Affairs Medical Center
10701 East Boulevard
Cleveland, OH 44106

Shadi Moghaddas

Division of Cardiology, Department of Medicine
Case Western Reserve University
Medical Services and Geriatric Research
Education and Clinical Center
10701 East Boulevard
Cleveland, OH 44106

Medhat O. Hassan

Department of Medicine
Case Western Reserve University
Medical Services and Geriatric Research
Education and Clinical Center
Louis Stokes Veterans Affairs Medical Center
10701 East Boulevard
Cleveland, OH 44106

Charles L. Hoppel

Division of Clinical Pharmacology
Department of Medicine
Department of Pharmacology
Education and Clinical Center
Louis Stokes Veterans Affairs Medical Center
10701 East Boulevard
Cleveland, OH 44106
Phone: 216-791-3800 x5657
Fax: 216-707-0254
Email: clh5@po.cwru.edu

Marsha P. Cole, Ph.D.
   Candidate

Graduate Center for Nutritional Sciences and
   Toxicology
University of Kentucky
800 Rose Street
444 Health Sciences Research Building
Lexington, KY 40536-0305
Phone: 859-323-6190
Fax: 859-323-1059
Email: mpcole00@uky.edu

Luksana Chaiswing, Ph.D.
   Candidate

Department of Pathology and Laboratory
   Medicine
William S. Middleton Memorial Veterans
   Administration Center
University of Wisconsin Medical School
Madison, WI 53705
and Faculty of Medical Technology
Mahidol University
Bangkok, Thailand 10700
Phone: 608-256-1901 x. 11715
Fax: 608-280-7087
Email: koymu@hotmail.com

Terry D. Oberley, M.D., Ph.D.

Department of Pathology and Laboratory
   Medicine
William S. Middleton Memorial Veterans
   Administration Center
University of Wisconsin Medical School

Madison, WI 53705
Phone: 608-256-1901 x. 11722, 608-265-6080
Fax: 608-280-7087, 608-265-6215
Email: toberley@facstaff.wisc.edu

Kelley K. Kiningham, Ph.D.

Department of Pharmacology
Joan C. Edwards School of Medicine
Marshall University
Huntington, WV 25704
Phone: 304-696-7314
Fax: 304-696-7391
Email: kiningham@Marshal.edu

Daret K. St. Clair

Department of Toxicology
University of Kentucky
363 Health Sciences Research Building 0305
Lexington, KY 40506-0305
Phone: 859-257-3956
Fax: 859-257-3955
Email: dstc100@pop.uky.edu

Joseph M. Rifkind

Molecular Dynamics Section
Gerontology Research Center
National Institute on Aging
National Institutes of Health
5600 Nathan Shock Drive
Baltimore, MD 21224
Phone: 410-558-8168
Fax: 410-558-8323
Email: rifkindj@grc.nia.nih.gov

O. O. Abugo

Molecular Dynamics Section
National Institute on Aging
National Institutes of Health
5600 Nathan Shock Drive
Baltimore, MD 21224

Enika Nagababu

Molecular Dynamics Section
National Institute on Aging
National Institutes of Health
5600 Nathan Shock Drive
Baltimore, MD 21224

Somasundaram Ramasamy

Molecular Dynamics Section
National Institute on Aging
National Institutes of Health
5600 Nathan Shock Drive
Baltimore, MD 21224

Andrew Demehin

Molecular Dynamics Section
National Institute on Aging
National Institutes of Health
5600 Nathan Shock Drive
Baltimore, MD 21224

Rajadas Jayakumar

Molecular Dynamics Section
National Institute on Aging
National Institutes of Health
5600 Nathan Shock Drive
Baltimore, MD 21224

Marco Cattaneo, M.D.

Hematology and Thrombosis Unit
Department of Medicine, Surgery and Dentistry
Ospedale San Paolo
University of Milano
Via di Rudini, 8
20142 Milano, Italy
Phone: 39-3497554504
Fax: 39-025516093
Email: fede.lussana@tisaclinet.it

Federico Lussana

Hematology and Thrombosis Unit
Department of Medicine, Surgery and Dentistry
Ospedale San Paolo
University of Milano
Via di Rudini, 8
20142 Milano, Italy

James M. May

Diabetes Research and Training Center
Department of Medicine
715 Preston Research Building
2220 Pierce Avenue
Vanderbilt University School of Medicine
Nashville, TN 37232-6303
Phone: 615-322-2197

Raymond F. Burk

Department of Medicine
715 Preston Research Building
2220 Pierce Avenue
Vanderbilt University School of Medicine
Nashville, TN 37232-6303
Phone: 615-343-7740
Email: raymond.burke@vanderbilt.edu

Brian M. Dixon

Molecular and Cellular Biology Program
Linus Pauling Institute
Oregon State University

571 Weniger Hall
Corvallis, OR 97331-6512
Phone: 541-737-8003
Fax: 541-737-5077
Email: dixonb@bcc.orst.edu

Swapna V. Shenvi　　　Molecular and Cellular Biology Program
Linus Pauling Institute
Oregon State University
571 Weniger Hall
Corvallis, OR 97331-6512
Phone: 541-737-8003
Fax: 541-737-5077
Email: shenvis@onid.orst.edu

Tory M. Hagen, Ph.D.　　　Assistant Professor, Editor
Department of Biochemistry and Biophysics
Linus Pauling Institute
Oregon State University
571 Weniger Hall
Corvallis, OR 97331-6512
Phone: 541-737-5083
Fax: 541-737-5077
Email: tory.hagen@orst.edu

Mark P. Mattson　　　Series Editor
National Institute on Aging
Gerontology Research Center
Laboratory of Neurosciences
5600 Nathan Shock Drive
Baltimore, MD 21224
Phone: 410-558-8463
Fax: 410-558-8465
Email: mattsonm@grc.nia.nih.gov

Advances in
Cell Aging and Gerontology
Series Editor: Mark P. Mattson
URL: http://www.elsevier.nl/locate/series/acag

Aims and Scope:

Advances in Cell Aging and Gerontology (ACAG) is dedicated to providing timely review articles on prominent and emerging research in the area of molecular, cellular and organismal aspects of aging and age-related disease. The average human life expectancy continues to increase and, accordingly, the impact of the dysfunction and diseases associated with aging are becoming a major problem in our society. The field of aging research is rapidly becoming the niche of thousands of laboratories worldwide that encompass expertise ranging from genetics and evolution to molecular and cellular biology, biochemistry and behavior. ACAG consists of edited volumes that each critically review a major subject area within the realms of fundamental mechanisms of the aging process and age-related diseases such as cancer, cardiovascular disease, diabetes and neurodegenerative disorders. Particular emphasis is placed upon: the identification of new genes linked to the aging process and specific age-related diseases; the elucidation of cellular signal transduction pathways that promote or retard cellular aging; understanding the impact of diet and behavior on aging at the molecular and cellular levels; and the application of basic research to the development of lifespan extension and disease prevention strategies. ACAG will provide a valuable resource for scientists at all levels from graduate students to senior scientists and physicians.

Books Published:

1. P.S. Timiras, E.E. Bittar, *Some Aspects of the Aging Process,* 1996, 1-55938-631-2
2. M.P. Mattson, J.W. Geddes, *The Aging Brain,* 1997, 0-7623-0265-8
3. M.P. Mattson, *Genetic Aberrancies and Neurodegenerative Disorders,* 1999, 0-7623-0405-7
4. B.A. Gilchrest, V.A. Bohr, *The Role of DNA Damage and Repair in Cell Aging,* 2001, 0-444-50494-X
5. M.P. Mattson, S. Estus, V. Rangnekar, *Programmed Cell Death, Volume I,* 2001, 0-444-50493-1
6. M.P. Mattson, S. Estus, V. Rangnekar, *Programmed Cell Death, Volume II,* 2001, 0-444-50730-2
7. M.P. Mattson, *Interorganellar Signaling in Age-Related Disease,* 2001, 0-444-50495-8
8. M.P. Mattson, *Telomerase, Aging and Disease,* 2001, 0-444-50690-X
9. M.P. Mattson, *Stem Cells: A Cellular Fountain of Youth,* 2002, 0-444-50731-0
10. M.P. Mattson, *Calcium Homeostasis and Signalling,* 2002, 0-444-51135-0
11. T. Hagen, *Mechanisms of Cardiovascular Aging,* 2002, 0-444-51159-8

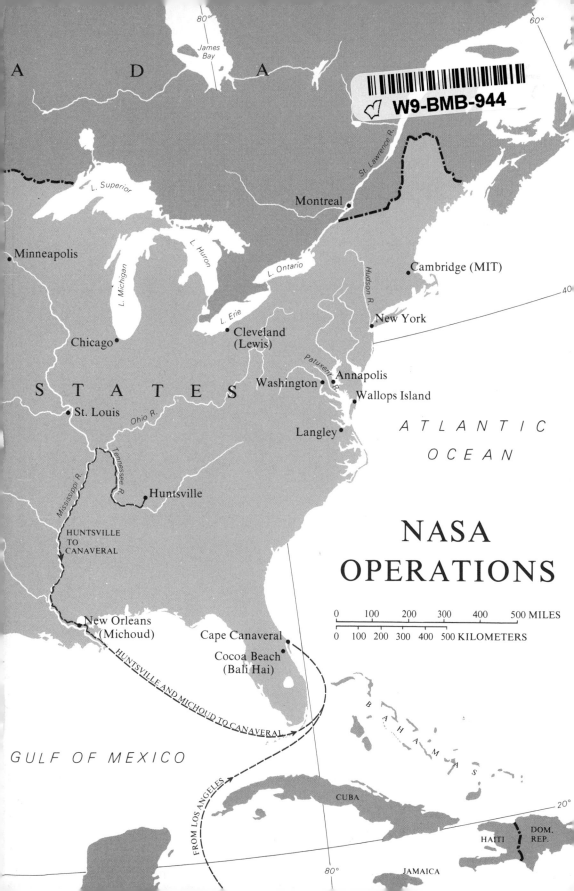

James Bay

A   D   A

L. Superior

Minneapolis

L. Huron

L. Michigan

L. Ontario

Montreal

St. Lawrence R.

Hudson R.

Cambridge (MIT)

L. Erie

New York

Cleveland (Lewis)

Chicago

S T A T E S

Patuxent R.

Annapolis

Washington

Wallops Island

Ohio R.

St. Louis

Langley

ATLANTIC

Tennessee R.

Mississippi R.

OCEAN

Huntsville

HUNTSVILLE TO CANAVERAL

NASA

OPERATIONS

New Orleans (Michoud)

Cape Canaveral

HUNTSVILLE AND MICHOUD TO CANAVERAL

Cocoa Beach (Bali Hai)

0	100	200	300	400	500 MILES

0	100	200	300	400	500 KILOMETERS

B A H A M A S

FROM LOS ANGELES

GULF OF MEXICO

CUBA

DOM. REP.

HAITI

JAMAICA

SPACE

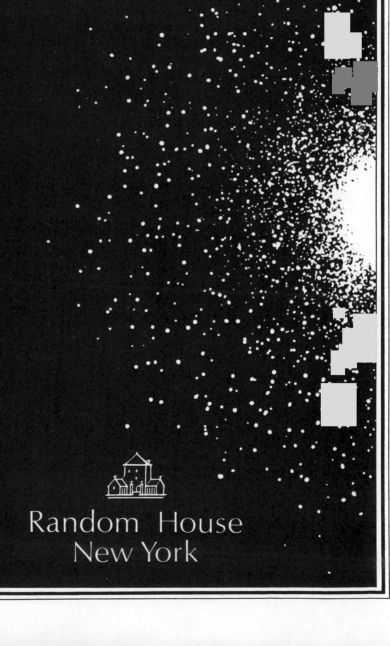

Random House
New York

S P A C E

JAMES A.
MICHENER

Library of Congress Cataloging in Publication Data

Michener, James A. (James Albert), 1907–
Space.

I. Title.
PS3525.I19S6 1982   813'.54   82–40127
ISBN 0–394–50555–7
ISBN 0–394–52764–X (lim. ed.)

Manufactured in the United States of America

2 4 6 8 9 7 5 3

FIRST EDITION

Cartography by Jean Paul Tremblay
Book design by Carole Lowenstein

ACKNOWLEDGMENTS

On 4 July 1976 I was invited by Dr. Donald P. Hearth of the National Aeronautics and Space Administration to participate in a round-table discussion of the meaning of America's Viking landing on Mars, and with that heady introduction to the greatest minds of the space age I began my serious study.

In the spring of 1979 I was appointed to the NASA Advisory Council, which advises NASA, and there I met repeatedly with men who conducted our space effort, and visited several times the great NASA bases at which the work was done. I was allowed to participate in the full life of the agency. I did this uninterruptedly for four years.

Lacking specialized training in science, I was disadvantaged, but my long experience with mathematics and astronomy repaired some of the deficiency, and my work with various aspects of our program repaired other gaps. Most of all, I talked incessantly with experts, visited laboratories, and studied procedures.

My acquaintance with NASA engineers and scientists was extensive, and to them I owe a great debt, especially those at Langley, Wallops, Ames, Houston, Huntsville, Goddard and the Jet Propulsion Laboratory.

My acquaintance with astronauts was more spotty, for I met only those who bumped into me as I went about my other duties. Deke Slayton was most helpful. John Young was an inspiration. Donn Eisele, a neighbor, gave me many insights. Because the Shuttle dominated the horizon in the years of my incumbency, I knew its pilots: Robert Crippen, Joe Engle, Dick Truly. Ed Gibson was extremely helpful in my study of the Sun, about which he has written brilliantly. Joe Kerwin, a medical astronaut with weeks in orbit, was unusually helpful on four different occasions. I had brief but rewarding interviews with Mike Collins, a graceful writer about space, and the two elegant women astronauts Judith Resnick and Anna Fisher.

At headquarters I was accorded courtesies by Dr. Robert Frosch, the administrator, and by Dr. Alan Lovelace, his assistant. They made available the consultative services of General Harris Hull, Dr. John Naugle, NASA's chief scientist, Nat Cohen, the executive secretary of our council, and Jane Scott, who supervised my movements. Before his untimely death in the Himalayas, Tim Mutch met with me many times to discuss scientific and managerial points.

Certain experts were recommended to me as unusually informed and helpful in their fields, and to these I am indebted:

Battle of Leyte Gulf: Admiral Felix Stump, who commanded one of the baby flattop squadrons in that historic naval engagement, and Bill Lederer, his witty assistant.

Peenemünde: Dr. Ernst Stuhlinger and Karl Heimburg, both of whom made the hegira from Peenemünde to El Paso to Huntsville.

Patuxent River: Marshall Beebe, USN, who explained the area in 1952. Admiral John Wissler, who showed me around in 1981.

Operation of a Large NASA Base: The following were especially instructive during my extended stay at the Marshall Space Flight Center in Huntsville: Dr. William Lucas, James E. Kingsbury, Thomas Lee, Robert Lindstrom, John Potate, Harry Watters, Joe Jones.

Mission Control Operations: Dr. Chris Kraft, the distinguished expert who handled the major sequence of flights; Gene Krantz, in charge of present flights, who allowed me to to sit in for an entire day to watch how it was done.

Astronomy: Dr. George Field, Dr. A. G. W. Cameron, both of Harvard; Dr. David L. Crawford, Kitt Peak; Dr. Jacques Beckers of the Multiple Mirror Telescope Observatory, Tucson; Dr. Anthony Jenzano, University of North Carolina.

Communications: Dean Cubley of Houston.

Lunar-Orbit Rendezvous: Dr. John C. Houbolt of Langley, who led the fight for this mode.

Supersonic Flight: John V. Becker of Langley, who pioneered this field.

Wind Tunnels: William P. Henderson of Langley, who twice demonstrated his 16-foot tunnel.

One-Sixth Gravity: Donald E. Hewes of Langley, who invented the device for creating an approximation of Moon gravity on Earth.

Interplanetary Navigation: Frank Hughes, Richard Parten, Duane Mosel, all of Houston. Frank Jordan of JPL. Dr. Philip Felleman of MIT was especially instructive.

Image Processing: Torrance Johnson of JPL.

Space Telescope: Dr. C. R. O'Dell, of the University of Chicago and Huntsville.

Earth Handling of Messages from Space: William Koselka and Chuck Koscieliski of the Goldstone Station in California; at the NASA stations in Australia, Lewis Wainright, Thomas Reid and Kevin Westbrook were helpful, and Bill Wood in Canberra provided living quarters.

Interplanetary Exploration: Charlie Hall and C. A. Syvertson, both of Ames, who were responsible for developing and supervising several pioneer missions to Jupiter and Saturn.

Life on Other Planets: Dr. Carl Sagan of Cornell, who has written brilliantly on this arcane subject.

I am particularly indebted to the following distinguished scholars and administrators who agreed to read portions of the manuscript to help me weed out error. They gave help beyond the call of duty or friendship. Such errors as remain are my fault.

Korea Air Battles and Patuxent River Test-Piloting: Captain Jerry O'Rourke, USN, who taught me dive-bombing in 1953 for my early novel *The Bridges at Toko-Ri* and who conducted a seminar for me in 1981 regarding Patuxent River and test pilots.

Wallops Island and Atmospheric Research: Abe Spinak, long an official on the island and a formidable research man.

Photo Imaging on the Mars and Saturn Expeditions: Dr. Bradford A. Smith, University of Arizona, who served as Imaging Team Leader during the Voyager missions to Jupiter and Saturn.

Solar Flares: Dr. Jack Eddy, High Altitude Observatory, one of our leading authorities on solar physics.

Circadian Rhythms: Dr. Richard J. Wurtman, Massachusetts Institute of Technology.

Technical Communications between Flight Control at Houston and the Astronauts of Gemini 13 and Apollo 18: Joe Kerwin, who served as CapCom during the fateful aborted flight of Apollo 13.

Medical Data Regarding Apollo 18: Joe Kerwin, astronaut and medical doctor.

Movement of Earth and Sun: Dr. A. G. W. Cameron, Harvard University, kindly read the brief but important section on multiple movements.

The Entire Manuscript: John Naugle, who lived at the heart of NASA operations for many years and who first suggested that I try to write this book. He taught me a great deal.

I shall always remember with affection and envy those brilliant men who served on the Advisory Council or who participated in our various seminars, and who gave me so much help in understanding the things they were talking about: Freeman Dyson of Princeton, Arthur Kantrowitz of Dartmouth College, John Firor of the National Center for Atmospheric Research, Daniel Fink of General Electric, George Field and A. G. W. Cameron of Harvard, who helped especially in advanced astronomy, and the three aeronautical experts who proved instructive in this field which concerns me deeply: Robert Johnson of Douglas Aircraft, Holden Withington of Boeing, and everybody's friend and counselor, Willis Hawkins of Lockheed. My special appreciation to William Nierenberg, Director of the Scripps Institute of Oceanography, who chaired our group. I never had an abler group of colleagues.

JAMES A. MICHENER
St. Michaels, Maryland
February 2, 1982

CONTENTS

This is a novel and to construe it as anything else would be a mistake. The Mott, Grant, Pope and Kolff families are imaginary and are based upon no real prototypes. The Solid Six group of astronauts did not exist, nor was there any Gemini 13 or Apollo 18.

However, the great NASA bases, the Patuxent River experience, the battle operations in Korea and the general activities of the astronauts are realistically presented.

Certain historical personages do appear briefly, such as Lyndon B. Johnson, President Eisenhower, Secretary Wilson, the astronauts Deke Slayton and Mike Collins, and the scientists Jack Eddy, John Houbolt and Carl Sagan, but they are not given fictitious roles or inflated speeches.

The Battle of Leyte Gulf and the behavior of the admirals, American and Japanese, are faithfully reported. There was no destroyer escort *Lucas Dean,* but there were warships like it, and its exploits are not exaggerated. The major bombing of Peenemünde occurred as stated in August 1943 and was an exclusive British affair, but there were follow-up bombings the next year and I have expanded one of these. Generals Breutzl and Funkhauser are imaginary, but of course, Wernher von Braun was real and even more powerful and impressive than I state.

SPACE

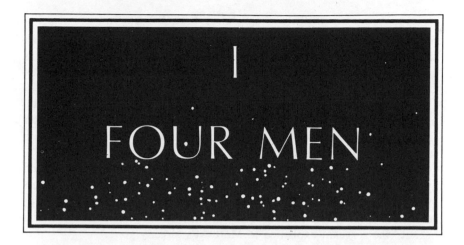

I
FOUR MEN

ON 24 OCTOBER 1944 PLANET EARTH WAS FOLLOWING ITS ORBIT about the sun as it has obediently done for nearly five billion years. It moved at the stunning speed of sixty-six thousand miles an hour, and in doing so, created the seasons. In the northern hemisphere it was a burnished autumn; in the southern, a burgeoning spring.

At the same time, the Earth revolved on its axis at a speed of more than a thousand miles an hour at the equator, turning from west to east, and this produced day and night.

As a new day broke over the Philippine Islands, two navy men, one Japanese, one American, were about to perform acts of such valor that they would be remembered whenever the historic battles of the sea were compared and evaluated.

Later, when the ceaseless turning of the Earth brought high noon to the island town of Peenemünde on Germany's Baltic coast, a small, quiet mechanical genius working for Adolf Hitler would find himself in the middle of an ordinary day which would have a most extraordinary conclusion.

A few hours following, when midafternoon reached London, a youthful American engineer, not in uniform, would see for himself the power of Hitler's vengeance weapon, the A-4, and would take steps to destroy it but not its makers, because even then the American government could foresee that when the war ended, they would need these German scientists.

And toward the close of that long day, when the Earth had revolved the western region of America into the hours of sunset, in a small city in the state of Fremont a boy of seventeen would experience three resplendent moments, and would realize as they were happening that they were special in a way that might never be exceeded.

.   .   .

In the early afternoon of that October Tuesday, Stanley Mott, an American civilian twenty-six years old, displayed a sense of almost frantic urgency as he watched the radar screen at a tracking station thirteen miles south of London.

'It's coming!' an English sergeant cried, trying vainly to keep the excitement out of his voice. And there on the screen, as Mott watched, the sinister signal showed, a supersonic, unmanned monster bomb coming at London from some undetermined spot in Holland.

Even on the radar it displayed its silent speed, more than two thousand miles an hour. It would not be heard at this station until some moments after it had passed. Then sonic booms would thunder through the air, reassuring the listeners that this bomb at least had passed them by. 'If you hear it,' the sergeant explained to Mott, 'it's already gone.'

In the fragile moments of final silence, everyone in the room listened intently for the tremendous sound which would indicate that the rocket bomb had struck, and sensitive devices were pointed toward London. K-k-k-krash! The bomb had fallen. The listeners turned antenna to new directions and soon an ashen-faced young man from Oxford University announced: 'The heart of London. But I do believe east of Trafalgar Square.'

'Hurry!' Mott snapped, and within three minutes he and the Oxford man and a driver were speeding toward London with a set of red cards showing on their windshield, allowing them to pass roadblocks and salute policemen who barred certain thoroughfares. 'Bomb squad,' the Oxford man called as the car sped past. This was not exactly true. He and Mott were not qualified to defuse unexploded bombs, as the real squad did; they collected data on the damage inflicted by these new and terrible bombs which Hitler was throwing at London in what he boasted was 'our act of final revenge.'

From the manner in which confusion grew as the car approached the area leading to Trafalgar Square, it was apparent that the trackers had been correct; the rocket had landed in the vicinity but well to the east. This was confirmed when wardens shouted, 'It landed in the City.'

Then apprehension doubled, for this meant that the crucial business heart of London, termed the City, was once more in peril. The Bank of England, St. Paul's, the Guildhall, from which Churchill spoke—how Hitler would gloat if his spies wirelessed tonight that one of these enticing targets had been struck, how smug Lord Haw-Haw would sound as he ticked off the losses on the midnight radio.

But when the weaving car entered Cheapside—with the driver crying 'Bomb squad! Bomb squad!'—Mott and the Oxford man saw with relief that the symbolic targets had once more been miraculously spared, but this discovery gave them short comfort, since they must now inspect the hideous consequences of wherever the bomb had fallen.

'Many lives gone this time,' muttered an elderly warden with pale face and drooping mustaches. He led the way through to a gaping hole where a short time before a small news kiosk had served businessmen working in the City. It and the shops near it had been eliminated—erased and fragmented as if made of sticks—with all their clerks and customers dead.

'I don't know which is worse,' Mott said to the Oxford man. 'That ghastly hole in the ground or the splinters of wood and bone.'

'Thank God, that monster in Berlin doesn't have fifty of these to send at us every day,' the English expert muttered.

'How many have hit London?' Mott asked.

'If my count is correct, this is only number seventy-three. Since September, when they started. Something's badly wrong with the German supply system.'

'Our bombing of Peenemünde is what's wrong,' Mott said. 'Your boys have wrecked their hatching ground.'

'Let's be grateful for that,' the Englishman sighed as he poked among the wreckage for any shreds of the bomb. His team was still not quite certain how the horrible thing operated. 'You know, Mott, before they started to arrive, we calculated Hitler could throw a hundred a day right at the heart of London. One hundred thousand civilians dead each month. We've been lucky. We've been terribly lucky.'

'How many dead here?'

The two experts consulted with wardens and came up with a figure of less than fifty, and when Mott repeated the number, almost with a sense of gratification, the Oxford man gave a convulsive sob. 'Look at one of the fifty,' and he pointed to the body of a young girl who had been serving in the shop of a tobacconist. She was torn apart, but her head was untouched and her pretty face was still smiling, or so it seemed.

Mott looked away. Seeking out a member of the real bomb squad, he asked professionally, 'Did you recover any metal parts? Any at all?'

'Total fragmentation,' the man said.

'Damn. Always we work in the dark.' He kicked at some rubble, gave a last survey of the wreckage, and stepped aside as hospital orderlies moved in to start recovering bodies.

'Shall we go on to Medmenham?' the Oxford man asked.

'That we shall,' Mott said. 'We'll hit those Nazis tonight with such a rain of destruction they'll forget London.' He looked up at the sky and said, 'Moonlight will be good till ten o'clock. Stand back, Hitler, you bastard.'

They sped from London on an emergency route leading to the west, and three times they crossed the winding River Thames, beautiful in its autumn coloring, with great trees crowding its rural banks. Heading in the direction of Windsor Castle and Eton, they could make excellent time, since the roads were free of traffic, and soon they were turning off onto a country lane that led to a remarkable site at which a remarkable meeting was about to take place.

Medmenham, a rustic village, was the site of England's ingenious Air

Force Signal Center, where data on the bombing of Germany were evaluated. Some of the brightest men and women in the world, English mostly but with a cadre of Americans and French, grabbed at aerial photographs as the plane crews delivered them and then made sophisticated calculations of the damage that had been inflicted. At Medmenham, as one watched these clever people at work, one got the feeling of a Germany that was being slowly strangled and reduced to rubble.

Tonight, the brightest of the Allied minds had assembled in a temporary shed to study just one set of photographs: those showing the German rocket site at Peenemünde, in former times a trivial summer resort located on a small island facing the Baltic Sea. If the German wizards at Peenemünde were allowed to proceed freely with their experiments and their manufacturing genius, London would be destroyed—and after that, New York and Washington.

'It could be the major target in the world,' an American Air Force general was saying when Stanley Mott joined the group. 'What's the word from Washington?'

'I bring a straightforward commission. Peenemünde is to be erased. Forget the other targets.'

'That we can't do,' an English general interrupted. 'You Americans with your heavy bombers are free to go at Pennemünde. We encourage you to strike at the breeding ground. But we British, with London in such peril . . . We must try to eliminate the actual launch sites. What news of the latest rockets?'

Mott said, 'About an hour ago one landed in Cheapside. Almost equidistant from the Bank of England, St. Paul's and the Guildhall. Hit a tobacconist's.'

'God must be with us,' the general said, then quickly: 'How many dead?'

'Less than fifty.'

The room fell silent. These men knew what the word *fifty* meant, the tragic reverberations outward to the families of the dead.

'So you will appreciate,' the English general said, 'when I insist that we must continue to seek out and destroy the launching sites.'

The American general, who seemed to be acting as chairman of the meeting, nodded. 'You do your job, we'll do ours. And tonight ours is Peenemünde.'

'Before we start on that,' an English civilian said, 'I'd like to show you these latest photographs of the area just north of The Hague. This little town is Wassenaar, and we feel sure that those shadows indicate a rocket-launching site. If we can knock that out within the next few days, we think we can drive the rocket operation back out of London range.'

'What is the effective range?'

'We don't know, of course, but we calculate two hundred and twenty miles, maximum.'

A different American general asked contemptuously, 'You mean Hitler has wasted all his energy—Peenemünde . . . the whole snakes' nest—on a rocket that can strike only two hundred miles? The man must be an idiot.'

'We know he's an idiot,' the English general said, 'but a damned lethal one. Our planes must concentrate on Wassenaar.'

An English civilian coughed. 'There's a problem. Wassenaar is a residential town. If we saturate . . .'

'I know,' the English general said. 'I know damned well what the problem is, and frankly, it's a cruel one. Advice?'

A different civilian interrupted an officer who was about to respond: 'We've consulted the Dutch government—secretly, of course. One of their men is waiting outside.'

'Bring him in,' the American general said.

A fifty-year-old Dutchman appeared in civilian clothes. Seeing the generals, he saluted. 'My name is Hegener. I go in and out of the Netherlands. Regularly . . .'

Mott thought: It's like saying I go in and out of New York. Regularly. By the Hudson Tunnel. But what a hell of a difference. He wondered how Hegener went in and out. In by parachute? Out by darkened motorboat?

'My government has studied the problem,' Hegener said, 'and we believe Wassenaar must be saturated.'

No one spoke. There was nothing to be said. Permission had been granted to take radical steps that might save the English city of London, but everyone in the room knew what penalties the Dutch town of Wassenaar must pay. It was a total war, which these men were determined to win because to lose would mean total hell. And now Wassenaar had moved into the front lines.

'Thank you, Mr. Hegener,' someone said, and the Dutchman rose to go.

'Do you live near Wassenaar?' an American asked.

'Oh no! I live well to the north in a fishing village on Texel. But it would be the same.'

When he was gone, the American general said, 'Agreed. Your planes to knock out Wassenaar. Ours to take care of Peenemünde. And we start tonight.'

'Is the raid set for tonight?' Mott asked. He seemed unusually young to be questioning a four-star general, but he worked in a field of such recent origin that most of its practitioners were young. Mott, for example, was by no means an expert in either rocketry or the work being done in atoms, but he was a solid engineer with a marked capacity for adjusting to any radical scientific developments.

'Yes, we're launching three hundred and ninety-four bombers at Peenemünde at 2100 hours. From sixteen different airfields. Led by four highly trained British pathfinders who've been there before. Tonight we knock out Herr Hitler's rocketry.'

This news presented Mott with so many problems that for the moment he could not sort them out, so he sat silent, studying his fingertips. He was about to ask that the room be cleared of all but the very top generals and experts, when the British leader said brightly, 'Gentlemen, I believe they're ready for us at the mess. To those of you who haven't been here before, we have a surprise in store. Fletcher, will you explain?'

As the men gathered their papers, almost every one top secret, an attractive woman in uniform stepped forward and said in beautifully arranged words, 'A patriotic gentleman has given us his estate for our mess. Danesfield his house is called, just a stone's throw down there. It's rather something and not at all what we have regularly, I assure you. It was built in the 1890s by a Mr. Hudson, who had the good fortune to invent and sell our most popular soap, Sunlight.' At this name several men chuckled.

'When Mr. Hudson grew tired of his mansion, he passed it along to a Mr. Gorton, who was also lucky. He invented and sold H. P. Sauce, and he was even richer than Mr. Hudson. He had twenty-one gardeners and forty-six servants. Gentlemen, you are going to dine in one of the stately homes of England.'

Stanley Mott, son of a Methodist minister in a small New England city and a graduate of Georgia Tech, was not prepared for Danesfield. The gray-stone building was immense, with a garage area larger than most mansions; ten apartments stood over what had been the stables; they were now occupied by Air Force drivers and mechanics. The hall itself contained forty-six bedrooms, in which the bright young men of the Signal Center slept, but it was the pair of rooms in which the officers would dine that stunned the Americans.

The first, a kind of reception-hall–dance-hall–living area, had a ceiling thirty feet high, a gigantic fireplace and a minstrels' balcony from which a six-piece military band played English airs as if a duke and his duchess were entertaining in 1710. Officers assigned here led the visitors through this enormous room and into the dining hall, a place of such brilliance that Mott could merely shake his head in wonder.

It was sixty feet long, with a green marble fireplace at one end, each part carved like a work of art. One wall contained four enormous bay windows that gave a view of the Thames below, but the extraordinary feature was the dining table. It could seat as many as seventy if the chairs were close together, and every item on it seemed to gleam: the napery, the china, the silverware. Forty-six men and four women sat down to dinner, served by enlisted men who had been waiters in private life.

The pace was leisurely, the talk civilized, the food reasonably good and the music from the minstrels' balcony lively. It was impossible to believe that these diners were dedicated solely to the defeat of Adolf Hitler.

But as the evening progressed, Stanley Mott began to get his ideas organized, and before the dessert was served he knew what he must do. Moving to the side of the American general, he whispered, 'I think you and six or seven of the top brains—'

'Not before the toast to the King.'

'Sir, I have the gravest information—'

'It can wait fifteen minutes.'

'Sir, it pertains to tonight's raid.'

The general turned abruptly, looked at Mott, whom he had never seen before this evening, and asked, 'That serious?'

'It is, sir.'

The general coughed. 'Archie, I wonder if we could speed this up?'

'Assuredly.' The English general indicated that the waiters should bring the dessert without clearing the table entirely, and when this was done, hastily, the men ate the quivering jelly with dispatch and leaned back as the American general rose and said, glass high, 'Gentlemen, the King!' When the toast was drunk, the British general rose, raised his glass, and said, 'Gentlemen, the President of the United States!'

As soon as the ceremonies ended, Mott said, 'Not more than eight of us.'

'Good,' the American general said, and forthwith he nominated the team, including three British civilian experts. The seven men and one woman—four military, four civilian—returned to the hut where the maps were and began their solemn discussion.

Mott spoke first. 'Gentlemen and madam, it is absolutely essential that we destroy Peenemünde.'

The English general interrupted: 'In the big meeting I kept my mouth shut. But actually, with the destruction we've already done to Hitler's rocket-building capacity, we think that Peenemünde has been fairly neutralized.'

Now Mott was on the griddle and he squirmed. His task was most difficult, for he was privy to data which no one else in this room knew or could appreciate. That Peenemünde as the cradle of German rocketry had been pretty much sidetracked by the swift progress of the war, he had to concede. The massive English raids of a year ago had wrecked it temporarily, and tonight's follow-up was intended merely to keep it off balance. The fearful rocket menace that Peenemünde had once threatened had been moved to other sites, and these men knew it.

But Peenemünde as the center for research in heavy water was a much different matter. Peroxide, as the English insisted on calling it, might prove to be the material which would enable the Germans to construct a bomb of radically different character, an atomic bomb if you will, one of which could destroy all of London in a single, searing blast. Mott could not be sure that Germany actually had a process for making heavy water, a most important agent which resulted when hydrogen atoms were displaced by deuterium. He only suspected that if the process did exist, it was functioning at Peenemünde, and he was not at all sure that if the Nazi scientists had the water, or peroxide, they would know how to convert it into a bomb.

So he opened the discussion gingerly: 'Gentlemen, we have reason to think that the Germans have developed at Peenemünde a process for making heavy water.'

'Oh dear,' one of the British civilians said. 'Not that silly-water nonsense again?'

Another said, 'I thought we'd disposed of that monster-bomb theory a long time ago.'

Mott said, 'I grant you, we have nothing positive on this. But our people think that if even the remotest chance exists—'

'Mr. Mott,' the American general interrupted with some impatience, 'I've already told you, we're going to bomb the living hell out of that place. What more do you want?'

Mott was a member of an adroitly assembled team; when they met in the White House, President Roosevelt chuckled. 'You look properly nondescript. All types. All ages.' Only five had specific scientific backgrounds: two university professors of atomic physics and three bright fellows from something called The Manhattan Project. The other six were a mixed bag: two businessmen, two military men in uniform, an FBI man, and to confuse enemy spies, Stanley Mott from Georgia Tech, youngest and by far the most disarming.

Roosevelt had told them two things: 'America is about to produce a master weapon. And we have reason to believe that at Peenemünde, Hitler is doing the same.'

Concerning this basic secret the eleven were forbidden to divulge anything, but all were quietly at work. Some had already been parachuted onto the Continent. Others were being moved about by submarine. And Mott was in London, where he would probably not be noticed. On this important night he began cautiously, revealing only permitted data: 'President Roosevelt has sent my team to Europe with a simple directive. We must destroy Peenemünde, whether it has a rocket capacity or not. And in doing so, we must under no circumstance allow our bombs to strike the living areas.'

The English general threw up his hands. 'Damn it all, in our early raids, they were the principal targets.'

'And thank God you missed,' Mott said sharply.

'Yes, we did,' the Englishman said. 'We had bad luck with our pathfinders. They laid their flares too far north.'

The American general looked at his watch. 'Our men take off in two hours. The living areas are heavily targeted.' He dropped his head slightly, so that his eyes stared straight out from under heavy eyebrows. 'Why are we to avoid them this time, Mr. Mott?'

He almost spat out the last words, displaying the contempt which an older military man usually felt for any intruding younger civilian, and one of the English civilians noticed this. 'Professor Mott, please explain.' And another civilian, catching the problem, said, 'Yes, elaborate, Professor Mott.'

Mott never used his title, earned with distinction in graduate work at Lousiana State, where he had taught the fledgling science of aeronautics, and he certainly avoided mentioning his undergraduate college, for he was tired of clever men who chanted:

'I'm a rambling wreck from Georgia Tech
And a hell of an engineer.'

But now when these accusing generals, so much older and heavy with braid, heckled him, asking if he was really a professor, he felt he must inflate his record. 'Indeed I am, in advanced aviation theory.' Actually, he taught the beginners' course.

'Clarify your point, Professor.'

Slowly and carefully Mott looked at each of the seven. He must say enough to convince them, not enough to betray his major secret. He coughed and clasped his hands nervously, all his actions calculated to gain him a respectful hearing. 'There are three men living in the Pennemünde camp tonight whose safety is absolutely vital to the free world. I think you can guess why.'

'Let me try,' an older English civilian said. 'You Americans and we English are pitifully far behind in rocketry. We're seeing what can be accomplished with the first generation of German rockets. And we fear the Russians are far ahead of us. So that in the postwar world . . .'

'There are three German scientists we must keep alive until they reach our lines,' Mott said. 'Count Wernher von Braun, a relatively young man who seems to be the genius of the rocket operation. My job from here on out is to get him safely to our side. Then we badly need General Eugen Breutzl. He's the managerial genius. We have reason to believe he's not a Nazi, just a technical wizard who could move our program ahead by generations. And the third man is a shadowy fellow. Name seems to be Dieter Kolff, if we have it correct. He's about thirty-five years old, and the reason we must get him is that he may prove to be the real genius of the team. He's their expert on the A-10.'

'What's that?' a civilian asked. 'Our information doesn't go beyond the A-6.'

'Well,' Mott said, as if consulting with a seminar of extremely gifted graduate students, 'you're the world's experts on the A-4, which you call the V-2. You know about the next in line, the bigger versions up through the A-6 and perhaps A-7. But we have fairly solid information that this quiet expert Kolff, if he really exists, is specializing on the A-10.'

'And what is that?' the same civilian pressed.

'It's the one that can hit New York. Fired from Germany.' There were several gasps, after which he said, 'Yes, A-10 or something like it is only a short time down the road.'

'I should think you'd want to wipe out the living quarters above all else,' the English general said. 'Exterminate such vermin.'

'No! No!' Mott protested. 'Because neither you nor we know how to make a rocket that will carry a bomb even ten miles. And we have reason to believe that the Russians are about to come up with one that will fly a thousand.'

'So you think that we must keep these three men alive?' the American general asked.

'It is vital.'

'Then why in hell do we bomb the place at all?'

And that was the question which could not be answered openly. Mott retreated rather lamely to the heavy water. 'To eliminate a short-range danger, we've got to knock out the heavy-water capacity. To protect our long-range security, we've got to save those three German scientists.'

'Professor Mott,' the general snorted, 'you sound like a damned fool. To break this on us at takeoff time for a major strike.'

'I feel like a fool,' Mott conceded. 'But have we a safe phone? Please instruct your pathfinders to lay their guidance flares well away from the living quarters.'

'We can do better,' the English general said. 'Young Merton, who will fly as tonight's coordinator, is waiting outside.'

Master Bomber Merton was twenty-three years old, a blond young man weighing less than a hundred and forty. He would have been out of place as a junior master in a classroom of unruly boys, but tonight he proposed to fly unaccompanied across the North Sea to Peenemünde, where he would circle aloft for nearly two hours, radioing instructions to the four English pathfinder planes as to where they should drop their flares, and then to the oncoming American bombers as to how they should launch their devastating bombs. The fate of three hundred and ninety-eight planes would rest in his hands; he would be responsible for the future of German rocketry, German heavy-water bombs, if they existed, and the security of the free world. He grinned boyishly and seemed shy in the presence of so many experts.

The woman photographic analyst moved to the wall and pulled aside white linen sheets that hid the target maps for Peenemünde, the little island nestled along the Prussian shore. It resembled a fetus, a monstrous thing brought to birth by mad scientists, and at the far northern end stood the launching sites for the great rockets that had alarmed the world. The test stands for the engines were clearly designated, as were the command headquarters and the army barracks. In green, well down on the island, clustered the buildings labeled SCIENTISTS' HOUSING, and it was to these that she pointed.

'We have solid evidence from both our photographs and prisoner interrogations that the scientists you seek do indeed live here. We believe their housing was moved south after our big raids of last year.'

'If there were heavy-water experiments under way,' Mott asked, 'where would they center?'

'When we had the abortive peroxide scare a year ago—'

'It was not abortive,' Mott said sternly.

'We found nothing,' the woman continued, unruffled. 'But we guessed that it would have been up here.'

'That's where we're concentrating tonight,' Master Bomber Merton said.

'And that's what must be avoided,' Mott said almost pleadingly.

'We can place the bombs anywhere you like,' Merton said enthusiastically. 'But you must tell us.'

Before Mott could respond, the American general stared at the two young men from beneath his heavy brows. 'Is Washington committed to this strategy?'

'It is,' Mott said quietly. 'I'm one of eleven men directed to spend the rest of the war trying to salvage those three Germans. Von Braun, Breutzl, Kolff. General, we must have them.'

There was a protracted silence, during which Mott wished that he could divulge what he had learned on the sand flats of New Mexico: that the United States had progressed far beyond the heavy-water principle and was in position to construct an atom bomb even more powerful than speculation had predicted. World terror was possible. It might arrive at any moment, from Russia, from Germany, from New Mexico. All things were in flux, and any nation that managed even a week's lead over the others would have an advantage of stupefying magnitude. The bomb that these men scoffed at was a reality, or almost so, and the likelihood that Germany might be first to launch it, and with rockets that could not be intercepted, was so awful to contemplate that everything possible must be done to interdict it.

Please, please, Mott thought, make these men accept partial evidence. They'll see the actuality all too soon.

'It sounds like an asinine proposition,' the American general said. 'Bomb hell out of an island, but don't touch the bottom half.'

'Sometimes,' the English general said consolingly, 'we're forced to adopt half-measures. To keep the whole in balance.'

'What do you mean?' the American asked.

'Surely I don't want to waste my heavy bombers striking at a temporary target like the Wassenaar launch site. You know we should be concentrating on knocking out the heavy industry. But Churchill has to give evidence to the citizens of London that we're doing everything we can to protect them from Hitler's rockets.' He paused and turned to Mott. 'How many people was it we lost today?'

'About fifty.'

A Royal Air Force man shook his head. 'If we know about it, all London knows about it. Fifty more dead. And the other day smack into a cinema. Two hundred dead that time. So we have to bomb Wassenaar.'

'Is this line safe?' the Master Bomber asked.

'Yes.'

Merton spoke with his people at Benson Air Force Base in the direction of Oxford, and Mott could hear him planning the night as if it were a game: 'Four pathfinders will find me already over the target. You'll drop your flares well away from the living quarters marked in green. Plenty of moonlight. Plenty of visibility. Ten minutes after you leave, the Moon will set and it will be dark. Then the Yanks come on. I'll vector them in, but they must not overshoot the flares. Is that understood? Roger and out.'

Visualizing both the German A-4 rockets and the monstrous American bombers, Mott wondered at the curious and self-defeating decision made by Adolf Hitler. One of his famed rockets could deliver about a ton of explosive, and never on a precisely determined target, while an American bomber, which cost about the same as a rocket, could drop six tons within a closely defined area.

At first glance it seemed that Hitler had made a hideously wrong choice, but Mott also knew that before long the Germans would have stouter rockets capable of delivering eight and ten tons of explosives, and his secret briefings had caused him to fear that within the year someone would have a new kind of bomb which would be calculated in the million-ton range, and someone else would have rockets which could deliver such a bomb across the Atlantic.

These were the days of awesome decision, and he watched with relief as Master Bomber Merton put down the phone, tapped the map, and said cheerily, 'Whatever they have hiding at Peenemünde, it gets a thrashing tonight.' And off he went to direct his hornets to a target which might or might not be fabricating heavy water to be used in an atomic bomb which might or might not be completed in time to annihilate London within the near future.

When he departed, Mott sighed. The hiding place of Von Braun, Breutzl and Kolff would be spared for one more night.

'Was it really so important, Professor Mott?' one of the American generals asked.

'The security of the world might well depend upon what we accomplish this night.'

On this same afternoon of 24 October 1944 the remnants of the Japanese Imperial Navy, badly battered by incessant American pressure, launched one of the most daring ventures in the history of naval warfare. It was a do-or-die effort made inescapable by General MacArthur's recent surprise landing in the Philippines. Japanese intelligence saw quickly that MacArthur's forces were not well secured and that a bold strike might drive them from the Philippines, bloody MacArthur's nose, and give Japan a year's respite to strengthen its homeland defenses.

This stupendous effort of throwing every available fighting ship and airplane against the Americans was called Sho-Go (Operation Victory) and its success depended upon the resolute performance of three war-hardened admirals who had been asked, each one separately, to perform a miracle. The top planners had every reason to believe that Sho-Go would drive the Americans from the sea, and humiliate MacArthur once again.

Sho-Go had three simple principles, the intermeshing of which would ensure a surprising victory. The entire surviving fleet would be divided into three parts, each with a totally different responsibility. The North Fleet, under the command of Admiral Ozawa Jisaburo, would sail down from Japan, allow itself to be seen, and then toy around north of the Philippines in hopes that Admiral Halsey would be tricked into rushing north with the bulk of the American fleet. These ships constituted a decoy which, because it would be outnumbered if Halsey fell into the trap, could expect to lose many of its major components. To make the bait more alluring, this fleet brought with it four huge carriers on the principle that 'Admiral Halsey can never resist going for our carriers.' They would be especially vulnerable.

The South Fleet drew the suicide mission. It would form off Borneo, well to the south of the Philippines, steam north, keeping to the coast of Asia, and then come sweeping east to pick its way through a narrow strait, which, if negotiated, would throw the great battleships and cruisers right onto the lap of MacArthur's shorebound men. But to accomplish this, the South Fleet would have to break through a relatively small American defensive fleet that would probably be alerted and waiting at the exit from the strait. That a naval battle of tremendous magnitude must take place, there was little doubt, and the Japanese admiral in charge of this fleet had good reason to suppose that by nightfall on 25 October he and all his ships would be dead.

He was Nishimura Teiji, a man without fear. He had fought his ships bravely in many battles and expected to continue doing so, whatever Sho-Go directed him to do. With consummate skill he sneaked his battle line up from Borneo, around the southern Philippine Islands and into the narrow strait that would lead him to MacArthur's beachhead. As dusk fell he prayed to his Shinto gods of war that no American fleet would be waiting for him at the exit, but as a sensible man he realized that this was a forlorn hope.

The two feints, one to the north, the other to the south, and each extremely dangerous, had been set in motion in order to spring free the redoubtable Central Fleet, which would leave from Singapore, steam north at flank speed, cut boldly east, and come crashing through the formidable San Bernardino Strait, which the American command had long ago decided was too perilous for any warships to negotiate. The job of bringing a major fleet—five massive battleships, twelve heavy cruisers, fifteen destroyers, all with enormous firepower—through waters deemed impossible to navigate was given to the boldest admiral of the three, Kurita Takeo, a man of medium height and modest weight, with a close-cropped bulldog head. On the eve of battle he told his commanders, 'I expect every one of our ships to steam through San Bernardino Strait without incident, and then to fall upon the enemy and drive him from the Philippines.' He led the way, moving at a speed that would have been incomprehensible, in these narrow waters, for a small fishing boat. Thirty-one major warships followed in line. If they broke through and if the American Halsey was lured north with his major fleet, and if Admiral Nishimura used his South Fleet to divert the other warships in the area, Admiral Kurita's powerful force would find only a phantom American fleet to confront it: a few baby aircraft carriers, a few small destroyers. These could easily be sunk, and then General MacArthur would be driven from his beachhead and perhaps even carried as prisoner to Tokyo.

Dusk on 24 October was a time of silent apprehension, for one of the greatest naval battles in world history was about to erupt: three separate Japanese fleets against three separate American fleets. A capricious fate had determined that no one of the Japanese fleets would meet an American force of comparable size and power. The individual battles were going to be terribly unfair, and not always in favor of the Americans. By dawn on 25 October, General MacArthur's fingerhold on the Philippines could well be in mortal peril.

It fell to Admiral Nishimura, leading the South Fleet, to feel the first taste of battle. Curiously, the Americans, despite their superiority in air power and their prudent use of scouting planes, did not detect the movements of either the Central Fleet or the South, and these massive forces were left free to move into their straits as they wished, but two American submarines, always on the prowl, by the sheerest luck were loitering along the very path that Admiral Nishimura was following, and with skill and courage they pumped torpedoes into one of his big ships. Before the battle was engaged, he had suffered a dreadful loss, but a much worse problem lurked at the exit from the strait.

Since the beginning of naval warfare, admirals had known that there was one condition to be avoided, and every ensign learning the rules of war had memorized the truism: 'Never let the enemy cross your T.' The same young men, when they had mastered this lesson, dreamed of the day when by clever maneuvering they could cross the enemy's T, for then victory was assured. Don Juan of Austria, half brother of Philip II of Spain, had crossed the Turkish T at the battle of Lepanto in 1571 and altered the history of the Mediterranean. Lord Nelson had crossed the French T and saved England. At Jutland in World War I the British crossed the German T to save Europe.

Of course, in 1944, with battleships having airplanes to scout for them, it was preposterous for naval men to still dream of crossing the enemy's T,

but some did, and among them was Admiral Jesse Oldendorf, commander
of the American battleships prowling the other end of Admiral Nishimura's
strait on the slight chance that the Japanese might be attempting to force
it.

As the bombers heading for Peenemünde on this night had discovered,
there was a half-Moon casting considerable light, but at dusk it stood right
at the apex, and before midnight it would disappear, leaving the sky dark.
Admiral Nishimura, heading straight for the waiting Admiral Oldendorf,
counted on this darkness to obscure the Japanese warships, and it did, so
on he plowed at a speed which terrified some of his subalterns.

The crossing of a T consisted of this. The enemy fleet must be in file,
one behind the other and in such position that its ships cannot easily or
quickly move up one beside the other. They form the stem of the T, and
for reasons which will be explained, are cruelly vulnerable. The attacking
fleet must be in line, which means that every gun on a given side of the ships
can bring to bear upon the lone enemy ship at the head of the file, whereas
this exposed target can bring its guns to bear on only one of its tormentors.
And as soon as the first enemy ship is sunk, which it will surely be when
facing such concentrated firepower, the next ship in file moves into the lead,
where it finds fifteen or twenty enemies waiting.

In the hours before sunrise, when the sea was dark and the Japanese ships were in file, one behind the other, Admiral Oldendorf crossed
their T.

Not often in naval history had there been a major battle in which the
forces were so ill-matched. Admiral Nishimura would exit the strait with
only seven ships: two major battlewagons, a cruiser and four destroyers. He
would be faced by overwhelming American strength: six major battleships
with terrifying names like *Maryland, West Virginia* and *Tennessee,* four
heavy cruisers, each more powerful than some battleships, four light cruisers and an amazing twenty-eight destroyers. This meant that the Japanese
were outnumbered 42 to 7. In addition, the Americans had forty-five small
and lively PT boats to sting and harass the enemy, forcing him to break up
his orderly approach.

The battle was joined in pitch-darkness, beginning at three o'clock in the
morning, a condition which Nishimura preferred because he knew that in
previous night battles the Japanese had usually bested the Americans, who
did not seem to know how to conduct themselves in darkness.

This time they did. As Nishimura led his small fleet toward open water,
American destroyers, bewildering in their abundance, slashed at him,
throwing his ships once more into confusion, slowing some down and
crippling others.

Then, from a distance of eleven miles, without seeing the Japanese fleet
and guided only by radar, the mighty guns of the American battleships
opened up, and whenever they paused, the eight cruisers took over, including the Australian *Shropshire.* Among them, the six battleships carried

more than three thousand heavy shells, which they threw with deadly accuracy until the night sky was illuminated with gunfire and towering explosions from the doomed Japanese fleet.

Nishimura Teiji died with his ships. From the moment Sho-Go was explained, he had known that when he exited from the strait, something would be waiting for him, but even in his most pessimistic moments he had not dreamed that his T would be crossed by six major battleships and eight monstrous cruisers. He lost six of his seven ships; the Americans lost none. It was a loss without parallel in recent naval history, but it was also a suicide venture which amounted to victory, since Nishimura had accomplished precisely what had been required of him. He had kept the big American warships bottled up at the south, leaving General MacArthur's troops on Leyte exposed to the Japanese Central Fleet when it broke through. A survivor from Nishimura's flagship reported that the little admiral had stood calmly on the bridge of his ship as it sank, obviously content that he had done his job.

The North Fleet had also gained a victory, in a manner of speaking, for Admiral Ozawa Jisaburo had tricked Admiral Halsey into running far to the north to take the bait which the Japanese had dangled before him, leaving the Leyte landings unprotected.

It was a tempting lure that Ozawa offered: a major Japanese fleet consisting of eighteen warships, including four of Japan's greatest aircraft carriers. Had Halsey refused this challenge, even though responding to it did imperil MacArthur's landing, he would have been a naval idiot. So after the most delicate weighing of alternatives, and fully aware of what he was doing, Bull Halsey roared north, taking with him an American fleet of staggering size: six great battleships like the *Iowa,* the *New Jersey* and the *South Dakota;* ten aircraft carriers like the *Essex,* the *Enterprise* and the *Lexington;* eight cruisers; and forty-one destroyers. Once more the Japanese were outnumbered, 65 to 18, but this had been intended.

What was not intentional was the lamentable fact that the four great Japanese carriers, deadly terrors in the early days of the war, were now without planes. This vast fleet could put into the air only fifteen airplanes, and since they were manned by untrained pilots, even these would soon be shot down; whereas the ten American carriers had a plethora of planes with superbly trained pilots to fly them. So in the second battle here at the north, like the first at the south, the imbalance between the two fleets was staggering, and Admiral Ozawa knew as day broke on 25 October that he, too, was engaged in a suicide mission. His task was simple: keep Halsey engaged, while sacrificing as few ships as possible.

Then came the slaughter. Halsey, convinced that the outcome of the Pacific war depended upon his knocking out the Japanese carriers, fell on them remorselessly. The battle had scarcely begun when the swift carrier

Chitose absorbed a hellish concentration of bombs, sinking at 0937. At 1018 the battle-hardened *Chiyoda* lay dead in the water and had to be abandoned; she would sink at 1630. At 1414 the monstrous *Zuikaku,* one of the most powerful carriers in the world, rolled over and sank. At 1526 the mighty *Zuhio* was attacked by twenty-seven American planes and sank under the weight of their bombs.

The guts of the North Fleet had been eviscerated, and Halsey's big warships were free to move close and finish off the remaining fourteen Japanese ships. It was apparent that only a naval miracle could save the Japanese fleet, and now just such a miracle occurred.

Admiral Halsey, gloating in his flag command quarters, began receiving anguished messages from Leyte Gulf, where a disaster of such enormous dimension had overtaken the American forces that General MacArthur's position was in mortal danger. Halsey was confronted by a cruel choice: stay north, finish off Ozawa's fleet, and terminate Japan's naval threat; or speed south to help avert disaster. His whole inclination was to stay north and destroy Japan's capabilities, and this would have been the correct decision. Left to himself, he would surely have chosen that alternative.

But now one of the sardonic mischances of warfare intervened to trick him into the wrong decision: he received a garbled interrogation from Honolulu. When sending important coded messages it was the custom in the United States Navy to preface crucial details with nonsense words and to close with others. This yielded a twofold advantage: it required the enemy to waste time trying to decipher the entire jumble, and when the operation was ended and its details known, it prevented him from making clever guesses as to which coded word had meant which salient fact. A well-constructed Navy message might read CHICAGO WHITE SOX FOUR CLEVE-LAND INDIANS TWO LANDING ON BOUGAINVILLE AT 0730 ZEBRA GET THEE TO A NUNNERY.

Admiral Nimitz, in Honolulu, watching the course of this great battle —to be termed later by historians as 'the greatest sea battle in the long history of naval warfare'—realized that Halsey's flight to the north had imperiled the operation, leaving MacArthur in jeopardy, and when he saw the danger imposed by Japan's Central Fleet, he rushed Halsey an urgent message: WHERE IS TASK FORCE 34?—referring to the portion of Halsey's fleet that was supposed to be guarding the center. The sending signalman properly opened the message with nonsense words: TURKEY TROTS TO WATER, which was traditionally digressive, but unfortunately he ended with a flourish acquired in some English class, and this could be read as part of the message: THE WHOLE WORLD WONDERS.

The unfortunate addition would still have been harmless if the receiving signalman had done what he was supposed to do, knock off the irrelevant beginning and ending phrases, but he was confused by the close relationship of the last two phrases and handed Admiral Halsey this message from headquarters: WHERE IS TASK FORCE 34? THE WHOLE WORLD WONDERS.

Halsey could interpret this only as a rebuke and possibly as a veiled attack upon his honor; because of his headstrong behavior, he had left a detachment of the American fleet in mortal danger.

In disgust and dismay, he turned away from the crippled Japanese North Fleet, which could now escape to safety, and sent his battleships south on what he knew would have to be a futile mission. If conditions in Leyte Gulf were as perilous as the messages reported, his battleships would arrive far too late to be of any good. At this sad point in the great battle he realized that he had been tricked; Admiral Ozawa, that canny master of naval deception, had dangled before him four aircraft carriers that were largely useless, with no planes, pilots or aviation gasoline. Even if Halsey had not attacked them, they would have died of their own strangulation.

So the Japanese won the first two engagements in this running battle, even though the cost had been suicidal. Nishimura had tied down the American battleships in the south, Ozawa those in the north. Now everything depended upon Admiral Kurita Takeo of the Central Fleet, and rarely in history did any admiral enjoy such an untrammeled opportunity to crush a major adversary.

Admiral Kurita launched his triumph in high style. After fighting off numerous American aviation attacks without losing one ship, he personally led his huge, powerful fleet in one of the notable maneuvers in naval history, bringing it safely through the narrow strait which the Americans had deemed impassable, considering it far too narrow and dangerous to permit the passage of a destroyer, let alone a battleship.

But Kurita was lucky, bringing with him a most formidable string of warships: five of the most powerful battleships, whose guns were of greater caliber than the Americans', eleven massive cruisers and fifteen destroyers. This fleet of thirty-one sturdy, well-manned ships could confront any adversary.

It was amazing what they did confront. With Halsey taking his six battleships north, and Oldendorf taking his six south, none was left for the middle. Nor were there any cruisers. Nor any large aircraft carriers. Nor any of the really big new destroyers.

What was there? A ragtail collection of small, thin-shelled, lightly armed, slow-moving baby aircraft carriers, called 'Jeeps' or 'baby flattops,' intended for unopposed antisubmarine patrol or the support of Army troops ashore. There were sixteen of these, each with one futile five-inch gun and a limited supply of all-purpose ammunition, which meant that it suited no specific purpose at all. To protect the defenseless baby flattops, there were nine moderate-sized destroyers and twelve sharply undersized craft called destroyer escorts, whose name correctly defined their duties. They were not intended for major battle.

In the DE *Lucas Dean,* built in a hurry in Bremerton nine months

before, the captain was Norman Grant, USNR, actually a thirty-year-old
lieutenant commander and a beginning lawyer from the western state of
Fremont, a man who had never seen the ocean before he volunteered for
the Navy to escape being drafted into the Army. Grant was the first American officer to spot the oncoming Japanese fleet as it moved through the early
dawn. Controlling his emotions, he signaled the admiral in charge of the
Escort Carrier Group: 'Major Japanese fleet exiting strait. Battleships,
cruisers.'

When planes confirmed the report, at 0647 on the morning of 25 October 1944, everyone in the little American fleet knew what was at stake.
Without heavy guns, without adequate torpedoes, and with no hope of
reinforcements from anywhere, these fragile ships must try to harass and
heckle and outguess a massive collection of warships and cruisers any one
of which had more fire power than what the Americans together could
muster. If the North and South Fleets of the Japanese had faced difficult
odds, this American fleet faced worse.

Nineteen-year-old Yeoman Tim Finnerty took down in shorthand what
Captain Grant said to the crew of the *Lucas Dean:* 'Men, we sailed all the
way from Seattle to take on the Japs. Here they come. Let's give a manly
account of ourselves.' And then, as the notes indicate, he gave his first order:
'Hard right rudder.' Since he and nine-tenths of his crew of 329 were
landlubbers, it was customary aboard the *Lucas Dean* to use simple *left* and
right instead of *port* and *starboard;* hardly anyone aboard the little DE
could have explained those nautical terms, or any others.

The sixteen little carriers were spread far apart, in three groups, each
with its own destroyers to protect it. Captain Grant's DE was attached to
the first group, the one nearest the oncoming enemy, so, as part of the
screen, he would be among the earliest to encounter Japanese fire.

Then came the order: 'DDs move out.' This meant that the three heavier
destroyers, those with the best chance of surviving hits from the Japanese
guns, would make the first runs, discharging their torpedoes into the path
of the oncoming fleet, then hoping to retire.

The men of the *Lucas Dean* lined the decks of their ship to watch the
opening maneuvers, and were disgusted to think that they were being held
in reserve while the bigger DDs sped directly at the enemy, throwing a
smoke screen to hide themselves from the Japanese gunners. But as the
Dean's men watched, they heard a mighty sigh of wind, saw briefly four
monster shells come at them and land resoundingly in the water, throwing
such giant concussions that the little DE was thrown about as if it were a
leaf on a turbulent lake.

'Look!' a sailor named Parker shouted. 'They're coming at us in tech-
nicolor.'

He was right. To aid in spotting the effectiveness of fire, each side used
heavy dyes of six or seven different colors. These first ones were red and
green, their splashes leaping fifty and sixty feet in the air.

'It's Christmas!' Finnerty shouted, and men looked strangely at one another as the red and green water came down upon them.

In a kind of glazed trance that might have been identified as cowardice, Captain Grant watched the DDs as they headed directly at the Japanese cruisers that led the enemy attack, and it staggered him to think that those small DDs should volunteer to throw themselves at all this might in order to give the American carriers just a few more minutes to escape southward. Since he spoke to no one, his men could not guess at his thoughts, nor predict what he might do when orders came for them to speed out to face the enemy.

There was no time for such speculation, because another salvo of four gigantic shells bracketed the *Lucas Dean,* throwing it about, and then Captain Grant came to his senses.

'Hard right,' he said in a calm voice, and when the third salvo from one of the Japanese battleships landed well aft of the *Lucas Dean,* he gave the order to swing in a tight circle and head directly for where that salvo had struck, on the principle that when the Japanese spotters saw the fountains of red and green marker-dye, they would correct their sights and not fire at the same spot again.

'Chasing salvos,' it was called, and Grant displayed an uncanny sense of when to move exactly into the middle of the last splash, and when to veer well away in some radical direction.

Then came the thrilling command: 'Small boys, move out!'

Over his intercom Captain Grant said, 'Here we go, right at them. Every man.' He did not finish his exhortation, for he knew it was not needed.

The *Lucas Dean* and three other small, fragile DEs leaped forward, abandoned the baby flattops, and sped directly at the oncoming battleships. It was preposterous, an act of insanity, boats so small against the mighty *Yamato, Musashi* and *Kongo,* but if the DEs could divert the battleships even momentarily, the American carriers might have a remote chance of escape. The gamble was that elements of Admiral Oldendorf's southern fleet would come roaring north, or some part of Admiral Halsey's big fleet might steam back to the rescue.

Because a constant rain of shells came at the *Lucas Dean,* the lead DE, Captain Grant had to dodge and duck, chasing salvos all over the sea, and this took him away from the other three little ships, so that when he was in position from which he might launch his torpedoes, he was alone, one small craft with three battleships coming at him in file.

'Gentlemen,' he announced quietly, 'we shall cross their T.' And that is exactly what he did. Starting from a point well to the east, he took the *Lucas Dean* on a course that carried him directly across the bow of the lead battleship, and when he had the three in the position he wanted them, he fired his entire spread of torpedoes.

Then came the most agonizing twelve minutes the crew of his DE would ever know, for it would take that long for the torpedoes to reach the battleships, and all the while the glorious fountains of color—red and green and blue and golden yellow—spouted about the little ship as the infuriated battleships fired at it. Ducking this way and that, Captain Grant evaded the salvos, keeping one eye always on the wake of his torpedoes.

'It takes a long time, sir,' Finnerty said, standing by with his notebook.

'Full speed astern!' Grant ordered, and the ship quivered as it halted in midflight, hesitated, and backed off while a mighty salvo landed a few yards ahead.

Now the *Lucas Dean* was doomed, for two cruisers had moved up to aid the battleships, and the bombardment became so intense that further escape was impossible. But then a low rain cloud swept in, coming from the west like a victorious runner. 'God, I hope it reaches us!' Finnerty cried.

'I hope it stays away till we see the torpedoes,' Grant prayed, and ignoring the incoming shells, he stared at the vanished wakes. 'Eleven minutes. Soon twelve.'

Peering under the clouds, he continued to stare at the Japanese ships. 'The BBs see our torpedoes,' he announced calmly, and the men watched as the big ships turned in what seemed like wild confusion. Turning to Finnerty, he directed him to write: 'All torpedoes ran hot and true. All missed.'

'Look!' the sailor Parker shouted. 'We hit a cruiser.' For only a second there was a distant roar, a towering geyser, and then the dark grayness of the saving cloud.

'We may have hit a cruiser,' Captain Grant told Finnerty, and Executive Officer Savage went among the men, shouting, 'We crossed their T.' He was right. One small ship with minuscule guns had driven the battlewagons into disarray, giving the baby flattops a few minutes of respite.

The four DEs turned in large circles and headed back to the flanks of the carriers, whose safety they were bound to defend, but they were rather useless there, so again came the command: 'Small boys, move out!' And once more Captain Grant and his men left the cover of their clouds, sped north, and engaged the great fleet bearing down upon the carriers.

Two of the DEs were promptly sunk by a hellish concentration of fire from the Japanese battleship and cruisers, and this left the forward carriers completely undefended, and unable to defend themselves. 'Bare ass to the wind,' it was called, and these carriers were just that. Each had one five-inch gun whose shells could not begin to pierce the steel plates of the Japanese ships. But in hopes that the meager weapon might do damage on deck, the baby flattops fired.

What happened in return was another miracle of warfare. The Japanese battleships turned their heaviest guns on the carriers, and the most exposed, the *Chesapeake Bay,* took four eighteen-inch shells at various parts of her deck, all within six minutes. But because the Japanese had expected to encounter American battleships, their guns were loaded with armor-piercing shells which would have created havoc had they struck the heavy plating of an American battleship, for then the steel-hard nose would cut through the deck, arm the fuse, and cause a gigantic detonation below.

When the same shells struck the paper-thin *Chesapeake* they screamed right through the ship, finding nothing hard enough to activate their fuses. When the sailors of the *Chesapeake* realized what was happening, one man cried, 'They're making Swiss cheese!' Four of the most powerful shells in the world had struck a Jeep carrier without causing a single casualty. There were, of course, eight gaping holes in the flattop, four where the AP shells entered, four where they left.

The *Lucas Dean* was not so lucky. With no more torpedoes to fire, it was only a partial warship, but Captain Grant was determined to use that part to maximum advantage. Throwing a heavy smoke screen, he dodged and zagged his way far forward until the ship reached a spot from which he could fire with some effect upon the smaller Japanese destroyers whose skins would not be thick enough to repel his shots. He fired sixteen times and accomplished nothing. But because he had taken a position close to the main Japanese fleet, the *Lucas Dean* had to be dealt with, and two cruisers came right at it, blazing harshly. Now there were no colored splashes, for the Japanese gunners could see their target, but there was still the game of chasing salvos, and Captain Grant played this to perfection, staying alive long enough to find shelter in another rain cloud.

But as he hid there, the Japanese cruisers could see what he could not: the cloud was extremely small, and the ship must be crouching somewhere within. Laying down a creeping barrage, the cruisers scored two hits, both fore, both devastating. However, the cloud remained long enough to give Grant sufficient time to survey the damage, and now he learned the rare quality of Mr. Savage, the executive officer, for this newly arrived Texan, who had never seen any ocean a year ago, took such complete command of emergency repairs that within half an hour the *Lucas Dean* was able to move under its own power, not fast but quite securely.

'What now?' Mr. Savage asked.

'Back to the wars,' Grant said.

'What else?' Savage replied.

Their DE could make only half-speed, and they had only a small portion of their ammunition left, but it was obvious that if they could in any way divert or harass the enemy warships, they might contribute slightly to the American position. So moving under protection of the rain clouds, they returned to the front and saw with extreme delight that American planes from the little carriers had begun all-out attacks on the Japanese ships. If the *Dean* could cause only a trivial confusion, it might be enough to make some Japanese ship falter, and slow down, and become a better target for the aviators. So Grant threw his little craft right at the heart of the oncoming Japanese fleet.

In the legends of many people one finds accounts of how the gods favored men of extreme bravery. The American Indians, the ancient Greeks, the Romans and the Goths all believed that if a man displayed unusual heroism, he would receive unusual protection . . . up to a point.

Norman Grant, a beginning lawyer with a wife he loved back in the small Western town of Clay, was such a man. When Finnerty asked him, as the *Lucas Dean* limped haltingly north, 'Do you intend to take on their whole fucking fleet?' he said, 'I do.'

For thirty-eight minutes this DE worked and wove its way as if it had a whole nest of torpedoes to discharge. It lobbed its few shells onto the decks of the much heavier warships, then walked the salvos back to safety. When it was clearly doomed, it found a rain cloud, and when two other equally heroic destroyers were shot out of the water, it somehow survived. It was a charmed ship, for the gods had taken it under their protection.

Every man aboard the *Lucas Dean* realized that their captain was proving himself to be a man of remarkable heroism, and some sensed that they, too, shared his courage. But heroism aboard a moving vessel is quite different from that required of a foot soldier, who can, if his spirit fails, run away. It requires true courage of monumental character for a soldier to stay and fight when he might flee, but aboard ship the captain merely points the bow in a certain direction, and no man on board can do a damned thing about it.

What caused Captain Grant to behave as he did that October morning? What produced in an ordinary lawyer from a small land-locked town in the West an impeccable sense of naval maneuvering? A chain of trivial incidents had linked together to make him the man he proved to be that day of battle:

> 1921, aged 7: His father speaking: 'You mustn't lie about the box of candy. If you took it, say so. No punishment I give you will ever be as bad as the punishment you will give yourself if you become a known liar.'

> 1932, aged 18: Mr. Stidham speaking: 'We are most pleased, Norman, that you're taking Elinor to the dance. Remember that we're placing her care in your hands. Home by one. And you don't have to prove that you can drive down a darkened road at seventy miles an hour.'

> 1941, aged 27: Head of the firm speaking: 'I tell each lawyer who joins our firm only once. Over the past two decades four lawyers in this county have gone to jail for misappropriating funds with which they were entrusted. And I've testified against three of them.'

> 1943, aged 29: Navy bo's'n speaking: 'By the old standards there isn't one of you men prepared to take charge of a Navy vessel. But I'm convinced you have character and courage, and that will suffice.'

. . .

Kurita's fleet contained one battleship the Americans desperately wanted to sink, the *Haruna,* veteran of many battles, and because of its emotional challenge, always a prime target. In the hideous days of late 1941 when America shivered in humiliation after Pearl Harbor and the Philippines, the nation sorely needed a hero, so enthusiastic public relations men concocted the doctrine that Colin Kelly, braver than most, had sunk the *Haruna.* Photographs of Kelly, his airplane and the destroyed Japanese battleship flashed across the world. But to the embarrassment of the Navy, in the next sea battle *Haruna* was there, spreading devastation.

But in that battle she was sunk again, after a vicious fight which the public relations men described in vivid detail. Of course, in the next battle she was present, her guns belching. Again and again she was sunk, and then again, but here, in late 1944, she was steaming menacingly right at the little carriers. A score of aviators, learning of her presence, vowed to sink her . . . for real.

'*Haruna* is mine!' one pilot from the carrier *Chesapeake Bay* shouted into his radio as he peeled off to smash her with his heavy bomb. In fact, he was so determined to do so that he followed his bomb almost down to the deck, and saw with pleasure that he had delivered a mortal blow.

'I've sunk the *Haruna!*' he shouted in plain speech. But the *Haruna* sailed on, directly at the *Lucas Dean.*

When Finnerty saw the monstrous battleship bearing down, about four miles distant, he gasped, 'Good God! Look!'

There was no way that the men of the *Dean* could determine that this was their hated enemy, and there was also no way that they could damage the perpetual survivor. But they could pretend that they had torpedoes, and if the oncoming battleship believed them, it might turn away and fall prey to the American airplanes aloft. So while shells fell about the damaged *Dean,* Captain Grant turned her broadside to the *Haruna* as if his tubes were filled with deadly fish.

He succeeded and he didn't succeed. The *Haruna* did turn aside, but as it did so it launched a fourteen-inch shell that landed just aft of the *Dean*'s tower, creating havoc.

The *Dean* was not blown apart, and it was in no immediate danger of sinking, but it was so sorely damaged that it had to retire, seeking what cover it could, and as it turned back in flight, as if it had been whipped by bigger boys, Captain Grant covered his face. He could visualize the terrible destruction the Japanese battleships would now wreak upon the baby flat-tops; he wanted to weep for the dead of this day, for the gallant hopes that had died with them. He and his men should have been able to hold back the enemy, protecting their part of the vast battlefront, but they had failed. There must have been something more he could have done, and in his failure he did not now want to see the destruction of his fleet. He was not a sailor. He was not a Navy man. He knew none of the traditions. But he did not want to lose his ship. He did not want to know the ignominy of defeat.

Then he heard one word. It was uttered in a Texas accent: 'Jesus!' He assumed that Mr. Savage had seen some final Japanese warship bearing down on them, and quickly he looked up to decide what steps to take in this last extremity, for he was determined that this little DE go down fighting.

'Look! Look!' Finnerty cried, and soon Savage was bellowing, 'Look at the bastards!'

When his eyes focused on the northern horizon, he saw a sight he could not believe. Admiral Kurita, with the entire American fleet defenseless and standing by for the slaughter, which would leave General MacArthur's forces on Leyte unprotected, had given the order for a general retreat. With victory assured, he fled the dangerous seas in which little ships had kept coming at him, no matter how many times they were hit.

'Finnerty,' Captain Grant said quietly. 'Mark this. At 0949 the Japanese fleet turned north and left the battle. The *Lucas Dean* has absorbed four major hits and can make only three knots, but she is still afloat.'

And then the gods had had enough. From out of the clouds to the west appeared a new type of warfare. It consisted of a Japanese dive bomber, manned by a single aviator wearing a white scarf decorated with a red rising sun. It was the first of a special breed of warrior, never before seen in warfare, and it came on and on, heading directly for the *Lucas Dean*.

It was a kamikaze, a plane and a man blessed before takeoff from a nearby land-based airfield. It was on a journey of no return, for the Japanese high command realized that if Sho-Go, their master plan, failed, they would be forced to rely upon other tactics.

'Shoot him down!' Mr. Savage screamed, but the bullets missed, their tracers showing high and low.

'Get that son-of-a-bitch!' Finnerty yelled at the gunners, but they could not adjust their guns to the resolute speed of this plane.

On and on it came, one small plane, one small man. In the end, just before the pair crashed into the *Dean*'s tower, the men of the *Dean* could see their enemy, a young Japanese, his face frozen into a horrible mask, his hands frozen to the controls.

There was a massive crash and an explosion of flame, which Mr. Savage's men might have controlled except that from the north came another kamikaze, headed straight for the *Dean*. It, too, avoided the gunfire, and at the last moment the sailors on the *Dean* could see its pilot's face, smiling, shouting, exultant, but they could hear no words, for almost instantly plane and man crashed into the port side of the DE, which exploded violently, broke in half and started sinking.

· · ·

When Captain Grant climbed into Life Raft Number Three he made a swift automatic survey of what was now his command station: Some food, less water, the three guns, no radio. When this was completed he started an assessment of the crew's condition, assisted by Pharmacist's Mate Penzoss, who had a clear understanding of what had happened during the wild two hours of the DE's rampage through the Japanese fleet: 'Original complement, 329. I counted at least forty dead before that last plane hit. Let's say ten more when she exploded. That makes fifty gone, 279 somewhere in the water.'

'How many went down with the ship?' Grant asked over his shoulder as he helped a swimmer climb aboard.

'Let's say fifty. So cut the number of swimmers to 229. How many here?'

Making a hasty count of the tangled bodies, Grant supposed that he had thirty aboard, including a dozen who were near death. Among those with lesser wounds was Tom Savage, the executive officer, whose face was very white.

'Where'd it get you, Tom?'

'A little fragment, must have been, here on the left side.'

Grant asked Doc Penzoss, a high-school graduate who dispensed aspirin and Atabrine, to look at the wound. 'Did it break a rib?'

'Don't think so.'

'Rescue craft'll pick us up before noon. We'll have a doctor look at you within the hour.'

Penzoss was called away from Captain Grant by cries from seamen who saw their comrades dying. He had one small bag of disinfectants and Syrettes and was determined to use them efficiently.

His place was taken by Yeoman Finnerty, who jotted in his notebook the figures that Captain Grant recapitulated: 'If all six life rafts got into the water, and if each contained forty men, we'll have saved the complement.' But Grant could see only three rafts afloat in the oily waters, and none contained more than thirty.

So the hurried search began, and from the waters Grant and his men pulled those who would otherwise have drowned. Once they came upon a seaman floating face downward, obviously dead, and Grant began to haul him aboard, but Penzoss took his arm quietly and whispered, 'We haven't enough space to stretch out the wounded,' and trying to keep the others from seeing, the pharmacist allowed the body to drift away.

Finnerty's notes said that the *Lucas Dean* had broken apart at 1007 on the morning of 25 October, in the sight of at least two dozen American ships, so it was likely that rescue would be swift, but midday came without any signs of such help. Kurita's fleet had disappeared, ignominiously, and new American ships were beginning to arrive from the south, but none came to where the abandoned men of the *Lucas Dean* drifted in the sea.

In late afternoon the men in Raft Three rescued a seaman from the DD *Hoel* who said that his destroyer had taken one hell of a beating: 'We lost one engine and half our guns. Then we lost our other engine and the rest of our guns. In the end they moved in close and blew us out of the water.'

'Many survivors?' Penzoss asked in his high voice.

The *Hoel* man turned and said, 'You talk just like my sister.'

As dusk approached, the floating men had to acknowledge that they would not be rescued this day, and since they had only two frail flashlights, it seemed unlikely that help would reach them this night, either. When darkness fell, some of the badly wounded died, and at regular intervals Penzoss supervised the throwing away of bodies. With the first burials prayers were said, but toward midnight this stopped.

Now the skies cleared, allowing a beautiful half-Moon to show high in the western heavens, and the stars came out, incredibly beautiful, and a farm boy from Minnesota was able to recite the names: 'Three of the loveliest stars in the sky. Vega, Cygnus, Altair.' A boy from New York who could rarely see the stars corrected him: 'Cygnus isn't a star. It's a constellation.'

'You're right,' the Minnesota boy said. 'But that star has such a difficult name, I always forget it.'

'Deneb,' the New York boy said.

The ship's navigator heard this conversation, and moved awkwardly to join the two men. He knew all the navigational stars, and through the long night he explained which ones would be setting in the west, which rising to replace them in the east: 'Alpheratz, Hamal, Aldebaran.' Shortly before midnight he told the listening men, 'Soon we'll get the finest bunch in the heavens. Orion.'

When the multiple stars of that constellation did appear, Lieutenant Savage began to groan, and both Captain Grant and Penzoss moved to his side. 'What is it, Tom?'

'Something's moving. I have one hell of a pain.'

Grant wanted to touch the wound to see if a shell fragment of some kind was exposed, but Penzoss restrained him. When they were well away from Savage the medic whispered, 'Gas, I'm afraid. The heat yesterday. The motion tonight.'

The raft was not of wood. It was a rubber affair, thick and greasy and heavy, and because it had no keel or stiffening, it rose and fell and twisted with the motions of the sea, so that even some men who had been at sea for two or three years became nauseated and a few newcomers really seasick.

'If you must vomit,' Penzoss said repeatedly, 'do it over the side.'

Toward dawn, when the skies were filled with bright stars, shining even more brightly because the moonlight had long since vanished, one man who had never really seen the heavens before, told the navigation officer, 'This is a night I'll never forget.'

'Look to the east,' the young astronomer said. 'Dawn. Planes will soon spot us, and we'll be picked up.'

But this did not happen. And no rain clouds appeared to protect the rafts from the Sun. Now the merciless heat was beating down upon the stricken sailors, and more badly wounded started to die at an appalling rate; even some men with only minor wounds began to experience dreadful pains and the fear of death.

No matter what the condition of the men, the burden of their suffering fell on Penzoss, who crawled from one to another, apportioning his precious medicines as he deemed best. He was twenty-one years old, a boy with almost no education from a small town in Alabama, but he performed like a doctor of sixty from Massachusetts General.

'You must do something for Lieutenant Savage,' Grant said at noon, but there was nothing Penzoss could do. A fragment of shell, which could easily have been extracted in a hospital with proper instruments, had worked its way poisonously toward lung and heart. The pain was agonizing.

'Can't you give him something?' Grant asked.

'I have a few Syrettes of morphine.'

'No better time to use them. There'll be a rescue before dark.'

The medic's frown indicated that he had given up hope of rescue on this day, but a scream from Savage drew his attention to that direction, and at Captain Grant's command he administered the Syrette, breaking off the tip professionally and inserting the needle deep in a blood vessel of the left arm.

It was, as he had suspected, useless, for at 1300, when the heat was at its fiercest, the Texan died. Then began Captain Grant's near approach to loss of self-control. Holding Savage in his arms, he started to tell Finnerty 'write that he was the most efficient officer . . .' but when the words were spoken he realized how inadequate they were to describe this glowing stranger who had boarded the *Dean* so late and with such distinction.

Looking aloft at the empty sky, Grant shouted, 'Where in hell are the planes?'

'Sir,' Penzoss whispered. 'The men.'

Grant cleared his head, but kept hold of Savage until Penzoss whispered in his high voice, 'Sir, we better bury him.'

'You mean, throw him overboard?'

'We must. We may have to spend another night.'

Reluctantly, Grant surrendered the body to Penzoss and Finnerty, who with some difficulty raised it onto the slippery edge of the raft, then dumped it overboard. Before it had disappeared, the raft moved toward a cluster of men who had kept themselves alive for more than twenty-four hours without the aid of any life raft. They were waterlogged and near death.

Captain Grant was first to dive overboard to rescue them, but soon he was joined by two other good swimmers, and with their help he hefted the tired survivors into the raft, but when sixteen had been added in this manner, Penzoss called down quietly, 'Sir, we mustn't overload.'

'And we mustn't leave these men.'

'Then we'll all go down.'

'Then we'll all go.' And he threw aboard the last of the swimmers.

They were from the baby carrier *Chesapeake Bay* and they had wild tales to share with the men from the *Dean*: 'Yep, we took four eighteen-inch shells from the *Yamato,* probably, right through the ship without exploding. It was miraculous.'

'But the holes did sink you?'

'No! No! We floated just as good as ever.'

'What did sink you?'

'This Jap airplane. Flew right into midships. Intentionally. Blew us to hell.'

So crews from the first two ships to have been sunk by kamikazes, a word none of the men yet knew, met on the swells of Leyte Gulf, a chance encounter which Finnerty noted.

'What are you writing there?' Captain Grant asked, and when Finnerty would not answer, Grant took the notebook and read:

> From 0700 till 1007 when the *Lucas Dean* broke apart, Captain Grant fought his ship with a gallantry that had no equal. Against odds that would have terrified the ordinary captain, he took his DE right at the heart of the Jap battleships and cruisers, and even when he had no torpedoes or ammo he maintained position in order to confuse the enemy, even though they could do twenty-seven knots and the *Lucas Dean* three because of lost power. In the life raft his courage manifested itself through two hot days and one cold night . . .

Grant tore the page from the book. 'There were no heroes in this fight,' he said. 'The crew was the hero. And especially Savage.' His voice came close to breaking.

Then came the sharks. The survivors from the *Chesapeake Bay* spotted one of their mates clinging to a floating chair of some kind, and they shouted reassurance, but as the raft drifted slowly toward the downed man, everyone saw with horror that two sharks were about to attack him.

'Shoot them!' somebody called, but before those with guns could act, the lethal fish tore at the man, ripped off his legs, then returned to shred the torso.

In the late afternoon, as the raft moved through the waters where other American ships had sunk, the men saw a score of corpses, arms and legs missing, and some watchers became so violently ill that they vomited, even though the raft was by now fairly stable.

'They could all have been saved,' Grant said, and this was the beginning of his great rage. How many of the incredibly brave men who in their little ships had withstood the might of the Japanese navy, how many of them were to die because some imbecile at headquarters had forgotten to dispatch rescue missions?

'Where are they?' he raged at the merciless sky and at the cruel waters. And then the stars came out, distant beacons shining impartially upon the remnants of the Japanese fleet, driven forever from the seas, and upon the victorious Americans drifting forgotten in the tropic waters.

'If you have good eyes,' the navigation officer said, 'you can see differences in the color. Saturn is whitish. Jupiter is red.'

'For Christ sake, shut up,' an enlisted man shouted.

'I'm sorry,' the officer said. He and the lad from Minnesota huddled together, and soon they were joined by the young man from New York. Through the long night they would console themselves with the stars, to keep from thinking about their comrades who would die before dawn.

Penzoss, endeavoring to recall what his Great Lakes instructor had taught about sharks, told the other men, 'Sometimes they let a man drift right past without touching him, especially if he's moving his arms and legs a lot. But like we saw, they can also attack with terrifying power. One thing we know for sure, let them smell blood from a wounded man or fish, they go crazy and tear him apart.'

'Are they still out there, followin' us?' a farm boy asked.

'They come, they go. They could be a dozen miles from us right now.'

'I'm gonna say a prayer on that.'

'You people there?' It was a voice from the sea.

One of the flashlights probed the darkness: 'There's a nigger out there.'

The raft was maneuvered to where a big black man swam without the assistance of any spar or floating chair. He was less than fifteen feet from rescue when flashlights showed that the water about him was being churned by huge dark shapes, and several men shouted, 'Sharks! Sharks!'

Penzoss, remembering a tactic his instructor had advised, cried, 'Shoot the bastards! Draw blood!' And the three riflemen blazed away.

The stratagem worked, because when one of the sharks took three heavy bullets he began to spurt blood, which sent the other sharks insane. With great slashing swipes of their furrowed teeth, they tore the wounded one apart.

Amidst the fury the black man swam closer to the raft, but when he reached it, the sides were so slippery and he so exhausted that he simply could not hoist himself aboard, so Captain Grant leaped into the dark water while Penzoss screamed, 'Use anything. Scare the sharks away if they start to move in.'

As Grant started to slip his right arm about the swimmer's torso to give an upward thrust, a stray shark, inflamed by the melee in which the others were attacking a second bleeder, swept toward the raft, smelled the black man's right foot, and snapped it off in one swift motion. Blood gushed over Grant's face as he hoisted the wounded man into the raft, but he ignored it as his men reached down to pull him to safety just before two wildly thrashing sharks swept in, then veered away, their mighty jaws empty.

'What happened to you?' Penzoss asked the black man as he applied a tourniquet.

'*Chesapeake Bay* went down . . . I was cook's helper . . . I swam.'

'Jesus! You were in the water all that time? And the sharks waited till the last minute?'

'Am I going to lose my foot?'

'You already lost it,' Penzoss said.

'Oh, oh! A colored man with no leg. A cripple. A beggar.'

'You didn't lose your leg. And the Navy takes care of heroes like you.'

The man made no reply, for in the moonlight he saw Captain Grant's insignia. 'You a lieutenant commander?'

'He's captain of the ship,' Penzoss explained.

'And you jumped in to rescue me? Among the sharks?' He dropped his head into his hands and wept.

To distract his attention, Finnerty asked, 'What's your name? I got to record it.'

'Gawain Butler.'

'That's a hell of a name.'

'My mother read Tennyson.'

Penzoss looked up. 'I didn't know that niggers read poetry.'

'We did,' Gawain said.

At midnight, when darkness engulfed the castaways, and the stars shone with terrible brilliance in a sky untouched by soot or the lights of civilization, the men of the *Lucas Dean* heard voices in the night, and they came upon other swimming sailors from the *Chesapeake Bay,* and a harsh decision had to be made. 'This raft can't hold no more,' a bo's'n said firmly, and Captain Grant had to agree.

But the swimming men, survivors through sheer courage for forty hours, had to be saved, so Captain Grant dived into the water, swam to the men, and led them to the raft. Before he hefted them aboard he said, 'Four volunteers requested to swim down here with me till morning.' Finnerty volunteered and three other seamen. Through the long night they would hold on to ropes that rimmed the raft, relieving it of their weight.

In the dark waters, Finnerty clutched Captain Grant's right arm and said, 'When we're rescued, I'm going to write all I wrote before, and a hell of a lot more.'

Grant said nothing. He was torn apart with fury that his men had been required to exhibit such bravery in their DE, and now were drifting, abandoned, after the fight. His guts were fiery with disgust, and only the fact that he was in charge of this pitiful bobbing craft kept him from screaming at the gods who had treated his men so shabbily. The rampaging sharks had moved well away to inspect other groups of survivors, and mercifully they did not return.

Never was the Sun hotter than when it rose on the morning of 27

October 1944, and as soon as it was high, seven moderately injured men succumbed, and only when their bodies were tossed overboard did Captain Grant consider the raft sufficiently lightened to warrant his climbing back aboard. He lay exhausted in the awful heat, but his mind was churning, and it was in these three dreadful hours of morning that he saw with wonderful clarity the course he must take if he survived.

He had been reared in the small city of Clay in the state of Fremont. He'd attended the state university in his hometown and the University of Chicago law school. He'd married Elinor in 1940 and had attended a crash course for prospective naval officers at Dartmouth College in the cold winter of 1943. Never brilliant, he had received in all his schools what professors called Plodders' A's, and some had recognized him as a better prospect than those who received such marks through their sheer brilliance.

His father was a merchant, and his wife's father a farmer, so he had no inheritance to look forward to. From 1939, when he acquired his law degree, to 1942, when he volunteered for the Navy, he had earned only a meager living in Clay as a general lawyer handling routine cases, but in his last year he had been approached by the Republican party to run for the state legislature, and he had given serious thought to that possibility.

Now he remembered the words of Yeoman Finnerty as they swam together in the shark-threatened waters: 'You're the greatest hero I ever heard of, Mr. Grant, and I'm going to say so.' He had told Finnerty to shut up, but now the words echoed, and he thought: In the world that exists after this war, men who are known as heroes will be valued. Look at Colin Kelly, who sank the *Haruna,* or thought he did. What a fuss they made over him. The state of Fremont can find a place for me. In his near-mania he gritted his teeth and muttered, 'It damned well better.'

'What's that, sir?' Finnerty asked, his own head reeling from the heat.

'Finnerty, what you said in the water . . . What I tore out of your book . . . You saw things better than I did.'

'What do you mean?'

And Captain Norman Grant, USNR, formulated his philosophy: 'Finnerty, the world is a shitty place. Leaving us to die out here. If we get back . . .'

'We'll get back.'

'You and I are going to take the world by the balls and squeeze till it screams.'

'A partnership?'

'Till death.'

'I think it's a plane, sir.' And it was. After forty-eight hours in the raft, with the Negro Gawain Butler sloshing his right stump with salt water to prevent infection, the survivors of the *Lucas Dean* and the *Chesapeake Bay* were rescued. They were flown to Manus, where skilled doctors and considerate nurses performed the saving operations which had been denied the many who died.

Captain Grant spent his first two days at Manus casting up accounts, and to the best of his knowledge, supported by what data Finnerty and Penzoss could supply, the facts were these: *Lucas Dean* known complement, 329; killed while aboard ship, 49; died while on rafts, 57; died floating in the sea, 92; known survivors, 131. When he looked at the deaths, many so needless, his rage returned.

But then he commandeered shore-based officers to help assemble the figures for the three-part battle, and its magnitude staggered him: Total number of Japanese warships, 69, including 13 under an Admiral Shima who trailed along behind; total number of American warships, 144; total Japanese ships lost, 28; total American ships lost, 5, to which should probably be added the DD *Albert W. Grant,* which was almost sunk not by Japanese guns but by American warships firing in the dark. Total number of Japanese sailors who died that day, probably 10,000. Of course, the Americans also lost numerous planes, the Japanese almost none—except the suicides. But at this time all the figures had to be tentative.

As the officers worked on this report, they heard rumors of the extraordinary heroism of Norman Grant and his *Lucas Dean,* and questions were asked among the survivors, with three enlisted men volunteering amazing reports: Finnerty the yeoman; Penzoss the medic; Gawain Butler, the black cook's helper from the *Chesapeake Bay.* So on a November day at the Manus field hospital, a cordon of war correspondents and photographers surrounded the bed in which Butler lay, ostensibly to watch him receive a medal for swimming alone for nearly thirty hours and losing his right foot to a shark at the last moment.

'It was quite a feat,' one of the newsmen whispered to his photographer. 'But why summon all of us?'

Then the admiral in charge of the ceremony said, 'Seaman Butler has asked permission to say a few words,' and in the precise English his mother had taught him, Gawain said, 'When I had lost hope, this man here, Captain Grant of the *Dean,* swam to rescue me, even though he knew sharks were about. And when he lifted me into his raft, he realized it was too loaded, so he swam all night, outside.' It hadn't happened just that way; Grant had got back into the water to provide room for *other* seamen from the *Chesapeake,* but that was the way the legend was recorded.

Then Finnerty spoke, telling of the wild-man way in which Captain Grant had fought his little destroyer escort. 'You mean,' he was asked, 'he said he was going to cross the T of the whole Japanese fleet?'

'That's what he said,' Finnerty replied. 'And he did it.' From his waterlogged notes he read out the quotation that was flashed across the wire services, properly edited:

YEOMAN FINNERTY: Do you intend to take on their whole fleet?

CAPTAIN GRANT: I do.

When the questions were finished, and the photographs snapped showing Grant at the bedside of Cook's Helper Butler, with Yeoman Finnerty and Pharmacist's Mate Penzoss at his side, Grant stayed with his men from the *Dean*. 'I didn't want this. Finnerty here can tell you I didn't want it. But it's happened, and by damn, we're going to use it for good purposes.' And then his resolve, so carefully nurtured since the battle began, vanished, and he broke into wild tears.

'The dead! The dead in the water!' He looked at his men and said, 'There isn't a man here who could equal Tom Savage. His death is on our hands, and we can never discharge it.' But with grim force, totally concentrated, he would try.

At the precise moment when Lieutenant Commander Grant was preparing to throw his DE at the oncoming Japanese fleet, the football players of his hometown of Clay in the northern part of the state of Fremont were preparing for the second half of their game against arch-rival Benton High School from the much bigger city which served as state capital.

Because of the war, the game could not be played at night, and because travel was limited, no one had expected a large crowd, especially since the game would be taking place on a Tuesday, when the playing field was not being used by the local university for its ROTC drill. However, since entertainment and sporting events had been cut to the minimum, townspeople had flocked to watch the hometown team.

Since Benton was almost twice as large as Clay, sports fans always assumed that it would win, and it usually did. But this year word had circulated through the state that Clay had a wizard, 'as good a halfback as Norman Grant was at his best, back in 1932.' The young halfback was good, and men at the store lamented: 'Danged shame we aren't playing a regular season, against these good teams from Kansas, so that John Pope could show his stuff against the best.' No one ever called him Johnny, because from his earliest days he cultivated a serious mien, as if he already knew he was intended for important duties.

He was seventeen that autumn, not tall, not heavy, but handsomely constructed for American games as they were then played. In basketball his lack of height was only a minor handicap, because once the whistle blew, his speed, his body control and his deftness made him a premier player. Of course, in later years, when players customarily resembled skyscrapers, men of his build would be at a severe disadvantage and might not even make the squad, let alone a team.

In football it was the same. He weighed only a hundred and fifty-one, and would never weigh much more, but again his extraordinary control and his ability to change speed and retain his balance when it appeared that he had been knocked down made him a high-school phenomenon, so that even when the players from Benton seemed gigantic, the Clay supporters could whisper sagely, 'Don't worry. John Pope will tie them in knots.'

And that was what he did. When Benton had the football in the first half they moved it pretty much as they wished and scored heavily, but occasionally on their march down the field they would make a mistake and Clay would recover the ball on a fumble or fluke, depriving them of yet another score. Even so, by the end of the third period the husky Benton Capitals had scored twenty-five points, with every prospect of adding to that total in the final period.

However, John Pope was having an exceptional day, for on those lucky times when his team obtained possession, he did as he was supposed and ran deftly through the big Benton line, twisting and turning to great effect. At the end of the third period he had scored all of Clay's points, twenty, a feat he had performed several times before.

At this point the game was temporarily interrupted by a ceremony which should have occurred at half-time, except that the speaker had encountered difficulty in breaking away from an important strategy meeting in Washington. Senator Ulysses Gantling was up for reelection this year, and as an outstanding Republican he had assumed responsibility for Tom Dewey's statewide campaign for the Presidency. Gantling's own reelection was hardly in doubt, but he had learned to take nothing for granted and was touring the state frantically for both himself and Dewey.

As a farmer, he had proposed the most effective counterthrust to Roosevelt's claim that 'you never change horses in midstream.' He toured Fremont, Kansas and Nebraska, shouting, 'If your horse is winded, lacks courage and shows signs of drowning when the water gets rough, you damned well better change . . . especially when a much better one is ready to take over.' That made sense to rural audiences, and there was talk that when Dewey was elected, Gantling of Fremont would find a place in his Cabinet. It was impossible for the voters of this region to believe that a majority in corrupt places like New York and Boston would want to give a dictator like Roosevelt a fourth term.

So the game was halted while Senator Gantling, saying never a word in favor of either his candidacy or Dewey's, stood tall and gray beside the flags while an honor guard from the ROTC held their guns at parade rest. He spoke with great feeling of the young men of this region who were at this moment fighting the enemy on far-flung battlefields. Then he asked that the spectators and the players of both teams bow their heads as Reverend Baxter from the Baptist Church read a prayer, after which the honor guard would fire a salute.

Some two thousand citizens of Clay did bow their heads and pray for the safekeeping of their volunteers who were at that moment in Italy, in France, in Africa, on Guadalcanal and at the gates of Germany, but no one in that crowd, not even Senator Gantling, who pondered such matters because he tried to govern well, could imagine what it was like to be in an icy ship with a frail bottom on its way to Murmansk or in a writhing metallic tank on its way across Belgium.

Five members of Norman Grant's family lowered their heads, praying for his safety, and if they had been told then of the heroic acts he was performing or the perils he was about to face in the dark waters of Leyte Gulf, they would have been unable to raise their heads, for they would have been frozen with horror.

One young man, a member of the Clay football team, did not lower his head in prayer, for as he was about to do so he happened to look at the eastern sky, where he saw something which astonished him. 'Look,' he whispered to Pope, who stood nearby. 'The Moon is shining at the same time as the Sun.'

'It often does,' John said without looking up.

When the prayer ended and the ROTC guns rattled, Senator Gantling said with what a reporter would call unusual felicity, 'As a loyal son of Calhoun in the western part of this state, and as a football player who used to contend against each of your teams, I believe I would be forgiven if I said that I hope you both lose. But I could never utter such words, because like all good Americans, I constantly pray that the best team will always win, for only then can we be truly strong.' Saluting the flag and marching out with the ROTC, he left no doubt as to which was the better team in the forthcoming election. But as he passed the lined-up players, he stopped briefly in front of John Pope to say, 'I'm keeping my eye on you, son. And what I hear is very reassuring.' He was famous for his garbled metaphors and also for his flashing smile, which he now directed at the young football star, who could mumble only, 'Yes, sir.'

The fourth period started with Clay trailing by five points, and Benton quickly made it eleven by scoring on a long run. But then John Pope took over, and with a series of brilliant plays, carried the ball down the field toward the Benton goal line, where the Clay fullback punched it across.

On the ensuing kickoff, Benton looked as if they would score again, but miraculously the smaller Clay line held, and Benton was forced to surrender the ball. Now it became a contest between John Pope and the clock, and on every series of downs it seemed as if the clock would win and that the game would end before Clay could score again. On first down, Pope would be dragged down by the Benton tacklers. On second down, he would gain nothing. On third down, someone else would carry the ball and fail. But on the fourth-and-desperation, Pope would somehow break loose and give Clay one more gasp.

As the final seconds ticked away, he carried the ball, and most of the Benton team, right down to the three-yard line. Then, when the Benton tacklers were concentrating on him, the Clay fullback again rammed the ball across the goal line. Clay had won, 33–31.

John Pope would never forget that game, not because of his outstanding heroics but because of what happened in the locker room afterward. Of course there was raucous celebration, and some of the Benton players did come in to congratulate him, but the significant thing was that a heavyset man in a dark suit sought John out and said, 'I used to play for University of Colorado. Son, if you go to Boulder with all the national publicity that team gets, you could be the next Whizzer White.'

'I've been thinking about the Naval Academy.'

'Navy? What's a halfback from Fremont doing thinking about the Navy? We're a thousand miles from any ocean.'

'Norman Grant, he's from this town, you know. He's in the Navy.'

'Son, let me level with you. If Norman Grant had gone to Colorado instead of Fremont, he'd be immortal.'

'He is immortal . . . around here. But thank you for your interest.'

'Son, things change. New ideas replace old ones. This time next year— You're a junior, aren't you? You may have forgotten all about the Navy. If you do, remember Colorado. When you go Colorado, you go first class.'

John did not linger to celebrate his performance. He knew he'd been good, and he felt gratified that a former player at a university like Colorado had praised him, but he had never allowed football or any other game to dominate either his current behavior or his long-term set of values. His interest at this moment was far removed from football, for as he left the gym alone he looked up into the evening sky and saw to his satisfaction that the half-Moon was visible high overhead and stars were beginning to appear, and he thought of two objects which had recently assumed great importance.

The first was a book which he had owned since July, the only one he had ever purchased with his own money. It had been published in Edinburgh by a firm called Gall and Inglis, and the university bookstore had needed ten weeks to secure a copy. When he reported to claim it he had been waited on not by a student clerk but by a full professor, who introduced himself formally: 'I am Karl Anderssen of Norway. I wanted to meet the young man who was purchasing this book. Who are you?' When Pope explained, the professor had asked, 'But why would you want this particular book?' And he held John's book in his two hands.

'I thought it was time I learned something about the stars.'

'This is one of the loveliest books in the world,' the professor had said, still clinging to the large flat volume. 'Norton's *Star Atlas*. Half the great astronomers living in the world today started with this as boys. Do you know it?'

'I've never seen it,' John had replied, so the professor opened the book that charted the heavens, but not to the fascinating diagrams that John was so eager to see. He turned instead to the many pages of small print that summarized most of astronomy as it was then understood.

'If you use only the charts, young man, you'll drop astronomy within six weeks. But if you start with these pages, and digest even a part of them, you'll always be a prisoner.'

'A prisoner?'

'Yes. The stars reach out and grab you. They infect your mind. They change your entire perspective.' Reverently he had handed the book over, then asked, 'Have you ever seen the stars?'

'Not really. But my father is borrowing a pair of field glasses for me, and when he does . . .'

'What a wonderful experience! You'll never forget it.'

'Do you operate the telescope at the university?'

'I do.'

'Could I look through it? Sometime?'

The professor hesitated. He was in his sixties and had transferred to Fremont because the atmosphere was so unpolluted that he could spend hours at his telescope instead of the minutes available in a smoke-ridden city like Cambridge or New Haven. 'No,' he had said that July afternoon, 'you can't look through the telescope.' When he saw John's disappointment he added, 'Look at the stars now with your naked eye and make them familiar. When you get your field glasses, see the enormous number that spring into view. Do it right. Step by step. When you've done these things and digested them, come to the observatory and ask for me. Because then you'll be ready.'

The second object that captivated young Pope this night was the pair of binoculars which his father was borrowing from a hunting friend. If things had gone well, the glasses should be in the drugstore now, so instead of going directly home, John headed in the opposite direction toward the center of town, where his father managed a drugstore which *his* father and grandfather had operated.

'They tell me you ran quite a few yards today.' His father always spoke this way, formally, half whimsically, never praising his son outright because he realized that the boy received more than enough adulation at school.

'I had a good day. The Benton linemen were clumsy.'

'I got the glasses.'

'Are they as good as he said?'

'They're German. Very expensive, so don't lose them. The writing says 7-X-50 and I judge that's pretty powerful.'

John took the glasses, then asked for the case and studied how they fitted into it. He hefted them, inspected the mechanisms to satisfy himself as to their operation, and smiled at his father. 'Thanks.' Quickly he added, 'How long can I keep them?'

'Paul's off to Detroit for the duration. Says he won't need them at the tank assembly line.'

'You mean . . .'

'Yes. They're yours for a year . . . a couple of years.' He watched his son's face, then asked, 'Don't you want to go out and try them?'

'No,' John said slowly. 'Not in the middle of town, where there's so much light and dust. I want the first sight to be perfect.'

His father nodded.

Throwing the strap across his shoulder and settling the heavy glasses against his body, John walked slowly home, glancing at the sky from time to time.

It was now approaching six, advanced war time, so that the noble stars of summer were about to appear for one last time this year in the deep west. From his intensive summer study of *Norton,* he had identified the star which he hoped would be the first that he would see through the binoculars; it was Arcturus, the golden-red giant that would soon be breaking through the fading daylight: Follow the curving handle of the Big Dipper, and there will be Arcturus. I'll see the great summer triangle, Arcturus-Antares-Vega. And when they disappear, there'll be another triangle just as good, Vega-Altair-Deneb. He thought of the stars as if he knew them individually.

But he had to hurry if he wanted to see Arcturus this year, for he knew that it would be dimmed by the earth's atmosphere because it would stand so low in the sky; and several times as he hurried home he was tempted to see if the glasses could pick up the star through the fading light, but he was restrained by what Professor Anderssen had said: 'Do it right. Step by step.' After supper, he thought, when the sky was properly darkened, he would launch his investigation, but almost immediately he realized: I started my investigation the moment I looked up at the stars with that book at my side. The binoculars are only the next step.

At the supper table he irritated his mother by propping *Norton* against his glass and studying one last time the chart which showed where Arcturus would be, but when Dr. Pope returned from the drugstore he said sharply, 'Down with that book. You're eating supper now.' So the book was laid aside, but even before his first bite, John asked: 'Can I please be excused? I want to be there when a certain star—'

'You'll eat your supper,' Dr. Pope said, but his wife laughed and said, 'He'll never have another chance to use his glasses for the first time.'

'He played a football game. He must be hungry.'

Mrs. Pope indicated that John could leave the table, for she knew that he was assailed by a hunger that comes rarely in a human life, and after he left the room she told her husband, 'I'll take him a sandwich later.'

In a few minutes John, wearing a heavy jacket against the cold autumn air, hurried through the kitchen. As he passed her, his mother said, 'Mrs. Kramer called to say you did wonderfully in football.'

'I had a good game,' he said, heading toward the backyard.

The elder Popes rarely attended the various games in which their son starred, Dr. Pope because he was needed at the store, Mrs. Pope because she could not convince herself that games were important in the long scale of human values. Physical exercise, yes. But organized games with cheerleaders, no. They were helpful in building strong bodies, and she certainly believed in that, having seen much sickness at the drugstore, where she had served as clerk before she married. But she never planned for her son to be a major athlete, and definitely not a professional of any kind.

The elder Popes, with three children to educate, the other two older than John, trusted that their offspring would be good citizens, and that was about it. The older son was going to be a doctor; the daughter gave signs at the university of wanting to go for her master's and then to teaching on the college level; John had shown no specific propensity, for he excelled at everything. His marks were never lower than B, and not too many of them. He was good at math, better at physics and chemistry, but he could also express himself adequately in either term papers or public speaking.

He was by no means an ideal child, for he had a fiery temper which he sometimes had difficulty in controlling, but in most things he bespoke the intelligent care his parents had spent in his upbringing. He was a Baptist, a Republican, a Boy Scout, a football star who did not take his acclaim too seriously, and now an amateur astronomer. He had not a single cavity in his teeth and was a lean, wiry six pounds under the normal weight for his age and height.

He was opening the door when his mother said, 'By the way, John, Penny phoned and asked what time you'll be over to study math with her tonight.'

'She just wants me to do her problems for her.'

'That's ungracious. If you promised to see her, call and cancel your date like a gentleman.'

'Mom, I don't want to bother with Penny tonight. Please, you call her.' And before his mother could protest any further, he was out the door.

When he first stepped into the night he did what astronomers had been doing for some two million years before the invention of the telescope: he stood in the middle of the open land behind his house and slowly surveyed the heavens, orienting himself as to the stars at this latitude, at this longitude and at this hour. He thus became one with the ancient Assyrians, with the wondering men who erected Stonehenge, and with the Incas of Peru. He looked only briefly to the north, for he had long since mastered the polar stars that never set; there was Polaris, friend of mariners, the two Bears, and the Dragon that wound its tortuous way between them. He knew each of the stars in the Big Dipper by its Greek designation and its characteristics, but his interest tonight was in the stars of the west, which would soon be setting, to be lost for half a year as they moved into proximity with the Sun, whose light would obscure them during the daytime hours.

And as he stood there, face up to the sky, he savored that mysterious moment when the glow of twilight disappeared into true darkness, allowing light from distant stars to reveal itself. Low on the horizon stood Arcturus, glowing red like some mighty furnace, and he wanted desperately to bring it first into his glasses, but he realized that the flickering atmosphere would diminish the star, so he turned his gaze higher, and after a while the whole panoply opened up, stars innumerable in brilliant configurations and colors.

Curiously, he did not bother with the bright half-Moon, for he judged correctly that this was a garish nearby phenomenon which he could always study at will; what he yearned to see were the stars, those scintillating messengers from immortal distances. So for some moments he surveyed his heavens, looking now at one high star, then another, until finally he settled upon the one which he would first see with his new glasses.

It was Altair, a gleaming white star in the constellation Eagle: 'You can always locate it. Track down from Vega and Deneb. You'll know it by its two bright guardians.' There it was, Altair, one of the brightest stars, one of the first to have been awarded a specific name by the ancients; in all societies it had been associated with birds, with flying, and now it flew through the dark prairie sky.

Slowly he brought his glasses to his eyes, cocked his head backward, and pointed the binoculars toward Altair. At first it seemed disappointingly blurred, but as soon as he twisted the central knob that moved both barrels his left eye saw the star in perfect focus. Then with a light touch on the knob that activated only the right barrel, he brought his right eye into focus also. And then he gasped, 'There are so many stars!'

What the chart had shown to be a moderately populated area turned out to be a veritable jungle of stars, and in that precious moment he deduced the nature of the universe: With my unaided eye I could see only a few stars attached to Altair. Now I see hundreds of them. And if I could use the university telescope, I'd see thousands. And if we could somehow lift that telescope up above the interfering atmosphere, I'll bet we'd see millions. Out to the farthest edge of the universe.

That is what happens when a boy of imagination looks seriously at his first star. But he was also a practical lad, and always his eye came back to brilliant Altair with its two distinctive guardians, and he realized that as long as he lived he would be able to look casually at the autumn sky and identify Altair. It was his forever.

In school John Pope was not a literary boy, but like his well-educated parents he could speak in complete sentences when grappling with ideas; when playing with his peers in athletic contests he mostly grunted. But now he said aloud, 'A human mind is limited only by the power it has at its command.'

When his arms grew tired from hefting the heavy binoculars, he sat on the ground, as the ancient Assyrians must have done when plotting their heavens, and rested his elbows on his knees, and he was in this posture when he became aware of someone behind him. Turning quickly, he saw his mother coming toward him with a sandwich.

'It's very beautiful, John.' When he grabbed the food and showed his football hunger, she pointed to a brilliant star overhead and asked, 'What's that one called?'

'Vega,' he said without hesitation, and suddenly he wanted his mother to see that star, for the books said it was particularly beautiful. After finding it himself, he handed the glasses to his mother and showed her how to progress from the horizon upward to the point overhead, and when she had done this she cried with pleasure, 'John, it's lovely.'

'It's called Vega, after some girl, I guess.' It never occurred to him that a star so exquisite could be anything but feminine.

He did not know much about girls; he often said that his sister was 'a real peach,' but what he meant by this he could not have explained. He had taken several different girls to school dances and was vaguely aware that many others in school considered him rather special, but he had done nothing about it. At seventeen he was not allowed to run about at night as some of the other football players did, and both his mother and father had asked him pointedly not to associate with the faster girls who had access to automobiles. Three young people from Henry Clay High School had been killed in hideous crashes, and the older Popes had told their son that he could not have a car until he was eighteen. He understood. There were numerous hard-and-fast rules in the Pope household, and each of the three children had played a role in determining what they should be, and had then accepted them.

'We don't want you to be prigs,' Mrs. Pope said. 'And we certainly don't want you boys to be sissies. But we do want you to grow up to be responsible young people. We want you to seek out others like yourselves. Young people who go to church, get married, have children who are decent.'

Mr. Pope said, 'I know you'll drink a bit, but I pray that you won't smoke. I'm convinced from what I see . . . men hacking with coughs that never end . . . Don't smoke.'

Mrs. Pope felt that fried foods twice a week were just about enough, and while this part of the West did not go in for salads, she was a stickler for vegetables: 'They give the stomach something tough to work on, and there will be no desserts in this house until your vegetables are eaten.'

Three times this autumn he had dated a girl in his class who was becoming important to him. Penny Hardesty lived in a frame house four blocks away, but in the wrong direction. The Popes lived on Ash Street, which itself wasn't one of the best. Then came, in alphabetical order, Beech, Chestnut, Dogwood and Elm. The Hardestys lived on Elm, a rundown thoroughfare housing the day laborers and hardy workmen of the town. Sam Hardesty worked for a trucking firm, his wife in a hairdressing salon. They had four children of good reputation, but none of the first three had gone beyond high school, and it was generally understood that Penny would not. The family was well regarded, but those better-positioned often asked among themselves, 'I wonder why Sam Hardesty never made more of himself?'

Penny was a B-minus student. Her teachers said repeatedly that she could be straight A if she applied herself, but they noticed in her a flippant manner associated with girls who became boy-crazy. She didn't. If she was driven off the straight-and-narrow that teachers loved, it was not because of boys; some deeper malaise affected her, and what it was not even she could have explained. Vaguely, she wanted to better herself, because she saw clearly that her two sisters and her brother had severely penalized themselves by not continuing with their education. 'They've put themselves in a box,' she told John on their second date, 'and I think it's awful to be the cause of your own punishment.'

He enjoyed being with Penny because she talked of serious subjects. She was not at all like the other girls, and as he met with her in classes and the informal life of school, he began to realize that his football prowess made little impression on her. She called the team 'those great animals' and teased him when the coach laid down rigorous rules 'for his little darlings.'

Penny was exceptionally good in history and civics and would have drawn down A's if she had been more consistent in writing her papers, but sometimes she would produce brilliant work, at other times the most sloppy and haphazard reasoning. In mathematics she was not good at all, and it was while coaching her in this subject that John Pope first realized that she thought entirely differently from him, for either she grasped an abstract concept at first confrontation, or she dropped it completely and would have nothing further to do with it. She could not, for example, fathom the principle of negative numbers, and when John drew the basic diagram— vertical line (Y-axis, ordinate) cut by a horizontal line (X-axis, abscissa)— and tried to explain the four quadrants, she understood the upper right, where everything was normal, but when she got to the lower left, where things were negatives which yielded positives, she placed her hands across that part and said, 'For me, it doesn't exist,' and she would not allow him to proceed.

Later she told him that when you lived on Elm Street you experienced so many negatives that you went blotto unless you blocked them out of your life and concentrated on the positives.

On their two recent dates they had, more or less at her instigation, engaged in some prolonged kissing, which John enjoyed immensely, and several times they had studied together at night, doing math or arguing history problems. Mrs. Pope liked Penny and was pleased that John had found himself such an acceptable girl to take to the dances. She noticed that Penny was especially helpful about the house, a trait she exhibited at home, too, where she had assumed responsibility for keeping the entire lower floor neat: 'I don't want to live in a pigpen.'

Mrs. Pope told her husband, 'There's nothing really serious between John and Penny,' and he replied, 'There would be with me and Penny, seeing she's so pretty.'

She was a most attractive young lady, almost as tall as John, with shimmering dark hair which she often wore in two pigtails and appealing bangs, wiry rather than fat, and unusually alert. She had a fine complexion and a face that was not strikingly beautiful but highly satisfying. She had a knack for wearing clothes that suited her and often favored neat dresses with crisp white Peter Pan collars, a costume which allowed her to look at the same time pert and irreverent.

So when John Pope first looked at Vega, the glorious summer star of the northern heavens, gleaming blue-white like the fairest diamond, it was natural that he think of Penny Hardesty . . . and then of their kissing . . . and then of what some of the other football players had been saying recently about their adventures with their girls.

John could not think of Penny 'in that way' because he well knew that she was made of much more serious stuff than the casual girls who knocked around with the team, girls who had their own cars and who lived in homes where the parents were often absent. He and Penny had talked about this several times and had both known that life held a good deal more than high school and Saturday nights in autumn. Penny, for example, was determined to go to college, somewhere, somehow, and John had confided to her a secret which not even his mother knew yet: 'Pop knows Senator Gantling from Calhoun, and he promised Pop that if I did well in school, he'd appoint me to Annapolis. About twice a year he checks on how I'm doing and last time he told Pop, "Your son looks like a shoo-in." '

'Annapolis? You'd go so far away?'

'You'd be invited. For the big dances. The uniforms and all that.'

'Annapolis!' She had seemed much more impressed, or perhaps bewildered, by the possibility than he was. But she had said a strange thing: 'My vision doesn't go beyond this town. I can't even think of going to nurses' school at Webster. And certainly not to Nebraska the way Charlene did. And you're thinking of Annapolis!'

The night was advancing. In England the tremendous fleet of American bombers had crossed the North Sea and were over Peenemünde, where the pathfinder planes had set their flares. In Leyte Gulf, Lieutenant Commander Grant bobbed in the water, trying to assure himself that American rescue planes would soon spot him and his men, not yet aware that the sharks were destined to find them first. In the quiet skies over Fremont, Vega had begun her descent, and an enchanted young man searched a neighboring constellation for the miracle about which he had been reading for some weeks.

It lay in Hercules, and with his sharp eyes he could just barely discern it, a faint hazy discoloration. Placing it carefully, he raised his glasses and vectored them in. And there it was!

M-13 it had been named, the great globular cluster in Hercules, one of the staggering phenomena of the heavens. It lay 34,000 light-years away, a massive glob of individual stars throwing enormous quantities of light across the two hundred million billion miles that separated it from earth. Look at it! John thought with reverence. Half a million stars in one cluster.

He could not see it well and could certainly not differentiate any of the individual stars, but he could discern the massive cluster and approximate its significance, a part of the celestial system so brilliant that it glowed across that immense distance.

'How wonderful it is!' he cried into the night air.

'What is?' a voice asked. A hand was placed on his shoulder and a head moved close to his.

It was Penny. John had promised that he would help her with her math tonight, but then had canceled the date without even having the courtesy to call her himself. His mother had said over the phone, 'John has a new toy, Penny, binoculars, and I'm afraid he'll be out of circulation for a while.'

When Penny heard this alarming news—that a pair of binoculars could be more important than a promised date—she had glimpsed a vision of the years ahead. She and John would date casually through their senior year, and off he would go to Annapolis, where he would find new horizons and new obligations; they would never meet again. Her opportunity of allying herself to a really first-class person would be lost, and she would be restricted to the third-class men and boys she saw all around her. Rightly or wrongly, she had identified John Pope as her only logical avenue of escape from a life which she knew to be extremely drab and limited, the life allotted to her sisters and brother. Appalled at that prospect, she had come quietly through the back streets to the Pope house. Arriving unnoticed just as Dr. Pope returned home from closing the drugstore, she had remained behind a tree until he entered, then listened as he called into the backyard, 'Don't wear those glasses out the first night.'

'I won't, Pop.'

When all was quiet she slipped past the house and into the yard, where in the light of the fading Moon she saw John, seated on the ground, his elbows on his knees, peering northward. When she moved closer she heard him talking to himself, and this tempted her to join the conversation as if she had always been there.

John, overcome by the emotion of seeing a perfect star, one of the subtlest in the heavens, allowed his binoculars to fall to their strap, turned quickly, and took Penny in his arms. They kissed for a long time, then launched into explorations they had never risked before, until finally they moved purposefully into some low bushes where they could not be seen from the house, and there they more or less undressed, using their clothes to protect themselves from the cold ground. With great thrusts and clutchings and yearnings they completed the adventure, then lay cold and shivering until they began again. The stars, which had once seemed so imperative, passed overhead unnoticed.

It was past one when they put on their clothes. They were shivering so furiously that Penny said, 'Sex. I'll always think of it as stone-cold.'

'Not me!' John said.

From an upstairs window Mrs. Pope called, 'John, leave the stars. You'll catch your death of cold.'

'I'll be in soon, Mom.' He walked Penny home, again through the back streets, with the binoculars banging at his side, and as they moved through the silent town she did a very unwise thing, or perhaps the wisest thing she would ever do. She revealed her strategy: 'John, you must understand this night.'

'I could never forget.'

'I didn't say remember. I said understand.' For just a moment she wondered if she should speak her thoughts, but it was her nature to do so: 'I can see the future, John. You'll go away. Annapolis. The war will still be on. Normally, I'd never see you again. But you're far more important to me than wars or colleges or anything at all. I wanted you to know that. Indelibly. I wanted to bind you to me, because I know you're a young man who's not afraid to be bound.'

'I was ready,' he said.

'You're the finest thing I'll know in life. I'm the best girl you'll ever know. I live up there among the stars. I wanted you to know.'

At her door they lingered, both aware that something very special had happened under the stars. They had looked far into the future, past the wars and the alarums that they read about in Shakespeare, and they knew that in the whirling space of which they were a part, they shared now and would always share a special relationship. They kissed goodnight.

On his way back home, John followed the more open streets, and this allowed him to see that in the university observatory someone was working with pale night lights, so on the chance that it might be Professor Anderssen, he turned away from the street that would have taken him home and hurried to the door of the observatory. It was open, so he entered. Hearing sound from the second floor, he ascended the rickety stairs and found to his delight that the man at the telescope was indeed the professor.

'I'm the one who bought the star atlas,' he explained.

'Yes! Yes, it's you. I see you've been working with your binoculars, as I advised.'

'They're not mine. A friend of Pop's. He's making tanks at Detroit.'

'Have you been following the heavens as they drift by?'

'Yes, sir,' John said, hoping to give the impression that he had used the glasses night after night.

'And what have you seen?'

'Well, I haven't bothered with the Moon very much.'

'The Moon can always wait. It's of little consequence, really. What about the stars?'

'I was thrown off my rocker by Altair. So many little stars I never knew existed.'

'What power are your glasses?'

'7-X-50.'

'You can see a lot with that.'

There was an awkward pause that betrayed the professor's desire to get back to his own work, and John knew that he ought to leave, but this night had been so extraordinary, so unbelievable, that he longed to extend it. 'Is there any chance that I . . .'

'Might look through the telescope?'

'Yes.'

'You've never done so before?'

'These are the best I've done,' he said, tapping the binoculars in a familiar way.

'It can be quite startling.' He looked at the big machine, then at John. 'But are you ready?'

'I think I am,' John said. Last night he would not have had the courage to say this.

'Let me ask you a few questions. What time zone are we in?'

'Greenwich minus six.'

'What time is it in London now?'

'Seven o'clock in the morning.'

'What's our longitude as we stand here?'

'Ninety-seven degrees West.'

'Our latitude?'

'Forty degrees North.'

'In orienting a telescope like this one, which of these two measurements is the more significant?'

'The latitude.'

'And why?'

'Because to build an equatorial mount—'

'You know what an equatorial mount is?'

'Yes. It allows you to point your telescope at a particular star and then have the whole telescope move with the exact motion of the earth, so that the star always remains in the center of the scope.'

'You're ready,' the professor said. Not many of his university students could have answered so precisely. 'But what should you see first, young man? What's your name again?'

'John Pope, my father's the druggist.'

'Of course, you're the famous football player my son talks about.'

'I play.'

'And you know this much about the stars?'

'I can scarcely credit the things I've seen.'

'What have you seen?'

'M-13.'

Professor Anderssen raised his chin as if he had been struck. 'You know the Messier numbers?'

'Some of them.'

'Would you like to see something rather extraordinary in Perseus?'

'You mean 869-884?'

Professor Anderssen clasped his hands and said, 'Son, how would you like to test yourself in real astronomy? Register as a special student for my course in January?'

'Could I? I'm only a junior in high school, you know.'

'When men like me grow old, we search for lads like you. Register.' He coughed, then said brightly, 'And now you shall see your first real treasure in the heavens. The double cluster.' Slowly he swung the telescope away from the area he had been studying, and John assumed that he was supposed to step forward and look through the eyepiece, but as he started to do so, Professor Anderssen cried, almost harshly, 'Stand back. This is an instrument of dignity, worthy of respect.'

He came to stand beside John, pointing in the dim light to the extraordinary beauty of the telescope, its polished wooden segments, its burnished brass fittings. 'The telescope was made by Alvan Clark of Massachusetts. In 1886. He was the best America ever produced, a profound astronomer and a better mechanic.'

'If it's so important,' John asked, 'how did it get here?'

'Son, this is the leading observatory in this part of the world. If it were not, I wouldn't be here.' He touched the telescope lovingly. 'Back in those years the university graduated a truly stupid man. I've seen his letter of application to study astronomy. Every word misspelled. *Astronnimy.* He was refused admission, so he went out and earned four million dollars bartering railroad stocks. First thing he did with his money was buy this Alvan Clark, and the building to house it. Used to come here night after night to look at the stars, and couldn't name one of them.'

Professor Anderssen pressed his hands against the gleaming woodwork and said, 'Before you look through a great telescope, you must look with your eyes. What do you see up there in a line between Perseus and Andromeda?'

Through an aperture in the ceiling John studied the cluttered heavens and came slowly to see a slight but fixed haziness. 'Is that it?' he asked.

The professor said, 'Now look at it with your binoculars,' and when John did, he saw to his satisfaction that it was a distinct aggregation of something, but precisely what, he could not determine.

'Now you're ready to see the famous double cluster through an Alvan Clark,' the professor said, and with some difficulty he searched for the pair, uttering pleased grunts when he finally focused upon it.

Stepping back, he invited John to look, and when the boy had adjusted the controls to accommodate his eye, he saw that what had seemed a confused haze was really a balanced pair of magnificent clusters, teeming with stars and vitality and nocturnal beauty. They seemed to be in competition, west against east, a staggering collection of great stars engaged in some kind of combat. Some were grouped tightly, as if locked in struggle, others were far-flung, but all were enchantingly interrelated, as if the torment of the heavens kept them associated against their will. It was the complexity and implied movement that made these clusters so appealing.

'How many stars in each cluster?' Anderssen asked.

'Do all the stars we see belong to the clusters?' John asked.

'An admirable question. No. Some stand between us and the clusters. Some form a distant background. In the left, three hundred individual stars. In the right, four hundred.'

'It seems impossible.'

'And now for the gem. Messier 31. Can you find it without the glasses?'

'Oh yes. I look for the Great Square of Pegasus, project the diagonal toward Cassiopeia, and halfway there, a bit to the west . . . I see it now.'

'What do you see in your binoculars?'

'A faint, hazy mass. Very stable. Very big.'

'It's the most remote object in the heavens that ancient man could see with his unaided eye. Do you know how far away it is?'

'No.'

'About two and a quarter million light-years. That means that if you and I send a message to Andromeda tonight, at the speed of light, and if they understand it and want to reply, we can't possibly receive their answer for four and a half million years. How far away is that in your calculations?'

'I'd need a pencil.'

'Here's one.' So John sat at the wooden desk used by the university astronomers, and by a darkened light put down his figures, reciting to the professor as he did: 'Two and a quarter million light-years multiplied by about six trillion miles per year.' He did the multiplying and adding of zeros, then reported: 'I get something like one followed by nineteen zeroes.'

Professor Anderssen was conducting his own calculations, using precise values, and he said, 'Remarkably close. The actual distance seems to be thirteen billion billion miles away from us.'

The two sat silent in contemplation of this stupendous distance, and John looked at the shadowy form with new reverence. 'Now see it in the telescope,' Anderssen said, and John moved to the eyepiece, staring across that immense distance to where M-31 glowed majestically in the night.

'See its magnitude,' Anderssen whispered. 'Note its shape, exactly like that of our galaxy. See the glowing core at the center, the immense radius of the fiery gases. Can you detect the swirling arms, the wild violence? Can you guess what mysterious control holds it all together?'

For eleven minutes, while the telescope subtly followed the movement of the distant galaxy through the heavens, John Pope stared at its multiple wonders. And then he heard again the quiet voice of the Norwegian professor: 'Tonight you've been introduced to two wonders. The beautiful and the stupendous. There are, we judge, one hundred billion other galaxies out there. And if we ever lift a telescope above our atmospheric interruption, I'm sure it will reveal an additional hundred billion. For space is limitless.

It goes on forever. Always remember, John, that you and I live on a minor planet attached to a minor star, at the far edge of a minor galaxy. We live here briefly, and when we're gone, we're forgotten. And one day the galaxies will be gone, too. The only morality that makes sense is to do something useful with the brief time we're allotted. I would be most pleased if you would report to my class in January.'

Slowly, through the starry night, with much more visible than when he started after supper—for the sky was now dark, allowing the weaker stars to shine through—he walked homeward, his binoculars hanging at his side. In Leyte Gulf it was four in the afternoon of the first day, and Norman Grant was baking in fierce sunlight on his raft, while at Peenemünde the German rocket experts were spending the early daylight hours endeavoring to assess the damage done by the tremendous American bombing.

John Pope knew he had experienced something rare and precious—his first journey into the heavens, the glimpse of perfect beauty in the star Altair, the awakening of love with Penny, and the vision of that galaxy infinitely remote: There can never be another night like this. My job is to make all nights good within their own limits.

'Damn it all!' his father shouted as he came in the door. 'Two-thirty! Just who in hell do you think you are?'

John was startled. He had never before heard his conservative father swear. 'I was at the observatory,' he apologized. 'They let me use . . .'

'John,' his mother called from the foot of the stairs. She was in her nightgown and it was evident that she had been crying. 'You should have telephoned.'

'I just stopped at the observatory.'

'You are not to roam the streets like rabble, John Pope,' his father said, jealous of the good reputation that name carried. 'And if you do go somewhere like the observatory, have the decency to telephone us. We care deeply what happens to you, son.'

'The professor invited me to attend his college classes. Starting in January.'

'That's gratifying,' his mother said.

In his bedroom he could not sleep, for the majestic universe seemed to be exploding about him, shattering and illuminating.

An hour before dawn the elder Popes heard their son's alarm clock, and they stepped into the hallway in time to see him disappearing down the stairs. 'Where in hell are you going now?' Dr. Pope swore for a second time.

'I want to see how the night ends.'

'John,' his mother said quietly, 'you must put on something more.' When her son hesitated, she added, 'We watch your health. Put on a jacket.'

When he reached the yard he saw above him the unequaled panoply of winter constellations: Taurus, Orion, the Twins, the group with great Sirius, and in the east the Lion and the outriders of the Virgin. He stood enraptured, using his glasses on one after another of their splendid stars, but it was not until just before dawn that he saw what he had left his bed to view. It was red Arcturus rising from the prairie, and as it climbed higher, fighting to sustain itself against the increasing light, he accepted as reality the fact that his Earth actually did revolve in a twisting path around the Sun. At dusk he had seen Arcturus slip away from him; at the conclusion of the same night, he was witnessing its return to the heavens.

'We do revolve in space,' he whispered to himself. Again he longed to capture this great red star in his binoculars, but again it lay too low for sensible viewing, so he waited, but by the time Arcturus had risen enough to clear the atmosphere, day had come and there were no stars.

At three o'clock on the afternoon of 24 October 1944, when Professor Stanley Mott was investigating the damage done by the rocket that landed in the heart of the financial district of London, and when Admiral Nishimura was placing in his private safe the Sho-Go instructions which required him to take his small fleet on a suicidal foray into Leyte Gulf, Dieter Kolff, a rocket technician of indeterminate rank, was pushing his bicycle onto a small ferry that would convey him from the top-secret island of Peenemünde in the Baltic to the mainland of Germany a short distance to the west.

He was thirty-seven years old, a small, thin, shy man with an ineffectual mustache. He wore heavy glasses which he took off when trying to impress people but replaced rapidly if a document or piece of equipment was handed him. He spoke softly but revealed a fierce willingness to defend his judgments; his inner convictions he shared with absolutely no one, not even Liesl, whom he was leaving the island to visit.

Developments in Nazi Germany had taught him this distrust. As a boy from an impoverished mountain area south of Munich, he had encountered scorn, for he was not from some hereditary warrior family in Prussia, or clever in business like a Ruhr German, or intellectually gifted like a Berliner. He had only one gift: he could look at a piece of machinery and see what was wrong with it. He had been able to do this on his family's farm and later when he worked in the factory in Munich. But because he was not university educated, or able to express himself well, he gained small profit from his gift.

When drafted into the army he remained a mute private, first on the French front, then on the Russian, and officers with infinitely less ability in keeping their machines of war functioning walked past him a score of times without ever asking for his assistance. But he was clever enough to see, in the spring of 1942, that any German armies which went deeper into Russia were apt to encounter tragedy, and he devoted all his energies to escaping from those gray, forbidding steppes.

His chance came in early 1943 when he was serving with the unlucky General Paul von Kleist in the Caucasus. During a vast retreat Von Kleist's tanks started to break down, and when the general hastened among his men, goading them to make repairs that were impossible, he spotted one taciturn mechanic who doggedly mended anything that was brought before him, and on the muddy repair field Dieter Kolff was commissioned a lieutenant and placed in charge of overhauling the great tanks.

Two weeks later Hitler dispatched an urgent request to the Wehrmacht, asking it to send him responsible young men with impeccable records to work at a demanding task. That was all that the order said, but discreet inquiries established that men with mechanical ability were needed, preferably not from large cities. Von Kleist pondered this cryptic statement and concluded that what Hitler sought were strong farm boys who had not been contaminated with city radicalism.

His quota was eleven, and after he had nominated nine promising lads his eye fell upon Lieutenant Kolff, the most reliable officer in the headquarters company, and a wily tactic evolved: I'll send the Fuehrer my best man and maybe . . . Just perhaps Hitler would overlook the disasters on the Caucasus front.

'Where were you born?' Von Kleist asked, and when Dieter gave the name of his rural village, the general said, 'Your papers say Munich. We don't want anyone from that trouble spot.'

'I'm from a farm,' Dieter replied, and that evening he was on his way out of Russia, rejoicing with every clackety turn of the train wheels.

He had not worked with the heavy installations at Peenemünde for two weeks before his extraordinary native ability was recognized, and late one afternoon he was brought before a tall, silent man with deep-lined face and funereal voice. 'This is General Eugen Breutzl,' an orderly said. 'Don't you salute generals?'

Kolff saluted awkwardly. 'They tell me you are very good with machines,' the general said. He was fifty-three that year and obviously harassed by the urgent demands constantly pressed upon him.

'I can fix things,' Kolff said.

'Education?'

'I worked in a factory. Fixing things.'

'Family?'

'Farmers.'

Breutzl frowned, then asked brightly, 'Big landowners?'

'No. A little chicken farm.'

'How did you become . . . well, an officer?'

'In Russia. I knew how to fix tanks. General von Kleist . . . a field commission.'

'You think you can fix the things we're making?'

'I can.'

'Do you know what they are?'

'The men say they're rockets. For hitting London.'

'Do you know anything about rockets?'

'From what I've seen, I can fix certain things.'

That had been almost two years ago, and now Lieutenant Kolff was one of General Breutzl's most valuable men. The general, an engineer and not a scientist, was in charge of building the great A-4 rockets which the scientific genius, young Wernher von Braun, had devised, and the job was not an easy one, for whenever General Breutzl had a production line nicely started, Von Braun altered the specifications, requiring a complete reorientation of machines and men.

'Why doesn't he make up his mind?' Kolff asked one day in desperation.

'Because it's an entire new world, Dieter. There are no rules to go by.'

Kolff was no longer an officer in the Wehrmacht. He was one of the anomalous breed that infested Peenemünde, men of no stripe but of great ability in grappling with the problems of a coming world. Out of respect, Breutzl was accorded his old title, but he was no longer a general in the military sense; he was a genius at perfecting engineering solutions which enabled rockets to fly, and in the early days when they had failed, twenty-three out of twenty-nine exploding on the pads or shortly after takeoff, it was usually because the scientist had ignored Kolff's practical advice. Once he said laughingly, 'And when I fail it's because I didn't listen to Dieter Kolff.'

The little farmer had an almost mystical sense of what an engine could do, or not do, and when the rockets became increasingly complex, he was often the only one who could unravel their mysteries. He was a kind of German Thomas Edison, and both Von Braun and Breutzl knew that they were lucky to have found him. 'He is,' said Von Braun, 'an untutored genius. How did we get him?'

'Number ten in a detachment of eleven,' Breutzl said. 'I wonder how many more we have out there we haven't identified.'

'We'll need them all,' Von Braun said.

The rocket program had not gone well in those first years. Again and again the leaders of Germany had come to Peenemünde to ascertain when the A-4s could be launched against London, and repeatedly there had been debacles, with rockets disintegrating in midair, but the three men had plodded on, convinced that what they had envisaged could fly, could carry a massive load of explosive to London and deliver it on target.

Now, as he unlimbered his bicycle at the far end of the ferry, Kolff reflected on how lucky he had been: If I was still a private, without my battlefield commission, Von Braun would never have looked at me. He doesn't care much for privates. He thinks I come from some important family. But he knows I can fix his rockets. Indeed, the rockets that were now falling on London reached there in large part because of innovations and corrections initiated by Kolff, and the fact that as a mere lieutenant he was permitted to leave Peenemünde at three in the afternoon to visit his girl was proof of the regard in which Von Braun held him.

When it was recognized that he had valuable skills, he had been removed from the A-4 and assigned to a project of ultimate secrecy, and it would have surprised him to learn that both Moscow and Washington had compiled dossiers on him, for each was determined to capture him when the war ended. Up to now he had been unwilling to concede that Germany might collapse, and the reason for his optimism was that he knew what tremendous weapons he and General Breutzl were about to perfect.

When he was detached from the A-4, he did not move to the next sequence, the A-5 through the A-9, each of which was planned to accomplish some tremendous thing. He was assigned to the A-10, last in line and the mightiest. It represented a concept so dazzling that he was allowed to discuss it only with Von Braun and Breutzl.

The A-10, and it was very close to solution, with production not much more than a year in the future, was a rocket that could be fired from Peenemünde with a colossal head of explosive, and land on Boston, New York or Washington. Dieter was not angry at the citizens of any of those cities, no more than he was angry at the people of London, who were being struck daily by his bombs. He was a technician, a man trained to apply his skills to whatever task loomed, solve its complications and move it to completion. If the aerial bombing of New York was desirable, regardless of motive, he would devise ways by which it could be accomplished. And it was on this task that he now concentrated.

So it was a very important man who mounted his bicycle and pedaled westward as the American bombers prepared to strike a mortal blow at Peenemünde. He was headed for a farm north of the mainland town of Wolgast; it was owned by the family of Liesl Koenig and was conspicuous for only one thing. It stood adjacent to an expensive summer resort with gorgeous water views on three sides: east to the channel separating the mainland from Peenemünde, north into the Baltic Sea, and west into a bay containing a very large island.

Liesl worked at this establishment, caring for rich Berliners during the high summer season and for modest Pomeranians during the truncated winter season. She was not a pretty girl, nor was she any longer young. Indeed, she might have been passed by altogether had not Dieter Kolff come to the island and met her during a walking trip on the mainland. She was now twenty-eight and would probably have moved to Berlin as a domestic had not the war intervened. She was a hard-working woman with a pleasing if subdued disposition, and Kolff felt that he was lucky to have found her.

On the highway west of the ferry he was stopped three times by guards, and his bicycle was well searched, even though the older guards were familiar with his visits to the Koenig farm. They nodded in friendly fashion as the younger men searched him, for nothing could move on or off Peenemünde without scrutiny.

Dieter spent a quiet afternoon with Liesl, had supper with her family, and walked in the autumn evening to the grounds of the resort, from which he could see the antiaircraft guns that lined the mainland shore. 'We've grown afraid,' Liesl said, 'since the big raid last year. Father saw scouting planes overhead this afternoon.'

'We saw them, too. They were Luftwaffe.'

'Not the ones Father saw.'

There were so many things that Kolff wanted to share with this responsive girl. She was, he was ashamed to tell anyone else, a lot like his mother, a good, reliable farm girl who would bring her husband stern qualities and much devotion. She understood whatever problems he was allowed to share with her, especially his fear of the Russians: 'You should have seen their villages. They let their farmers live like animals. If they were ever to come here . . .' He shuddered.

'Is there a chance they will?'

He hesitated. In Germany one was prudent never to say what one thought, unless it conformed to some rote requirement, but it was also necessary for every human being to reach out and confide in someone. Liesl could well be a spy conscripted in this particular spot to trap Peenemünde workers like Kolff, so he must say nothing about the A-10, nor about any of the lesser bomb systems for that matter. But about Russia he could speak. He had to speak.

'Two years ago, when I was there, our officers were confident the Russians could never turn the tide on us. That was a poor country. A land of peasants. But now . . .'

'They're moving closer, Dieter.'

'Are you afraid?'

'Yes, I'm afraid.'

They said no more that evening, but each knew that now the agenda was clear and overwhelming: somehow they must avoid capture by the Russians. All that they did hereafter would be predicated upon that imperative.

When darkness fell, they retired to a barn on the resort premises and made love, a practice they had fallen into when they became aware that Russian armies were descending upon Germany and that terrible uncertainties might soon engulf them. Each depended upon the other in these perilous days, and each knew that salvation lay only in the other's love. Liesl's suspicious father had asked four questions: 'Does he own his own farm? Was he ever really an officer in the army? What's he doing on that island, anyway? And whatever happened to that Detterling boy? He owned a good farm.' Under the circumstances, she felt it unwise to discuss anything important with her father, who so far had made only one substantial observation about the visiting stranger: 'He eats like a pig. Don't they feed him over there?'

He had identified Kolff's major peculiarity: despite his frailness, he could consume unlimited quantities of food without affecting his girth, but as Liesl pointed out, 'You have no right to complain, Father. He usually brings us far more food than he eats.'

On a normal visit Dieter stayed with Liesl until about nine at night, when he cycled back to catch the last ferry, which crossed at ten, but on this night he was agitated by so many conflicting bits of gossip circulating on the island that he longed to stay, not to discuss the possibilities openly, but simply to talk with someone.

So they lingered on the grounds of the summer resort, discussing trivialities, until Liesl stopped their walking and took him by the hands. 'What is it, Dieter?' When he looked surprised, she added, 'What big thing disturbs you?'

In silence he contemplated in order the seven major developments that disturbed him, not one of which could he openly state or even intimate: There was a rumor that Himmler's secret police were going to make another move against Von Braun. There was another that General Breutzl was to be demoted and exiled to the Russian front. There were constant fears that Peenemünde would be closed down entirely, because the Russians were moving too close. And so on, plus an eighth one which he himself had generated, and this he could share with Liesl.

'The general has aged . . . badly. They blame him for everything that goes wrong, but I can tell you that nothing goes right without him.'

'You like him, don't you?'

'I wish all Germans were like him. I wish all fathers were.'

'Mine's complaining again.' She hesitated, then said softly, 'We should get out of here, Dieter. Both of us.'

'Yes.' After a long while he said, 'It will be up to me, Liesl. I'll tell you when.' And after another long reflection he changed the subject. 'I promised Baron von Braun to look after the general. I must go back.'

'But you've missed the ferry.'

'I steal chickens for them from our mess. They'll lift me over.'

It was ten-thirty when he bade Liesl goodnight, kissing her breasts at the gateway to her farm. 'What's that?' she asked, pointing to the sky.

The Moon was bright, deep in the west, and it glowed upon a lone aircraft that flew fantastically high. They watched it for some minutes, guessing wildly as to what it might signify. And then two streaking pathfinder planes came in very low, dropping not bombs but flares of different colors which glowed in the night.

'Oh God!' Dieter cried. 'It's a raid. With those flares it'll be a major raid.' And he pedaled furiously toward the ferry, keeping his eye on that plane mysteriously high in the heavens, wondering what it could be, not realizing that in it rode Master Bomber Merton, who would direct the oncoming Americans to the targets illuminated by the flares.

He had not reached the ferry when the first bombers came roaring in, much lower than he expected. They were huge, and dark, and the Moon disappeared just as they reached Peenemünde. 'Someone planned this exactly,' he told the men at the ferry, and then the great explosions began.

'I've got to get across,' he said.

'Not in this,' the ferrymen said, seeking cover. And for almost two hours the men huddled there, listening with growing horror to the tremendous load of explosives being dumped upon the island.

'Where did those first yellow flares land?' Dieter asked the ferrymen.

'Down by your quarters,' the man said.

'Oh Jesus! They're trying to kill General Breutzl.'

'And your Von Braun.'

'He's in Berlin. Listen, I've got to get across.'

'Not now.'

Other planes moved in, German fighters this time, and some of the enemy bombers began to burn and fall into the Baltic. One came right at the empty ferry, kept aloft and crashed in the direction of the summer resort at which Liesl worked.

Now he had two worries, his general and his girl, but when the bombardment ceased, and the German fighters withdrew, Dieter hurried not to the Koenig farm but to the island, to see what had happened to General Breutzl. Wherever he went, guards stopped him, for the destruction was massive and buildings of all kind were afire. Commandeering a guard with a motorcycle, Dieter abandoned his own vehicle and rode pillion to the scientists' quarters, the ones that Professor Mott had ordered spared.

The first set of flares had overshot their mark, not landing on the manufacturing and research facilities as intended, but directly on the living quarters of the scientists. The monitor aloft had warned each incoming flight of the imprecision, but the target was so tempting and the flares so distinct that whole sticks of bombs had struck the area.

Dieter, approaching from the north, could see the devastation, the gaping, burned sections, and he realized that had he not gone to visit Liesl, he would now be dead. But what of General Breutzl?

'Over there!' Dieter yelled into the ear of the driver, but the cyclist said, 'Not me.' So Dieter dismounted and ran toward the shattered buildings. He did not have to enter, for on the lawn outside the dormitories were laid the thirty-one bodies, and toward the middle of the row, calm and kindly even in death, lay General Eugen Breutzl, whom the Nazis had never trusted but on whom they had been forced to depend.

When no one was looking, and for reasons of secrecy which he could have explained to no one, not even to himself. Dieter waited till all the others were preoccupied with the devastation caused by the raid, then moved to the concrete vault in which the general's plans for the A-10 were kept. These work sheets, usually the result of long consultations among Von Braun, the general and Kolff, were safe. Allowing no one to see him, he removed them, carrying them to his own wrecked quarters, where he set fire to a few inconsequential ones, snuffed out the flames, and intermingled the charred pages with a few of his own diagrams. At that moment he had no clear idea why he was taking such precaution; it was instinctive and had something to do with the rumors that Von Braun might soon be arrested again by Himmler's men.

. . .

Two nights later, at three o'clock in the morning of 27 October, when Norman Grant, wallowing in the waters of Leyte Gulf, had about decided that his dwindling crew of heroes would never be rescued by a forgetful Navy, Dieter Kolff sat upright in bed, awakened by an idea which flashed through his canny mind like a thunderous explosion of lightning: Chickens! That's what will save me—chickens!

He had a right to be apprehensive about his security, because as soon as the bombs stopped falling, an old adversary, ominous and persistent, returned to the island, eager to pursue past suspicions. He was Colonel Helmut Funkhauser, forty-eight years old, a somewhat overstuffed would-be Prussian with no neck and pinched-together eyes. Son of a modest butcher in Hamburg, he had been an early volunteer for Hitler's Brown Shirts, not because of any philosophical conviction but because membership was exciting and a glimpse of the future. By extraordinary obedience to any orders from above and by attention to detail, he had risen to become one of Heinrich Himmler's lesser aides, and it was then that he began claiming Prussian ancestry. His present assignment had been handed him by Himmler himself: 'Bring those damned scientists to heel. Get rid of Von Braun. And make sure that our SS men take charge of everything.'

When Kolff saw Funkhauser step out from the black sedan he realized that trouble had returned, for several times in the past he had encountered this colonel, finding him to be an insecure petty dictator, subservient when superiors were present, arrogant when they were not. He was not a murderous Nazi acting from deep principle; he was merely one of the functionaries who carried out orders.

Kolff had first met Funkhauser in mid-1943 when the colonel swept down on Peenemünde from his headquarters in Berlin, one hundred and ten miles to the south, to arrest Von Braun, General Breutzl and Kolff, whisking them away, without Hitler's knowledge, to a secret SS prison camp near Stettin. There he had grilled them for six days, building against them charges of disloyalty which could lead to their execution.

His charges were threefold: 'You've been guilty of disloyal thoughts. You have used Peenemünde as a base not for military revenge against the English but for future space travel. And you have made secret plans to escape to England, where you think you will be free to work on your rockets without the Fuehrer's supervision.' Any one of the accusations, if proved or even strongly suspected, would warrant death.

Colonel Funkhauser's supporting evidence was ingenious, and illustrated the paranoia which Himmler was relentlessly introducing into German life: 'Four of my spies, inserted into the Peenemünde work force, have heard you, Von Braun, wonder out loud in bars and the like whether the A-4 will bring England to her knees, despite the fact that the Fuehrer has publicly stated that it will do so. You, Kolff, have been heard predicting that the monthly quota of nine hundred rockets cannot be met.'

'Until we solve the problem of why they explode just as they're about to come down—'

'Silence. There's grave suspicion that they explode because you personally have sabotaged our war effort. And all three of you are known to be planning for the years after the war, when your rockets can be used for travel to the Moon, or the planets.' Here he became livid with bitterness, bending his fat body forward and staring with beady eyes at the three men. 'You are traitors to the Fatherland! You are disloyal to the Fuehrer! Your job is to destroy London now, not worry about space travel later on.'

There was much to this charge, Kolff admitted to himself at the time, not on General Breutzl's part, for he was a military perfectionist, dedicated to the job of producing A-4s in the most effective manner. Von Braun and Kolff, however, had often speculated on how their mighty machines could be utilized in peacetime, and they saw clearly that with the power and control they were developing, man could be thrown far into space and brought back to safe landing. 'It could be done,' Von Braun had once said, 'within four years of when we make our serious start. And if we don't make it, Russia will.'

'How about America?' Kolff had asked.

'They had the best start of all—their genius Goddard. But no one listened to him, and now they find themselves with no capacity whatever.' During the remainder of his life Dieter Kolff would recall that when Von Braun first voiced such thoughts about the future—Russia's advances, America's retreats—the baron had fallen silent, as if he had revealed much more than he intended, and it was obvious that he had more he wished to predict. But he did not dare to speak, for he, like everyone else in Germany, had to be afraid of who might be listening, or where the spics were planted. And Dieter remembered that as soon as he uttered those words, Baron von Braun stared at him, as if calculating whether he might be the spy planted by Himmler to trap him.

Colonel Funkhauser's guess that the Peenemünde personnel were dreaming not of the present war but of the future peace was shrewdly correct, but his suspicions about his prisoners' plans for fleeing Germany were paranoiac: 'Von Braun, you've been seen twice. When you took off in your little plane, you headed not toward Berlin but out to sea. Did you know that I gave orders to the air force that if you ever did it again, you were to be shot down? No questions, no warnings.'

'I fly my plane to get to the meetings your people keep convening,' Von Braun said softly. He was a big man, ample in all dimensions, with a large head and a very large face which seemed to be younger than its thirty-one years. Indeed, he looked like some enthusiastic university second-year student, and much of the animosity he encountered stemmed from the fact that he appeared insultingly youthful to be exercising the great responsibilities given him. He was arrogant, too, and for three good reasons: had he wished, he could have called himself Baron von Braun, for his father had held that title; as a putative baron, of Prussian heritage, he had a certain uncontrollable insolence, especially when meeting with the lumpen-proletariat that filled Himmler's force; and indubitably he was a genius whose mind worked so swiftly that assistants were left behind and gaping.

General Breutzl, for example, never tried to keep up. When young Von Braun flew off into the scientific empyrean, he nodded, waited till the flight was over, then attended to the instant problems. One day Von Braun had explained how Albert Einstein had proved that if a man could travel outward from the earth at the speed of light to some remote star and then come back at the same speed, he would age from thirty-two to forty-seven, but when he returned to Berlin, that city would be eighteen thousand years older than it had been when he departed. This had agitated Kolff, for it went against reason: 'How can there be two times running at the same moment?' But Breutzl had merely nodded, saying, 'So now our man is back home, and he still faces the problem of why these damned A-4s are exploding just before striking their target.'

In this 1943 confrontation Colonel Funkhauser did launch one substantial charge against the three Peenemünde experts, and he delivered it with bitter sarcasm: 'You are supposed to be the ultimate brains in this operation. You're supposed to draw up the plans for a rocket which will destroy London, then give those plans to the engineers and stand back while they make thousands of bombs which we can fire across the Channel. Professor von Braun, do you know offhand how many last-minute changes you've made in your rocket plans? Since you started two years ago, that is?'

Von Braun fidgeted, for he knew that this was a weak point in his performance. More than a hundred times, and this was not a figure of speech but an actual count, General Breutzl had pleaded: 'Wernher, you must settle upon one plan, no more changes. Then let me go ahead and show the factories how to duplicate those plans.'

But rocketry, with its insatiable demands for new metals, new fuel systems, new guidance controls, new everything, could never be easily nailed down. Changes were inescapable for the solid reason that unforeseen malperformances dictated them. If Von Braun had proposed a few changes, Hitler should be grateful that he was on hand to identify them, because in the end—say the beginning of 1944—Germany was going to have a massive rocket that would destroy London and end this war.

Colonel Funkhauser produced a piece of paper, which he waved before Von Braun. 'Make a guess, Professor. How many changes have you sent to the factories?' And there the ridiculous figure was: 65,121. It was accurate. It was inevitable. To make a monster rocket from scratch and to ensure that it could perform a chain of intricate maneuvers was a trial-and-error process. Von Braun himself had retreated, lunged ahead, wobbled, stumbled in confusion, and at the end had come up with a rocket that looked fine but which failed in twenty-three of twenty-nine tests.

So he had sent 65,121 alternations to the workmen, and he could foresee another five thousand before the rocket functioned. It was in light of this that one day in 1943 he made in Kolff's hearing his second reference to America: 'It takes sixty-five thousand errors before you're qualified to make a rocket. Russia has made maybe thirty thousand of them by now. America hasn't made any. Therefore, men like you and me and the general, we'd be a hundred times more valuable to the Americans than to the Russians.' When he showed no inclination to expatiate on this, Kolff asked no questions, but the comparison lodged in his mind, and not exactly in the way Von Braun intended. Kolff thought: If the Russians are so far advanced, they'd recognize the value of men like the general and me. Good God, that means the Communists will be out to capture us. And he began to watch nervously the progress of the Red Armies along the eastern front, for with every victory over Hitler's troops, they moved a mile, a league closer to Peenemünde.

'So you are all guilty of sabotaging our war effort,' Funkhauser had said grimly, 'and I'm sure you will be shot as soon as I submit my report.'

Obviously, they had not been executed, even though Funkhauser had recommended it. Powerful friends of Von Braun, and he had them everywhere, intervened with Hitler himself, and the Fuehrer spared him. Breutzl and Kolff were sentenced to death, but Von Braun would not allow this. For six days he devoted every minute to their rescue, when it might have been to his advantage to let them be executed on the spurious grounds that they were indeed saboteurs while he was 'pure.' But he could not do it, and in the end he carried his campaign to Hitler, convincing him that the A-4 would never fly successfully without the help of these two experts.

Dieter Kolff owed his life to Baron von Braun, as he took pleasure in calling him, since it was reassuring to be working with a baron, and he never forgot it.

So on the night of 27 October 1944 when he thought: Chickens! That's what will save me . . . he was a man with a right to be terrified of what Colonel Funkhauser might do to him once he fell outside Von Braun's protective shelter.

His strategy was this. Deep in his autonomic system Dieter realized that as long as he could retain control of General Bruetzl's papers, he had a bargaining power with whoever won this war, Germany, Russia or America, because it was easier for Von Braun to conceive fantastic concepts than it was for someone like Breutzl to translate them into practical manufacturing operations. And the combination of Breutzl's plans and Kolff's ingenuity might actually surpass what Von Braun was capable of, especially in countries like Russia and America, which had a plethora of imaginative theoreticians but not too many skilled in practical application.

Dieter Kolff knew that he was a valuable human being, one of the most valuable in the world at this moment, but he also knew that with his unimposing appearance and his lack of formal education, he could achieve little without the charismatic leadership of his hero Von Braun. He was welded to this brilliant baron, now and forever, but until he discovered what Von Braun was going to do in the aftermath of war, he must prudently protect himself.

I must act today, he told himself before dawn. Funkhauser and and his SS men will start looking into the Breutzl case: 'How did the general die? Where are his papers?' Kolff would be interrogated, and he would be wise to have those papers far from Peenemünde in some safe place. He had no minutes to spare.

Waiting until dawn, lest he arouse suspicions, he took a large knapsack, went to where he had hidden the Breutzl papers, and stuffed them inside. Knowing that he would be shot immediately if these papers were found on him, he walked casually to the bomb-damaged kitchen, where he nodded to the helper with whom he had established a system to defraud the regulations—beer to the cook, chickens to Dieter—and in this way got hold of three dressed fowl, which he tossed casually atop the papers.

On his bicycle he pedaled his way to the Peenemünde end of the ferry, where he gave the SS guard one of the chickens, trying his best to appear noncommittal about everything and in no particular hurry: 'I'm going to see my girl. She must have been terrified by the bombing.'

'Anyone in your buildings hurt?'

'Killed. Dozens of them.'

'Those bastards. When do we blow up London?'

'Any day now.'

At the far end of the ferry he was warmly greeted by another contingent of SS men, to whom he handed his second chicken.

'What's in the knapsack?' they asked.

'Chicken for my girl,' he said, displaying no anxiety, no desire to be on his way.

'Are you . . .' The SS men made the common gesture indicating sexual intercourse.

'Why do you think I'm taking the chicken?' Dieter asked with a faint smile that made his little face with its inadequate mustache look quite ridiculous.

'I'd better inspect the knapsack,' the SS man said, pulling aside the covering. 'Orders, you know.' Dieter strained his throat to keep from gulping, and displayed no nervousness as the guard poked around the naked chicken.

'Good luck!' the other guards said. 'And thanks for our chicken.'

Trying desperately to do nothing that might attract attention, even though his heart was thumping, he pedaled down the road toward the summer resort, where he found Liesl working with three other girls at preparing the place for winter. Keeping his left arm over the top of his knapsack, he joked with the girls, then indicated that he wished to be alone with Liesl, and blushed when the girls teased him about his intentions.

When they were alone, in broad daylight but in a part of the establishment where they were hidden from the others, Dieter faced his first life-or-death decision. There had been other moments of importance, like his landing the assignment to Peenemünde, and his sitting in Stettin prison waiting to be shot, but in those affairs he had not had much choice. Now he was making the first in a series of decisions which would determine the remainder of his life, and he took each step with full cognizance of its peril.

'Liesl, we must go to your farm and do something of vital importance.'

'Yes.' Peenemünde had now been bombed several times, first by the British, now by the Americans, and in each raid errant bombs had come close to the Koenig farm, so that death had been imminent. Also, the Russians were moving always closer from the east, the Americans from the west. Decisions of great moment must soon be made by all Germans, and Liesl was ready. She knew no other unmarried man but Dieter and was prepared to follow his lead.

'I think we'd better go now,' he said, so she made excuses to the other girls, who teased her bawdily. When they reached the Koenig farm, he asked her to fetch a shovel, and when she produced one, he said, 'We must find a safe spot. I have important papers. If these papers are found, we'll both be shot. If they aren't found, they'll be our passport.'

'To where?'

He had hoped that she would not ask this question, for it was one he had not yet answered in his own mind. What was Von Braun going to do? Join up with the Russians, who were actively engaged in the rocket race? Or with the Americans, who were so far behind? Desperately he wished to know Von Braun's plans, but even without them he knew the right choice.

'To America. They'll be needing people like me. Somehow we must get these papers to the Americans. For the present, we must hide them.'

And after the hole was dug, he realized that he was placing his life in her hands. If she was a spy planted by Colonel Funkhauser, he was already dead, but he knew there was no alternative. He handed her his life, and she buried the knapsack.

When the ground was tamped flat she quietly returned the shovel to her father's barn, then came and stood before him. 'Does this mean you will marry me?'

'I've thought about that. You're the one girl I love. You know that. But it would be terribly risky to go before a magistrate now. Too many questions, and the SS might interfere.'

Her body sagged. He represented her only chance to escape this farm, to escape the Russians, and now he was refusing to marry her. She did not voice her resentment or even think of retaliating against him, for she realized that she was in a perilous position from which she could escape only with his help. 'If you're afraid . . .' she began.

'I am,' he said with great force. 'Everything's in chaos. I was damned lucky to get past the guards at the ferry.'

'I know,' she said with a bitterness not entirely masked, but Dieter was too self-occupied to recognize her scorn.

'But I know that you are my life, Liesl, and I think we should be married right now.'

'How? If you're afraid of the SS.'

'By our own will. Here, under the sky.' She stood there, silent, so finally he asked, 'Would you be willing to marry me, right now?'

'Will it be a real marriage?' she asked with peasant caution.

'The minute you touched the knapsack we were married,' Dieter said. 'God knows when a minister will be free to confirm it.'

'How shall we do it?' Liesel asked, as if she were a little child needing instruction.

Dieter took her left hand in his, but forcefully she changed this, aware that her right hand should do the pledging, and when she was satisfied, she looked at him, a twenty-eight-year-old farm girl placing her life in his care.

'I take you as my wife,' Dieter said, standing near the buried knapsack, which would be their wedding ring and documentation.

'I take you as my husband,' Liesl said, breaking into tears as she visualized the marriage she should have had, with the girls from the resort dressed in white. After an awkward pause, she asked, 'Aren't you going to kiss me?' And Dieter did. Then she maneuvered him cleverly toward the barn, where they consummated their unusual marriage.

'You must always be ready to leave at any moment,' he warned her. 'And if I send a message to meet me somewhere, you must bring the papers.' When she nodded dutifully, he said, 'You know they're our only passport to a new life.' And she said she knew.

On his way back to the ferry he was assaulted by the sick suspicion that she might indeed be one of Funkhauser's spies, and he could hear the colonel's words in the Stettin prison: 'Four spies that I inserted into the work force at Peenemünde . . .' But even if she were a spy, there was nothing he could do about it now. He must live the next critical months in treble anxiety, for the world was falling apart and he was already dizzy from trying to hold on.

Such speculations were driven from his mind when he reached the ferry and learned that the SS troopers were about to launch a search party for him. 'Colonel Funkhauser has been demanding that you report to him . . . immediately.'

He pretended surprise and indignation. 'When did he arrive? I should have been informed.'

'Flew in unexpectedly to check the damage.' Two guards from the mainland end entered the ferry with him, and when they reached the other side they were joined by two more, who mounted their motorcycles to form a cordon about his bicycle, and in this austere manner he traveled south to the bomb-ravaged dormitories, where he found Funkhauser's men rummaging among his private possessions.

'What happened to General Breutzl?' the colonel asked. He was an untidy man, thirty pounds overweight, who always wore his SS uniform two sizes too small on the specious grounds that if it was kept tight, it would also be kept neat.

'He was killed. By one of the first bombs.'

'And what did you do about it?' Funkhauser asked in his silky public voice.

'As planned. I tried immediately to save him, but that was hopeless. So I assumed responsibility for his secret papers.'

'And what did you do with them?'

'They were destroyed in the fire. I rescued just a few sheets and . . .' He looked toward where his envelope had been planted and saw with satisfaction that Funkhauser's men had discovered it and turned it over to the colonel.

'I see that you found something,' Funkhauser said, staring at him with his pinched-together eyes. 'These charred bits. But I wonder if they're what you really found?' He changed his manner abruptly and asked, 'What were you doing on the mainland?'

Dieter felt trapped. Did Funkhauser mean on the night of the bombing, or now? Did he even know that Dieter had been away from his post on the night when Breutzl was killed? After just a moment's hesitation he replied, 'My girl. I wanted to see if her farm had been hit during the raid.'

'Had it?'

'No, thank God.'

There would have been deeper questioning had not the colonel been interrupted by a disheveled messenger with startling news: 'The Fuehrer's aide telephoned. You're to fly to Wolf's Lair immediately . . . with Dieter Kolff.'

Funkhauser looked in amazement at the man he had been interrogating. 'You? What would Hitler want with you?'

Hurriedly, Kolff picked among his scattered belongings, finding bits of clothing proper for a visit to Hitler's retreat hidden three hundred miles to the east. 'Have I time to shave?' he asked, and Funkhauser grumbled, 'On the plane.' So the same convoy of motorcycles rushed the two men back to the north end of the island, where Funkhauser's plane stood ready.

Once before Dieter Kolff had met his Fuehrer, in the spring of 1944 when Hitler pinned the silver medal on his quivering chest: 'For valiant services to the Third Reich.'

Dieter's performance had been of great merit to the Nazi war effort, for when the precious A-4s continued to blow up while aloft, he went almost directly from the prison cell in Stettin to a watch point on the Baltic coast northeast of that city, and there, in the heart of the area on which the defective rockets fell, he stationed himself with binoculars and camera, awaiting the next test shots.

For the first time he saw the mighty machine from the recipient's point of view: a monstrous silver torpedo, beautifully proportioned, leaping through the sky as if impatient to reach its target, silent at first, then with resounding cracks as it broke through the sound barrier, disappearing as quickly and mysteriously as it had come, for it was traveling at a speed of one mile per second. It was therefore nothing like an airplane, and eyes that were adjusted to planes had little chance of even seeing an A-4.

But it was Dieter's job to see, and since the rocket slowed perceptibly when it started its erratic dive, bearing in its nose a ton of Trialen, many times more destructive than TNT, it was just possible to watch its performance. And as he did so, he identified the trouble. 'What seems to happen,' he told Von Braun, 'is that when the engine cuts out, enormous pressures accumulate in the chamber, and the sides blow out.'

'What can be done about that?' the master asked.

'Simple! We wrap a steel band around the rocket at the critical point. Bind it together.'

'Won't that slow the speed? Aerodynamically?'

'Slightly. Very slightly. But that's the price you pay for safe delivery.'

When Kolff's simple device was installed, eighteen out of nineteen trial runs succeeded, and the A-4 was ready to strike at London. Hitler had been overjoyed, because he had foreseen in a dream that this instrument of destruction was going to win the war for him. First London, and when the English were battered to their knees, fifty even more powerful rockets every day into the heart of Moscow, or whatever other city the Russians held.

'And this is the little fellow who won the war for us?' Hitler had said when facing Kolff at the Berlin ceremonies. It had been a stupefying period: one day facing death in a Stettin prison; the next receiving a silver medal from the hands of Hitler himself. Now, engaged in traitorous activity against the day of Germany's defeat, he could not even guess what might lie in wait at Wolf's Lair.

The little plane sped eastward, keeping well north of Stettin, then along the very coast which Dieter had guarded, waiting for the next A-4 to explode before his eyes, then south of Danzig, which had once borne the shameful Polish name of Gdańsk but never again, and out into one of the romantic and secret places of Europe, the vast Masurian Lakes, each with a shoreline of radiant beauty and mystery.

In the heart of this region, not far from the Prussian town of Rastenberg, Adolf Hitler had built the gigantic subterranean center from which he intended to conquer the world. It was called, in German, Wolfschanze and was indeed a lair from which ferocious beasts could prowl, destroying society's flocks.

Nothing had been done by accident. Near Wolf's Lair there was no airfield, nor was there any conspicuous railroad. No big roads were allowed, with the result that Allied scout planes had searched for the hiding place a hundred times without ever identifying it. Yet hidden in the woods was a complete city, constructed of gigantic concrete cubes with steel-reinforced ceilings sixteen and seventeen feet thick. Had the enemy scout planes spotted the place, the following bombers would have done little damage, for not even the famous Tallboys of the RAF could have penetrated those ponderous shelters.

Colonel Funkhauser's plane landed at a well-camouflaged airstrip many miles from the Lair, and in a small car he and Kolff were whisked down country roads hidden by trees. When they reached the center of the establishment, a concealed city of some twenty thousand, Kolff recognized the infamous bunker in which, a few months earlier, the dissident generals had tried to assassinate Hitler. He was familiar with the monstrous structure because after the attempt, Colonel Funkhauser had assembled all the workmen at Peenemünde to warn them: 'Now you're going to see what happens to traitors who try to take action against the Third Reich.'

Funkhauser had screened the newsreels made by Goebbels of the conspirators' trial: a three-man banc of judges, all Nazi stalwarts without legal training, had screamed at the accused, reviling them and castigating them day after day. In the end, all were found guilty and some were hung from rafters like carcasses of mutton, with jagged hooks piercing their necks and brains. The film showed them struggling as the cattle hooks worked their way in. Others were suspended with piano wire about their necks; when they squirmed, the wire cut their heads off. Kolff had been one of the men who had vomited. Now he was at the center of this madness.

But when Hitler appeared, smallish, thin, dramatic in general appearance, Kolff, like all other Germans present, was eager to assist him. They saw him as a leader in trouble, a man endeavoring to do his best for Germany, and he merited the love of his people. All the monstrous misbehavior of his underlings was forgotten and forgiven when the man himself stood forth, quiet, hesitant, smiling in his weary way, pleading for support.

'Kolff, tell me. What is the future of the A-4?'

'My Fuehrer, you know that with the ones that we're firing on London from Wassenaar in Holland—'

'I know about that. So do the English.'

'We're getting twenty-nine out of thirty excellent firings. I do believe the problems that halted us for so long—'

Hitler, weary of the continual excuses, abruptly ordered that lunch be brought: for the others a rich chicken stew with dumplings; for himself mixed vegetables lightly cooked and a large bottle of Fachingen mineral water. As they ate he asked in a sudden change of subject, 'Kolff, have you ever been to Nordhausen?'

'Not yet, sir.'

'I want you to go. With Breutzl dead, you know more about production than any of the others. See if they're on the right track.' When he rose to stride up and down beneath the protective ceiling, the others rose, too, but he bade them be seated.

'Now, General Funkhauser . . .'

'General?'

'Yes. You're now in charge of all A-4 rocketry. Peenemünde, Nordhausen, Wassenaar. We've had enough of scientists. Now we need warriors.'

'I'm ready,' General Funkhauser said in clipped accents that boded much trouble for scientists like Von Braun and his fellows.

'Now tell me honestly, what's been happening with the A-4,' Hitler said, resuming his massive oaken chair.

From his pocket General Funkhauser produced a slip of paper: 'Excellent news! Five days ago, an A-4 hit a London cinema, 287 dead. Last week an A-4 hit Stepney at marketing hour, 197 dead . . .' On and on he went, detailing the chance landings of chance rockets. Taken altogether they did not add up to a thousand deaths, nor to the interruption of one industrial operation. Yet the men in the subterranean center consoled themselves with the fact that the horrible English bombings of Germany were at last being revenged. General Funkhauser's family in Hamburg had been wiped out in the terrible fire bombings of 24 July 1943, when fifty-five thousand civilians had died, and now with grim satisfaction he recited the retaliation: 'Two weeks ago an A-4 landed in a small village near London—I had the name but forget it now—and more than ninety people were killed.'

Hitler rose from his chair, moved about with obvious delight, and cried, 'We shall be revenged. Funkhauser, for every German soul that perished in your Hamburg, a thousand Engishmen will die. When we get the rockets flowing, that is.'

He looked directly at Dieter Kolff and asked, 'They will keep flowing, won't they?'

'That's my job,' Kolff said.

'See that they keep working at Nordhausen,' Hitler said, and the conference was over.

General Funkhauser wanted very much to stop at Peenemünde to inform the insolent scientists that for the rest of the war he would be in charge, but Hitler had been so insistent that Kolff inspect Nordhausen that he deemed it prudent to fly directly to that extraordinary site, and within two and a half hours they were landing at a secret airstrip on the southern rim of the Harz Mountains. Small cars were waiting to carry them to the mouth of the tunnel that led to the underground works.

It was like descending into hell, Kolff thought, and when he saw the appalling conditions in which the thousands of slave laborers worked—dark cells with no sunlight or ventilation or toilet facilities or food—the grandeur of Adolf Hitler at Wolf's Lair dimmed. This was hideous, the portrait of a beleaguered nation gone underground, snarling like a pursued animal. The

French prisoners who worked here, the Poles, the Dutch, the thousands of Russians, were slaves who would never again know freedom.

It was remarkable that such an installation, more than a mile deep, with branches running in all directions, cut into the stone by other slaves now dead, could produce the intricate parts needed to make an A-4 fly, but thanks to the dictatorial control of Himmler's SS men, it did. Slaves who would never again see the light of day forged parts which carried messages to the stars.

'Can our production be maintained?' Dieter asked, judging it to be prudent for him to show interest.

Without attempting to answer this question, Funkhauser summoned the local manager, a brutal, scowling man who had once served as a policeman in a rural town: 'We experience sabotage now and then. Can't be prevented.'

'How do you handle it?' Dieter asked.

'We line all the men in the section against that wall and machine-gun them.'

'Don't you lose skilled labor?'

'These are minimal jobs. We get replacements by the truckload. We can teach them in one afternoon.' He laughed. 'They learn or we shoot them.'

At this moment Kolff chanced to see Funkhauser's face, and for the first time he realized that the new dictator of the A-4 program did not approve of conditions at Nordhausen, but before either of the visitors could speak, the local man said with obvious pride, 'Look at the high quality of work we do here,' and Dieter had to agree that it was miraculous: 'You wonder how men in such conditions can do such fine work.'

'Discipline,' the manager said. 'We wouldn't dare assign German workmen to a hole like this. And the slaves we do get have to be guarded by SS men. We couldn't trust anyone else.'

He was eager for his new commander to see Dora, the camp where the replacement slaves were kept, and when Dieter saw this miasma, this abhorrent place with its rows of shacks, its wall where saboteurs were shot, and its incredibly filthy kitchens, he wondered why the war did not halt tomorrow, but even as he protested inwardly, it occurred to him that the conditions under which German prisoners would in future live under the Russians were apt to be equally bad, and he resolved that if he escaped he would run to the west rather than to the east.

When the tour ended and he was alone with Funkhauser he was afraid to say what he thought of the infamous things he had just seen, but the general felt no compunction. 'As soon as we knock out England, places like this must be eliminated. Too much wasted human capacity.' And still Kolff kept silent, for he was thinking that any sensible observer of this war must know that throwing casual and almost accidental single rockets at London was never going to subdue that city or its allies. Good God, he thought, this is almost November, and only seventy-three rockets have hit London, with twenty-six of them landing in remote suburbs. Really, nothing had been accomplished, or would be. Wernher von Braun was right in thinking, if he did so think, that the major justification of the A-4 would be in its peaceful application, in its offering man the chance to travel outside the limitations of Earth.

In the meantime, he would return to Peenemünde, no longer the major center of the rocket effort, and do whatever was required to stay alive under General Funkhauser's monitoring eye. In his spare time he would continue his experiments on the A-10, which in years to come would be able to bomb New York and Washington, for he shared the emotions of the men at Hitler's headquarters: Allied bombers had pulverized German cities, so Allied cities must be terror-bombed in return. It was illogical, considering his basic concern about escape, but it was understandable. He, too, wanted revenge.

These contradictions were eliminated shortly after the turn of the year, for Russian troops moved ever closer to Peenemünde, while the Americans and English applied heavy pressure along the western front. One day Von Braun appeared unannounced at Kolff's research hut, announcing a meeting of the leading scientists at a time when General Funkhauser would be absent from the island. It was a grim assembly, made more so by their leader's ominous words: 'Russian troops will be here soon. It's inevitable. Our task is simple. Keep our cadre together. Take our papers with us. And move west to be captured by the Americans.'

One young scientist, terribly frightened, asked, 'Won't we run the risk of being shot by Funkhauser?'

Without flinching, Von Braun turned and smiled at the young fellow. 'We run four risks of being shot. In the closing days the SS may shoot us to prevent the spread of our knowledge to other countries. Out of sheer hatred the Russians may shoot us when they arrive. The Americans may shoot us if we can't explain things fast enough when they overrun us. And wherever we move, some damn-fool sentinel may shoot us by accident.'

'But why do you choose the Americans?' another asked.

'I have never understood how the English do business. They seem to despise anyone who works for them, even their own people. I have no feeling for the French at all. They'd be too stingy to support a real space effort. The Russians? They're abominable, and those of us who side with them will do poorly. The Americans have the money, and after they see what we're able to do with the A-4, they'll be willing to let us spend it in building a real space program.'

Amazingly, more than a hundred scientists, fully realizing the risks they were taking, agreed that when the distant guns began to echo at Peenemünde, they would put together a cavalcade that would wander the face of war-torn Germany trying to find Americans to whom they could surrender. They could not know, at this painful stage of Germany's impending defeat, that in France, Professor Stanley Mott, a practical engineer like themselves, had put together his team of experts whose job it would be to scour Germany in search of Wernher von Braun, General Eugen Breutzl and Dieter Kolff, trusting that the Germans would have sense enough to bring their papers with them. Mott had heard rumors that General Breutzl had been killed in the big air raid of 24–25 October, but he hoped that this was not correct, for it was the managerial genius of this man that would be most sorely needed during the first stages of America's effort to build a rocket.

When the rolling thunder of Russian artillery barrages could be heard in the south, announcing that Stettin was about to fall, the scientists of Peenemünde made their move. In large convoys of trucks, small cars and anything else that could run, they headed west toward Nordhausen and the underground horror in which their A-4s were stubbornly being fabricated, in the last wild hope that some miracle would enable them to destroy London, or at least Antwerp.

On the day of departure, with doom darkening the sky and the mind, Dieter Kolff faced a series of difficult decisions. He realized that once aboard one of the trucks leaving Peenemünde's island, he would have no chance of disembarking on the mainland side to pick up Liesl. It might be practical to leave the area with the others, then double back to fetch her, but this seemed illogical. Or he could simply ride with his colleagues and forget her, but that he could not do; he loved Liesl and appreciated her heroism in sharing with him the dangers of hiding the papers. Overriding these personal considerations was the fact that whereas the trucks carried tons of documents, to keep them away from the Russians, he better than anyone else, better even than Von Braun, knew that what they carried were the simple equations, the easy solutions that any Russian or American scientist could reconstruct in a few weeks, given a real A-4 to analyze. The knapsack that Liesl had buried on her farm contained the secrets of the A-10, the rocket that could soar four thousand miles across oceans to attack other continents. These papers were irreplaceable, and to leave the area without them would be insane, so when the big trucks rolled away they left Kolff standing alone.

After Von Braun's team disappeared in the west, he stuffed a few valued belongings in his knapsack—a slide rule, a drawing compass, an S curve—and went to his bicycle, but before he could leave the island a member of the skeleton SS Troops commandeered him for a painful duty: 'Himmler says we're to blow up any remaining A-4s.' So with great concentrations of Trialen, Dieter had to destroy the majestic engines he had helped create. Those lying partially completed on the ground were easily pulverized, but when the SS men came to the last rocket, standing upright on its pad, they did not know how to handle it, so the job was given to Dieter.

There it stood, the last A-4 at Peenemünde. It rose sleek and silvery forty-six feet in the air, like some monstrous artillery shell waiting to be loaded. Beautifully proportioned, aerodynamically perfect, it looked as if it longed to be on its way to some distant target, its fins ready to keep it stable as it slashed through the atmosphere. It was magnificent, and it was doomed.

'We'll fire it,' Dieter said. 'Out over the Baltic. The Russians must never get a rocket like this.'

He was the only one who knew how to prepare it for firing, and when the controls were set, he advised the SS men to take cover behind the log-and-stone revetments, for, as he warned them, 'The noise and flame will be terrific.'

He was the last man at the launching pad, a mere five feet four inches looking up at the rocket nine times taller than he. As he stood there he could see marks from the hundred improvements he had made, the thousand that Baron von Braun had suggested. This was one of the noblest instruments yet made by man, a messenger to a new age, and it would soon fly aimlessly.

Throwing the switches, running from the launching area, he leaped behind a bulwark as the mighty engine exploded. Upward through the autumn sky rose the last rocket, out toward the Baltic it roared, and far from Germany it plunged harmlessly into the dark waters.

Dieter feared that the northern ferry might be guarded by new SS men who would not let him pass to the mainland, so when the rocket disappeared he pedaled south to the bridge where the guards would recognize him. When they asked where he was going he said, as always, 'To see my girl,' and as soon as he reached the Koenig farm he announced, 'Time to dig up the papers.'

'Are we leaving?' Liesl asked.

'Haven't you heard the Russian guns?'

'I've been terrified.'

She did not seem like a woman who could be easily terrified, yet it was clear that she had for some weeks been obsessed by the approaching enemy and was now relieved that steps were to be taken. It was she who produced the shovel and started digging; it was she who knelt down to retrieve the knapsack.

Her father and mother, tied to the land their ancestors had farmed in Pomerania for generations, preferred to trust their fortunes with the Russians; they had despised what they had seen of the Nazis and judged that things could not be much worse under Communism. The farewells were not tearful; all over Germany families were being torn apart, and most took solace from the fact that their members were at least alive. Herr Koenig did not kiss his daughter but did shake her hand, as if she were a stranger from the village. Frau Koenig, standing in the doorway that led into the barn beneath the bedrooms, wept. She, too, shook hands first with Liesl, then with Dieter. At the last moment Liesl ran to the cow she had raised and kissed it on the side of its placid face, embracing it with her arms.

So they started on their hegira, he walking, she on the bicycle with the precious knapsack strapped into a large bundle behind. They headed south for Berlin, but whenever they came to a crossroads, armed guards kept shoving them north and away from the capital, which was already over-crowded.

'We are ordered to Nordhausen,' Dieter explained again and again. 'They are waiting for us in Berlin.'

'Blocked,' the guards said. 'You must keep to the north.'

If they did this, Dieter realized, they must sooner or later come into conflict with the SS units guarding the Baltic coast, so with all the energy he had he pressed for a southerly direction, and it was this stubbornness that caused the perilous shooting.

They were on the outskirts of Neustrelitz, a small city halfway between Peenemünde and Berlin, when an SS guard, determined to protect his post, even against Russians, directed them to stop pressing south and head west-ward. Dieter pointed out, quite correctly, that to do so would take them in the Lake Müritz region, which would be difficult to negotiate.

'West!' the guard ordered, and later when he spotted the Kolffs trying to sneak down a lateral road, he took aim at Dieter and hit him in the left shoulder. When the guard saw his target go down in a heap, he was satisfied that he had killed him, so he took careful aim at Liesl, but as he did so, she saw him, and in a flash fell to the ground, encouraging him to assume that he had killed them both. For a moment he contemplated running over to pick up their bicycle, but he knew he himself might be shot if he abandoned his post, so he thought no more about the matter.

On the ground, Liesl saw that her husband was bleeding copiously, so keeping low, she tended his wound, satisfying herself that he was not about to die. When she had the blood stanched, she turned her attention to the bicycle, pulling and hauling until she could work it into a position outside the line of sight of the trigger-hungry SS man. When she succeeded in getting both her husband and the loaded bicycle in safe terrain, she slapped Dieter's face several times, challenging him to get on his feet and out of Neustrelitz.

He could do neither. His wound was more serious than she had detected, and after a few steps he fainted dead away. Now she had to make grave decisions.

Lugging first him, and then the bicycle, she worked her way almost to the outskirts of the town, but by then she was exhausted. Sitting under a tree, she breathed heavily and listened to her husband's irregular panting. When a farmer came by she commandeered him: 'Good fellow! My husband has been hurt. Can you find a doctor?'

The man had his own preoccupations: 'The Russians are coming. Who cares about doctors?'

'My husband is dying,' she pleaded.

'I'll watch him. You fetch the doctor.'

'You'll steal my bicycle.'

'The Russians will steal it if I don't.'

'Will you fetch the doctor?'

'What is he, a spy or something?'

'He is my husband.' The forceful way in which she spoke convinced the farmer. Placing his own bundles beside the bicycle, he said, 'See, I trust you, even if you don't trust me.'

When the doctor arrived, a pale thin man, he asked, 'Are the police after him?'

'An SS man shot him for no reason.'

'God damn them,' the frail doctor said. He inspected Dieter's wound, then looked up at the farmer. 'This man could die if he's not attended.'

'He can come to my place,' the farmer said, so he and Liesl watched as the doctor skillfully extracted the bullet and medicated the resulting gash. Handing Liesl a vial of medicine, he said, 'Three days' rest, he'll live.' Before leaving, the doctor looked in all directions, then returned home by a different route.

For three days the Kolffs hid with their bicycle at the farm west of Neustrelitz, talking incessantly with the owner, a sardonic man who had seen many fortunes rise and fall in his lifetime: 'Germans down now, never lower. The war's lost. Somebody will shoot Hitler soon. Then we'll get the Russians and the damned Allies.'

'Why do you hate the Allies?' Dieter asked, not confiding that he was in search of them as saviors.

'The bombings. Have you seen Berlin? Hamburg? I hear rumors that Dresden has been wiped out. One hundred and fifty thousand dead in one night. The Allies, too, are monsters.'

Then he became reflective. 'I know what you're doing. Running away from the Russians in hopes that the Allies will capture you. And I wonder what you guard so carefully in that bundle on your bicycle. I'll tell you what it is, documents you hope to sell to the Allies. I'll bet you're from Peenemünde, aren't you?'

When Dieter refused to answer, he asked, 'What awful things were you up to? I never saw such secrecy. But don't worry about running away to join the Allies, because I'm going to do the same thing. They're bastards, all of them, but at least they aren't Russian.'

His wife would not leave the farm, but he had no hesitancy in leaving her, and on the last night he explained why: 'I know Germany, the good Germany. Can you believe, sitting here tonight on the edge of ruin, that within ten years we'll be one of the most powerful nations on earth? And why? Because of people like you two. The husband very intelligent. The wife very courageous. I liked the way you looked after your man, little girl. You could run this country. A damned sight better than Hitler ran it.'

They were off, a wounded man, an elderly farmer, a would-be housewife and two bicycles. The farmer insisted that the Kolffs ride the bicycles, at least until Dieter recovered from his wound, and in this way they tried to move south to Berlin, but always they were stopped. At the interrogations the farmer said, 'This is my son, wounded on the Russian front, and my daughter. We're joining my brother in Frankfort.'

'You can't move down this road,' the guards said, so, invariably, the trio were shunted westward until they came to the outskirts of Wittenberge, a small town on the right bank of the Elbe River.

'This is a famous place,' Dieter told his wife. 'Martin Luther started here . . . at the doors of the cathedral.'

The farmer, a good Lutheran, burst into laughter. 'All you bright boys say that. And you're all wrong. This is Wittenberge with an *e*. Wittenberg without the *e* is miles and miles upriver. Martin Luther never saw this Godforsaken place.'

When they were inside the town, walking about to see how best to spend the few marks they allowed themselves each week, Dieter suddenly stopped in horror and leaped behind a pillar, for there, coming straight at him, was General Funkhauser, attended by three SS men. When the pompous, pudgy commander lost Peenemünde, having allowed its principal scientists to escape, he was demoted to officer-in-charge of the Wittenberge District, which the Russians would soon be attacking. It was his task to conscript every able male and arm him for the defense of the town, because if Wittenberge fell, Berlin would be exposed on the north. Dieter, guessing that something like this was afoot, sank deeper into the shadows, allowing the powerful and vengeful man to pass.

When he returned to Liesl and the farmer, he was shaking, and they thought he had been attacked by a fever, but after he took a drink of wine and sat for a moment he informed them of their peril: 'General Funkhauser is in charge of this town, I'm sure of it. I saw him striding along with three of his SS men, and if he even hears of us, we're dead.'

With the greatest circumspection, the farmer went into the heart of town to make inquiries, and he returned with doleful news: 'Every male is now a member of the defense army, under command of General Funkhauser. We must all report at once or be shot.' In the silence he studied Dieter, then asked bluntly, 'Are the papers valuable?'

'They can save our lives,' Dieter said.

'Then we must sneak out of here.'

With great ingenuity the farmer organized a plan whereby the three of them, with their two bicycles, could edge their way to the south of Wittenberge, but as they moved through the dark night an SS guard detected them and fired. The farmer was killed. The Kolffs were arrested.

In the morning they were hauled before General Funkhauser, and Dieter was astonished by the changes he saw in the man: because of anxiety and meager food he had lost more than twenty pounds and now had a neck like ordinary humans; also, his eyes seemed more compassionate, and Dieter remembered how Funkhauser had been repelled by conditions at Nordhausen. He's becoming a human being again, he thought. He knows the war's lost, and will soon be quitting Himmler and his gang. Alone with Liesl he whispered, 'Do everything possible to keep him confused. He may save our lives.'

The interrogation started badly: 'Well, our hero from Peenemünde. The little man who has a silver medal from Hitler himself. What evil tricks are you up to this time?'

Dieter stood silent, remembering that since this unpredictable man had once tried to have him executed, there was a likelihood that the sentence would now be carried out. Funkhauser, obviously uncertain of himself, was encouraged by Dieter's cowering. Tapping the knapsack which lay on his desk, he asked sardonically, 'And what is our little man stealing from the Third Reich? Secret papers? Could they be the ones I was looking for after the death of General Breutzl?'

Keeping his eyes fixed on Dieter, he shoved the knapsack at him. 'You open it. Show me what secrets you were going to sell to the enemy.'

With fumbling hands, Dieter dug into the knapsack, producing a few papers. 'What are they?' Funkhauser asked in his silky voice. When Kolff made no reply, the general screamed, 'Are they the secret papers of General Breutzl? Of course they are. And what do they deal with? Germany's secret weapons.' Whenever he said the word *secret* he lingered over it, as if, like Hitler and Goebbels and the German public, he believed that some mysterious force would still save the nation.

Dieter, realizing that Funkhauser had incriminating proof of everything he charged, could only remain silent, awaiting judgment. It was harsh: 'He and his wife. Spies and traitors. Shoot them.' He stomped from the room, leaving Dieter alone with two husky SS guards, who led him out into the hallway, where they grabbed Liesl, throwing her behind her husband as the death march to the courtyard began.

It was a warm day at the beginning of March and the sky was that wonderful Prussian blue which seemed half-dawn, half-midnight. Staring at it and remembering the days when he first bicycled to the Koenig farm to court Liesl, he wanted to take her hand, to console her, but the guards, now augmented by three riflemen, kept them separated. So he had to be content to look back at her, and he was relieved to see that she was marching to her death without panic. She even smiled at him as if to say that since they had been goaded into making their choices, there should be no lamentation.

When they were stood against the wall, Dieter asked in a quivering voice, 'May I kiss my wife goodbye?'

'Go ahead.'

'Liesl, it was short . . . but very good.'

'I love you, Dieter.'

They kissed, and then of their own accord, as if their punishment was the inevitable consequence of their own actions, they resumed their places against the wall, and the three soldiers planted their feet wide apart and hefted their rifles. For an awful moment Kolff and his wife looked into the shining barrels, and Dieter, the engineer-mechanic, wondered: How can three shoot two? Something might go badly wrong. Then he saw, kneeling on the gravel, a fourth man with a machine gun, and in a curious way he was satisfied. The SS were doing it right.

But in the split second before the command 'Fire!' General Funkhauser ran into the courtyard, sweating, and shouted, 'Take them back to their cells.'

'We have no cells,' an SS man shouted back.

'Keep them in a closet. And guard them.'

The closet in the town hall of Wittenberge was seven feet wide and three feet deep, with no light and very little air. They had to find a place for themselves among brooms and mops, but there were several workmen's smocks on which they could sleep. They were kept in this dismal place for what seemed like a week, although it could have been more. They were fed miserably, never had enough water to drink, and were allowed out only to go to the bathroom, one at a time, under heavy guard.

'He's confused about the papers,' Dieter guessed.

'A guard told me as we went down the hall, "Germany's defeated. Everyone is closing in upon us." He was almost crying, as if it were unfair.'

'We must do nothing to anger them, Liesl. They're in a trap, too, and they know it.'

On what seemed to them the eighth day, General Funkhauser brought them both to his office, an ornate affair, rather handsome in its display of the symbols prized by a provincial town. There was the engraving of Bismarck, crisp and clear in its fine black lines, the colored portrait of some local general, and the huge photograph of Hitler, menacing and fatherly at the same time. And there, on his desk, was the knapsack.

'Are these papers what I think they are?' Funkhauser asked, and instantly shrewd Liesl deduced two facts: the General was in desperate trouble, like all of Germany, and he had grown to believe that somehow these papers could save him.

Calmly she said, 'They could save your life when the Allies come. But they have meaning only if Dieter is alive to explain them.' She would hook their lives to his, for she knew that otherwise he would shoot them in the back when the Allies approached.

'They look like plans for a rocket,' Funkhauser said, riffling the papers.

'Sssssh!' she warned. 'They cover a weapon so secret that only Hitler and General Breutzl knew the full details. And Dieter.'

When Funkhauser looked at the inoffensive little man he could not believe that Kolff could have been privy to some great secret, but then he remembered that when he and Dieter had visited Hitler at Wolf's Lair . . . 'He did take you aside at the end, didn't he?'

'This is something entirely different,' Dieter said.

'You think the Allies would want to bargain for these papers?'

'That's why Von Braun sent them out secretly,' Liesl said. 'With the one man who could explain them.'

'Wait!' Funkhauser snapped, his beady eyes narrowing. 'Von Braun and all the other leading scientists are at the underground works at Nordhausen. Why aren't you there, with them, if you're so important?'

'I'm not important,' Dieter said, 'but the papers are, and Von Braun knew that I was the only one who could deal with them.'

In some irritation the general instructed his guards, 'Lock them up,' but when they were alone in the darkness Liesl assured her husband: 'He's worried. The Russians have him worried. And we have him worried. He won't shoot us now.'

Early next morning General Funkhauser summoned them to his office and dismissed the guards. Without preliminaries he moved from behind his desk, stood with the Kolffs as if they were his equals, and pointed to the knapsack. 'Could we deliver these papers to the Americans?'

'Those were my orders,' Dieter said.

'From whom?'

'From Baron Wernher von Braun,' and as he uttered this influential name, he automatically reached for the knapsack, bringing it to his chest as if it were something he must cherish. Funkhauser jerked it away and clutched it himself.

'We'll take it through the lines to the Allies,' he said. Then, looking with some contempt at the Kolffs, he added, 'I can speak a little English, you know.'

They were a curious trio as they wound their way toward the triangle formed by Hamburg, Bremen and Hanover. General Funkhauser was always in the lead with a small bicycle which he had commandeered and to which the precious knapsack was tied. He had been afraid to use an SS automobile lest it attract too much attention and perhaps cause his arrest, and it never occurred to him to let one of the Kolffs use his bicycle, for he was a general, made so by Hitler himself, whom he was now abandoning.

Usually Liesl rode the Kolff bicycle, but she kept close watch over Dieter, and whenever she detected that the wound in his shoulder was causing serious discomfort, she dismounted and made him ride. They ate poorly, slept wherever they halted, and smelled horrible, but they noticed with some amusement that General Funkhauser was quite vain of his appearance, so that no matter how dusty his uniform became, he took pains to keep it as neat as his fatness would permit.

He was proving to be a remarkable man, able to adjust to anything. Such food as they obtained was due to his ability to forage on land that seemed completely barren. He would eat anything—a stray duck, fish caught by some farm boy from the family pond, a sheep shared with sixteen, crusts of stale bread from a village bakery—and was willing to concoct whatever story was necessary to cover the situation. Dieter was his younger brother and they were heading to the family shop in Bremen. Liesl was his daughter, searching for the husband who may have survived the bombing of Hamburg. But wherever they went, he listened to the rumors of war, and when he learned that British troops were advancing in the north, he led his refugees south: 'No German is ever smart enough to deal with an Englishman.' When villagers told him that a French unit was about to take Bremen, he scurried away: 'The French eat well and live miserably.'

But no matter where he led his dusty entourage, they saw the ruin that had overtaken Germany. It was heartbreaking, whole towns wiped out in one night's bombing, a village on which three accidental bombs had fallen, farms burned and deserted. Once they stopped at a scene of desolation, and Funkhauser screamed at the heavens, 'Goering, you fat beast, you promised me we would never be bombed.'

Tears came to his eyes as he thought of Hamburg. He had not actually seen his devastated city but had heard from those who had watched the Funkhauser homes bombed to fragments and then burned. Sniffling, he looked at the Kolffs beseechingly and asked, 'What country deserves punishment like this? What did we ever do wrong?' And each day, more firmly, he turned against both Hitler and Himmler, even cursing them when he saw some especially hideous wreckage.

He had always been a man to change his loyalties quickly. As a lad he had listened approvingly when his liberal father praised the German Republic, but in 1931 he had switched easily to the youthful Nazi party, seeing in it the salvation of his Fatherland. He had served for a while in the army of Ritter von Leeb, whom he then considered to be the finest German he had known, but when differences arose between Hitler and his generals, he sided completely with the Fuehrer and assured his associates that the generals, especially Von Leeb, who had failed to capture Leningrad, were asses lacking in military genius.

When the bad days of the war approached, he saw clearly that Heinrich Himmler was the only man who had a clear vision of both the past and the future, and he threw his energies totally into the service of that master conniver. Most eagerly did he work to undercut the army and the regular police, and now, at last, when isolated units of the SS were supposed to hold forlorn outposts like the town of Wittenberge, he awakened to the fact that Himmler was really a psychopathic megalomaniac, a phrase he had heard one of his young assistants use to describe Winston Churchill, and he was abandoning him, as proper Germans should.

On two different occasions he had ordered Lieutenant Kolff to be shot, and for good reason, yet here he was with Kolff and his peasant wife, ducking and dodging through the rural bypaths of a defeated Germany. It was insane, but he felt sure that something would work out, as it seemed always to do.

He was not careless where the Kolffs were concerned. Always at night or at the beginning of any crisis he kept his bicycle close to his side, the knapsack where he could touch it. He also kept his revolver on the ready, and he had begun to contemplate various clever ways by which, in the moments of surrender to the Americans, he could dispose of these two. The more he saw of Liesl the more he distrusted her, a silent, inscrutable type who could be plotting anything. And as for Dieter, it was clear that he was a South German oaf with a sparse mathematical ability and not much more. It was inconceivable that the Americans would want that one.

But until he reached the Americans, he needed the Kolffs, and so he was generous with them. If he refused to share his bicycle, he did divide all food equally with them. He was jovial when the weather turned bad and they had to plod through mud, and incredibly ingenious in devising stories which brought them always closer to the American lines.

On one such foray he heard that an American army had captured Nordhausen, and for some time he sat disconsolately on the ground beneath an evergreen, apart from the Kolffs. Then he turned to face Liesl: 'Did Dieter ever tell you about Nordhausen?'

'He said it was horrible.'

'It was. A taste of hell. When did I first realize that Germany was doomed? When I stood in those caves at Nordhausen.'

'Why did you permit them?'

'It was Himmler's idea. The industrial city of the future. Poles and Russians to work underground.'

'I grew up on a farm,' Dieter broke in. 'So did Liesl. We need the sky.'

'Where was your farm?'

'A village not far from Oberammergau, south of Munich.'

'Really!' Funkhauser leaped to his feet, quivering with excitement. 'I heard in the village that Von Braun and his top scientists have been moved to Oberammergau! Maybe we should work our way south to join them. They'll be protected by the Americans.'

Without further reflection he headed his party south toward the mountains, but on the second day he called a halt, deeply confused. 'If the scientists moved south in a group, Himmler must have ordered it. When he has them all safe in one spot, he'll machine-gun them, all of them, to prevent them from taking their secrets to the Allies.' He became so convinced of this that he changed course completely and headed due west, grumbling, 'Lakes or mountains, Himmler or Hitler, to hell with them all. We've got to reach the Americans. Now!'

He was relentless in pursuit of this policy, forging ahead toward the sound of distant battle, and one night as the three lay down to sleep, completely exhausted, Liesl whispered to Dieter, 'The general is making up his mind about many things,' and she left Dieter's side and crept away.

In the morning Funkhauser bellowed, 'Where's my revolver? Where are my papers?' and Liesl said, 'I took them,' and he shouted, 'Why do you betray me?' and she said coldly, 'Because you planned to shoot us . . . today or tomorrow.'

The bluster faded; with a contrition that might or might not have been authentic, Funkhauser said, 'At Wittenberge, when we set out, yes, I did think of bringing you close to the Americans and shooting you. Anyone would have. But as we've traveled these dangerous miles . . .' He paused and held out his hands. 'I've said so many times that you were my family that I've come to believe it.' Keeping his hands out, he begged, 'Do not shoot me, I beseech you.'

'We never planned to shoot you, General,' Liesl said. 'Now lead us to the Americans, for you are an excellent guide.'

He led them into a much different kind of confrontation, for as he crept like a cunning badger through a woods, with the Kolffs trailing, he stumbled right into a contingent of the German army, and in the confused gunfire that ensued, Liesl took a bullet through her left leg.

'Down!' Funkhauser bellowed, and the three travelers fell upon pine needles.

When they looked up, Liesl clutching her leg, they saw an amazing sight. Their assailants were a disorderly gang of boys, fourteen and fifteen years old, but in full military uniform. One of them was sobbing, 'I shot a lady. Oh my God, I shot a lady.'

General Funkhauser, realizing that he had come upon one of the desperation units commissioned by the Nazi high command, began to storm at the children, 'What are you doing in these woods? Why are you shooting women who are trying to save the Fatherland?'

When he announced that he was a general in the SS and in command of this section of Germany, some of the boys saluted, and he tried to console the little boy who was weeping: 'You couldn't have known it was a woman. Now you help bind her wound.' And he lectured the older boys on how they must maintain better control when on maneuvers.

'What are your orders?' he asked.

'We are to stop the Americans.'

'Where are they?' he asked eagerly.

'In the next town. We expect them soon, and we're to hold these woods against them.' He looked at their feeble rifles, their thin arms barely able to manage the guns effectively, and saluted: 'Protect the Fatherland.' And he called to the Kolffs, 'Hurry, hurry! This is the day that determines everything!'

As they emerged from the woods to seek the town of which the boys had spoken, it became obvious that Liesl could neither walk nor pedal the

Kolff bicycle, so in a burst of generosity Funkhauser performed an act which would in years far distant be remembered with charity: 'Liesl, my daughter, you must sit yourself on my bicycle so that I can push you into town.' And with a fatherly eye he kept watch on Dieter, who teetered along on the Kolff cycle, and in this way they struggled toward the fateful meeting with the Americans. 'Hurry, hurry!' he encouraged his charges. 'Our trusted allies will soon roar down this road.'

Halfway between the exit from the woods and the entrance to the town the three fugitives met their first Americans, a patrol roaring out to locate the enemy. 'Honored sirs!' Funkhauser shouted to the motorcycle vanguard. 'I am General Helmut . . .'

'Get your ass off this road!' a rude voice shouted.

'Honored sirs! I am General . . .'

A big man in a dirty uniform wheeled his motorcycle, placed a foot in Funkhauser's belly and shoved him off the road; the American did not have to discipline the Kolffs, for they had jumped into a ditch.

When the patrol passed, Funkhauser resumed his approach to the town, and he was pleased to see that a regular marching unit was now coming toward him. Hands up, he ran toward the American captain, shouting in clear English, 'Sir, sir! I have papers which your generals will want.'

'Out of the way, you fucking Krauthead,' a soldier grunted, shoving him back into the ditch as heavy guns rolled by.

'Please, listen!' he cried from beside the road. 'I have important papers which your generals . . .'

The semitanks rolled past, and when they reached the woods Liesl could hear agitated gunfire, and she was about to weep for the little boys when she saw that General Funkhauser was standing transfixed, staring at the woods as he contemplated the awful tragedy his one-time leaders had brought to Germany. 'Children with little guns! Defending against motorized cannon. And Hitler's men promised us that no enemy foot would ever step on German soil. Damn them all.' He remained staring at the woods as the heavier American guns exploded into action; then, in total despair and silence, he helped Dieter mount his bicycle, then went back to the ditch to rescue the bleeding Liesl, and pushed her humbly into town.

As they turned a corner leading to the main square, they found themselves face to face with another American, this one in dusty civilian clothes. At first he was as startled as they and began to call for troops to protect him, but then he peered inquisitively at Dieter's face and took a deep breath.

'Dieter Kolff, I believe,' he said in German.

'From Peenemünde.'

'Did you bring the papers on the heavy water?'

'I brought the secret papers,' Funkhauser interposed, tapping Liesl's knapsack and introducing himself. 'General Helmut Funkhauser, Commandant General of Peenemünde, at your service, sir.'

The American ignored him and asked Kolff again, 'Did you bring the papers on the heavy-water installations at Peenemünde?'

'Heavy water? What's that?'

'You had no . . .' Mott hesitated to say the crucial word, but he could not restrain himself. 'You had no atomic works there?'

'What would they be?'

'No papers?'

'Sir, these are the secret papers of General Eugen Breutzl.'

'Where is he?'

'Dead. In the great bombing.'

Mott shook his head. 'He was a good man. Before the interrogation—'

'I knew Breutzl well,' Funkhauser interrupted, pressing himself forward.

'You will all be properly interrogated,' Mott assured the three. 'But Breutzl, what was he working on here?' and by his gestures and his interest he indicated that now the papers in the knapsack were his.

'On a rocket that will fly from Peenemünde to New York.'

The search was ended. For two years Mott had sought this little man, had studied diligently the one photograph available. Now he was found. Germany had produced no atomic bomb. But it had been on the verge of discoveries equally important, a rocket that could fly between continents, and the secrets were to rest with America, not Russia.

Intuitively Mott did something he would later recall with astonishment, something that bespoke his stern New England upbringing. Seeing in the much-damaged street the gaping doorway of the village church, its seventeenth-century façade blown away by American bombs, he said, 'I think we should pray . . . give thanks . . . for our deliverance.'

He led the three Germans into what was technically their church, and he sat on one of the old benches, depleted spiritually by his long search, and as he closed his eyes he heard General Funkhauser intoning, first in English, then in German, 'We thank you, God, for directing us to make all the right choices.'

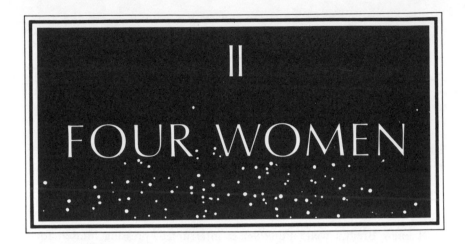

II

FOUR WOMEN

FROM THE MOMENT IN THAT SPRING OF 1946 WHEN THE REPUBLICAN leaders of Fremont telephoned their war hero Norman Grant, asking if they could drive up to consult with him, his wife, Elinor, became apprehensive, and she showed it.

As a loyal Republican she realized that Fremont was crucial to the Republican cause; it would be a linchpin in the off-year drive to purge Congress of the Democrats who supported the incompetent Harry Truman. Through some aberration, fanned no doubt by the recent war hysteria, Fremont had in the last election sent one Democrat to the House of Representatives, and it was imperative that he be thwarted in his bid for reelection.

Elinor was eager to see this correction made, and had her husband lived in that congressman's district, she would have encouraged him to contest the seat. Unfortunately, the Democrat represented the big industrial city of Webster on the Missouri River, which made Grant ineligible.

What the politicians wanted, as they explained when they convened in the local headquarters, was some young man of good reputation who could head that statewide ticket in the race for the United States Senate. And therein lay the difficulty, as Elinor saw immediately: 'Senator Gantling considers that seat his . . . for as long as he lives.' Some of the visitors showed their impatience at having to discuss such matters with a woman, but Grant had insisted upon his wife's presence: 'She's always given me sound advice.'

'Gantling's an old man. He weakens the ticket.'

'He's only sixty-two,' Elinor protested.

'Sixty-four,' one of the downstaters said, 'and he looks eighty.'

'He is sixty-two,' Elinor said primly. 'I looked it up.'

'You guessed what we wanted to talk about?' the downstater asked.

'Yes, and I must point out that my father has always been a close personal friend of Senator Gantling. Ran his campaign for him when he first went to Congress.'

'We all supported him then, but he's had his day, Mrs. Grant.'

'And I would remind you that my husband's father also worked for Gantling. This family simply cannot serve as the spearhead to defeat that fine man.'

'Mrs. Grant, I think we should take a very careful look at the state of Fremont,' and the downstater spread the map on the table. 'You summarize our thinking, Lewis.'

A burly gentleman who regularly delivered a heavy Republican majority from the sparsely settled northwest section of the state jabbed at corners of the map as he spoke with considerable force. 'Four areas matter, and mine's not one of them, so I'm free to speak realistically.'

Fremont was the most typical of the great Western states. Named for the flamboyant explorer John Charles Frémont, it had honored in its four major cities those outstanding politicians of the early nineteenth century whose interest in the West had helped that vast area become an integral part of the nation. In the east the commercial city of Webster; in the west the regional capital of Calhoun; in the north, with the state university, Grant's home city of Clay; and in the center the capital city, named after the man who may have been the best of the lot, Thomas Hart Benton.

'Senator Gantling is an important man in his home district of Calhoun,' the big man was saying. 'But the whole damned town has only nineteen thousand people. Over here in Webster, where the votes really concentrate, Gantling is known as a fool.'

'That's too strong,' Grant protested.

'Tell him, Henry.'

And Henry did. 'Senator Gantling has run his course, Norman. And you, too, Mrs. Grant. You must wake up to reality. He's insulted our people, ignored them, passed them by when goodies were distributed. It's the old fight of the eastern end of a state versus the western end. It happens everywhere. Philadelphia versus Pittsburgh. St. Louis versus Kansas City. And right on your doorstep it's Webster versus Calhoun, and I warn you right now. If we Republicans run Gantling again at the head of our ticket, Webster and the whole eastern half of the state is going to vote Democratic. I warn you.'

As the discussion continued, even Elinor Grant had to concede that her antique favorite, Ulysses Gantling, had probably worn out his welcome in the state of Fremont. The little town of Calhoun still favored him as a local boy, but the big city of Webster was fed up with his posturing ways.

Then the big man from the northwestern district revealed the deeper purpose of this meeting: 'Norman, you must keep your eye on the bigger target. 1948. Tom Dewey will pretty surely be our man then, experienced, one national campaign under his belt, a born leader. He'll run against that goddamned haberdasher from Kansas City, and you know and I know that if the election were held today, Truman wouldn't get ten electoral votes. Even Senator Fulbright of his own party advised him to resign, the country's so against him.

The manufacturer from Webster laughed. 'Did you hear Truman's reply to that one? Said he needed no advice from Senator Halfbright.'

'We all know he's a disgrace, totally unfit to sit in the White House, and our job is to get him out. Returning this state to its proper stance in 1946 is the best thing we can do in preparation for 1948. A good strong senator. Knock off that damned Democrat in Webster . . .'

'That's why I'm here,' the manufacturer said. 'Grant, I need your help. Enormously. With you heading the ticket, I can defeat that Democrat. With Gantling, I'll not only lose the House seat but also the Senate.'

'Is he really so weak?' Grant asked, and as soon as he uttered these words Elinor realized that he was beginning to visualize himself as savior of the party, as a man standing before the voters with fresh new ideas, and she was frightened.

Elinor Stidham had been born in 1917, when her father, a well-to-do farmer from north of Clay, was absent fighting in France. She therefore never knew him as the robust, simple man he had once been; she saw him only as a frail person, badly damaged by the war and unsure of himself. She was two when he was finally released from the hospital, and she could not recall his ever playing with her, or bouncing her on his knee; he certainly never spoke of the war or of the adventures she imagined him as having.

She developed into a quiet, stately girl who always seemed much older than those in her class. She did extremely well in school, and at the university, too, and could have become quite popular had she sought that kind of approval. Her marks were mostly A's and she joined one of the good sororities, but she was elected to no office, not even in Kappa Alpha Theta, and most students were ignorant of her presence on campus.

Boys always noticed her, but after chilly rebuffs they allowed her to move alone, which she did, from sorority house to library to classrooms to the gymnasium. She was tall, slim, attractive, with very dark hair which she kept tight about her head, and it pleased her that several of the more serious male students, especially the bookish types, signified a serious interest in her, even though the rowdy element no longer did.

The campus was astonished, therefore, when its premier football player, Norman Grant, suddenly started dating her. Half a dozen campus beauties had invited him to their dances, and several dozen others would have liked to do so, but it was obvious that he'd settled on Elinor Stidham.

A wealthy alumnus, proud of Norman's football skills, had casually given him a Chevrolet on the sensible grounds that 'any football player as good as Norman Grant is entitled to a convertible.' In it Norman drove Elinor up to the Stidham farm, where he spent long hours talking with

Frank Stidham, who still refused to mention his experiences in the war but who was eager to talk about the nature of a good society.

Stidham was a Republican, of course, as all responsible citizens of Fremont tended to be, but he had an extremely wide social comprehension which encompassed Burke, Jefferson, Lincoln, Woodrow Wilson and especially the Frenchman Alexis de Tocqueville, whose ability to identify the fundamentals of the American system astounded him: 'If a young man wanted to grasp the true nature of this country, the only book he would have to read is De Tocqueville.'

'Professor Bates says the same thing about Lord Bryce.'

'Well, now . . .' Stidham twisted in his chair as if his back hurt, then smiled. 'Bates has something there. Yes, he has. But when I was in England, I felt that men like Bryce, and I met a lot of them, ponderously elaborated the obvious, which is what Bryce does, I'm afraid. But in France the brilliant mind cuts right into the heart of a problem, laying waste the verbiage, and that's what De Tocqueville does. Have you read him, Norman?'

'No, I've been too busy trying to keep up with my classes. Pre-law is no snap.'

'Why do you play so many games, Norman? Isn't football enough? Do you really need basketball, too? And then baseball?'

'I'm just geared that way, sir.'

When two of the football players asked Grant why he bothered with that Stidham broad, seeing that she never put out, he smiled and said, 'Elinor and I've known each other since high school. We dated a couple of times then.'

'Did she put out then?'

'It's none of your business—but no. But one thing kept sticking in my mind.'

'What?'

'When I drove up to the farm in a borrowed car for our first date, her father spoke to me as if I were his equal. Maybe you've seen him. Smallish fellow, seems to be in pain a good deal. And he told me that his daughter was very precious to him—'

'All fathers say that. I went with a dame—'

'And he added that it wouldn't be necessary to impress his daughter by driving seventy miles an hour around the curves of a dark road.'

'What the hell has that got to do with anything?'

'The more I thought about it, in later years, that is, the more I realized that he was letting me know that the Stidhams take life seriously. And so do I.'

He had left the university with eight varsity letters and a high B-plus, which made it easy for him to enter law school in Chicago. When he left Clay, Elinor had two more years to go for her degree, but she never doubted that he would be back, to see her father if not her. Once she said sardonically, 'I sometimes think that Norman comes here to eat your pies, Mother, and to have Father tutor him for his law exams.'

Mr. Stidham was not a lawyer, but he was an acute student of American history, especially its foreign policies relating to war, and Elinor could remember clearly the night in 1938 when her father told Norman, 'I'm deeply worried about Mr. Roosevelt's actions vis-à-vis Japan.'

'We could handle Japan, if anything happened,' Grant assured him.

'I don't mean that. It seems to me that war in Europe is inevitable. Things are so unstable that even the slightest disruption . . .'

'What has Europe to do with Japan?'

'Don't you see? If war does break out there, attention will be diverted from Japan, and their war lords will feel free to undertake the most daring ventures. Sooner or later they will do something which will infuriate America, and then the fat's in the fire.'

'Why are you blaming President Roosevelt?' At his law school Grant was discovering to his astonishment that most of his better professors defended Roosevelt, whereas no one in Fremont did.

'I simply think he ought to do nothing that drives a wedge between us and Japan.'

'Is he doing so?'

'I'm afraid everything he does is antagonistic.'

'Maybe we should be antagonistic. The way those yellow devils have been treating China.'

'The point is, Norman, that if Roosevelt continues, this nation must be prepared to fight Japan on a very broad front indeed.'

'It's a small island. We can handle that island, I'm sure.'

'You should look at your map. It's a group of islands, and they will not be the battlefield.' When Norman asked what would, Stidham took down an atlas which displayed the Pacific in a large double-spread. 'The battlefield will be the entire ocean. Java down here. The Philippines up here. Malay even. Hawaii no doubt.'

Such reasoning was preposterous, and Norman said so: 'Japan is a tiny place, sir. They're not capable of an effort like that. Our Navy would knock the hell out of them.'

In 1940, when he was back in Clay with a law degree and a foothold in a good local office, Norman proposed to Elinor Stidham, as she had always been sure he would. The wedding was held in the Baptist Church, and the honeymoon was by train to Niagara Falls. Because of Norman's sports achievements, newspapers as far away as New York City chronicled the marriage, and while they were staying at the newlyweds' hotel at the Falls, an admiring older couple showed them the wire-service announcement in the Buffalo paper, then ordered a bottle of wine to help them celebrate.

In 1942, when all of Mr. Stidham's remarkable prophecies had come

true, Norman Grant was sent to Dartmouth College for a six-week course
that would make him an officer in the United States Navy, and the problem
arose as to what his young bride ought to do for the duration. The two men,
Stidham and Grant, discussed the matter thoroughly and decided that
Elinor should stay at the Stidham home and engage in such/patriotic work
as might develop, but when they informed her of their decision she surprised
them by saying that she had already written to the hospital in Hanover,
New Hampshire, where Dartmouth was located, and had obtained a job as
helper in some menial capacity.

The men were outraged, with Norman making the most sensible objection: 'I'll be busy twenty hours a day. There's no way I could . . .'

She would not listen. Better than any young woman in the state of
Fremont she understood the nature of this war. For years she had listened
as her father patiently identified the major strains that must produce the
conflict, and if he had been unable to convince the members of the Clay City
Rotary Club, or his new son-in-law, he had certainly convinced her.

She had followed Norman to Dartmouth and had served as nurse's
helper in the local hospital. Then she had moved to the Patuxent River in
Maryland when it looked as if Norman was going into naval aviation. When
BuPers suddenly switched him to the badly understaffed destroyer unit on
the West Coast, she found a job in Seattle helping to run a restaurant, and
from there she had sent her husband off to what became, in 1944, the great
Battle of Leyte Gulf.

Now, in 1946, she looked much as she had in high school and college:
still slightly underweight, still smartly dressed, still distinguished by her fair
skin and very dark hair. As each year passed she became more beautiful,
and although during the war she had given ample proof of her courage, she
seemed always to become a little more frail, a little more vulnerable.

She did not want her husband to challenge Senator Gantling. She did
not want him to move to Washington if perchance he did win: 'Norman has
fought his war, gentlemen. It's unfair to make him repeat.'

'Wouldn't it be a good idea,' the man from the northwest asked, 'if we
called Paul Stidham in here? He knows Gantling. He knows Grant. He'd
give us all sober advice.'

So Stidham was called on the telephone, and shortly he was among the
men with whom he had conducted many campaigns. Tight-lipped, with his
forefingers pressed against his lips in a kind of church steeple, he listened
as the politicians spread their problems before him, and after his daughter
had expressed forcefully her opposition to Norman's candidacy, he said
very quietly, 'I agree completely that Ulysses Gantling has run his course.
If you offer him to the voters again, we will lose his seat and the Democrats
will retain their hold on that House seat. Gantling's time is up, and he must
face that harsh fact. He must step aside for a better, younger man, and I
know no one more qualified to make the challenge and serve in the Senate
than Norman Grant. I've followed his course of self-education for the past

fourteen years, and he's ready. You men will serve the state and the nation well if you nominate him and see that he wins the primary.'

'Will you serve as state chairman? Grant for Senate?'

'Certainly not. I shall support Senator Gantling, as always.'

'But it would look dreadful . . . Norman's own father-in-law . . .'

'And his wife,' Elinor said crisply.

'Good God!' the man from Webster growled. 'Are we a bunch of insane children?'

The politicians jumped on the Stidhams, pointing out the scandal that would inflame the state if a young man challenging a well-known incumbent found his wife and his distinguished father-in-law supporting the opposition.

'You're entirely correct,' Stidham said quietly, 'it would be scandalous. But I'm beholden to Ulysses Gantling and could not possibly desert him, especially since I believe that Norman can win despite my stand.' He could not be moved. Honor-bound to continue defending a man he had helped into the Senate years ago, he refused to abandon him in the last stages of a career which had not been outstanding but which had been defensible. Ulysses Gantling had never been a first-class senator and would never be, whereas Norman Grant had at least an outside chance, so logic demanded that Paul Stidham shift his allegiance to his son-in-law. But honor required that he stand by his old friend, and this he would do.

'What about your daughter, then? Shouldn't she campaign for her husband?'

'I campaign for nothing,' Elinor said.

'Will you at least keep your mouth shut?' the man from Webster asked.

When Elinor refused to reply, the man from Calhoun, on whom would fall the heavy burden of opposing Gantling, the honored citizen of his own town, asked, pleadingly, 'Don't you admit that your husband is much the better man?'

'He's a superb man,' Elinor said, moving slightly toward where her husband sat.

'Wouldn't he make a fine senator?'

'The best.'

'And don't you want to see Tom Dewey elected in '48?'

'Anything to get rid of Truman.'

'Then will you please keep your mouth shut?'

Elinor looked at her father, who stared straight ahead. Finally she said, 'My family has always supported Ulysses Gantling, who has proved himself to be honest and trustworthy . . .'

'And damned dull,' someone interjected.

'So I must vote for him. But I will keep my mouth shut.' With that she patted her husband slightly on the shoulder and left the room.

· · ·

During the campaign Elinor took an intense dislike to Tim Finnerty, the brash young newspaperman from Boston whom Norman imported to help run his Benton office. After one glance at Finnerty, she warned her husband: 'I don't really care whether you win or lose, but if you care, you ought to get rid of that young monster. In this state a Roman Catholic Irishman from Boston will do you more harm than good.'

When Norman insisted upon keeping Finnerty, she never again went near the Benton office and showed her resentment whenever the young Irishman visited their home in Clay. She did hear, however, that Finnerty was an asset among the rougher element in the riverfront city of Webster, and she had to take notice when he unveiled the stratagem which more than any other accounted for her husband's sudden spurt in the polls.

During the first four weeks of the primary Senator Gantling had played adroitly upon the emotions of his state, pointing out his years of faithful service and the damage being done to the Republican party. To the surprise of many, the old warrior was proving a much abler antagonist than predicted, and three weeks before the voting he looked like a sure bet for reelection.

It appeared to many voters that Norman Grant was running principally on the ground that he had been a football star at the university; there was a good deal of sports talk, and cheerleading, and nostalgia. And it was after one such rally that Finnerty read the riot warning: 'We're going to cut out all this shit.'

'Young man, watch your words,' one of the locals said.

'Do you want to win this election, or don't you?'

'Young man, I've written to Boston about you. You're a registered Democrat.'

'I'm employed as an honest workman to see that my old buddy gets elected to the second highest office in this land. I take no credit for what we're going to do from here in. A friend of mine's come up with a strategy that's a beauty. So from tonight on we'll knock off the old shit.'

He spent that night on the telephone, and two days later, before an audience in the critical swing district in Webster, he revealed the new strategy. It consisted of having Norman Grant pose in front of a mock-up of a destroyer escort, while three good-looking young American men— himself, Pharmacist's Mate Larry Penzoss of Alabama and Cook's Helper Gawain Butler from Detroit—stood at attention in their Navy uniforms, bedecked with ribbons and medals.

He spoke first: 'I am in the paid employ of Norman Grant. It's my job to get him elected to the United States Senate. So anything I tell you is suspect. But Larry Penzoss here, from the great state of Alabama, he came at his own expense. He's not getting a penny from Norman Grant, and he has something important to tell you.'

With a marvelous Deep South drawl Penzoss re-created the scene on the raft, and with a pathos that brought tears to many, told of Captain Grant's heroism and compassion. He astonished Grant by recalling in wrenching detail the death of Executive Officer Savage and Captain Grant's deportment during the burial at sea.

In the silence that followed his speech, Finnerty indicated that Gawain Butler, now a restaurant man in Detroit, should speak, and the tall black, moving on a prosthetic right foot, stepped forward to tell in impeccable English the story of how Norman Grant had pulled him from the shark-filled waters and had then volunteered to spend the night in the water, at infinite risk to his life, so that a nigger, as he phrased it, might be saved. Gawain ended: 'It's up to you to decide whether Captain Grant will make a good senator. I can assure you he made a fantastic captain.' He saluted and stumped back to his place in line.

Then Finnerty took over: 'I warned you before that anything I might say would have to be suspect. So I'm not going to say anything. But with your permission I'm going to read you from the notes I took that day of battle. They were written in 1944, when I was a green kid of nineteen, noting as was my duty the behavior of the bravest man I have ever known, the bravest man the entire state of Fremont will ever know.'

From an inside pocket, fumbling as he did so, he produced a water-stained book, not the real one, of course, for that formed part of the Navy historical record, but a good imitation, soaked in the washbasin of a Fremont hotel two nights ago and dried over a groaning radiator. Turning the pages carefully, he came to the morning of 25 October 1944 and in a low Irish voice he read:

'Yoeman Finnerty (That's me). "Do you intend to take on the whole Japanese fleet?"

'Captain Grant (That's him): "I do." '

Cleverly the young Irishman broke the tension: 'In this world a lot of men say "I do," but no matter how badly the marriage works out, it never involves the consequences that hit us that morning.' When the listeners stopped laughing, he fumbled with the notebook again, confiding details of overpowering effectiveness:

'Immediately after the battle ended, I wrote in my log as required a report of what I had seen that morning. Later, when Captain Grant had a chance to see it, and read how I had praised him, with his customary modesty he tore the page out and threw it away. I should now like to read you my report as I reconstructed it later, when the United States Government wanted to give him the highest medals this nation can give: "Against odds that would have terrified the ordinary captain, he took his DE right at the heart of the Jap battleships and cruisers, and even when he had no more torpedoes or ammunition, he maintained position in order to confuse the enemy. In our life rafts his courage continued, for he voluntarily placed himself in waters which only a few minutes before had contained sharks in order to save others." '

Here he pointed with his left hand at Gawain Butler; with his right hand he closed the notebook, returning it to his pocket.

A political reporter from the *Chicago Tribune,* eager to see Fremont get itself organized in preparation for the Dewey victory in 1948, wired an enthusiastic account to his paper:

> Four days ago this reporter was satisfied that the aging warhorse Ulysses Gantling was a shoo-in for a sixth term as senator from Fremont. Even the challenger's father-in-law was supporting the tested old warrior.
>
> But in Webster and again last night in Benton, Norman Grant disclosed a strategy that gained him frenzied, hand-clapping, soul-wrenching, throat-choking support, and since it seems likely that he can repeat this act throughout the state, I now predict that he will sweep Fremont in a landslide.
>
> What is his trickery? Simple. He telephoned three young heroes who had served with him on the destroyer escort *Lucas Dean* in the Battle of Leyte Gulf, and these simple men, without coaching of any kind or prompting from Grant, narrated scenes of his heroism. Especially effective was a tall Negro from Detroit, a cook with one leg missing, who told the voters how Captain Grant had pulled him from the water after a shark had chopped off his foot. Many heroes have done things like that, but what Grant did next, in the cook's own words, established a new criterion for heroism: 'To make place for me on the raft, he quietly jumped down into the water himself, even though he knew sharks had just been there.'
>
> One minute after Gawain Butler of Detroit finished telling his story, the people of Webster were willing to elect Norman Grant President of the United States. That they will elect him senator seems assured.

It was not until the fifth repeat of the heroism act that Elinor Grant saw it. The three sailors had motored from the northwest corner of the state to Clay, and at a huge rally in the university auditorium, with no mention of Grant's football prowess, and certainly no pompon girls, the three men stepped forward to relate their experiences during the Battle for Leyte Gulf. When they were finished, and the roaring cheers had died away, Elinor told her husband, 'Revolting. How in God's name could you allow that miserable Finnerty to arrange such a travesty?'

'I didn't allow him,' Norman said. 'I encouraged him.'

'Did you summon those three men? Those exhibitionists?'

'I was too dumb to think of it. It was Finnerty's idea.'

'And you don't feel ashamed? Humiliated?'

'Elinor, an election between honest men is like a battle between sovereign nations. You better win.'

'You'd do anything to win, wouldn't you?'

'Only if it's honest. Only if it's necessary.'

'You think an obscenity like that fake patriotism is necessary?'

'Last week I was losing. Thanks to Finnerty's brilliant idea, this week I'm winning. And I will encourage Gawain Butler to tell his story across this entire state. Because it's good for Fremont to hear a black man speak. It's good for them to hear someone from Alabama. Or an Irish Catholic from Boston.'

'You feel no shame?'

'There's something you will never be able to comprehend, Elinor. When we finally crawled out of that raft . . . Hundreds of men needlessly dead because no one at headquarters had remembered to send out rescue teams . . . I told those three men that the world was a shitty place . . .'

'I don't want to hear such language.'

She fled to her father's house and asked him what he thought of Norman's blatant flag-waving, and he had to reflect some moments before answering: 'America has an enormous propensity for electing military heroes to offices they're not capable of filling. William Henry Harrison, Ulysses Grant, William McKinley. I have no doubt that Dwight Eisenhower will be laureled with the Presidency any time he wants it, on either ticket.

'But you must remember that we also got a couple of rather good men this way. Andrew Jackson and Teddy Roosevelt among others. And best of all, George Washington, whom we so desperately needed. Every one of those men was elected not for his capacity, but because the public perceived him as a military hero. This nation will always be eager to believe that a military man is more intelligent than he really is. Now it's your husband's turn.'

'Is he a bright, good man? I no longer know how to judge.'

'He's a football player,' Stidham said. 'A fine, strong, honest football player. And if he had been something different, we might have lost the Battle of Leyte Gulf and sacrificed an additional half a million young men.'

'Will he be a decent senator? After such a despicable start?'

'Norman has a fighting chance to be a fine senator, but I expect he'll turn out to be only average. Never a distinction, never a scandal. That was the best I could get out of Ulysses Gantling. I'll be satisfied if we do as well with Norman.' He hesitated, trying to strike a balance concerning his fragile daughter. 'It's you I'm afraid of, Elinor. I suspect you'll make a very poor senator's wife.'

'So do I,' she cried, running to her father's chair, and kneeling beside him. When her convulsive sobs quieted, she whispered, 'It's never been Norman I've been afraid of. It's always been me. I'm not suited for this job. I simply am not.'

'What makes you think I was suited to be an officer in France? A pathetic farce, really. Or Gantling's campaign manager? I very nearly lost him that first election. We do what we have to do, Elinor. And now I think it's time for you to appear on the podium with your husband. He's fighting for one of the premier jobs in the world and he deserves your help.'

At the climactic rally in Benton, five nights before the primary, she sat on the stage beside her husband and, at Finnerty's insistence, even said a few words. But when the three sailors appeared in their freshly pressed uniforms, with ribbons neat and medals polished, she wanted to throw up.

Rachel Lindquist believed that one test of a woman was how she organized space: 'Whether it controls you, or you control it.'

When her roommate at Wellesley had asked what she meant by this, she had said forthrightly, 'A kitchen at home. Do the plates and forks command it in disarray, or do you instruct the ugly things where they belong and see to it that they keep their place?'

'What's the great virtue in that?' asked her roomie, a slovenly girl from Virginia, pouting.

'Because it establishes who's boss, that's why. Because when the space is ordered, you're free to live creatively.'

'Are you lecturing me?' the fluffy girl asked.

'This room proves to me that you allow space to dominate you. Everything is in chaos. Your clothes spread everywhere.'

In the weeping spell that followed, the roommate announced her intention of quitting the room and finding another girl to bunk with, and Rachel encouraged her to do so. The upshot was a visit to the dean, who listened to the roommate's weepy recitation of accusations, smiled and said consolingly, 'Betty-Anne, I agree with you. You'll be much happier with a girl more like yourself.'

The change was approved and each girl was happier. Rachel, of course, had to room alone for several months, but in that time she instituted a system of beautiful orderliness, so that later, when a Jewish girl from Scarsdale moved in with her own neat clothes, things progressed with no strain.

Rachel Lindquist's father was a member of one of those hard-working, gifted Swedish families that settled in Worcester, west of Boston, in the late years of the past century. Her grandfather had invented a process whereby Carborundum particles could be attached to fabric, producing an excellent abrasive for use in manufacturing, but since he was unusually cautious in financial affairs, he missed his opportunity to convert his small operation into a massive corporation the way some of the other Worcester Swedes did, but his four patents were so original and so carefully protected that he and his descendants did collect gratifying royalties from the big combines.

Rachel was carefully educated in a private school near Worcester and then at Wellesley, where, after her unfortunate experience with her first roommate, she had an unbroken chain of successes. Her parents expected their only daughter to excel in her classes, which she did, and the friends who had known her in the lower schools were sure that her lovely blond hair and elegant figure would ensure a good marriage.

She was repeatedly invited to dances at Harvard and Amherst, and in her junior year, 1941, she met a senior at Yale named Stuart. A graduate of Groton, he represented one of the fine milling families of New Hampshire, and it was assumed by everyone, especially her parents, 'that Rachel was safely settled.'

That was before Pearl Harbor. Toward the middle of December, when the world seemed to be falling apart, she attended a political seminar at MIT and there met Stanley Mott, a young professor from Georgia Tech. He was so alert, so vividly interested in what aviation could do for the world that she was immediately attracted to him, and at the end of the three-day session, with Hitler and Tojo and Mussolini on the agenda daily, she real- ized that she was intended for something in life more exciting than young Mr. Stuart of Groton and Yale, and New Hampshire milling.

Her parents were distraught: 'Who is this Professor Nobody?'

'He teaches at Georgia Tech.' She might as well have said that he came from Arkansas.

'An illiterate plantation owner, I suppose,' Mrs. Lindquist said. Al- though she belonged to only a minor branch of Boston's great Saltonstall family, she felt a burning obligation to protect the superiority of that revered name.

'He's the son of the Methodist minister in Newton.'

'I didn't know there were Methodist ministers in New England . . . in the better suburbs, that is.'

'Graduated with honors from the local high school, one of the best in the country, and he won a science foundation something or other. A full scholarship.'

'If he's as good as you say, why in the world would he have elected Georgia? If he was really first class, that is?'

'I wondered about that, too,' Rachel confessed. 'If he's as bright as he seems . . . I mean, the men with him said he was a genius in aviation. Why wouldn't he have gone to a real university? Like Harvard or MIT?'

The question was so perplexing that Mr. Lindquist launched a chain of telephone calls, to bankers, lawyers, educators, and the police of Newton. He learned that Stanley Mott came from a standard lower-class family of good reputation, that he had been a wizard in science at Newton and had ranked high in all national test scores. He had gone to Georgia Tech because he was interested in engineering as a practical science and had done at least as well in his classes as Rachel had done in hers, but as Mr. Lindquist observed: 'No one in his right mind would equate Georgia Tech marks with those from Wellesley.'

'How did he ever become a professor?' Mrs. Lindquist asked, and her husband explained that he wasn't a real professor, only an assistant: 'He has no more than a master's degree, you know. Something to do with aviation.'

'Did he get his master's at MIT?' his wife asked.

'Louisiana State, I'm afraid.'

'He seems always to shy away from the first-class schools.'

The Lindquists were displeased when their daughter wanted to invite Professor Mott to Worcester, and were relieved when he reported that he could not come: 'I've got to give and grade my exams. And the Army Air Corps has been talking with me.'

They did not see him until May of 1942, for he was kept busy teaching crash courses for the military, and when he did come north he was ten pounds underweight and rather haggard. He did not create a good impression, for he was distressingly nervous: 'The Air Corps has been badgering me.'

'Are you to be a pilot?' Mr. Lindquist asked.

'No. I can't fathom what it is they're after.'

'Would you prefer the Air Corps to the Navy?' Mr. Lindquist, as a courtesy to his daughter, felt obliged to keep the conversation moving, even though he understood few of the answers. This Mott was a rather tedious young man, not at all like that Stuart chap from Yale, but he could talk coherently, which was more than some of Rachel's young callers were able to do.

'You must be proud to know the Air Corps wants you,' he said.

'That signifies little, Mr. Lindquist. There are so few of us trained in aviation engineering.'

Rachel was obviously attracted to him, and when she insisted upon taking the train all the way to Atlanta to see the Georgia Tech graduation, her parents awakened with a shock to the fact she intended to marry him.

'At least bring him back to Worcester for a proper wedding,' Mrs. Lindquist pleaded.

'It's only reasonable,' Mr. Lindquist added. 'His people would be just as eager as we are.'

'He doesn't have people,' Rachel said. 'Only his mother.'

'Was she deserted?'

'Widowed.'

Under pressure, the young people consented to a formal wedding in Worcester, but it was a rather drab wartime affair. Mrs. Mott came out from Boston, ill-at-ease and barely presentable. Two of the real Saltonstalls graced the party and many of the Swedish establishment, but the bright young men and women who would normally have added radiance to such a wedding were absent, the men in training camps, the women dashing about the country to keep up with them. And as soon as the Motts were married, Stanley had to report to Wright Field in Ohio—attached to the Air Force, but with civilian status.

In true military fashion, he was assigned not to aviation work but to an advanced study group endeavoring to deduce what the German scientists at the secret Baltic base of Peenemünde were up to. His work was classified top secret, which meant that he could tell his wife nothing.

Rachel understood. She had been attracted to Stanley by his obvious brilliance, and the more she saw of him during their catch-as-catch-can courtship and marriage, the more she appreciated the solid qualities of his mind. Whatever he was free to tell her, she understood, and sometimes his silences were more instructive than what he said.

She had one more year to go on her Wellesley degree and was reassured when he encouraged her to complete it, no matter what the hardships. Like him, she rushed normal procedures, taking a criminally heavy program right through the academic year and into the summer as well. As soon as she graduated, she hurried to Dayton, where she took a job helping in a day nursery filled with children whose mothers were doing manual labor at the air base. When the older woman who attempted to run the vastly enlarged nursery collapsed from overwork, Rachel took complete charge, and even when she informed Stanley that she was pregnant, they both agreed that she should continue her work.

It was now that she exhibited her devotion to the principle she had expounded at college: The test of a woman is how she organizes space. In the Mott rooms at the motel she established a place for everything and rigorously discarded any object that was not essential; as a consequence, the Motts lived in constructive order, whereas most of the other young couples, many from places like Vassar and Harvard, lived in chaos.

She applied the same rule to her personal appearance. She had thick blond hair which she wore drawn back in a severe Grecian style. She was pleased with the effect this created, for it framed her placid Swedish beauty handsomely and worked well with the simple clothes she preferred. She brought with her four conservative suits, all light in color to match her complexion, and four blouses with no frills.

She felt it indecent ever to live without art; at college she had had an expensive record player but no stacks of popular single records, like the other girls. She told Stanley: 'I've always felt that eight or ten really good complete albums were enough.' She abhorred anything later than Beethoven and would allow him only his Seventh Symphony and Razumovsky quartets: 'There's great vulgarity in Beethoven.' She had a gorgeous piano concerto by Mozart and one of his lilting violin concertos. But mostly she liked Bach and Vivaldi, holding that composers like Schubert, Schumann and Stravinsky were violent exhibitionists. When she found a composition she liked, she played it constantly, but it was always something like the Brandenburg Concertos.

In their early marriage, when her records all sounded alike to Stanley, he said, 'One of the fellows in graduate school had a marvelous record. Ravel's *Bolero.*'

'Oh my God!' she said.

In art it was also less-equals-more. Stanley, having had several good civilization courses at Georgia, wanted to spend part of his first paycheck for a nicely colored photograph of the Cumaean Sibyl by Michelangelo: 'The professor explained how elegantly it fitted the architecture of the Sistine Chapel.' He drew an illustration of the converging areas.

Rachel took one look at the obscene reproduction, a horrible affair of improper colors and forced foreshortening, and refused him permission to bring it into their limited quarters: 'Art must command. It must fill its area on its own terms. It must say something fresh to you every day.' For two weeks she studied all the reproductions in the Dayton area, finding nothing that satisfied her.

'What's the big deal?' Stanley asked.

'It's all *Monks Fishing,*' she said.

He did not understand, but wanted to, so even though he was fatigued from the demanding work on rocketry and atomic energy, the devices the Germans were working on at Peenemünde, he asked if he could accompany her on her next visit to the reprint galleries, and it was on such a trip that she explained *Monks Fishing.*

'Have you ever noticed that in really bad novels, when the author wants to present an artist, it's always an architect? Why do you suppose that is? Because to the average readers a poet would be insufferable. To them a novelist is a man who lies about the house doing nothing. A painter is a mess. But an architect wears a nice suit. He can be shown drawing in a clean office. And when he goes out to supervise the builders he can wear tweeds and smoke a pipe. Best of all, you can see the end product. And it's useful. You can imagine offices in it and electric light companies. Architects are the salvation of the middle class.'

'What in the world does this have to do with *Monks Fishing?*'

'Because in painting it's the same way. You want a cheap copy of Michelangelo because you know the original's in the Sistine Chapel, and that makes it acceptable. Well, rich Americans and Europeans who travel all over and want to buy a work of art always buy *Monks Fishing.*'

She took him to a store she had located which specialized in such art, and there she showed him some fifteen big, expensive, colorful reproductions of paintings by unknown French and Italian commercial artists. In one a group of monks in colorful robes sit about a long table, dozing disrespectfully while a cardinal in bright red tells an interminable story. This was titled 'The Boring Story.' In the next the monks watch admiringly as the cardinal in red drinks a substantial draught from a beautifully painted goblet. This was titled 'The Toast.' The third, fourth and through the thirteenth showed the same monks at the same table reacting in various amusing ways to the cardinal, or sometimes two cardinals.

Masterpiece number fourteen was what Stanley Mott had been awaiting. It showed four monks beside a river, two drinking from a bottle which they pass from hand to hand, one snoozing under a tree while the bob on his fishing line indicates that he has caught an unattended fish, and one fishing with no results. It was called 'Monks Fishing.' Number fifteen carried the same title but showed one of the monks having fallen into the stream while trying to land a rather large fish.

'Don't ever buy *Monks Fishing,* Stanley.' In another store she showed him the one painting she had been able to approve. It was a Piet Mondrian, all clear and crisp and beautifully organized, with a few simple lines and highly effective colors.

As soon as he saw it he realized that this was a portrait of his wife. The simplicity matched her overall appearance. The few black lines represented her sparse attitude toward decoration. The perfectly adapted coloring of the enclosed spaces was the coloring of her blond hair, her flawless complexion, her subdued suits. The Mondrian was Vivaldi translated into visual imagery.

It was too austere: 'I sort of hoped we'd get a Van Gogh 'Sunflowers' . . . or maybe—'

'Don't tell me,' she interrupted. 'You wanted an Orozco.'

'Is he the Mexican? Yes, one of the professors at Georgia Tech had a marvelous copy of women bandits during the Mexican revolution.'

'Orozco would be big in Georgia,' she said, but as soon as the words left her lips she was apologetic. 'I don't mean that, Stanley. Really I don't.'

She rummaged through the reproductions till she found a copy of the Van Gogh and a very garish attempt at the Orozco bandoleras. 'Don't you see, Stanley? These are unutterably trite. If we had them on the wall a week, we'd grow tired of them.'

'I looked at those women through a whole semester. They stood right behind the professor's head, and I still like them.'

'Later on you won't,' she said, and since she would be paying for the framing with her own money, he encouraged her to buy the Mondrian. In their cramped quarters it proved to be exactly right, and when the orderliness of the Brandenburg Concertos marched through the room, the picture seemed destined for that space, with these two people, and this music.

Rachel allowed only one aspect of her life to deviate from this norm: in her bedroom, where no one but her husband could see, she kept a collection of seven wonderfully carved wooden figures of human beings, each about nine inches tall. There was one group of two related figures, a mother combing the hair of her daughter, and one of three, an elderly couple dancing while a grouchy lean man played his accordion, and two superb single figures, a farmer mowing with a stubby scythe and a woman looking at the sky. Six of the figures stood forth in plain, untouched wood; the lanky accordionist wore a colored cloth cap and played a blue accordion.

The figures were obviously folk art, but where they came from, Stanley could not at first decipher. To him they had the sentimental quality of Orozco's marching women; indeed, they were identical in spirit. Yet Rachel loved them, and finally she told him what they represented. Perched on the bed, her head cocked alluringly so that her hair hung free, she said, 'When I was thirteen my parents took me to Sweden. Mother deplored the place, finding it so different from Boston, but Father was deeply moved at seeing the bleak impoverished village from which he had sprung.' It was called Döderhult in the southeast province of Småland, and after a brief stop Mrs. Lindquist had wanted to hurry back to the civilization of Stockholm, or preferably London, but her husband had insisted upon staying, and it was during the second day that Rachel discovered the wonder of this little town:

> 'I was walking aimlessly along a road that led to the Baltic when I saw a shop window containing a congregation of these little wooden figurines carved by a local man, and immediately I realized that they were the equivalent of the Tanagra figures of Greece. An enthusiastic teacher had taught us about them in our fifth-grade unit "Greece and Modern Man." I went right into the store and selected these seven. I hadn't enough money, so the shopkeeper said he'd hold them for me till I could persuade my parents to anticipate my allowance. Mother was furious, called the little things junk, but Father was deeply touched. When he saw them he began to cry. Later he told me that the woman looking at the sky was his mother. "She looked exactly like that," he said. And there they are.'

The artist, Stanley learned, was an untutored Swedish peasant named Axel Petersson, an intuitive genius who could make wood sing, and in time Mott grew to regard the little wooden people with even more affection and understanding than did his wife: 'They make you human, Rachel. They tell me that you yourself are a Swedish peasant . . . trying to act sophisticated.'

In her intellectual tastes she was far from a peasant. On Sundays, when they had a few free hours, it was she who suggested that they read aloud one of the plays being produced in these years. Once under a tree in an Ohio valley she read him the entire *Murder in the Cathedral;* she had been to Canterbury during her sophomore year and was thus able to set the stage for him. He could see the assassins coming toward Becket, and for days thereafter he found himself thinking of medieval England.

The most memorable reading was one she had insisted upon: 'It's very long, Stanley, but I think we need it.'

It was *Strange Interlude,* and it occupied them for most of a long afternoon. When it came time for Stanley to take the book, he found positive delight in altering his voice for the asides, and in the midst of one unusually expressive passage, Rachel kissed him passionately. 'You're really very good, Stanley. You could have done well at a school like Yale.'

'I did well at Georgia Tech,' he said defensively. 'We knew who Eugene O'Neill was, you know.'

'I didn't mean it that way, really I didn't.'

'What did you mean by saying yesterday that we needed this play?'

She smoothed down her dress, coughed and said, 'Because for the last few months we've been talking in posed sentences, just like these characters. Our worlds are drifting dangerously apart, Stanley, and that's perilous.'

'You know what my work is, Rachel. I simply can't talk about it.'

'That part I know. I believe FBI men are watching you. At least I have good reason to think so. And they should. But we mustn't be like the characters in this play, never speaking our minds.'

'What do you want me to say—that I'm allowed to say?'

'Europe? What do you think's going to happen to Europe?'

'It's inconceivable to me that Hitler can retain control of all Europe. It goes against all reason.'

'And if he fails, will Stalin control it all?'

'You have to face one problem at a time.'

'But if the other man is looking far ahead, he may be able to solve two or even three problems at the same time.'

'Even one defeats me, sometimes.'

'Is your work so difficult?' Before he could respond, she said brightly, 'Scratch that, Stanley. What I really wanted to ask was this. How do you see us living after the war ends? And I don't even mean that. What I mean is, how long do you think the war will last?'

'Four more years.'

She gave a little cry: 'Till 1947! Oh God, can we survive so long?'

'We have to,' he said, and with that he resumed his reading.

A few days later he informed her that he would be leaving Wright Field and moving to London. 'No, you can't join me there. Absolutely impossible.'

'What do you think I should do, Stanley? Till the baby comes . . . no, what I really mean is, after the baby comes?'

He thought about this for a long time, then kissed her tenderly. 'You know, the best thing we've done in years was to read *Strange Interlude.* He wrote that play about us.' He kissed her again. 'But to answer your question, I don't have a clue. I don't know how long I'm going to be gone. It's a vital mission and it could take years. Darling, I just don't know.'

The next morning, when she was preparing one of his suits for the cleaner, prior to his departure for London, she found in his coat pocket a photograph of a small man who, from the cut of his clothes, appeared to be German. The only noticeable thing about him was a mustache that wandered ineffectually over his upper lip, and he had on the kind of cap factory workers in England often wore. The picture bore no name, no identification of any kind, but she surmised that her husband was heading for Europe to find this man.

She pondered a long time as to what she must do about this photograph, and she sensed that she had not been intended to see it. She could even have committed a crime of some kind in doing so, and she supposed that the best thing to do was return it to its pocket and leave the suit as it was, without a pressing. But her compulsive sense of neatness would not permit this, and for the last two days of their time together in the Dayton motel she kept the photograph to herself. When the time came for him to leave for London, she kissed him ardently, then handed him the photograph.

'I hope you find him,' she said.

When in the summer of 1945 the colonel from the Air Force arrived in Worcester, where Rachel Mott was maintaining quarters for her son Millard while she worked at a nearby war production company, he informed her that her husband had been commended for his role in finding and rescuing several important German scientists. When she asked what kind of scientists they were, the colonel told her truthfully that he did not really know. 'I think we can assume they had something to do with weapons, but exactly what kind I wouldn't even dare guess.'

She then asked whether one of the scientists had been a small, rather thin man with a scraggly mustache, and he said, 'Ma'am, the fact is, I don't know anything. Except that your husband is alive, and the Air Force thinks very highly of his work.'

'Will he be coming home soon?'

'I would surely think so.'

Stanley arrived in the United States in November 1945, but was not even allowed free time to visit his wife in Massachusetts. He called her as soon as the military transport docked and said, cryptically, 'It's vital that you take yourself and Millard immediately to Fort Bliss in El Paso, Texas. Ask for a friend of mine named McCawley'—he spelled the name twice. 'And I leave it to you to get us the best damned quarters in the fort. I love you, and I want to talk to you directly, not like in *Strange Interlude*.'

That was all he said. Fort Bliss; El Paso, Texas; McCawley. She supposed that he had spelled the man's name incorrectly, but when she reached Fort Bliss she found that it really was McCawley. He was a sergeant with unusual powers in the assignment of quarters, and when, dead tired from her mysterious trip, she told him that she was Stanley Mott's wife, he beamed. 'One of the best. I served with him in France. Tireless.'

'What was he doing, Captain McCawley?'

'I wish to hell I was a captain. It's sergeant. And I was a sergeant then, doing his paper work.'

'Which was what?'

'Top secret then, top secret now.'

'Then why am I here?'

'Because your good husband, God bless his musclebound ways, is going to arrive on Thursday.'

'For a long stay?'

'Years, I should think.'

And that was all she could discover. Her husband was still a civilian, still engaged in some top-secret business. But he was on his way to Fort Bliss and would be stationed there for a long, indeterminate period. She sighed and proceeded with the three-day job of wangling from the military in charge of the fort the gear she would need in order to convert their barracks quarters into a decent home.

In this assignment she received much help from Sergeant McCawley, who had a thieving mind and a cynical approach to military life: 'Get all you can the first week, when they're glad to have you aboard. Because later on, invariably you become dirt.' Because the main flood of whoever was arriving had not yet appeared, she and McCawley had their choice of rooms, furniture, kitchen equipment and bedding. He wanted to force upon her a whole roomful of junk she knew she did not need, and when he saw how sparsely she had furnished the quarters, he said, 'Mrs. Mott, I would advise you to accept this crud, whether you need it or not. Because maybe later on you can trade it off with your neighbors, whoever they are.'

'I think this is adequate,' she said, but he looked so hurt at having his advice rejected that she asked him gently if he would mind baby-sitting Millard while she went in to El Paso to purchase a special gift for her husband.

'How long since you've seen him?'

She counted up the dreadful years of lonely train rides, of giving birth to a baby when one didn't know if the father was still alive, the spells of heartbreaking loneliness. 'It was a long time, Sergeant, and I hope it's never repeated.'

In McCawley's car she went from one art shop to another, until she found a fairly good silk-screened copy of Orozco's marching women. By good luck it had been framed austerely, not California-style, and she bought it for twenty-eight dollars. The man gave her the wire and pinned hook for hanging, and when she returned to her quarters McCawley helped her find just the right spot over the davenport, where Stanley would have to see it as soon as he entered the door.

'This room does look pretty nice,' McCawley admitted, 'but I have a surprise for you.' He had sequestered a storage locker in the basement of the barracks, a large wired-in cubicle with a newly printed sign: STANLEY

MOTT. Inside was enough military furniture to accommodate two families. 'Believe me, Mrs. Mott, you can use this in artful trading.'

On Thursday, as promised, the long train pulled in to El Paso station, where carefully guarded military trucks, with their canvas sides in place to prevent observation, rolled up in long lines to receive the military prisoners assigned to Fort Bliss. Rachel was not permitted in the station area, so she did not see the German scientists debark: General Helmut Funkhauser giving orders, Wernher von Braun's principal assistants stepping gingerly onto Texas soil, inconspicuous Dieter Kolff coming forth in a huge American hat that obscured his face. No women had been allowed to accompany their husbands to America, but there were over a hundred men, confused and insecure, assigned to a fort they did not understand for duties which had not been explained.

At Fort Bliss the Germans were unloaded first from the trucks, and now Rachel could see for the first time her husband's prey, and that one-time photograph had been so deeply engraved on her memory that when she saw Dieter Kolff come down the steps of the truck, she recognized him immediately and uttered a small prayer: 'Thank God, Stanley found him.' She knew that these words made no sense; she had not the slightest comprehension of why Kolff had been so eagerly sought, but as the daughter of a well-disciplined Swede and a Saltonstall of Boston, however remote, she knew intuitively that men and women felt better when they fulfilled the task set them.

'Stanley!' she cried, and there from one of the last trucks stepped her husband, looking precisely as he had when he left, no heavier, no thinner, no mustache, no scars. When he saw her he walked properly toward her, then broke into a run, embracing her furiously. She refrained from crying, but after their fourth or fifth kiss she did point to where Dieter Kolff was marching to his new quarters: 'I see you found him.'

'Took two years.'

'Was it worth it?'

'We were all screwed up about Peenemünde, but . . .'

'What's Peenemünde?'

'I'll tell you when we get home. Where is home?'

When she led him to the apartment and opened the door, the first thing he saw was Sergeant McCawley standing there with Millard, and he called for the two-year-old boy to run to him. McCawley had trained the lad to cry out 'Daddy,' and there was new embracing, but as Stanley clutched his son he saw over the boy's shoulder the Orozco, the painting he had so admired at Georgia Tech. Placing Millard in a chair, he went to the wall and took down the painting. Handing it to his wife, he said, 'All the time I lived in confusion I remembered our apartment with the Mondrian . . . the order . . . the neatness. I've outgrown Orozco. Let's trade it in for something simple and clean.'

But when he tossed his duffel into the bedroom he saw the little wooden figures of Axel Petersson, especially the older man dancing with his wife, and the pair were so real, so instinct with the humanity that binds lives together, that he grabbed them in his hands and danced about the room, smiling at his wife and shouting, 'This is what we waited for, all of us,' and he caught his wife and they fell on the bed.

Later in the day, after they had slept and showered, McCawley drove them to the art shop, where Stanley himself traded the garish Orozco for a fine Mondrian, a vertical rectangle with black lines delineating handsomely proportioned blue and red and yellow spaces, and when he hung it in his new living room he kissed his wife and said, 'Very sensible, Rachel. In here, where we present ourselves to the world, crisp neatness. In the bedroom, where we live our true lives, the dancing figures.' And that's the way it was to be.

At the end of one week Rachel Mott told her husband, 'I'm in love with these crazy Germans. I can't believe Hitler ever touched them.'

She respected the manner in which the scientists organized their living space. Each man assumed responsibility for bringing order into whatever corner was assigned him, and each kept his area impeccably neat. She noticed also that each man devised for himself some work space on which he could spread out his papers, or make his tools.

She was both amused and impressed by General Funkhauser, for he was an obvious fraud but one determined to please his new American masters. He perfected his English and explained things for her, telling much more about Peenemünde than her husband had felt free to do. He was first to volunteer for any arduous duty and seemed to know more about the A-4s than even Von Braun, and he explained several times how he had rescued, at no slight danger to himself, the papers summarizing the top-secret work being done at Peenemünde. She smiled at his pretensions but continued to listen to his blandishments.

From her talks with General Funkhauser, who now weighed thirty pounds less than he had at the rocket base, she learned that if the war had continued a few months longer, or if on the other hand Funkhauser had been placed in command of rocketry a few months earlier, Germany might have won. One afternoon she asked him if rockets could indeed carry men to the Moon, and although he had once condemned Von Braun and Kolff to death for having suggested this, he now revealed himself to have been an ardent space enthusiast: 'I always said that with rockets we can go anywhere—the Moon, Mars, Venus, even directly to the Sun.'

About the fourth week Rachel began to suspect that General Funkhauser was not entirely disinterested in his courtship of Stanley Mott's wife, because at the conclusion of any particularly long discussion, he managed to bring up the subject of that basement storage cubicle where there were several pieces of furniture he could use, and gradually the surplus found its way to Funkhauser's quarters, until he had a kind of eighteenth-century Prussian overstuffed castle right in the heart of Fort Bliss.

At the end of one meeting, General Funkhauser lingered to say, 'The men admire your beautiful hair, Mrs. Mott. It's so blond and German.'

'Swedish,' she corrected.

'Swedes are mainly German,' he said. 'Completely Nordic.' To this she made no response, so he added, 'But you'd look ever so much prettier if you wore your hair in braids. The way my sister did.'

'Where is she now?' Rachel asked.

'Killed by American bombers.' When he saw her wince, he added, 'The men talked about your hair, Mrs. Mott. They agreed it would look better —more German, that is—if you wore braids.'

The idea of sacrificing her carefully devised Grecian coiffure for a pair of dangling Saxon braids delighted Rachel and she broke into laughter, but General Funkhauser was not amused. 'Later, you will see.'

He then changed his attitude completely, becoming a sweet Rhenish peasant. 'The men think you are beautiful, Mrs. Mott. You remind them of their wives.' Before she could respond, he added, 'That little table, the one where the leaf drops down. I could use that very capably for my papers, Mrs. Mott. Do you think . . .'

She laughed and said, 'Any man who tells me I'm beautiful can have any table he wants,' but the general frowned at this suggestion that he had praised her only to get one more piece of furniture.

At a later meeting she asked Funkhauser about the little man her husband had been seeking, and the general said expansively, 'I saved that one's life. A minor mechanic at the rocket base.'

'Could I meet him, please?'

'Your wish is my command,' Funkhauser replied, using a phrase he had learned at the cinema, and when he returned with Dieter Kolff walking respectfully behind, she found the latter to be a quiet man approaching forty, who spoke sadly of his wife wandering somewhere in Germany. He was the first prisoner to mention his wife, and he did so with such obvious affection that Rachel asked her husband, 'When will the Germans be allowed to bring their wives over?' and it was then that she discovered that these scientists existed in a legal no man's land.

'They have no papers,' Stanley explained. 'None of any kind.'

'How did they get in the country?'

'We slipped them in.'

'A hundred and ten! Some slip.'

'No one knows officially that they're here. The records say simply "With the knowledge of the President." '

'Why does he want them here?'

'That I am not free to say.'

So she went back to General Funkhauser, and he was eager to talk: 'You watch the railroad yards. Soon great trains of stuff will begin arriving. I suppose you know what.'

'No, I don't. My husband is more military than most military. He simply will not tell me anything.'

'Proper. Highly proper. I demanded the same of my troops.' He caught himself. 'I was an engineer, mostly.'

'What will be in the trains?'

'Things,' and he would say no more, for he suspected that in his enthusiasm he had said too much.

Rachel developed a considerable respect for the care with which the Germans protected and advanced their intellectual interests. Like good men of all societies in all ages, when they found themselves in forced constraint and forbidden to carry on their normal occupations, they organized themselves into a kind of university in which each man taught, without books, the subject he knew best. The Fort Bliss university was exceptionally rich in that most of the Germans in the barracks were highly trained specialists: mathematics classes were brilliant; physics the same; and mechanical engineering, some of the best in the world. The humanities were more difficult, although two men did organize a good course in German political thought which attempted to explain German history from Bismarck through the Weimar Republic and down to the collapse of the Third Reich.

Preeminent among the students was Dieter Kolff, the farm boy with a rudimentary education and magical fingers that could mend machines. Grasping the empty months as an opportunity to catch up with the trained men about him, he delved into mathematics and science with such a dogged persistence that he caused chuckles: 'There goes Dieter with his trigonometry notebook like it was a Bible.'

Curiously, he learned the big words of his new-found knowledge in English rather than German, and he began inserting phrases like *reciprocal ratio* and *level of minimal return* in his long German sentences. History, philosophy and literature were non-essentials whose vocabulary he avoided; calculus, astronomy and physics were his delight, so that by the time he graduated from Fort Bliss University (Pragmatic) he was going to be lopsided but very solid.

He did cultivate one intellectual diversion. At Peenemünde he had learned to enjoy symphonic music, borrowing records from Von Braun, and when he learned that Mrs. Mott had a supply, he asked if he could borrow some. 'No,' she said. 'My records are precious and they must not be abused on bad machines. But you're welcome to come listen.' She arranged informal concerts, which were attended by many of the Germans, and in this way Dieter became familiar with the classical music of his native land.

It was because of this university that Rachel was drawn more deeply into the German orbit. When Dieter Kolff told her that a frail handsome man named Ernst Stuhlinger was instructing those who were interested in radical new principles governing an ion ramjet, she said, 'These must be some of the brightest men in the world,' and Kolff replied, 'They are.' Then he added, 'But if . . .' He could not phrase his thoughts in English and had to depend upon her faulty knowledge of German. 'What we need most is someone to teach us English.'

So she became an instructor in the German university. The scientists liked her teaching, and General Funkhauser volunteered to serve as her assistant, correcting her now and then when she used the wrong word for some scientific principle.

As she worked she became worried about the bleak lives which most of her Germans were leading. They seemed not to be used in any constructive way; only the top men ever got to the testing range at White Sands. The others moped in the barracks, perfecting their scientific education, but little else. Once when she asked one of the Germans to give a little talk, he astounded her by saying, 'At night we study the stars. There is a hole in the fence that keeps us in. We slip through that hole and wander on the prairie, looking at the stars and feeling the free wind on our faces. We think the soldiers know about the hole in the fence, but they also know we need space to move in, as if we are not prisoners. I go through the fence every night. Even in the rain.'

When she asked another prisoner to give his talk, he said, 'Better I speak German,' and before she could protest this waste of the educational period, he indicated that General Funkhauser could interpret for him. 'Every day we study hard to make our rockets better, so that when the United States wants seriously to catch up with the Russians, we will be ready to help. Kolff here has new machines to make the engines. Bergstrasser has a new fuel system. I have, in my own modest way, a new plan for inertial guidance.'

'What is inertial?' Rachel asked.

General Funkhauser started to explain, but it was obvious even to Rachel that he didn't know what he was talking about, so a very young man rose and said in broken English, 'A new system . . . like the compass . . . no needle . . . three gyroscopes.' Of this, Rachel could make no sense whatever, but after class Dieter Kolff stayed behind and said, 'Me too . . . I don't understand inertial . . . a better compass . . . much better.'

'But what's a gyroscope . . . three gyroscopes?'

He whirled his right forefinger rapidly. 'Give stability.'

'Oh, yes! We had that in physics, I'm sure.'

'When will come our wives?'

She liked men who were hungry for their wives; she had been so terribly hungry for her husband. In subsequent days she saw a lot of Dieter Kolff, and once asked him why her husband had sought him so diligently.

'Professor Mott . . . I looking for him, too . . . very good man, very sensible man.'

'But why was he looking for you?'

Kolff's mustache twitched. He wondered if he dared speak. He wondered if this woman was an American SS planted in the fort to trap him. But then he concluded that from all that he had seen, she was remarkably similar to Liesl Koenig, and he said, at some danger to himself, 'Do not speak husband. He is very secret. I work on some important weapon. Not important man like General Breutzl, but . . .'

'Is he here in Fort Bliss?'

'Dead. I his helper. I know everything.' He stopped. 'Please not to speak.'

Those words were enough to clarify her husband's two years of anxiety, and when she sat with Stanley that night, with their son between them, she felt an overwhelming appreciation for what he had been doing, and the manner apparently in which he had done it: 'I'm very proud of you, Stanley.'

He reached across his son to embrace her, fervently. 'I've been able to guess what you must have gone through. Alone all those months.'

'When will the German wives be allowed to come over?' she asked.

'We don't even know whether the Germans will be staying in this country.'

'Really, you ought to make up your minds. This isn't human.'

He leaned back and stared at her. 'Has Dieter Kolff been talking with you?'

'No, but in my class I talk with him.'

Occasionally the German scientists were granted permission to shop in El Paso, and on festive days they were even allowed to cross the international bridge into Ciudad Juárez on the other side of the Rio Grande, provided they were accompanied by American soldiers. Some of the younger men used this as an opportunity to visit the Mexican brothels, where they were welcomed because of their good looks and their generosity with money.

The serious scientists sometimes preferred to visit Juárez with their English teacher, and often Rachel led groups to the bazaars and the good food. She had grown to like chili and tamales, and especially the crisp tacos fried in deep fat. 'It's murderous food, really. But I think one can stand it from time to time.'

Now things at Fort Bliss grew serious. A secret report arrived via Paris to the effect that the Peenemünde men who had been captured by the Russians were enabling the Soviets to make quantum leaps in their rocket program, and belatedly the American military began to appreciate the treasure they had in Von Braun's group. The prisoners began to spend a good deal of time at White Sands, where Dieter Kolff supervised the assembly and testing of the A-4s which Professor Mott's team had gathered from various storage sites in Germany.

Much work was done on refining the engines and the guidance systems, and Baron von Braun was often absent from the fort, discussing potentialities with American military men in Los Angeles or Washington. Classes at the informal university met less frequently, except for Mrs. Mott's instruction in English, and even that was no longer urgently needed, since so many of the scientists were now speaking quite passable American.

The Germans were startled when the fort authorities announced that they could now purchase automobiles and use them within restrictions. Twenty-two younger men banded together and bought a used Plymouth. General Funkhauser, with funds borrowed from five other older men, bought a large Buick, which he then used as a taxicab, earning substantial profits—which he shared, half to him as manager, half to the other five as owners. It was he who obtained permission to take six Germans and one American with a machine gun all the way to California. When he returned he told everyone, 'That's the land of opportunity. When they set us free, which will be any day now, we must all head for California.'

There was still no news of when the German wives would be allowed into the country, but as a further measure to keep the scientists happy, Stanley Mott was designated to fly to Germany with greetings from the men and to ascertain how the women were doing and whether they were obtaining the meager funds their husbands were sending them from the allotments paid them by the United States Army. He located most of the wives in a barracks at the town of Landshut, northeast of Munich, but when he asked about Liesl Kolff, he was told she was not there, and the commandant said, after searching his files, 'We have no record that Dieter Kolff was ever married.'

And then the fortunes of the German scientists took dramatic turns for the better. The American military belatedly recognized that these brilliant men were sorely needed if the United States was ever to catch up with the Russians in rocketry, and it became apparent to everyone that the Germans would be required to stay in America for many years to come. But how to provide them with legal papers of immigration without disclosing to the world, and especially to the citizens of the United States, that America was using Hitler's scientists, who were hiding in the country illegally?

One part of the problem was rather easily solved: eventually the wives assembled at Landshut were quietly placed aboard military transports and shipped to Boston, where they were entered as ordinary immigrants with provisional papers. In due time they would reach Fort Bliss.

Meanwhile, at the fort, some high shenanigans were under way, and it was due largely to the wit of Rachel Mott that the logjam about the paper work was broken. On her frequent trips to Cuidad Juárez she had made friends with the customs officials, whom she persuaded to be lenient with the Germans when they brought back armfuls of cheap Mexican purchases, and in these negotiations she had also come to know the chief immigration authority.

One afternoon she went to him and placed her problem honestly before him: 'We want to regularize our Germans. It's very important for the nation's security.'

'I've been wondering what we ought to do about them. Clearly, they're here illegally.'

'Illegally, yes. But with the knowledge and approval of the President.'

'I've been told that, and I'm damned if I know what it means.'

'It means we need them, badly.'

'Why?'

'Top secret.'

'Then why are you meddling in it?'

'Because no official wants to deal with this through ordinary channels.'

'What do you want me to do?'

'Tomorrow morning, at nine forty-five, we want you to be here, but to be looking upstream. At ten sharp we also want you to be here, inspecting every bus that comes in from Mexico.'

'And then?'

'You make all the Germans get out, one by one, and you give them ordinary visitors' passes. In three months they can exchange these for permanent permission, and in however many years it takes, they can apply for citizenship.'

'Tomorrow?'

'Yes.'

So on a bright Thursday morning one hundred and ten German scientists who had never been in the United States, officially, climbed into buses at Fort Bliss, entered the international bridge at 0945 and drove into Mexico. Once in Cuidad Juárez, the buses circled about a statue of some Mexican general and came immediately back across the bridge, where they were halted peremptorily by the chief of immigration. The scientists filed out of the buses and marched into the immigration offices, where they solemnly swore that they had, for some months, been living in Mexico City. They petitioned for entry permits, which were granted, after which they filed back into the buses and drove to the prison at Fort Bliss, legally entitled to be there.

One scientist, looking at his stamped paper with the silver eagle, said, 'It was so very German, that whole arrangement.'

A few days later the wives arrived, and when Rachel watched them disembark she burst into tears, for their patient, aging faces reminded her of her own, and of the years of absence, and of the endless journeys back and forth. When the women embraced their husbands she had to turn away, and she was weeping when Dieter Kolff came to her: 'My wife did not come. What can I do now?'

. . .

In that chaotic spring of 1945 when Stanley Mott had wandered into yet another German village, searching for scientists, and had stumbled upon one of the men he sought most avidly, he carried with him memorized instructions as to how he must handle Dieter Kolff and any unnamed men, like General Funkhauser, who might be fleeing with him:

> Because there is a strong likelihood that Himmler's SS Troops will seek to machine-gun the entire Peenemünde cadre to prevent them from bringing their secrets to us, speedy efforts must be made to move any captives to the secure area which will be established near Munich.

But these careful plans had made no provision for handling wives, especially those with no legal proof of their marriage.

So Liesl Koenig Kolff was left stranded in central Germany, with no papers, no wedding license and no knowledge of where her husband might be, her only consolation being that she had escaped the Russians. When stories began to filter out concerning conditions in East Germany, she was grateful that Dieter's resolve had saved her at least from that fate. Rumors circulated that men from Peenemünde were being kidnapped right off the streets of West German towns, so highly did the Russians value their knowledge, and for some months Liesl trembled with fear, convinced that she was about to be snatched because she knew that secret papers regarding future rockets existed.

She became one of the millions of women of this period who had no meaningful past that could be certified, no papers to prove her identity, no sensible hope for the future. In her wanderings she became much like Elinor Grant and Rachel Mott in their years of ceaseless travel without their husbands. Men went away to the excitement of war; women were left to meander with ration books and babies, and neither would ever understand the miseries of the other.

When Liesl learned that the scientists' wives were congregating at the barracks in Landshut, she traveled across much of Germany to join them, but since none of them had known her as Dieter's wife and since she had no papers or anyone to certify her, the American guards would not permit her entrance, and she drifted off to Hamburg, where city-wide rebuilding provided opportunities for almost anyone who would work.

Even so, she found it difficult to land a job of any kind and had to be content with a frowzy night club near the waterfront, not as an entertainer or a hostess, for she was neither pretty enough nor young enough for such glamorous work. She did not qualify even as a waitress or a kitchen helper; the best she could get was a job as a cleaning woman. She reported seven days a week at nine o'clock in the morning, and worked till ten or eleven at night; in time the new German government would halt such exploitation, but in this time of crisis she was glad to have a job of any kind and did not complain.

She roomed with two other girls, much like herself, whose husbands had either died or absconded, and because Liesl knew how to hoard pfennigs and buy always at the cheapest places, they managed. When she tried to correspond with her parents at the farm, she received no reply, and this worried her, but when one of the girls suggested that she cross over into East Germany to see what had happened to the farm, she shuddered.

She had better luck with her husband. Through authorities with the American occupation forces, she learned with difficulty where the German scientists were imprisoned. 'That's altogether the wrong word,' a major from California said. 'They're being kept together because they work well as a team.' He gave her the address of Fort Bliss, to which she sent a stream of letters advising her husband of her plight as a displaced person with no documentation.

She sent five letters before she received a reply, and when it arrived, all stamped and censored by two governments, she sat down in the night-club kitchen and held it unopened in her lap, just staring at it and trying to estimate what plan of salvation it might contain. That Dieter would somehow rescue her, she had no doubt, and this was justified, for when she opened it, she found it full of the most soaring optimism. It was the first letter she had ever received from him, so she could not claim to recognize his handwriting, but she did recognize the competence with which he wrote:

> Life here is good. Professor Mott's wife is a fine, decent person who teaches me English. We work as you can guess, and although we are in a fort we are not in prison. I have been to Mexico three times.
>
> I have discussed with both Professor Mott and Mrs. Mott ways by which you can get to the United States. Do everything possible to get here. It is not heaven, but it is certainly not Russia.
>
> There are three ways we can do it. First, go to the collection center at Landshut near Munich and join the other wives. I am surprised you haven't done this. Second, see if there is any way you can get from the church in Wolgast where we were married by the Lutheran minister a copy of our wedding certificate, which will authorize you to join me when the time comes. Third, if all else fails, I shall hurry back to Germany as soon as the law allows and fetch you. Von Braun and Stuhlinger say they will return to Germany to marry their childhood sweethearts.

As soon as she read Dieter's second suggestion she understood his tactic; they would have to convince the authorities that they had been married in a church in Wolgast, the small town opposite Peenemünde's island, and that the papers had somehow been lost when the Russians arrived. Her sixth letter to Fort Bliss covered this point nicely:

> Two times I have traveled to Wolgast to see if I could get a copy of our marriage certificate, but when the Russians reached there, they tore our little church apart, and all the records are lost.

Husband and wife corresponded thus for many painful months, building a careful history of their past lives, and Liesl eased Dieter's mind when she reported that she had quit her job in Hamburg in order to move closer to the other wives at Landshut 'so as to be ready to join them when the time comes.'

The time came, but she was not allowed to accompany them on their journey to the United States, for the American authorities, well versed in such problems, concluded that she was merely one more prostitute trying to slip into the States on the spurious claim that she was married to somebody. In despair she watched the legal wives move out, then found her way back to West Berlin, where she was lucky to get another job cleaning up the kitchen of a cabaret.

She was there one night, sweaty, tired, bedraggled and hopeless, a drab thirty-year-old German woman given to plumpness, when the manager informed her that an American man wished to speak with her. Realizing how dismal she must appear, she started to tell the manager that she could not go into the cabaret, but he anticipated her: 'Not in there. I took him into the alley.' After wiping her hands, she met him, Professor Mott, with whom she had spent three wonderful days at the time of her deliverance.

'I've been sent over to investigate—' he began, in good German.

'And Dieter ask you to find me,' she interrupted in English.

'How did you learn English?' he asked.

'I know some day I be going to America. People everywhere speaking English these days.'

He wanted to take her immediately to his hotel and give her a good wash and a meal, but she said she must finish her work, so he waited, and when they were alone he spoke rapidly and frankly: 'I am quite sure that you and Dieter were never married, and this raises all sorts of difficulty.'

'We were married in a little church in Wolgast, but the Russians—'

'Drop the Russians! You're a woman without papers, and Army Intelligence will spot you a mile off.'

'I was married in Wolgast,' she said stubbornly, 'and when the Russians—'

'Here's what we'll do. I will go before a notary public at the American embassy in Bonn. And I'll swear that when I rescued Dieter Kolff and General Funkhauser in 1945, you were there as Dieter's wife and it was you who possessed and delivered to me the papers we so badly wanted.'

'I did,' she said quietly. 'Did Dieter tell you how I got them?'

'He told me two things, Liesl. How you saved them at the farm. How you got them from Funkhauser.'

'It's strange,' she said in German. 'Funkhauser is there safe, and I am a fugitive.'

'From the way Funkhauser's starting, he'll be president of something one of these days.'

On his return to Bonn he made the deposition, and Army Intelligence sent men to Berlin to investigate the case of Liesl Koenig, who claimed she was the wife of Dieter Kolff. It took them about six minutes to decide that she was lying, but when they also went to Hamburg and Landshut, they found that she had left a trail of good remembrances: 'Hard-working. Studied English. Saved her money.' Her roommates, when questioned, proved that they were of the same type, not prostitutes at all, but merely women left adrift. Not many interrogations produced so consistent a record, and the investigators reported: 'About her marriage, many questions. About her character, none.'

The clerk at the Bonn embassy who handled such routine matters was a black man, assigned there to prove to the Germans that America did not want to go the way of Hitler's racism. He was, of course, the only black in the embassy and vastly overeducated for his job, but he was effective; any German who wanted a visa to visit America, or a permit to emigrate there, had to satisfy this black man as to credentials, and he was very canny. Looking only at the reports of the field investigators, he was inclined to deny Liesl Koenig a visa, but when he studied Professor Mott's report of the woman's behavior at the time of Germany's surrender, he realized that here was an exceptional case.

Summoning Mott, he said, 'Bring that woman in. She merits closer attention,' and when he saw Liesl and heard her stubborn insistence that she had been married, in a little church . . . 'I know about Wolgast,' he said, 'we've made inquiries there. No such church ever existed. The Russians left Wolgast untouched.'

'I was married in a small church—'

'Fraulein Koenig,' the consul interrupted, 'because of your great service to the United States, I am issuing you a visa. It refers to you as Mrs. Kolff. When you reach Fort Bliss you may want to get married legally, but at any rate, you're entitled to join your . . .' He stopped, cleared his throat and ended, 'You are herewith given entrance so that you may join Mr. Kolff in El Paso.'

At the fort, Liesl was amazed at how quickly the German wives had adapted to American ways: there was a school, from kindergarten to the fifth grade, a kind of hospital, garages for the family cars. They had already made a shrewd analysis of the El Paso stores. The women were all learning English, and some wrote long reports to young girls back in Germany whom the unmarried scientists were planning to import as wives.

Liesl was even more impressed by the Motts. They looked after the entire German contingent, and she discovered that she was not the only drifting wife that Mr. Mott had succeeded in getting into the States. When Wernher von Braun was called to Washington to give advice to the American government, Mott went along to protect and advise him, and in all the work at White Sands, Mott served as intermediary between the American military and the Germans. In addition, he was a constant friend, and when General Funkhauser was arrested for running a public taxicab without a license, it was Mott who explained to the Texas Rangers that the voluble general was both legally in the United States and well on his way to becoming a citizen.

'That's all well and good,' the Ranger said. 'But he's operating that damned Buick of his as a taxi.'

'He's helping out the men here who have no cars. And he's doing it at the Army's suggestion.'

'Who suggested it.'

'I did.'

'Are you Army?'

'I'm liaison. I represent the Army.'

'Well, Professor, you tell that fat-ass German that if the El Paso traffic cops catch him one more time driving Mexican women over to Juárez in his taxicab, he's in jail.'

The way Mott handled such matters won him the affection of the German wives, but it was his work on scientific problems that gained him the respect of their husbands; originally he had known little about rockets, but his solid work in aeronautics had enabled him to learn rapidly, and before long he was almost as capable as Kolff in anticipating and solving problems.

'He is very good, that one,' Dieter told his wife. 'In daytime he keeps General Funkhauser from being arrested by the traffic police. At night he helps men like Stuhlinger get permission to do the things that are necessary.'

One night both Mott and his wife came to visit the Kolffs, and it was Rachel who said, 'I've been visiting with a minister in El Paso, and he assures me that he would be most happy to arrange a wedding for you. He's Lutheran.'

Dieter and Liesl looked at each other, then she turned away and went over to a desk, pulled open a drawer, and rummaged till she found her passport, visa and qualifying documents. Handing them to Mrs. Mott, she pointed to the various lines that identified her as Mrs. Dieter Kolff. 'I swear many times I married. You, Professor, do the same. And Dieter swear, too. If I change my story now, I go to jail. You and Dieter go to jail.'

There was much legalistic discussion of this, until Liesl grew angry.

'Listen, you! It matters not whatever you say. Because I truly married. In a field near Wolgast. Just as I have said.'

When the Motts looked at her in amazement, fearing that the years of hardship had somehow addled her, she stood there angrily and said, 'When the world falls apart, when this man'—and she indicated her husband— 'knew not what to do with his papers, he comes to me and asks my help. We take our lives in our hand. We fight the whole SS, and I bring the shovel and we bury them. And I ask him, "Dieter, will you marry me?" and he say, "No, it is too dangerous." And I almost die with shame. And then he say, "Much dangerous we do it public in church. The SS ask about papers. But I marry you here under the eye of God." And in an open field near Wolgast we marry ourselves. And always I am his wife. I don't need no El Paso church.'

After a long pause Mrs. Mott, who was never deterred from a course she believed was right, said, 'Liesl, the German wives here in camp . . . they say the American authorities at Landshut turned you back because they knew you were never legally married. If you allow me to arrange a wedding now . . .'

Liesl spoke solely to Mrs. Mott, in German: 'Every woman in this camp, you and the German and American wives, we all got through the years of war somehow, and the years of destruction that came after. And I do not now ask you how you lived during the long years when your husband was away. I do not ask how the German wives lived before they reached El Paso. For myself, I found work in night clubs, not singing, not dancing with the customers. I was the lowest helper, not even washing dishes in the kitchen. I worked in the toilets, scrubbing floors. So I do not give one damn what the others say. I survived, and that's enough.'

Her own problems faded into insignificance when Stanley Mott informed the Kolffs that he had heard there would be an investigation of General Funkhauser. 'The Army and the FBI aren't stupid,' he said. 'They know that some of the German scientists we brought here were committed Nazis, and they're going to keep digging them out until they're all back in Germany.' The Kolffs seemed stunned by this. 'You'll be questioned, I'm sure,' Stanley went on. 'But don't worry. We'll be right there with you.'

From the first day the Peenemünde men arrived in the United States, there was constant agitation against them. Politicians who had served in the Allied armies at Salerno or the Bulge were little inclined to extend a cordial welcome to their former enemies. Some Jewish veterans who had seen Buchenwald and Auschwitz were repelled by the thought that now their country was depending upon former Nazis for its military might, and occasionally ugly incidents had occurred in El Paso when the Germans went shopping. Some veterans were especially outraged when the women spoke German in the stores, and the FBI received numerous anonymous complaints that the Nazis at Fort Bliss were communicating with Communists in Mexico.

It fell to Stanley Mott to defend his charges, and he did so faithfully. He told Congress, the local newspapers, the weekly magazines and the area Rotary Clubs that the most careful screening had been conducted, and that every individual guilty of criminal behavior or even suspected of it had been weeded out and sent back home. As for the remainder, and particularly Von Braun's inner team, he assured his listeners that they had been as much endangered by the Nazis as any other Germans who had been destroyed:

> 'On the morning that I rescued General Funkhauser, Dieter Kolff and his wife, with their ultra-precious secret documents which they had been endeavoring to deliver into our hands, I learned that in a different part of Germany, Heinrich Himmler's SS troopers had massacred eleven scientists they suspected of sabotage. And we had frightening proof that Himmler's men intended doing exactly the same to the brilliant men who are now housed at Fort Bliss. Gentlemen, it was touch and go. And if Himmler's men didn't get them, the Russians were going to.
>
> 'I spent three years of my life trying to work it so that these men got to America and not into an early grave. I know every one of them. I know every record, every black mark and every white. And I certify that they were needed. They're needed now. And they will be needed in the future. Without them we might have stood naked in space.
>
> 'What is more important in the matters that you have been discussing today—the question of their loyalty now and their cleanliness in the past—I also certify these men. I know them better than I know my own son.'

It was because of testimony like this, often repeated, that Stanley Mott became known throughout the government and the Army as Professor Krauthead. He laughed when his wife told him of the nickname, and admitted that he deserved it: 'At college—no, even in high school—I was often laughed at because I always had single objectives. I was known as a straight arrow. With some people that's a term of criticism. Not with me.'

'Where is the arrow pointing now?' she asked.

'Out there,' he said, indicating the heavens.

'You think it's that important?'

'Even more than you can guess.'

'Isn't it because you were assigned the job of finding these men?'

'It goes much further back than that.'

'You certainly didn't read science fiction as a boy?' she asked, amusement echoing in her voice.

'I've never read any. But I did study aeronautics, you remember. And what I study, I tend to believe. If it stands inspection.'

'You really believe that aviation and rockets and space are critically important?'

'In our lifetime we'll leave El Paso at nine in the morning and have late lunch in Paris. I or somebody like me will walk on the Moon.'

'What nonsense.'

'Von Braun doesn't think so. Nor Stuhlinger. Nor Dieter Kolff.'

'Sit down, Stanley. I want to ask you something very important.'

They sat near the window, staring out at the row of low buildings that housed the Germans, most of whose men were up at White Sands testing an improved version of the A-4. Of the hundredfold Peenemünde rockets that had been assembled in New Mexico, only five remained; all the rest had been shot into the air northward toward Carrizozo, often exploding, as they had in the Baltic, sometimes performing miraculously.

Rachel shot her question: 'Stanley, do you think it prudent to defend the Germans as vigorously as you do? In public, I mean.'

'You told me you'd grown extremely fond of them.'

'I have, and I've tried to help them. But how do you know they weren't all dedicated Nazis? How can you certify their credentials so unhesitatingly?'

'Some of them I refused to certify, and they're back in Germany.'

'But Von Braun and Kolff, weren't they Nazis, too? Don't we have proof that Hitler gave Kolff a medal, personally?'

'We've been all through that. Dieter Kolff traveled halfway across Germany to hand me the secret papers. In helping us to avoid simple engineering mistakes, I would judge Kolff to have been worth about three billion dollars to this country.'

'I'm not talking about money. I'm talking about you, making a fool of yourself if this blows up in your face. If they all turn out to have been Nazi criminals.'

When he started to defend his judgment and his tactics, she cut him short with the one question he could not easily answer: 'All right, I'll give you Von Braun and Kolff. But what about General Funkhauser?'

'I thought he was your buddy.'

'He is. I've grown to like him very much. But I also suspect he was a Nazi and maybe even a storm trooper.'

Mott pressed his hands against his temples, a gesture he had acquired in Georgia when test questions were unusually perplexing. 'I've studied every aspect of the Funkhauser problem, and I come up with this. He obeyed but he did not initiate, and at the first opportunity he quit the sorry business.'

When congressmen pestered him about Funkhauser he reiterated that sentence until he came to accept it as the fundamental judgment regarding all his Germans. Jewish groups had come to Fort Bliss with solid complaints, and he had reasoned the same way with them. And the FBI, extremely careful in such matters, had compiled a rather damaging dossier: 'These papers prove your man Funkhauser was a Nazi criminal.'

'They do nothing of the sort,' Mott snapped. 'Look at what the papers say. He was a reasonably good administrator who bumbled along from one job to the next, altering his colors whenever necessary. Study the record and you'll conclude that he can be characterized as absolutely anything.'

'How do you characterize him, Professor Mott?'

'As a man whose courage and determination enabled us to get hold of documents we sorely needed for the safety of this nation. If I defend him, it's because I appreciate the great good he did us.'

'Would you be content if we shipped him back to Germany?'

'I would oppose it with my life. In very risky times, Helmut Funkhauser chose our side. If caught, he would have been shot.'

'A rat deserting a sinking ship.'

'Exactly, but, gentlemen, he brought with him one whopping piece of cheese.'

The day came when two Army generals and an FBI team appeared at Fort Bliss. As was expected, the Motts were asked to summon the Kolffs, and when the party assembled, a young FBI man said succinctly, 'We have solid evidence on every stage of Helmut Funkhauser's life in Germany. We know the date on which he sentenced you to death, Herr Kolff, the date on which he flew you to meet Hitler. We know that he was appointed to supervise the rocket works at Peenemünde, and what he did at the caves of Nordhausen. There is nothing you can tell us, except for the few months that are blank.' He stopped, and was about to conclude his statement when one of the generals took over.

'The period between when you left Peenemünde and when you met Professor Mott.' He waited. 'Tell us what happened in that period.'

Dieter and Liesl Kolff looked at one another, and finally she spoke, in broken English, and she was so nervous that one of the FBI men said in good German, 'You may speak German.'

She looked at him but did not smile appreciatively, as he thought she might. She frowned, for she saw in this young man with the close-cropped hair, the dark blue suit, the highly polished black shoes, America's version of the perpetual policeman: the SS who knocked on doors at night; the French Sûreté men she had known while waiting for her boat at Le Havre; the Russians whom she had escaped. They were the same in all nations, essential but to be avoided. If General Funkhauser, regardless of his record, was in trouble with these young men, she had to be on Funkhauser's side.

Slowly, and with great care, she told of hiding the papers, of her marriage to Dieter in the little church at Wolgast, of their flight after the bombing and their encounter with Funkhauser. She did not disclose the sentence of death passed in Wittenberge or the emotions she felt when facing the firing squad, but she expounded at some length on the courage shown by Funkhauser in getting them across Germany and his resourceful-ness in finding them food and safe passage, and places to sleep at night.

'He was a very brave man,' she said. 'Without him we would have been dead.'

'Did you know him to be a Nazi?'

'My father was a Nazi. He had to be or he would get no barley.'

'But wasn't General Funkhauser a hard-working Nazi?'

'I never knew him at Peenemünde. First time I saw him, he was city commander at Wittenberge. Trying to do a good job. But he gave up that important post to flee with us . . . to take the secret documents to the Americans.'

'Herr Kolff,' the FBI man said abruptly. 'You haven't answered my questions. Did you and your wife agree that she should do the talking?'

In English, Dieter said, 'She always speaks first. She's a farmer's daughter.'

'Is what she said accurate?' The FBI man studied his papers. 'Were you really married in the church at Wolgast?'

'A woman ought to know where she was married.'

'About Funkhauser. Was he an ardent Nazi?'

'He was. I was present when Hitler promoted him to general.'

'And gave you a medal?'

'Hitler appreciated me for the same reason your people do. I can fix rockets, that's all.'

'What did you think when General Funkhauser sentenced you to death at Stettin?'

'He was a colonel then. I thought I was dead.'

'Why weren't you?'

'Because Germany needed rockets. The way the world needs them now.'

'If you were an American official, would you allow General Funkhauser to remain in this country?'

Before Dieter could reply, his wife did a surprising thing. 'Pardon me, misters. But you must see what General Funkhauser did for us.' And she pulled up her skirt, revealing on her left leg above the knee a deep, jagged scar. 'In a small battle I was shot through this leg, and the general could have grabbed the papers and gone ahead and escaped without us. But he put me on his bicycle and pushed me the last miles, and Professor Mott can say so, too, for he lifted me off the bicycle.' Looking directly at each of the FBI men in turn, she said, 'I would give him refuge.'

It was irrelevant, really, what the Kolffs testified, because the matter of *The United States* v. *Funkhauser* was taken out of the hands of the little group in Fort Bliss. On one of his trips to California, General Funkhauser had met with leaders of the aviation and rocket industry that was centered in that state, and he was so impressive in his knowledge of rocketry and its manufacture, so modest in his account of how he had steered Von Braun around seemingly insuperable blockages, that very soon three different companies wanted to hire him.

California senators tend to be powerful, and when they went to the White House to say that their constituents, five or six of them, wanted to employ this master scientist Funkhauser, he was cleared immediately. The general left Fort Bliss in a private DC-3 and returned some years later in his own Beechcraft. He was a troubleshooter for Allied Aviation, specializing in their rocket and space ventures.

Liesl Kolff submerged herself in the reassuring routine of El Paso, and one morning she was told, 'Mrs. Kolff, you may accompany your husband to White Sands today. Something special.'

She was present, at a goodly distance, when the last complete A-4 in the world was launched with an infinity of recording devices aboard. She saw the enormous flames shoot out and heard the echoing roar. She watched as it climbed perfectly into the high blue of the desert sky, then sped off to the north. How different this treeless desert is, she thought, from the green woods of Peenemünde. What a far way we have traveled, Dieter and I.

She gave birth to a son, whom she named Magnus, after Von Braun's younger brother, and surprised everyone at Fort Bliss when she spoke loudly and forthrightly in defense of Wernher von Braun when newspapermen in Washington accused him of having been Hitler's right-hand man: 'We are all Americans now, even General Funkhauser, and I want to hear no more about the past. The last A-4 is gone. Now we must occupy ourselves with other matters.'

She and Dieter remained close to the Motts; she baby-sat for them whenever needed and refused compensation. She recognized the fair-haired Rachel as a most generous and sensible woman, and of course, both Kolffs looked on Mott as their savior.

The four were together, veterans of Fort Bliss and completely acclimatized to life in the Texas-Mexican Southwest, when news came that the Army had decided to experiment with rockets in a massive way. Dieter and Mott were delighted, for they saw this as a breakthrough in the field they had elected for their life's work, but the two women were apprehensive when they learned where the Army intended sending them.

'Alabama,' the soldier on the phone said. 'A place called Huntsville, Alabama.'

'Why there?' Mott asked in amazement.

'Because Senator John Sparkman lives in Huntsville,' the soldier said. 'And in Army life that's a damned good reason.'

Further investigation showed that a huge arsenal had been activated there during World War II, Redstone it had been named, and it had served well. But with peace breaking out it had been no longer needed; the Huntsville people who had worked there were thrown into the cadres of the unemployed, and it had fallen to Senator Sparkman to find them something to do. He had found them a challenging new job: these Alabama farmers, cotton pickers mostly, would build the machines that would throw men out to the stars. But to accomplish this feat they would need the help and guidance of the Peenemünde men like Dieter Kolff.

'It's what I dreamed of,' Kolff said. Like General Funkhauser in decaying Germany, he was prepared to move wherever he was needed, and now he was needed in Alabama.

In the dark days of the 1946 senatorial campaign, when Fremont's naval hero Norman Grant was discovering that no mere amateur was going to defeat the practiced old warhorse Ulysses Gantling, he became aware of a rather pretty freshman girl from the university who was working as a volunteer in his headquarters, savagely determined to see the old senator defeated.

Once when she was stuffing envelopes with obvious fury, he asked her, 'Why the frown?' and she replied, 'I hate that double-crosser.'

'Who?' he asked, and she snapped: 'Gantling.'

'I never allow myself to speak of him that way,' Grant said with a disarming smile, and she snapped again: 'Well, he hasn't done to you what he's done to me.'

Grant had sat down beside the agitated girl to ask what Senator Gantling, a rather kindly man even though a political enemy, could possibly have done to a pretty college freshman, and the girl explained: 'He didn't do it to me. He did it to John Pope, the mealy-mouth.'

'Pope?'

'No. Gantling,' and she pretended to spit at the corner.

Grant, after looking carefully at the flushed girl, made a shrewd guess: 'And you hope to marry this John Pope some day?'

'If he gives me a chance.'

Grant smiled and reassured her: 'He will. Who is he? Who are you?'

The girl drew back, her bright eyes flashing. 'You don't know who John Pope is? You're not ready to be a United States senator.'

Now Grant laughed. He was losing the primary but not his sense of humor. 'On my word, I've never heard of the young man.'

'Where were you when he was setting all kinds of football records around here?'

'Oh, that John Pope? I was away at war.'

It was extremely fortunate for the future senator that he said these words, because after Penny Hardesty had introduced herself and wished the hero well, she had a bright idea: 'If you were the hero people around here say you were, Mr. Grant, you ought to appear before the crowds in uniform. Get their sympathy.'

'I'd never do that. The war's over.'

'And so are you if you don't pull out the plug.' She felt so strongly about the necessity for some dramatic impact in his flagging campaign that she took her concern to the bright young Irishman who seemed to be in charge of strategy, and told him, 'Finnerty, this campaign is dying on its feet, and you know it. We've got to capitalize on the boss's military heroism, or we're going to lose.' She shook her finger in Finnerty's face. 'And I don't want to see that foul-ball Gantling back in Washington.'

'I'm quite sure Norman Grant would never consent to trailing around this state in his naval uniform. That is definitely out.'

She stood by Finnerty's desk, biting her nails, obviously agitated by this daily erosion of what should have been a winning position. Then the idea struck her: 'Finnerty! He doesn't have to appear in uniform. You do.' She became excited, and with flashing hands, arranged the imaginary podium: 'Grant stays over here in whatever he chooses to wear. No, make it something dark blue that might be taken for a uniform. You stand over here. Buy yourself a new uniform if necessary. And you read the two citations that appear in this brochure.'

She was so enthusiastic about the possibilities that she babbled on, predicting Gantling's sound defeat, but Finnerty stopped her: 'What would you think if I could import a tall colored man who lost one foot to the sharks. Very handsome, speaks very well. I mean, in a state like Fremont, would it help or hurt?'

It took Penny one second to answer that question. She leaped around the desk and kissed Finnerty on the cheek. 'You should be running against Gantling.' When he recalled the incident later, it occurred to him that Miss Hardesty never referred to the campaign as a crusade to elect Grant, but always as a vendetta to defeat Gantling, and one day when things were moving handsomely he asked her why. They were in a diner with their candidate, grabbing a hurried meal between stops at factories, and Penny, with her mouth half filled with cheeseburger, said, 'I despise Gantling because he's a spineless weasel.' Finnerty told Grant, 'We better keep this one away from the press.' But she continued: 'For four years Gantling promised John Pope that he would assign him to Annapolis. Did so twice in my hearing. But last year, even though John graduated with all sorts of honors, Gantling could see this campaign looming ahead, and he gave his appointment to the son of that crapper who's running his campaign in Webster. On a scale of ten, John Pope is a nine-point-nine, that son-of-a-bitch in Webster is a two-point-three—'

'Penny,' Norman Grant interrupted. 'I wish you'd not use profanity. Some newspaper person might hear it.'

'He's a newspaperman,' Penny said, pointing to Finnerty.

'And I agree with Captain Grant. Knock it off.'

'I never swore till I met Gantling. He is really a—'

'Start now,' Grant said. 'My opponent is what you say. He has the character of a weeping willow, and it looks as if we're going to retire him. Thanks to Finnerty . . . and you.' He added this last phrase so lamely that Finnerty had to say, 'Captain Grant. You better know now. It was Penny who dreamed up the idea of us three veterans.'

Grant nodded severely, then asked, as if he were her father, 'Where is young Pope now?'

'Who knows? He was so disgusted when Senator Gantling reneged on the appointment to Annapolis that I think he just sat in a corner and cried. Then someone told him that each year the Navy sends a handful of superior enlisted men on to Annapolis. He's in the Navy somewhere, and before long, if I know him, he'll be selected for Annapolis.'

'If I'm elected . . . I really don't know much about this, but if I'm entitled to, I'll appoint him.'

'John would not rely on that, Mr. Grant. He's been deceived before . . . by a senator.' Her lips trembled and she came close to tears, but then she stuffed the last of her burger into her mouth, looked at her watch and said, 'We're due at the glove factory.'

When Grant won the primary in the early summer of 1946, Penny Hardesty moved to his statewide headquarters in Benton, where she assumed, with Finnerty, command of that office. From everything she read, she became convinced that this was the year for a Republican triumph, and it was she who coined the phrase that helped Grant cast scorn and ridicule on the rather drab ward heeler the Democrats had nominated to oppose him: ONLY ONE MAN IS FIT TO SERVE IN THE SENATE. She also invented the slogan that helped the entire state ticket defeat the Democrats: HAVEN'T YOU HAD ENOUGH? She drafted sharply worded statements explaining how Truman's ineptness and the fumbling of the Democratic Congress had caused meat prices to rise while delivering little profit to the farmer. She ventilated three regional scandals in which Democratic bureaucrats had abused the Western states, and to cap her achievement, she went personally to the home of Ulysses Gantling and persuaded him, for the welfare of the party and the nation, to make a ringing endorsement of 'our great naval hero, Captain Norman Grant.'

On election night, when Grant saw the magnitude of his victory and realized that he had won six secure years in Washington in one of the finest jobs the nation had to offer, he told Finnerty and Penny, 'I want you to come to Washington with me.'

He encountered two objections: his wife, Elinor, deemed it most unwise to take so young a girl to the capital; and Penny herself pointed out that she did not yet have her degree from the university. To his wife, Grant replied, 'That bright little girl is forty years old right now. It's Washington that had better watch out, not Penny Hardesty.' And to Penny he said, 'I've called the people at Fremont State, and they've arranged to transfer your credits to Georgetown University. It's all been done.' Then he added the clincher: 'And if Mr. Pope does get into Annapolis, there you'd be.'

So Penny Hardesty, nineteen years old and the fourth child of a working-class family that had never sent a member beyond high school, went to Washington to help establish a newly elected senator in his offices and to pick up a full scholarship at Georgetown University, arranged for by her employer. She resembled the thousands of other young girls who left distant states to build their careers in the nation's capital; they were all bright, all ambitious, all moving into a city where eligible men were outnumbered by nubile women ten-to-one.

On that score Penny had no worries. In fact, she was so fearfully busy attending to her senator twelve hours a day and cracking her books at night that she could not have dated had she had the opportunity. Tim Finnerty, through his association with her in the Fremont campaign, appreciated what a brilliant, coordinated person she was and was ready to escort her anywhere. Indeed, he was so eager to do so that she had to clarify things: 'Look, Finnerty. There're two reasons why we're not allowed to get serious. A Midwest Baptist is not the girl for a Boston Catholic to take home to his mother, and his sister in the nunnery, and his uncle Francis Xavier, who is a priest. And somewhere out on the bounding blue I have a sailor.'

Senator Grant showed Penny his memorandum to officials in the Navy in which he asked their advice as to whether he was legally entitled to appoint to Annapolis a young man who had already enlisted as an ordinary seaman. The Navy, inordinately proud of having one of its heroes in Congress, called immediately to assure Grant that they would look into the matter and reply shortly. In the meantime Penny received a letter from her sailor, proving that this young man did not wait for others to solve his problems for him:

> Marvelous news. I've been appointed to Officer Candidate School. It won't be Annapolis, but it will give me a chance to go into flying later on. I've already told Mother and Dad, and I want to tell you, too, but nobody else. I stood either at the very top of all the men who took the exams, or close to it. It's going to come true, Penny.

Just as she was kissing the signature, Senator Grant came by with the good news: 'Navy tells me to go ahead.' And on this assurance she sent the telegram: SENATOR GRANT HAS APPOINTED YOU TO ANNAPOLIS. I AM PROUD OF YOU. PENNY.

She would always remember the ensuing years as among the richest of her life—not the most exciting, for they were to come later, but the most rewarding. She worked in the office of a fine man, whom she could respect increasingly. She worked beside a brilliant man, Tim Finnerty, whose shrewd insights into political maneuvering she envied. She was attending a fine university whose professors, Finnerty pointed out acidly, 'are exactly the kind of Catholic subversives you yokels from the West ought to come up against.'

She was beginning to see, from the inside, that the Democrats were not the inept slobs she had said during the campaign and that Harry Truman was a rather more substantial President than she had at first perceived. 'Watch out, Finnerty. That man won't be a pushover in 1948.' But both Grant and Finnerty were satisfied that Dewey would win easily.

Because she was taking pre-law courses at Georgetown, she became Senator Grant's liaison with the Justice Department and developed a burning admiration for the manner in which the Supreme Court of the United States served as a buffer between the various branches of government and especially between the forty-eight sovereign states.

On four different occasions she had an opportunity to meet Justices of the Court: twice she carried papers to Chief Justice Vinson, who seemed austere and preoccupied. Justice Burton she liked immensely, but Justice Douglas made her suspicious; she agreed with Senator Grant that some of his dissenting opinions were asinine. But the Court as a whole, especially the stalwart conservative judges like Burton, Reed and Jackson, satisfied her that the system evolved by the founding fathers was a good one, probably the best known to any nation.

But when the work was done, and her explorations finished, it was to the lovely town of Annapolis that she repaired, always delighted by the first sight of its towers, the stateliness of the Naval Academy, the delicate charm of its little streets and Southern mansions. Sometimes, as she drove her Plymouth in from Washington on Friday evening, she would draw over to some curb and simply look at the beauty of this rare town, checking the old brick houses she had not seen before, then driving slowly down to the enchanting harbor that crept right into the heart of town, with small craft lining its shores. It must be, she thought, the most beautiful state capital in America.

To her left, as she studied the harbor, rose the old gray buildings of the Naval Academy, where John Pope was learning the rules of his profession. In his plebe year he was allowed few privileges; sometimes Penny made the trip to Annapolis and wasn't even able to see him. But she came to know the widow of a naval captain who ran a small boardinghouse on colorful Pinckney Street, and when John was not available, there she nestled down to study her law books. When he was given freedom he joined her there for dinners which the widow delighted to prepare, after which John took over the Plymouth for a drive through the Maryland countryside.

Once when he had a full day off, they boarded the ferry and rode across the bay to the Eastern Shore, where they entered a strange and beautiful world that seemed locked by history into the eighteenth century. They ate crabs and oysters and beaten biscuits and told each other how different this was from Fremont and Nebraska. On one drive back John spotted an ice cream stand, from which he purchased a pint of rum raisin ice cream, and as they finished the last bites, licking the wooden spoons, Penny whispered, 'I was going to say that I wished life could go on like this forever. We don't have to wish it. You and I can make it continue.'

After their first sexual experience in the autumn of 1944 it had been understood between them that they could repeat it whenever an opportunity occurred, and during John's senior year in high school they had found many occasions for relaxed and extended explorations. They were in love and there was every expectation that some day they would marry; they both wanted this, equally, and no attractive girl that John met as a football hero diverted him from Penny, and not even a man as gifted as Tim Finnerty distracted her.

In the week before John enlisted in the Navy, they had made love every night, as if trying to store up memories sufficient for the long years ahead, and whenever he managed to snatch a leave, they did the same. Once she traveled to Chicago to be near the Naval Training Station when he was granted two days of freedom, but now that he was a fully registered mid-shipman at the Naval Academy he felt constrained: 'The Navy would knock the devil out of me if they found I'd been registering with you in some cheap hotel.' This they refused to do, so their love-making was restricted to the Plymouth, parked in some dark Eastern Shore lane, or in the home of some girl friend in Washington. But their affection for one another increased with each meeting, whether they were able to go to bed or not.

Mostly they talked, neither ever growing weary of learning what the other was engaged in. 'They have some of the brightest professors at Georgetown. Really brilliant men whose teaching is entirely different from that at Fremont U. Question. Question. Question. They want to drive you in a corner, and if you can't fight your way back . . . goodbye.'

John said that his studies at the Academy were tougher than he had expected, especially in mathematics. 'You'd think the Navy ran on a slide rule. Sometimes I can hardly keep afloat, until I remember that the others are having an even tougher time with the formulas than I am. You know, Penny, we got a damned good education back there in Henry Clay High School.'

On one visit, when the widow either accidentally or prudently had to visit relatives in Baltimore, they hurried to bed, where John confided the good news: 'As you know, I put in for aviation training, and three days ago I received confirmation. I go either to New Mexico or Pensacola for real flight training. Not exploratory stuff, but the real thing.'

Before he could do this, however, he had to master small-craft sailing, and the Navy kept some nineteen two-man boats in the Severn River, where he learned to handle sails, cast off ropes and dock his little yacht, as he and Penny called it. Twice he was able to take her sailing, and on one glorious weekend he and six other novices, under the eye of a former Navy captain, were able to take their girls on a two-day cruise down the bay to the enchanting town of Oxford, which dated back to the 1600s. The men slept aboard; the girls checked in at the old inn on the waterfront, and at dusk they met for crab cakes and beer. On the quiet sail back to Annapolis, John whispered, 'The day I graduate, we get married.'

'I decided that three years ago,' Penny said. She was well on her way to becoming a lawyer, and told him, 'When you're flying off some carrier, I'll be fighting government cases in some town like Boston. You watch.'

Even though she had learned to respect the quiet, tough manner in which Harry Truman handled the perilous tasks of the Presidency, she was astounded when the 1948 election drew to a close with him still in contention. She had assumed, like all Washington people from the Western states, that Governor Dewey would win easily, and she had even played the game of who would be invited to join his Cabinet: 'There's a real chance that Senator Grant will be offered Secretary of the Interior.'

'And I'll advise him not to accept,' Finnerty said.

'Why in the world not?' Penny asked. 'When Dewey wins this year, he'll be good for eight years. That's better than being a senator.'

'There's nothing better than being a senator,' Finnerty said.

Together with Grant, they returned to Fremont to campaign for the entire Republican ticket, and when she saw once more that stable, solid group of Republicans she was reassured: 'Dewey has it. And you, Senator Grant, are going to have to make some tough decisions. How do you incline?'

At such moments she became vaguely aware that her boss and his wife were not having an easy time handling his new responsibilities. Elinor Grant was as attractive as ever, her dark hair still framing the pallid face austerely, her controlled smile still giving an aloof but pleasing impression. What seemed lacking was any conviction that she approved what her husband was doing. When Midshipman John Pope took his girl Penny to the Army-Navy game in Philadelphia, it was a total event: both of them wanted Navy to win, silly as it might seem to others; both of them cheered, and drank beer afterward, and yelled at their friends in a day of irresponsible delight. And whenever Penny negotiated a new milestone on her way to a law degree, John exulted with her. When Mrs. Grant refused to participate in any celebration of her husband's achievements, Penny said, 'Maybe she doesn't comprehend what an enormous thing it is to get a bill passed through the Congress. Especially one that will benefit the entire West.'

If Penny was confused by Elinor's indifference, she would have been appalled had she learned that Mrs. Grant still protested the fact that the senator had brought Penny to Washington. 'Mark my words, Norman, that girl has her cap set for you. Sooner or later, there's bound to be a scandal.'

Once, in the moment of victory over the hapless Democrat who had opposed him in the senatorial race, Norman Grant had kissed his ablest lieutenant Penny Hardesty; Elinor had seen this and it rankled.

She nagged her husband so incessantly that one morning in 1949—when Harry Truman was in the White House for four more astonishing years and big, friendly Tom Clark was on the Supreme Court—Senator Grant summoned Penny to his office. 'Penny, I'll let you have the bad news straight, and I don't want to discuss it. You're fired.' She gasped, and then he added quickly, 'And five different senators want to hire you. I'd take Glancey of Red River. He's a mover.'

'Why?' she asked, stunned by the two messages, one so devastating, the other so commendatory.

'I can't say.'

'It's Mrs. Grant, isn't it?' When he said nothing, she added, 'It's got to be.' When she carried the news to Finnerty he gasped, although he had been forewarned by the senator, and she said, 'It's got to be Mrs. Grant, doesn't it?' All he would admit was 'He doesn't have an easy time with that one.'

'He advises me to take the job with Glancey of Red River.'

'So do I.'

'Then you knew?'

'Yes, and that's all I'll say.'

'Well, I'll say something more. Elinor Grant is going to destroy her husband, you watch.'

'Nothing can destroy our boy, and you know it.'

She sat on his desk. 'Why is it that women hate other women? Every senator I know has a wife who despises all the women who work for him. Why can't women . . .'

'Frankly, this is the wrong time to discuss the problem with me. I'm getting married next month.'

'That's wonderful. Who's the girl?'

'An Irish girl. From Boston. A good Catholic, like you said.'

'Now I can kiss you!' Penny said, and suddenly she was lost in tears. She was being separated from two men who meant so much to her, Grant and Finnerty. She had helped propel them toward the stars and now she was being cut loose. 'You're buzzards, all of you. And I love you, all of you, even old double-dealer Gantling.'

Before she shifted jobs she was requested to join in a series of conferences, which determined many of her future attitudes. Paul Stidham, Elinor's father, now old and enfeebled, hurried to Washington to look into the problems that seemed to be immobilizing his daughter, and as soon as he arrived she appeared to improve, regaining her wit and her quiet competency.

Paul asked if he could meet with Penny Hardesty alone, and when they sat together in the senator's inner office he asked bluntly, 'Did my daughter have any justification in having you discharged?'

'Sexually, none, although I believe she feared that. Tim Finnerty in our office wanted to marry me. I've been engaged for some years, more or less, to John Pope, whom you probably remember as a football hero at Henry Clay High School. He's a midshipman at Annapolis, only a few miles away.' Speaking almost harshly, she said, 'I am not a sex-starved young secretary.'

'What was the problem?'

'You know better than I,' Penny said coldly.

'Her inability to get Washington in focus?'

'Or anything else,' Penny said with asperity. This man's daughter had damaged her grievously and she felt no inclination to treat him gently; had he educated Elinor better, this would not have happened.

'What's her trouble, Miss Hardesty?'

'You've surely known for a long time, Mr. Stidham. She's unable to face the reality of her world. So she engages in fantasies about people like me . . . and her husband. She has no concept of what his job entails, or the power he might command, or the good he might do.'

'What are you going to do?'

'I'm going to work for a real senator, a tough, brawling man who knows what he wants and who gets things done. A Democrat, God forbid.' She laughed heartily, then apologized: 'I'm sorry, Mr. Stidham, that I've been so blunt. But unless you get your son-in-law off dead center, where his wife has forced him to stand, he's going to be a very poor senator indeed.'

'My own opinion.'

'Oh, Finnerty will keep getting him elected, and he'll fill a spot. But that's not what he intended when he took that oath in the life raft.'

'What oath?'

'Finnerty and that wonderful Negro told me about it. When the second night ended and it looked as if they would all perish, Norman went kind of wild and swore that if he survived . . . Well, he was going to do something with his life. He's not doing it.'

A plenary session was called, to which, significantly, Mrs. Grant was not invited. It was held in the back room of a Washington restaurant, ostensibly to bid Penny Hardesty farewell. Grant attended, of course, and so did Finnerty and Paul Stidham. The head of Grant's office in Fremont was there, and to Penny's surprise, so was her new boss, Senator Michael Glancey of Red River, a ruddy-faced, boisterous Democrat from the oil fields.

'I have asked you all to join me,' Paul Stidham said in his soft, high voice, 'because my son-in-law Senator Grant needs your advice. Frankly, I long for him to pull a strong oar in the Senate, and he isn't doing it. What's wrong?'

Senator Glancey was not hesitant: 'When a freshman comes in here, he's wise to keep his mouth shut. Norman's done that. But he's also wise to start chopping out a niche for himself. And you haven't done that, Norman.'

'I've worked on agriculture.'

'And very well, too. But men seem to attain stature in this body not by attending to the issues that please the people in their home state. We're all obliged to do that. What counts is the way a man tackles the big issues, the ones that affect us all.'

'Meaning?'

'The biggest thing in the world right now is atomic energy. What we do with it. How it fits into the national and international defense posture.'

'You're handling that rather well. You and Lyndon Johnson.'

'Thank God for Lyndon; he has his head screwed on right. If he can hold his seat in the Senate, he'll be a force for good.'

'What has atomic power to do with me?' Grant asked.

'Not a damned thing,' Glancey snapped. 'But advanced aviation and rockets and what they're calling space are also going to be of major importance. I'm sure of it, and on my aviation committee we need a good man from the Republican side. A strong fellow likely to be reelected term after term.'

Finnerty said, 'I think we can guarantee the elections, Senator Glancey.'

'I think so, too.' As a successful senator, Glancey had learned to pay attention to what the field managers of other senators said, for he appreciated how much an elected official owed to the men who kept the machine rolling. Turning to the man from Grant's state office, he asked, 'Do you concur? Can you keep getting him elected?'

'There's not a cloud on the horizon.'

'There's always a cloud on the horizon,' Glancey corrected. 'It's just that sometimes we don't recognize it.'

This encouraged the Fremont man to speak more frankly. 'Our senator is safe for one more election, of that I'm sure. But if he has not established himself . . .'

'Exactly,' Glancey said. Then he chuckled. 'God knows I'm not here to elect Republicans. But the solemn fact is that we're never going to carry Fremont. So what we want is a good Republican rather than some clown. A feisty young Republican will knock you off one of these days, Norman. Not a Democrat. That is, if you allow yourself to become an old clown like Gantling. We all knew he was doomed.'

'And you think Norman will be doomed if he doesn't get off dead center?' Stidham asked.

'Definitely. What I offer you, Grant, in return for this very bright young lady that you're tossing my way, is full partnership on our aviation committee. We need you as a former military man, a hero if you will. We need a strong, continuing man in your party.'

'I've never piloted an airplane.'

'Nor have I. To tell you the truth, I'm what is known as a white-knuckle flier. I'm scared to death of the damned things. But I fly in them because my job demands it.'

Senator Glancey asked for another drink, then said, 'Our country's the same way. But we must learn to handle planes and all the things that'll come after. And you're the man to help us.'

. . .

So in the spring of 1950 John Pope and Penny Hardesty, not yet married, committed themselves to aviation, he at a naval air station in Pensacola, where he would master advanced fighter training, she to Senator Glancey's office, from which as a lawyer she would be encouraged to exert constant influence on legislation dealing with aviation and the burgeoning field of rocketry.

On graduation day at Annapolis, two United States senators appeared to cheer Penny when the newlyweds came out beneath the canopy of crossed swords—Grant, Republican of Fremont; Glancey, Democrat of Red River—and each kissed the bride for the delighted photographers. Mrs. Grant, who did not accompany her husband to Annapolis, was freshly disturbed when the pictures appeared in her hometown newspaper.

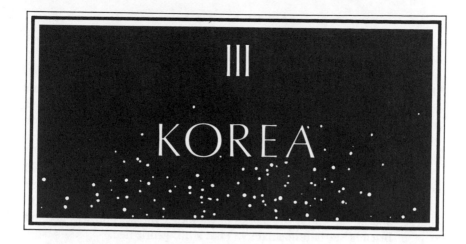

III

KOREA

LIEUTENANT (JUNIOR GRADE) JOHN POPE DREW THE WORST ASSIGN-ment of his career on a bitterly cold January day off the coast of Korea when a sailor aboard the carrier *Brandywine* shouted, 'Hey! Chopper coming in!'

Pope and other pilots on stand-by moved to the railing of the ship, stamped their feet to keep warm, and watched as an Air Force copter came low over the freezing waters, circled professionally, and dropped neatly onto the designated square. The bearer of bad news was a colonel in his forties, a no-nonsense type who strode across the deck to greet the captain of the ship, who passed him along to the Carrier Air Group commander. Within minutes all Navy pilots were called to the briefing room belowdecks.

'Problem's simple,' the colonel said as he stood with pointing stick before a map of the two Koreas. 'The North Korean air force consists of a few native pilots, a lot of Chinese and a handful of very good Russians who fly out of sanctuary up there beyond the Yalu River. We have no complaints. Our F-86s are knocking the hell out of them in one-on-one combat. Our only wish is they'd send more MiGs down the alley, because if they do, we'll crucify them.'

Pope thought: Standard Air Force doctrine. When do we get to the point? The colonel, as if he had heard the question, said, 'So why am I here? I'll tell you why I'm here. The damned Koreans have come up with a gimmick that's giving us real trouble. With the best F-86 pilots in the world, we can't handle it, and frankly, gentlemen, I've come here to enlist your help.'

With his wand he pointed to an imaginary channel leading down the west coast of Korea to Inchon, the seaport used by the American forces, a center of great cargo dumps and gasoline depots. 'The little bastards have built themselves what we call the Slow Boy, a small, cumbersome plane made largely of wood. Flies only at night, reflects practically no radar signal, carries a healthy load of small bombs, and operates on a Who-gives-a-damn? principle. That is, it flies very low, and if it sneaks through and bombs one of our dumps, fine. If it gets shot down, who cares?'

The colonel laughed at the crudity of this tactic, then grew serious. 'Trouble is, it works. They keep getting through. Our F-86s are no damn good trying to spot those plywood crates slipping in. Our gunners don't find them. So our ammunition dumps keep exploding. What we need is four or five of you Navy men who are practiced night fighters. With your heavier, slower planes. Police that corridor and knock hell out of the Slow Boys.'

He said no more, but the CAG commander took the podium and said crisply, 'Washington and Hawaii approve. We're detaching a group of four F4U-5NL night fighters to K-22 as of now. Lieutenant Pope will be in charge,' and he rattled off the names of the other three. 'You will take off at 1300. Briefing starts immediately. That's all, gentlemen.'

K-22 was situated only forty miles from where the *Brandywine* rolled in the heavy seas. It perched on the extreme eastern edge of snowbound Korea on a small peninsula jutting out into the Sea of Japan, and every American aviator who served there acquired a tricky little habit that would remain with him the rest of his life. It concerned airplane takeoffs.

It wasn't the perpetual fog which gave trouble, nor the proximity to the sea. It was the water in the gasoline; it gave no trouble once the plane was airborne, for then rapid fuel consumption permitted the engine to ingest the small amount of water without danger, but on takeoff it was hell.

Since a plane on taking off needed every ounce of forward thrust, even the slightest dilution by water could prove fatal, and that was no figure of speech, because the plane, just as it was about to lift into the air, would find itself choking. It would gasp, then stutter, then start that dreadful plunge, ending with a sardonic explosion. The rotten gasoline which had refused to lift the plane into flight now exploded in ghostly flame, burning the pilot to death.

At K-22 that winter five planes had burned on takeoff, and pilots not on flying duty sat in the rude mess hall tensed up whenever a fellow pilot was on the strip preparing to take off. Conversation would halt. The young men would lean forward. Everyone would listen to the engine as it revved up, trying to detect any stutter. When the plane started down the runway, the nervous pilots would try not to look at one another. They just sat there, tense, listening.

Roar-roar-roar! The pilots could visualize the plane as it sped toward the sea, gaining speed, reaching for the go-no-go point. The listeners waited. Roar-roar-roar! This time the supply of fuel continued unbroken. The plane sped north toward the waiting enemy at the Yalu.

No one mentioned the takeoff or its successful completion. Occasionally one of the grounded pilots would sigh, as if completing a prayer, but he refused to speak of the water in the fuel, nor did he congratulate the pilot who had made the roger-dodger takeoff. Bright conversation resumed. The acey-deucy games continued, until the next flight. And that was the tricky little habit John Pope acquired at K-22. He fell silent when a fellow pilot was trying to get his plane into the air.

Since K-22 was an Air Force base, lined with those sleek F-86 Sabre Jets, Air Force personnel manned the facilities, which meant that Pope's three Navy fliers were outsiders, and therefore at a disadvantage, but Pope was a master pilot now, cautious, brave, unusually capable, and he proposed to take no guff from anyone. His logbook showed more than nine hundred hours in seven distinct types of aircraft, with numerous entries in red indicating night flights.

He stowed his gear where the sergeant indicated, accepted the cot he was assigned, parked his F4U where told, and instructed his three associates to keep a low profile: 'Our job is to find those Slow Boys.'

He was not allowed to stay aloof, because with healthy curiosity the Air Force pilots wanted to know about his plane. 'It's a relic, really,' he said. 'World War II. You probably knew it as the Corsair, the ones the Marines used to shatter the Jap air force in the islands. Marvelous plane. Big, heavy, absorbs punishment like a tank.'

'Why the funny designation? All those letters and numbers?'

'You know the saying: "There's a right way, a wrong way and the Navy way." The F means fighter, and it was fearsome. The U is our way of indicating the manufacturer, in this case Chance-Vought, one of the best. The 4 means the fourth prototype in this series. I understand 2 and 3 weren't much, but with 4 they hit a winner. The 5 means the fifth major improvement in this version. The N means night fighter, and the L means it has de-icer boots and some other ingenious stuff to combat lousy weather.'

'Jesus!' a captain said. 'You have to be a graduate engineer to know the name of your plane. But why is it so heavy and so slow?'

Pope considered this logical question for a moment, then said, 'You fly the F-86? Well, it's a gazelle. My F4U is a rhinoceros. In the jungle, there's a place for both.'

'But the heaviness?'

'You land your F-86 on flat terrain. You can run three thousand feet before you hit the brakes. We land on a carrier. We stop within one hundred feet. In effect, we have no brakes.'

'How do you stop?'

'It's rather exciting. You're up there making about a hundred eighty knots. Midnight. Far ahead you spot your carrier. Lots of blue lights. The red wands of the landing officer glowing. You cut back to about a hundred knots, drop your gear, your flaps and especially your tail hook. And you put your plane right down on the deck of that plunging ship.'

'How can you see the landing area? At night? With no lights?'

'You can't. You trust the lighted wands and—slammo! Your hook grabs the wire and you stop with one terrific jerk. That's why our F4Us have to be so heavy. To withstand the shock of that grabbing wire.'

'And if your hook misses it?'

'Tough luck. You slam straight ahead into the barriers, a tangle of wires strung above the deck. They smash the plane but usually spare the pilot.'

'And if you miss?'

'You get swim pay. If you're around to collect it.'

His new assignment was a curious one. He slept all day, rose at dusk for breakfast, climbed into his F4U, and taxied out to the end of the darkened runway, where he assumed strip alert. This meant that he sat in his plane hour after hour, all lights out, pitch-black everywhere, getting his eyes accustomed to the night and waiting for the signal 'Slow Boy coming down!' Then he leaped into action, but mostly he just waited.

To civilian observers it seemed fearfully exciting, and one *New York Times* reporter wrote: 'A flight into darkness, a faint dim signal on the radar, a swift pursuit, the tap-tap-tap of the forward machine guns, an explosion filling the sky when the enemy cargo is hit, and then the flaming debris floating past like wounded butterflies at some misty lakeside.' The reporter had been to Harvard, and he had a good ear, a good imagination, but what endeared him to the pilots at K-22 was his appealing habit of paying for drinks at the mess, where he listened to aviator talk.

To Pope the night patrol was something quite different, as he said in a letter to Penny: 'You spend eighteen nights on strip alert and nothing happens. You go up four nights and find not even a shadow in the moonlight. Finally you spot something coming south, but it's a flock of birds. And on the rare night when you do intercept an enemy, the guy on your wing shoots him down.'

What Pope did enjoy were the orders that arrived occasionally: 'Tonight ignore the Slow Boys. Seek targets of opportunity and knock them out.' Then he ranged solo across all of North Korea like some swooping eagle trying with his keen night vision to spot enemy activity on the ground below. He loved the sense of freedom such activity produced, the sheer joy of flying through unencumbered space, enfolded in a darkness which he alone commanded.

He was seeking trains. Daylight attacks by the Air Force and Navy had so paralyzed Korean transportation that no train dared move when it could be seen; they crept out at night, running swiftly from one hiding place to the next, carrying an immense amount of war supplies to the various fronts.

'It's unbelievable what a Communist repair crew can do after we bomb the hell out of one of their rail lines,' the Air Force colonel had said in one of his briefings. 'At ten in the morning we can tear up five hundred feet of track, then strafe the wreckage all day, and next morning they have the thing repaired. That night, trains sneaking down as usual.'

Speaking directly to the Navy fliers, he said, 'It's not easy. Korea's a hilly place. A lot of tunnels in this land. So when you come roaring in and smash one of their boxcars, what do they do? Uncouple it, leave it standing, and speed the engine into some tunnel where you can't get at it. What you men have to do is knock out the engine. And that won't be easy.'

One night Pope did spot a train. The stars were brilliant in a moonless sky, and when he returned to K-22 he swore that he saw the train clearly in the starlight: 'I came in low, knocked two of the boxcars off the track. And you know what happened next.'

'The engine ducked into a tunnel?' a Navy flier asked.

'With fifty or sixty undamaged boxcars.'

After this had happened a few times, the F4U detachment held a think session at which they devised a bold strategy which, if it worked, would take care of any North Korean train caught between tunnels: 'We'll knock it so flat that even the blind photo birds will be able to find it.'

The photographs were important, because the armed forces had discovered that pilots were so enthusiastic, and such congenital liars, that little credence could be given their exaggerated claims. Confirming proof was essential.

'I came in low,' a blazing-eyed pilot would report, 'and dead ahead stood this train. Tat-tat! I knocked it twenty feet off its tracks.' But when more sober fliers went out to find the derailed train, they usually found nothing. So the custom grew that as soon as a pilot reported a kill, recco planes went out to photograph the scene, and when they got shots of an engine on its side or a string of boxcars burning at the mouth of some tunnel, the squadron celebrated.

Why were the photographs so important? Certainly the Air Force did not imperil reconnaissance planes merely to prove that some hotshot Navy pilot was a liar. The true reason lay deep within the psychology of the aviator: medals were awarded not on hearsay but on incontrovertible proof of performance. A pilot could sit in the bar of the officers' club night after night, claiming kills, and no listener took him seriously unless some other flier supported his report with substantial evidence. And that's why the photographs became so important, especially with the night fighters.

In daylight combat, a wingman could confirm, or a ground observer who saw an enemy plane come down in fiery parabola, but at night it was almost impossible for a fellow pilot to witness anything. There was, for example, the Air Force pilot at K-22 who returned to base morning after morning claiming that he had overtaken one of the plywood night invaders and had blown him out of the sky. No one saw these kills. No one could inspect the ground behind enemy lines to identify the shattered plane, but the high command was so eager to create the illusion in Washington that it was dominating the skies that it gave this windbag a medal with two clusters.

And that was the heart of the matter. Combat aviators hungered for medals. They took unparalleled delight in the ribbons, the glittering medals which testified to their heroism. Only rarely in the mess did an aviator say anything which indicated that he considered himself a hero, but even the quietest man wanted the decorations which silently proclaimed that fact. For an additional medal, men would lie, exaggerate, falsify, support friends in hopes that friends would support them on some later claim; above all, they would take the most outrageous risks in order to qualify for one more ribbon.

It was fatuous. It was juvenile. But it was also the essence of the heroic experience, for armies had found that whereas men would fight for many noble reasons—home, country, family, hatred of oppressors—the best men fought best for the good regard of their fellows, and the time-honored proof of their regard was the medal. In the years when John Pope and his fellow officers were flying their night combat missions against enemy flak and the hazards of weather and sudden mountain heights, each man was receiving $263.63 a month, lousy food and cheap whiskey. What compensated them for the enormous risks they were taking was the respect of their fellow pilots and their intense love of aviation.

That was why John Pope, when he went out one wintry night to test the new strategy of killing trains, was careful to inquire as to whether a photographic plane might be available next morning.

'A Marine from K-3 flew in this afternoon with a souped-up photo Banshee. Raring to go.'

'Tell him to be ready.' Pope did not predict garrulously that he was determined to bag a train; to do so would have been alien to his pattern, for he was the quiet type, efficient, even retiring. He knew that few men could fly an airplane better than he, or handle it more efficiently at night, but he never spoke of his skills. In a crowd of young men in civilian clothes he would be one of the last to be identified as an aviator, and even in military uniform he resembled an effective staff officer or a photographic reconnaissance interpreter, a photo bird.

On this night, as soon as dusk fell, he climbed into his F4U, with its massive load of ammunition for strafing and its bombs for heavy work, and taxied to the far end of the runway, where he assumed his position of strip alert. He waited. Staring at the Sea of Japan, he watched the grand procession of stars as they rose from the waters: the Bull reared his horns above the sea, followed by the huddling Twins. At nine the Lion crept out, and at midnight he had a clear view of the bold star he had studied so longingly in the hours before dawn on that first night with the borrowed glasses: red-gold Arcturus flaming like a beacon.

He slid open his window so that he could lean out and see the stars overhead, and there was Orion the great hunter: I'm a fair country hunter myself, and tonight I get me a train.

It was well after midnight when the signal came for takeoff, and when he checked the sky one last time to ensure his orientation, he saw that Orion was skidding toward the western hills and dragging with him the heavenly animals: They're getting out of my way. Thanks.

Steadily he applied power to his engine and listened approvingly to the swift acceleration of the propeller as it strained against the brakes. Suddenly he lifted his toes, the F4U surged forward, and as he roared down the runway he realized that every pilot within hearing distance was listening to his progress, even though apparently asleep; they were praying that the gasoline would be good and that he would soar aloft, but he was not the least bit uncertain, or afraid, or clenching his teeth. He was supposed to take off from K-22 at 0134 and he intended to do so. To fail would be unthinkable. If there was water in his gasoline, it could wait till he got airborne.

In more than a hundred precarious landings on the chopping deck of a carrier he had never once supposed that he might fail to engage the restraining cable, or plow into the parked planes on the deck, or plunge off the end of the deck and die trapped in his plane. His job had been to get the plane safely down, and he always did, night or day, storm or fair. His job this night was to prove the efficacy of the new tactic and he roared aloft to do so.

Since K-22 was positioned well below the battle line to protect its fuel dumps from intruding Communist planes, he spent his first minutes heading due north, which carried him well out to sea, but when his instruments indicated that he must be at least forty miles into enemy territory, he turned west, dropped to a thousand feet, and began searching the valleys.

In the darkness he saw little, even though his eyes were well accustomed to moonless nights: The Slopes aren't risking much this time.

Like many pilots, he referred to the enemy in impersonal terms. Slopes. Asiatics. Kimchi Kings. K-22 employed many able South Korean workers, and large segments of the front line were defended by Republic of Korea forces whose endurance under attack was legendary, and the pilots maintained amiable relations with these allies. But the North Korean enemy were Slopes.

He made six long sweeps, then reported in code: 'Nothing visible.' Occasionally he inspected the western alleyway leading from the Chinese border to Inchon, hoping to find one of the wooden Slow Boys sneaking south, but he detected nothing. He kept well away from Pyongyang, the North Korean capital, where antiaircraft fire was concentrated, and he maintained a prudent watch for Russian MiGs, which had recently been attacking the American night fighters, for as an aviation expert he was aware that the Russian plane was many times faster than his, better armed and capable of flying much higher. He was brave, but not foolhardy, and he recalled the doctrine of his squadron: 'If you meet a MiG one-on-one, run like hell, because you're outnumbered.' It was the job of Air Force F-86s to tackle the MiGs, and he was quite content to have them do it.

He realized that in his F4U he had a limited time in the air, and it seemed that on this night he would find nothing, but as he checked his fuel and thought about heading home, he saw in the starlight a moving object, deep in a valley, and when he roared down to inspect he found to his delight that it was a Communist engine pulling at least sixty boxcars. But it was heading at top speed for the safety of a tunnel.

With restraint he ignored the splendid target, so vulnerable to his guns, and disciplined himself to put into effect the strategy his men had agreed upon. Leaving the train with its antiaircraft guns popping away, he wheeled and sped toward the entrance of the upcoming tunnel. There, with fine precision he dropped one of his large bombs, tearing up the track and blocking that tunnel.

Still he ignored the train, swinging around to the other tunnel from which the train had just emerged. There he laid another heavy bomb smack on the tracks, blocking that escape.

Gunners aboard the train, realizing what he had done, fired into the night with fury, accomplishing nothing but the clear outlining of their train, which now stood trapped in open space.

Flying well to the west, Pope turned in a great circle, spotted the train, and roared back at low level, blazing his guns directly at the engine, which he seemed to miss.

Undaunted, he whispered to himself, 'Better luck this time.' He took a wide sweep back toward the west, came in purposefully ignoring the antiaircraft fire, and struck at the engine again. This time his aim was good, for there was an explosion and a vast release of steam, but he suspected that this might be a stratagem calculated to deceive him, and he remembered what the old-timers at K-22 had warned: 'The best railroad men in the world are those Slopes. They know trains. They can trick you a hundred different ways.'

Again he flew west, turned and came back, but this time when he lined the engine up he saw that the steam had been no ruse; the train was badly wounded but by no means destroyed. So, ignoring the flak, he came in hard and low, releasing a bomb at the right moment. With a gigantic flash, metal hit metal, the engine teetered, and the first three cars followed it off the track. This train was wrecked.

Pope wanted to stay on the scene to shoot up the fifty or sixty stranded boxcars, but he knew he had no fuel to spare, so he called K-22, giving other pilots the coordinates of the waiting target: 'Finish it off!'

But now, as he headed south, satisfied that he had performed well, he had two burning concerns: he wanted to find that Marine who had come to K-22 with his photo Banshee and he wanted desperately to see Altair come rising from the sea, his star, his omen to bless this night.

Just as he approached K-22 from the west, with his nose pointed out to sea, he saw bright Lyra dead ahead and then, low on the horizon, as its eagle wings dropped water, came Altair. He saluted.

. . .

The Marine captain who had brought the photographic plane to K-22 on temporary duty was two years younger than John Pope but some twenty years more experienced. A real football hero from a small Texas town, and not an ersatz underweight like Pope, Randy Claggett had gone to Texas A & M and had fought the entire establishment to get into the Marines rather than the Army, which A & M boys were expected to join. He was taller than Pope but not noticeably heavier, for in high school he had been a fleet end, adept at confusing the opposition. In college he had been too light for the varsity, but as a scrub he was outstanding because of his willingness to tackle even the biggest regulars.

He was profane, tough and make-believe illiterate. A first-team fullback had knocked a small corner off one of his big front teeth and the dentist had ground down its mate for symmetry, which gave him a raffish gap-toothed grin, which he delighted in flashing in the heat of any argument. His logbook showed that he had piloted fifty-nine different aircraft types and was expert in sixteen, including the best Navy types: F4U-4, AD-2, F9F-4 and the heavy F3D-2. He had a mania for airplanes, and if sober men like John Pope could justly be considered experts, he was three or four magnitudes more advanced, for in some strange way he *was* an airplane. When he sat in his cockpit he became attuned to its set engine, a part of its guidance system, an extension of its flaps; he did not fly the plane, he flew himself.

It was therefore a humiliation that he had been diverted into reconnaissance work: 'Goddamn baby-sitting, that's what it is. Y'all know that when I go up there, I got no guns, no bombs, no nothin'? Takin' pitchers like some clown at a carnival.'

The Marine brass had not been stupid in assigning Claggett to the Banshee, for it was a major asset in the American arsenal. Stripped to essentials and with no armament of any kind, it could ascend to 52,000 feet, and with miraculous cameras, photograph large sections of enemy terrain with an accuracy that seemed incredible: 'I can drive this bucket of bolts so high I can take a snapshot of God at work.' He had taken photographs from maximum altitude which showed North Korean soldiers working at a transport depot and he swore that a good photo interpreter with proper microscopes could determine the make of the automobiles, and certainly whether they were cars or trucks: 'Don't you bastards try nothin' down here, because I'll be watchin' you from up there.'

He was in bed when Pope broke into his quarters a few minutes before sunrise. 'Are you Claggett? The photopuke?'

'Who in hell are you?'

Like many serious pilots, Pope never swore and it startled him sometimes when a fellow officer let loose with a chain of profanity, but he needed

Claggett, so he said, 'I'm John Pope. Temporary duty off the *Brandywine*.'

'I'm Claggett. Perpetual temporary duty.'

'I just destroyed a train. We've got to have good photographs.'

'I know, I know. You destroyed a train. I fly my ass off to get a pitcher, turns out to be a two-wheel manure cart, shit all over the landscape.'

'This was a train . . . with at least sixty boxcars.'

'It'll be the first.'

'It is the first. We devised a new tactic. Block up the tunnels to prevent escape . . .'

Claggett sat up, running his thin fingers through his heavy, matted hair. 'You blocked 'em off?'

'I did.'

'That I must see. Those goddamned Slopes bombed our dump the other night.'

'One of the wooden Slow Boys?'

'The same.' He twisted his scrawny body out of bed, worked his shoulders as if they had recently been broken, and looked at himself in the mirror with disgust: 'I better shave.'

In the morning twilight, as Altair faded from view, the two pilots shaved, Pope heavy from sleeplessness, Claggett drowsy with too much, one ready for bed, the other for enemy skies. With precision Pope designated where the train must still be, unless the incredible North Koreans had cleared one of the tunnels and muscled the undamaged boxcars inside.

'I can find it,' Claggett said, and when the two men reported to operations they found great excitement because the dawn patrol had located Pope's train and had shot up the stranded cars.

'Everything's ablaze,' an intelligence officer said. 'Claggett, we want pictures.'

'You got 'em,' Randy said, and within minutes he had his Banshee in the air, headed northwest toward the valley where the boxcars were aflame, but the Russian pilots who flew some of the North Korean MiGs had anticipated that when the train was set afire, other American planes would stop by to confirm, and they were waiting.

They came at Claggett from due north as he was heading west, four of them with powerful armament and great speed.

It seemed that he was doomed. 'Jesus Christ!' he called to base. 'Four MiGs right at me. I'm headed upstairs.' Pulling the nose of the Banshee almost straight up, he poured on the juice and took off like a purposeful hawk. 24,000 feet with the MiGs closing fast. 28,000 and no escape. 32,000 and the first MiG makes a pass with tracers decorating the sky just ahead. 35,000 and three MiGs hammering at him. 37,000 and he has a fleeting suspicion that one of the MiGs has fallen behind. 40,000 and he breathes deeply, for all the MiGs are trailing. Up, up he goes, to well above 45,000 feet above the frozen hills of North Korea, and as he rests there for a moment, in absolute safety, for no other military plane in the world can fly so high, he watches a most beautiful sight.

Out of the morning sky to the east come three Air Force F-86s. For the moment they are well below the capable MiGs and they are outnumbered, but by the time the Russian pilots realize that they will soon be under attack, the F-86s have gained altitude, so that the battle will be an even one, and Claggett sees that the powerful American planes will have a good chance of bagging a couple of MiGs.

Before the battle can be joined, the Russians, under strict orders to bring their precious planes back safely, withdraw, retiring speedily and in good formation to their sanctuary north of the Yalu. Claggett can come down and finish his job.

The F-86s, suspicious of the Russians and aware that they might sweep in unexpectedly to down the photographic plane, signal to Claggett that he must stay with them, which he is quite willing to do: 'Don't want no MiGs up my ass.'

And so the four American jets fly out toward the Yellow Sea, drop low and come in at a perfect angle so far as sunlight is concerned. The sixty photographs, when developed, will show a T-69-type Chinese engine, heavily armor-plated, blown off the tracks near the entrance to a tunnel, followed by sixty-seven loaded boxcars, three off the track, twenty-one aflame, and all seriously damaged.

For this episode Lieutenant (j.g.) John Pope will receive his monthly pay of $263.63, a medal with ribbons, and a recommendation for promotion to full lieutenant, and the squadron will be satisfied that it has at last devised a tactic for knocking out Communist trains.

Randy Claggett, Marine captain, was a new experience for Pope, who had watched many braggarts wilt when demands were great, and many quiet men display great talent when called upon, but he had never before encountered a military man as loud-mouthed as Claggett who was in every respect a better flier than himself. At the bar, after the wrecking of the train, Claggett was especially effusive: 'Boy, I have seen many trains knocked on their ass, but never one better than this. Whoever hit that baby made the crap fly. I came in low and sweet to get the pitcher, when I see four MiGs comin' right up my bucket. What do I do? I shift gears and say, "Randy, son, you better get to Dallas before they do." At 40,000 they drop off. Remember that, fellows, you get to 40,000 they call it quits.'

He laughed rather noisily at this suggestion, because few American planes except his could approach that altitude. 'There I am at 50,000, eatin' gas like it was popcorn, with them four MiGs jess awaitin' for me, and I say, "Randy, you fart, them foxes down there got you treed and they gonna chew you up, if'n you come down." And then I see the sweetest sight ever, three F-86s comin' out of the sunrise. Bartender! Give every Air Force man in this bar a free beer.'

Claggett was not always so kind to the Air Force: 'This K-22, it's a cesspool. You ought to see K-3 down at Pusan. We live down there. We got Jo-sans.'

'What's a Jo-san?' Pope asked.

'Korean girls. They wait in the mess. Best screwin' this side of Fort Worth.' He rummaged in his wallet for a photograph of a Korean Jo-san, but came up instead with a fine color photograph of his wife, a handsome blonde.

'That's Debby Dee,' he said. 'Married her the day I got my wings and been flyin' ever since.'

The pilots drinking Randy's beer passed the photograph around and each man appraised Mrs. Claggett with professional skill. She was beautiful, no question about that, in a cheerleader way, but she seemed older than Claggett, perhaps because her beauty was the florid type that fades quickly. Pope wanted to ask how old she was, for she seemed infinitely older than Penny, but he said nothing.

In the days that followed he often found himself in Claggett's company, which was surprising in that Pope flew at night, Claggett in daylight, but Randy required so little sleep that he often went along on Pope's ground duties, talking incessantly: 'How did I get stuck with photographic duties? Man, you know I could fly fighter planes better than them Air Force clowns we have to put up with.'

'You spoke rather well of them the other day. After they saved your tail.'

'In an emergency they're useful. But to answer your question. I gave the Marines all sorts of hell till they allowed me to opt for flight training. You know, as a kid I used to take cars apart. Father came home one day, his whole Packard was strewed acrosst the lawn. He like to died. I got a real feel for engines, Pope.'

'Why aren't you in fighters?'

Claggett ignored the question. 'When I left Pensacola, I reported to VC-4 in Atlantic City. You ever fly off that field? Telephone wires right acrosst the end of the runway. We ast the government four times to take them down or we were gonna crash into houses. Said it was too expensive. So one night we cut 'em down.'

'We?'

'Well, I did. Everyone at the base knew who did it, so I got some fryin', but the command was glad to see them down. Only next day they put 'em up again and fined the squadron. Who gives a damn?'

Pope never did discover just how his rambunctious colleague had found his way into Banshees, but an older Marine who flew in from one of the carriers said, 'The Banshee requires the best judgment in the business. Or it did when we were testing it. And they chose Claggett because—'

'Were you in flight test?'

'Two years at Patuxent River.'

'Good duty?'

'Best in the world. I flew forty-seven different planes. Invaluable.'

'How do you get that duty?' Pope asked.

'One morning the Angel Gabriel knocks on your door. Strictly luck.'

'But don't you have to know airplanes?'

'Everybody knows airplanes. What you have to know is Gabriel and his cockamamie horn. Toot, toot, we shoot.' And he waved his right hand high in the air.

A few nights after this, when planes were grounded, Pope accompanied Claggett to a movie on the base. It starred an actress John had enjoyed in *Gone With the Wind,* Vivien Leigh, and an actor with whom he was not familiar but of whom he had heard much favorable comment. Claggett said, 'You've got to see this guy Brando. Terrific!'

The film was called *A Streetcar Named Desire,* which Pope thought ridiculous. His opinion worsened when he found that Brando played a sloppy, profane ignoramus who went around in a dirty T-shirt. 'This Kowalski is a bore,' he told Claggett during the first intermission when the reels were being changed. 'I'd kick him out of my house.'

But when Blanche DuBois began to act the irresponsible, addle-pated sister-in-law, Pope became uneasy and wondered why the Kowalskis didn't kick *her* out. As the seamy details continued to unfold, Pope became actually nervous, for the picture of family life being offered was not at all what he wished to see. 'That woman's impossible,' he mumbled.

'You'd kick her out, too?'

'Wouldn't you?'

'All she needs is a good screwin'.'

Pope never responded to such talk, not because he was prudish, but because he believed that when he married Penny Hardesty in his Annapolis days he settled once and for all any problems relating to sex, and he was always vaguely disturbed to find that other officers felt otherwise. He was extremely happy with Penny and was repelled by the harsh view of marriage being presented in this movie, and when the Brando-Leigh relationship became downright ugly he could not stay to watch.

'I'll see you at the hall,' he said as he slipped uneasily from his seat. Claggett could not understand his friend's behavior, but when half a dozen other pilots rose to leave the improvised theater, he grabbed one by the arm and whispered, 'What's going on?'

'I don't fly all day to see this crap at night,' the Air Force major snapped.

'What crap?'

'A dame like that.' The Air Force man pulled his arm free and stalked out of the shack.

Later, Claggett realized that this film had struck too close to the lives of the fliers, for as he heard them talk about it he learned that some had wives who were as flighty as Blanche DuBois; others had homes which were threatened by circumstances not unlike those that separated Kowalski and his wife. These pilots, who were risking so much against the MiGs and the darkness and the upreaching mountains and the watered gasoline, wanted films that showed placid family life: contented wives in picket-fenced gardens watching over well-behaved boys who were playing Little League baseball.

He sought Pope and asked, 'Did the movie really hit you so hard?'

'I walked out, didn't I?'

'But why? It was just a movie, and a pretty good one.'

'Did it get any better? After I left?'

'She continued her dance. Stupid, mixed-up broad.'

Now Claggett grabbed Pope's arm, a habit of his, for he never liked to see a friend walk away angry. 'Sit down, Pope. You mustn't take things too serious.'

'I don't understand you, Claggett. You show me this picture of your beautiful wife while you're looking for the photograph of the Jo-san you're shacked up with.'

'I found that pitcher,' Claggett said enthusiastically, and from his wallet he took the snapshot of a lovely Korean girl, sixteen or seventeen years old, in one of those appealing dresses in which the beltline came just under the breasts, with the rest of the dress falling free in one handsome, unbroken sweep.

'Ain't she somethin'?'

'Why do you fool around with her? If you have . . .'

Claggett now produced the familiar photograph of his wife, Debby Dee, and placed it on the bar table beside that of his Jo-san. 'Two superior chicks.'

'Where is your wife?'

'Iwakuni, I guess. She followed me to Japan, and I suppose she's livin' it up over there. She usually has somethin' cookin'.'

This was so distasteful that Pope rose abruptly and went to bed, but he was so accustomed to flying at night and sleeping in the daytime that he tossed in restlessness, and after about an hour of frustration he rose, slipped into his fatigues and returned to the officers' club, where Claggett still sat, this time with the Air Force major he had spoken to in the movie. They were talking about women.

'I don't care to waste an evening watching some sick babe making a fool of herself,' the major said, indicating a chair that Pope could use if he cared to join them.

'But most women are that way,' Claggett insisted.

'Rubbish! I'll bet you three-fourths of the fliers in this unit are married to perfectly normal women.'

'Granted,' Claggett said. 'But the normal woman is usually just as screwed up as that sister-in-law in New Orleans.'

'What in hell are you saying, Claggett?' the major cried.

'Statistics.'

'Not covering the people I know.' The major turned to Pope and said, 'You . . . I always forget your name.'

It irritated Pope that Air Force types, especially majors, feigned not to know the names of Navy fliers who joined their units. 'Name's Pope.'

'That's right,' the major said. 'Pope. Pope. You fly the special F6F.'

'F4U night fighter.'

'Pope, F4U. What we're arguing about, Pope, is women. Claggett here says that all women are pretty much like that mixed-up babe in the movie.'

'I know. He was selling me that line before I went to bed. But—'

'Now wait,' Claggett protested. 'You can't use Pope as evidence. He's a notorious straight arrow.' He said this with a kind of affectionate, patronizing sneer. Pilots were characterized by other pilots in brief phrases which summarized a whole constellation of attitudes, thus identifying the man without need for elaboration. Randy Claggett was referred to respectfully as a *front runner* or a *super stick,* the first referring to his known willingness to volunteer for any difficult flying job, the latter to his skill in performing it. Beginning fliers fantasized about earning either of these accolades; Claggett had both.

John Pope, as Claggett had warned the Air Force major, was a notorious *straight arrow* in that he didn't smoke or drink, he exercised to keep his weight down, he performed any task with rigorous perfection, he didn't use profanity, and he stayed away from Jo-sans. It was assumed by fellow pilots that one day Super Stick Claggett would be dead and Straight Arrow Pope an admiral.

'Yes,' the major said with a broad, welcoming smile, 'I've heard you were a true straight arrow, Pope. As such, you couldn't possibly agree—'

'Wait a minute!' Claggett interrupted. 'His wife's just made herself a lawyer. Puts her completely outside our argument.'

The major drew back and looked at Pope in obvious confusion. 'A lawyer? You mean, she works at it?'

'Yes, she's legislative assistant to Senator Glancey of Red River.'

No one spoke. Neither Claggett nor the major could comprehend how a pilot in military service could sustain a marriage to a woman who held her own job away from the base. Many wives often worked, military pay being what it was, but only as schoolteachers or secretaries to commanding officers, and always on the base or close to it.

'How do you handle it?' the major asked, but before Pope could answer, Claggett asked, 'You got a pitcher of her?' and Pope produced three snapshots of Penny, each quite feminine and lovable. The two fliers, studying with great care, deduced that she was a brunette, about a hundred and five pounds, petite, bright, witty, with flashing eyes and a strong sense of duty.

'No,' Pope corrected. 'She's not what they call petite. About five-four, but you're right, she does have drive. Votes Democratic sometimes.'

Again the two pilots were mystified, for the wives of young officers who hoped to become admirals were well advised to vote Republican, and their husbands were almost obliged to.

'With a solid, safe woman like her,' the major said, 'you didn't like the movie either, did you?'

'Why do they make films like that?' Pope asked. 'The dirty side of life?'

'War's a pretty dirty side,' Claggett observed, 'and they sure make movies about it.'

'But war's unavoidable,' Pope said. 'We're at K-22, three men, three different services because the Communists made us come here. You don't have to make a movie about a doomed woman like that one.'

'Shakespeare wrote his plays about doomed people,' Claggett responded. 'You ever see *Othello?*'

'Where did you ever see *Othello?*' the major asked with obvious surprise.

'We got little theater at Texas A and M.' He laughed. 'The big brass of ROTC on campus were disgusted with the plays bein' shown. All defeatism . . . downers. So they organized a special series. *The Problems of Command.* Ibsen's *Enemy of the People* to show the conflicts of public office. Shakespeare's *Coriolanus* to show divided loyalties. *The Caine Mutiny.* And *Othello.*'

'What was it supposed to show?' Pope asked.

'The sour relationship between a commandin' officer and some jerk on his staff. Best play of the lot.'

'Did Debby Dee see the plays?' Pope asked.

'I didn't know her then. She was varsity cheerleader at Texas Western.'

So many fliers protested the showing of a downbeat film like *A Streetcar Named Desire* that the K-22 commander summoned the education and entertainment officer and chewed him out: 'There will be no more films like that shown on this base. We want only patriotic, upbeat stuff like Ginger Rogers and Fred Astaire.'

A notice was posted in the officers' mess to the effect that henceforth all movies would be screened prior to showing and that undesirable films would be shipped back to the depot in Tokyo. Who would do the censoring was not indicated, but the entertainment officer told his friends that it would be himself, the chaplain and a colonel.

When Pope read the notice he chanced to see above it a mimeographed announcement which obviously came from the Bureau of Naval Personnel, and he supposed that it had been forwarded to K-22 by some aircraft carrier operating in the Japan Sea:

NAVY AND MARINE FLIERS

For the class starting on June 15 there will be a few openings at the Patuxent River Naval Air Station for pilots with wide experience who wish to become test pilots for the newer types of aircraft. Apply in writing with full credentials and recommendations to . . .

The phrase *newer types of aircraft* had been inserted with the specific purpose of attracting pilots like John Pope, and the bait was shrewdly placed, for that morning he drafted a letter to his commanding officer, still aboard the carrier, seeking permission to submit his application.

It would never have occurred to him to confide to anyone his secret ambition to become a test pilot; straight arrows proceeded strictly by the book, kept their aspirations to themselves, and either succeeded or failed according to their demonstrated abilities. It was an impressive dossier that he was able to forward to Washington: unblemished flight performance in nine different aircraft; no disciplinary action; three trains destroyed, with Claggett's photographs to prove it; two medals to substantiate the kills; and superior ratings from every commanding officer under whom he had served.

But there was one nagging omission which a casual reader of the application might overlook but which a Navy selection board would spot immediately: he had never engaged an enemy plane in combat, neither a Russian MiG nor a North Korean Slow Boy, and since he flew only at night, it was unlikely that he would ever encounter a MiG, for the Russians refused to squander these valuable planes on speculative missions. His only chance for aerial combat lay in tracking down a wooden Slow Boy, and this he was determined to do.

At two o'clock on the morning of 12 May 1952, when eagle-like Altair was flying toward the apex of the heavens, a radar watcher just south of the battle line detected a blip which had to be an airplane of some sort coming south toward the huge gasoline dump at Inchon. An alert was sounded and Pope's F4U leaped into the air.

The heavy plane climbed to 7,000 feet and headed northwest to intercept the intruder. In the starry night Pope spotted the enemy well below him, plodding along with its burden of TNT. Breathless with excitement, he swung into position well aft of the Slow Boy, shifted about in his seat till he found the best position, and zeroed in, his guns ready to explode on this perfect kill.

In fact, he was so intent on his mission that he failed to see the second half of this night's North Korean effort: a MiG flown by a Russian pilot whose job it was to shoot down whatever careless American pilot started after the Slow Boy. By the time Pope realized that he had stumbled into a trap, the MiG was firing its tremendous guns, and Pope, sick with fury at having been tricked, felt bullets striking his F4U.

It absorbed a hellish beating but tried valiantly to fly on. A wing trembled, half cut off at its base, and then a tank exploded. In flames the F4U spiraled toward the ground, crashing some fifteen miles north of the battle line. Americans and Koreans alike saw it come down, and by 0430, when sunlight was threatening to end the night, teams from both sides were converging on the wreckage, and it was an even chance as to which would reach it first. For some minutes they were aided by an immense burst of flame to the south: the Slow Boy had dumped its bombs on a gasoline depot.

The North Koreans came by foot from a nearby base, the Americans by helicopter from a field to the south, but all were preceded by a low-flying plane of tremendous speed, Randy Claggett's Banshee. As he photographed the wrecked plane he caught in his cameras the distinct picture of a downed aviator some distance away, his parachute beside him, his arms raised and waving.

In the officers' club at K-22 Pope and Claggett held a gloomy review:

'Sonnombeech, Pope, we came here in January to shoot down Slow Boys. It's June and we've accomplished nothin'.'

'I saw a Slow Boy. What I didn't see was his MiG.'

'We've scrubbed two F4Us and I didn't get any pitchers worth a damn. The Navy must be real proud of us.'

'You took on four MiGs that day.'

'And you did get three trains.'

'Hitting a train on the ground is not blasting a plane in the air.'

In their depression they fell ominously silent as a plane revved up for takeoff. They listened to it speed down the runway, stutter with soul-shaking terror, then catch its breath and soar into the air.

'Pope, I was intended to be a fighter pilot. I watch these F-86 clowns, I could die with envy.'

'I don't know. When I was down in that rice paddy waiting to see who was going to come through the trees, my side or theirs, I didn't have a single regret. I love to fly, and you know what I thought? War is the ugly price you pay so that you can have the fun of flying.'

Claggett drank his beer gloomily and took deep offense when Pope ordered a second ginger ale. 'Goddammit, how can a pilot drink that horse piss?' When Pope showed no inclination to defend his preference, the wiry Texan reached out and with a swipe of his hand knocked the ginger ale to the floor and said with passion, 'Pope, I been awatchin' you, and you know airplanes. I have deep respect for men who take planes seriously. Ain't many of us do. I got a proposition for you. Which I would be pleased if you took it seriously.' And from his blouse he produced the notice which had been posted on the bulletin board. True to form, as soon as he had seen the notice he quietly snaked it off the board, on the principle: 'I don't want no competition.'

'Navy's callin' for a few knowin' men. Would this application be of any interest to you?'

When Pope studied the form that Claggett extended, he saw something which amazed him: 'Randy, did you get a master's degree at Purdue?'

'Like the man says on the third line, "Number One in his class of sixty-seven." '

'Why do you talk that illiterate Tex-Mex?'

'I study hard so I can live the way I want. I want to talk Texican. I want to live tough.'

'With this record, they'll accept you for sure.'

'I hope so, and I wish you'd apply, too. We could be a team.'

With his right forefinger Pope pushed the announcement slowly back toward Claggett. 'I saw that the morning it was posted. Before you stole it so the competition wouldn't see it. My application's been in for weeks.'

'You sneaky sonnombeech! I'm convinced they'll select us both. And we're gonna take them planes higher and faster . . .' He jumped into the air, his arms waving. 'Pope, let's fly the wings right offen them beauties.'

In 1952 Senator Norman Grant, Republican, Fremont, was up for reelection, and his political mentor, Tim Finnerty, told him, 'Senator, in twenty years you can see two dozen new senators come to Washington, and many of them serve only one term. Do you know why? Because they don't run as hard the second time as they did the first. But if you can tuck that second term under your belt, you can be good for six terms. We better get to work.'

Finnerty did not want to risk this second election without the assistance of Penny Pope, who had been so effective the first time around, but as Grant pointed out, 'That raises a problem. Penny votes Republican, I suppose, but she's working for Senator Glancey, who's a Democrat. He might take offense.'

'Problem's simple. You ask Glancey for a loan of his Girl Friday.'

'No, Tim, I won't do that. Won't put Glancey in my debt, because who knows what quid pro quo he'd demand later on?'

'You mind if I ask?'

'Is her help that important?'

'Senator, this is your crucial second election. Everything's important. Even the color of your stationery. I want you to stop using that blue-ink letterhead. Trustworthy men use black.'

When Finnerty made his pitch in Glancey's office, the Red River senator required one minute to assess the problem accurately. 'Norman needs my girl but doesn't want to obligate himself by approaching me personally. Now, I need Norman to give me Republican help on certain things in aviation and defense that I want to accomplish. I want him to be indebted to me. I insist upon it. So there's no chance whatever that I will release Mrs. Pope unless Norman asks me personally.'

'That he won't do,' Finnerty said forcefully.

'That I will seduce him into doing,' Glancey said quietly. 'And when I outline my problems to him, he'll want to be obligated.'

'Norman Grant does not obligate easily,' Finnerty warned.

Glancey changed direction completely, something he was notorious for doing. One minute he was talking duck shooting in the Ozarks, the next an affirmative vote on a new bomber for the Air Force. 'What we're overlooking, Mr. Finnerty, is the attitude of the young woman in question. Had we not better consult her?'

He rang for Penny, and when she appeared he rose courteously and asked her to be seated. 'I'm sure you know Mr. Finnerty of Senator Grant's office. And I'm sure you can guess why he's here.'

'About Grant's vote on the bomber?'

'Not at all, Mrs. Pope. He solicits your assistance in the forthcoming election.'

With the directness that made Penny Pope attractive to many besides her husband and her employer, she said, 'But he's a Republican, and I work for you.'

'Precisely,' Glancey said.

'Of course, I'm more liberal than my husband.'

'Liberal enough to vote for Adlai Stevenson?'

'Maybe not that liberal.'

'Would you like it if I gave you my blessing? About working for Senator Grant?'

'I would appreciate it. Tim and I work well together.'

Glancey turned to Finnerty and said, 'So it's simple. For three good reasons I have no objection to my Girl Friday working for the opposition. I doubt that our man Stevenson can win nationally. I'm sure Grant can win in Fremont. And I need his help on my big projects.'

'Then it's agreed?'

'Not at all. I want Grant to come here. To ask in person.'

Mrs. Pope accompanied Finerty to Norman Grant's office, and when Penny saw her fellow townsman, thirty-eight years old, trimly dressed, with a nineteenth-century manner, she intuitively felt that he was entitled to reelection, for he looked the way a senator should.

'Senator Glancey says we can have Penny . . .' Finnerty began.

'If I ask in person?' Grant asked. When his aide nodded, Grant shook his head as if perplexed. 'That old swamp fox. He wants a deal of some kind.' Turning to Mrs. Pope, he asked, 'Can you be of substantial help?'

'We got you elected last time.'

'Aren't you giving yourself too much credit?' Grant said jokingly.

Penny leaned forward. 'There are only two kinds of senators. Those that get reelected and those that don't. The first are of great value to this country. The others we can forget.'

'I certainly intend to be reelected.'

'Your type is also divided into two. Those like Senator Glancey, who fight and scratch and gouge, God bless him, and cannot be kept from winning, and those good men like you who need a great deal of clever assistance. You need Finnerty and me. We do the gouging.'

So Norman Grant walked down two floors to meet with Michael Glancey, and the latter spoke without equivocation. 'I doubt if Stevenson can win, because this country is hungry for a military leader. Profound decisions will have to be made in the years ahead, and I'd rather see you representing Fremont than some dunderhead I couldn't trust. Since there's no chance the Democrats can win your seat, I'd be pleased to see Mrs. Pope helping you over the hurdle.'

'Then why did you insist that I come down here in person?'

'Because I want you to promise that you'll stay put on my aviation and defense committees. I'd be proud to see you the minority leader of those committees one day, and you will be, Norman, if you get reelected this time.'

'What big things do you see coming along?'

'I'm not sure about specifics, Norman, but I'm sure that the Russians are way ahead of us in certain areas. And if they are, we could be in trouble one of these days.'

'You believe I could help?'

'Vitally. You know what war is. You know what national danger is. You, me, Lyndon, Symington, a handful of others. As the leading Republican, you'll be crucially important.'

Grant had been in the Senate long enough to comprehend basic values, so he asked, 'What good would Fremont get if I stayed with the committee? I was planning to shift to Agriculture.'

'Fight like hell to get Agriculture, Norman. Your people will love it. See you as their champion. But stay with me, too, and if what I see developing takes place, there's going to be a lot of industrial expansion. I'll protect you.'

'Thank you for letting me have Mrs. Pope. She's a wonderful woman.'

'I know that better than you,' Glancey said.

For these intricate reasons Penny Pope spent the summer of 1952 organizing the state of Fremont as it had rarely been organized before. She applied everything she had learned in Glancey's election of 1950—he won by a landslide—plus some original ideas of her own, and in early October she flew to Alabama to talk with Larry Penzoss, then up to Detroit, where Gawain Butler was principal of a small black school.

She had no trouble with Penzoss, who was immersed in the dull job of dispatching trucks; he could break away for six weeks if needed. But with Butler, things were not so simple. Since his school was about to open he was needed on the job, and he had grave doubts about the voting records of Senators Grant and Glancey when black rights were involved. 'Why should I break my back to help men who never help me?'

'Mr. Butler, you've told me a dozen times about how Senator Grant helped you climb aboard that raft. Now he needs—'

'You seem not to know, Miss Penny—'

'Make it plain Penny.'

'When men leave the raft, they must continue to grow. Senator Grant is exactly where he was that morning we were saved. No better. No worse. Me, I've been to college. I've seen a whole new world. I've acquired high standards as to how men should behave.'

'Mr. Butler—'

'Call me Gawain.'

She hesitated, then laughed freely. 'That's a crazy name for a Negro principal.'

'It sure is. Know what the tough boys in my school sing? "He's Gawain and he ain't comin' back." '

'Gawain, if we can get you and Penzoss and Finnerty on the stage again, Norman Grant has this election sewed up.'

'But what do we Negroes get out of it?'

'You will have a friend in high places. You will have me to help you in Senator Glancey's office.'

'He will never vote for justice.'

'Why do you suppose he hires me? I heckle him every week we're in session.' Butler started to protest, but Penny cut him off: 'Gawain, I have a powerful nose for politics, and I can foresee situations coming down the road when the votes of Glancey and Grant might be very important to your people . . . to your school . . . to you. I may not be able to get you two votes, but I'm absolutely convinced that on a just bill I can get you one. That means a stand-off with my senators. It's your job to handle the other ninety-four.'

Penzoss spent four weeks in Fremont, appearing with a uniformed Tim Finnerty, medals shining, and they accomplished much, but Penny kept them in the smaller towns from Monday through Thursday. Over the weekends, when Gawain Butler with his limp and his cane flew in from Detroit, she scheduled the three heroes into the major cities and onto the more important radio and television shows.

They were handsome young men—Finnerty, twenty-seven; Penzoss, twenty-nine; Butler, thirty-one—and although Penzoss had had to have his uniform let out at various seams, they still created a heroic illusion. Their testimony to Norman Grant's good character bore weight, and by the end of October it looked as if the senator would be reelected, just as it seemed certain that General Eisenhower would win the state and probably the nation.

Grant and Butler had their serious talk in the western city of Calhoun. 'Looks like we're in,' the black man said.

'How's your school doing?' Grant refused to utter even one word which might indicate that he thought he was winning. He was running scared and refused to take any poll seriously.

'We have many problems, Senator.'

'Even in the North?'

'I wasn't speaking of Negroes. I was speaking of Detroit.'

'I'm sorry. That was thoughtless of me, Gawain. Tell me, are you pretty well launched in the Detroit system? You'll get a bigger school one of these days?'

'I'm afraid Detroit's going to face very serious problems.'

'I'm confused. You mean black versus white?'

'No! I mean things are changing so fast. Business moving out to suburbs. Off the tax rolls. Unemployment.'

'They tell me that's true of all cities.'

'It is, and you must do something about it.'

'Where do you come in?'

'I'm a citizen of Detroit. But I'm also a black man. And every wrong thing that happens in a big city has double impact on us Negroes.'

'What do you want me to do, Gawain?'

'Vote occasionally to help us.'

'Like what?'

'Fair employment practices, so that Negroes can join unions. Better schools in the big cities. Urban renewal.'

'That's a pretty broad spectrum.'

'That's why I'm working to help elect you, Senator Grant. With your background and your character, you ought to be able to handle a broad spectrum.'

The two men sat silent. Butler had said everything that he was concerned with, so there was no need for him to speak further. Grant was thinking that this was about the fiftieth urgent agendum that had been pressed upon him, each more crucial than the other, and he was becoming powerless to evaluate them, but he did acknowledge that he had two personal obligations which had to be considered seriously. Senator Glancey had been invaluable in launching him properly in the Senate, and if Glancey needed help on aviation matters, he would get it, and Gawain Butler was one of the finest men he had ever known, in uniform or out, and if he felt that Negroes in the big cities needed help, he would have to weigh that claim studiously.

'I think we have this election won, Senator Grant.'

'If we have, I'll want to hear from you.'

'You will.'

When Professor Mott received orders to move the Germans from El Paso in Texas to Huntsville in Alabama, he sent most of them by train, but Dieter

Kolff and seven other families wished to drive their second-hand automobiles across country, so a caravan was approved, and as Mott watched the efficiency with which Kolff organized the expedition, he was reassured: when the American Army got these men, it was getting a bargain.

Dieter had acquired a 1938 Oldsmobile touring car, the handsome one with the heavy chrome-steel bars across the grille and the overdrive which allowed the driver to shift the monstrous thing out of normal high gear, where the engine continued to grind, and into a superdrive in which the engine merely kept the momentum already in the car moving forward. It had not been much of a car when Dieter got it—twelve years old, a hundred and twelve thousand miles—but by the time he and a wizard engine man named Unger had rebuilt it with specially tooled parts, it was good for another two hundred thousand.

There would be nine cars in the convoy, counting the Chevrolet in which Mott, his wife, their son Millard and their baby Christopher would lead the procession, but on the eve of departure they were joined by a tenth: three soldiers under the command of First Lieutenant McEntee, whose job it was to see that the Germans made the transit to Alabama without saying anything to the press or straying about in idle sightseeing.

The soldiers were not needed, because Dieter Kolff had devised mimeographed plans that accounted for every mile and every minute of the trip: 'We shall go via Carlsbad, Dallas, Little Rock and Memphis. Each car will be numbered one through nine and will maintain position. Each piece of luggage in each car will be numbered and accounted for every night and morning. The cars will be kept clean, with large paper bags into which all litter will be thrown. At each stop throughout the day we will arrange for the next gasoline fill-up, and we will stop together.' And on and on.

Lieutenant McEntee had his own orders, but they were ignored, Kolff having anticipated everything.

The first clash of wills between the American Army and the Peenemünde Germans came at Carlsbad, where the safari stopped for gas. 'Since we are here,' Kolff said as if the arrival had been accidental, 'we should see the famous caravans.' One of the soldiers said, 'You mean *caverns*. You're not permitted to do that.'

'Since we're here,' Kolff repeated, his tense little body prepared to defend itself, 'why don't we just stop by?' He pronounced the innocent words *chust stopp py,* and when the Germans reached the entrance to the natural wonder, Mott found that the officials in charge were awaiting them with free passes and cold drinks. Kolff had written ahead, two weeks before, advising them of the exact minute his men would arrive.

Lieutenant McEntee protested again, but the government official already had Kolff out of the Oldsmobile and was distributing pamphlets to the other cars, so that a visit to the caverns became inescapable. Mott, in looking over Kolff's itinerary for the trip, had wondered why this day's stage was so relatively brief. Now he understood, for the excited engineers spent two hours underground, bombarding the Carlsbad scientists with a barrage of questions, especially about the myriad bats which used the caves as a daylight refuge.

'You go way down,' Kolff said to the attendants. 'We go way up.'

'Do you fly?'

'No, we—' Before Kolff could explain about rockets, Lieutenant McEntee intervened to forbid the conversation, so Dieter returned to the bats. 'They fly at night. So do we.' The guard could make nothing of this, but when the tour reached the lowest level, where the Germans could marvel at the limestone points whose imperceptible downward dripping through the eons had created a subterranean cathedral, Kolff whispered to the guide, 'Rockets,' and the man said, 'No, stalactites.'

Lieutenant McEntee, infuriated by Kolff's deception, assembled the Peenemünde families at the night stop and reminded them: 'No stopping. No sightseeing. Our job is to get to the Army base at Huntsville in good order.'

As the caravan headed for Arkansas, Stanley Mott reflected on the years he had known these Germans, and he said to Rachel, 'I wonder if there was ever a migration in this country of a more brilliant concentration of human power?'

Rachel could think of two possible competitors: 'Maybe the Pilgrims on the *Mayflower*. Maybe the Mormons moving west to Utah. They were powerful, too.'

'But those men up ahead and the ones on the train, they hold the future in their hands.'

'Do you really think so?'

'I do indeed. I've lived with them for six years now, and I'm constantly staggered by the clear vision they have.'

As they crossed the country he shared with her the dreams of these remarkable men, insofar as he had been allowed to know them: 'You know that quiet Ernst Stuhlinger? What do you suppose he's working on? No laboratory, no equipment but a pencil and a sheet of paper, and that incredible mind. An ion ramjet.'

'And what's that?'

'We think of outer space as empty. No gravity. No atmosphere. But there is this solar wind. Not blowing the way earthly wind does. Just particles of energy flowing out from the Sun. Constantly. As long as the Sun lasts. Stuhlinger thinks he could build a device of enormous size, a huge mouth really, which would speed through the upper atmosphere, gathering up these stray ions the way a whale gathers plankton in the ocean.'

'Can you see the ions?'

'Invisible. And almost nonexistent. One part in a billion, or something like that. But with an ion ramjet you could collect all there are in a given part of space, convert them to energy, and fly your machine for many years in the atmosphere.'

Mott was always distressed, when he spoke of such speculations, by the fact that his son Millard showed no interest, even though Mrs. Mott, not trained as a scientist, could follow his explanations. The boy was diffident, interested in nothing, disgusted with Huntsville even before he reached it, and Mott wondered what deficiency in himself had created this intellectual vacuum. The constant moving about, perhaps, had dulled the lad's capacity for enthusiasm, and when he watched the zest with which the Germans headed into new territory, he feared that Millard had failed to develop one of the most precious human attributes, wonder, and the ability to project oneself into unexplored dimensions.

Hans Unger, who had helped Kolff rebuild the Oldsmobile, was devising in his head a better guidance system for the rockets he was convinced the Americans must build. 'If we don't,' he said, identifying himself with his new country, 'we shall lose the race to the Russians.'

'Is the race itself important?' Mott had asked, and he remembered the colloquium that Unger had once convened in the barracks at El Paso: 'Chentlemen, Professor Mott hass asked a most benetrating qvestion. Duss it matter the Roosians, they are aheat of uss?'

Mott would never forget the intensity of the replies: Von Braun, Stuhlinger, Kolff, Unger hammered at him, driving home their conviction that within the next decades someone would command space, and the military advantage derived therefrom, and the ability to predict weather, and the possibility of stationing a device of some kind to throw back radio signals to any spot on Earth. 'But the most significant return,' Von Braun had insisted, 'will be the encouragement of the spirit of exploration . . . in all fields . . . in all arenas.'

Mott had asked point-blank, 'Are you satisfied that with the rockets we could build now, we could get to outer space?'

'Tomorrow,' Von Braun snapped. 'If we're set free.'

'And the Moon? And Mars?'

'Give us six years. Professor Mott, we're on the verge of tremendous accomplishments. But so are the Russians.' Mott remembered with chilling effect what Von Braun had said next: 'Your United States has about one hundred of us Peenemünde men. Russia must have captured four hundred. Do you think that by accident you got all the bright ones? Don't you think Russia got some able ones, too?'

'But did they get any geniuses?' Mott asked.

'In this business a genius is merely a good engineer. I'm a good engineer. So is Kolff over there. You set Kolff free, by this time next year he could have something orbiting in space.'

It was almost as if this caravan of used automobiles were heading purposefully to some powerful destiny. The fate of a good deal of mankind rode with these wandering scholars; one young man in a rebuilt Pontiac dreamed of throwing out from a potential spacecraft an immense gossamer construction made of the most delicate filament, infinitely finer than a nylon fishing line. As he explained it to Mott: 'In outer space, you understand, with no wind, no gravity, no disturbance of any kind, a piece of my filament would be just as rigid as a steel beam eight inches through.'

'I can't believe it, but what would be the purpose?'

'Collect radiation from the sun and convert it to electricity. Perpetual motion available at last.'

'Is that practical?'

'Would I work on it, otherwise?' *Odderveiss*, the young man said, returning to his sketches.

The boldest idea rode with the driver of the 1938 Oldsmobile, for Dieter Kolff had never surrendered his vision of the A-10: the immense rocket, which should have come off the line in early 1945, with the ability to launch from Peenemünde and deliver Trialen bombs into the heart of New York or Washington. Now that he lived in those cities, figuratively, he had diverted his imaginary rockets to other targets: Moon and Mars and Jupiter.

'It can be done,' he insisted to anyone who would listen. 'We can do it now, and we must.' In German he had often discussed the step-by-step procedures with Mott, hoping that Mott would report his conviction to the military, but nothing had happened, and he was bringing to his new job in Alabama not the equipment necessary for such shots into space and not even the plans, but only the moral conviction that whichever nation first mastered space might well master the world.

It would be said later in Huntsville: 'Over a hundred German scientists arrived here at eleven o'clock on an April morning and by nightfall more than sixty had applied for cards at the free library.'

They were housed temporarily at the former Redstone Arsenal, which had been a thriving installation during the war but which served no peacetime need, and the citizens of Huntsville, while vigorously opposed to accepting Nazi Germans, as they called the Peenemünde scientists, were nevertheless gratified that at least someone had moved in to keep Redstone active and inject money into the local economy. These conflicting reactions meant that the reception was uneven, social leaders of the old Confederate city standing aghast at the invasion, bankers and businessmen being rather glad to see it. Certainly, there were no untoward incidents. Magnus Kolff, like the other youths, was enrolled in the local kindergarten, and when he returned for lunch with the exciting news that band instruments could be borrowed without cost, his mother said, 'Get a trumpet, this afternoon,' and the early days at Huntsville were marked by loud and enthusiastic trumpet practice.

Liesl Kolff spent three days converting her new barracks into decent living space and then was seen about the camp no more. She spent her time in town trudging from one address to another, looking for a proper home in which to house her family: 'No more camps. No more tents. We're human beings now.'

Huntsville residents were considerate of her desires, and one family after another suggested houses that might be available, but some were not large enough and others were too expensive. At the end of two weeks Liesl had succeeded in helping six other German families to settle into their own rented homes, but the Kolffs were still in barracks.

And then one day, as she looked toward the north, she saw the beautifully wooded hills of a high area called Monte Sano, 'The Mountain of Health' a local woman explained, and Liesl went there, climbing the narrow footpaths until she reached a splendid plateau from which she could see the city below and the military installations beyond. From that moment she knew what she and Dieter must do, and next day she asked her husband to cut her a heavy walking stick from a sapling, and using this to knock aside brush, she explored the entire plateau until she found an almost perfect spot: sloping land that could be converted into a German-type wooded area with pine-needle base, cliff to protect the area from below, broad vista to delight the eye, and most important, tall, stout trees to give shade.

Next day she took Magnus to the hill with her, and while he practiced trumpet calls off-key, she piled stones at what she deemed would be the corners of a satisfactory lot. On the weekend she led Dieter and Magnus up the hill to see what she already called 'our house,' and when Dieter saw what she had uncovered he was satisfied that they must build here: 'After nearly five years of test shots in New Mexico, I'm hungry for trees.'

But how to get the money to buy the land, if it was for sale, and build an American house, which must be very costly? Dieter went to his counselor, Professor Mott, who was himself living in a rented home. 'How can we Germans get enough money to buy our homes? Or build ones?'

Mott explained that in America one went to a bank and pleaded with the banker for a mortgage, but that none would be available unless the applicant already had a nest egg of several thousand dollars. 'Could we see the banker, just in case?' Dieter asked, and an appointment was made with a Mr. Erskine, descendant of a well-regarded Confederate family, who listened attentively to Dieter's plea, then said with some warmth, 'Mr. Kolff, the city of Huntsville is truly delighted to have you Germans as our guests. You could be the salvation of this city, and we intend to offer you every consideration. But we cannot issue mortgages unless you have some down payment to protect us.'

That was final, and Kolff understood, but Mott asked if he could speak with Erskine alone. 'I assure you I've not said a word about this to Kolff, but would you drive out to the camp to see what kind of people they are?'

'I surely would. Let me assure you, Mott, I'm sick about refusing so many of your Germans, men and women of good character apparently . . .'

'Come see.'

So with Dieter sitting in the back seat, the banker and Mott drove out to the barracks, and there Erskine saw the cleanliness of the Kolff home, the trumpet on the sideboard and the extreme neatness of the place, but what impressed him most was the 1938 Oldsmobile standing beside the barracks. It was impeccable, well-washed and polished, with shiny black tires. Any family that would rebuild an antique like that and care for it with such obvious affection would repay a mortgage.

'What we can do,' Erskine said, back in his office, 'is grant you a mortgage—that is, all the German families—on the lowest down payments we've ever accepted. How much money would you need, Mr. Kolff, land and house?'

'If we can get the land . . .'

'Where?'

'I'd rather not say till we get the money.'

'That's prudent. But how much?'

'Land, maybe fifteen hundred. House, maybe five thousand.'

'Six thousand, five hundred—and no security? That's rather much, Professor.' He broke off the conversation to ask, 'Are you buying, Mott?'

'My future's very uncertain. I'm not military, you know. I'm renting.'

The banker asked Kolff if he would wait outside, and when he was gone, Erskine said, 'These are the kind of people we want in this community. Will they be here long?'

'I believe this is a long-term commitment. The government doesn't know it yet, but the whole push of experiment . . .'

'Does the Army agree?'

'The Army is fumbling, sir. But it knows it can't turn back.'

'I can only repeat what I said to Kolff—and you can tell all your Germans this. I can give them mortgages at the lowest possible rate, the lowest possible down payment. If your man Kolff can come up with . . . well, let's say two thousand dollars . . .'

'He can't. There's no way he can.'

'He drives an automobile.'

'He bought it for forty dollars. What you see is what he did.'

Erskine leaned back and drummed his fingers. 'We forget down here in Alabama that immigrants still come to our shores. With nothing. Wife, two children and nothing. It's amazing, really. Why don't you assemble all your Germans who want to buy homes, see how much money they can come up with, and come back and see me. We might be able to work something out en masse.' But when the Peenemünde men were assembled, they had almost no savings and their salaries were already allocated to furniture and food.

The solution came from a remarkable source. General Funkhauser, fifty-four years old and handsome, with graying hair and a gray worsted suit, flew in to check with the Army concerning rocket contracts obtained by Allied Aviation, and when he heard of the plight of the German scientists he said on the spot, 'I'll lend you fifteen thousand dollars, and Allied will guarantee another fifteen thousand against your salaries on our projects.'

When Mott heard this he insisted that Funkhauser leave his meeting at Redstone and drive immediately to the bank to assure Mr. Erskine that the funds would be available, and the general so charmed the banker, a trait Funkhauser had perfected in California, that a deal was arranged whereby the thirty thousand, some in hand, some guaranteed, could be used as a revolving fund which the Germans could then use as collateral to enable them to buy their own homes.

The first loan was made to Dieter Kolff, and ten minutes after it was assured, Liesl had a real estate man tramping over the plateau of Monte Sano, noting the rock-pile corners of her proposed lot. At the end of two weeks several German families had bought adjoining lots, and one of the most congenial settlements in northern Alabama was under way, a place of solidly built homes, wooded gardens and lanes marked with flowering shrubs.

A significant characteristic of Monte Sano was the amount of music that could be heard as the German children brought home their free instruments, and after a while the Huntsville band, accustomed to playing John Philip Sousa and American Legion marches, was offering Mozart and Beethoven.

At the arsenal things were not going so smoothly for the German scientists; they were now prisoners of the Army and were restricted in their work to those rockets which the Army alone was developing for potential military use—Corporal, Sergeant, Redstone—and were not free to participate in the exciting and competing work being done by the Navy, with their more scientific Viking research rockets, or by the newly fledged Air Force, which was developing missiles like the Bomarc and Matador to its own specifications. It seemed to Dieter that America was prodigal in its waste of talent, headstrong in allowing conflict among agencies, and lagging in its pursuit of the Russians.

'I don't see how this country ever gets anything done,' he told his wife as they worked together to make their home on Monte Sano always a little neater and better. 'You put Von Braun in charge of everything, he'd have rockets in six months.'

'America won the war, didn't she?' Liesl asked.

'That's a mystery also,' Dieter said, but at the same time he was continuously grateful for the asylum America had provided and, unlike certain of the Peenemünde men, never considered returning to Germany. He was especially gratified with the easy manner in which Magnus was fitting in to American patterns and was proud of the boy's fine marks at school. Once when Wernher von Braun came to Monte Sano for supper, the great scientist took Magnus on his knee and interrogated him about mathematics and geography, and the Kolffs were proud of how their son acquitted himself.

When the boy was in bed, Von Braun confided his fears, his large, usually placid face betraying real doubts about the Army program in which he was inextricably enmeshed. 'American generals are like German generals. If our team does a single thing that might be useful only to science, they scream and inspect us for loyalty.' He laughed. 'Remember how General Funkhauser was going to have us shot because we were thinking about space? They don't shoot you in Huntsville. They do worse. They cut off your funds.'

On the other hand, if the Germans applied themselves to military projects, they enjoyed remarkable freedom and constant encouragement. This was partly because the generals realized that in going before Congress in search of funds, they were restricted in what they could divulge; to the appropriation committees, they appeared as merely one more group of American military men, singing the same tired songs; but if they could throw the burden of testimony on Von Braun and General Funkhauser and specific experts like Dieter Kolff, all speaking in heavily accented phrases which carried an extra freight of scientific substance, they were apt to gain attention and grants.

Von Braun seemed to be away from Huntsville most of the time: in Washington to testify before Congress, in Chicago to speak before large assemblies of scientists, or in the smallest Tennessee town to explain to local businessmen the significance of the new science. He was a genius in meeting American voters where they were and leading them gently, amusingly, to where he wanted them to be. He was especially adept at using his German accent effectively, and Dieter once heard him say to a group of representatives from a House committee, 'When I left Alabama this morning to fly here to testify before you, my wife asked, "Wernher, do you have your speech prepared?" and I told her, "I know it backwards," and that's how I'm giving it, I'm afraid.'

Von Braun, from his painful experience with Hitler and the Wehrmacht generals, knew how effective models and displays could be when talking to non-scientists, and it was for this reason that he often took Kolff along with him when he wished to make an especially powerful presentation before President Eisenhower or Senator Glancey's committee: 'I have my prized assistant, Dieter Kolff, to demonstrate the four parts which will fit together to make a Saturn rocket.' And Kolff would take the carefully machined mock-up and break it apart, allowing watchers to handle the segments; then he would skillfully put them together again, as if he were a child playing with toys. Von Braun did not invite him to speak about the parts, for

Dieter's English could not be relied upon; Von Braun did the talking, and it was largely due to him that Huntsville continued to receive the funds necessary for basic research.

But he and Kolff could never understand the peculiar workings of the American system, in which the Army remained suspicious of the Navy and the Air Force combated both, on the grounds that space should belong to those who flew it. 'They could see, if they studied what happened to Germany's war effort,' Von Braun said one night at his home when Kolff and Stuhlinger and the visiting Funkhauser were discussing next steps, 'what happens when you allow generals to fight among themselves and make scientific decisions based on their own narrow interests.' He was recalling the devastating debates that had occurred at Peenemünde, where the German air force had used the north end of the island to build an unmanned airplane, which proved extremely effective in bombing large areas, while Von Braun's group filled the rest of the island with their competing rocketry.

'I defend the American system,' Funkhauser said. 'Everyone competing with everyone else.'

'It's so wasteful,' Von Braun complained.

'More so than even you imagine,' Funkhauser conceded. 'Because in my opinion, some of the very best work is being done by private industry. I sometimes think that Allied Aviation is ahead of all the services.'

The experts discussed this for some time, in German, and when Funkhauser told them what he had seen in the California and Texas aviation shops, they were astonished. 'What will happen, I think,' Funkhauser predicted, 'is that we will all drift along, going our own ways, until something big happens. Bang! Then we'll have to pay attention. In six weeks, Army . . . Navy . . . Air Force . . . private industry—we'll coalesce into one very effective instrument.'

'And if nothing big happens?' Kolff asked.

'Something big always happens,' Von Braun said.

The Germans were stunned after they and the Army experts had developed a set of rockets with enormous power and a body of compact scientific instruments to ride atop the rockets and send back to Earth data concerning the upper atmosphere. This beautiful and sophisticated arrangement of equipment came close to what Kolff had been dreaming of, and one afternoon he showed Von Braun a set of calculations: 'With this, and just a little more boost, we could throw that science package right out of the atmosphere and into Earth orbit.'

'Don't say that!' Von Braun snapped. 'Not where people can hear.'

But someone at Huntsville did hear, not this specific conversation but others which had idly speculated upon the power of the new rockets, and on the eve of test-firing the package, a harsh warning came down from the Department of Defense at Washington, signed by the Secretary himself:

In firing the test rocket you are to take every precaution to ensure that no part of the rocket or its payload escapes into outer space. International consequences would be grave if this were to happen. Every member of the team will be responsible to see that it does not.

So the American capacity to loft an object into space, where it would orbit the earth at an altitude of about a hundred and twenty miles and stay there for years, untouched by storms or rust or the decay of its power supply, was killed before it had a chance to demonstrate its ability.

The Germans did not despair. Quietly and with remarkable skill they turned their attention to that chain of almost insurmountable problems which would enable them to throw into the air not some small device weighing three pounds, but a monstrous space vehicle weighing twenty-five tons. The burning interest of men like Kolff could not be quenched by directives from Washington.

Occasionally, just occasionally, they had to face the fact that whereas their Peenemünde team was accomplishing miracles at Huntsville, at other bases about the nation American scientists, with no help from any Germans, were accomplishing equal results. 'I doubt that their rockets will fly,' some of the Germans predicted, but Kolff, having listened attentively to what General Funkhauser had reported about American industry, suspected that with or without the Germans, America was going to solve the rocket problem.

But when one after another of the American rockets fizzled, he noticed that the authorities kept coming down to Alabama to consult with Von Braun, and he realized that at last his leader, whom he admired so intensely, was recognized as essential to the American effort. And because he was Von Braun's engineering genius, he was essential also.

Therefore, when he finished his work at the Redstone laboratories, always moving his great design of a master rocket ahead inch by inch, he returned to Monte Sano and its neat German community with a sense of deep satisfaction. His wife had a secure home now, much better than the farmhouse she had shared with cows in Pomerania, and his son had a proud position in the school band: youngest member and best trumpeter.

And then one night he climbed the hill with disastrous news. Assembling the Peenemünde people, he told them, 'Professor Mott has been fired.'

Yes, the fine young engineer who had searched Europe for them, who had herded them to safety at the village near Munich and inducted them into American life at El Paso, was no longer needed by the Army. A delegation of Monte Sano Germans formed immediately and drove down into Huntsville to the house the Motts had rented, and there they found Stanley and Rachel sitting disconsolately in the middle of their austere living room, facing the Mondrian prints they had brought with them from El Paso.

'We'll go on strike!' Kolff said, and five men who had learned English because Rachel had been so generous with her time assented.

'Don't be foolish,' Mott interrupted. 'I've never been an Army man. Just a civilian employee. And now my employment's ended.'

'But you saved us all,' Liesl Kolff cried.

'And we will fight for you now,' her husband vowed.

The protests were prolonged and heartfelt. These Germans knew they were of value to America and were able to contribute that value only because Stanley Mott had championed them against enormous odds. He had found them, saved their lives, and delivered them to the laboratories of the New World. Now they would defend him.

Even Wernher von Braun made representations to the Army command, who replied that Mott was merely one more civilian whose job had been completed, and he must go. Frantic calls to universities and other learned institutions proved that the scientific explosion which was about to overtake America had not yet begun. 'We can't even find jobs for our doctoral candidates,' one graduate school reported. 'We're advising them to go into high-school teaching.' Mott, with only an M.S., had little bargaining power.

To his surprise, Rachel was remarkably philosophical about his dismissal. 'You know what the old general told us when he was ousted: "War promotes, peace demotes." ' She assured Stanley that if they did have to settle for a high-school job, no matter where, she was sure that she and the boys could adjust, and without knowing where they were to go, she started packing.

It was Dieter Kolff who saved them, or rather his wife, for Liesl heckled her husband incessantly: 'You cannot allow these good people who saved our lives . . . how many times . . .' At this point in her sentence she would stand with her heavy arms cocked at an aggressive angle, her stubby hands on hips that grew broader year by year, and demand to know what he proposed doing.

What he did was use the telephone at the base to call General Funkhauser out at Allied Aviation: 'General, the wonderful young man who saved us both, he's being fired.' When Funkhauser established that the man was Professor Mott he exploded, causing the phone to rattle, and three days later, in the Allied four-engine plane, he came roaring in to Huntsville. Within minutes he was meeting with the Motts and Kolff in the latter's office.

'I can't give you a job right now with Allied,' he said as he stalked about the room. 'But if we did have a job opening'—he pronounced it *chob*—'I thought you might like to know how highly we prize a fine engineer like you. Guess what our salary would be?'

Mott was too humiliated to play games, so he gave an abrupt, absurd figure: 'Fifteen thousand?'

'Eighteen,' Funkhauser said in volatile German. 'And I assure you of

this, young man. There is going to be a scientific awakening in this country
—aviation . . . atomic power . . . space. Things you and I haven't dreamed
of yet. And when that happens, men like you are going to be at a premium.'

He dropped into a chair, grasped the arms, and stared at Mott as if he
were a horse to be traded. 'You're a commodity. What can we do today with
a commodity?'

Suddenly he jumped up, pointed an accusing finger at Kolff, and cried
again in German, 'Stupid, why didn't you think of it?'

'Of what?'

'Those fellows in Hampton, Virginia! They're always looking for men
exactly like Mott.' He grasped Mott's arm and said, 'You are of enormous
value, young man, we'll prove it.' Grabbing for a telephone, he arranged a
meeting for that afternoon, then told Dieter, 'You're flying with us.'

During the short flight to Virginia the two Germans reminded Mott of
the extraordinary group of people he was about to meet: 'The National
Advisory Committee on Aviation—NACA, each letter pronounced—is like
nothing else in America. A board of twelve leading experts who serve
without pay. They hire eight thousand extremely bright engineers and
theoreticians to investigate flight—airplane engines, airplane design, airport
facilities, new metals, new fuels. If America is preeminent in aviation, it's
because of NACA.'

'Would I fit in?' Mott asked. 'I've never had advanced courses in aviation.'

'You'd be ideal, Stanley,' Dieter said, patting him on the knee. 'From
what I've heard of NACA, it doesn't go looking for aviation experts. It hires
the most brilliant engineers it can find and turns them loose. Your wide
background is what they're looking for.'

Funkhauser interposed an additional consideration: 'Stanley, we're entering the age of space. We need people who can think about bold new
horizons. Americans equal to Germany's Oberth and Russia's Tsiolkovsky.
You know who they are?'

'I do.'

'Good. You're far ahead of the others.' He winked at Kolff. 'NACA
doesn't know it needs this young man, Dieter, but we know it needs him.'

Mott's introduction to NACA was disarming: a clutter of unimpressive
buildings not far from the James River, a panel of four intense specialists,
a series of penetrating questions. 'You come highly recommended,' the
spokesman said. 'Was it really you who saved the Peenemünde documents?'

'It was,' Funkhauser said. 'I searched all over Germany for him, and
he searched for me.'

'And what were your main courses of study?'

'Mechanical engineering, materials, structures.'

'Excellent,' and the spokesman explained the philosophy of NACA, a
philosophy which had enabled the agency to pioneer far more than half

the discoveries that had made flight possible, profitable and safe: 'We like to bring in engineers who've had wide experience in general principles. Who know what a vector is, a slide rule. And we put them to work on every conceivable type of problem until they appreciate the complexity of flight, trusting that they'll apply what they know to what we don't know.'

'I'd like that.'

'When can you start?'

'Tomorrow,' General Funkhauser said.

'We could use you tomorrow,' the NACA man said.

'That sounds wonderful, sir, but I have to close out my duties at Huntsville.'

'Why? They fired you, didn't they?'

'I can't just walk out.'

The NACA men nodded, almost approvingly; if this man was loyal to people who had fired him, he would certainly be loyal to those who hired him. 'Agreed,' the chairman said. 'Start work as soon as you can get here. But by the way, where did you say you were educated?'

'Bachelor's, Georgia Tech. Master's, Louisiana State.'

With spontaneous enthusiasm the chairman rose, reached across and shook Mott's hand. 'That's a spectacular combination. We have seven superbrains in NACA. Three from Louisiana State, two each from Purdue and Georgia Tech.' When he led Mott toward the door, he added, 'We don't want you to come here just to work. We want you to become one of our next superbrains.'

Mott halted and his throat choked up, but after a moment he asked, 'Could I call my wife?' The NACA men heard him say, 'Better than you could have dreamed, darling. They're shifting us into the fast lane.' She must have responded with a question about opportunities in the new job, for he replied, 'Unlimited,' and hung up.

When Mott reported to NACA he was assigned to the operation that stood at the very heart of Langley's contribution to the nation, the vast wind tunnel in which models of the best airplanes in the world were tested and improved upon. It was a huge white building, two blocks long, of astonishing shape: 'Looks like a monster doughnut covered with confectioner's sugar that somebody squashed from two sides so the hole almost disappeared.'

The speaker was a white-haired engineer named Harry Crampton, who had worked in the smaller Langley tunnels for thirty-one years and who now supervised the masterpiece. 'We call it the Sixteen-Foot Tunnel,' he said, pointing to a diagram of the multimillion-dollar center, 'because here, where the wind reaches its maximum speed, beyond Mach 1, the cross section is sixteen feet. That's enormous. You can place your model in the center and it will avoid turbulence occurring along the walls.'

He led Mott into the tunnel itself, a cavernous affair with enormously thick and polished walls. Its crushed-doughnut design meant that it had two fairly long straightaways, four abrupt 90° corners, and two short connecting arms. 'A very narrow capital O might be a better description,' Crampton said, and Mott, in his desire to be cooperative, made his first mistake: 'Some scientist did a good job here.'

Crampton stopped, stiffened, and in the gloom of the great tunnel, said, 'Scientists are men who dream about doing things. Engineers do them. This was designed by engineers, built by engineers, and is run by engineers. You're an engineer, young fellow, and you're to be proud of it.'

'I'm sorry,' Mott said.

'You thought that if an engineer was real good, he became a scientist. It's the other way around. If you want to be an engineer but find you have ten thumbs, you become a scientist.'

He led Mott on a walk-through of his tunnel, counterclockwise from where it narrowed. At the first squared-off bend stood an axle from which protruded twenty-five huge wooden propeller blades, so exquisitely shaped that they cleared the tunnel walls by less than an eighth of an inch. When they revolved at furious speed they created a massive movement of air, and only a few feet farther on, a second set of blades caught this moving air, accelerated it, and whipped it down the back straightaway at a speed of over five hundred miles an hour.

'Twenty-five blades in the first set, twenty-six in the second,' Crampton said. 'Why?'

'To avoid resonance,' Mott answered quickly, and the old engineer was pleased, for if the sets had been identical, and rotating at their enormous speeds, the moment would come when they would spin in harmony and set up a vibration that would tear the building apart. With a 25–26 ratio, that harmonic resonance could be avoided.

The propeller blades were made of a handsome white spruce, and Crampton asked why, but Mott could not answer. 'I'll give you time to think about it,' the older man said as he led Stanley between the stationary blades and into the long straightaway. 'Here's the secret of any wind tunnel. The air comes roaring off the propellers, and you gradually broaden the diameter of the tunnel so that a huge mass accumulates, traveling relatively slowly but at high pressure. Now, here you suddenly constrict the diameter, so that the same mass of air has to rush through a sharply diminished opening. It must go faster. It reaches the speed of sound, and then as the diameter opens up, the speed of the air actually becomes supersonic.' And when Mott studied the interior of this great twisting worm, he realized that in no portion did the diameter remain the same for long; it was always either expanding or contracting.

'What we're doing is playing games with our mass of air. Slow it down, rush it ahead. The result? When it comes past the critical point, it's a monster gale.' Like a proud parent, Crampton looked at the test section, then laughed. 'But at the same time, the air is playing games with us.'

'In what way?'

'You understand what the sound barrier is?'

'Mach 1. About seven hundred and sixty miles per hour at sea level.'

'It varies according to temperature.'

'I thought temperature and altitude,' Mott said.

'Many people do. Only temperature. Now think a moment. The higher you go close to Earth the colder it gets. But the governing factor is temperature.'

Crampton leaned against the tunnel wall, polished like a jewel to allow the air to pass with minimum friction, and pointed to the handsome metal pylon to which vehicles to be tested were attached. 'Seems incredible, but three years ago we could move air past that stand at Mach 0.9, just under the speed of sound, or Mach 1.1, just over. But the tunnel would not allow us to study what happened close to Mach 1, which was where the mysteries happen in high-speed aviation. Breaking the sound barrier it was called. Many judged it to be impossible. Too many planes went haywire when they attempted it.'

'Three years ago you couldn't do it. Can you do it now?'

Crampton ignored the question. He tapped the carefully tapered sides and said, 'They must not allow any of the high-speed air to escape, because that's how we build up our miles-per-hour. But as the air approaches Mach 1 in this final constriction, so much accumulates in such a little space that it begins to vibrate, choke, flutter. It allows us to photograph nothing.'

'But just beyond Mach 1 it calms down?'

'Yes. We knew that if we could get the plane through that barrier, supersonic flight would be more predictable. This wind tunnel proved that. So the barrier became a terrible psychological and physical problem. I have some old schlieren photos in my office showing you how terrible. The whole tunnel seemed to vibrate and we honestly believed that no airplane could pass through and survive.'

'How was it handled?'

'Simple. A determined pilot named Chuck Yeager took his X-1 up to a great height, where the atmosphere wasn't too heavy, and flew right through the barrier, but in our tunnels we still couldn't analyze the science of it, and when other pilots tried to break through it, they crashed.'

'I always thought the English broke the sound barrier. I saw this movie in which Ralph Richardson's son . . .'

Crampton groaned and lowered his head, as if bearing a savage burden, one often borne before. 'Movies are going to destroy human intelligence. That damn-fool movie dealt with crazies who took their planes up and dived them, without control, until they accumulated speeds that tore them apart. Chuck Yeager took his X-1 up and flew it, under perfect control. All the difference in the world.'

'Did you get the wind tunnel straightened out?'

'Not me. A genius named John Stack.' He paused to consider how he could best explain to Mott. Then pride captured him. 'At NACA we solve everything, eventually. That's our job, and now it's yours.'

'This time, how?'

'Stack reasoned that if the tunnel was choking at Mach 1, it must be because it was receiving too much air. He concluded that we were feeding in much more than necessary, and it was his brilliant idea to come in here just before the throat and bleed off just enough of the supercharged air to allow the remainder to pass through without creating turbulence. Look at this photo.' And he showed Mott a high-speed schlieren photograph of an unsatisfactory model perched atop a narrow steel pylon, more than a hundred minute wires leading from a hundred sensors mounted on various interior parts of the plane. It stood in the midst of a wind roaring past at Mach 1, with the air eddies magnificently depicted as they swirled about the uneven protuberances. Even Mott, untrained in wind-tunnel analysis, could see that the wing on this model created far too much turbulence. And what was remarkable, the general body of air, even at Mach 1, was orderly and in no way turbulent. Mr. Stack, whoever he was, had solved his problem and opened the pathway to the development of airplanes that could break through the sound barrier almost as undisturbed as a horse-drawn carriage heading for a country picnic in 1903.

'At NACA,' the instructor said, 'there are no insoluble problems. Only time-consuming ones.'

And then as the two men stood in the throat of the tunnel, where the walls narrowed like the digesting portion of a python, Crampton placed his hand upon the chrome-steel pylon and said, 'You must treat Langley with reverence. It's a holy place, really, because without it we couldn't have proved that engine nacelles should be fused into the wing of the plane rather than stand exposed so that mechanics could service them more easily. We gave the plane forty additional miles an hour with that one. It was at Langley that we proved wheels drawn back into the fuselage after takeoff added another sixty miles. And it was here that we improved the bombers that subdued Hitler.

'The tunnel must be protected. And if you ever bring in a model with a loose bolt or a fragment of metal that might break off, you can destroy this tunnel.'

From his pocket he took a coin and placed it against the pylon. 'Let's imagine that you, Engineer Mott, have brought in a model which is defective. This little piece of metal is going to break loose. Now follow me,' and he walked swiftly down the darkened tunnel to the first set of twenty-five blades. 'We're traveling at six hundred miles an hour and we smash into these wooden blades. We shatter three, and their rubbish flies through here to strike the twenty-six blades, and the whole tunnel is rendered useless.'

Mott studied where two blades in the first set had been adroitly repaired, as if a jeweler had inserted small pieces of wood to fill the holes caused by some break-away piece of metal. 'Now you understand why we use wooden blades? If we used steel, which would in many ways be better, when a flyaway bolt struck them, their pieces would become bullets.'

Crampton touched the gigantic blades as a father might touch a son who had done well in games. 'When you work here, Mott, you work in a cathedral.'

It was a year before Mott got into the tunnel, for he was so good at designing models that Crampton kept him in that part of the operation. 'You're a real engineer, one of the best. You know materials and how to handle them. If I'd had you as my model builder fifteen years ago . . .'

'I'd like to start work in the tunnel.'

'And you should. I've been selfish, keeping you over here in the shops. But you'll be a better tunnel man for it.'

When he moved into the tunnel, one of seventeen creative engineers supported by twenty-three highly skilled model builders and mathematicians, he launched a series of experiments to identify the sometimes minute modifications that pinpointed improvements to be made in the full-scale prototypes of the aircraft before they were sent up the Chesapeake Bay for testing at the Naval Air Test Center at Patuxent River. He found his work totally absorbing, for it utilized all that he had learned at Georgia, Louisiana and New Mexico.

His life with his family, ensconced in a small white bungalow on the banks of the James River, with a small boat of their own, was the happiest he had ever known. His elder son, Millard, having been expelled from an exclusive school in New England, was idling his way through an ineffectual public school education, but he was behaving himself, and Christopher reveled in the waterfront, competing with other youngsters in one-man small-boat races. Rachel, indefatigably concerned about the problems of her society, had no Germans to teach English, so she directed her enthusiasm to black playgrounds around Hampton, where she served as a voluntary teacher's helper, taking over whole areas when regular supervisors called in sick.

The Motts, as a group, had found their niche, and even Rachel's mother, when she visited NACA, had to agree that her son-in-law had finally landed a job commensurate with his qualifications, but she did feel obliged to offer two criticisms: 'They're not paying you nearly enough, Stanley. And I hope that when you have a good hold on things here, you'll apply to MIT for a teaching position.' She could not believe that any really first-class intellect ever spent the productive years of his life at any place other than Harvard or MIT. Second-class men did rather nicely at Princeton or Yale, and for the others, there were the Western colleges that excelled at basketball.

Stanley and Rachel were amused by her mother's pretensions, and Stanley tried to explain that NACA was closely associated with the very Harvard and MIT professors whom she admired. 'Experts from those schools often spend weeks with us at NACA working on problems too abstruse for the university men to solve. In fact, last week I was working with two professors from MIT on the problem of how to bring a body traveling twenty-five thousand miles an hour in empty outer space back through the friction of the heavy atmosphere without permitting it to burn up from the tremendous temperatures generated.'

Mott had told the professors, 'If we ever send men into space, as Von Braun insists we will, the problem will not be getting them up into space. The Huntsville Germans are sure they can do that with rockets they already have. The difficulty will be getting them safely down. Through the atmosphere. At temperatures which cause ordinary metal to burn like paper.'

The three men studied this in abstract for three weeks, then conducted what experiments they could in the wind tunnel, but since it was obvious that they could never generate speeds of 25,000 miles an hour, they were again thrown back into speculation. They spent another six weeks drafting a report on the current status of bringing a metal body back through the atmosphere, and in the end made a one-paragraph recommendation:

> At the present state-of-the-art we do not know enough to make even tentative suggestions as to how this intricate problem should be solved, but we do know that our ignorance of the atmosphere above 65,000 feet will be a permanent disability unless immediately resolved. We recommend an intensive study of the atmosphere to a height of 200,000 feet and higher if present equipment permits.

This advice was so obviously sensible that when the MIT professors departed, the engineers in charge of NACA looked about for one of their men to head the study of the upper atmosphere, and because of Mott's excellent work in the wind tunnels, they gave him the job, and for the next two years he spent about half his time at nearby Wallops Island.

This was one of the low, marshy barrier islands of the Delaware-Maryland-Virginia peninsula, contiguous to Chincoteague, where the wild ponies thrived. It was a forbidding place, smothered in mosquitoes and buried in swamps, but its splendid beaches, curving like majestic scimitars, provided launching spots from which scientific instruments could be thrown high into the air by small, powerful rockets using solid fuels.

There were in these early days no commodious quarters for visitors, so that when one flew the relatively short distance from NACA installations at Langley to the frontier area at Wallops, one traveled from long-established order to disorder, from comfort to discomfort. However, the life on Wallops was so primitive, with great fishing and boar hunting and living in tents, and improvised meals heavy with carbohydrates, that most men enjoyed it: 'This is the Daniel Boone part of my life. My wife and kids sure as hell can't follow me here.'

At Wallops, America's fundamental research into the upper atmosphere took place, and the secret of the excellent results obtained—best in the world—was twofold: rockets and telemetry. The former carried sophisticated scientific instruments thirty and forty miles into the air; the latter reported what happened en route . . . up and down.

A specialist in telemetry explained his arcane art: 'Simplest way to get data, of course, would be to have the nose cone or payload of the rocket containing the instruments parachute back to earth so we could visually check them. Two problems: our rockets must fire out to sea to prevent land disasters; and the complexity and weight of the parachute system would negate the value of the shot. So we go two different routes.'

He took Mott to the radar range, where delicate instruments monitored every moment of a rocket flight so that speed, acceleration and atmospheric resistance could be determined. 'Look at the graphs the radar produces. They tell us everything.' The expert laughed. 'Everything, that is, except what we really want to know. So we fall back upon this final system.' And he showed Mott how the instruments sent aloft delivered electrical impulses to a kind of radio which relayed them back to earth. 'When we send this baby up, it can talk to us in code and report every slight change it encounters. We call it telemetry.'

Occasionally the instruments didn't work. A most intricate device would be placed atop a sounding rocket, complete with a score of telemetric devices, and it would soar the first five miles through the visible cloud layer, through the stratosphere and mesosphere, reporting perfectly on conditions there, but when it entered the ionosphere, where the data became critical, some small component of the instrument system, damaged by the physical stress of launch, would cease functioning and the shot would be scrubbed.

These failures irritated Mott, for he knew that he was on the verge of understanding the atmosphere, that mysterious ocean of air which seemed so evanescent on a summer's day but which was almost as solid as an oaken board when one wanted to penetrate it at one's own speed. He studied the best reports available, especially those of the Russians, who had done such good work, and he constructed the most beautiful diagrams of the atmosphere, using eleven different colors to indicate the bands which appeared to differentiate the varied characteristics of this great, unknown ocean.

He was captivated by two physical features that did not seem, at first glance, to be in any way associated with NACA's desire to bring a metal vehicle back through the atmosphere: the matter of temperature at various altitudes, and the spectacular manner in which pressure diminished as one rose higher and higher. He was not obligated to study these phenomena, but he was drawn to do so on the off chance that they might shed light on his basic problem.

He had always supposed, from his experience in climbing mountains and from what normal airplane flight proved, that the higher one went into the air, the colder one became, and his tests at Wallops confirmed this. At one mile up, it was cold. At two miles, it was noticeably colder. At nearly three miles in the Rockies, it was bitter. And on an airplane seven miles up, it dropped to −50°.

It continued this way to an altitude of about twelve miles, and then things went haywire, as if an entire new set of rules applied, for at sixteen miles, the temperature started to rise sharply until, at thirty miles, it was a comfortable +48°. But this soon changed, for at fifty miles, it dropped to a severe −110°, where it remained for some time.

But at about fifty-five miles, it started a dramatic leaping as if fire had been placed under the instruments; it reached more than +200°. And then at some point beyond which the Wallops machines could not yet soar, an almost unbelievable phenomenon would occur: the temperature of the atmosphere would be the same on all sides of the machine, but the side facing the Sun would accumulate so much radiation that it would heat beyond the boiling point, while the shadow side, only a few feet distant, would be −200°.

It was a crazy ambience, this vertical pillar of atmosphere, but it was the portion of the universe through which man must move if he wished ever to enter space, and its peculiar behavior was dictated by physical laws that could be unraveled if men like Mott had sufficient brains and enough rockets at Wallops Island to accumulate the data. There were, of course, other groups in various parts of the United States, as dedicated as he, working on similar problems related to space: How to build better rocket engines? How to combine more efficient fuels? How to navigate when there are no landmarks to refer to? How to construct suits in which men could live in a world of no pressure?

It was the latter concern which kept Mott focused on the problem of decreasing pressure as one rose through the atmosphere. At sea level it had been agreed that pressure was normal, 100 percent, but it diminished quickly as one climbed upward, until at the top of the Rockies it was only 50 percent of normal, and at five miles, it was so weakened that men required additional oxygen to breathe. If air pressure at sea level was judged to be 1, at sixty miles up, it became 0.000002, and so far as human breathing was concerned, oxygen and pressure both could be said to have vanished.

Mott spent several months analyzing this phenomenon and interpreting what it would mean to either a man or a machine, and he helped deduce the principles which would govern any flight into the upper reaches of the atmosphere. In doing so, he became so enchanted with this mysterious ocean of air that he would often stand on the beach at Wallops, not far from the primordial soup from which life had emerged three or four billion years ago, and watch with awe as one of his weather rockets soared into the air, bearing its precious little cargo of instruments which would send down arcane signals as to what was occurring aloft, and as it passed gradually from sight he would remain on the silent beach, imagining himself a passenger aboard that rocket, passing from cold to hot to burning hot and freezing cold, breathing normally in the first seconds, then feeling his throat constrict as oxygen became more rare, then gasping for one final breath of air that did not exist, before turning on the latest device of his imagination which would provide him with oxygen and proper pressure.

Like all such experimenters in these years, whether in the backwaters of America or the remote corners of Soviet Russia, Mott lived in a world of juvenile excitement, moving from one threshold to another like a boy with a chemistry set or a new collection of maps, always wondering, speculating, making wild guesses, and striving to thrust back a little further the frontiers of knowledge. One evening, as he watched the Sun already sunk throw its rays around the edge of the western earth to illuminate one of his radiosondes rising into the highest layers of the atmosphere, a hundred miles up, making it shine while Earth grew increasingly dark, he realized that with imperceptible steps he was making the transition from engineer to scientist, for with the skills of the former he was attacking the mysteries which preoccupied the latter, and he was increasingly proud to stand in both camps, a man who could at the same time control material things like metals and wind tunnels yet grapple with the ultimate mysteries such as life at incredible altitudes. His four published papers indicated the direction in which his mind was growing:

> Mott, Stanley and Crampton, Harry: *Effects on the Base, Afterbody and Tail Regions of Twin-Engine Airplane Model with Extra Low Horizontal Tail Locations at a Speed of Mach 0.7.* 1955.
>
> Mott, Stanley and Winslow, Elmer: *Aerodynamic Characteristics of a Delta Wing with a 75° Swept Leading Edge at Mach 2.36 to Mach 3.08.* 1955.
>
> Mott, Stanley: *Preliminary Tables for Estimating the Properties of the Upper Atmosphere as Derived from Telemetry Delivered by Rockets and Free Balloons.* 1956.
>
> Mott, Stanley: *Probable Structure of the Atmosphere at Heights beyond 350,000 Feet.* 1956.

As his work at Wallops drew to a conclusion, it was generally recognized by his associates that he knew as much about the upper atmosphere as any man alive, and they suspected that this mastery would serve as a plateau from which he would ascend to even greater understandings, not because of his undoubted ability but because the speed of change was so great that anyone who stood upon an eminence in these particular years would be thrown inescapably higher.

As often happened with men obsessed by abstract ideas, Stanley's mastery came at the expense of his family life. Because of his increasingly protracted absences from Langley, Rachel had to assume responsibility for the boys, and she witnessed daily how much Millard and Christopher needed their father. The older boy had become moody and insecure; the younger, assertive and rather difficult to handle. Judging that only a little fatherly care could bring the younger son, Chris, back into orbit, she directed most of her attention to Millard, now thirteen, and the more she saw of him the more disturbed she became, for he was definitely developing characteristics which, if projected ten years, would make him most unmanly.

The children of top-flight engineers and scientists, such as those one saw at NACA laboratories, were apt to be highly individualistic, and this did not disturb Rachel, but she did believe that boys should develop as boys and girls as girls, and it distressed her to see anyone confused about his or her status. Millard was definitely confused and she wanted her husband to do something about it.

As soon as the problem was presented to Stanley, in whispers upon his return from Wallops, he acknowledged that he must act quickly, and he suggested a camping trip to the undeveloped marshes east of Chincoteague, and the family responded enthusiastically. They borrowed a small truck from a NACA engineer, put together some informal camping equipment, including a Coleman stove, and were off, taking the ferry from Norfolk across the mouth of the Chesapeake to Cape Charles and then up the peninsula to an area as wild and forlorn as any in America, but also as powerful because of its relationship to the sea.

There they camped, netting themselves off at night from the ferocious mosquitoes and probing Assateague Island during the day for signs of feral pigs and strange birds. Young Christopher lost his boisterousness the first day and settled down to enjoyable explorations with his father: 'Look at the herons. Four kinds and the book shows only three.' With a heavy pencil he checked off each of the birds he saw, more than fifty, giving himself credit for some that not even Rachel could identify as they sped past.

Stanley spent many hours with the boy, leading the conversation when possible into the subjects of deportment and congenial family living. 'Are those boys the police arrested fun to be with?'

'The best.'

'What would you have done if you'd been arrested?'

'It wasn't serious. They didn't really steal anything.'

'They broke a window. They climbed into the store.'

'But they didn't take anything.'

'They were taken to jail. Have you ever been in jail?'

Mott called the local police for the address of the nearest jail, and one morning he took his sons to see what a stone-walled prison was like, and when they saw the heavy gates and the bleak corridors they understood a little better what their parents were talking about. Young Chris, in particular, was impressed: 'Mom, they ate from tin plates on long benches and every time somebody opened a door, somebody else locked it.'

'Boys who break into stores live in jails,' Rachel said.

The experience must have frightened Chris, for during the remainder of the camping trip he kept even closer to his father, so that by the time they packed for home Mott believed that he had reestablished contact with his younger son.

With Millard the problem was more serious, for the boy was not committing offenses against society which might one day land him in jail. He was at enmity with himself, and nothing that Mott senior could volunteer in an effort to penetrate the cloud in which the boy had immersed himself proved effective. 'Grandmother is still willing to pay your way into a good school.'

'I'll never go back.'

'Not to the same one.'

'They're all the same.'

'Millard, there must be a hundred schools—'

'They're all bullies.'

'One bad example.'

'Father, I don't want to hear any more about it. Let her keep her money.'

'It isn't a matter of money. When you grow up, do you want to be an engineer, like me?'

'I hate math.'

'All right, what don't you hate?'

Millard would confide nothing, so Stanley and Rachel together talked with him about the necessity of a college education, and she said, 'I know a dozen girls who grew up with me, really fine girls. They were like you, didn't want an education. Now they can do nothing.'

'They could do anything you do.'

'They could. But they don't.'

'What's stopping them?'

'College urges you forward to do things,' Rachel said, and in her case this had been true, for no matter where she had been assigned by good or bad luck, she had felt obligated to dig in, to do what was needed.

'To do what I do,' Stanley told his son, 'you have to have at least two different degrees. The men who move the firing stands around don't need any.'

'I'd like to move the stands,' Millard said defiantly.

'Of course you could,' Mott said quickly. 'It's a good job and those men are good men. But when a boy has the capacity . . .'

'I can't do anything that you're talking about,' Millard replied in an almost whining voice.

'Why don't we try this way?' Rachel suggested. 'You spend the rest of this year, Millard, thinking about the various things you might want to do. Tell us about them, and we'll tell you the steps you have to take.'

'For example,' Stanley said, 'if you want to be a policeman—'

'I hate jails.' And there the master conversation, the one that was to have unraveled difficulties, ended. Mott tried three more times to gain his son's confidence, but Millard had found in school or on the streets someone his own age with whom he preferred to discuss important matters, and this meant that his parents were permanently excluded.

Mott's attention to this vital concern was diverted when he was assigned by NACA to find the answer to the most fascinating question he had so far encountered in his adult life: 'Mott, you know as much about the atmosphere as any man we have. The Department of Defense is faced with a perplexing problem: How get a bomb or an aircraft back down through the atmosphere . . . before it burns up? They're assembling a top-drawer study group at our installations at Ames. We've nominated you because in the years ahead we've got to have someone here at headquarters who's conversant.'

The Ames laboratory of NACA was in California next to a naval air station south of San Francisco, and since Stanley's assignment there was not permanent, it meant that he could not bring Rachel and the boys west. They stayed at Langley and he saw them as often as he could on his trips back east to compare notes with men who were working on the reentry problem there. At Ames he occupied austere quarters, which satisfied him, for he was immersed in his challenging task.

'When you make the jump from aviation to space,' a scientist named Schumpeter said, 'you have to unlearn everything you've been taught,' and he held up the sleek, streamlined model of a Lockheed F-104, allowing the sunlight to play upon its needle-sharp stainless-steel nose and advance probe.

'Let's see this beauty in the air tunnel,' and he took Mott to the Ames tunnel, a vast affair, where they could watch how effectively this perfectly designed plane slipped through the air, its slim nose opening a path and its knife-sharp wings cutting through without making a disturbance.

'Perfect for its purpose,' Schumpeter explained. 'I worked on the provisional models and helped them eliminate the bumps and protrusions.'

Back in his laboratory, he laid the model aside, almost contemptuously. 'Not a single characteristic of that plane helps us with our problem. The F-104 flies in the air . . . we have to fly through it. It makes thirteen hundred miles an hour, we make twenty-five thousand. It spreads the air aside so that it can slip through, we build atmosphere up like a wall and have to batter our way through. And it flies through cold air, whereas we fly through friction temperatures so elevated we really cannot comprehend them.'

And then, with the aid of military rockets which climbed to great heights, he demonstrated the real problem: 'We're going to take this model up to more than eighty miles. Three stages. And when we get there, we're going to turn it around and fire two more stages to send it hurtling back through the atmosphere. Not as fast as a returning spaceship, but fast enough. And you watch what happens to that beautiful nose.'

Schumpeter led the entire team back to Wallops Island, and on a starry night they fired the three-stage Honest John + Nike + Nike almost vertically into the darkness, watching its first flames burn out at 20,000 feet when its second stage took over. It soared far out of sight, reached its apex, turned over, and began its headlong rush back to Earth. As it reached Mach 17 the two remaining stages were fired, driving the model thundering back into the thin but rapidly accumulating atmosphere at the blinding speed of Mach 20.

As the scientists and engineers awaited its return, Mott speculated: 'If we'd used those last two rockets to maintain our upward velocity . . .' He hesitated, for he was not secure in his knowledge of rocketry and did not wish to sound stupid in the presence of the team with which he would be working for a long time, but his proposal was so daring that he felt compelled to explore it.

A young engineer named Levi Letterkill anticipated him: 'Yes, if we'd maintained the upward thrust and goosed it with two additional rockets, we could have built up our speed to about eighteen thousand miles an hour, enough to throw us into low Earth orbit.' When Mott hesitated about making any response, the young man added tentatively, 'I've been told that if you can get up to twenty-five thousand miles an hour, you can escape low Earth orbit and go into orbit around the Sun.'

'Could our rockets tonight have produced such a speed?' Mott asked.

Letterkill stood silent, making calculations. 'Yes. We could have gone into orbit this night . . . or tomorrow night.' He hesitated, for as Mott was to learn, he was a cautious man working in unknowns where a miscalculation might prove disastrous. 'I think we might have wanted slightly more powerful rockets in the last two stages.'

'Are such rockets available?' Mott asked, and another member of the team answered, 'With big enough rockets, anything is possible.' Mott, remembering a dozen failures of the A-4s in New Mexico, concluded that it was going to be just a little more difficult than these men were saying.

When his team assembled all evidence on the vanished rocket and its payload—telemetric reports, optical observations, multiband radar records —Mott was startled by the conclusions a Department of Defense expert offered: 'Nine inches of the hardest metal we can fabricate burned away as if it was a dry board.'

Several experimenters asked for an elucidation, and he said, 'The thin leading point of the metal encounters molecules of atmosphere, battles against them, builds up a super heat, finds oxygen in the atmosphere and burns like chaff. When the point is gone, the next sixteenth of an inch faces the tremendous heat, and it burns, exposing the next point. And then the whole thing goes, one small point after another.'

'And remember,' Schumpeter said ominously, 'this model had to penetrate only part of the atmosphere and at only part of the speed our returning vehicle will have.'

A heat engineer said, 'If our model had encountered the true conditions, its entire substance would have been consumed.' In the night air a plane, its lights flashing, headed back to Patuxent River across the bay, and the men watched its progress. 'A plane like that,' the heat engineer said, 'could not possibly get back through the atmosphere. Every vestige except maybe the castings of the engine mounts would burn up.'

Back in California, the team went to work, always with the model of of the burned F-104 before it. 'We want something as different from that as possible,' Schumpeter reminded them, and the search centered upon that requirement.

The heat engineer established the three basic alternatives and disposed of two: 'We can come in with a pointed nose and burn up. Or we can use a heat-sink principle, which is entirely practical, except for one slight handicap.'

When members of the team wanted to know what a heat sink was, he explained easily: 'We construct a metal, an alloy of the most specific components featuring titanium, and we cover the entire leading edge of the vehicle with this alloy. When it comes thundering back through the wall of the atmosphere, the alloy accumulates the heat and doesn't burn at all. It simply absorbs it . . . dissipates it.'

'Even if the nose is pointed?' Mott asked.

'No, no!' The engineer laughed. 'You make the point sharp enough, the heat will burn anything, anything at all. So we've got to be talking about a blunter surface. But with a blunt surface, the heat sink will work.'

'What's the drawback?' someone asked.

'Weight,' and he put on the blackboard some figures. 'If we cover the leading edges of a blunt-nosed airplane with enough alloy to heat-sink the temperatures, the plane would weigh something like three hundred tons and would require fifteen or twenty of the engines we now use, which would in turn require fifteen or twenty times the amount of fuel. A heat sink is a marvelous idea . . . for a tank, not for an airplane.'

'And the practical alternative?' Schumpeter asked.

'Ablation,' the engineer replied, and for the first time Stanley Mott heard the miraculous word which would dominate his life for nearly two years. From his study of Latin at the high school in Newton, Massachusetts, he knew the word *ablative,* for it denoted a grammatical form much loved by Julius Caesar, a no-nonsense engineer himself. 'The ablative absolute,' his Latin teacher had explained, 'is used by men of action who don't want to waste words: *Ponte factō Caesar transit.* The bridge built, Caesar crossed it. Consider how effective this is. No bothering with who built the bridge or at what cost. The bridge was built, as a bridge should be, and Caesar crossed it.'

For some weeks Mott had concentrated on this amiable construction, using it correctly and effectively: 'Equation solved, I turned the page.' He did not crybaby about the difficulty of the chemistry equation; he solved it and got on with the job. In fact, the ablative absolute could be said to have become Mott's guiding principle in his education, and he was delighted to learn from a footnote in his Latin grammar that the ablative was one of the earliest cases in human language. It died out in Greek and the Teutonic tongues and did not even have a name until Caesar personally christened it. 'My case and Caesar's,' Mott said whenever he came upon a felicitous example.

But now he could not envisage any relationship between his grammatical ablative and the engineering one. 'An ablative material is one that merely wears away. It doesn't actually burn, although it looks as if it had charred. It boils away, or evaporates, one tiny bit after another, in the super heat. And it does so with astonishing slowness. Water, wind, fire, even heat can't destroy it in a hurry. But almost anything can wear it away . . . very slowly.'

The word in its two meanings was even pronounced differently: *ab'lative* in grammar, *a blayt'uv* in engineering. But Mott paid attention when the heat engineer demonstrated what might be achieved with a good ablative material: 'I have here a block of reasonably good material, two inches thick. With this blowtorch I'm going to produce extreme heat on this face. You'll see the material become white-hot, evaporate, and leave a residue which the air from this fan will blow away. But I'll hold the back of the thin block in my left hand, which will not even feel the heat.'

And he did exactly that. The blowtorch hissed its throbbing flame directly at the block of material, which behaved as the engineer had predicted: it charred but it did not burst into flame, and when the discolored material blew away, what lay underneath was not even discolored. Nor did the tremendous heat penetrate the block; it was carried away by the material as it was ablated.

When he completed his demonstration the engineer asked Mott to hold the block, and even at the point of maximum heat, Stanley could feel nothing, so effective was the ablation. 'What is the material?' Mott asked.

'Now here we have hope,' the engineer said. 'This isn't even a good material. It would last up there about one second. Char completely away. But I'm convinced that we can construct a material to our specifications—and it won't be just good, it'll be perfect. That's our job.'

For six months Mott worked with the Department of Defense reentry team and with experts from private business on the bizarre task of creating a new material that would fill a precise need in the space program, and after only a brief exploration of the problem and an analysis of what the various companies could provide, it became apparent that the contract for constructing the new material to specifications would have to be awarded to Allied Aviation, because their people had already begun investigating this problem. They had not by any means solved it, but at least they knew where the difficulties were going to lie, and it was in this way that Mott found himself once more working with General Funkhauser.

The man was amazing. Starting with a knowledge of ablation even more defective than Mott's, he was assigned by his company to supervise the project because the American managers had learned that this remarkable German could organize an effective team to attack any problem in either aviation or space. He had a general knowledge of everything and a specific skill in cajoling experts to work together, and when it came to serving as an interface—one of the bright new words—between private industry and government, he was a genius. 'After all,' he told Senator Glancey's committee in secret session, 'if I could work with a madman like Hitler and keep my head, I can certainly work with reasonable men like General John Medaris.'

The new material would be constructed of three components: a basic substance which burned slowly even under ordinary conditions, a fiber of some kind to provide tough resilience, and a binder. In the old days it would have been asbestos, flax-cord and glue, which together could have formed a fine sturdy material that would not burn in an ordinary gas flame, but now even better materials were required.

Each of the three components had to be invented separately, and the experts at Allied Aviation proposed some eighty different substances, each effective by itself but not particularly useful in combination. 'Two of them are always right,' General Funkhauser observed, 'but the third intrudes like an unwanted guest at a honeymoon.'

The search went on interminably, and so much superheated gas was wasted on burning away materials that were supposed not to burn that Mott began to wonder if the proper combination would ever be found.

While these studies were under way, Schumpeter was engaged in devising the proper profile for the space vehicle itself, not the giant structure that would sit atop Von Braun's rocket when it went up, but the small capsule in which the passenger would direct the flight, and the more he worked, with that shining F-104 on his desk, the bigger and bolder the ablative surface became, until one day in desperation he sketched on his blackboard a monstrous affair which looked not at all like an airplane but like a giant toadstool.

'It still has a protruding stem,' one of the team pointed out. 'That'll burn away.'

'We'll bring it in ass-backwards,' Schumpeter said, and for some minutes the team studied this remarkable proposal, which seemed to contradict everything known about flight, and gradually they began to see that what Schumpeter was proposing was really the only way to solve this difficult problem: if a pointed nose burned away, bring the damned thing home like the side of a barn, smear it with a foot of ablative material, and come bursting right down through the atmosphere with sparks flying as the material carried the heat away.

The team flew back to Wallops Island, where Rachel and the boys sat in their car off the base to watch strange blunt objects being thrown into the upper atmosphere by their father, who told them, after months of testing, 'We're on the verge of something great. The others have solved their part of the problem. I haven't.'

When Schumpeter's revolutionary structure proved that it could manipulate the upper atmosphere, the pressure on Mott and General Funkhauser to provide the proper protective material increased, and in the eighth month of their experiments they produced a masterful new material composed of silica-based granules in place of asbestos, a newly invented fabric instead of familiar ropes, and an epoxy in place of glue.

Schumpeter summarized the tests: 'This is a wonderful material. Perfect in every requirement, except one. It weighs five times too much per cubic inch.' And when he placed his calculations on the board they supported his objection: 'You've given me an excellent material for protecting Mack trucks on their way through Arizona. Now let's find something for a spaceship.' So Mott's team went back to work.

In many ways Mott epitomized his nation and his culture. Despite the fact that he had ignored the pioneering work of Robert Goddard, he had been forced by German successes in World War II to take rocketry seriously, and this had led him into making advanced studies of the upper atmosphere, and once he comprehended the nature of that mystical ocean he was driven to master it with rocket vehicles and imaginative instruments to measure the heating rate which would have to be neutralized before man could venture upward through the atmosphere, break loose from it, and then return through its fiery heat. His two most recent publications indicated the intensity of his study:

> Schumpeter, Karl and Mott, Stanley: *Controlled Rocket Experiments, Three Stages Up, Two Stages Down, Testing the Ablative Characteristics of Eight Alternative Configurations.* 1957.
> Mott, Stanley: *Nineteen Ablative Coefficients of Seventeen Fabricated Materials.* 1958. (Secret)

His speculation about the future had started with his innocent question on the beach at Wallops: 'If we'd used those last two rockets to maintain our upward velocity . . .' He had known the answer before he framed it; if his studies helped men to penetrate the atmosphere and return safely through it, the next step must be to shoot them into brief orbit, and after that to send them on sustained orbits, and from that platform to challenge the Moon, then Mars, then Jupiter, then the Galaxy, and on to the very edges of the universe.

How simple his first steps along this path had been: algebra in grammar school, trigonometry in high school, calculus in college, and now the majestic problem: If we should ever want to send a rocket to the Moon, what trajectory would we use? The questions, the possibilities were endless, and although he could not yet chart specific solutions, he saw with great clarity that the proper approach was to apply to each chance assignment his complete brain power, trusting that other men like himself were applying their power to their contributory tasks.

He worked nine weeks, incessantly, his glasses blurring from perspiration and from the fumes of his testing, and in the end he helped produce a master ablative material, light as soft wood, sturdy as hardened steel, quick to evaporate and carry away heat, but stubbornly averse to burning. When Schumpeter put *these* figures on his board he cried, 'We have it!' and one more step in the infinite process of commanding space was completed.

Funds for the kind of experimentation Stanley Mott was engaged in were provided by a grudging Congress, which often masked the purpose of the work by allocating the money not to NACA but to the military, for Schumpeter's studies of reentry applied equally to a ballistic missile of the Army, a rocket of the Navy, and a putative spacecraft of NACA.

NACA now had a staff of about 7,000, and with branch centers like Ames and Wallops Island, it controlled research facilities worth more than $400,000,000, so funding became a major problem. Fortunately, Lyndon Johnson, the power in the Senate, supported the aviation program and its ramifications in space, but he had to assign the difficult task of shepherding the necessary bills through Congress to the two Western senators, Glancey and Grant, and it was for this reason that Senator Grant saw less and less of his fragile wife, Elinor, who often stayed behind in Clay when he attended the sessions in Washington. As for visiting the NACA bases, which her husband had to do with increasing frequency, this she refused to do, whether she was in Clay or in Washington, yet she continued to protest whenever she saw a photograph or news story which indicated that Mrs. Pope had accompanied the committee.

Her principal concern, however, was not her husband's probable infidelity with the secretary of his committee, but the ominous fact that little men from outer space had been visiting Earth for some time and were about to make themselves generally known prior to assuming control of world government.

She had come upon her knowledge of impending invasion in a curious way. While waiting in her hairdresser's salon in her hometown city of Clay, she had idly picked up one of the lurid magazines provided the clients, but was repelled by the crime and sex it reported and was about to put it aside when toward the back a well-prepared advertisement caught her eye.

It featured the photograph of a world-famous scientist, Dr. Leopold Strabismus of Uppsala, a distinguished-looking man with large head, neatly trimmed black beard, and penetrating eyes which transfixed the reader. Mrs. Grant immediately liked this learned man, for he radiated assurance and knowledge, and she could almost hear him speaking his message:

WILL YOU BE READY WHEN THEY COME?

President Eisenhower knows about them. So do his Joint Chiefs of Staff. So does the Airlines Pilots Association. So does J. Edgar Hoover, and it is his job to keep this dramatic knowledge from the public.

Who are they? The Visitors from Outer Space. The little men behind the Flying Saucers you've heard about. You know, of course, that they have already landed at numerous places in America, but what you don't know is that they have organized a program for taking over our government and bringing sanity to our troubled world.

The advertisement went on to promise that if the reader joined Universal Space Associates—in California, of course—and paid its modest yearly dues, she or he would receive monthly reports on the activities of the Visitors and advance information on their future plans: 'You will be saved and the others won't.'

When Mrs. Grant returned to her home, her hair neatly arranged after her weekly visit, she was so haunted by the memorable features of Dr. Strabismus, and so concerned about his warning, that when she rose the next morning she hurried back to her hairdresser's with pad and pencil to take down the California address. When she wrote to USA she not only asked for information about the little men in their space machines, but also confided her abiding fears to Dr. Strabismus, hoping that he might give consolation.

I am a woman with a college education who endeavors to keep abreast of what is happening in my world. My husband is engaged in some kind of mysterious work with the government, and I am certain it concerns the Visitors from Outer Space that you speak of.

He refuses to tell me what his business is, and I am growing fearful that very bad things are about to happen to us and would appreciate hearing from you.

When the letter reached headquarters in a suburb of Los Angeles, a young woman, who represented one-third of USA, was about to address an envelope and mail back the glossy promotional literature that showed the actual landing of a flying saucer, when the name of the correspondent in Fremont caused her to hesitate. 'Dr. Strabismus, you'd better look at this! I think this woman's husband could be a senator on the Space Committee.'

From the second of the two rooms which constituted USA a tall, heavy, youngish man with a beard came to inspect the suspicious letter, which he held to the light at various angles. He asked to see the envelope, which his secretary retrieved from the wastebasket, and then he telephoned the reference desk at the local library. Elinor Grant, of Clay, Fremont, was indeed the wife of Senator Norman Grant, a leading member of the Space Committee, and the letter was obviously a transparent attempt to entrap USA. Dr. Strabismus was too clever to be caught in that bind. 'You haven't mailed her anything?'

'I was just about to.'

'Do nothing. Let me keep this.' And he took the suspicious correspondence into his office, where he placed it on his desk—to be studied gingerly as if it were a triggered bomb.

From his early days in Mount Vernon, New York, when he was Martin Scorcella—Jewish mother, Italian Catholic father—he had kept running only a few steps ahead of the police, and at one of the universities enlarged by the state of New York to accommodate the flood of World War II veterans, he had actually been arrested by campus security forces for retrieving the discarded mimeograph forms from which examinations for large classes had been printed, and had escaped punishment by brazenly confronting the university's authorities: 'Can you afford a scandal? Do you want the papers to know how many students bought copies of my exams?'

'Exams?' the dean of instruction had asked.

'Yes, exams. I've been doing it for three terms.'

The university calculated that young Scorcella had earned some $9,000 from his stolen pages and sent him flying. He landed in a small room in New Haven, Connecticut, where he wrote term papers for Yale undergraduates and sometimes graduates, an easy task, for he had a wide acquaintance with scholarly literature and a facile pen for adapting it. 'Creative plagiarism,' he called it.

He was never arrested by the New Haven authorities, for they could think of no local ordinance on which to charge him, but after he had composed some ninety different papers and theses, he awakened to the fact that he was working very long hours to help brainless young men compile the grades that would enable them to earn a great deal of money without working half as diligently as he, and he became quite irritated by the unfairness of such a system.

His numerous papers in physics and geology, including three doctoral theses, had generated a sincere interest in science and an appreciation of its limitations. When excitement over flying saucers became a national fever, he foresaw that with the intellectual climate in such turmoil any bright young man capable of manipulating it was going to earn himself a fortune, so he grew a beard, which lent force to his powerful face, took down his sign DIPLOMA BY YALE/EDUCATION BY SCORCELLA, and awarded himself the name Leopold Strabismus, borrowing the first from Leopold Stokowski, whose Bach transcriptions he liked, and the second from a medical term he had used in a thesis.

For about five months he brooded in Mount Vernon, trying to visualize some operation that would place him at the center of the scientific revolution which he knew was coming, and consistently his mind reverted to the word *space* as used in the popular newspaper stories about 'the little men from outer space.' He saw that this was going to be the charismatic word which would unlock enormous possibilities, but his first attempts to capitalize upon it in New York were unproductive; he then realized that the really effective manipulators of such projects were headquartered in California: 'They have an unlimited supply of whackos out there.' He kissed his mother goodbye, moved to Los Angeles, and hired a secretary who loved the nonsense of life and an adroit Mexican-American named Elizondo Ramirez, who was exceptional in handling both minor forgeries and major business deals.

He spent three months preparing the advertisements that would appear in the cheaper magazines, choosing each word to achieve major appeal, but at the end it was Ramirez who gave him the most effective ideas: 'Chief, the best ads in this field I've ever seen, you standing in front of a wall containing six or seven framed diplomas, only the name of the university showing and best if it's in Europe.' Ramirez visited offices throughout the area, taking surreptitious photographs of surreptitious diplomas, which he delivered to an ingenious printer for copying. When the handsome documents were stood along the wall, and the time came to select Leopold's major degree, the one to be featured in the ads, the two men vacillated between Utrecht, the Sorbonne, Vienna and Uppsala. Strabismus inclined toward the middle pair, but Ramirez warned: 'Chief, half the quacks out here use either Sorbonne or Vienna. Stay away from them.' In the end they chose Uppsala because its double *pp* produced a fine scientific ring.

When it came to naming the great research center, Strabismus found that he was not happy with any proposed so far and started over. Ramirez applauded this decision: 'Everything depends on the right name, like a story I saw the other day,' and he produced a clipping about an elderly lady who had given UCLA three million dollars. When asked how she had accumulated so much, she said, 'I knew I knew nothing about stocks, so I just ordered Merrill Lynch to put all my husband's insurance money into Americans and Generals.' When the reporter said he was still confused, she explained: 'I knew that any company that was allowed to have American or General in its name had to be good.'

The problem was solved by the secretary: 'So what are the best initials in the country? USA.' And Strabismus cried, 'The S could stand for *Space.* What are the others?' The three conspirators tried many solutions, but again it was the girl who produced the winner: 'Universal Space Associates. I like the *Universal* because it sounds big and out there. And *Associates* gives the sense you're in the middle of the operation.'

Many of the agency's most effective financial devices were contrived in these group brainstorming sessions. 'Chief, best trick I ever saw, a doctor doing the cancer bit in Long Beach. Had a cure, seafood and walnuts, which brought him a lot of dough, but then we organized a circle of subscribers all across the country, and for seventy dollars extra a year we'd send them four personal telegrams reporting on last-minute breakthroughs. You'd be amazed how much extra those telegrams brought in.'

USA proved much more profitable than Strabismus had anticipated, and he could have moved into more spacious quarters, with another four or five secretaries, but he took delight in running the research institute from the two cramped offices and with only his two original helpers: 'I love the power of words. I get a real thrill out of sitting here and drafting the material that's going to bring us millions one of these days.'

The approach, as perfected by Ramirez, was simple: 'Send us $44 and we'll share with you our secret discoveries.' For an additional $52, anyone really interested in the future of the world would receive every month an urgent letter signed by Dr. Strabismus himself, advising on recent activities of the little visitors. And for $76 more a year, one could receive telegraphic communication when events of shattering importance were about to happen.

The three scientific investigators garnered over $80,000 that first year, aided by the flurry of flying saucers landing across the country, and when a hungry press invented the name Unidentified Flying Objects, Strabismus grabbed onto the acronym UFO and used it in all his advertisements, which made him a world authority on UFOs. It was then that his oratorical and television notoriety began to blossom.

He learned that the United States contained several centers which could always be relied upon to produce major paid attendance for any symposium on UFOs: Boulder and the Denver area were very reliable; Dallas and Houston were high on the list; Miami was reliable and for some reason Seattle was good; New York was unreliable and cities like Philadelphia and Washington were disasters, showing little real interest in serious scientific experimentation; but the best of all was Boston, because meetings held there could be depended upon to attract skeptical professors from Harvard and MIT and also bright young men from Route 128, the Highway of Genius on which many of the nation's major scientific firms were located, and these men sensed that they must be attentive to all ideas circulating in their society, no matter how abstruse or downright crazy. Many of their most effective discoveries had begun with ideas no less insane than those promulgated by Leopold Strabismus.

In four years the outfit, still consisting of only three people, was clearing $190,000 a year, with unlimited possibilities, and it was therefore no trivial investment that Strabismus sought to protect against the danger represented by Mrs. Grant's letter. When he discussed the matter with his associates he warned: 'This is probably masterminded by her husband. Tempting us to commit fraud through the mails. Let's sit tight on it.' But three weeks later USA received an even more urgent letter from the senator's wife, begging for assistance because her husband still refused to divulge what he was up to.

'When am I scheduled into Boulder?' Strabismus asked his secretary, and when she said that he had a major speech at the university four weeks hence, he directed her to send Mrs. Grant a carefully couched letter informing her that unfortunately the doctor was absent for consultations with leading scientists from Europe, but that he would be in Boulder on April 16 and would be most happy to consult with her, should she care to make the short trip from her home in Clay.

She attended the speech, listened with intense interest as he fended off critics from the Denver scientific community, and realized that she had at last come into contact with a man who understood what was happening in the world. She surprised him by suggesting that he drive back to Clay with her in her car, and when she heard the secret details of how little men had already landed, assumed human form, and infiltrated the highest levels of government, she was terrified by the danger not only to the United States but to humanity in general.

'Ah, no!' Strabismus reassured her. 'We have every reason to believe that these visitors are amicable. With their superior intellect and technology, we should expect only the most beneficent assistance . . . if we listen to what they say.'

'Are we listening? I mean, men like my husband, in positions of power?'

'No, we are not.' As he stared at the empty plains, overpowering to one raised as he had been in crowded New York, he confided: 'These plains remind me of what the little men told me about parts of their planet.'

'You've seen them?'

'Of course! My first contact with them launched my dedication to research on other worlds.'

'Were they indeed kindly, the ones you met?'

He explained how they had sought him out because of his advanced work on extraterrestrial societies. 'It was in a valley north of San Francisco . . . well authenticated in the literature. They landed about three hundred yards from the highway and signaled me to join them.'

'What were they like?' Her curiosity was insatiable, and Strabismus seemed always to use just the right words to sustain it. He sounded plausible and generous, and the fact that the little visitors had selected him as a major emissary to the people of Earth did not make him either arrogant or selfish.

'I intend sharing all I know with people like you, Mrs. Grant, so that when the visitors take their first steps in controlling our government, they'll find reliable support.'

He stayed at the Grant home for three days, a tall, distinguished scientist with a dark beard, and when he departed for California he took with him Mrs. Grant's joining fee of $44, her $52 for the monthly special report, and her $76 for the telegram service, which he especially urged her to subscribe to: 'It'll happen like the bursting of a bomb at dusk on the Fourth of July. Poof! They'll announce themselves. You should be prepared.'

And because USA was about to enter negotiations with the little men which might prove determinative, Strabismus left Clay with a special check for $2,000 to cover expenses of these meetings at various spots around the world. A widow in Dallas had contributed $125,000 to cover some of the expenses, and a retired Army officer in Seattle, who had married well, had given $23,000.

When Senator Grant returned home to mend his political fences during the summer recess, he found to his dismay that his wife had mailed four checks to an outfit in California for a total of $5,360.

'What in the world is this for?' he asked.

Elinor was evasive: 'While you've been wasting time on your precious committee and its pretty secretary, I've been working, too.' He inquired on what, she showed him some of the Strabismus literature, and after he studied it carefully he satisfied himself it was fake. He was shocked to think that his wife had fallen prey to such nonsense, but when he tried to discuss the matter seriously, she rebuffed him with a series of arguments she had heard Strabismus use with great effectiveness when silencing his critics at Boulder.

'You don't believe, Norman, because you've been conditioned to ignore psychic evidence.' When he asked what psychic evidence had to do with flying saucers, she said, scornfully, 'Because you haven't seen them yourself, you reject the reports of great scientists who have actually met and consulted with the visitors.'

'What great scientists?'

'Dr. Strabismus, for one. He's met with them and is privy to their plans.'

Elinor's use of such precise and almost learned phrases as *privy to their plans* when discussing such nonsense disturbed the senator, and he called friends in the FBI to obtain information on Strabismus:

A harmless quack thrown out of New Paltz for stealing examination papers and out of New Haven for writing graduate theses for Yale students. Runs a three-man so-called research operation into outer space from a two-room storefront in Los Angeles, from which he sells by mail services relating to the arrival of little green men. Also solicits personally, but the postal department can find no evidence of fraud, nor can we. Preys upon frightened women especially.

The senator could not confront his wife with these actual findings, for his relationship with the FBI had to remain confidential, but he did ask Mrs. Pope to employ a detective to investigate Strabismus, and when that operative uncovered many of the same facts, he was free to place them before his wife.

'The man's name is Martin Scorcella. He was a cheap thief in college, a plagiarizer at Yale. He never saw Sweden, and I'm sure he never saw any little men in California.'

With a power that Grant had never suspected in his wife, Elinor rebutted everything the detective and the FBI had reported. 'He told me all about his early years. New Paltz was the college you're speaking of. The professors were against him, and he outsmarted them. Yale University begged him to become a full professor, because he knew more than any of the undistinguished men on their faculty. And he did see the little visitors who confided their plans to take over this country. It may surprise you to know it, but one of President Eisenhower's closest advisers is a man from another planet in disguise. They're in your precious Navy, too, in positions of high command and in most of our leading banks. You're in for an awakening, Norman Grant.'

When $3,000 more of their savings fled to California, Grant realized that he must enlist the help of someone outside his family to convince Elinor of her folly, for he was obviously powerless to do so, and he asked Mrs. Pope if she knew any reliable scientist in the NACA community with whom he might talk on a matter of extreme importance. 'I want a stable man of excellent background and wide knowledge of the space field.'

She suggested several names but could recommend none without reservation, for some were too old to be informed on recent developments, and some were too specialized, but at this point a visitor from the Virginia headquarters arrived in Washington with a report on what the experts at Ames in California had decided about the problem of ablation, and Mrs. Pope decided on the spur of the moment that he was precisely the man required. 'I've never seen him, Senator, but I do know his record, and it's superb.'

When she slipped into the meeting room in which General Funkhauser and Stanley Mott were demonstrating to the committee the qualities of the material they had confected, she saw, standing behind the lectern, a slim, youngish man with glasses, and when she whispered to a staff scientist she knew, he assured her that that was Mott. She listened to Mott's complete presentation, his precise, clipped New England manner of speech, always finishing every sentence, and it was easy to believe that he was as capable as her informants had said.

She listened to his difficult vocabulary, both as an intelligent layman and as an employee of the Space Committee, and what she heard was pleasing: 'I believe that with this material, which is expensive per cubic inch but not excessively so, we have solved the problem of reentry.'

'Any practical use in everyday life?' Senator Glancey asked.

'It's very light. It could be used to insulate airplane engines, I would think.'

'Who will own the patent?' Glancey asked.

'Allied Aviation,' General Funkhauser said.

'I should think that if the government, through NACA . . .'

'Senator,' the general said, 'we have paid most of the developmental costs.'

'But who provided the basic concepts?'

While the discussion continued, Mrs. Pope signaled to Professor Mott that she wished to see him, and he left the podium to join this attractive brunette, who said, 'Senator Grant would like to speak with you in his office.'

'Me?' He followed her, wondering what kind of error he might have made, and was completely unprepared for what followed when he was alone with the senator, whom he had never before seen.

Grant was now a heavyset man, but very straight in bearing and military in manner. 'Sit down, please. Mrs. Pope tells me that you have an excellent record in NACA.' He pronounced each of the letters separately rather than as an acronym, the way others often did.

'I'm grateful for the chance to work with such an exciting organization.'

'Mrs. Pope tells me you know a great deal about space . . . outer space, I think they call it.'

'Others know more.'

'But you are keyed in? I mean, you do know what you're talking about?'

'I've studied.'

'Good.' The senator rose and stalked about his office for some minutes, then stopped before Mott and asked abruptly, 'You will swear to keep what I say confidential?'

Since most of what Mott heard these days was confidential, he found no trouble in nodding.

'Professor Mott, tell me the truth. Are there any little green men?'

Mott was stunned. He had often read with contempt newspaper stories of people who saw ordinary things like the planet Venus or an escaped balloon and called the police to report a ship from space. Whenever his rockets were active at Wallops, he could depend upon someone's having seen a UFO that had landed just down the road to unload little men who had fanned across the countryside. He was perplexed as to why the invaders were always little, always men: 'If you consider our Galaxy, our Sun is rather small, so there's about a sixty-forty chance that if some planet did have people, it would be attached to a very large sun and might be quite large itself. The chances are therefore better than fifty-fifty that newcomers would be not smaller than us, but larger.' But always, he went on, the invaders were little, because the first postwar reports had said so, and as for the *green*, that description came not from observers who met the little people, but from the eager imagination of the first newspaper reporters who had recognized a good story when they heard one.

'So far as we know, Senator Grant, no living human being has seen a visitor from another planet, and we have no believable record that anyone in past ages saw such visitors, either.'

The senator breathed deeply. 'My wife says she has seen them, landing on a mesa in Arizona, and she's talked with a man in California who has met and spoken with them.'

Mott was trapped. If he laughed, he might infuriate a senator of paramount importance to NACA, and if he supported the crazy wife, other scientists would hear of it and brand him a fraud. As an engineer he favored blunt speech, and as a scientist he had to respect evidence and condemn fraud; he could not bewilder this troubled man who had sought his advice. 'Senator, your wife is being hoodwinked. Has she given this man good money . . .'

'Nearly half our savings.'

'Definitely fraud.'

'No. The postal department says the man makes no criminal claims. And it isn't extortion because she gives him the money willingly.' He produced a small bundle of material from California, much of it bearing the charismatic bearded countenance of the great scientist. One quick glance assured Mott that this was typical pseudo-science rubbish.

'This would be amusing, Senator Grant, if it weren't so persuasive . . . so capable of doing damage. Could I meet your wife?'

'She's back home. Doesn't like Washington too much.'

'She's fallen into rather ugly hands, Senator. When I return to California, I'll look into this.'

'No scandal, Mott.'

'It's already a scandal if this man is persuading your wife to hand over your savings.'

'I mean, no publicity.'

'I would never tangle publicly with a man like this. But I'd like to see what he's up to. Gives science a bad name.'

When Mott returned to Ames, and the clean-up work on ablation, he excused himself for several days, and with travel orders provided by Mrs. Pope, dropped down to Los Angeles, where he located in a nondescript suburb the national headquarters of Universal Space Associates, only to learn that Dr. Strabismus was absent, giving a lecture in Boulder. His questions about the intellectual research projects of the Associates were neatly fended off by the secretary, a bright young woman, and those dealing with finances by Mr. Ramirez, who seemed especially quick with figures. However, Mr. Ramirez could not recall what bank USA used for the deposit of the funds: 'That's all left to Dr. Strabismus, and he's on a lecturing trip.'

'When will he return?'

'Not till Thursday,' the secretary said.

'Good. I'll be working at the Jet Propulsion Laboratory in Pasadena, and I'll be back Thursday.'

'Are you government?' the secretary asked.

'Yes.'

'I just remembered, he'll be heading directly to Seattle.'

'I shall meet him in Seattle, and if you and Dr. Strabismus play tricks on me you'll go to jail.'

'Have you any credentials?' the young woman asked brazenly.

'I do,' and he produced his NACA identification.

'He's at home,' she said evenly. 'If you can wait . . .'

'I'll wait.' And within a few minutes the distinguished head of USA appeared, tall, well-dressed and shrewd.

'Come into my office,' he said, and when he led Mott into the second room, Ramirez disappeared. It was a messy place with a large flat table on which Strabismus worked on the printed materials which provided his fortune. 'Who sent you?' he asked.

'A gentleman high in government,' Mott said, and he expected his words to have a sobering effect on the scientist, but Strabismus laughed.

'Isn't it obvious, Mr. Mott, that if you take any intemperate steps, Senator Grant will be hurt much more than I will?'

Mott swallowed. This was going to be much more difficult than he had foreseen. 'There are ways to investigate men like you . . .'

'The postal department, the FBI investigate me regularly. I'm completely clean.'

'You're stealing from gullible women.'

'Half my members are men, Mr. Mott. Some are men just like yourself who are sick and tired of the pretensions of established science. I advise you to go back to your duties in Virginia. Don't be tricked into doing the dirty work of a befuddled senator whose brilliant wife sees the new light.'

Indicating the brightly colored pamphlets on the table, Mott asked, 'How many contributors do you have?'

'Fellow explorers? Mr. Ramirez would know that . . . he's out.'

Mott proved unable to unnerve Strabismus, for the doctor had learned at New Paltz and Yale that the law protects the abuser much more than the man abused, and since he had been ultra careful never to transgress the laws of solicitation by mail, there was little the government could do about him. He was selling dreams to bewildered persons, and that was no crime.

'Don't you see?' he asked Mott as he engineered him toward the exit. 'I depend on you. It's the explorations you men at NACA conduct, the pronouncements you make, that agitate my clients and send them running to me. The more you succeed, the more confused the world becomes, and the more I'll be needed. Now you go back to your test tubes and rockets and do my work for me.'

Mott was so angered by the man's insolence that he left California determined to combat the fraud, and when Mrs. Grant next returned to Washington he hurried up from NACA to show her how callously the California guru was abusing her. For reasons he could not have explained, he insisted that Senator Grant be present at the interview, but when he stood before these two leading citizens he felt quite out of place, a rather small man with eyeglasses confronting a handsome senator and his well-coiffed wife, but he had work to do.

'Mrs. Grant,' he began hesitantly, 'I've looked into Universal Space Associates and I must advise you that it's a cheap operation of three irresponsible people in a pair of dirty rooms. I have photographs of the place.'

When he produced his snapshot of the mean quarters, Mrs. Grant refused to look at it; instead she smiled slightly, her lips primly together, as if she held a secret that these two men could never comprehend. And as he proceeded with his deflation, introducing more and more evidence, her smile persisted. No matter what he said, she had anticipated it and erected her defenses against it; in the end he accomplished nothing.

He was flabbergasted, for he was in the presence of an intelligent college-trained woman who simply refused to accept evidence. But this was not the heart of the matter, for when he finished—humiliated by this woman's calm belief—she clarified her reactions by handing him two publications from Dr. Strabismus. The first was entitled *If They Try to Attack Me* and was as clever a bit of writing as anything Mott had ever encountered; in beautifully phrased paragraphs with the shrewdest headings possible, the California charlatan had refuted in advance every line of reasoning an ill-spirited critic might advance, and Mott blushed to see how completely Dr. Strabismus had forestalled him:

> They will say I was arrested at Yale University.
> They will tell you that the Air Force has never seen a Flying Saucer.
> They will try to convince you that Visitors have never been seen by
>   reliable witnesses.
> They will say that we do not do reputable research.
> They will deny that Visitors are among us right now.
> They will abuse you if you tell them that Visitors are participating
>   in President Eisenhower's Cabinet meetings.

After Mott read this masterful pamphlet, he laughed and said, 'I wish NACA had writers this good.' But when he looked at Mrs. Grant she was not laughing. She merely showed that complacent smile, pleased that she had routed her two enemies.

It was the second publication which shocked the two men, for Elinor had never previously shown her husband the kind of frenetic letter Dr. Strabismus mailed at the start of each month to his $52 subscribers:

> Alert! We have learned definitely from a meeting of Visitors held aboard a spaceship in the South Atlantic to which they invited two of our associates, that the Visitors have grown distrustful of the behavior of the Eisenhower Administration and are going to reveal themselves and take over the United States government next Tuesday.
>
> The historical event will occur at eleven o'clock EST and you will find in every community, and especially in your own, citizens whom you have known favorably who will disclose themselves as Visitors who have been working among you to test you. Be as cooperative as humanly possible, for upon their good opinion of us in these early hours will depend the safety and continuance of this nation.
>
> LEOPOLD STRABISMUS
> *Universal Space Associates*

When the two men finished the communication, Mott reading over Grant's shoulder, they looked up to see Elinor smiling triumphantly. 'It all ends Tuesday,' she said, 'this charade you've been playing.'

'Are you one of the Visitors?' her husband asked gravely.

'You will be astonished,' she said. 'In every community men will step forward and disclose their true character. You will be astonished.'

'Elinor . . .'

'You and your silly little Senate. You, Professor Mott, and your make-believe investigations at NACA. One snap of a finger and the Visitors will reveal more wonders than you could dream of in a thousand years.'

The men kept close watch on Mrs. Grant over the weekend, and saw that by Sunday she was in a state of euphoria, for the old world had only one more complete day to run, and she was preoccupied in planning for the new. She speculated aloud as to who in the Senate and Cabinet would step forward at eleven o'clock EST to reveal himself as having been an agent of the Visitors, and she could think of only a few Republicans worthy of that role and no Democrats. Never for a minute did she consider her husband a possibility: he had condemned himself through his love affair with Mrs. Pope.

And then, about noon, on the fatal Monday before the changeover, she received a telegram from Dr. Strabismus:

Reprieve. At a last-minute meeting aboard the spacecraft I and my assistants were able to persuade the Visitors to grant President Eisenhower additional time to get the affairs of this nation organized in accordance with the dictates laid down by the superior planets.

The Visitors will not repeat not take over at eleven tomorrow. The Visitors working among us will not repeat not reveal themselves. They have agreed to be patient and watch how we handle this extra time. Everything now depends on Washington.

LEOPOLD STRABISMUS
Universal Space Associates

When she showed the telegram to the men they could not believe that she accepted such transparent nonsense, month after month, but after she gave them time to digest the tremendous news, and its implications for the future, she retrieved the message and clutched it to her, smiling gently at her critics as if she were privy to some profound secret denied them.

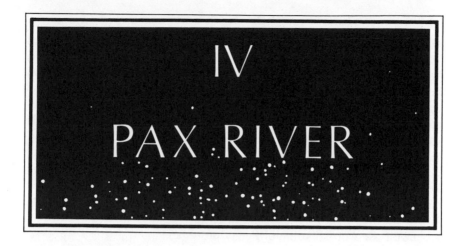

IV
PAX RIVER

NEITHER JOHN POPE NOR RANDY CLAGGETT WON ASSIGNMENTS TO
Patuxent River with their 1952 applications, and after the Korean War
ended they lost contact, Claggett going to a Marine squadron at El Toro
in California, Pope to the Navy installation at Jacksonville, on the opposite
side of the continent.

But the Navy command had spotted Pope as one of their most promising straight arrows, and after he had served at Jacksonville for only seven
months he received orders to report to the University of Colorado in Boulder to try for a Ph.D. in engineering, with minor attention to astronomy.
Naval officers, if they wished to progress in the service, had to have three
entries on their record: combat experience if a war was under way, advanced
education, and command of a fighting unit. Pope had performed his combat
duty with medals, and it was now assumed that he would do the same with
his next obligation.

But when he reported to Colorado's dean of engineering, that scholar
said, 'They've proposed a schedule for you that looks impossible.'

'I'm not afraid of work.'

'Engineering alone's a full-time program. So's astronomy.'

'I already know a little of each. I'm ready to try.'

The dean gave him an impromptu quiz, then telephoned for a professor
from the astronomy department to do the same, and Pope rattled off his
answers so confidently, not being afraid to say 'I don't know anything about
that' when the questions became too difficult, that the men agreed: 'You can
attempt it, if you wish.'

Like many successful men, Pope believed that whatever was required of
him to do at the moment represented the happiest experience of his life.
When he was playing football in Clay at age seventeen and first felt the
power in his body, he thought: This is the best thing I've ever known. The
four years at Annapolis, when he was courting Penny, 'were maybe the
happiest years I'll ever have.' The flying days at Pensacola, when 45 percent

of his associates dropped out because of deficiencies and nine men died because of faulty judgment, 'were maybe the most exciting days of my life, because it was then that I learned I could fly with the best.' Korea would be unforgettable because it tested his courage, and no man is entitled to an armchair opinion about that. Of the forty-three fliers most closely associated with him, eleven had perished and three were crippled so badly they had to leave the service. 'They were precious days,' he told Penny. 'Days like that come only once in a lifetime.' He rarely spoke about his experiences in battle, but one autumn night when he was touring Fremont, he sat in a Webster bar with Finnerty and his wife and said, 'Got a letter today from this Texan Randy Claggett. When I was downed in North Korea and the Slopes were closing in on me . . .'

'Don't use words like that,' Penny protested.

'Well, the Commies. It was a foot race. The baddies or the goodies. And Claggett spotted me from his Banshee. That's an airplane. And he vectored in the helicopter. I understand, Finnerty, why you feel attached to Senator Grant. I feel the same way about Claggett.'

Often at Colorado, when snow dusted the Rockies behind the campus, or elk came down to the lower levels to graze, or the principles of engineering and astronomy began to clarify, Pope would exclaim, 'These must be the best days a man will ever know!'

A succession of such judgments did not mean that the speaker was deficient in ability to discriminate; it meant that life was providing a series of graded adventures, each appropriate to its moment, and the recipient sensed this. Or as Claggett once said, 'I'm growin' up lucky.'

For Pope the days grew even better when Penny flew out from Washington to spend a weekend with him at some lodge high in the mountains where snow covered the trails, and where she sat with him before the fire, telling him of battles within the Eisenhower administration.

Their peculiar pattern of marriage, first with John's service in Korea causing separation and then her work in Washington keeping them apart, seemed to intensify their love, for they were certainly more dedicated than most military couples. They found each other interesting intellectually and more than pleasing sexually; their long absences built up desires which flamed when they did finally get together, and when they were forced by their demanding schedules to part, they did so with renewed assurance that their next meeting would be even more incandescent.

They were a fortunate couple, and they knew it, their sharp differences in political opinion merely heightening their sense of individuality. Every bit of evidence John saw strengthened his conviction that only Republicans could be trusted to organize society; every superior officer he had served under had been a Republican; all the men in the Senate who could be trusted to support the military had been so, too; and the few outspoken Democrats among the aviators he knew tended to be troublemakers with limited career possibilities.

Penny, on the other hand, watched in Congress as tough-minded Democrats like her Senator Glancey did the hard work and initiated the important bills. She felt that the Republicans she knew, even Senator Grant, for whom she had campaigned, tended to be cardboard cutouts of real men, and while they served a useful and precautionary purpose, if they alone were allowed to govern, the country would stagnate.

They discussed such matters frequently, and John took considerable umbrage at Penny's downgrading of Senator Grant: 'If you think so poorly of him, why did you bring me to Fremont to vote for him?'

'Because he's an honest man, much better than the imbeciles, Republican or Democrat, who ran against him. Besides, we need him on the committees. He does good work there, I will admit.'

'First you drag him down, then you build him up. Make up your mind.'

'Norman Grant is a space-filler. We have forty senators like him, on both sides of the aisle. But he fills his space with dignity.'

'I suppose your Glancey is the true hero?'

'He's a prime mover.'

It was amusing the way in which both the military and the politician sought glib phrases to summarize human experience—*front runner* in aviation, *prime mover* in politics—and when the phrase was apt, it served as a convenient intellectual shorthand. In the Navy these days the operative word was *outstanding,* with a long, heavy emphasis on the *stand;* one no longer used words like *excellent, very fine,* or *first class;* everything superior was categorized as out*stand*ing. In Penny's political world the in-phrase was *bottom line,* especially when used as a verb: 'It's a seductive idea which the voters will like, but first let's bottom-line it,' which meant that the profit-or-loss summary, which appeared on the bottom line of financial statements, had to be estimated.

'I think Norman Grant is out*stand*ing,' John Pope said.

'But when you bottom-line what he accomplishes, it isn't much,' his wife replied.

Their love reached its apex in a curious way. John, like all aviators, was infatuated with automobiles, and when a 1949 Mercury convertible crashed on the Boulder–Denver speedway, he bought the wreckage for $75, and with the help of two other officers taking advanced courses at Colorado University, rebuilt it into a fine, sturdy machine with a homemade canvas top weatherproofed by an expensive liquid concocted for the Air Force.

He used the Mercury primarily to run down to the new Air Force field at Colorado Springs to protect his flight status. If he flew thirteen hours a month, he received $185 extra pay, and he had come to depend on this money. Also, he needed to keep himself proficient in night flying, a demanding skill for which he felt he had a special aptitude.

He had never flown over terrain that was more exciting: to the east, the vast plains leading to his home state of Fremont; to the west, the mighty Rockies with fifty peaks higher than 14,000 feet and majestic plateaus bigger than some states. On days when the plains basked in sunlight and the mountains stood below him clothed in snow, the contrast was stunning, but on nights when the moon was full and the Earth below resembled the drawing for a fairy tale, he experienced a sensation of grandeur and unlimited national power which caused him to exult. It was a marvelous sky, a majestic land, and he felt himself master of both.

His studies were going well. As an adult now, with a wife he loved, he was able to avoid the wrenching dislocations which attacked many younger students, so that his unusually heavy burden of classwork became simply another hurdle to overcome. He worked about fifteen hours a day, concentrating on his slide rule in engineering, on the stars in astronomy. Early in his studies he realized that his overriding task was to handle the engineering courses well, and this he did, devoting most of his study hours to them, but he found that his early experiences in astronomy had given him such a solid foundation in that science that every minute devoted to the stars seemed to yield multiple dividends.

Their identification he had long mastered; now he was learning their mechanics, and every lecture or demonstration revealed new wonders that delighted him. He knew the color, size and distance of the most of the major stars and the significance of these measurements. He also knew the peculiarities of certain important stars invisible to the naked eye but of crucial meaning to the structure of the heavens: Barnard's star, which might be the only one in all the billions in the sky which could one day be proved to have planets like the Sun; Proxima Centauri, closest star to Earth; Epsilon Eridani, the near star most resembling the Sun in its characteristics.

What pleased him most, however, was his increasing knowledge of the mechanical structure of the Sun's planetary system, for he now had sufficient mathematics to follow the analyses of the great astronomers. He was especially delighted with the deductions of the French scientist Joseph Louis Lagrange, who, with the simple mathematics available to him in 1780, had deduced that when one massive object orbited another, five points developed in remote space at which very small celestial bodies could find refuge and remain stable despite the pull of the larger bodies. He spent some time calculating the five Lagrangian Points for the Sun and Jupiter, then tried to visualize what tiny heavenly bodies might be lurking there.

The reason why John's Mercury convertible became a significant factor in his love for Penny became apparent when spring vacation provided him with nine free days. Calling Penny to be sure she could arrange a brief vacation of her own, he jumped in his car, and with only a few dollars and a Conoco road map, sped eastward—eighteen hours a day, with a little sleep in the back seat when the convertible was parked beside the road with the improvised top up.

He roared into Washington remarkably fresh and rested, picked Penny up at Senator Glancey's office, went in to wish Senator Grant well, and headed back to Colorado.

He and Penny delighted in traveling like this: they rose at 0400 in the morning while it was still dark, dashed a little water over their faces, combed their hair, and zipped into the clothing which they had left piled on the floor when retiring. By 0415 they were on their way westward, watching the stars retreat before them as the Sun came up.

By 0930 they had covered nearly three hundred miles, for they drove steadily and at top speeds. They were hungry now, so they pulled up at some gas station and asked for directions to the best hash house in the district, and usually they received good advice. They were also tired from the five-hour dash, so they ordered a substantial breakfast and relaxed. John usually slipped into the men's room to shave while Penny read the local paper to see what this region thought of Washington, and after a leisurely meal of pancakes, scrambled eggs, hash browns, sausage, toast, jam and two glasses of milk, they returned to the rested Mercury and sped westward.

They followed interesting highways through West Virginia, Ohio and Indiana, where they picked up Route 36, which carried them into St. Joseph on the banks of the Missouri, and from there into Fremont, where they spent the night at their homes in Clay, John sleeping with the Popes, Penny with the Hardestys. From Clay it was an interesting gallop to Boulder and the vacation glories of the Rockies.

They never stopped for lunch, grabbing a few apples and cookies en route, and expected to cover something like seven hundred miles a day, except that when they hit the free and open spaces of the West they revved the convertible up to ninety miles an hour and sometimes reached eight hundred miles for the day. They stopped at 1930 for a bite of dinner, wherever they happened to be, and finished off the day's driving beneath the evening stars. At 2200 they stopped at whatever motel was available, kicked off their clothes, and went right to sleep. At 0400 the next morning they were wide awake and eager to be on their way.

The thing that made such travel rewarding was its cheapness—gas, 31¢; motel, $4.50; breakfast, $1.45—and the fact that they were seeing new aspects of America; it was also spiritually refreshing in that during the long drives they were free to talk. In fact, the best conversations the Popes conducted occurred on these trips, for the car became a cathedral-in-motion in which two worshippers convened to settle family questions of the highest moment.

'Where will the Navy send you after Boulder?' Penny wanted to know.

'Not overseas, for sure. I've done that duty.' She was relieved. 'But it could be Germany.'

For John, overseas consisted of only two things: a war zone like Korea or shipboard duty, especially in the Pacific. Germany was mainland and relatively close to home.

'We could manage Germany,' Penny said.

'You ever think about leaving Washington?'

'Not really. You know, John, I believe that if an important job opened up . . .' She paused, then said, 'I've worked with enough senators now to feel sure they'd confirm me for any job to which I was entitled.'

'The way you talk sometimes, you won't get an appointment with a Republican President in office—and after Eisenhower has two terms, Nixon'll have two.'

'Don't you be too sure of that.'

'Eisenhower's sure to be reelected. Best president we've had in a hundred years, and the voters know it.'

'I suppose he'll make it,' Penny said, 'but I'm not at all sure about Nixon being able to follow on.'

'The men I work with . . . Colorado . . . the Air Force . . .'

'They're all Republicans, John. But that's beside the point. What I mean is, I could very well be selected as legal counsel for some influential committee.'

'That would be swell!' John said with real enthusiasm. 'You could handle such a job, better than most.'

'None's on the horizon, you understand, but these things have a way of suddenly popping.'

'You ever think about children?'

'All the time. I wish we could have some.'

'You ever think about adopting some?' When Penny made no reply, her husband said, 'It's perplexing how things work out. Of all the men I know in uniform, I think I love my wife more than any of them, but we have no children. I know this skinny ape from Texas . . .'

'You mean Claggett?'

'Yes. He had this dipsy-doodle wife. College cheerleader or something. He shacked up with any Korean Jo-san who would have him, and I figure from what he told me one night that his wife did the same with anyone at Iwakuni. And they have three children. Beats all.'

'John, if a good job does open up in Germany, grab it. I'll spend my summers with you.'

'I'm quite sure it'll be stateside. We'll have a bundle of opportunities to work things out then. And if a really fine appointment should open up, make Glancey and Grant support you. And I mean really support.'

'I'll do that. Symington owes me a lot, and so does Mendel Rivers.'

'What do you think it might be, Penny?'

She sat close to him as the afternoon landscape rolled past, and for some moments she kept her forefingers to her lips. Then she said, 'Glancey is one of the very brightest men in America. I mean, this Red River hillbilly has radar. He always knows where the money is, where the skeletons are buried. But he also has a fantastic sense of what's happening in the world, and he's convinced that stupendous scientific miracles are about to happen. What scares the devil out of him, he believes it's the Russians who'll produce them.'

'Like what?'

'Like he doesn't know. But I'm infected with his enthusiasm, if that's it, or maybe his fear. I think we're on the verge. Commercial planes flying faster than sound. Some new kind of television. I don't know. But I do know that throughout world history . . .'

'You been reading a lot?'

'When you work for a man like Glancey, you want to read a lot. And what I've read convinces me that whenever there's a yeastiness in the air, great things happen.'

'You think we're in such a period now?'

'I'm convinced of it. Aren't you?'

'I did have a glimmer one night in Korea. After Claggett took his Banshee to fifty-six thousand feet, much higher than the specs said he could. You know how he did it? He had his mechanics hammer his tail pipes into a much more restricting outlet. Squeeze it down. This gave him greater thrust but also greater heat. When I warned him about it he said, "This bundle of bolts either breaks sixty thousand or explodes." '

'But you say he only got to fifty-six thousand.'

'Yes, he showed so much heat he knew he was going to explode.'

'What has that to do with the future?'

'That night Claggett told me he knew in his bones that man could fly anywhere, any altitude, any speed.' He drove in silence across the great prairie of the West, the land which early explorers had predicted could never be settled—Grand Island, North Platte, Julesburg—then added, 'He told me that every muscle in his body wanted to keep on flying upward. Only the machine faltered.' There was a long pause. 'He said our job was to devise equipment that didn't falter!' He laughed. 'You've never met Claggett. He talks like an illiterate. But when he's sharp on target he talks like a professor. "Devise equipment" was how he said it.'

When they came down out of the mountains after five days of probing the upper trails, sunburned and chap-lipped, they found a letter awaiting them from Claggett:

> Up the ass of them clowns in Korea. Back home I wangled an appointment to Patuxent River, which is three times as good as they told us. You fly everything, everywhere. Real frontier stuff, wild blue yonder and up your bucket. John, break your ass to get here. You're twice as good as anyone here except me.

When Penny read the letter tears showed in her eyes and she whispered, 'Get that job, Pope. It's so close to Washington, we could be together every weekend.'

So he wrote letters from Boulder, she from Washington, and just as John was completing his doctoral thesis he received notice of his next assignment: Test Pilot School, Naval Air Test Center, Patuxent River, Maryland.

· · ·

In Huntsville, Alabama, the family of Dieter Kolff was happier than any of its members had ever been before. There was enough food, assurance that the stay in America could be permanent if the Peenemünde people so elected, and much work to be done. Liesl tended her home, her garden and about ten acres of other people's woods with a peasant joy that enriched the lives of those who came in contact with her.

She did not appear much in public, for she realized that her dumpy figure and the odd way she wore her clothes set her apart from the rather well-dressed Alabama women and even from the younger German wives, who were adjusting easily to life in their new land. She was approaching forty now and had put on considerable weight, as German farm women did, and she felt that her place was in the home or in the woods of Monte Sano.

Her husband had carved a handsome walking stick for her, a heavy one cut from some local tree like oak, and with it she commanded her little forest, which she kept meticulously neat in the German fashion. Any fallen twig had to be picked up and piled in one of the spots from which her neighbors could obtain such firewood as they needed. Paths were to be raked and each spring the winterkill had to be broken into usable lengths, so that by the end of two years she had created not a woods but a park in which flowers were free to grow where before only pine needles had accumulated.

Her garden and her home were equally neat, equally fruitful, and sometimes whole weeks would pass without her thinking about her family farm opposite the island on which Peenemünde stood. Her English was so halting that she did not yet think or dream in that language, and she doubted that she ever would, but she did do her calculations in English, and German systems of money were forgotten.

She tended the family finances, especially the savings, and whenever her husband and her son brought her extra money from unexpected sources, she hurried it down to the bank and handed it to Mr. Erskine in discharge of the Kolff mortgage. Once when she entered the gray-stone bank building Mr. Erskine invited her into this private office, where he told her, 'I loaned money to ninety-one German families, almost no security. Not one has failed to pay me back on time, and you're ahead of schedule.'

This emboldened her to ask, 'If I pay all back, yes? Mr. Kolff and I borrow again, yes?'

'Of course! That's what I'm here for, to lend money, and your credit is A-1.' Then he asked what she wanted the money for, but she was embarrassed to explain. 'As a matter of fact,' he said while she fumbled, 'you could extend your loan right now.'

'What you mean, extend?'

'Well, instead of waiting to pay off the small balance outstanding, you could borrow what you need now, and make the balance that much larger.'

'You say I could have the new money now?'

'Right now. But the directors would have to know for what purpose.'

'I want to buy the woods.'

'How many acres?'

'Ten.'

'Do you need them?'

Mrs. Kolff considered this for such a long time that Mr. Erskine suspected she might not have understood, but she was thinking of how human beings hungered for land, and of how they never had enough land, and of how states and nations always lusted for more land, and how in the end men and women returned to the land, their dust to become part of the great inheritance, and she recalled what her father had often said: 'If a man is safe with ten acres, he's a lot more safe with ten times ten.'

'I mind the woods,' she said. 'I build the paths. I would like to be sure.'

'Do they stand next to your house?'

'They're part of it, and I like to be sure.'

'I'd like to see them,' and he drove her up the hill in his own car, and as soon as he saw the lovely park he realized the trap into which this woman had placed herself: by cleaning the ground and making the woods so attractive, she had increased its value to a point at which she could not afford to buy; with her hard and voluntary work she had destroyed her own dreams.

'I'm afraid you'd never be able to afford these ten acres,' he said.

'How much?'

'I could ask, but they would be very costly,' and later when he told her how much the owners wanted in comparison to what she and Dieter had paid for their original plot, she was appalled.

So she surrendered her dream of owning the park, but this did not deter her from tending it as before. Her major interest, however, became her son Magnus, only eight years old but such a strong trumpeter that he was asked to play in the school band and in the Huntsville orchestra as well. He was by no means a genius, but he was exceptionally good, with a knack for reading music at sight; it was as if he had some inner decoding device which enabled him instantaneously to translate lines and dots on a sheet of paper into clear notes on his trumpet, and his mother was delighted. Even the sound of his practicing pleased her, and she would often ask him to accompany her to the park when she did her work there, fancying that the birds listened approvingly as he played.

Music was important to Magnus but it did not preempt all his interest, for he loved to play rowdy with the boys at school or participate in soccer with the German boys on Monte Sano. He was freckle-faced, rather heavy for his age, with thick blond hair cut straight across his forehead, and although he did reasonably well in school, he found most of his subjects depressing. What he preferred was music and sports, and he was becoming outstanding in each.

He did not like to speak German even though he understood when it was spoken to him, and when his parents coaxed and bullied him to retain his mother tongue, he stubbornly refused: 'Nobody at school speaks German.'

'You will be happy one day that you know this language,' his father predicted.

'I'll learn it then,' he said with adult shrewdness.

He was a good boy, and when others in school got into serious trouble, he watched from the sidelines, too prudent to be lured into situations which were bound to result in punishment: 'If they catch you American kids, it's all right. Your father talks to you. If they catch me, my father beats me.' There was another deterrent voiced repeatedly by his mother: 'Remember, Magnus, you're not an American yet. They can send you back to Germany at any time . . . if you're bad.'

Liesl was not sure of her facts. Some of the German wives had explained that Magnus and their children, having been born in America, were automatically citizens, but she was certain that she and Dieter were not, so she assumed that if the parents were expelled, the children would be, too, and she used this threat to keep her energetic son in line.

But the day came in the fall of 1955 when the immigration commissioner and the local judge decided that it was in the interests of the United States for these Germans to be brought securely into American citizenship, so an impressive ceremony was staged, with Army officers in uniform and state dignitaries present to give speeches. As the solemn ritual began, the immigration man asked each of the applicants routine questions about the Constitution and the President, then certified them as having completed satisfactorily their course of prescribed study. The judge then asked everyone to stand, and in brief, emotional words, conferred citizenship upon these unusually valuable newcomers, and a woman in charge of the ceremony signaled that the town band should play. Stubby little Magnus Kolff, youngest member of the band, blared his trumpet sweetly to the strain *Mine eyes have seen the glory* and many eyes were moist.

Dieter Kolff himself was not doing well during these days when his wife and son were so happy; it was not that he was delinquent but that his superiors, especially Dr. von Braun, could not get their priorities sorted. No one could be sure, week to week, what the mission at Redstone was, or what the Army was proposing to do next, or whether there would be any money on hand come the first of the month. It was chaos, really, and sometimes the more thoughtful Germans would whisper at night, 'How did this nation ever defeat us?' And although they did not openly voice their next rhetorical question, they did ask it of themselves: How could this nation stand up to Russia?

The situation was this. Under the guidance of a Pentagon that did not understand rocketry or space—and which intuitively distrusted the field because it posed difficult new problems—and while the generals and admirals were composing glowing accounts of how they had won the last war with weapons they did understand, a deadly battle developed among the three major services, and whenever the specialists in one looked as if they might spurt ahead, authorities in the other two conspired to haul them back, which would not have been unproductive had the Pentagon provided a referee to adjudicate among the contestants, selecting the best of each set of proposals. But the man at the top was Charley Wilson, trained in building automobiles and tanks, and to him the whole prospect of expensive missiles which he would never comprehend was distasteful, so instead of receiving firm direction from the Pentagon, the engineers at Army's Huntsville and NACA's Langley got only confusion and at times downright ineptitude.

The Air Force, in whose hands the whole mix should probably have been left, was putting its hopes in the Thor and the Atlas Intercontinental Ballistic Missile (ICBM), which if it worked as planned, could be modified to serve almost any mission; some dreamers visualized seven or eight different kinds of Atlases, splendid American-devised machines which would throw objects clear to the Moon. But with incredibly bad luck, the Air Force ran into constant difficulties, and their first ten attempts to fly their rocket ended in disaster.

The Navy backed its Vanguard, an unclassified rocket designed to place scientific satellites in orbit as the American contribution to the International Geophysical Year, when all the nations of the world would cooperate in vast new explorations of the upper atmosphere and space itself. The Navy solution was not a good one, but the top Navy officers were among the best politicians in the world, so their faltering experiments were protected.

The Army, betting on Von Braun and his Germans at Huntsville, was offering the Jupiter, a magnificent-looking offspring of the Peenemünde A-4, fifty-eight feet tall, nearly nine feet in diameter, with enough rocket power to launch either an atomic warhead or a scientific payload to the Moon. But it was not immediately recognizable as superior to the Air Force and Navy solutions, so it had to fight its way insecurely to a position of dominance.

'It's vital,' Kolff told his assistants, 'that we make every item in this Jupiter foolproof. It has got to work, pray God, it has got to.'

In the summer of 1955 Kolff's team spent sixteen and seventeen hours a day perfecting each step in the intricate, monstrous system: miles of thin wire; hundreds of electrical connections; nine different kinds of metal; tons of gear. In the winter of 1956, when they test-fired the gigantic contraption, binding it to Earth with bands of steel, lest it soar aloft without its guidance mechanism, the whole rotten thing collapsed and the team had to go back to the laboratory and try to deduce what had gone wrong.

Von Braun was distraught, for he knew that agents in Huntsville were reporting each disaster to Air Force and Navy, and for a while investigators from Washington hinted that the whole Army show might be closed down because of inefficiency and the team dissolved: 'You could surely find jobs for your men in private industry. Reliable mechanics are always needed.'

'They called you "a reliable mechanic," ' Von Braun said disgustedly when he reported the interview to Kolff. Then he laughed, boisterously, his massive head bobbing with sardonic disgust. 'You, who have worked on the world's greatest rockets. How old are you, Dieter?'

'Forty-nine, almost fifty.'

'Do you think of yourself as "a reliable mechanic"?'

'I'm a rocket man. Waiting till we get a chance at the big one.'

'I wish to God you were a reliable mechanic, so we could get that damned thing in the air.'

'We've analyzed everything and still don't know what went wrong.'

'Can we hope the next one will go?'

'We'll make it go,' Dieter said, and he recalled the days of despair at Peenemünde. 'Remember when Hitler invited eight leading generals to see the invention that was going to win the war? Phhhhht. I wanted to die.'

'We nearly did, both of us.' Von Braun laughed again. "And if we fail next time, Dieter, we'll die again. In a different way.'

Now Kolff found difficulty in sleeping, for he perceived that a great deal more than Army prestige would be riding on the next Jupiter: America's posture vis-à-vis Russia, potential future flights to the Moon, and indeed, the entire space program of not only America but perhaps the entire world. There were a hundred men, Kolff estimated, who wanted to see this multi-faceted program go forward; there were a hundred million, it seemed, who wanted it to fail.

In September 1956 Kolff flew to Cape Canaveral in Florida, an Atlantic Ocean offshore island almost exactly like Wallops but seven hundred and fifty miles farther south, and there on the desolate dunes he supervised the positioning of the huge rocket. When he saw it secure in its gantry, pointed slightly out to sea, he tried to visualize the complex innards, any one of which could malfunction to cause a failure, and he shuddered.

The waiting time was agony, and he could see perspiration forming on Von Braun's face. Finally the signal came. The engines ignited and a monstrous blast engulfed the launch pad. Slowly the great machine lifted into the air and with tantalizing motion started to climb away from the gantry . . . up . . . up, not in a titanic upward explosion, but still slowly, as if it were crawling. It continued, its engines bursting flame, and then its speed increased, slowly, purposefully and always upward, until at last it attained a stupefying power that carried it high into the air, flames following, and out over the sea.

Radar and telemetry signals showed that it climbed to the unbelievable height of 682 miles, which carried it 3,335 miles down range before it plunged into the dark Atlantic.

'We've provided America with a majestic tool,' Von Braun exulted, and when he saw Kolff sitting limp upon a stool, all emotion drained, he went over and sat beside him. 'We've taken our first step toward our Moon.'

The sensational flight had one curious aspect which only the top experts appreciated: an object thrown into the air could go into orbit at a rather low altitude, say one hundred miles up, and this one had soared almost seven times that height without doing so. What was the matter? When Mrs. Pope asked on behalf of the committee, Von Braun explained: 'Height has nothing to do with it, really. It can soar a thousand miles straight up and still fall right back to Earth. But if it gets out of the atmosphere and has enough speed, it will always go into orbit.'

'How much speed must it attain,' she asked, knowing that her senators would grill her on details.

'Mathematically, it works out to 16,029 miles an hour. To cover variations in conditions and the effectiveness of our machines, we work with the figure 17,500 mph. I can assure you this, young lady. If it's less than 16,029, it doesn't matter how high it flies. Earth's gravity will always pull it back into the the atmosphere. But even if it goes only one hundred miles up and attains 17,500, it must go into orbit and remain in it.'

Before Penny could comment, he broke into a chuckle. 'Oberth used to tell us, "If you could drive an automobile at 17,500 mph, it would have to climb to orbit." '

Now Penny asked the vital question: 'But when you had your machine a hundred miles up, why didn't you goose it sideways and throw it into orbit?'

'Ah, my dear! That extra speed, that's what requires the extra energy.'

'Can I tell the senators that you'll be able to apply that extra energy?'

'One of these days, yes.'

When Dieter returned joyously to Huntsville, Liesl presented him with further good news: 'At last the owner appreciates that I make his woods better and he's willing to sell us two acres . . . a decent price. Tonight I am very happy.' But before Dieter could congratulate her, she produced a letter whose contents made the land purchase debatable:

Mr. and Mrs. Dieter Kolff,

Your son Magnus is so exceptional in playing the trumpet that the management of the National Music Camp at Interlochen, Michigan, would like to invite him to play in our Youth Orchestra for seven weeks this summer.

The letter went on to explain that although this was a full scholarship, granted in recognition of Magnus' unusual musical ability, there would be travel and incidental expenses which the Kolff family would be expected to meet. This would use up the money that Liesl had intended applying as down payment for her cherished woods.

It was the kind of problem which enriched family life: two options, either of which would justify an entire year of family labor. The Kolffs studied the matter at supper, with Liesl confessing that although she wanted the woods, she felt that Magnus' education should come first, and the boy saying that whereas he did want to go to the music camp and play real symphonic music, he liked the woods just as much and wanted the family to own its share. Dieter, obviously, would have to make the decision.

Before he could do so his attention was diverted by a frantic telephone call: 'Kolff, get down here immediately! Four men we can't identify are raising hell.'

When he reached the base he found enormous agitation but no solid facts: 'All the Germans are being deported. Nazis.' That, of course, was fallacious, but when he entered his office he found his secretary in tears and two strange men shuffling through his papers.

'All in German?' one of the searchers asked.

'Rocket work is mostly German,' Dieter said. And then he learned that the Pentagon had reached a portentous decision regarding the future of Huntsville, and before it was divulged these operatives from Army Intelligence were checking to see what arcane work the Germans were up to. Kolff, because of his notorious interest in long-range rockets, was especially suspect.

At 0900 the next morning everyone assembled to hear the directive prepared by Secretary of Defense Charley Wilson, as avowed an enemy of rockets and space exploration as the German generals who had given Von Braun so much trouble at Peenemünde. The instructions were entitled *Roles and Missions Directive,* and the engineers gasped when a brigadier general glumly summarized them:

> 'Gentlemen, as of 0800 this morning the United States Army, and particularly the personnel at this base, is ordered to stop work now and permanently on any rocket or other piece of ordnance with a range greater than two hundred miles. Such work henceforth will be the responsibility of either the Air Force or the Navy.
>
> 'This means that practically all projects currently under the supervision of Dr. von Braun and his associates will be terminated. An effort will be made to find work for all members of the staff, either here at Huntsville or in private firms elsewhere which may be interested in space technologies. These orders are in effect now.'

When the meeting dissolved, shocked men stood in groups speculating on what might happen, and someone started the rumor that the Germans would be collected in a concentration camp at El Paso, but that was quickly squelched by the general, who told the men, 'You're legal American citizens, with as much right to stay here in Alabama as I have,' but when the men asked whether they could keep their jobs, he was evasive.

The tension was broken when Kolff's secretary ran up, crying, 'You better get to the field. The Pentagon men are going ape.' And when Kolff reached the storage area he found that the engines on which he had worked with undeviating devotion for nearly twenty years were being dismantled: 'We can't run the risk of any hanky-panky. This base is now limited to two hundred miles and these Jupiters are under wraps.'

By the time Dieter could get back home Liesl and Magnus knew of the disaster, but even before they could offer condolences, he said, 'We'll buy no woods. We'll send no one to camp. In fact, I don't know what we'll do.'

'Can we stay here?' Liesl asked.

'I think we shall have to sell the house and move.'

Liesl stifled a sob, then asked, 'Where?'

'I don't know.'

When Lieutenant John Pope, USN, reported to Patuxent River for training as an advanced airplane test pilot, he found his Korean fly-mate Captain Randy Claggett, USMC, living in a helter-skelter paradise.

Pax River was one of America's finest military installations, a set of airfields located at the far tip of a peninsula jutting out into the Chesapeake Bay and roughly equidistant from Richmond, Annapolis, Washington and Wallops Island. The last two relationships were important because if administrators of the base got into trouble, they could always have easy access to the high command in the nation's capital, and if airplanes on test flights had really difficult maneuvers to perform, they could fly out over the Atlantic, using Wallops Island as their point of reference and their refuge if emergency landings or refuelings became necessary. Pax River was a beautiful, well-run base staffed by some of the world's most expert fliers.

Because of its enviable location, incoming pilots could choose among four locations in which to live: barracks on base which only the squares elected; miserable private digs just outside the gate which everyone tried to avoid; an attractive group of newly built homes at a settlement called Town Creek, where married couples could raise their children safely; and a remarkable frontier area across the Patuxent River at a Navy small-boats base called Solomons Island, so inconvenient, primitive and rowdy that only the toughest pilots married to the most resilient wives elected to live there.

Randy Claggett lived at Solomons, and in order to report for duty in the morning, he had to either drive thirty miles upriver, cross over and drive thirty miles back or take an old motor launch run by the Navy between its two bases. This launch could take no cars, so a pilot who lived at Solomons had to own three automobiles: a real one for the wife and kids, a broken-down hack to carry himself from barracks to the launch, and another crate parked across the river to use for getting from the opposite landing to the test center. Only the first was licensed.

As soon as Pope reported, Claggett took over: 'Amigo, no self-respectin' front-runner ever lives on base, and the town rentals are unspeakable. Only horses' asses live in suburban grandeur at Town Creek, so the only possible place is Solomons. Come with me.'

They went to a parking lot, where Claggett jumped into a Chevrolet fourteen years old. 'I paid me a hundred and six dollars for this affair, but with a little work I got it to run.' It barely held together, but since it was needed only to get Claggett from the landing to base and back, plus runs to the liquor store now and then, it sufficed. The launch looked as if it would positively sink in midstream, but it chugged across the river to the left bank, where an unbelievable 1939 Chevy waited.

'This'n cost me forty dollars and three weeks of work, but hell, it only runs two miles each way, no plates, no nothin'.' This astonishing vehicle carried the two pilots to a row house on the Navy base where toys and various children's vehicles covered the sandy weed-grown lawn.

Banging his way into the house, Claggett shouted, 'Debby Dee, the sonnombeech is here!' And from the kitchen appeared a handsome, blowzy blonde who appeared to be a few years older than her pilot husband. Like Randy, she was from Texas, and like him, she had an infectious good will toward the world, large eyes which smiled enthusiastically and an obvious windblown charm. She used an exaggerated Texas drawl and did her hair in a preposterous way. She was careless about her dress and even more indifferent about the raising of her children, so far as Pope could discern, because she alternately bellowed at them or consoled them passionately if they came to harm. She had two sons and a daughter, but as she explained right at the start: "The boys aren't Randy's. He was good enough to marry me when Frank was killed in flight trainin'.'

'The sonnombeeches are mine now,' Claggett said, as he belted one of the lads for hauling a pedicycle into the room. Both he and Debby Dee assured Pope that there was only one place to live. 'Solomons has everything. Wonderful neighbors. Great parties Saturday night and a pretty good Methodist church for Sundays.'

Randy insisted on taking Pope to a garage off base where the owner had a pathetic Ford for thirty dollars—'Hell, John, you and I could rebuild this bale of bolts in five days, run you perfect home to the landing.' The man also had a rather better Ford at ninety dollars—'I'd recommend it, John, because you'll need something reliable to move about the base.' But what Pope appreciated, then and years later, was another discovery Claggett made: 'John, isn't that a 1949 Mercury over there?'

The body of the convertible had been wrecked beyond repair, but the canvas top looked as if it had escaped serious damage, and when the two pilots inspected it, they found that with some care it could be removed from the wreck and installed in place of the self-made job Pope had been using on his car. The owner would not sell the top, absolutely refused, but he would sell the whole car for twenty-five dollars, and when the pilots had transferred the top he bought back the rest of the hulk for ten dollars.

'With epoxy to touch up the scars, you've got a new top, good for decades,' Claggett said. And then Pope delivered the unwelcome news: 'I'm going to live in quarters . . . on base.'

'Oh, for Christ sake!' Claggett exploded. 'Only worms live on base. At least buy a decent house out at Town Creek.' The Claggetts felt so strongly about this that they called several of their pilot friends and lined up two rather nice houses, but even when Pope saw how attractive they were, and how congenial the military families who lived nearby seemed to be, he stood firm: 'My wife's working in Washington, for the time being, and we won't need a house.'

It was Debby Dee who took him aside, cigarette dangling from her full lips. 'Pope-san, if you're strapped for cash, Randy and I could . . .'

'It's not cash at all, Debby Dee. It's just that I don't need a house.'

'But the owner'll sell this excellent— Look, clown, this house has three bedrooms. It's only thirteen thousand dollars and he'll give you a twenty-year mortgage at five point three percent.'

'I don't want a house. All I want to do is test planes.'

She stepped back and saluted. 'Join the brotherhood, you sonnombeech. And I suppose you know the password? Professionalism.'

It was certainly Randy Claggett's beacon. He could horse around at home on Solomons, or at weekend parties, or when tinkering with his three cars, and he could talk Tex-Mex, but when he approached a new airplane whose characteristics were unknown and to be proved, he became a kind of self-contained god, a being totally immersed in the task at hand, and he believed with reason that no one on Earth could discharge that job better than he, for he was a professional, best in the business.

Everyone at Pax River aspired to that reputation, and when Pope's incoming class of fifteen assembled in the Test Pilot classroom, Captain Penscott, who would be their supervisor for five months of basic training, greeted them without emotion: 'Gentlemen, you've been chosen because you're the best military pilots in the nation. You know far more about airplanes than those you served with, and by this time next year two of you will be dead because you didn't know enough.'

And during the fifth week the sirens sounded, because a Navy lieutenant with 1,400 hours in his *Aviator's Flight Logbook* had augered in an F7U-3 —flown it nose-first right into the tarmac at three hundred miles per hour. He had one of the new houses at Town Creek, and Debby Dee was the first wife to come across on the launch from Solomons to take care of the widow and her two kids.

When Pope was handed his first *Flight Test Procedures for Stability and Control Evaluation,* mimeographed by Douglas Aircraft to guide military pilots in testing the A4D-3, a light attack bomber which might or might not go into full-scale production, he was astonished by the complexity of the tests he was supposed to conduct and about which he was obligated to furnish written reports. The booklet identified thirteen almost unrelated aspects of the airplane which had to be tested under flight conditions, such as:

> How does the plane behave in a stall?
> Does it have dynamic longitudinal stability?
> What are the characteristics of its high-speed dive recovery?
> How do its lateral controls respond in critical situations?
> What is its dynamic stability?

In simpler terms, the test pilot was supposed to put his plane into every conceivable kind of jeopardy, bring it out safely, and record precisely what happened before, during and after the crisis. It was in this written reporting that many test pilots failed, and Pope was profoundly impressed by the meticulous care with which Randy Claggett wrote his reports. He might sound illiterate during a Solomons beer bash, but when he brought a test plane back to Earth, he wrote with the precision of a writer for *Scientific American:* 'The company engineers have to know exactly what happened, and only you can tell them.' When he saw Pope's first reports, he showed his contempt: 'Too wordy. Too imprecise. How? How much? How long before the response?' And always he wanted to know how Pope had *felt* when the strange things were happening: 'That's a better guide than all the telemetry the engineers invent. Not what you thought. Not what the instruments showed. But how your guts felt when the plane yawed unexpectedly. How did your ass feel when it started to slide? Did you feel your eyes drifting? Goddammit, Pope, you're the most expensive instrument they'll ever put in those planes, and the most complicated, so trust your reflexes.'

At one party Claggett reverted to this theme, and with a beer can in one hand, he directed a conversation with six other pilots; they were in the kitchen, of course, while their wives were in the front room discussing shopping markets and kindergartens. 'We're the end of a long line, gentlemen.' (He was imitating Captain Penscott.) 'The end of a long process of Darwinian selection.' And he invited the pilots to offer their guesses as to the statistics he wanted.

'If you got into Annapolis or West Point, you were one in five hundred who thought they were eligible. If you graduated, only thirty percent were allowed into flight training. Only sixty percent of that number made it to completion. Advanced training washed out a good twenty percent. And a hell of a lot didn't live through the squadron. MiG guns or their own carelessness did them in. I understand that about a hundred of the best fliers in the world apply for test-flight training every class, here or Edwards, which leads me to think that each of us represents something like one in two hundred thousand.'

'How in hell did you get that?' asked one of the pilots who had been doing his own figuring.

'Because it's a good round number. Now let's look at the costs. High school, four thousand dollars. Annapolis, four years, forty-eight thousand dollars. Flight training, including the smashed SNJs, a hundred and fifty thousand. Advanced flight and peacetime squadron, three hundred thousand dollars. Korea, three years, the banged-up planes, a million eight hundred thousand dollars. Pax River, three years all told, another five hundred thousand dollars. What's that add up to? A lot of mazoola.'

Pope studied with interest the dogged way in which Claggett pursued his career, and he listened carefully to his suggestions: 'I heard Captain Penscott say you were one of the best. If so, make your moves with the most careful attention. You must get into Flight Test. That's where we do the real work, testing the hottest things that fly . . . in the abstract . . . philosophically. If you can't make that, Service Test is acceptable, but it's a step down. You take the plane when I'm through with it and see how it fits Navy requirements. If you're obviously not a first-class stick man, they'll put you in Electronic Test, which is all right if you grew up wiring Heathkits. Armament Test is the same thing—avoid it. A guy like you, known as a straight arrow, faces one fatal temptation. They'll want to keep hold of you as a teacher in the Test Pilot School, and if you let them . . . farewell, poor Yorick, I knew him in the old days when he was a pilot.'

'Can I get into Flight Test?

'You have to get in, it's that simple.'

Claggett had two other bits of advice which he deemed vital, for when he shared them he kept hold of Pope's arm, bringing him close as if he were whispering recondite information shared only by the professionals. 'John, never become too close to the manufacturer's field representatives. They're business. We're military. And if you're seen suckin' up to them, the rest of us will figure you're trying to land a civilian job when you're through here, and men who do that are beneath contempt.

'Also, John, never hobnob with the VR types, the pilots testing the transport prototypes. It'll be obvious that you're hoping for a later job with Pan American or United. To hell with them. They fly boxcars. We fly airplanes.'

And when Pope's five months of intensive training drew to a close, Claggett cautioned him again: 'I think you're gonna be one of the great ones, John. Normally I despise men who bunk on base just to save a few bucks, and I really don't like straight arrows, but dammit, you know airplanes as well as I do. You really do. The one unforgivable sin in your work for the next two years is to crack up a prototype aircraft. Kill yourself, that's okay, and screw the commander's wife, that's okay, too. But you're here to protect that aircraft, and if you auger one in, you've failed your test.

'And don't allow yourself to become too attached to one type. Remember, the airplane has no affection for you. To it, one pilot's as good as another. Test the goddamned thing and walk away from it.' Proudly he showed Pope his *Aviator's Flight Logbook,* which recorded his pilot's experience in seventy-one different kinds of aircraft, even some of the despised VR types, and in the final days of his own preparatory training Pope watched with admiration the brazen way in which Claggett gained access to the newer planes as they arrived at Patuxent River.

He would wait till someone landed a prototype, go over to it, kick the tires and ask casually, 'How do you start this bundle of bolts?' A pilot could have 3,000 hours in the air with all types of planes and still not be able to guess how the next manufacturer had decided to hide the ignition system on his new plane. When Claggett found out, he would ask the returning pilot, 'Anything oddball about this one?' And always one pilot would help another, warning him of special problems.

Off Claggett would go, sometimes with only the vaguest permission from the tower, but after he had put the new plane through its maneuvers and made voluminous notes as to its performance, he would land and seek out one or two pilots who had flown it before and spend perhaps three hours comparing notes on the most intimate details of this plane's behavior. Only then would he meet with the team in charge of the plane and with the manufacturer's representatives to report in astonishing detail on the strengths and weaknesses of their product.

'I have one failing you should avoid,' Claggett confided on the evening before Pope's graduation from the school part of the Patuxent River program. 'I'm a sucker for any kind of cross-country flight. I'll even go commercial. So I take every trip that comes along, and pilots who do this put themselves in grave danger. Fly out to the big factories in Los Angeles. Edwards Air Force Base to test their new planes. Maybe over to England to meet with the British at Boscombe Downs.'

'What's the danger?'

'You become known as a giddy-biddy, a goody-grabber, and when you come home you find that someone who's been tending to his knitting has drawn all the good assignments, and you're no longer in the mainstream. You get none of the new planes.'

'How do you protect yourself?'

Claggett looked around him as if fearing spies, then said, 'By being the best damned pilot on the lot. By writing the best reports. By flying the ass off anything they let you climb into.' He laughed. 'I'll never be cured. I love that Pax-Jax-Lax routine.' He was referring to the field designations of Patuxent River, Jacksonville, Los Angeles. 'My heart grows double when the engine revs up and I'm on my way. At thirty thousand feet the world is mine.'

Next day John Pope graduated as a full-fledged test pilot, and Captain Penscott, recognizing his ability, invited him to become head of instruction in the training school: 'It's a long-term job, Pope, one that carries with it real distinction. You could purchase a house and live well.'

'I would be honored,' John said. 'But you know my wife works in Washington, and I was hoping I'd get Flight Test.'

'Has Claggett been poisoning your mind?' Penscott asked amiably.

'Well, he has said two things,' Pope lied. 'That to become a permanent instructor was about the best a man could hope for. And that hard drivers tried to get into Flight Test.'

'I was afraid you'd say that,' Penscott said. 'Flight Test it'll be.'

That night Randy and Debby Dee Claggett threw a graduation party at Solomons, with the ancient launch working overtime to carry the people from Town Creek across the river and young Tim Claggett driving the broken-down Chevy round-trip from the pier to the three row houses his mother had borrowed for the bash. By this time Pope was well enough acquainted with the Pax River people to know what to expect: no alcoholism whatever in the entire crew, no talk of books or art, the loudest possible hi-fi music, politics never mentioned, men in the kitchen, wives in the front room, models of aircraft fastened to all the walls, and the warm-hearted camaraderie of men who had spent the last dozen years risking their lives and who hoped to spend the next dozen doing exactly the same.

What Pope was not prepared for was that when he left his austere bachelor quarters on the base and drove his Mercury convertible to the ferry, crossed it and climbed into Tim Claggett's Chevy, he found Penny waiting for him in Debby Dee's front room. Randy had driven hell-bent to Washington to bring her down for the gala night.

His heart stopped when he saw her—straight, neat, hair trim against her well-shaped head, her eyes wide, her broad face glowing with delight at seeing her husband again. 'Penny,' he cried. 'How did you find this place?'

'The Flying Gorilla,' she said, pointing to Claggett, who was once more playing the Texas beetworker from Central Mexico: 'I breeng you Señorita, sir. My seestair, very pretty, very clean, three dollars.'

The Navy wives made a fuss over Penny, who with her working experience in Washington was able to fit in immediately with women whom instinctively she liked: 'I have no children, dammit, and I think it's that clown's fault.'

'No, no, memsahib!' Claggett shouted. 'In Korea our boy Pope had three children. The fault ain't his'n.'

The Navy wives liked Penny and spent much time trying to discover what it was she did in Washington, and she explained that because of her law degree she had been able to land this demanding job as secretary to the Senate committee that dealt with aviation and space: 'You might say that I help men like Lyndon Johnson and my boss Michael Glancey find the money that keeps places like Patuxent River functioning.'

'Bless that girl!' Debby Dee cried, and she asked Penny if she wanted anything to drink.

'A beer,' Penny said, and Debby Dee shrieked, 'Us beer drinkers got a new convert.'

The party continued till dawn, and as the sun came up over the Chesapeake, Debby Dee led the Popes to one of the borrowed houses, told all the late drinkers to scram, and put the new test pilot and his beautiful Washington wife to bed. 'Get some kids,' she told them. 'It ain't legal to be a test pilot without kids.' Her own son Tim was still driving the ramshackle Chevy back and forth to the landing as the test pilots made their way across the river and back to their jobs.

Penny was so delighted with Pax River, and especially with the Claggetts, that she made plans to leave Washington on most weekends, sleeping over at either Solomons or Town Creek, and the more she saw of the orderly yet frenzied life of the test pilots, the more she loved it and the more she respected the men and women who participated in it. She was very proud of her husband and saw that most of the other wives were proud of theirs, and she was staying with one of the families at Town Creek when one of the new test pilots who had graduated with John augered in, reducing a great plane to a compact mass of metal and bone and blood. He was the first of the fifteen to die.

Then she appreciated doubly the meaning of her husband's occupation, for the entire base—admiral in charge, Captain Penscott in charge of the school, tech reps from the manufacturers, young men who had come aboard as beginners in the new class—coalesced about the stricken home to make death bearable, if not understandable.

On her weekends Penny came to know the older test pilots, who were either still working on the base or returning to it to compare notes or drink beer with their earlier associates, and she saw that John Glenn, quiet and sober, was much like her husband, a true straight arrow, and from watching Glenn, she came to know John better. Al Shepard was all dignity and power, while Scott Carpenter was relaxed and amiable. She had difficulty believing Pete Conrad had ever gone to Princeton. She was overawed by Bill Lawrence, perhaps the ablest flier, all things considered, that Pax River was to produce—if she excluded Randy Claggett and her husband—but she was grateful for a rowdy, talkative type like Gerry O'Rourke, who kept things moving with his irreverent comedy. It was a splendid group of men, and she could not believe rumors that the Air Force parallel types at Edwards in California excelled. 'They may fly higher,' she told the Senate committee, 'but they cannot fly any better.'

She was sleeping at the Claggetts' one Friday night, tired from her week's work and the speedy trip south, when she heard a loud explosion across the river and awoke to see flames leaping toward the sky. She was terrified, because her husband was engaged in night flying that week, and for a dreadful half-hour she supposed that it had been his plane which had 'bought the ranch.'

Claggett was not doing any night flying, so he and Debby Dee were present to console her, and the latter said, from long experience, 'We'll get a phone call. We always do.'

'You mean they'll tell me about it over the phone?'

'Good God, no!' Debby Dee blurted out. 'They send the chaplain, or one of the fliers in uniform. If nobody comes up that walk— You'd be able to hear the launch, too.'

They waited a long time, talking of inconsequentials, with Penny Pope starting even when a cricket's rasping legs gave noises that could be interpreted as the start of a phone ringing, and then they waited longer still for the sound of the launch, but in the end it was John Pope on the phone: 'Hello, kiddo. You get down here all right? Just called to see.'

When Penny replaced the phone she looked for a moment at her companions, sitting there in the semi-darkness, not exulting with her, for her gain was the dreadful loss of someone equally precious. And then she collapsed. 'Oh, Debby Dee! I love him so much.' And in a flood of words this capable, self-directed committee secretary told of their courtship under the stars in Clay, when John was already interested in astronomy, and of their nights together in the university observatory with Dr. Anderssen, and of their courtship while John was at Annapolis, and of the generous way he encouraged her, and of her love which grew deeper with every year.

'You have kids,' she told the Claggetts, 'and so do all the others. John and I have tried, and maybe failure cements us even closer.'

'Why don't you quit your job and move down here?' Debby Dee asked, hoping to ease her into less-hysterical conversation.

'Whatever you do, it's never right,' Penny said, so they gave her two stiff drinks and put her to bed.

Now, when she visited with her husband over the weekends or during a Senate break, she loved him increasingly, for at last she understood what impelled him: 'You want to be the best, don't you? You want to drive yourself always to the maximum performance.'

'I'll never be the test pilot Randy is.'

'You're twice as knowledgeable about airplanes,' she said forcefully.

'Specifications, yes. But what makes one fly and another falter, no.'

'Are you making a mystery of it, a religion?'

'It is a mystery. At the farthest edges when you're up there with a plane that's never been really tested, it is a mystery.' He hesitated, for he must next speak about things that the test pilots would usually voice only to other test pilots, but he loved this strong-willed girl from the plains as none of the other pilots loved their wives; she was part of him, the measure of his life—and he wanted to share everything with her.

'Since we started our tour, three men just as well trained as I am have flown their planes into the ground, and statistics predict that four more will before we're through. Every one of them knew his plane. Every one talked slowly and clearly into his mouthpiece as things began to fall apart. And every damned one of them did the first right thing, and then the second and then the fifth and sixth, and nothing worked, and they were still trying to figure things out when they hit. Randy Claggett would have saved every one of those planes. At step three he'd have figured something, something never in any book. And that's the difference.'

She drew in her breath, then asked, 'You? Would you have brought them down?'

'I might have figured it out by step five, but then it could have been too late. But I promise you this, Penny, if they do come up the lane one day, the chaplain and the others, you can be positive that I was about to try step six.'

Once he allowed her to see the mimeographed instructions Grumman sent to the men testing the F11F-1, a plane in which the Navy had placed great faith when it issued the original contract, but which was proving a dismal disappointment:

LATERAL CONTROL

Purpose: To determine aileron force gradient.

Procedure:
1. Trim out in the desired condition.
2. Roll into a left or right turn to an angle of bank 45°.
3. When the turn is stable hold the rudder fixed in the trim position and abruptly apply a given amount of aileron and hold it until the airplane has reached a 45° bank in the opposite direction.
4. Record the time to roll the 90° and note aileron force required.

Important Note:
Make this check at 1/4, 1/2, 3/4 and full throw aileron displacements, first left, then right.
Further Application:
Make checks at various altitudes and air speeds to determine rate of roll at various Mach numbers and their equivalent air speeds.
Caution: Watch out for flutter. If it occurs, lower speed instantly.

When she leafed through the booklet she found that her husband was obligated to perform more than eighty such tests with their *Further Applications* and *Cautions* as to when the wings might fly off. 'How many planes are you men testing?'

John rattled off the names of twenty-six on the field at this moment, including many that would prove useless when subjected to tests like the above but also those noble workhorses of the fleet, those planes upon whose predecessors the safety of this nation had once depended: the Douglas dive bombers, the Grumman fighters, the great Chance-Vought F4U series, which the Marines had used to repel the Japanese and which Pope had used in Korea against the Chinese.

He shared with her, as a virtual member of the Senate committee, the two scandals at Pax River: 'There never was a plane more difficult than the old F4U. Birdcage so high the pilot couldn't see to land it on a carrier. Had a really nasty way of snap-rolling at high G's. But we never had a better plane. It was made of concrete. Could not be shot down by anything but a three-inch shell. An absolutely marvelous plane, and I flew it all through Korea, the Chance-Vought Corsair, my love.

'So now the same company with the same engineers builds the Navy the F7U, the Cutlass. And it's a disaster. There doesn't seem to be a thing right about it, especially the engines. Pilots call it the Gutless Cutlass, and men like Claggett have sent in a dozen reports on what has to be done, and they can't seem to fix it. You know, I suppose, that Claggett refuses to fly it any more. Calls it the Widow Maker.'

'Do you fly it?'

'I fly anything.' Without further comment he told her of the F3H planes, first and second series. 'The poor old F3H-1, maybe the worst disaster of modern times. The Ensign Killer. Had a J-40 engine, I think, and performed so dismally they sent the last forty of them down the Mississippi on barges. Too dangerous to fly. So they brought out an improvement—F3H-2 with an Allison J-71 engine. We named it the Screamin' Demon, and it broke our hearts to see how at so many critical points it failed. A great plane on paper, it never quite made it. I found its air-to-air missile system elegant. First in the world that will kill an oncoming target head-on, But dammit, both the plane and the engine failed us. Claggett and I have sent in dozens of reports. But most of the faults can't be corrected.'

'But you still fly it?'

'That's our job. We're testing them. And if we don't test them, the Navy buys them and then the young pilots get killed expecting them to perform properly.'

'Is it really rough?'

'Thirty days, thirty flights, maybe fifty, not a thing happens. Plane goes into a spin, you note the numbers, you bring it out of the spin, you note the numbers.'

'Are spins dangerous?'

'Not if you bring the plane out.'

'And if you don't?'

'Then you try something, and something else, and always you find something.'

When she returned to Washington after discussions like this, she had increased admiration for the men all down the line who made aviation possible: the big companies that made the planes, the Senate committees that paid for them, the generals and admirals who fought to get the right ones, the gallant young men who flew them, and then that special breed of quiet supermen who drank beer in the kitchen on Saturday night and tested the untried planes on Monday morning.

In recent months two more men in their thirties had been killed: one testing a plane that should never have left the factory; the other in a plane which was as good as any nation in the world was making, but which on this particular day over the Chesapeake Bay behaved erratically, and the young fellow in it panicked and lost his life and a plane that any of the other pilots on the test line could have brought down easily.

The more Penny saw of the pilots, the more reassured she was about their essential sanity: there were no daredevils in this group, and any youngster who sought to achieve that reputation was either dropped completely or disciplined by the oldsters like John Glenn or Randy Claggett, and it was peculiarly effective when the lanky Texan assumed the role of taskmaster. He never attacked the young show-off directly, or in front of others, for he realized that a test pilot required all the self-esteem and bravado available, nor did he denigrate the man's basic ability, for the young man would not have been chosen for Pax River if he was not competent, but what he did do, and most directly, was challenge the man's professionalism.

'You know, Forbes, this ain't much of a report.'

'The facts are there.'

'But ifn a report ain't done good style—I mean slam-slam-slam, one point directly after the other—and I mean in order, goddammit, just like the book says . . .'

'It's all there.'

'It ain't all there, goddammit. It ain't there ifn I cain't find it.'

'What do you want me to do? Become a professor of English?'

'Exactly,' Claggett would say with great warmth. Then, putting his arm about the man, he would say, 'Forbes, you're one of the hottest pilots on this here line. I reckon you can be the very best in your group. Ability? Unbounded. But whippin' that plane around the sky is only one-third of this job. The other two-thirds is feedback. You tellin' the brain boys what's what. And this you must do in precise . . . orderly . . . fashion. I spend one hour testin', two hours reportin'. It's called professionalism, son, and ifn you ain't got that, you ain't got nothin'.'

Penny studied with amusement the various ways in which these men proved their professionalism. The preferred automobile was a meticulously polished two-seater black Thunderbird. The family car had to be the largest possible used Buick station wagon, although an Oldsmobile would also be acceptable. A house had to have a high-fidelity sound system, but not a bookcase, for the men did enough reading on the job, and their wives had neither the time nor the interest. Beer was the drink, rarely whiskey, and some families who had served overseas were addicted to Tuborg, Heineken or Asahi Black, even though those imported brands cost more.

The families were curious affairs, close-knit emotionally but wildly divergent socially, in that members, from long experience in military families that moved constantly, even from continent to continent, had learned to shift for themselves and each individual for himself. Thus, the young fathers tried to play the role of the stern paterfamilias, and a reasonable discipline was maintained in the home, but the youngsters found their own diversions and went their own way in many things.

There was a wide variety in family styles, from the rigor of the Marine colonel and his Michigan wife to the slap-happy freedom of the Claggetts, but in the entire group, so far as Penny could discern, there was not one crybaby wife, not one would-be superman husband. They were not necessarily well adjusted, but they were . . . well, she could only borrow her husband's favorite word—professionals.

It was almost laughable, however, to watch these wandering families, these rootless pilots, suddenly trying to play Horace Homeowner, with carpenter's tools, paintbrush and lawnmower. Pax River, at the time, had seventy-one test pilots, and only four of them had ever owned a house before. Now two-thirds of them did, and the transformation was a shock.

Penny was joking about this one night during a weekend visit, when she suddenly burst into tears, her trim businesswoman façade racked by sobs. 'John, I want us to buy a house. There's one for sale at Town Creek, and I want us to have it.'

'Why? We'd never live in it.'

'John,' she blubbered, 'it's the normal thing to do.'

He drew her into his chair and kissed her many times, stroking her pretty legs and saying, 'We won't be here long, Penny, and—'

'None of the others will be either, but they all have homes.'

'And when we're reassigned it'll be difficult to sell—'

'It's difficult for the others. But I notice they always find a buyer, somehow.'

'It would be a waste of our money, with you in Washington—'

'I've saved the money,' she said grimly, leaving his chair. 'I'll buy the house. I'll sell it, and I'll make money doing it.'

'With you in Washington—'

'Stop saying that! You and I are a family. And a family should own a house. And even if we do have to move around, we'll keep the house. It'll be our permanent anchor.'

John could not prevent a guffaw. 'You ever lived in southern Maryland in the summer? You ever live here in the winter, for that matter? Now get to bed.'

When they were under the covers she snuggled close to him and whispered, 'I have enormous respect for Debby Dee Claggett. I'd want to be a better housekeeper than she is, but I could never be a better mother. Do you know that she's three years older than her husband?'

From Monday through Saturday noon, week after week, John Pope experimented with planes about to be purchased in large lots by the United States Navy, and he came to be recognized by the high command as 'the guy who will fly anything.' He was especially appreciated by the manufacturer's representatives for the extremely thoughtful reports he submitted after each flight, for he seemed to become one of them, a man desperately interested in the success of every model he tested, and after one long spell of intense application, even Claggett, the most professional of the test pilots, had to warn him: 'Remember, John, the plane doesn't love you. If it's a clinker, say so, reject the damned thing.' But Pope felt that any plane which had matured to the point of having actually been built, even if only three prototypes were in existence, was worth saving.

His attitude was tested one morning when Captain Penscott asked him and Claggett to give two problem planes a workout. 'Pope, you take the F3H up for maximum maneuvers, and you, Claggett, take the F7U, to serve as the target plane.'

'I don't fly the F7U,' Claggett said in a low, respectful voice.

'Why not?'

'Because it's pitifully underpowered and has killed too many good men.'

'Are you afraid to fly it?' Penscott asked, and deathly silence engulfed the ready room, because for anyone to challenge Randy Claggett's courage was preposterous. He had flown more different types than anyone on the base, and in more different kinds of dangerous assignments and weather. He had taken the most tentative planes aloft and given them the most punishing analysis, often finding himself in perilous situations from which only his iron will saved him, and if three new planes arrived tomorrow on a barge, too dangerous to fly, he would want to give each a whirl.

But he had satisfied himself that the F7U, this bastard son of a heroic father, was unacceptable, and he would bother with it no more. His friends had lost their lives in this plane for reasons which he had outlined before their accidents occurred, and one of the finest squadron commanders the Navy had ever produced had been broken because of his rebellion against sending his young men aloft in this Gutless Cutlass, and Claggett felt that this was enough. Now he was being asked if he was afraid to fly it.

'Yes,' he said. 'I am afraid.' And without permission he walked quietly from the ready room.

Captain Penscott faced an extremely difficult decision; at Pax River a man could be a full Navy captain in charge of testing, with all the power that that implied, yet be less significant than the top pilot who was actually taking the questionable planes aloft. Penscott could dismiss a new-comer who showed signs of weakness, but he could not discipline the best pilot of them all because he refused to fly a plane that had been proved to be a killer.

He made a command decision: 'Pope, will you fly the F7U as target?'

'Yes, sir.'

'Find Claggett and tell him he's to fly the Screamin' Demon.'

'Yes, sir.'

So over the Chesapeake, two of the finest test pilots in America, in two fearfully disappointing planes, performed every prescribed maneuver, with the target F7U performing like a masterpiece and the pursuing F3H attacking it with vigor, but in the routine return to base, Pope's F7U began to lose stability, and the first to notice it was Claggett in the pursuing plane.

'John, this is Randy. I had that once. Pull back, old man.'

When this failed to produce the necessary correction, Claggett said, 'John, it looks like your left aileron. Adjust!'

Again there was no improvement, and now the F7U was in real trouble, heading for a disastrous spin at only a thousand feet above the water.

'John,' came the quiet voice, 'try a tight turn left.'

The headstrong plane ignored this correction and gained speed in a pronounced spin to the right, a vertiginous and twisting drop, and now Pope heard nothing, not Claggett's voice, not the tower, not even the plane itself. Patiently, methodically, without a shred of panic, he ran down the final items on his mental checklist, the one prepared months ago after long discussions with men who had fought this wayward plane, and as it was about to crash into the Chesapeake, he made the last corrections, pulled its nose up, and set it level for safe landing at Pax River.

When he delivered the F7U to the ground crew, he walked soberly to the ready room, where he and Claggett wrote seven pages of summary comment on the deficiencies of this plane, betraying no hysteria but specifying fact after fact which condemned it. And when Claggett was finished with that job, just as thoroughly and just as negatively, he spent two more hours reporting on his F3H. For duty of this caliber they received $429 a month.

If John Pope tried to ape the high professionalism of Randy Claggett, he also found delight in adopting the Texan's major bad habit. He had become a goody-grabber, eager to take the Pax-Jax-Lax route to anywhere, so he was delighted one Sunday evening when Claggett called him in bachelors' quarters with the news that General Funkhauser, one of the honchos at Allied Aviation in Los Angeles, wanted a consultation on the F6Q-1, which was approaching the time when prototypes would be coming into production.

'Pick you up at the landing, 1900,' Pope said, and when in the evening darkness a special run of the wheezing launch brought Claggett across the river, John was waiting in his Mercury convertible. With the top down, the two pilots roared along dark Maryland roads to Washington National Airport.

'I don't like asking you to fly commercial, especially a night trip,' Claggett apologized, 'but all I could get was Government Transportation Request, so we're taking United.'

They boarded one of the last flights out of National and droned westward to St. Louis, where they would change to a more powerful four-engine job that would carry them to Los Angeles. Pope dozed on the flight west of Denver, but Claggett excused himself: 'I'm gonna make a serious run at the redheaded stewardess.' And toward morning, when Pope looked toward the vacant seats at the rear of the plane, he saw Claggett and the redhead necking.

They landed at Los Angeles at 0600, grabbed a rented car, and stormed along the superhighways toward Pasadena, where General Funkhauser and his aides would be waiting. They stopped for a leisurely breakfast of coffee and eggs, then pushed ahead to Allied Aviation.

They talked with tremendous concentration all morning, ate a lunch of salad and rye crisp, then worked with the engineers all afternoon. At 1700 they were back in their rented car heading for the airport, where they had a fish dinner before boarding the United Airlines Red-Eye Special for the all-night flight back to Washington. There they jumped into the convertible at 0800, roared down to Pax River, and reported to the airfield.

Claggett spotted a new arrival, a WFZ, about which he was curious, so he walked quietly over to the plane and asked the pilot, 'How do you start this bundle of bolts?' After he had checked the intriguing new system he asked, 'Any peculiarities I should know about?'

With that he took the new plane into the air, flew high over the blue waters of the Chesapeake and far above the Atlantic at Wallops Island. When he landed, he asked for the original pilot and compared notes for about an hour. Then he wrote his report, entered the new plane in his *Logbook,* jumped in his ancient Chevy, drove to the landing, crossed in a rainstorm, got into his even more decrepit second Chevy, drove to the Solomons barrack, kissed his wife, and fell asleep for sixteen hours.

The two men would accept any chance to travel, but what they enjoyed most was any trip to Edwards Air Force Base in California, because they knew that when they landed at that vast salt flat they were in the presence of their peers, the finest Air Force test pilots. Here Chuck Yeager had broken the sound barrier in powered flight and Joe Engle had flown the X-15 almost out of the atmosphere to a height of 280,600 feet.

One had to respect the work done at Edwards, but at the same time one had to be always alert to defend the equally fine accomplishment at Pax River. The difference was this: an Air Force airplane, taking off and landing on fields of immense dimension, could be an ultimate flying instrument, the only consideration being the ideal combination of flight, altitude, speed and maneuverability. Wings could be wide or narrow, as the probable mission of the plane dictated. Weight could be minimal, every component honed to the vanishing point. Anything could be altered to provide greater combat effectiveness, and the speed at landing could be 250 mph if that's what the combination produced.

But as Pope explained one night in the mess at Edwards: 'A Navy plane is bound by so many restrictions, you wouldn't believe it. Weight? Not a single Air Force plane I've seen could be used aboard a carrier, because if we soldered a restraining hook to the bottom of one of your birds, the girders necessary to absorb the shock of that sudden stop would be missing. When she lands, bottom of the plane gets torn off.'

Claggett, who loved his excursions to Edwards, enjoyed especially this arguing with the Air Force types: 'You take the F4U, that marvelous plane the Marines used in World War II. Did you know that its wings folded? So it could be stacked on deck. You put folding wings on an F-105 and you couldn't get it off the field.'

The two Navy men rarely made much headway in their arguments with the hotshot Air Force fliers, and one night Claggett, in some irritation, said, 'I'm not sure that many of you clowns could qualify for landing on the deck of a carrier.'

'We can fly anything with wings,' a taciturn man from Tennessee called Hickory Lee said, 'or even nubs of wings.'

The argument grew furious, with Claggett describing the difficulties his Marines had experienced in transferring their high caliber of land flying to the carrier *Essex* off Japan in 1945. 'I want you apes to listen, and Pope can verify what I'm sayin' because it's history. The Marines sent one of their best contingents, nineteen fliers with top records and three weeks' carrier familiarization. At the end of nine days flyin' without ever seein' an enemy plane, what were the results? Seven pilots dead, one more drowned off the bow end. Seventeen F4Us lost at sea or completely wrecked.'

The Air Force men were attentive, and Claggett added, 'In those same nine days Navy pilots, making far more takeoffs and landings, lost not a single man. Dented not a single fender.'

At this point the argument grew so heated that Claggett stomped out of the mess, uncharacteristically leaving the fight, but after he had made a quick deal for some large cans of white paint, he returned quietly to summon Pope, and together the two men went out to a hard-surface runway and sketched in bold sloppy strokes the outlines of the landing deck of a medium-sized carrier. The work was arduous, requiring much stooping over, and far from accurate, but toward midnight, when they were satisfied with the results, they returned to the mess, where this fellow Hickory Lee was still arguing. Smeared with white paint, the two Navy men challenged the locals to a contest: 'I want you apes out there at 0600. I got me two colored paddles and I'm gonna be your landin' officer, and I wanna see if you clowns can even hit the deck, let alone land on it.'

At dawn the pilots assembled, and the Air Force men were astonished at how minute their target was going to be, but Claggett bellowed, 'All right, Lee, take her up!' And when the Tennessee captain sped his F-104 down the runway and high into the clouds, he made a sweeping turn, straightened up, and came roaring down at the simulated carrier at whose stern Claggett waited with two paddles to represent a landing officer. Several things happened: the F-104 was so much lighter than the rugged Navy types that Lee could not slow it down the way Navy pilots did; he came in high and fast, searching for a long landing area on which to brake down after his wheels touched. Also, Claggett complicated things by jiggling his paddles more than necessary and flashing the okay-to-land signal just a trifle slow.

Lee slammed onto the imaginary carrier, applied his brakes heavily, and ran about a mile and a half off the bow end. 'You failed, you dumb sonnom-beech!' Claggett shouted. 'You're in three thousand feet of water.'

He invited the others to try their luck, and when they landed, brakes screaming, and overshot the carrier, the Air Force men appreciated what a tremendous shock they would have had to absorb in order to stop their planes in the indicated distance. Grudgingly they admitted that there might be something about carrier flight they had not fully appreciated, but the trials continued, a gang of grown-up kids playing with toys that cost $3,000,000 each.

'You all flunked,' Claggett said at breakfast, 'and even so, it wasn't a fair test, because I couldn't simulate one thing. On a real carrier, just as you approach the stern, the ocean lifts the ship thirty feet in the air, you fly right into the rolling edge, and we never see you or your plane again.'

The Air Force men liked Claggett; they respected the intense profession-alism he displayed in all he did, so that Pope was not surprised when, at the conclusion of one test period at Edwards, some of the older Air Force types rose formally at the end of an evening meal and informed Randy that he had been selected for membership in the most exclusive flying club in the world, the Society of Airplane Test Pilots. Claggett, obviously proud of the honor, reverted to Texas hillbilly, to the delight of the pilots: 'To peripherize the words of a great Confederate gineril, "If nominated, I ain't gonna run, and if elected, I ain't agonna serve, and if you-all try to put me in one of them newfangled F-100 series, I'm agonna gallop right acrost that there desert." '

But the Pax-Jax-Lax tour that Pope remembered with greatest pleasure came when he finagled a four-week reciprocal visit to England's test center at Boscombe Downs, which lay southwest of London near the cathedral towns of Salisbury and Winchester. There, in the gray clouds that hung over the English Channel, he tested the sophisticated aircraft being developed by the English experts, and whenever he discovered something he did not like or which seemed second class, he noted it but was hesitant about voicing his negative opinion too strongly, because he remembered that it was on this field and others like it that the Spitfire was tested; it had everything wrong about it except its fantastic maneuverability and its stubborn capacity to absorb punishment and still shoot down the Luftwaffe in staggering num-bers.

He liked the British pilots, with their painstaking and sometimes creak-ing traditions, and he had to respect the severity with which they went about their work, but the highlight of his tour came when Penny cabled that her committee was sending her to England to look into negotiations regarding shared British-American facilities, and after her work in London she would be heading for Boscombe Downs. John consulted with his English pilots as to where she might stay, and they recommended the Boar and Thrush, a small inn from which the tower of Salisbury cathedral could be seen across the plains, and there the Popes spent one of the happiest weeks of their lives. Using her committee expense account, Penny rented a sports car, and in it they explored the glorious countryside: Salisbury, Winchester, Plymouth, the Hardy country, the prim majesty of Bath, and the spot that moved John most deeply, that circle of massive monoliths at Stonehenge, for when he saw this mysterious relic of four thousand years he imagined himself one of the ancient astronomers who oriented it, and he insisted that they wait there among the rolling hills until the evening stars appeared, so that he could check the accuracy with which the great stones were aligned.

'I have never been happier,' he said. 'I have the best job in the world. I work with the best men. And I sometimes imagine it will go on forever.'

Penny replied that she felt that she had the best job possible: 'To be at the center of things. To feel the changes coming on so fast. I suspect that Glancey and Grant will be reelected forever, and I'll stay at their right hand doing the work.'

They were an unusually handsome pair, there in the shadows cast by the great stones; they were both thirty years old, both slightly underweight, both of medium height and fine appearance, and they were both straight arrows, attuned to jobs which they took seriously and which demanded their best. Their future prospects were illimitable; they were in love; and they were spending their vacation in one of the gentlest areas of the world.

Penny saw in the English papers that three choral societies were uniting for a program in Winchester Cathedral, and with the help of women at the air base she arranged tickets for the Popes and an English couple whose husband flew with John. Somehow they jammed themselves into the sports car and trundled off to Winchester, where the united choir was a delight: boys of fourteen and elderly women of seventy, old men and round-faced young girls, singing the ancient songs of England and the best religious music.

John had little appreciation of the music but could enjoy the soaring architecture of the cathedral, and during intermission he found special pleasure in noting the numerous plaques set into the walls in commemoration of this or that English regiment which had served in India or Khartoum, but at the close of the second half of the program the choirs offered two encores that brought Pope right out of his seat. He had never heard either piece before, but with the aid of the brief explanation by the choir leader, he could immediately recognize their importance. The first began as a show piece for the baritones, who were then joined by all the voices; the words were a poem he did not know by a poet whose name he did not catch:

'And did those feet in ancient time . . .'

The majestic thunder of the song made him want to cheer, and when the voices died away in prayer for a better day, he led the applause, hoping the chorus would repeat the song. Instead they closed with what the announcer said was one of the finest operatic choruses, which, like the first encore, had a solid religious base. It was the chorus of Israelites lost in their Babylonian captivity, dreaming of their homeland:

'*Va, pensiero, sull' ali dorate . . .*'

It was a perfect musical setting to words of deep emotion, and again Pope led the applause, watching with delight as the mixed choir bowed again and again.

Back at the Boar and Thrush he commissioned Penny to find copies of the two encores, and at the first music store she entered, an enthusiastic woman clerk interrupted as soon as Penny started humming. 'Oh,' she said, 'that's a grand hymn. Words by William Blake about 1800, music by Sir Hubert Parry about 1900, and the rousing arrangement by Elgar around 1915.' She blushed, then added in a whisper, 'It became the marching song of the Labour party. My father's Labour and he made me learn it.' She had three good versions of the hymn, but neither in this store nor in the others Penny visited could she find a recording of the second encore.

However, an older clerk who seemed to know a good deal about music told her that the chorus was from Verdi's *Nabucco,* an opera almost never given. He thought that perhaps the chorus might have been put on discs by an Italian company, but could find no proof of this in any catalogue.

So the Popes had to be content with the William Blake song and a record player borrowed from the landlord at the Boar and Thrush, and for the last two mornings in England, Penny could hear her husband bellowing in the resonant bathroom:

'Bring me my Bow of burning gold:
Bring me my Arrows of desire: . . .'

When they returned to Patuxent River they found that Claggett had completed his tour and was taking command of an F8U-1 Marine squadron at Beaufort Air Base near Parris Island in South Carolina. At the farewell party on Solomons, after he had sold his two Chevys for $30 and $65, he took Penny aside. 'You have a big job to do, Penny. When I leave, John becomes Numero Uno. Every pressure will be put on him to stay here at Pax River. Good living quarters. Great assignments.'

'Where do I come in?'

'You must drive him out of here. Don't, don't let that fine young man accept another tour here. That's the graveyard. That stigmatizes him as a man without real drive. Get him busted free.'

'For what?'

'Goddammit, don't give me that simple school-girl crap. You know damned well for what. For command. To get in line for the big jobs. Captain of a carrier. An admiral's stripes.' He gripped Penny firmly by the arm. 'You see it in the Senate. Some of the men forge ahead. Most stay on the minor committees. Your man is destined to be a mover and a shaker. Don't let him be sidetracked.'

'Are you destined to be a mover and a shaker?' she asked sarcastically.

'You bet your ass I am. And so are you.'

Claggett's warning had been perceptive, for when he left Pax River, John Pope became the front runner, the true airplane driver admired by the incoming classes. He got the best assignments, worked most closely with the better manufacturers, but most important was the joy he continued to find in taking a new aircraft high above the peaceful Chesapeake and out over the turbulent Atlantic, testing it, pushing it, feeling it respond to his commands, and sometimes identifying terrible faults which would forever prevent the plane from gaining acceptance into the Navy's arsenal.

Another man augered in, and John Pope was sent to notify his widow, then almost immediately thereafter still another, a young man who seemed destined to follow in the Glenn-Shepard-Claggett-Pope hierarchy of solid test pilots. Now he was gone, a white fish-gnawed corpse dredged out of his crashed plane at the bottom of the Chesapeake.

For some days Pope stayed off by himself, reflecting on the tremendous price the nation paid and would continue to pay so that it might have small, complex airplanes that could carry fighter pilots safely in defense of the country, or large, simplified aircraft that could transport huge numbers of people from place to place. The attrition was fearful, sometimes even sickening, so that Captain Penscott was safe in warning any incoming class of fifteen that 'by this time next year two of you will be dead,' because invariably they were. In his gloom John wanted very much to talk with Penny, or to spend an evening with the Claggetts, but he was alone, and perhaps this was best because it forced him to sort out his ideas, and after three bad days he came back onto the line, choosing for himself the newest and most difficult planes.

He had one extremely close call, when the ailerons on a prototype failed to perform properly and he feared he might have to eject over the Chesapeake, but to do so would mean the loss of an aircraft, and this he could not permit. So with sweat standing on his face, he wrestled the difficult plane into obedience, then brought it savagely back to base and slammed it onto the tarmac.

That afternoon, teeth grimly set, he took control of the area in which outlines of an aircraft carrier had been neatly painted on the tarmac, complete with landing signals and restraining gear submerged beneath the runway, and there he watched the new students bring their planes in for landings as near to the real thing as possible.

They would fly a long leg to the west, turn over the Patuxent River and come banging eastward toward the bay. At the proper moment they would begin their swift descent, watch the landing lights at the rear of the simulated carrier, drop very low, cut their engines and slam onto the deck, where cables stretched taut would catch at the dangling hook, stopping the heavy plane with a force of G's that was unimaginable to one who had never experienced it.

After heckling the newcomers for two hours, Pope took one of the F6Q-1s up himself, made the long circuit, and came thundering down to the make-believe carrier. Reading the signals perfectly, he dropped his plane precisely on the deck, felt his hook grab, then experienced a wild sensation as the hook tore loose from the undercarriage, allowing the plane to skid at great speed down the tarmac on its damaged and collapsing wheels.

With automatic reflexes, Pope did everything possible to keep his plane from crashing wildly or turning over in flaming wreckage. Nine of the routine procedures proved useless, and he thought: We bought the ranch on this one. But when he wrenched the wheel violently to the left, some sorely damaged hydraulic system caught for a moment; the left wheel stayed upright and the plane came to rest in the middle of the tarmac.

Coldly, Pope climbed onto a wing, worked his way aft, and dropped to the ground. After surveying the wrecked plane for about half an hour, checking the points of failure, he let somebody drive him to the ready room, where he spent two hours writing his report on exactly what he thought had happened, with pen-and-ink sketches of where in his opinion the metal had failed. He concluded his report:

> The F6Q-1 is a fine airplane, very responsive under all conditions in flight and with remarkable maneuverability along all axes. If the hook can be strengthened, especially where it joins the empennage, I believe the plane will give a good account of itself.

He then spent four hours with the distraught representatives of Allied Aviation, and on succeeding days he devoted so much time to the field representatives that some of the old-timers, who had witnessed this phenomenon before, started the rumor: 'Pope's had it. Seven, eight near-misses. Now he's sucking up to Allied for a desk job in industry.'

One of the young fliers who had great regard for Pope's impeccable record went to him with the rumor, at which Pope snapped: 'You think I'm a desk type?'

'No.'

'Neither do I.' And when General Funkhauser flew in to check personally on the bad performance of his plane, Lieutenant Commander Pope refused even to see him, saying that his written report had to suffice.

Captain Penscott made apologies: 'I've seen it a dozen times, Helmut. It's called "end-of-the-skies syndrome." A young tiger, flew anything with wings. His days here are numbered and he's scared to death that from now on he'll do no more flying. Desk job. Executive on a carrier.'

'A man like Pope can still fly, even at such jobs.'

'There's flying, Helmut, and there's real flying. They know the glory days are over. And it makes them edgy.'

For the past four years Norman Grant had been having a lonely time in Washington, for his wife no longer came to the capital even for brief visits, saying that she preferred staying in Clay, where she could supervise the education of their daughter, Marcia, now a headstrong high-school senior. It had been Mrs. Grant's correct suspicion that Marcia would not thrive in Washington, and this became an added reason for avoiding the capital, but primarily she wanted to stay home to receive the urgent messages sent by Universal Space Associates, and the more deeply her husband became involved in space, the more she rejected everything he was doing, for she knew that the Visitors were going to assume control any day now; their advanced technology, Dr. Strabismus warned, would make obsolete anything being attempted.

The senator dealt increasingly with what might be called 'the space program,' even though no one in government had officially acknowledged that America needed a space program. Thoughtful men like Lyndon Johnson, Michael Glancey and Wernher von Braun did speculate on what the next practical steps ought to be, but their work had little real focus because most of the experimentation was being conducted in secret by the military.

In their discussions, the leaders were always apprehensive lest the space program become identified with the Democratic party, then in control of both houses despite the fact that the Republican Eisenhower had been reelected President by a huge majority. So whenever a consensus had been reached as to what must be done next, the men brought Norman Grant into their confidence and depended increasingly upon him for bipartisan support. At one informal meeting, when they disclosed some of their hopes for the future, Grant asked, 'What cost figure would you propose for such a program?' And Majority Leader Johnson said, without apology, 'About two billion.'

'Billion!' Grant exploded. 'You'd be lucky if you could get two hundred million over a three-year period.'

'Norman,' Johnson said in his expansive Texas style, 'we're talking about a man-sized budget for a man-sized project for a man-sized nation.' And he outlined roughly his turbulent vision of the future: 'New machines, new types of men flying them, new materials, new problems. It's all going to change, Norman.'

It was at this meeting that Grant dug in his heels. Pointing his finger at Von Braun, he said sternly, 'I'm not going to serve as errand boy to the Treasury to finance your grandiose playthings.'

With the suavity that had always marked Von Braun's relationships with any authority which might have the power to veto his grand design of putting men into space, the German said quietly, 'Senator Grant, it isn't my plaything. It's the world's obligation, and there can be no turning back.'

'Simply because a thing can be done is no justification for doing it,' Grant said, 'and certainly not at the cost you men propose.'

Von Braun laughed warmly and said, 'You're entirely right, Senator. We never have to do something merely because it can be done. But you and I aren't going to be the judge of that.'

'Who is?'

'Russia,' Von Braun said with iron in his voice. 'Every report we get from behind the Iron Curtain confirms our fears that Russia will soon amaze the world with some bold move.'

'Like what?' Grant asked.

'I don't know. But I think they have a capability of putting a nest of scientific instruments into earth orbit.'

'I can't see that as revolutionary,' Grant said.

'And I would not be surprised if they followed with a man in orbit.'

'To what purpose?'

'To astound the world. To gain an enormous propaganda victory.'

When Grant demurred still further, Lyndon Johnson broke in: 'Von Braun's convinced me that if Russia succeeds . . .'

'What do you want me to do?'

'Be prepared, Norman. I want you to think about these problems, because if Wernher is correct, and the Russians do perform some spectacular feat under the gaze of the whole world . . . hell, we could be in hot water.' And then he lapsed into the Texas drawl he used when making a folksy point: 'They was this rancher on the Pedernales and he didn't have much of a herd, so he got his two sons to make imitation cow flops outen brown papier-mâché, and he placed hunnerds of 'em aside the highway, and when my Uncle Sam Houston Richards asked the old man, "What you doin', Clem?" the old man said, "Whether you got a herd or not, the neighbors better think you do." When Russia makes its big move, Norman, we better be prepared to prove to the neighbors that we can match her.'

When Grant showed that he was not convinced about Russia's capacity, the men convened another meeting at which two experts from the Russian desk at the Central Intelligence Agency made reports on the current state of their information, and both Glancey and Grant were astonished by what they heard:

'We have good reason to believe that Russia right now has the capacity to throw a man into space and keep him there for several days.'

'How can you know that?' Grant asked.

'Workmen who report to us about launch and landing sites in Siberia.'

'Are they reliable?'

'Always have been. Also, we speak with scientists in Sweden who monitor the skies, and with the world's best detection devices at Jodrell Bank in England. Bits and pieces, but each confirms the other.'

'And you think Russia has the ability to do what Von Braun predicts?'

'We can reach no other conclusion.'

Grant rose and moved about the room, as if preparing himself for his next question. 'Tell me in simple terms, what would it mean if Russia did put a little machine in space? Or a big one with a man?'

Intuitively, everyone turned to Von Braun, who had been contemplating just this situation for nearly thirty years, and a bland smile came over his large features. 'The world will be turned upside down. It will be told by Moscow that this proves the superiority of Communism, and where space is concerned, Moscow will be right, and the world will know it.'

Grant asked the CIA men what they thought, and they agreed that the propaganda victory would be immense. 'We'd be on the defensive in every country in the world. Can't you hear them chiding us? "You said you were world leaders, but in reality you're world followers." I assure you, Senator, it would be a disaster.'

'And the very next day,' Johnson predicted, 'you and I and Glancey would rush into the Senate and approve a House bill for five billion dollars . . . to catch up. That's why I plead with you to help us now, before the event.'

Grant was a conservative Western senator with broad experience in the military, and he suspected that this was all part of a tactic to scare and get funds, so he asked, 'If Russia is so far ahead of us, and we've been spending so much money these last few years, why in hell are we so far behind?' He glared at Von Braun.

'But we aren't!' Von Braun cried. 'Two years ago we could have propelled an object into space. At Wallops Island our multiple-stage rockets—'

'Wait a minute!' Grant interrupted. 'There's an expert from Wallops Island in Washington right now. I think Mrs. Pope will know how to catch him.' And when Stanley Mott was presented to the informal committee, Grant said, "Mott, we've been told that Wallops had the capacity, some time ago, to loft a device into earth orbit. Is that correct?'

'We think so, sir.' And he told them of that Wallops launch the previous January when Levi Letterkill voiced his guess that if all five rockets of the Honest John + Nike + Nike had fired directly upward, orbital velocity of 16,029 mph would have been achieved.

'That was Letterkill's guess,' Grant snapped. 'Anyone can make a guess.'

'But later he ran his figures through the computer. Three days' intensive analysis. And he proved conclusively that Honest John could have done it.'

'And America would have had a satellite in orbit?'

'Yes, sir.'

'How sure are you of your data?'

'Letterkill's one of our best men.'

'Were you satisfied with his figures?' Grant asked.

'Gentlemen,' Mott said with his customary caution, 'I can only give an opinion.'

'That's why we asked you here,' Grant snapped.

'We could have gone into orbit.'

Grant threw down his pencil. 'Damn it all, if Von Braun in Huntsville knew we could do it, and this Letterkill at Wallops knew it, and you knew it, Mott, why in hell didn't we do it?'

Von Braun did not speak, nor did Mott, although each knew the answer. Grant, disgusted by what he was hearing, glared at Lyndon Johnson, who deferred politely to Glancey, who frowned and said, 'So you nominate me to be the bastard? All right.' Clearing his throat, he said, 'If Dr. Von Braun was not a good soldier, he would tell you, Norman, that your Secretary of Defense, Charley Wilson, issued secret orders that no American rocket was to be thrown into space.'

'Good God, why not?' When no one answered, Grant fumed: 'If a Russian space shot is so all-important, why haven't we been first?'

Mott replied, 'Direct orders from President Eisenhower.'

'I don't believe it,' Grant said, and he stormed out of the office, shouting at Mrs. Pope, 'Tell the White House I'm on my way over.'

By good luck Charley Wilson, whose retirement from Defense had already been announced, was still in Washington and Grant had a chance to talk with both men. 'They inform me, Mr. President, that Russia may be about to loft a scientific package of some kind into outer space.'

'Those fellows at NACA, they're always dreaming something.'

'They're like the military commanders,' Wilson said. 'Using Russia to justify their request for more money.'

'They assure me, Mr. President, that if Russia gets there first, it'll be a huge propaganda victory.'

'I'm sure they think so, Grant,' Eisenhower said with a look of gentle amusement. 'But I can't believe the world is going to get very excited over something not much bigger than a football going around the Earth.'

'I've learned two things in this town,' Wilson said. 'The military always wants more hardware and the scientists always want more money to study things like why dogs bark and why grass is green. You can't ever satisfy them, and they never accomplish a damned thing.'

'Have orders been given to our team not to put anything into space?'

'They certainly have,' Wilson said. 'We don't want that can of worms opened up.'

'I judged it best,' Eisenhower concurred, 'that we not trespass into areas about which we know so little. And if you think about it, Norman, you'll agree.'

The two leaders, each so impressive in his early field of war or business, each so stalwart and responsible in his later work as a leader of government, walked Grant to the door, assuring him that Lyndon Johnson and Wernher

Von Braun were fine men, but never to be taken too seriously in this matter
of space. At parting, Eisenhower said, 'Norman, keep a cautious eye on
your committee. One of these days it'll be needed, but it mustn't go off
half-cocked.'

So Senator Grant returned to the room where Mrs. Pope was collecting
stray papers to be burned, and told her, 'It's reassuring to talk with the
President. He puts things in perspective.' And at that moment, late afternoon at Jodrell Bank in England, a British scientist who specialized in
monitoring Russian activity telephoned one of the CIA men who had
testified earlier in the day with information that 'something happened in
Siberia this morning, Position L, nothing big. We can't decipher it, but for
sure, something was tried.'

That summer of 1957 was, in Elinor Grant's judgment, one of the most
exciting periods of world history, for as she explained to her eighteen-year-
old daughter Marcia: 'The Visitors have been extremely displeased with the
way President Eisenhower has dragged his feet in the takeover, and on three
separate and distinct occasions they've been about to invade Washington
and have been stopped only because Dr. Strabismus has intervened.' She
had the telegrams to prove it. The most recent stated:

> Last week the Visitors held a plenary session in a spaceship off
> Morocco, which I was privileged to attend. Two members of Eisen-
> hower's cabinet, who are in reality Visitors implanted there long ago,
> joined me in persuading the Visitors to delay for one more brief
> respite their planned takeover. I can state with ultimate authority
> that it is now scheduled to take place the first week of October. The
> precise date will be sent you later.
>
> LEOPOLD STRABISMUS
> *Universal Space Associates*

Marcia recalled with amusement that the implanted Visitors had originally
been 'one Washington official with access to President Eisenhower,' but had
quickly become 'one of the President's intimate advisers,' then 'a member
of the Cabinet,' and now 'two members of Eisenhower's Cabinet,' and she
speculated on what kind of charm Strabismus might possess to enable him
to seduce her mother so outrageously, but in mid-July the world-famous
scientist, as his brochures described him, came personally to Clay to solicit
further funds for the impending plenary session of the Visitors, the one
which would determine pretty much how the United States would be governed after the takeover.

He was heavier now, thirty-two years old, with a beard increasingly
handsome. He wore his black hair combed straight back and it emphasized

the white suits he preferred in summer, and this offset his dark eyes, whose effect he strengthened by a judicious use of mascara. But his salient characteristic was the growing self-confidence that surrounded him like an aura; experience had shown that he could do anything, defend even the most outrageous fraud, and gain increasing support from the very people he was bilking. He had charisma, as carefully nurtured as delicate plantings in a spring garden, and his only problem now was how best to capitalize upon it.

'It's essential that I be in attendance,' he told Marcia and her mother as he sat with them in their sunny reception room, 'because the fate of outstanding citizens like the senator will hang in the balance. It stands to reason, doesn't it, that superior though they are, the Visitors will have to depend upon some of our citizens to help them govern, and it might as well be Senator Grant as some boob from New Jersey.' And then he turned his dark eyes full upon Mrs. Grant. 'Or you, Mrs. Grant. The Visitors are certainly not going to discriminate against able women.'

Brazenness like this captivated Marcia, and speculating on just how brazen he would dare to be, she started to watch him intensely, and he decided that the target on this visit was not the mother, whose limitations he understood, but the very pretty daughter whose capabilities were as yet unknown. Marcia was a petulant girl that summer, entered in the university but displaying no unusual promise except for her striking beauty. She was taller than her mother and slimmer, and her unblemished complexion testified to the care she gave it. She wore her hair attractively long, with two plaited braids behind her ears, and these she decorated with small blue ribbons that matched nicely her blue peasant's skirt—which flared, when she moved suddenly, to display her fine legs.

Dr. Strabismus noticed the legs, and with never a word spoken between them, the great scientist and the senator's daughter launched a courtship which proceeded with deepening import as the three talked about the impending invasion. The doctor was meeting with financial disappointment, for as Mrs. Grant explained: 'The senator has closed out our joint account. He became quite infuriated over that last check, so I no longer have access to money which is half mine, by rights.'

'Indeed it is,' Strabismus agreed. 'But didn't you tell me last time that you had personal funds . . . from your father? Wasn't he a distinguished . . .'

'Farmer. Yes, he did leave me an inheritance, but I'm saving that for Marcia when she marries.'

Dr. Strabismus smiled at Marcia and said that this was an excellent idea, most prudent, but in view of the culminating importance of the impending meeting, and its special importance to them through the position in the new government which her father might obtain, did they not agree that a contribution now might be the best way to protect Marcia's future?

While Mrs. Grant flustered this way and that, trying to find an answer,

Marcia stared directly at Dr. Strabismus in her sultriest manner, as if to say: 'I know you're a fraud, an outrageous fraud, and if I had you alone for two minutes, I'd have your pants down.' He smiled right back, as if to say: 'Well, we know one another, and if I had you alone for two minutes, I'd have your panties off completely.'

It was Mrs. Grant's opinion that she and Marcia could spare, at most, $1,500 of the latter's inheritance, and for this Strabismus thanked them profusely, then with masterful skill maneuvered so that Marcia could drive him back to his motel in her Pontiac, and six minutes after he got her there, they were in bed, wildly, joyously.

'You're the most cunning fraud,' she whispered into his beard.

'And you're the sexiest kid on the block. You're ready for California, Marcia baby.'

'My parents would never let me . . .'

'You don't have to tell them.'

'They are a pitiful pair of jerks, aren't they?'

Strabismus preferred not to answer, because he knew that Mrs. Grant was no worse than other flighty women who supported him, and that while Senator Grant was largely ineffective, he was not a public disgrace like some congressmen he had heard of. Most of the girls who flocked to California to share in the adventures of space with him were convinced that their parents were imbecilic, and he supposed that this was a national sickness upon which a clever man could capitalize.

She laughed. 'In effect, I'm paying you fifteen hundred dollars of my own money for this toss in the hay.'

'And it's worth every penny, isn't it?' Marcia agreed that it was, and when next day Dr. Strabismus met with Senator Grant's two women, he warned them: 'Remember! The takeover occurs without any chance of postponement during the first week of October.'

When the senator returned from Washington, Mrs. Grant showed him the October letter from USA, mailed in mid-September to speed donations, and he slumped into a chair to read every word of this amazing document, trying desperately to fathom how his wife could believe such transparent rot. When she told him that her cooperation had assured him a job with the new government, he exploded: 'Are you losing your mind, Elinor?'

'No. And when Dr. Strabismus visited here Marcia liked him, too.'

'Where is she?'

'She's gone to California. To visit school chums.'

'Where in California?'

'Los Angeles, I think.'

'Good God! Don't you see what's happened? He's enticed her out there, and you know what that means.'

'Norman, that's unworthy! Just because you can't see what's happening about you . . .'

He called the FBI in Washington, and within two hours had confirmation that one Marcia Grant, rumored to be the daughter of Senator Grant, was living with Dr. Strabismus and helping address letters in the two-room office of Universal Space Associates.

'What have you done to your daughter?' he cried when he told his wife the ugly news.

'Spies,' Mrs. Grant snorted. 'They're trying to protect an old regime from the revolution that's about to overtake the world, and they'll say anything to save their skins.'

In the middle of September, Marcia returned sheepishly to Clay, entering her university classes two weeks late; when her mother tried to interrogate her about Strabismus, she broke into tears, then entered into a series of passionate dates with a football player.

The three Grants were at home in Clay when the urgent telegram arrived on the first of October warning them to be extra attentive during the coming week because the intentions of the little Visitors were not at all clear:

> But I can assure you that events of supreme importance threaten, and we must all be prepared. I wish I could be more specific, but the Visitors are extremely impatient with President Eisenhower, and I cannot predict what they might do.

The senator was so disturbed by this nonsense that he called the Secret Service to see whether it constituted a criminal threat to the President, and they dispatched from their Chicago office an operative wise in American ways to consult with Grant:

> 'America's full of kooks, probably three in every hundred. Political, economic, religious, the world-is-ending gang. You ought to see the stuff that reaches our desk. Unbelievable. If we tried to track down all the wild ones in orbit, we'd need a force ten times as large, and even then we'd cover only the fringe. This is a nation of zanies held precariously in check by the sane majority.'

When Grant showed him the actual telegram, the Secret Service man laughed. 'This is tame. We know Strabismus well. Compared to the others, he's sane. Works rackets on widows. Has a sweet tooth for girls one day older than sixteen. He provides amusement, I suppose, and does minimum harm.'

'Can he be held in any way for stealing money? A good deal of money?'

'From your wife?'

'Yes.'

'She gave it to him of her own free will and accord, as the legal saying goes.'

'How do you know?'

'I could guess what it was when you called, and I checked the bank records. Twenty-one thousand dollars plus, and every cent legal.' Then he spoke as father to father. 'Senator, your girl came home, didn't she? If she's free of VD and not pregnant, you're a lot luckier than some families. Take my advice, drop the case.'

When the first three days of October passed without incident, Mrs. Grant grew apprehensive, for she had convinced herself that this time the Visitors really would arrive, and she believed that because of her faithfulness, they would invite her to help in governing. She was forty that year, with a long life ahead of her, and she welcomed the arrival of the little men and the better world they promised.

Family problems reached a crisis on Friday when the three Grants dined together and the senator proved powerless to combat his wife's reckless slide into unreality. 'I forbid you to give that charlatan another penny of Marcia's money.'

'I'm doing it to protect her position in the new world . . . and yours, too, I might add.'

'Can't you see he's a charlatan?'

'Don't keep parroting that word,' Mrs. Grant screamed, and she would have rushed from the table had not her daughter reached out to take her hand.

'Mother,' Marcia said, 'we all know he's a fraud.' And while she continued to hold Elinor's hand she recited the facts: the two mangy rooms, Mr. Ramirez and his forgeries, the young girls who trekked in from various parts of the nation. 'You might as well know the truth. He kicked me out when a girl sixteen years old came in by bus from Oklahoma.'

Mrs. Grant drew her hand away and stared straight ahead, refusing to hear these calumnies, but Marcia was now relentless. 'Research? He dreams up everything. He has a staff of one, himself. And as for travel to Morocco, the only trips he takes are to towns like this to steal money from women like you.'

Mrs. Grant remained very erect, hands in lap, then said gently, 'I hope you'll be forgiven when the Visitors arrive tomorrow or Sunday. God knows, I've done all I could to protect you.'

At that moment the phone rang. It was Michael Glancey from Washington with news that would soon astound the nation: 'Norman, turn on the television. Hear it for yourself.'

'The Soviet Union has announced, and observers at England's Jodrell Bank confirm, that Russia has today placed in orbit about the Earth a satellite they call Sputnik. It makes a complete circuit of the

Earth every ninety minutes and is broadcasting a series of clearly heard radio signals in code as it moves swiftly through the sky. It is the world's first adventure into space.'

'The world has nothing to do with it,' Elinor said rhapsodically. 'It's the little Visitors . . . on the day he predicted.'

Marcia had to smile. 'Strabismus! That lucky son-of-a-bitch!'

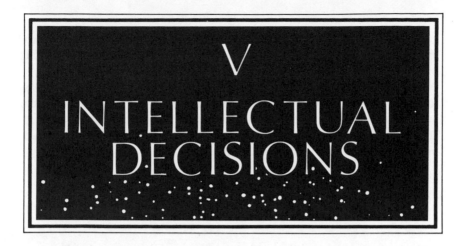

V
INTELLECTUAL
DECISIONS

IF AMERICA HAD BEEN LAGGARD IN ITS EXPLORATION OF SPACE, DESPITE
the recommendations of its premier minds, it displayed an astonishing
determination to catch up once the Russians had led the way, but before
effective steps could be taken, intellectual choices of the most excruciating
complexity had to be made in the areas of management, finance, personnel,
and above all, engineering and science. From October 1957 through June
1962 some of the best intellects in the nation grappled with these matters
and strove desperately to make the right choices.

President Eisenhower and Congress faced three tremendous problems:
Should space be controlled by the military, since they could use it effectively
against an enemy? Should it be financed by creating a bold new agency like
the Atomic Energy Commission, which had masterminded the atomic
bomb? If men were to fly in space, from what pool of volunteers should they
be chosen?

The nation's scientists and engineers had their own mind-breakers to
solve: What kind of machine should be launched into space? Since ordinary
compasses would be of no use, how could this machine guide itself to the
Moon or the planets? Was the Moon a solid body on which men could walk,
or was its surface composed of dust into which they would disappear? And
suppose the round trip proved feasible, how could the returning vehicle
make its way back through the terrible heat of reentry without burning up?

Penny Pope started to tackle her duties one minute after she heard the
news report about Sputnik. Dashing in to Senator Glancey's office, she
called Senator Grant in Clay, and by conference phone the two senators
talked with Lyndon Johnson, who had been informed by the CIA. Hurried
meetings were arranged, which Grant joined as soon as an Air Force jet
could fly him to Washington.

After the committee consulted by telephone with Dieter Kolff in Huntsville, Stanley Mott at NACA laboratories in Langley, and General Funkhauser in Los Angeles, the most urgent strategies were devised. Especially

helpful was Wernher von Braun, who assured the senators that 'America can have its own satellite orbiting the Earth in sixty days,' and when the committee checked with Kolff, this big-rocket man cried, 'Thirty days.'

Accordingly, Penny scheduled a score of meetings whose purpose was to make decisions regarding America's first flight into space, and each meeting was attended by the beep-beep-beep of Russia's Sputnik as it sped across the United States in amazing obedience to the schedule announced in advance by the Moscow propagandists:

> 1932 hours: Above San Francisco, California
> 1933 hours: Above Reno, Nevada
> 1939 hours: Above Clay, Fremont

The Soviets had included the last location because they knew that Norman Grant, a major force in aviation and space groups in the Senate, lived there.

In these meetings, at which she served as rapporteur, Penny had a chance to observe the considerable differences that individualized Johnson of Texas, Glancey of Red River and Grant of Fremont. The first was a folksy wheeler-dealer who believed that absolutely anything was possible if reasonable men sat down to find a common ground from which to proceed; he simply would not accept defeat and could conjure a dozen dirty deals to avoid it; he had a personal vision of what the next few months would produce and an unquenchable faith that things would evolve as he wanted them to. Penny found his attempts at humor unbearably corny and she did not like the suggestive way in which he put his arm about her: 'Now, honey, you jus' call him and reason with him. He'll come around.' But she developed an enormous respect for the man, for she realized that on him—and at times, on him alone—depended America's space program.

Senator Glancey was her man, a hefty manipulator in his rumpled pin-stripe suits, his unkempt hair and his jutting Irish jaw bespeaking a bulldog tenacity. He had the ability to give rich people, whom he admired immensely, everything they wanted to ensure their financial support, while protecting the little people on any emotional issue, for their voting support. He was not a demagogue, but he did have an amazing aptitude for being highly visible on any issue which promised votes and deftly concealed on those which were likely to produce controversy. Like many Southwestern Democrats, he voted Republican most of the time but gave resounding speeches filled with references to Thomas Jefferson and Franklin D. Roosevelt. He had what many self-educated men like him acquired, a sure sense of American history and an abiding belief in the destiny of his country.

In the dark years when America accomplished nothing in space, he was convinced that this condition could not continue indefinitely, and Penny knew that it was due mainly to his prescience that the engineers at NACA and the scientists at Huntsville received the funds they needed to continue their work in obscurity. By now Penny recognized everything that was wrong about her senator—his drinking, his obsequiousness toward anyone with wealth, his pitiful eagerness to get even the smallest government installation located in Red River, and his willingness to trade away any position if it would gain him votes on something he profoundly believed in —and she had concluded that he was, all things considered, the best man in the Senate and the kind of politician she would probably be if she ever got the chance.

For Senator Grant, whose presence in the Senate was partially due to her inspired assistance, she had both awe and contempt. She knew from what Finnerty, Penzoss and Butler told her that he was a hero beyond compare, and she had observed his incorruptible deportment in the Senate: grave, thoughtful, fearfully conservative, always reluctant to take a major stand on anything, and totally supportive of any bill that might aid the military, while remaining generally indifferent to the kinds of social-engineering bills which sometimes ignited Senator Glancey. Grant was a fine senator but his horizons were severely limited, and her contempt for him derived solely from the fact that he refused to grasp the opportunities which a secure seat in the Senate provided. Knowing him personally, she felt no hesitancy about challenging him on issues which she felt he misunderstood or on which he should have taken a stronger stand, and he felt no embarrassment in fending her off with an indulgent smile. It was on committee work that Norman Grant and Penny Pope formed a sturdy team, he the conservative Republican with growing leverage within his party, and she the superefficient young lawyer whose spiked heels beat a rat-tat-tat as she hurried from desk to desk with essential papers.

It was significant that both Glancey and Grant thought of Penny as 'my girl,' and each relied on her for major decisions, but whenever they used the word *girl,* she immediately corrected them: 'You are not my boy. You're a grown man and a United States senator. I'm a grown woman and the administrative director of a very important committee.'

It was Penny who convened six rocket experts, who cautiously decided: 'We should be able to launch an American rocket during the second week in January with a strong likelihood of success,' and she circulated a memorandum establishing 14 January as the target date, but on 3 November 1957 Russia lofted into orbit Sputnik II, much larger than the first and containing a passenger, the dog Laika.

In panic, those preparing America's response insisted that the launching be rushed forward to December or even the end of November, and they received lively support from those in charge of Vanguard, who assured them that their rocket was ready. But when the compromise date of 6 December was announced, Penny warned her senators: 'Don't be surprised if it flops. I know we're not ready.'

However, the entire Senate committee, accompanied by their executive secretary, flew down to Cape Canaveral in Florida for the auspicious entry of the United States into the space age. They watched five miles away when the Navy's thin, frail Vanguard stood poised at the edge of the Atlantic Ocean, ignited with a roar, rose upward for one second, then collapsed in a wild and fiery explosion. And the radio, which should have been soaring into space, lay on the ground uttering a feeble beep-beep-beep while the whole world watched and listened in dismay.

'A shameful disaster,' one of the committee members wailed, and everyone who spoke to the senators reflected the same attitude. Even Glancey was disgusted, but Norman Grant, with that stubbornness which had characterized his behavior at Leyte Gulf, tightened his neck muscles and said, 'Schedule the next shot as soon as possible.'

He was watching, grim-lipped, some weeks later when the second rocket collapsed with a pitiful moan, after a flight of six inches, and he listened bitterly when a naughty joke began to circulate: 'How does an American space scientist teach his son to count? 7, 6, 5, 4, 3, 2, 1, oh . . . hell.'

In Huntsville, Dieter Kolff heard the taunts and kept his mouth shut, but at night when he climbed the hill to his sanctuary on Monte Sano he hammered at the table and told Liesl in German, 'It's heartbreaking! They insist on showing the world the failure of their Vanguard. And all the time I have the Juno rocket that will do the work. It's insane! Liesl, I'm chasing butterflies.'

She stopped what she was preparing for dinner and made instead a dish of salt pork, onions, caraway seeds and sauerkraut, but he was so distraught that he could not eat, and then she knew that he was assailed by severe depression.

These humiliating disappointments had no visible effect on Grant, and even less on Wernher von Braun when he appeared before the committee: 'In one sequence at Peenemünde we tried to fire seventeen rockets, and fifteen failed. Often you learn more from a failure you can analyze than from an accidental success.'

'I'd settle for an accidental success,' Glancey said, but he knew that what Von Braun said was correct.

Penny Pope was impressed by the methodical way in which Senator Grant grappled with his chagrin over the televised collapse of the Vanguard, and she applauded when he announced President Eisenhower's determination to conduct the forthcoming tests in full scrutiny of the taxpayers who were financing it: 'We'll make our next attempt exactly as we made the last. All the television the networks want. All the foreign press that wish to come in—'

'There's a Japanese reporter asking special privileges,' Penny interrupted. '*Asahi Shimbun.* Shall I encourage him?'

'He's welcome,' Grant snapped. 'Our war with Japan is over.' Then he turned to basic matters. 'If we failed so badly with the Navy's Vanguard, we won't repeat that folly. We'll go with that Juno rocket Huntsville's been advocating, and the heads of NACA will inform the Alabama team immediately.' When Dieter Kloff learned of the decision he threw his hands in the air and exulted: 'At last we have our chance!'

On 29 January 1958 the senators and Mrs. Pope were again in Florida, examining from a distance Kolff's massive Juno rocket atop which sat the Explorer spacecraft, and as they watched through binoculars, they noticed that the palm trees nearby were beginning to bend in a heavy wind and they learned that at 40,000 feet up, this wind was blowing at such a speed that it would divert the rocket and make any ascent impossible. 'A hundred and eighty miles an hour up there,' the meteorologists reported, so reluctantly the flight was scrubbed, and the disheartened committee returned to its motel.

On 30 January they were out again to study Juno and her historic cargo, but this time the winds rose to the savage speed of 235 miles an hour, enough to blow the rocket and the Explorer apart, so again the mission was aborted, and at dawn when the senators returned disconsolately to their motel, they saw that Penny Pope had tears in her eyes.

'It's so damned unfair,' she said, pointing to a headline in an early newspaper she had collected: *American Space Shot Phhhhhts Again.*

Senator Grant took her into the motel bar, where he ordered a tonic water for himself, plain, and a beer for her. 'Have you ever tried to guess how many failures the Russians must have had before they succeeded?'

'Do you like to wash your dirty linen in public?' she asked.

'Failure in a technical process is not dirty linen. It's inescapable.'

'You like our way better? This public ridicule?'

'I'm never afraid of public ridicule if I'm going to win in the long run.'

'And are we going to win?'

'Without a doubt.' He took a sip of his tonic water, then added, 'Isn't it reasonable to believe that our Germans are as good as their Germans?'

'You think men from Von Braun's team did it for the Russians?'

'Who else?'

On the night of 31 January the winds subsided, and at 2030 hours word flashed through the Canaveral area: 'Tonight we go!' But when the countdown reached 2145 hours, Dieter Kolff noticed a leakage of liquid fuel on the launch pad, and rumor circulated: 'The launch is scrubbed,' and Penny could hear groans from the press area.

Dear God, she prayed, please let it go off on schedule. She felt that America could not tolerate another fiasco; the senators who backed the project with their reputations could not survive endless disasters. Please, God, she prayed.

The countdown was halted and it appeared that the launch would indeed have to be scrubbed, but suddenly Kolff broke from the blockhouse, ran forward, dropped face down, and started inching toward where the mighty rocket was throwing its fuel.

'Get back!' the safety crew bellowed.

'Kolff! It could blow at any minute!'

Stubbornly he kept crawling forward until he was directly under the massive engines. Then, tasting the spill, he returned to the blockhouse and smiled broadly. 'Condensation. Nothing's broken. Resume countdown.'

At 2245 hours the Peenemünde experts reached the pregnant sequence, 10, 9, 8, 7, 6, 5, 4, 3, 2, 1 . . . There was a titanic flash as Juno's engines roared into action, a mighty gasp as the multipart instrument rose in the air, and then a second burst of flame as those in charge signaled Kolff to arm the upper stages.

'There she goes!' Glancey shouted, and members of the committee started to dance. Senator Grant caught Penny by the waist and lifted her in the air as she cried, 'Thank God, thank God.' But late that night, when it was certain that the American satellite had attained orbit and was functioning even better than predicted, Senator Grant asked Penny to draft a cautionary note to President Eisenhower:

> The policy you so wisely promulgated of doing everything under public scrutiny has succeeded admirably, but it is my duty to point out that we have put one satellite in orbit weighing 31 pounds, but Russia has put two, Sputnik I weighing 184.3 pounds, and Sputnik II weighing a huge 1,121 pounds. Most important of all, Sputnik II proved that a living thing could survive in space, so one must suppose that a Russian man will soon follow.

> We are far behind, Mr. President. We are in military peril and we had better catch up. I am eager to talk with you about these matters.

Satisfied that it could get something into orbit, the nation turned its attention to the problem of how the space effort should be organized, and Senator Grant leaped eagerly into the debate: 'The entire project must be turned over to the military. At installations like Redstone Arsenal in Alabama they have the capacity to do all that's needed. Furthermore, they have the personnel and the managerial capacity to take giant leaps forward.' Many congressmen with military service supported his arguments, and one pointed out: 'It'll be easier to fund the effort through the military budget, because Congress is always eager to vote whatever military funds are needed and damned reluctant to give money to civilian science.' Grant made a final telling point: 'President Eisenhower, himself a military man, will opt for military control.'

A group of powerful Western senators, having observed at firsthand how ably the Atomic Energy Commission handled large projects and even larger budgets, recommended that America's space effort be governed by such a body: 'We'll have no scandals if we go that route.' And each of these senators had two or three personal friends they were eager to nominate as members of the commission when it was formed.

Senator Glancey spearheaded a third group, ably supported by General Funkhauser, civilian leaders of the aircraft industry and many champions of private enterprise. These men argued that the entire project should be placed in the hands of existing private firms, since it was clear that the great industries of California had the expertise to do the job and the know-how to keep costs down. When Glancey became vociferous in his support of such thinking, he was sharply challenged by Grant:

GRANT: Why do you oppose the military?

GLANCEY: Because I'm in favor of the American way, private enterprise.

GRANT: When the security of the nation's at stake, the military's the one to be trusted.

GLANCEY: You control costs better if you rely on private enterprise. They have to make a profit.

GRANT: Cost is not a consideration when the safety of the nation—

GLANCEY: The same men are going to be making the decisions, whatever we select. If the Army fires Von Braun and his gang today, private industry will pick them up tomorrow.

GRANT: I am especially impressed by the need for security, secrecy if you will, in this field. The military knows how to handle that, the private sector doesn't.

GLANCEY: You make too much of security. On most things we can work in the open.

GRANT: In this field, one of these days, security will be of the utmost importance. Believe me.

GLANCEY: For a few brief months, or even weeks. Then the whole world knows.

GRANT: But it could be precisely those weeks that might determine the fate of the world.

While such debate fermented, a group of scientists gathered to argue that the whole project could best be left in the hands of those who were going to provide the answers, and they urgently proposed that a national scientific foundation of some kind be formed to assume control. The outstanding part played by certain university laboratories in developing the atomic process was cited, and it was proposed that a consortium of MIT, Cal Tech, Chicago and Stanford could easily and effectively bring the space age into being, but the possibility that a gaggle of scientists could organize anything, let alone supervise a budget, was so roundly ridiculed in the press, in Congress and in industry, all of whom depended upon science for their safety and advancement, that this proposal was quietly dropped.

That left a fifth possibility. Often in the early stages of the debate each of the four major claimants conceded that NACA was a possibility, with its three excellent centers at Langley in Virginia, Lewis in Cleveland, Ames out in California, but they always spoke with disparagement: 'Of course, we have good gray NACA, but it's never been capable of managing much.' The fact that NACA had always been governed by an unpaid board of dedicated scientists and engineers, without a visible and voluble spokesman, had worked against it. Also, its tradition of rarely spending all the money budgeted because its quiet leaders believed that any project ought to be cost-efficient, raised suspicions, for Washington felt that any agency which did not have huge overruns could not be doing serious work. And finally, since NACA worked closely with three segments of the society—the military, the private airplane industry, the academic community—it was perceived to be subordinate to all three and not a viable entity of itself. In the great debate, NACA did not have to be taken seriously.

When the contending parties threatened to disrupt the nation with their angry debate, one man stepped quietly forward and in his unpretentious way made a series of spectacularly right decisions which established the patterns for the space age. President Dwight D. Eisenhower had not shown much perception in his initial reactions to the space age, for he pooh-poohed the frenzy into which some Americans, including Glancey and Grant, had fallen: 'Why be afraid of something not much bigger than a football?' But as the crisis deepened, so did his understanding, and he now summoned all parties to the White House, where he confided that he was about to send a message to Congress that would settle the debate once and for all:

'Gentlemen, it's decided. We'll have a civilian space agency. But not private industry. Not a consortium of scientists. And not NACA. It will be a new agency built upon the old, using the best of everything we've got.

'We'll send a signal to the world that we intend to use space for peaceful means. We'll work in the open, finance everything in the open, and accomplish wonders with the men and equipment we already have.'

Back in his office, Senator Grant was appalled by this decision: 'The general can't be thinking straight! I've got to head this off before a terrible mistake is made.' He asked Penny to arrange a private meeting with the President, at which he vigorously defended the military's right to control space, and Eisenhower, knowing how important this hero could be in the months ahead, did his best to console him. 'Norman, under my plan the military continues its secret work, as always. And if our civilians uncover anything of significance, your people will be the first to know. But I'm convinced that the exploitation of space must be left in civilian hands, and if you think about it, you'll agree.'

With this assurance, Senator Grant became the Republican leader in shepherding the President's proposal through Congress, and he and Mrs. Pope worked long hours through the spring and early summer, hammering out details and doing the kind of tedious work which underlies any good legislation. During one long weekend, when they worked with Senator Glancey over what they assumed were the last alterations in the bill, they were shocked when Lyndon Johnson stormed in with nineteen refinements he deemed necessary, and Grant was disposed to ignore them, but Glancey warned: 'I've learned one thing in the Senate. Don't ever ignore Lyndon Johnson, or he's gonna nail your pelt to the barn door.' Seven of Johnson's proposed changes protected the interests of Texas, one way or another, and all seven were adopted.

Since the Democrats had only a 49–47 margin in the Senate, the votes of Republicans were important, and now Senator Grant became a focal figure. When certain jingoists tried to force the proposed agency back into the military, he stood forth as the acknowledged military hero in Congress: 'Ike's the best commander in chief we've had since Teddy Roosevelt, and if he wants it in civilian hands, so do I.'

'Six months ago you were all for the military,' his critics pointed out.

'Six months ago I didn't know what I know now,' he said.

'Six months ago Ike hadn't twisted your arm.'

'I suppose God gave us arms so they could be twisted,' Grant said.

Often at the end of the day he would be so exhausted that he wished only to wash his face in cold water, grab a quick sandwich somewhere, and plop into bed, but Penny, who worked even longer hours, would catch him heading for some fast-food outlet and argue: 'Senator, you'll destroy your digestion if you eat that junk. You must get yourself a decent meal—with vegetables and a salad.'

At such times he would suggest that she eat with him, and they were often seen in the unpretentious restaurants near the Capitol where senators, congressmen and staff from the Library of Congress ducked in for hurried meals. One evening, during an unusually leisurely meal, Penny noticed that Grant's face seemed suddenly more lined, as if the burdens of office were weighing too heavily on him. 'Senator, if you keep frowning like that, you're going to be an old man . . . next year.'

'I'm worried about Russia,' he said.

'Senator Glancey's worried about Russia, too. But look at his face. Open, bland, not a wrinkle in the world.'

'All he worries about, really, is Red River.'

'He knows how to relax. You should learn.' When no comment was made, she asked, 'More trouble at home?'

'That damned Strabismus. Mrs. Grant insists upon sending him all kinds of money.'

'Why don't you stop it?'

'I have. My money, that is. But now she's sending him her inheritance.'

'Isn't there a law about fraud?'

'He commits no fraud. We're powerless.'

'What's going to happen?'

He pushed back his plate, tried several times to formulate a reply, then asked, 'How do you and John work things out? I mean, with him not at Patuxent River any more?'

'Navy wives have always devised ways. Our men are gone, then they come back.'

'I think a good deal about marriage and home these days, Penny. Is the way you live any kind of solution? I mean, the two careers? The long separations?'

Penny was now thirty-one, as compelling in appearance as when she first worked for him, and she could visualize the long decades that lay ahead. Speaking very slowly, she said, 'John's career would always come first, I'm sure. But it's a broken one. Here, there. Asia, Mediterranean. I'll adjust to it. But my career with you and Senator Glancey, that's important too, and I feel sure that John will adjust to it.'

'It seems to me you're trying a very difficult game.'

'For sure. And aren't you doing the same?' When Grant evaded the question, she added, 'You in Washington. Mrs. Grant in Clay. Are John and I any more separated than you?'

He picked at his food, then indicated to the waitress that she should take the plate away. 'It's not the same. Not at all. You two are working at major jobs . . . making major contributions. Elinor and I are working at only one job, and she's actually trying to tear down the sensible work of this nation.' He was not proud to be talking like this to an attractive young woman who was the executive secretary of his committee, and he knew the poor impression he must be making, but in recent weeks he had grown quite desperate —he overworking in Washington, his wife frittering away her life back home—and he needed help.

'Penny, would you consider flying out to Clay and talking sense to my wife?'

Without even a pause, Mrs. Pope laughed. 'Senator, how foolish can you be? Surely you know that Mrs. Grant despises me. Charges me with having an affair with you. Or trying to.'

Grant clasped his hands over his belt and studied the restaurant table: 'That's one of her saner ideas. And not to be taken seriously.'

'I have to take it very seriously.'

Impulsively Grant asked, 'Penny, how did you grow up to be so sensible? So strong?'

'I had a good, tough father and I married a good, tough man.' As soon as she said this she realized that her words were a condemnation of the senator, and she started to apologize, but he forestalled her: 'Elinor had a fine father, one of the best. As for me, I'm damned if I can see what I ought to have done differently. Except maybe stay at home and run a small office on Main Street.'

'I've thought about this a good deal, Senator. So have all the girls in your office.'

'And what have you gossips concluded?'

'That sometimes nothing can be done.' She shrugged her shoulders, then added, 'Except throw this Dr. Strabismus in jail.'

'Did you know that Marcia's out in California with him again? They're building a big new center, and she's a consultant. Nineteen years old and she's an architectural consultant.'

'Now you have reason to go out and shoot him.'

'When I asked if you would go to Clay to talk with my wife . . . of course I didn't mean it. But would you fly out to Los Angeles and see if you could . . . well, I mean . . . save my daughter?'

'I'll go tomorrow,' Mrs. Pope said, and although the battle for the space bill was nearing its apex, she arranged for others to do her work, taxied to the National Airport and flew to Los Angeles.

The address she had in her notebook led to the two shabby rooms from which Universal Space Associates held forth, but Dr. Strabismus was not there. Mr. Ramirez, supposing her to be one more silly woman in love with his employer, handed her a slip of paper directing her to a suburban hillside, where she found an imposing white building near completion:

University of Space and Aviation
Dr. Leopold Strabismus
Ph.D., LL.D., D.H.L. Chancellor

From the dusty roadway Penny watched as trucks rumbled in for the building she was sure would be called Old Main, and she was amused to discover that Strabismus, fraud though he was, longed for legitimacy. He was making a financial killing from his two shabby rooms but he wanted the respectability that would come from what others would accept as an honest university. She smiled, and her feelings toward him softened a little. Placing her hands to her mouth, she shouted, 'Marcia Grant? Are you there?'

Instead of the senator's daughter, a tall, bearded, heavyset man appeared from one of the unfinished doorways, and as soon as he saw Penny, in her trim business suit with its white collar, he assumed that she was someone from Oklahoma or South Dakota who had been sending him money, and he stepped forward with a gracious smile and a big extended hand.

'Come right along, ma'am. This is where the university will be.'

'Dr. Strabismus?'

'Yes, indeed. And this will also serve as headquarters for our space research.'

'It's quite grand, really.'

'And where are you from?' he asked solicitously.

'I'm here to speak with Marcia Grant, and if you'll call her . . .'

'Miss Grant is not here, unfortunately.'

He looked at Penny, suspicious now, and his manner changed abruptly.

'I think she is,' Penny said coldly, 'and I'll go find her.'

'This is a hard-hat area,' Strabismus warned, stepping quickly forward.

'You're not wearing one.' She brushed past him and called, 'Marcia! Marcia Grant!'

From a second door the slim, leggy young girl stepped forth in a kind of slouch, her beautiful face marked with a disapproving scowl. 'What's happening out here?'

'Marcia,' Strabismus shouted. 'Go back!' But before the girl could obey, she recognized the visitor and cried, 'She works with my father!'

With a powerful grip Strabismus caught Penny's arm from behind and whipped her about. 'What are you, a spy?'

'I'm an employee of the United States Senate,' Penny said quietly, 'and if you don't take your hands off me, I shall summon a federal marshal.' With her right hand she brushed him away, then proceeded through the dust to where Marcia waited, and when she reached the extremely attractive young woman she greeted her warmly. 'I think we must talk.'

'Don't go with her,' Strabismus cried, trying to intercept Marcia, and when the two women ignored him, he said menacingly, 'Don't touch my car!'

'We'll go over there,' Penny suggested, pointing to a roadside diner frequented by workingmen, and when they were seated at the oilclothed table she said forthrightly, 'Marcia, quit this nonsense and come home with me.'

'Did Father send you?'

'He did.'

'Does Mother know?'

'I doubt it. There's not much communication, you know.'

'You're sleeping with Father, aren't you?'

Penny was shocked by what she did next. With a wide sweep of her right arm she brought her hand forcefully across Marcia's face. 'You're talking with me now, not some damned fraud.'

The suddenness of the attack so astounded Marcia that she could not determine how to react, but Penny's fierce integrity demanded a response: 'I'm sorry.'

Penny was even sorrier. She took the girl's two hands in hers and said, 'I'm the one who's sorry, but I work in a tough world where any challenge to honor must be met . . . right then.'

'I didn't mean to insult your honor.'

'It was your father's that was offended.'

'May I ask a reasonable question without getting my head knocked off?'

'Shoot.'

'Are you in love with Father?'

Penny chuckled, then looked with real warmth at the confused girl. 'I think all women who work for good men like your father grow to love them . . . in a detached sort of way. But have you ever seen my husband?' She took from her small handbag a cellophane folder in which she carried three photographs of Lieutenant Commander Pope, one in tennis shorts, one in dress uniform, one as test pilot seated in a jet. 'I really don't need to romance older men.'

'He's neat,' Marcia said. 'Where is he?'

'He's not running a racket . . . not living off the contributions of addled women.'

'Be careful. Strabismus may wind up a much more powerful force than Father, or your husband.'

'What's this university bit?'

'California lets you get away with anything. It has good laws on the books but never enough manpower to enforce them. They've made us a registered university. We're going to start classes any day. Well, to be truthful, there aren't going to be any classes. All we do is sell degrees.'

'Aren't you ashamed of letting Strabismus get away with this?'

'What do you mean, Strabismus. I'm in it, too. I'm Dean of Faculty.'

'My God! You didn't even finish freshman year!'

'In California, anything goes.'

'Marcia, last year Strabismus kicked you out for some Oklahoma teen-ager. Next year he'll kick you out again. You've seen what your behavior's done to your mother.'

'Mother is a horse's ass, and you know it.'

Again the arm came up instinctively, but this time Marcia intercepted the slap. 'We've had enough of this charade, Mrs. Pope,' she said, and rose from the table, stalked back across the road and informed Dr. Strabismus in a loud voice: 'She struck me—twice.'

'We'll sue her for assault, that slut.'

Penny, just behind Marcia, heard him, and now in a rage, she shouted, 'You say that to me, Strabismus, and I'll get someone to slap you around.'

'You can be sued!' he cried. Calling out to workmen, he said, 'You heard her. She threatened me.'

When Strabismus and the workmen pushed her bodily off the grounds Penny went to her car, slumped behind the wheel, and was thoroughly ashamed of herself, for as a lawyer she knew that in verbally threatening Strabismus, she had committed an assault, and in actually slapping Marcia, a battery—for either of which she could be thrown into jail. But she was now fighting mad and refused to leave California without seeing whether she could in any way deflate this impossible man. When she presented her credentials at police headquarters she was turned over to a Chinese detective, who listened patiently, then said, 'We've studied his case eight or ten times. Complaints from all over the country. Impossible to prove fraud.'

'But the little green men?'

'Half the country sees little green men. My mother does.'

At the local FBI she asked, 'The young girls? Aren't they below age? Isn't that statutory rape?'

'He's very careful on that score. Young girls he sends back home. For example, how old's your case?'

'Nineteen.'

'Legally an adult. She can sleep with anyone she wants.'

'How about the Mann Act?'

'Now there you might have something. If Strabismus sends these young women air fare, or buys them a car in their home state . . .'

'Will you check it? I suspect he did send her the money.'

'Not in our jurisdiction, but we could alert the Vice Squad of the local police.' But when the detectives went to the modest house in which Strabismus and the Grant girl were sharing quarters, they found that Marcia had receipts which proved that she and not Strabismus had paid for her transportation to California. 'Definitely not chargeable under the Mann Act,' the police said.

There was no legal way by which Penny could attack Strabismus, for although he had mulcted citizens of more than a million dollars, he could not be punished because his advertisements had told contributors exactly what they would be getting, and he delivered. The fact that he was peddling arrant nonsense was not actionable, because in comparison to other ideas circulating in California his little green men were downright normal. Nor could anything be done to force Marcia to leave the bed of this outrageous man—she had climbed in willingly, and if she left, six or seven other young women would be most pleased to take her place. Mrs. Pope accomplished nothing.

On her last day in California she made a final appeal to Marcia, but the beautiful girl who should have been studying Biology 103 in some real university would not listen. 'Leopold and I may be on to something very big with this university idea. No one can tell where it'll wind up, but I'm staying with it. The young girls, they come and go. As for Mother, I doubt I'll have any further contact with her. She's quite batty, you know. But you can promise Father that I'll do nothing to embarrass him in public. He's nowhere, but he'll be all right if he can ever get another war started.'

During the flight home Penny sat brooding, endeavoring to unravel the mystery of why these women behaved as they did: Elinor Grant occupies one of the enviable positions in this nation, and she's blown it. Her daughter is bright enough to have any job she wants and pretty enough to have any man, and look what she does! And how about me? She thought about herself, her skills, her ambitions, her solid love for her husband, her lack of children: I haven't cooked a decent meal in three months.

From her purse she took out the photographs of her husband, and for a moment she wished that he would quit the Navy and settle down in some good town like Clay, at which point she would surrender her job with the Senate and care for him and any children they might adopt, but when the plane landed at St. Louis she bought a paper and found that the space bill was encountering opposition from both the military and the scientific community, so in a rush she called Senator Glancey's office, and was told, 'Get back here. Everything's in the balance.'

She worked the last two weeks of July in a frenzy, helping her senators fend off last-minute amendments that might cripple the national effort, and often at night when the arm-twisting had to be done, she gained the impression that only one man in the United States appreciated the awesome possibilities of space, and that was Lyndon Johnson. Once she told Senator Glancey of her belief that Johnson was willing to use even the most nefarious means to gain his ends, and the Red River man laughed. 'You got it backwards, Penny. He isn't willing to use nefarious means. He prefers using them.'

On 29 July 1958 Grant and Glancey stood behind President Eisenhower when Public Law 85-568 was signed, giving the nation a mighty new agency whose job it would be to catch up with the Russians. Behind the two senators stood Penny Pope, hair drawn neatly back, blue suit belted around her slim waist, smiling as Senate Majority Leader Johnson whispered, 'Honey, you wrote more of this damned bill than any of us.' NACA, the National Advisory Committee on Aviation, with a budget of $117,000,000 and a staff of 8,000, had become NASA, the National Aeronautics and Space Administration, with a budget soon to be nearly $6,000,000,000 and a staff of 34,000.

When the details of the new bill reached Huntsville, the gloom which already engulfed that base became actual panic, and the Germans, who had been living on the edge of a dark precipice, not knowing how they were to be disposed of, now saw that their Alabama work had no future at all, for as Kolff explained to his men: 'The new agency is embracing all the strong branches of NACA. They're taking Langley. Ames in California. Lewis in Cleveland.'

'And us?'

'They don't want us. We continue under Secretary Wilson's directive: "Develop no vehicles that might be used in space." '

'What can we do?'

'We can fire our rockets two hundred miles down range.'

'And if they go two hundred and ten?'

'We'll be arrested.'

'How can we live with that?'

'I don't know,' Dieter said. 'Perhaps we'll be dispersed. The old gang, all scattered.'

At home he was disconsolate, and so was his family. Liesl, still mourning her dead dream of creating a beautiful park, watched now as the land was being subdivided into ordinary building lots, its natural beauty ruined, its fine footpaths torn up by bulldozers. Monte Sano was still the most attractive place in Huntsville, so that the local residents often complained: 'How did we let those damned Germans come in here and steal it right from under our noses?' But the noble place it might have become had Liesl's plan been adopted was forever lost, and she grieved, not for her personal disappointment but because this seemed a thoughtless way to treat natural beauty.

Young Magnus Kolff tried not to show his disappointment at having twice been denied permission to attend the music camp at Interlochen. He compensated by being the best trumpeter in northern Alabama, and his parents were delighted when he was invited to play in several different orchestras and even to try out for the summer band at the University of Alabama—but when Dieter discovered that this was a marching band, a football band with emphasis on funny gyrations and exercises which emphasized not music but the spelling out of A-L-A-B-A-M-A, he put his foot down: 'Music has nothing to do with football. You can't go.'

The university, still hoping to get the boy, invited the whole Kolff family to Birmingham to see one of the less-important football games, Alabama versus Tennessee, and during the first half of his first American contest Dieter did get excited by the drill-like precision of the teams, but what happened at half-time killed both the event and any chance young Magnus had to play with that band.

'What we offer next,' the band leader announced in a voice filled with pride and excitement, 'is nothing less than a musical tribute to three great composers, Beethoven, Tschaikovsky and George Gershwin.' Dieter had never heard of the last, but he was fascinated by what the band might do to honor the first two masters.

'Da-da-da-tah,' the band played, offering about ten bars of the Fifth Symphony. Then, without piano, they played twenty bars of a Tschaikovsky piano concerto, after which they played one minute of *Rhapsody in Blue,* with eight clarinets doing a respectable job of indicating the piano part. The entire tribute to three fine composers required one minute and twenty-three seconds, after which the band returned to its marching maneuvers.

'You cannot become part of that insult to Ludwig van Beethoven,' Dieter said firmly when the family returned to Huntsville, but he was soon to discover what peer pressure could be in American life. His son's teachers, his band instructor and the school principal climbed Monte Sano to plead with Dieter to allow the boy to attend the university music camp.

'To march with that band, on an autumn afternoon, when Alabama is playing Auburn,' said the principal, his voice quavering, 'is one of the finest experiences a boy can have.'

'They don't play music,' Dieter said stubbornly.

'But, Mr. Kolff,' the principal said gently, 'we hear that your part of the arsenal may be closed down. Your family may have to leave here. It would be important to Magnus when he moves to another school—if he could say with pride, "I played at the Alabama-Auburn game." '

With a stubbornness born of ten generations of farmers determined not to succumb to improper blandishments, Dieter resisted the entreaties of his son and the boy's uneducated allies, including the faculty members and the school principal. 'You will not march about some silly field.' he said in German. 'Please, Poppa,' came the plea in English. 'All the other boys do it.'

Dieter sought to divert his son's attention by borrowing a seductive catalogue of the G. C. Conn Band Instrument Company of Elkhart, Indiana, and showing Magnus the glittering photographs in color of a real silvery trumpet, saying, 'Look at this, Magnus. On this you can play real music, and we'll send away for it.' But Magnus replied, almost scornfully, 'If I join the big band, they give me free the next size better over on this page.'

Dieter was now fifty-one, gray-haired, his narrow face betraying his apprehension about the future of rocketry under NASA domination, his eyes deep-set and still glowing with the ambition which had dominated the years of his imaginative and constructive life: he still wanted to build the great rockets that would carry payloads to the stars. What kind of instruments were in the payload he would leave to others: NASA, the Army, some new science agency, anyone. His job, and one which he felt only Von Braun and he could discharge, had been simply to build the vehicle, and now he was being forestalled.

'Hell,' he told his wife in German. 'They're strangling us.' He was not eating well, and one night at the table he came close to tears. 'Two hundred miles Mr. Very-Bright-Charley Wilson limits us to. Liesl, in 1943 we were throwing the A-4 two hundred miles. So many years later and we're back where we started.' Grimly he reminded her that the only significant triumph the Americans had known had come from his Juno rocket and its Explorer payload. 'And this is the thanks we get.'

When a dignitary from Washington came to define the new restrictions, the Germans were assembled to hear the distressing news, and it turned out to be much worse than the rumors. Any project of even superficial interest was to be taken out of Alabama and positioned at one of the NASA centers, but the really significant efforts which might alter the thinking of the world, like Dieter Kolff's potential rockets, were to be scrapped entirely. The Army at Redstone was not to be limited to two hundred miles; it was to be gutted and put back on the ground, where it ought to be.

The scientists and engineers were so stunned by this obvious miscarriage of intelligence that they made no protest during the meeting, but that night when the leaders gathered at Kolff's for a wake, angry resentments were voiced and men in their sixties asked, 'Where will we go? How will we find work?'

Others were more preoccupied with the fallacious strategy of such a decision, and one man said angrily, 'No wonder the Russians are ahead of us. It might be better if they dominate the field. Teach the Americans some sense.'

But Dieter could not permit such thinking. 'Don't ever say that! You'd already left Peenemünde before the final days. Each morning rumors as to what the Russian armies were doing to the population . . . how soon they would reach us. I can tell you, it was a terrible time.'

'But in Russia they encourage men like us to do our work. We have proof of that,' and he pointed toward the sky.

'Don't say that!' Dieter repeated. 'Not one of us here would rather be in Russia, and you know it.'

'I would rather be working on something sensible,' the man said, and all agreed, but what that something could possibly be under the new rules, no one could guess.

Not even General Funkhauser, when he flew in from California to hire the services of four Germans needed for special work Allied Aviation was doing, could be hopeful. 'We've been told the Army can't afford to keep this base now that its major mission has been proscribed. And each of the other services has its own plans. No one will touch this place, but an office will be opened to see if we can find jobs in other parts of the country for you Germans.' One thing was certain: like Adam and Eve before them, the Kolffs would go into exile from the lovely Eden they had created atop Monte Sano. 'They can rename it Monte Insano,' Dieter growled.

Packing had actually begun, when an extraordinary occurrence in the White House saved them. It had nothing to do with Huntsville, Alabama, or even the space program; it dealt with shame and remorse.

Never in recent American history had there been any action more despicable than that of President Eisenhower when confronted by the rabble-rousing of Senator Joe McCarthy, for at the height of his campaign of vilification McCarthy had found it expedient to accuse General George Marshall not only of stupidity and ineptness, but of treason. It was a time of inflamed passions, and the senator's wild charges gained such currency that the reputation of one of America's finest patriots was dragged in the slime.

Those who knew the three men—Eisenhower, Marshall and McCarthy —expected the President to spring to Marshall's defense, and for a very valid reason: Marshall had been Eisenhower's superior, had vaulted him into command of the Allied forces, and had supported him unquestioningly at every crisis. If ever one man owed another a debt, it was Eisenhower.

But when the attack came on his old leader, an attack without a shred of substantiating evidence, Eisenhower scurried for cover; not only did he refrain from springing to the defense of Marshall, he also excised from speeches already typed any favorable references to a man who had been the architect of his, Eisenhower's, glory. It was a shameful period in presidential history, and when critics later pointed out his pusillanimous behavior, Eisenhower must have winced.

He did have a defense: the crucial problem of the nation at that time had been how to muzzle the Senator from Wisconsin before he wrecked the Union, and almost any tactic that would remove him from public life was defensible. Eisenhower's problem was McCarthy, not Marshall. The latter was expendable, so the President had turned his back upon his mentor and his friend.

Now, in 1959, with Marshall and McCarthy both dead, President Eisenhower wished to make amends, and when he learned that the Army base at Huntsville was about to be phased out, it occurred to him that if NASA could use this once-productive base, it might appropriately be renamed in honor of the old friend he had treated so shabbily. Dieter Kolff was among the experts summoned to the White House, and in impassioned, heavily accented language he defended the work he and the other Germans had been doing there:

'Mr. President, your honor, believe me that the Germans who were captured by Russia in 1945 were just as brilliant as Dr. von Braun here or workmen like these. If we here in America are on the verge of building rockets which will carry men to Mars or the Moon, I am sure that our cousins in Russia are capable of the same accomplishment. [He pronounced his words as *Chermuns, Rrroshia, vertch* and *aggomplishment,* which gave his statement an added, almost scientific, weight.] Please, Mr. President, put this great installation to some fruitful use.'

Such pleas, repeated many times, satisfied Eisenhower that the rocket site could be adapted to service in the new age of space, and forthwith he directed that it be christened The George C. Marshall Space Flight Center, and on the day the transfer was completed—with a speech to remind the locals that General Marshall had been a powerful soldier, a fine Secretary of State, the creator of the Marshall Plan, which had helped save Europe, and a winner of the Nobel Prize—Dieter and his engineers perfected their plans for the gigantic rocket which they had named Saturn I, suspecting that there would be many improved versions later: Saturns II, III, and who could predict how many more.

A few months later they rigged their first Saturn to a test stand, tying it down so that it could not soar into the air, and with some trepidation, ignited the first of the monster engines. The mighty roar of America's entry into the space age could be heard across state lines; the earth was scorched; the imprisoned power was terrifying as it shook all of Huntsville; and as the liquid fuels burned away, challenging the Sun in their power, Dieter Kolff stood with his hands folded over his chest, as if in prayer, and his eyes were moist.

The long perilous journey from a farm village near Munich to the Russian front to Peenemünde to El Paso to Huntsville to Cape Canaveral to the stars was back on track.

That night young Magnus, sensing his father's euphoria, broached for the umpteenth time the possibility of his playing trumpet in the University of Alabama marching band, but to his dismay his joyous father showed no inclination to surrender. 'Son, never use Beethoven in a poor way.' Dieter, however, was pleased, sometime later, when the best orchestra in the area, a pitiful thing by German standards, asked Magnus to play with them and offered him the use of one of the finest Conn instruments. As the leader said when he talked with Dieter, 'Your son is the best trumpeter in Alabama.'

When little NACA exploded into gigantic NASA the effect on the conservative, penny-pinching engineers who had been running Langley was so drastic that it was almost amusing. Men had to expand their vision a thousandfold overnight, and experts who had been pondering problems a hundred miles into space were now encouraged to visualize operations occurring two billion miles away.

A new breed of managers appeared, too, men alerted to the necessity for good public relations, so that where secrecy and hesitancy once prevailed, with NACA engineers terrified of even uttering a theory before it could be proved, the NASA men delighted in throwing up into the wind of publicity the wildest statements to titillate the general public. One such imported expert, former editor of a newspaper, studied the rosters of all the branches taken over by NASA and saw to his dismay that only a few of the practical engineers who had perfected the marvels of this age possessed doctorates, and he was quite blunt when he faced the management with his data:

> There is no major agency in this nation with as few men with doctorates as NASA. It's a disgrace, and it places you at a severe disadvantage when you testify before Congress or in public. If I can issue a press release which says that Dr. Stanhope of NASA predicts this or that, it gets attention. If I have to rely on Claude C. Stanhope, who holds this or that position and, for God's sake, isn't even a professor, I get no hearing at all.

> Watch carefully what the Army and Air Force do. It's all General this or Doctor that. Navy plays the game better than anybody. They're lousy with Doctors. Now take my advice. You get yourself

some Doctors who can go before Congress and win us some appropriations.

A committee reviewed the entire personnel of the new agency and winnowed the possible candidates into two groups. The first were those younger men who had already demonstrated outstanding intellectual capabilities in getting their master's degrees in various good engineering schools and who could be relied upon to handle the advanced work for a doctorate. High on this list was Stanley Mott: B.S., Georgia Tech; M.S., Louisiana State; IQ 159; lifetime grade average, 3.89.

'We've talked with the men at Cal Tech,' the older man in charge of the Program Doctor Rush informed Mott when the latter came to Washington, 'and they tell us that their program normally takes three years.'

'Beyond the master's!' Mott gasped.

'This is the top school in the nation, maybe the world. They don't throw doctorates around.'

'I don't want to drop out for three years. In that time we could be on Saturn.'

'That's what we said. We showed them your record. The nine research papers you've already done—on the upper atmosphere, ablation, bringing a blunt-nosed body back through the friction belt—satisfied them that you're well beyond the average doctorate level right now.'

'Did they listen?' Desperately Mott wanted to spend a year at Cal Tech, for in his advanced work at Langley and Wallops Island, and especially during his studies of ablation in California, he had seen that much of the really powerful thinking being done in these intriguing fields stemmed from this small, tight, distinguished center of learning in Pasadena. To share in this high intellection, to stand beside these brilliant men as they wrestled with the most arcane new concepts, would be a privilege, and he would undergo any hardship or embarrassment to get such an assignment. He would even plead for a chance.

'The difficulty is,' the personnel man said, 'that what we want you to specialize in is the most arduous field they have, celestial mechanics, what holds the universe together and makes it run.' He stopped to allow this startling assignment to sink in, but as soon as he heard the phrase *celestial mechanics* Mott's heart skipped a series of beats, for this was precisely the field in which in his spare time he had been educating himself. It seemed to him that this was the highest external field of knowledge to which a man could aspire; internally there was gene structure, of equal import and about to reveal secrets just as noble as those of the outer universe, but his mind had always soared outward, so it was inevitable that he would be preoccupied with the mechanics of the universe.

To be allowed to grapple with those secrets! To be one of the handful who comprehended the structure of a galaxy or the behavior of atoms at the outer edges of space!

'I'd volunteer to spend the three years for that,' he said quietly.

'Maybe there's no need.'

'Oh, but I'd like to try!'

'We've had substantial discussions with them . . . emergency and all that . . . national interest . . . and they're willing to make a concession. If you work hard and are able to maintain the level of studies you've already done with us . . .'

'I will.' He was a learned man, one of the best in his field, forty-one years old, but he was pleading like a Boy Scout who wanted to attend summer camp. 'I can work, you know.'

'They say that perhaps you could handle the material in two years.'

'Oh!' Mott had nothing else to say. He was being offered a belated chance to catch up with the most advanced thinking of his age, and all that was asked of him was that he apply himself. When the personnel man waited for an answer, Mott mumbled, 'They'll have to redefine the word.'

'What?'

Mott laughed, the hearty guffaw of a man released from tension. 'I said that when I get through, they'll have to redefine the verb *work.*'

Rachel was enchanted by the news that her husband was going to get his doctorate; she had often felt that he was far more learned than most men who had the degree, but her brief time at NACA had demonstrated how even a good man could find himself at a disadvantage because he lacked the doctorate. The two boys were delighted at the prospect of living in California and studied maps to see how far Cal Tech was from the beach; they were disappointed.

Real disappointment, however, was voiced by Rachel's mother, Mrs. Saltonstall Lindquist, in Worcester, Massachusetts. It was the custom in American social circles for women who were divorced, but who preferred keeping the family name of the former husband, to use as their first name not their given name, Mary or Esther, but their own family name. To refer to one's self as Mrs. Armstrong Cheney was much more polished than to appear in the social columns as Mrs. Mary Cheney.

Rachel's mother, being a widow rather than a divorcee, really had no right to adopt this pleasing convention, but with a family name like Saltonstall, she could not withstand the temptation, and as Mrs. Saltonstall Lindquist she retained the social prestige to which she felt herself entitled. When she heard of her son-in-law's implied promotion to become one of NASA's senior scholars, she told the social leaders of her city:

'Rachel tells me that NASA realized it needed some of its own men to be trained in celestial mechanics . . . what holds the Sun in place, and wouldn't we be in a fix if it lost its place and dragged us around the universe in its fiery tail?

'Well, it's a relief to me, I can tell you. I mean Stanley, not the Sun. It's not pleasant to have to admit you have a son-in-law who went to Georgia and Louisiana. But I do wish he was taking his doctorate at a school of real distinction, like Harvard or MIT. Who ever heard of Cal Tech?'

The second group of NASA leaders identified by the inspection committee comprised those older men of undoubted brilliance who could use the title *Doctor* with good effect when testifying before Congress, but who had neither the time nor the energy to go back to the study halls of some university. NASA solved their problem rather neatly by quietly suggesting to the universities from which they had graduated that it might be rewarding to the academic community if So-and-So, a pillar of the space community and a brilliant scientist, could be invited back to give the graduation address and receive an honorary doctorate as compensation. Some very good men were decorated in this manner.

That left eight or ten able Europeans, including Dieter Kolff, who had no American university which could be gently blackmailed, but their special situation was resolved rather neatly by a NASA administrator at Ames in California: 'We have this new institution in Los Angeles, the University of Space and Aviation, which was properly licensed by the state of California to provide a college education, but which now issues spurious mail-order doctorates in any imaginable subject for a fee of five hundred dollars, whether the recipient has ever set foot in California or not.' It would have proved embarrassing if NASA had tried to send its engineers like Kolff to that campus, for until the new building was completed, there was no campus, no faculty, no library and no classrooms. There was, however, still that excellent printing press on the side street producing a catalogue much superior to that of the Sorbonne and an engraved diploma more impressive than that of Oxford, Yale or Louisiana State.

The diploma was signed, just under the eagle, by the provost of the new university, Dr. Leopold Strabismus, who also offered the M.A. at $300 and the ordinary B.A. at $200.

When Dieter proudly showed his diploma, and his admiring family saw that their father was a full-fledged doctor, just like Wernher von Braun, a rousing celebration was launched, and although everyone present knew that something quite preposterous had happened, no one knew quite what, and it was assumed that if Americans placed even more emphasis upon a doctorate than did the Germans of 1933, and if Kolff was demonstrably brighter than most of the Americans who held one, it was only appropriate that he be given his.

Word spread that Dieter's was an honorary degree, awarded for his outstanding contributions to the space program. He accepted with grace, referring to himself as Herr Doktor Kolff and intimating to his associates that they might prefer to address him by his new title, too. In his testimony before Congress he was now Dr. Kolff and his words were listened to with added attention.

Stanley Mott and John Pope were alike in three respects: each was a straight arrow, each loved space and the stars, and each tended to believe that whatever he was doing at the moment represented a highlight in his life and possibly the maximum excitement that he would know. Leonardo, Immanuel Kant and Albert Einstein had probably felt the same way, and none of them had ever felt any necessity to apologize for his enthusiasm.

For Mott to enroll at Cal Tech, to walk the olive-lined brick paths, to meet with the top analytical professors in the world, and to pore at night over the reports of theorists from Cambridge in England and Pulkovo in Russia was the most demanding intellectual exercise he had ever engaged in. At the end of six months he understood exactly where he stood, as he reported to his superiors at Langley:

> Up to my neck in things I don't comprehend. Only one eye and one nostril above the waves. I've been asked to participate in a gripping problem. Once every 175 years the planets arrange themselves in a formation which permits us to launch a spacecraft that could wander among the planets, picking up propulsive energy from the gravity of each in turn. We could go to Venus, Jupiter, Saturn, Uranus and Neptune, each planet whipping us along to the next.

> This alignment occurs in the period 1980–1982. We calculate that if we launch in 1977, we could reach Saturn in 1981 and Neptune in 1989. I'm not yet equal to the task of helping to plot this journey, but I'm certainly sweating to catch up.

During the next six months, with the assistance of professors who lived among the planets as if the professors, and not some primal force, controlled their motion, he began to grasp the laws which governed even the tiniest particle of dust in the farthest reaches of the universe. Mars and Jupiter became merely the outriders of the massive galaxies that dominated both the remote distances and man's imagination.

As he worked he began to wish that his assignment to Cal Tech had indeed been for three full years, for there were many minor avenues he wished to explore, but NASA kept quietly prodding him to attend to what the directors assumed would be their priority for the next decades: 'Remember that your major concern is not wandering among planets, but how to plot the course of a manned satellite on its journey from Cape Canaveral to the Moon and back to some kind of splashdown in the western Pacific.'

Accordingly, he turned his back on OQ-172 the farthest object, 117,-000,000,000,000,000,000,000 miles distant, and began to focus sharply on the Moon, a mean of only 238,890 miles away (nearest 226,000; farthest 252,000). In fact, that distance seemed so abbreviated when compared to those he had been studying, he came to think of the Moon in familiar terms, as if it rested over the next farm. He was assisted in this thinking by the scientific shorthand he had mastered at Georgia Tech: for example, the large number, representing the distance in miles to OQ-172, could be stated in powers of 10, in this case 1.17×10^{23}, the superscription 23 designating the number of figures following the decimal. The distance to the Moon was a simple 2.3889×10^5, and the frequently used million was 1×10^6. The beauty of the system was that if one wished to multiply two huge numbers, say three trillion (3×10^{12}) by two billion (2×10^9), one simply multiplied the 3×2 and then added the superscriptions $12 + 9$ for the answer 6×10^{21}, which meant 6 followed by 21 zeros. The universe was organized in powers of 10.

One peculiarity of the system delighted him. It was difficult for even an astronomer to remember how many miles light traveled in a year, yet this was a measurement fundamental to space. The figure was easily obtained: seconds in a minute, times minutes in an hour, times hours in a day, times days in a year ($60 \times 60 \times 24 \times 365 = 31,536,000$ seconds in a year), which you would then multiply by the speed of light, 186,000 mps. Some early student had realized that the total number of seconds, 3.1536×10^7, was practically identical with Pi, 3.14159265×10^7, so that astronomers often said that the miles in a light-year were Pi $\times 10^7 \times$ C, the last letter being the symbol for the speed of light. This produced a rough approximation, which caused the astronomers to joke: 'Close enough for use in NASA,' which customarily carried tolerances to seven decimal places.

That rockets could cover the relatively brief distance to the Moon, 2.3889×10^5, Mott never doubted, and now he began to construct those magnificent charts which showed how it could be done. A rocket would lift off from the Cape, enter low Earth orbit, stay there for several revolutions to confirm orbital data, then fire another set of engines and take off for the Moon. Of course, both the Earth and the Moon would be engaged in following their own orbits, so that the relative relationship between the two would be changing from second to second; the trick would be to aim the rocket not at where the Moon was, but at where the Moon was going to be in the number of days, hours, minutes and seconds it would require the rocket to traverse the 238,890 miles. It was an elegant problem regarding the motion of a body with six degrees of freedom, but one that could be solved, and he directed all his attention to it.

However, when the brain of an individual is fiercely concentrated on a given problem, it is sometimes diverted by accident into an unexpected channel, which proves more significant than the one being followed, and this now happened to Stanley Mott. He was attending a night seminar at the great telescope on Mount Wilson east of Cal Tech when he chanced to see an amazing photographic plate which showed one of the most distant galaxies, invisible to the unaided eye and to most telescopes, but absolutely perfect when caught in a giant telescope and held in focus on the photographic emulsion for eight hours.

The galaxy was seen edge-on, a thin, beautiful sliver of stars innumerable and clouds of primordial dust, but in the dead center, as in our own Galaxy, there stood a gigantic ball of generating fire from which the energy which informed the galaxy had originated and was still originating, and Mott realized that when he studied this remarkable plate, he was being vouchsafed a glimpse of his own Galaxy. This was what the universe was like, this incomparable beauty, this inconceivable multiplicity.

As photographed from Earth, this epic galaxy, this poem of the heavens, stood at an angle of forty-five degrees from the horizontal, the most effective possible presentation, as if an artist had positioned it for maximum effect. But it was the implications of the photograph which enraptured Mott: That band of shadow along the near edge, what could it be, cosmic dust? The spicules of flame leaping from the rim, how high into the perpetual darkness did they fly, a billion miles, five billion? The wonderfully tapering tips so far from the central bulge, what would the life of a star be at that remote point? And finally the thing itself, this collection of a hundred billion separate stars, perhaps two hundred billion, this unity, this diversity, this terrible fracturing violence, this serene loveliness, this image of mortality which was surely destined for flaming destruction, what did the thing itself signify?

Like any sensible man who is suddenly struck by a vision ten times greater than any he had anticipated, Stanley dropped all his work on the Moon and spent three weeks trying to understand this photograph, one of the most completely successful ever made, one worthy of his digression.

He learned that because it was invisible and not discovered till late, the galaxy bore no name. It was referred to simply as NGC-4565 (*New General Catalogue of Nebulae and Star Clusters,* compiled by a Danish astronomer and published in 1888). It lay along an edge of the constellation Coma Berenices and was about twenty million light-years distant, which meant that what Mott was seeing in 1961 was what the galaxy had looked like 2×10^7 years ago, and it awed him to realize that in the multiplex of years since that moment, the galaxy could have modified totally, or moved into conflict with another galaxy, or vanished altogether. He was seeing an echo of some great thing that had once existed, and wherever he looked in the outer universe he was seeing the same type of thing: evidence that greatness had once been, but no proof whatever that it still was.

NGC-4565 held him captive for three long weeks, as if its gravitational pull were asserting itself over the 117 billion billion miles that separated it from Earth, and he was bedazzled when he learned that it was traveling through space at a speed of almost three million miles an hour. When he finished his study and returned to his work on the Moon, he knew that he had directed his intellect permanently into orbits so vast, so infinitely far beyond the Sun's planetary system, that he would be forced to spend the remainder of his life not on Earth, not on target Moon, not on Mars or Saturn and not even in his own Galaxy, inexhaustible as it was, but out in the infinitely cold, the infinitely remote distances of the farthest galaxies. He acknowledged that as a faithful servant of NASA, which paid his bills, he would have to perform his routine duties and make the mundane calculations for the Moon trip—note how he brought the Moon down to Earth by describing its distance as *mundane*—but his mind and his imagination would be elsewhere.

Rachel Mott was not liking California. Her severe New England upbringing had not prepared her to accept the free-and-easy life of the Pacific coast; even her disciplined hairdo, each strand in its assigned place, seemed to protest the windblown excesses of the West. And she was not at all happy about the reactions of her sons to their more relaxed environment.

Millard, now eighteen, with a slim, blond, athletic figure, was spending most of his time on the beach, learning to surf; his shins were scarred from losing battles with the board, his face was tanned and his hair windblown. He had associated himself with a group of handsome young men much like himself, and they seemed well behaved, but the two or three girls in the gang, as Rachel called it, were a rougher type, and she often wondered how any of these young people succeeded in school, since their sole preoccupation appeared to be surfing.

One morning she asked one of the girls, 'How are you doing in school?' and the girl replied, accurately, Rachel thought, 'It's a bore.' When she inquired among the boys, she was surprised to learn that two of them were already in college, and when she tried to check on how difficult the studies were in a Western university, the boys replied, 'The professors are all jerks.' She was tempted to dismiss these replies as the shorthand of youth, but when she probed deeper she found that Millard really did consider his teachers jerks and their lectures a bore.

Rachel's upper lip grew tense at such moments, not in anger but in regret that these fine young people were missing what had been so important to her and Stanley: the challenge of new ideas. When her upper lip tightened her lower lip protruded somewhat, lending her an air of hardness which she did not have, really, and when the surfers saw this, they retreated, for they did not care to waste their golden hours on anyone over thirty who might hassle them.

Rachel's displeasure with California did not extend to the university where Stanley had immured himself. As she wrote to her mother:

Your last letter was far too harsh, Mother. Cal Tech is a fine school and in certain limited areas it would approach either Harvard or MIT, but it hardly has the refined scholarship of either of those outstanding universities. Stanley seems to thrive on his heavy work-load and Christopher grows browner each day. I sometimes worry about Millard, as he has apparently surrendered completely to California life, and I do not appreciate its slovenly ways. I'll be delighted to leave here and return to the relative sanity of Virginia, and I'm assured by visitors from headquarters that when Stanley lands his Ph.D. he'll be in line for an important promotion in the burgeoning NASA. Brains do pay off, though not apparently in the case of women.

One May morning she saw California at its worst, and it terrified her. She had taken young Chris to a store in one of those appalling malls, hoping to find bargains in the loose-fitting slacks and shirts boys his age preferred, and at first she was pleased with the selection such stores offered, but when she had bought several items and had taken Chris to a sandwich shop for lunch, she had an opportunity to inspect the workmanship in the shirts and was dismayed by the shoddy goods she had purchased.

As she stuffed the shirts back into their package, her gaze wandered to the next booth while she waited for the fresh salad she had ordered for herself and the savory western sandwich Chris had wanted, and she saw at the untidy table a little panorama of California life. A mother with curlers in her hair and a tight sleazy blouse across her ample bosom was whispering to her daughter, who looked to be about ten years old. She was a rather pretty child, with hair done in high style and manicured fingernails flashing bright red polish. The child's face was made up with mascara, rouge and a fine powder, which did create a delicate balance and an appearance suitable for a college girl of twenty. Her dress must have been very expensive, for it was marked by the simplicity of a couturier; it seemed most inappropriate when displayed on a child.

'My God!' Rachel muttered to herself. 'That child's wearing a bra!' That was correct; to fill out the expensive dress properly, the little girl had been given a bra—Young Miss Special—with padded cups, and to anyone but a conservative mother from Boston, the effect was pleasing: a little girl of ten had leapfrogged more than half a dozen years to become a heartbreaker of seventeen.

What really disgusted Rachel, however, was the manner in which the blowzy mother was feeding her daughter: a Double Grand Malted, a large plate of Fritter Fries and a bottle of West Best Ketchup, which was being doused vigorously over the greasy potatoes, after which enormous quantities of salt were applied. Rachel, looking at the wretched combination—all calories and not a vitamin in the lot—thought: It's all right to contaminate a child's dress style, because that can be altered easily if the person acquires any sense as an adult, but to damage the body, which can't be repaired, that's criminal.

She finished her own salad so slowly, wondering whether children were being equally abused in suburban Boston, that young Chris left the table to wander among the shrubbery that landscaped the sandwich shop, and her attention moved from her attractive son in his clean outfit to the plants which lined the street, and she thought: Maybe California doesn't look after its children, but it certainly knows how to tend a lawn or a line of shrubs. They know how to make good salads, too, she conceded. It hasn't all been a loss.

She had been daydreaming in this manner for some minutes when the little girl, who had also left her table without Rachel's noting that fact, came screaming back into the restaurant. 'Mummy, Mummy! He showed me his you-know-what!'

At first Rachel was unable to interpret this jargon, but when patrons in other booths began to stand in order to see the wronged child and the boy who had committed this sexual assault, she realized with horror that they were staring at her son Christopher, who had slipped back into the sandwich shop, his face red with confusion and shame.

'Goddamned degenerate,' a woman snarled at Chris as he slinked past.

'Mummy!' the little girl continued to scream, not unpleased with the commotion she was causing. 'He showed me his you-know-what.'

On the fourth repetition of this unfortunate phrase, Rachel wanted to sink into the floor, just disappear, die maybe, and she thought that if the child uttered that stupid sentence once more, she, Rachel, would strangle her. But then, in the agonizing pause while the flustered waitress tried to add her check, Rachel thought of another man in her family, Uncle Donald, who had never been able to control himself where women were concerned. He loved them, respected them, but never discovered a sensible procedure for living with them. There was the awful scandal when as the happily married father of three he ran off with a pretty clerk in the drugstore, and the worse affair when he exposed himself to four little girls, not forgetting the time he was horsewhipped outside a bank.

Rachel, her face beet-red, thought of Uncle Donald and wondered if young Chris was destined to follow in his flamboyant steps, and she could hear her mother informing all the neighbors: 'Donald's not a Saltonstall, thank God.'

For the fifth time the little girl explained to the patrons what Chris had done, and then mercifully the check arrived. Rachel paid it and was about to stalk out of the restaurant when she instinctively stopped, reached for her son's hand, and brought him to her.

'You ought to take that one to a good psychiatrist,' a customer snarled, and it was this that infuriated Rachel most. In the street, beside the shrubbery in which the crime had occurred, she thought: In California they think they can solve everything with a good psychiatrist. And she was about to apply the simpler cure of Massachusetts and swat her son, right there in the street, when he said, not in self-pity, 'She asked me to.'

'I'm sure she did,' Rachel said eagerly, embracing her son in sight of the customers.

At home that afternoon she sat in a darkened room, trying unhysterically to sort out not only this messy affair but also the general relationships within her family. She was bored with her mother's simplistic, social-climbing ways and felt little rapport with her; the decades had passed too swiftly and Mrs. Saltonstall Lindquist had not kept up. She was relieved that Uncle Donald had scuttled away after one of his episodes and was now living in Minneapolis, where the colder climate seemed to have defused him. She was deeply in love with Stanley and appreciated increasingly the intelligence and judgment of this bespectacled wizard; curiously, she enjoyed trying to follow him in his abstruse exploration of the stars and she understood when he asked her to frame the glossy photograph of NGC-4565 which he now kept over his desk. From time to time she had intimations that Stanley might even be a genius, not in the Einstein class, of course, but at least the equal of any of the professors at MIT, for whom she had enormous regard.

But now she could think only of their sons, and her feeling that they were heading into deep trouble. And she realized that it had been Stanley's weakness, and hers, too: over the years, as her husband had become increasingly immersed in his work, he had drawn further away from his children, and she had made little effort to challenge this.

Millard's surfing friends were, well, dubious. They were bronzed and trim, but they weren't what one might call healthy, and this was proved by the weird assortment of girls they seemed to prefer. In thinking of these strange girls, she used one of the California words she disliked most heartily: None of them are *cuddly*. She couldn't help laughing: You've got to hand it to California. Sometimes it does come up with the right word. And not one of those girls is cuddly.

She wondered if she had been. She wondered if any living human being ever saw herself as she presented herself, sexually, to the world. She was quite sure that the little girl gorging her Fritter Fries and ketchup now thought of herself as a prim, reserved child who had been wronged; her mother thought of her as a virgin angel; and Rachel thought of her as a little degenerate in training to become a prostitute.

And then she had a really ugly thought: I would rather that Millard be mixed up with that pitiful little girl, when she gets a few years older, than with the sterile things Millard's been bringing here. And finally she saw clearly the corroding situation that faced her family: Millard's a homosexual. I think he'll always be.

At last the composure fled, and in the darkened room she wept. She had said, long ago, that the measure of a woman was how she organized her space, and she had accomplished miracles: the neat rooms, the Mondrians on the wall to establish the standards; her unflinching support of her husband regardless of what luck he was in; her repeated work with others less fortunate; and her constant concern with political problems. All these had given evidence of her good intentions. How, then, could her sons be stumbling into so much trouble?

Christopher's escapade with the Fritter Fries girl, as Rachel was already calling her, was no light matter; it bespoke a young lad who gave multiple signs of becoming just like his great-uncle Donald, an unstable, bewildered male who fell prey to anything in skirts. And it wasn't only the sexual problem that caused Rachel's apprehension about her younger son; like his older brother, the boy seemed absolutely drawn to the weaker members of his class in school, and he had already been detected twice in doubtful performances, not the rowdy exhibitionism of young males but the sneaky destruction of property and the flouting of authority.

This time she would speak sternly to her husband about these matters and demand that no matter how urgent his work at Cal Tech, he must become more concerned with his sons and take steps to try to ensure that they developed into responsible persons. There's time, she assured herself. Even the Fritter Fries girl could be rescued if someone snatched her away from that impossible mother. Millard and Christopher can both be saved.

So when Stanley Mott returned to his rented rooms that afternoon, 25 May 1961, his attention should have been concentrated on what young Chris had done at noon, but instead he burst into the apartment aflame with excitement. 'Have you heard the news? Where's Millard? We must all listen to the television.'

Millard was spending the night with one of his surfing buddies, but the rest of the family gathered for the six o'clock news to hear a replay of President Kennedy's message to Congress:

> 'Now is the time to take longer strides—time for a great new American enterprise—time for this nation to take a clearly leading role in space achievement, which in many ways may hold the key to our future on earth.

> 'I believe this nation should commit itself to achieving the goal, before this decade is out, of landing a man on the Moon and returning him safely to Earth. No single space project in this period will be more impressive to mankind, or more important for the long-range exploration of space; and none will be so difficult or expensive to accomplish.'

When the President finished speaking, Stanley leaped out of his chair. 'They told us at the laboratory, but I couldn't believe it. "Before this decade is out." That's only nine years. Rachel, do you realize the work that will have to be done!'

She tried repeatedly to divert his attention to their sons, but she could see that he was inflamed by wild visions of what impended, and once she was even foolish enough to allow herself to be momentarily distracted from her mission. 'If it happens, what role would you have?'

This allowed him to speculate, all through dinner, on the possible channels into which his career might flow. 'Thanks to Cal Tech, I know about as much about the Moon as anyone else on board. But if we accomplish what the President outlined . . . Don't you see? As soon as we reach the Moon we'll be drawn irresistibly to Mars and Jupiter. Inevitably. And that's where I'll really be able to contribute.'

When his enthusiasm had spent itself, and he returned from Saturn windblown and bearing the dust of stars, she sent Christopher to bed and asked her husband to turn off the news program and sit attentively while she said something of considerable importance. Whenever she spoke like this, perhaps twice a year, Stanley dropped whatever he was doing and said, 'Yes?' for he knew that his wife was not a frivolous woman.

She was forty-one that night, a handsome, disciplined woman who had tended herself and who looked sternly competent as she said, 'Your older son is spending the night with that dreadful Clarendon boy, who I know is a homosexual. Your younger son distinguished himself in a public restaurant by exposing himself to a ten-year-old girl who had been gormandizing on greasy Fritter Fries. Stanley, you have a problem with your sons. We have a problem.'

It was unfair to drag a man down off the stars, and on a night like this, to make him survey the condition of his sons' lives, and Stanley Mott was not equal to the challenge. 'Ten-year-olds! Rachel, didn't you ever play doctor when you were young?'

The last six months of Mott's residence at Cal Tech would be remembered as the most difficult period of his life, because he was deeply engaged in completing his doctorate—*Theoretical Treatment of Several Multibody Influences on Procedures for Launching a Manned Flight to the Moon and Returning Its Passengers Safely*—and he allowed nothing to divert him. But when NASA realized how directly his doctorate impinged on the challenge thrown out by President Kennedy, it was inevitable that he be asked to participate in some of the most crucial debates ever engaged in by America's scientific community. Great scholars of the most exalted reputation, two with Nobel Prizes, were scrapping with one another, not over some erudite refinement of a concept but over a practical matter on which depended the reputation of the United States: What strategy should be adopted to land a man on the Moon and get him back safely . . . now?

The administrator himself stopped by Cal Tech to impress upon Mott the gravity of this debate. 'Everything hangs on our making the right choice. Your field of expertise qualifies you to join the committee.'

'I'm honored, sir, but I have my thesis to complete.'

'If you help us get our men on the Moon, you'll have a real-life doctorate any man would envy.'

'Could I do your work, and finish my work here at Cal Tech at the same time?'

'A superman could. I'd probably have tried in my day, and fallen flat.'

'Can I try? I mean, may I try?'

'You may.'

He would never forget those months. In the heat of committee debate he would boldly oppose two revered academicians, knocking down their recommendations with his new-found knowledge, then return to the campus, where he would listen meekly as the Cal Tech professors lambasted the analytical procedures in his thesis. It was a game of such vivid intellection, such cyclonic changes of concept that he could scarcely keep all the facets in view, and sometimes he feared that his brain might simply call a halt and cease to work, but then some completely wild suggestion would be made, forcing him to reorganize all his data and speculative ability, and just as he had taken three weeks off to digest that immortal photograph of NGC-4565, he would quit whatever he was doing and attack this new problem.

Such a digression now arose. A group of distinguished astronomers presented NASA and, by means of a press conference, the nation, with grave doubts about the feasibility of actually landing a man on the Moon; they did not mean the engineering difficulty of getting him there or the scientific mystery of enabling him to find his way without a compass; they meant the terrible dangers that might arise when a man tried to step down upon the Moon.

'There is a strong likelihood that the surface is composed of lunar dust about fifteen feet thick into which the man would disappear,' argued three of the experts

'Judging from preliminary analyses, the surface might be composed of materials in such delicate balance that they could well ignite or even explode when subjected to pressure from a human foot,' another group said.

'The real danger will be the heat beneath the lunar surface, enough when agitated to melt metal,' submitted one man.

'No,' said another, 'what photographs we have indicate the possibility of deep crevices into which machine and men alike will tumble.'

One scientist, whose self-imposed task it was to keep conversant with European studies, informed the committee that an Italian astrophysicist of impeccable reputation had conducted experiments which proved conclusively that a human being could not walk—could not manipulate his body joints—in any ambience with gravity less than one-fifth of that on Earth. 'And you're proposing that our man walk in gravity as low as one-sixth, on the Moon. It can't be done.' This confused even Mott.

And the medical men whom the dissidents consulted identified the real fear: 'There is a strong probability that the Moon contains diseases unknown on Earth. They will either strike down the humans who land among them, or attach themselves to those humans and run riot if brought to Earth where no counterstrains are known.'

These fears became so pervasive that NASA had to institute a commission to confront them, and Mott, as a leading selenologist, was invited to participate; so for some months his major attention, when not completing his doctorate, was focused on these challenging problems, and it was he who drew up the conclusions which would govern procedures until the moment when men actually stepped upon the lunar surface:

> We are entitled to operate on the principle that the Moon has a solid crust which will support the weight of a man. Crevices may well exist, but the principal part of the surface, especially in the belt which most concerns us, appears to be free of them. The risk of stumbling into an undetected one is so small that it can be taken. We find no evidence that the surface is or will become inflammable. We have no experience with one-sixth gravity, but experiments are under way to simulate it. With our present knowledge, we see no impediment to free movement.

> We are aware of the Italian studies which prove that man cannot walk in a gravity of less than one-fifth, but we are loath to accept these findings and shall conduct our own investigations immediately.

> Speculation that the Moon may harbor virulent strains of unknown viruses must be taken seriously, and our medical team is going to recommend three weeks of quarantine for any human or object returning from the Moon.

Setting aside all other matters, including even work on his doctorate and speculation about farthest space, Mott concentrated on this practical question of whether a man could control his joints and body movements in one-sixth gravity, and the place he turned to for instruction was Langley, where he found two men who had anticipated this curiosity, attacking it in a way that illustrated the inventiveness of the human mind. As the senior investigator said, 'The problem was forthright. How do you place a man in one-sixth gravity? The solution was simple.'

What they had done was go to a very high gantry, already in existence, from which a cable 155 feet long could be suspended. At the ground ingenious body supports were attached to the supposed astronaut's head, shoulders, hips and legs. A wall was leaned back 9.5° off the vertical, and when the astronaut, suspended by the cable so that five-sixths of his weight was carried by the wires, walked against this inclined board, he experienced only one-sixth gravity. It was imaginative and perfect.

Mott insisted that he be placed in the gear, and as soon as he was suspended and allowed to stand against the inclined wall, he understood the mathematical principle. If the wall was inclined 90° to the ground, his entire weight would be held by the cable and he would experience null gravity. If the wall was laid flat on the ground, the cable would carry none of his weight, and he would experience the normal gravity of Earth. At 9.5° off the vertical the geometry was such that he discovered what one-sixth gravity meant.

In this condition he ran, jumped, bent down, twisted, climbed a ladder, leaped from a height of thirty feet, and fell slowly, comfortably back to the wall, and then, running as best he could in the dreamlike ambience, he marshaled all his strength and leaped right over a twenty-foot fence—an astonishing feat. The experience was so exhilirating that he wanted to remain in the gear long after the experiment ended, and watchers took photographs of this slender man in steel-rimmed glasses, forty-three years old, running like a gooney bird on Wake Island and leaping great fences like Aladdin or Buck Rogers.

When he submitted his final report, conceding only that there might be malignant viruses, which, however, he felt could be controlled, he was attacked on all sides, but he stubbornly refused to make any concessions: the Moon was approachable, it was not deadly, and men could walk upon it. For three weeks following the release of his conclusions he was required to defend them before scientific bodies, groups of reporters and television cameras, and with every recitation of his findings he became more obdurate in his support of them. He became NASA's Moon man, and having cleared the way intellectually for the great experiment, he now worked assiduously to make it succeed. All his daylight hours and many of his dinners were devoted to Moon problems, and often it was not till eleven at night that he found time to work on his doctoral thesis, and he would sit hunched over his desk till two or three in the morning, when Rachel made him come to bed.

As a member of the Moon Committee, Mott was told that five major solutions to the problem of lunar landing had been proposed, and it was impressed upon him that if a landing were to be accomplished by 1969, as Kennedy had promised, a choice among them had to be made quickly and correctly. 'I can never determine which obligation is the more important,' one scientist said, 'speed or accuracy.'

The five proposals were easy for Mott to grasp, since he had already analyzed four of them in his thesis, but to choose irrevocably among them was difficult, for it meant staking the nation's reputation and the lives of its astronauts on a process that might prove disastrous. At the first meeting he heard proponents defend each suggestion.

'The first and easiest way is what we call the Jules Verne Approach, since he described it in surprisingly relevant detail back in 1865 in his novel *De la terre à la lune.* He even predicted that the journey would start at Cape

Canaveral in Florida, where ours will. His method? Simple. You build one hell of a big cannon, shoot a capsule to the Moon, carry power with you, and when you're through exploring, shoot yourself back to Canaveral.'

The speaker, an old hand from the NACA days, assured the committee that the Verne Approach was practical, and reasonably safe, in that the gigantic rocket could let itself down gently on the Moon because the force of gravity there would be only one-sixth of that on Earth, which also meant that the power required to lift the rocket back into space would be only one-sixth the amount required to lift off from the Earth.

There was one difficulty. The rocket would have to be so big and heavy, if it were to launch from Earth, carry men and equipment to the Moon, and then retain enough power to leave the Moon and return to Earth with heat shields in place, that no rockets then in existence could do the job. A prospective superrocket called Nova might do it, but the experts warned that it could not be operative before 1975, and there went President Kennedy's promise that we would make the landing before 1970.

'The second way,' said one of Von Braun's men, 'has been studied exhaustively since 1930. It's called Earth-orbit rendezvous and it's really quite simple. You lob a rocket that we already have into low Earth orbit and let it ride there, carrying the machine that will land on the Moon. Then we send a second rocket aloft, join it with the first, supply the first with all fuel and equipment, and from this stable platform the Moon rocket will fire and be on its way.

'The beauty of this assembling in orbit is that it requires only small rockets, the total weight is less, and the journey to the Moon is made in a small, easily maneuvered machine.' The difficulty was that rendezvous would be perilous, the joining doubtful, and the successful lift-off from the Moon with a well-worn vehicle extremely problematic. But the Von Braun man insisted that it could be done.

Now, for the first time, Mott spoke in the meeting. 'How does Von Braun's major assistant view these matters? Dieter Kolff?'

A specialist from Alabama stammered, then confessed: 'Dr. Kolff supports the first alternative. Use one of his gigantic rockets and blast right to the Moon.'

'Does he think he could provide such a rocket within the next four years?'

'He says he could do it next year.'

'Do you think he could?'

'No. And not in ten years. Dr. Kolff is mad about rockets . . . big ones . . . he's to be forgiven.'

The third proposal was sponsored by some geniuses from California: 'Build the lightest possible rocket. But use two in tandem. Rocket One carries the men and their food directly to the Moon. Rocket Two follows with all scientific gear, all the fuel necessary for the return trip. They land within a quarter of a mile of each other . . .'

'And if Rocket Two lands on the other side of the Moon?' a scientist asked.

'With inertial guidance, that doesn't happen.'

'And what is inertial guidance?'

'A modern miracle which you must take on faith . . . for the present.'

'And the men in Rocket One, must they also take it on faith?'

'That's how they found their way to the Moon in the first place.'

This proposal merited the most critical attention, and when the proponents circulated beautiful drawings and cleverly made miniatures of Rocket One, Rocket Two and the Transfer Vehicle that would carry fuel from the latter to the former, the august committee became a group of schoolboys, moving their toys this way and that across their polished table.

'Can a vehicle like this travel on the Moon's surface?' an academician asked.

'We think so. The rest would have to be taken on faith.'

Alternative Four was a most attractive proposal made by a group of private engineers who believed that a manageable rocket, with maximum power and size, should be launched toward the Moon, and when it had exhausted its fuel, a second rocket would overtake it with a monstrous load of fresh fuel, which it would deliver to the first rocket, sending it and its astronauts on their way to the Moon landing and a subsequent return to Earth.

'And what happens to the empty rocket?' one of the committee asked, and the engineers looked at the great scientist in disbelief.

'It's in orbit. Absolutely nothing affects it, neither wind nor rust. It just keeps going forever.'

'In orbit about the Earth?' the scientist asked.

'It no longer has anything to do with Earth. It wanders through the planetary system and remains in orbit about the Sun as a small man-made asteroid.'

Mott had already studied the weights, fuel requirements and payloads for these four systems, and his knowledge proved valuable when the discussions started. Invariably the proponents of the alternatives challenged his figures, for theirs were always more hopeful, but between them they did agree on parameters, the new word this year, and sensible discussion became possible.

The fifth proposal was astonishingly different, and as it was being offered, the committee members leaned forward. It was made by an Air Force colonel in his late forties, a real super stick, a true believer, with piercing eyes that darted from one member to the next when his chin thrust forward in that person's direction, as if he knew he had to convince these brilliant men one by one.

'My plan is simple and daring. Using a relatively small rocket currently available, we will shoot a man and three years of food and oxygen to a flat site on the plain near Copernicus. We're absolutely certain that he can get there, and land, and survive with equipment and compressed foods we already have.'

'How does he get back?' Mott asked.

'He doesn't,' the colonel said. And when the gasps subsided, he added, 'Not right now. Not this year. But we have every right to anticipate that within three more years of night-and-day research we *will* have rockets equal to the task of going to the Moon and rescuing him.'

'Good God!' one of the scientists snapped. 'Do you mean you're willing to risk the life of a human being on a chancy venture like that?'

'I've risked my life on lots worse.' His arrogance offended the scientists, but he continued, 'I flew to eighty thousand feet when we had rudimentary oxygen systems. At Edwards, I sent men up to a hundred and fifty thousand feet when every component was debatable. To have the honor of being the first man on the Moon, return or not . . .'

He paused and looked around the table. 'To establish the discovery rights of the United States to a surface area bigger than Asia? To go down in the history books of the world? Gentlemen, I could get you twenty test pilots in our services who would take off tomorrow.'

'Even though they would have to wait there three years, alone?'

'They would have a radio. Think of what they would broadcast to the world.'

'And at the end of three years they might hear on their radio that the rescue rockets were not functioning . . . that there would be no rescue rockets. Would you send one of your men on such a trip, Colonel?'

'I told you, twenty would leap at the chance.'

'Would you?'

'I came here to volunteer.' He stood very erect, a man not much over five feet six, weighing about one hundred and forty pounds, and as he waited in the silence it became apparent to the committee that they were dealing not only with fascinating proposals, but with a problem of life and death and the history of the world.

The Moon Committee came down strongly in favor of the Jules Verne Approach: 'A hell of a big rocket, up, land, and come home.' When Dieter Kolff in Alabama heard the decision he was overjoyed, because this was what he had been preaching for twenty years, and even though his ardent support of this proposal put him somewhat in opposition to Wernher von Braun, who favored Earth-orbit rendezvous, he was jubilant and assigned his men a score of studies which would enable the tremendous Nova rocket to leave the sheaves of paper on which it had been theoretically planned and become a titanium-and-steel reality.

But Mott was now working in a world of superintellection, and as soon as a decision of any kind was promulgated it became the subject of intense analysis, with the most tenacious brains in the world snarling at it to expose its weaknesses. This was essential to the process, for Mott's committee would ultimately spend some $25,000,000,000 to support their decisions, which would merit all the close scrutiny they could get.

When the debate about straight-up-and-straight-down was at its blazing apex, he happened to visit Chance-Vought, the well-regarded company that had built those remarkable airplanes for the Navy, the F4Us and the F8Us —and the fiasco in between, the F7U—and there he was accosted by a quiet man who had spent his life contemplating the intricate problems of hoisting enormous weights into the air and keeping them there in forward motion. During a memorable night at the edge of a test field this man carefully indoctrinated Mott with the concept that would ultimately save the space program:

> 'Keep your eye on the simple problems. Solve them, and everything else falls into place. And the greatest problem is this. You have to lift a ridiculous weight into the air to carry enough fuel to get you off the Earth, through space, off the Moon and back to Earth.
>
> 'If it's this weight that's holding you back, why not get rid of the weight? Yes, that's exactly what I mean. Get rid of the damned stuff.'

When Mott asked sardonically which part of the weight the man proposed dispensing with, the part that carried you up or the part that brought you back home—and considering himself rather clever to have posed the question so succinctly—he was surprised by the Vought man's response:

> 'I mean all of it. Not just the rocket stages, as we do now. I mean the whole damned bundle except the tiny little chamber in which you ride the last forty miles of the journey. I mean you're to do on a large scale what you've been doing on a small scale at Wallops. Use the first batch of fuel, then throw away the engines that burned it. Let that whole organism fall back into the ocean and sink. Just as we do the Atlas.
>
> 'Then use the next batch of fuel, and throw away the engines that burned it. I mean cut them loose completely and let them fall into the ocean. Then throw away all the instruments and electrical gear required so far. And when you land on the Moon, throw away most of the vehicle that got you there. Just leave it on the Moon. And when you get off the Moon and back to your mother craft, throw away the cabin that took you down to the Moon.
>
> 'Throw everything away, Mott, and on your return trip to Earth, you throw away even the machinery that brings you home, until at last you're a thin little man in a very small capsule suspended from

a parachute, and when you hit the water you throw away the capsule and the parachute.

'You're to think of yourself as launching into space in a complex vehicle consisting of eight or nine components weighing thousands of tons, and at the end of your flight you land naked in Mother Ocean, where you started from in the first place. All the rest you've thrown away. You have become the spaceship.'

This became Mott's operating principle, so that whatever proposal was placed before him was analyzed as to how much of it could be thrown away and how quickly, and it was his application of this great truth that doomed the Jules Verne Approach. 'But, sirs,' he argued with the Verne proponents, 'in your plan you carry an immense machine to the Moon and then you spend all your energy to bring it back to Earth.'

'Is there any other way?'

'Von Braun and his Germans at Huntsville propose a very sensible plan. Assemble the Moon rocket from components lofted into low Earth orbit. No gravity, no strain.'

One by one, Mott discarded the other alternatives: they were too heavy, too costly, too speculative, or, in the case of the Man-on-the-Moon-and-Let-Him-Rot, too inhumane. The only practical way to reach the Moon, he was convinced, was by the approach devised by Wernher von Braun, who knew more about rockets than anyone else on Earth.

Accordingly, when NASA established a new committee to make a hard final decision regarding an actual flight to the Moon—'And no more fooling around'—Mott led the fight to kill off, once and for all, any further discussion of the Jules Verne Approach. 'We've moved into a new century with new capabilities. Let's use new techniques.' And he became such a vigorous exponent of Von Braun's Earth-orbit rendezvous that committee members started calling him Our Little German.

He told one of the engineers, 'You meet only a few men in your lifetime who are geniuses. If you're smart, you cling to them.' And the engineer snorted: 'Von Braun's no genius. He's an engineer.' Mott thought of several sharp retorts, but none seemed likely to be effective, so he said lamely, 'I suspect it'll be Von Braun who takes us to the Moon.'

By dint of much midnight work he qualified for his doctorate that summer, and with his own money he invited his mother-in-law out to Cal Tech to be with the family at the stately ceremony. Mrs. Saltonstall Lindquist noted with approval the quiet dignity of the university, the charm of the olive-girt walks and the grandeur of the faculty club, perhaps the finest in America. 'It's better than Harvard's,' she admitted grudgingly.

· · ·

Because of the stupendous surge in space ventures following President Kennedy's challenge, and particularly because of the inflated NASA budget —well through the first billion dollars, and galloping toward the fourth and fifth—some dozen industrial firms offered Mott choice appointments with salaries that dazzled, but he thought of himself as a government servant engaged in the world's most exciting decisions, and he rejected them all, except that on the eve of graduation General Funkhauser motored over from his headquarters in Los Angeles with some shrewd observations:

'You haven't been listening, Stanley. NASA is not going to make anything. It's going to let everything out to commercial contractors —us, Chance-Vought, Grumman, North American, Douglas, Boeing. We're the ones who'll build the space age, not NASA. You join our firm and you'll build the vehicles that go to the Moon. I am the space age, not Dieter Kolff at Huntsville or your friends at Langley. Join me and you join the first team.'

And when Mott did stand back and look at what was actually happening, instead of what the neat flow charts said was happening, he saw that General Funkhauser was painfully correct. The long-time airplane companies—Grumman, Douglas, Boeing—were really running the space program while the NASA bigwigs toured the country making speeches and testifying before Congress.

When Funkhauser offered him $37,000 a year to help Allied Aviation make proper decisions in the space age, Mott felt he had to discuss the tempting opportunity with his wife, and since Mrs. Lindquist was visiting, with her also.

The women were divided in their counsel. Mrs. Lindquist said, 'Stanley, you've worked like a dog, and what do you have to show for it? A miserable rented house with one bathroom. Unless MIT offers you a full professorship, with a house thrown in, join the company and earn a decent salary.'

Rachel saw a different vision: 'You've made yourself one of the top brains in the country. The world is wheeling around to your point of view. Stay with it, Stanley. You could be the American Von Braun.'

Just as his committee was about to announce that America would adopt Von Braun's Earth-orbit rendezvous, he received a cryptic call from Mrs. Pope in the Washington office: 'Senator Glancey wants you to fly directly to Huntsville. Dieter Kolff seems to be making waves. Has strong objections about something.'

When Mott checked in to the Huntsville motel and called Dieter, he sensed tension and assumed that as soon as Kolff could drive down from Monte Sano to pick him up, the German would launch his complaint, but young Magnus was in the car with him. Mott was pleased to see the boy because despite his absorption in his work, there was an ever-present worry in the back of his mind as to what he and Rachel ought to do about their sons, and it was helpful to observe another boy of about the same age for comparison.

'How are you doing in school?' he asked the square-faced blond, and the answer he received was so different from what his own sons might have given that he was astonished: 'I still do poorly in English, but I'm really learning something in mathematics and science, but what I like best is music.'

'What music?'

'We have an orchestra in town. I play trumpet.'

'He's only fifteen,' Dieter said as he drove the Volkswagen up the steep roads leading to Monte Sano, 'but he's been accepted at the university. Scholarship in music.'

'Do you drive your father's car yet?' Mott asked.

'Oh, no! That comes when I'm sixteen. Special permit.'

'But can you drive?'

'Oh, no! That comes when I'm sixteen.'

'I wouldn't want him to touch the car till it's legal,' Dieter said.

At the cottage on the hillside Dieter was impressed by the clever additions the Kolffs had made to their home—a room here, an added storage space there, and since their continued stay at Huntsville had been endorsed by the President, a screened-in porch on which they could sit and survey the city lights gleaming below them.

The meal was one of Liesl's best, an inexpensive cut of beef marinated in a strong vinegar and cooked for an extra period in a pressure cooker; this broke the tough fibers and allowed the marinade to penetrate all parts. With the sauerbraten she served potato dumplings and a homemade dark bread, and the meal was so appetizing and so obviously nutritious that Mott asked for seconds, his hearty appetite belying his thin, wiry frame.

While Mrs. Kolff cleared the table and Magnus went to his room to study, the two engineers sat on the porch and began a conversation which challenged all that Mott's committee had been doing:

MOTT: What's eating you, Dieter?

KOLFF: The decisions you're about to make. They distress me.

MOTT: I was told you now supported Von Braun's proposals.

KOLFF: I do. I'm always a loyal soldier. You know that.

MOTT: I'm sorry your simpler plan couldn't be accepted. But the Jules Verne Approach . . .

KOLFF: I argued. I lost. That's finished.

MOTT: Then what's the problem?

KOLFF: The idea itself. It's corrupt with error.

MOTT: Going to the Moon? You've talked to me about that for years. In El Paso . . .

KOLFF: To the Moon, yes. But never to the Moon as a major target.

MOTT: What's wrong with the Moon as a major target?

KOLFF: Because when you hit the wrong target you congratulate yourself. As if you'd accomplished some great thing.

MOTT: Do you doubt we'll land on the Moon?

KOLFF: We'll land there. Trouble is we'll never get off.

MOTT: Now wait! Just wait! I've spent months reviewing every step of our procedure, and I'm morally certain we can get our men safely off.

KOLFF: The men, yes. The nation, no. Once we land on the Moon, we'll remain imprisoned there.

MOTT *(soberly)*: What do you mean?

KOLFF: I mean the terrible error of sending astronauts there. The terrible error of making the Moon shot a circus event.

MOTT: The men are the heart of this adventure.

KOLFF: And that's what's wrong. We do not require them for a Moon landing. They'll be in the way. They'll make the adventure less significant than it should be. They'll cheapen everything. And in the end, Stanley, they'll be the reason why we stay imprisoned on the Moon.

MOTT: Explain.

KOLFF: Look at the Moon, coming like a gray goddess in the east. Then look at the stars over there where the moonlight doesn't fade them out. The Moon is a vagrant thing. It comes and goes. The stars are forever, and our obligation is not with the temporary Moon . . . that's easy to grasp. Our obligation is with the stars . . . and they're not easy to comprehend.

MOTT: Would you scrub the Moon shot?

KOLFF: Not at all! It's a logical first step. But I would get it over in a hurry. I'd not send any men there, to avoid the circus effect. And I'd get on with the job of real exploration. Out there, where the battleground of the mind awaits us. *(And he pointed in a direction far from the Moon.)*

MOTT: Why do you object to the astronauts?

KOLFF: Now we come to the heart of the matter. The men are not technically necessary. You know that and I know it. But to accommodate them, we have to make the capsule enormous when it should be quite small. Then to lift the capsule we don't need, we must have rockets twice normal size. Then we must have fuel for the oversize rockets. And we have to have support systems for all the things we don't need. And most dangerous of all, when we get there the attention of the world is diverted to the men and away from the significance of our adventure.

MOTT *(very slowly)*: Dieter, I know what's eating you. You're a man who can build very big rockets. At Peenemünde, you dreamed of one that could cross the Atlantic. At White Sands, it was always bigger, bigger. All you want to do is fire great big rockets and to hell with their purpose. You're an engineer who's gone mad.

KOLFF: And you're an engineer who's lost sight of the big goal. Science has corrupted you.

MOTT: You believe we could explore the Moon and Mars without men in the machines to guide them? To react to emergencies?

KOLFF: And better. Give me the money we're wasting on the manned part, we could complete the basic exploration of the solar system in three years. We could land our machines on the Moon and bring back samples tomorrow. We have the devices to photograph the universe, to land on Venus, to fly out to Saturn to inspect the rings. We could do it faster and better and obtain twice as much information.

MOTT: Why don't we?

KOLFF: Politics. For political reasons President Kennedy said 'We'll fly a man to the Moon and bring him home.' *(Here he paused to laugh at himself.)* All my life I've been the plaything of politics. Adolf Hitler has a dream, and I'm summoned from the Russian front. Helmut Funkhauser wants to wipe out the stain of Nazism, so he leads me into your arms. Now it's the business politics of *Life* magazine.

MOTT: What in hell do you mean?

KOLFF: *Life* has a contract with the astronauts. Exclusive. No other magazine. So it has to make them notable, how you say, *newsworthy*. Fifteen writers spend all their time converting seven ordinary young men into gods. And look at the newspaper! Abandons all critical judgment and writes about Al Shepard as if he were Columbus. And what did he do? He rode in a machine like the one we made at Peenemünde a quarter of a century ago. And neither *Life* nor the *Times* perceives the real significance of these flights.

MOTT: It's news. It's tremendous news.

KOLFF: It's the wrong news.

MOTT: You can't stop it, and Von Braun can't stop it, and I can't stop it, so what are you going to do?

KOLFF: I'm going to watch quietly while the circus triumphs, and then watch sadly as the meaningless parade grinds to a halt. And when we are doing nothing I shall sit here on this porch and look at the stars and weep.

Kolff was so impressive in his analysis that Mott impulsively altered his travel plans, remaining in Huntsville to talk with the other experts about the implications of what Dieter had said, and although the Germans were loath to disclose anything counter to government policy, it was clear that they shared Kolff's apprehensions about manned flight as a dead end. Von Braun was not in residence at this time, so Mott sought permission to wait until he returned, for he suspected that the German leader must also see the essential uselessness of including human beings in the package being sent to the Moon, and in the two extra days he had to wait he talked guardedly with many people.

Von Braun proved an enigma. He was delighted that Mott's committee had eliminated the Jules Verne Approach, and had pretty well dismissed the three other options, for this meant that his recommended assembly in Earth-orbit rendezvous would have to be adopted, and this would require his continued management. He was in a strong position, and he knew it.

He did not want to discuss, even fragmentarily, the possibility of making the Moon shot without the involvement of human beings. 'That's all been settled at the top. We can live with it, quite easily. Besides, the men they've chosen are so highly trained they'll be an asset during the flight.'

'But wouldn't it be simpler . . .'

'The matter's settled,' Von Braun said, and it was obvious that he did not intend saying anything which might reopen it. As at Peenemünde, authority had spoken, ending speculation, but as Von Braun ushered Mott to the door he did say two things. 'I hear you were one of the strongest champions of my Earth-orbit rendezvous. Thank you. You were not only courageous. You were right. And don't let Dieter Kolff disturb you with his speculations. He'll never be happy till he fires one of his rockets right out of the solar system. And when that time comes, he'll be right. But for the present, he's not.'

Two hours later, as Mott was preparing to fly back to California, he received an urgent phone call from the Space Committee in Washington. It was Mrs. Pope: 'Senator Glancey wants you in his office this afternoon at four. Bring Kolff.'

The meeting was short and brusque. On one side of the table, like a condemnatory grand jury, sat Senators Glancey and Grant, accompanied by their chief of staff, Penny Pope, who took no notes. The meeting had been called by Glancey, but it was Grant who started the discussion:

'Just what in hell do you two men think you're doing?'

'What, sir?' Mott asked.

'Stirring up trouble about the Moon shot. Goddammit, we have trouble enough without men in our own organization adding to it.'

'What do you mean, sir?' Mott asked, with no sign of subserviency. The many invitations to join major companies that had been offered since he had achieved his doctorate gave him a confidence which he had not known before.

Norman Grant, with sixteen years in the Senate, had also lost the hesitancy which had marked him at his first election. He was now accustomed to knocking down adversaries if persuasion failed, and he judged that in this crisis some knocking down was needed. 'We have reports that you two men have been agitating at Marshall Space Flight Center against our proposal to have astronauts man the capsule when we land on the Moon.'

'Dr. Kolff and I discussed it, sir,' Mott said, using Dieter's cherished designation to impress the senators. 'Dr. Kolff is a world expert in these fields and I sought his opinion.'

'Well, I can assure Dr. Kolff that in this matter his opinion is not worth a damn, and he had better keep it to himself.'

'All opinions demand attention, Senator Grant. Have you heard some of the crazies we've honored with a hearing?' When he told the senators about the Air Force colonel who wanted to be set down on the Moon with a three-year supply of food and oxygen against the day when more powerful rockets might be invented to come save him, Senator Glancey shook his head, but Senator Grant said grimly, 'I'm sure we could get volunteers to try it. If I were younger, I'd go in a minute.'

Glancey said, 'The problem is this, Mott. Grant and I have to justify before Congress the God-awful budgets you NASA people hit us with. Five billion dollars a year. We cannot justify this if we go before the Senate and say, "This is for scientific exploration." But if I stand before the Senate and say, "This is to put a brave American boy on the Moon and bring him back safely," the senators will wipe the tears from their eyes and approve twice what Grant and I ask for.'

'But you know,' Mott said stubbornly, 'that it could be done cheaper and better without the men.'

Grant banged the table in disgust. 'Dammit, Mott, when Mrs. Pope brought you in here a few years ago I thought you were one of the brightest men we had in NACA. Now you sound downright stupid.' As soon as he said these harsh words he apologized. 'Withdraw that. If there's one thing you're not, it's stupid. I'm told you did wonders at Cal Tech. Congratulations. But you are obtuse. By God, you are obtuse.'

'Yes, you are,' Glancey said, and now the tense session got down to cases.

'It's like this,' Grant explained. 'The NASA program is terribly expensive. It depends on people like Glancey and me and the Vice-President to keep it funded, and the best thing we have going for us is not Wernher von Braun, good as he is, or brilliant men like you and Kolff. It's the astronauts, God bless 'em, because the people of this country have taken these men to their hearts. If you were perceived as saying one bad word against John Glenn, you'd be driven out of NASA by nightfall. He's sacrosanct, and so are the others. On them rests the whole defense of NASA. We're not sending a monkey to the Moon. That was a terrible mistake. Ran the risk of people laughing. And we're not sending a machine, because people can't love machines. And we're not sending scientific instruments, because people are interested in them only in Boris Karloff movies. What we are sending is brave young American heroes, and don't you forget it.'

'What we're really doing,' Glancey said amiably, 'is muzzling you two. You can talk between yourselves about next steps and better steps, but in public, you keep your mouths shut.'

'If you don't,' Grant said, 'you could imperil the very program that you've worked so diligently to set in motion.' Turning abruptly to Mrs. Pope, he said, 'You may bring him in now,' and when she left the meeting room, Grant said, 'We've invited a gentleman to join us. To explain facts.'

The newcomer was a handsome, meticulously groomed man of about fifty, dressed in an expensive gray whipcord and wearing imported shoes fastened not by ordinary laces but by lengths of leather ending in soft Italian tassels. 'I'm proud to introduce Tucker Thompson,' Grant said, 'long-time editor of *Folks* magazine. His corporation's been awarded an exclusive contract for covering the special group of astronauts we're about to select, and I've asked him to outline the gravity of the situation.'

Thompson spoke in a Vermont dialect, twangy, subdued, extremely confidential; every sentence he uttered conveyed the impression that he wished to take the particular group of hearers and none other into the secrets of the space age:

> 'I suffer from two grave disadvantages. Our company has won this contract in opposition to *Life,* so we're newcomers. I don't wish to say a word against *Life,* because they've done an out*standing* job presenting the astronauts to the public. But we're convinced we can do better. Also, my job makes me a kind of public relations man, and you'd have a right to be suspicious of anything I say.

> '*Folks* magazine does not interpret the great space adventure as a circus. We're not in the business of creating instant heroes. And I truly believe we'll never overplay our hand in presenting our astronauts as anything supernatural . . . just the finest young men our nation has produced and their wives as prototypes of what young American womanhood should be. We are not selling dreams, we're selling realities.

> 'And the reality is this. America sees its space program as identical with the astronauts. And their families, I might add. Their families are a significant part of this mighty program. It would be impossible to imagine a bachelor astronaut, because half his significance would be missing. I think I could say without fear of successful contradiction that without its astronauts, America would have no space program.

> 'What's the bottom line? No one must print or say or circulate in any way even the slightest hint that any part of the space program could go forward without the astronauts. We have an enormous investment in these fine young men and it simply must not be imperiled.'

Mott found it offensive to be lectured by someone who apparently knew so little about the scientific difficulties of the space program—the mind-breaking anxieties which kept even the best astronomers agitated for months—and he decided the moment had come when he must speak as a scientist.

'Our two senators remind us of the political realities. This distinguished editor tells us of the public relations aspect. Dr. Kolff and I are here as engineers and scientists responsible for the crucial decisions, and I remind you that the Moon shot is only part of our program. Either before or after its success, we'll be sending a probe to Mars. Unmanned.'

'And the nation will know nothing of it,' Tucker Thompson predicted, 'because writers like me will have no human beings on which to hang our story.'

'You think the story is everything?' Mott asked.

'I do.' Then, sensing that he was being put into opposition to these two brilliant scientists, he told a joke. 'Public relations men, which I am not, have to be watched. When Moses was leading the children of Israel out of their captivity in Egypt, he gathered them on the banks of the Red Sea and told them frankly, "Children, we're in trouble, deep trouble. The sea ahead of us. The desert around us. The Egyptian army bearing down upon us. Tell you what I'm agonna do. I'm gonna separate that Red Sea and make a pathway of dry land. We'll march across, and when the Egyptian army tries to follow, I'll tell you what I'm agonna do. I'm gonna close up that pathway and drown 'em all." The Israelite PR man who heard this was ecstatic. "You do that, Moses," he cried, "and I can get you three pages in the Old Testament." '

Grant said, 'With our astronauts we get three pages in *Life* every week, three columns in the *Los Angeles Times,* three pages around the world. Never forget, you scientists, what a colossal beating our nation took when Yuri Gagarin was parading country to country proving that Communism was superior to democracy. I want John Glenn and Virgil Grissom to be doing the parading, and on the happy day we land one of our men on the Moon, we back Russia right off the map. It's as simple as that.'

To Stanley Mott, ideas were the noblest manifestations of mankind, and he felt that in this room his ideas were not being accorded the dignity they deserved. He had spent his lifetime wrestling with these majestic concepts and responsibilities, and he was not disposed to allow two senators who had entered the field only recently, or a writer who had been handed an assignment, 'Astronauts & Space,' to dislodge him peremptorily from his reasoned positions, and he was about to speak rather forcefully when Mrs. Pope caught the set of his jaw and said brightly, 'Well, I think that winds this up.'

But the two senators had detected Mott's displeasure, and after Mrs. Pope had led Kolff back to the waiting room, Mike Glancey put his arm about Mott's shoulder and said, 'The difference between a politician like me and a scientist like you is that to hold my job I have to get elected . . . every six years. You only have to be appointed . . . once. And what you learn from elections is that man is the measure of all things. If there's not a man in the picture, it ain't a picture.'

'He's right, Stanley,' Senator Grant said. 'I had enough engineering in the Navy to know you're right in your basic argument. Of course we could proceed without the astronauts. But it would be terribly wrong to try.'

'The taxpayer, the man who foots the bill, would walk away from our program. Your most creative dreams would be dead.'

After they had talked this way for some time, Glancey told a story about the first day of his first election campaign. 'Stanley, I was the brightest kid in Red River. And I'd studied all the proposed legislation to make myself even brighter. But when I went out to make my speech in an Italian section, the first question was, "How do you stand on House Bill 21-957?" I'd never heard of it. Had to do with Italian immigration. They didn't give a damn about all the hot issues—war, taxation, medical care, the new dam—they wanted to know about 21-957, and when I didn't even know what it was, I lost any claim to their support. I didn't get fifteen votes in that district.

'Point of the story,' Glancey said, 'is that you must listen to the people on whatever terms they care to speak. In space it's astronauts . . . Tucker Thompson photographing the anguished wife behind the white picket fence.'

Mott listened, and the more he considered the phenomenon of the astronauts, the more he was driven to the conclusion that the senators were right and he was wrong. Dieter Kolff's enthusiasm for the big mechanical rocket had blinded him to the social persuasiveness of the astronauts and their wives. Man was the measure of all things, and although it was correct that machines could perform miracles, they could not enlist the emotional support of the public. Astronauts could, and he left this confrontation committed to the role of human beings in space, for without them as a measure, a criterion for meaning, the program had no viability.

At the door, Grant asked, 'What news from Los Angeles?' and for a moment Mott could not decipher what the senator was talking about. He first assumed that Grant was referring to some member of the study committee who had voted against Earth-orbit rendezvous, and started to fumble for an answer, but then he remembered that Grant had once commissioned him to check out the nefarious Dr. Strabismus, and recalling Dieter's handsome diploma, he burst into laughter, and said, 'Haven't you heard? USA is no longer a research institute. It's now the University of Space and Aviation.'

'Good God!'

'And even NASA bought six or eight doctorates for the older NACA hands. To give our outfit a touch of class.'

'You've got to be kidding.'

'Not at all. I saw one of the diplomas on Dieter Kolff's wall three nights ago. It was signed by the chancellor of the university, Dr. Leopold Strabismus, and by his dean of faculty, Marcia Grant, Ph.D.'

Senator Grant sat heavily on one of the meeting-room chairs. 'Ph.D.? She didn't even finish freshman year. And now she's the dean of faculty.'

'It's not as bad as it sounds, because the university has no faculty.'

When the last objection to Earth-orbit rendezvous had been disposed of and the special committee was on the verge of recommending that flight to the Moon be conducted according to Von Braun's solution, a nagging feeling assaulted Mott, and after three days of trying to suppress it, he knew that he must in prudence consult one final time with the men he had worked with longest, those stalwart engineers at Langley who had kept advanced programs alive during the bleak years when they had scarcely a penny, and when he reached there some of his cronies suggested, 'Why don't we fly up to Wallops where no phones can reach us and hold an old-time think tank on the beach?'

They commandeered a NASA plane and flew the short distance to Wallops, where they spent the morning inspecting the striking changes made possible by the acquisition of a nearby naval base. The launching sites had concrete bases now, and there were roads through the spacious, sleeping marshes. There was a commissary instead of cold beans out of a can and a general air of prosperity, but several of the men voiced the doubts which perplexed Mott but which he did not wish to discuss in public: 'I wonder if they do as much work as we used to, when we slept on the beach and waited for the results of our little rockets?'

In the afternoon they carried chairs to the beach and sat looking out across the Atlantic, that splendid body of turbulent water into which so many of their experimental rockets had fallen in years past, and after a while one of the men said, 'They're making a big fuss about the Mercury men, but none of them has been higher than we sent our rockets from this very beach.'

'Yes, but one of these days they'll go straight up, two hundred fifty thousand miles, and by damn, there won't be any atmosphere to measure up there!'

'What's it going to be, Mott? Straight up and on, or some kind of rendezvous?'

'We've dropped the straight-up bit. That's dead.' But when he told them that it looked as if NASA would adopt Von Braun's plan for Earth orbit, one of the men said, 'We have this super-brain at Langley, chap named John Houbolt, who's trying to convince people that it's folly to use Earth-orbit rendezvous. He claims it should be lunar-orbit rendezvous.'

'You mean, fly the whole works up to the Moon, but don't land it? Separate it into components and let one of them do the work. Then reunite and come back down?'

'Exactly what he preaches.'

'I don't think much of lunar-orbit rendezvous,' Mott said, and he revealed that in his doctorate he had not even considered it. 'But in our committee, of course, we did have this half-baked presentation, but I can't recall we spent fifteen minutes on it. There'd be no advantage.'

And then one of the Langley men said something which caused bells to ring in Mott's head. 'You miss the whole point of what Houbolt's proposing; he claims there would be a weight advantage. As the rocket ascended, you would throw off the parts that were no longer needed. It would get constantly lighter, until at the end you'd have only this little bundle. I think he says you'd leave even the landing machine on the Moon. Or most of it.'

'How's that?' Mott asked abruptly, for he could hear the Chance-Vought man speaking that night beside the test field in California: 'Throw away everything, Mott . . . even the machinery that brings you home . . . You have become the spaceship.'

'It's his plan, not mine. But he has studies showing that under his system, the weight would grow constantly less . . .'

Another engineer broke in: 'Mott, are your people visualizing what Moon vehicles will look like? I mean, are you constantly aware that because there is no atmosphere, no nothing to create friction, your machine can have as many protuberances, odd angles, whole faces jutting out . . . You know, it can look like anything you want it to look like. Don't get locked in to some streamlined beauty. You streamline an airplane to get it through the solid atmosphere. With no atmosphere, you don't need streamlining.'

He suggested that the men move inside. 'Give me a place to draw.' When they were settled with their beers, he sketched what he thought a Moon lander might look like, and it was good that he did, for even these practiced engineers were prone to forget that in an ambience without an atmosphere to cause friction or constraint, a vehicle could indeed be built of the flimsiest material and configured in the most bizarre ways. 'If you want a place for a celestial monkey wrench, you just tack it on the side.'

But when the engineer was finished with his dramatic presentation of what *his* spacecraft would look like, a big square bundle with fifteen or twenty projections, Mott returned to what the other man had said on the beach: 'Tell me about this throwing away of components,' and the men played a brilliant game of ideas-and-space: 'You start with this gigantic rocket, the biggest Von Braun can build, and in let's say fifteen separate steps, you discard item after item. After its utility has been discharged. You wind up in lunar-orbit rendezvous with let's say six components, and only the light ones. This one breaks away and takes you down to the Moon. You never see it again. This one, this one, this one. In the end you come home in a basket. That's the advantage of lunar-orbit rendezvous.'

'You know,' Mott said reflectively, 'an engineer from Chance-Vought made exactly the same pitch. Throw everything away. What are the facts?'

Without firm data, but with sophisticated guesses, the excited men began a study. The stars appeared, the Moon rose, the Earth in its incessant revolution caused the heavens to look as if they were turning, and the constellations climbed into position. One of the men dashed off in his car for sandwiches and beer and another for additional scratch paper, and gradually the rough dimensions of the problem were established, and toward three in the morning, when every aspect had been analyzed, Mott came up with these figures:

At launch, a vehicle which would carry three men to the Moon would weigh about 6,600,000 pounds. In a flight of about 200 hours, everything possible would be jettisoned, maybe nine components in all. At final splashdown, there would be no fuel, no food, no oxygen, no nothing, just three men in a capsule with an ablative front all burned off. Total residual weight, not more than 11,000 pounds.

'Jesus!' one of the Langley men said. 'It could be done.' They spent the next hour checking the data, and at 0400 in the morning, when Altair was climbing above the eastern horizon to inspect the workmen in the porch, Mott agreed: 'It could be done.'

He hurried back to Langley to meet with this man Houbolt, who seemed the typical specialist whose ideas were being rebuffed by his superiors. 'Thanks a million for coming, Mott. The others simply will not listen when I try to tell them that lunar-orbit rendezvous is superior to any other. If the scientific community of this nation will not listen to reason . . . They won't even look at the comparisons.'

Mott talked with him for two days, reviewing in detail his excellent data and diagrams, and came away convinced that whereas Wernher von Braun's Earth-orbit rendezvous was workable, lunar rendezvous was far superior, and he began quietly to campaign for it. His advocacy had to be muted because he had already been rebuked for having butted in on the astronaut-versus-machine argument, and he was not sure he could survive another head-on collision with the Senate committee; indeed, there was reason to think that it might have been Von Braun who alerted Senator Grant to the earlier subversion being practiced by Mott and Kolff.

So Mott had to move gingerly, but now he found an unexpected and extremely powerful ally: Lyndon Johnson, in a series of maneuvers so complicated that none could follow, charmed Texas millionaires into ceding land near Houston to a university, which in turn offered it to NASA as a possible site for the nation's major space center, and with a chain of forced-draft studies which supported the Houston location, Johnson persuaded NASA to locate its Manned Spacecraft Center there and to staff it with most of the brilliant men from Langley. Thus Lyndon Johnson's Texas center became the arch rival of Von Braun's Alabama center, and the war was on.

If Alabama backed EOR, Texas had to back LOR, and Mott found himself automatically allied with the flamboyant Texans against his original German allies in Huntsville. It was a fight which continued for almost a year, with politics, finances, regional pride, fundamental ideas and the great drives of the space age intermingled, and in the end a stalemate existed between Earth orbit and lunar orbit.

Senators Glancey and Grant became so uneasy with the impasse that they summoned Mott to testify before their committee, but he was so involved with the fighting that he asked to be excused, and they agreed that he should be saved for a rescue operation. Mrs. Pope did schedule hearings at which Alabama pleaded for EOR and Texas for LOR, and when the acrimonious debate ended, without conclusions, she telephoned Mott to appear before her two senators in the morning.

He drove through the night from an inspection he had been conducting at MIT and appeared before the senators bleary-eyed. Once more their words were harsh: 'We've got to have a decision before the end of the month. See if you can knock heads.' He asked them which mode of landing they preferred, and Grant snapped: 'We have no knowledge. All we have are the bills to pay.'

Mott flew first to Texas, where a colossal space center was rising from marshland, and he had to admit: 'If you're going to do it, this is the way. Presto-changeo! Let there be a space center!' He found the Texans adamant in believing that the Langley alternative was the only practical one: 'Fly it high, throw everything away, orbit around the Moon and take minimum gear down to the surface, even less when you leave the Moon.' It could be accomplished with rockets then in existence, or about to be, and it was an elegant solution.

As a one-time engineer, Mott loved that word *elegant,* for it implied an entire scale of values: an elegant solution had to be simpler than its adversaries, it had to be easily assembled, it had to be cost-efficient, and it had to be instinctively satisfying to the engineering mind. Lunar rendezvous was elegant.

But it had to be sold to Alabama, which would be providing the rocketry, and when Mott reached Huntsville he sensed immediately that the Germans felt he was about to betray them. He had mournful meetings with Von Braun and Kolff and long-drawn-out sessions with the lesser engineers, who tried unsuccessfully to drive him into corners. When he talked with Kolff he found no concession whatever; a year ago the square-faced little man had placed his entire career and reputation on the line in favor of the Jules Verne Approach, and when his beloved big rockets were shot down, he transferred his loyalty to Von Braun, defending his leader's EOR. Now he was being heckled to change again, and this he refused to do.

He asked Mott to dine with him on Monte Sano, and again Stanley met with Liesl and Magnus, who was preparing to play Telemann's Concerto in D for Trumpet with an Alabama-Tennessee orchestra. 'The solo part, you understand,' Mrs. Kolff said. 'Five cities. He will travel in a bus and see places Dieter and I have never seen.'

'He's very young for such an assignment,' Mott said.

'He's been playing since he was four,' Dieter said. 'A great tribute to America. You gave him the instrument, and the instruction.' After supper the parents persuaded their son to play the cadenza from the first movement of the concerto, and the stocky lad stood with his feet slightly apart, his head high, and played the limpid, rippling music, displaying his skill at triple-tonguing and sustaining a long series of sweet, rounded notes. When he finished, he bowed and went upstairs to study.

But the Kolffs had not invited Mott to hear their son play; they wanted to talk with him about the great decisions soon to be made, and to his surprise Liesel joined him and Dieter when the chairs were placed on the porch so that the stars of summer could be seen. She said nothing, but she did listen intently.

KOLFF: I must talk frankly with you, Stanley.

MOTT: Not about manned flights. That's settled.

KOLFF: Agreed. I know when my team has lost.

MOTT: And not about the Moon as target. We're going there, and nothing can stop us.

KOLFF: Agreed. I tried to talk sense with you and failed.

MOTT: *(with slight impatience):* So what is it?

KOLFF: A problem with the most serious repercussions. (He spoke alternately in German and English, using simple words in the latter language, complex ones in the former, but he betrayed no preference, switching from one to the other in a lively flow of ideas.)

MOTT: Our decisions are nearly final. There can't be much—

KOLFF: But there is, and this time you must listen, Stanley. I beg you, I pray you not to commit NASA to lunar-orbit rendezvous.

MOTT: You astonish me. Lunar orbit's a marvelous solution.

KOLFF: Yes, but to a problem not worth solving.

MOTT: It'll land us on the Moon. And get us off.

KOLFF: It's a one-time spectacular. It's a brilliant accomplishment with no constructive follow-on.

MOTT: With this technique we can go anywhere.

KOLFF: No, no, Stanley! It will carry you only to the Moon. And then its utility is dead . . . vanished . . . a costly dream wasted and down the drain.

MOTT *(soberly):* What do you see as the error, Dieter?

KOLFF: Von Braun's solution of Earth-orbit rendezvous is infinitely superior because it gets you to the Moon almost as efficiently, but in addition, it erects a platform from which all the universe can be explored later on. Will we want a space station in permanent orbit? We can do it from Earth rendezvous a hundred miles up, maybe three hundred, no more. Do we want to explore Mars and Venus? We'll start from our space platform in Earth rendezvous. Mine the asteroids? Put great telescopes in space? Establish settlements on the Moon? All these things can be done if we start with a solid space platform constructed in Earth orbit. Your way we can do none of them.

MOTT: And we may refuse to do them all.

KOLFF: The sweep of history will not allow us to refuse. We must do each one.

MOTT: And if we do refuse?

KOLFF: If we prove irresponsible, other nations will carry on—Japan . . . India . . . France . . . and always Russia.

MOTT: Are you badgering me because Von Braun asked you to?

KOLFF: Do you know the phrase *sub specie aeternitatis?* Under the eye of eternity? I am neither for Wernher nor against him. I only want this nation to do the right thing. I am acting as if eternity was watching over my shoulder.

MOTT: I'm afraid the decision's gone against you, Dieter. We're going to choose lunar rendezvous.

KOLFF: Then I shall have to oppose you. I'll support Von Braun as vigorously as possible. Because I want to prevent you from making a tragic error . . . from selling out cheaply when you know better. Something I never thought you would do.

But Dieter Kolff and the other Germans he enlisted in his crusade, men determined to go down fighting on this clearly perceived moral principle, received a staggering shock when Von Braun convened a meeting of the entire Alabama team and announced without emotion that at last he appreciated the reasoning of the men in Texas and was joining them. He said that his Alabama plan of Earth-orbit rendezvous was dead and that everyone should now rally behind the Texas lunar-orbit rendezvous and make it work.

Some of the Germans gasped when the announcement was made and a few challenged him to state his reasons, which he did, and after the hubbub had subsided he invited Mott to explain how the Texas-Alabama cooperation would work: 'It could be seen, I suppose, as a crass political surrender to the might of Texas and Lyndon Johnson, but that would be only partially true. It's also the scientifically right choice. And there's a third aspect which may override both the first and second. By doing it this way, we ensure all the major bases, and Cape Canaveral, of equally important assignments. We'll break the instrument down into seven or eight parts. Huntsville will take responsibility for a couple, California for two or three, Mississippi for one, and Houston for its two, plus the astronaut program itself.'

'And how,' asked a practiced engineer, 'can we possibly fit together seven parts made in seven or eight different shops?'

'By precision,' Mott said, and he started to explain how the specifications of each part would be so exactly drawn that it would abut against its neighbors below and above with tolerances of a thousandth of an inch. But then he saw with dismay that Dieter Kolff, infuriated by what he held to be a wrong decision, had risen to his feet, red of face, ready to blast the program while members of the press were in the room taking notes. He must be forestalled.

'And our good friend Dieter Kolff,' Mott said blandly, 'will at last be able to build his monster rocket which will carry us to outer space.'

The Germans working under Kolff cheered, but Dieter, aware of the trick that had been used to silence him, glared and sat down. He and Mott would not speak to each other for seven years.

. . .

It was said previously that President Eisenhower, never an advocate of wasting money in space and almost an enemy of the program, made a series of crucial decisions and made them right. The first was when he placed the program in civilian hands and then protected it from military encroachment. His second may have been even more determinative, for when he learned that the fledgling NASA was about to broadcast a Civil Service Notice inviting civilians to apply for astronaut training at a salary of $8,330 a year and a rating of GS-12, he hit the roof, warning the administrators that such a blanket solicitation would bring crazies out of the woodwork, or as one jaundiced observer phrased it: 'We'll be deluged by all the matadors, scuba divers, hot-rod racers, hopheads, Mount-Everest-because-it's-there gang and half a dozen women who will demand that the Supreme Court enforce their right to fly.'

Eisenhower stopped such nonsense in a hurry. Summoning the NASA command, he said bluntly, 'The men we need for this job are already in our armed forces. Our test pilots. They've been doing work like this for years and they'll jump at the chance.' By that simple device he ensured that the first seven astronauts would be competent, disciplined types who would never embarrass the nation. Besides, as a military man, he knew he could hire the best Navy captains and Air Force colonels for $560 a month 'plus a few perquisites here and there.'

Commander John Pope had been with his Air Group squadrons aboard the *Tulagi* off the coast of Asia, supervising intelligence flights over trouble spots like Korea and Vietnam when the first BuPers announcement was posted inviting any Navy fliers with test-pilot experience to volunteer for the pool from which a small group of men would be chosen for astronaut training. Since he was happy with his job, evaluating it correctly as an essential step to any position of high command, he could express no interest in this new career possibility, but he did notice that had he wanted to get back to that kind of work, he would have been eligible: 'Two years experience as test pilot in at least twenty major types of aircraft, not over forty years of age as of 31 December, not over 5 feet 11 inches, not over 177 pounds,' He was vaguely pleased to see that he would have qualified on every point, and then he forgot the whole affair.

But in April 1959, when he became aware of the furor caused by the presentation of the first seven astronauts to the public, he checked carefully to ascertain whether any of his test-pilot friends were in the group, and for two days he moved about the *Tulagi,* telling anyone who would listen, 'Hey, I know these guys. Al Shepard and Scott Carpenter were with me at Pax River. Great guys. I flew with John Glenn in Korea, him in daylight, me at night. At Edwards they told me this guy Slayton was a hotshot.'

From a distance he followed the press releases about the Sacred Seven, as an irreverent Navy pilot called them, and read with interest and a little envy the splendid stories *Life* ran about them and their wives. When the first Mercury shots took off with monkeys as passengers, this same Navy pilot took to calling the overpublicized astronauts 'Spam in a Can,' an allusion to the fact that they would be not aviators in the old sense but passive cargo in an intricate machine controlled by computers and ground-based directors.

Pope did not share this contempt. He argued that in the first stages of any new development the mechanics took priority, and he predicted: 'Give men like that one flight, and they'll take over. I know those characters. They're take-charge guys.' And he assumed that they would be quickly leaving the Earth on their historic missions, but he had grossly miscalculated the difficulties the American program would encounter.

He was aboard the *Tulagi* that day in April 1961 when the Russian Yuri Gagarin made man's first flight into space, and was depressed for several weeks by what he held to be a personal defeat: 'Where were our Navy men? Why weren't they up there first?' And his disappointments were not alleviated when Alan Shepard finally made what Pope had to describe as 'a pathetic counter-gesture,' and after the details were made available he wrote a discouraged letter to his wife:

> Don't let your senators go around making speeches about the glorious triumph of our space program. Shepard's flight was like a child's sparkler when compared to Yuri Gagarin's meteor. Shepard rose 116 miles in the air, Gagarin 203. Shepard was in the air 15 minutes, Gagarin 108. Our man traveled 303 miles, theirs 25,000. Shepard was weightless five minutes, Gagarin, 89 minutes. Tell your men to get busy.

John Glenn's real flight into space, a three-orbit triumph, excited Pope enormously, and he began a collection of major stories about the astronaut and his reception in various nations. He learned the name of Glenn's wife and the fact that she had a slight stammer 'which she bravely overcame, proving that the wives of the astronauts have just as much courage as their husbands.' And he began to think seriously of volunteering for the astronaut corps when the next group was chosen from the military test pilots.

But when the announcement was posted on the bulletin board at Jacksonville, where he was checking new planes to assure that they could land easily on the carriers stationed off the coast of Florida, he was forestalled from submitting his name by Admiral Crane, commander of the district, who gave him a sharply pointed fatherly talk:

> 'Pope, avoid this temptation. It looks enticing—to be an astronaut and to have your picture in the newsreels. And we can be proud of our Navy men. They've done a better job than any of the others. You know, of course, that John Glenn's a Marine.

'But I assure you that every one of these men who leaves the service, Navy or Air Force or Army, will be surrendering his career in the service, whether he thinks he is or not. He'll have the glamour for a while, the excitement of parades, but when he wants to come back and help run the Navy, he'll find the doors quietly closing against him. The great job of running one of the nation's armed services will be denied him.

'Pope, it's well known in the Navy, and I'm sure you've suspected it, but you stand high in everyone's opinion. We have no position to which you can't aspire. You saw my last fitness report on you. The next one will be stronger. Don't fritter away this golden opportunity by grasping at some temporary bauble. Leave the Moon to the wild-blue-yonder boys. The real job is down here on the oceans of the world.'

Pope did not volunteer for the second selection of astronauts, and he had put the matter pretty much out of mind when several things happened. In September 1962 when the new selections were announced, with the nine young men displayed on television, he shouted to Penny, who was visiting him from Washington, 'Hey, they took Pete Conrad! You knew him at Pax River. You slept at his house one night, after the big party.' And when Penny ran into the room she found her husband shouting with an excitement she had rarely witnessed, 'That's Frank Borman. I flew with him at Edwards. And I'm sure that little guy on the end was John Young. He's a terrific flier. If it's the Young I knew, he's a hard driver.'

Now Pope began to follow with real longing the careers of the original Sacred Seven and the new Nifty Nine, for these were men his own age, men he had flown with, men with whom he had conducted simulated dogfights in untested planes over the silvery waters of the Chesapeake or the barren flats at Edwards. He remembered going up to Pete Conrad one morning at Pax River and asking, 'Anything odd about this crate?' and he could almost hear the Princeton man instructing him: 'Very delicate when you try to land at low speeds.'

But his sudden interest related in no way to any dissatisfaction with his own career. Admiral Crane had guessed right about Pope's good standing with the Navy hierarchy, because shortly after his perceptive observations at Jacksonville, John received notice of his promotion to full commander and an assignment as executive officer aboard his old carrier *Tulagi,* still stationed in the Pacific. This nipped any personal interest in space that might have been germinating, for as he prepared himself for his new duties, Crane stopped by to talk to him: 'Aren't you glad you stayed with the fleet? Discharge this duty with distinction and you'll earn yourself captain's stripes. After that, you're eligible for any job we have.'

Penny was delighted to hear of his promotion and arranged to fly down to Pensacola for the party for which he would don his new stripes, and John was pleased to see how she radiated her pleasure. As they were dressing for the celebration she uttered a little yelp of glee as he donned his new uniform. 'You're even more handsome as a full commander.' Then she tried to talk about her job, but he was too preoccupied to follow the details. Later she said, 'I told you something about ten minutes ago, but you weren't listening. Senator Glancey's had me busy getting authorization for a special selection of astronauts. The program's moving ahead faster than we anticipated. Would you have any interest in volunteering?'

'Nope. I did, briefly, a few months back. But things have opened up better than I could have expected in the Navy chain of command. I'm set.'

She kissed him ardently and cried, 'I'm so relieved, John. As I watch the space program unfold, it seems so damned . . . well, hysterical. Politicians using it to get bases for their districts. Newspapers using it to up their sales. And this man from *Folks* laying his oily plans. In the end, many of the astronauts will be short-changed.'

'Admiral Crane said the same thing, months ago.'

'And I've a strong feeling that when it's at its height, the country will drop it like a bad tomato!'

When John said he doubted that last statement, she said, 'I already see signs that Glancey is beginning to back off, and he's an absolute litmus paper. He and Lyndon Johnson see things ten years before they happen.'

'How about Grant?'

'He's a dear, John. Red, white and blue right through the center of his limited brain. I love that man.' She laughed uneasily, then added, 'I mean, my heart breaks for him sometimes. His dipsy-doodle wife. That crazy daughter of his. He really deserves better.'

'What's his daughter up to now?'

'Haven't you heard? She's a Ph.D. and dean of faculty at a university in Los Angeles.'

'I don't think that's so crazy.'

'But the university has no faculty. It sells beautifully engraved diplomas for five hundred dollars each. We can get you a second Ph.D. anytime you say the word.'

They had a passionate celebration in Pensacola, a treasured meeting of two people whose love had grown each year since high school, but an embarrassing moment occurred during the rowdy speeches in the officers' club. John had said how much he appreciated his promotion, even though he wasn't sure he deserved it—loud protests—when Penny rose, rattled her knife against her glass, and said, 'Promotions everywhere in the Pope family.' Facing her husband, she said, 'I didn't want to intrude on your celebration, but I'm the new permanent counsel of the Senate Space Committee.'

Amid cheers and whistles, wives gathered around her with kisses, and John, watching from his end of the table, had the ugly thought: That flush of excitement when she arrived was caused by her promotion, not mine. What he did not remember was that she had tried to tell him of her good luck but was prevented from doing so by his inattention. Then, dismissing such speculation as unworthy, he jumped from his chair, elbowed his way through the wives, caught Penny by her two hands, and drew her toward him for a kiss.

'Does *permanent counsel* mean you can't be fired?'

'Not unless I steal funds.'

'Hooray! We can afford a new car!'

Commander Pope's career would probably have proceeded according to Admiral Crane's predictions had the carrier *Tulagi* remained in Pacific waters, but it did not, and when Pope reported for duty as executive officer he learned that his immediate assignment was to accompany the carrier out of Jacksonville and into the Caribbean, where it would serve as the principal recovery vessel for the three-orbit flight which Astronaut Scott Carpenter was about to make in his Mercury capsule Aurora-7.

The briefing book for the recovery procedure contained one hundred and forty-one pages, with a biography of Carpenter which showed that he had learned his test-piloting at Pax River. From a first rapid reading of the instructions, Pope deduced that about two dozen Navy ships would be in position to monitor the flight and pick Carpenter up from whatever part of the ocean he landed in, Pacific or Atlantic, and that about 125 airplanes would be in flight to lend assistance.

> At the heart of everything [he wrote to Penny] will be the *Tulagi,* waiting with helicopters, powerboats and rescue frogmen to see that our boy gets down safely. We'll spot the capsule on radar first, track it into our location, then pick it up visually so that we can vector our copters into the exact point he hits. It's an amazing exercise in tactics and I'm proud to have my ship play a part in it.

He studied each page of the briefing book and became acquainted with what everyone along the flight path would be doing at each moment: the lonely watchers on Ascension Island, the remote listeners in Australia, the men in the fail-safe destroyer near the Antarctic Ocean, the hundred-odd experts at Cape Canaveral who would follow each mile of the flight. And always he would come back to the duties of his carrier *Tulagi,* whose operations would close the circle and bring Scott Carpenter home safely.

It was an intricate role the carrier had: to position itself properly so as to track the capsule as it descended under its parachute, then dispatch helicopters at the proper signal, deploy frogmen to rescue Carpenter if his system fouled the way Gus Grissom's had endangered him on the second

Mercury flight, arrange for the orderly transfer of the astronaut to the carrier, and dispatch the proper messages to assure the world that the flight had ended safely.

Much of this detail focused on Pope, and to ensure its proper execution he drilled his teams repeatedly, both in dry runs and in real-time simulations. Insofar as he could determine, the *Tulagi* was going to perform competently, quietly, very forcefully, and when the great carrier steamed out of Jacksonville with sixteen newspaper and television reporters aboard, he told everyone, 'This is a military assignment. I shall expect out*standing* performance.'

The *Tulagi* assumed its station in the Caribbean on the afternoon of 22 May 1962, with the expectation that Carpenter would descend out of the skies in the late morning of 24 May. Helicopters were tested, radio circuits to the mainland were checked, and the frogmen were sent into the water on both the twenty-second and the twenty-third to be sure that they were familiar with temperatures and currents.

Shortly before dawn on the morning of the twenty-fourth the *Tulagi* was hit by a chain of squalls that deposited a great amount of rain and caused some of the reporters to file disheartening stories, but by 0900 the storms had departed and the ocean had assumed a character so benevolent that one newsman said, 'Hell, he can water-ski over to us,' and at that moment the powerboats that would deliver the frogmen to the capsule flashed by, throwing spray. It was a glorious morning, the kind that Columbus must have known when sailing these waters.

Now the *Tulagi* began to receive reassuring messages from the control center at Cape Canaveral: 'Aurora-7 on target. All systems go. All stations reporting favorably. Splashdown as scheduled.'

But when the flight was about an hour from its completion, ugly little uncertainties began to intrude, and once Pope heard Cape Canaveral asking: 'How much fuel?' He did not hear the answer, but the Cape said: 'Check again. How much fuel?'

Thirty minutes out it became apparent that something had gone badly wrong, because the Cape was signaling ships far distant from the *Tulagi* to prepare for possible recovery maneuvers, and when Pope checked to see where those vessels were—although he knew perfectly from his studies— he saw that they were two hundred and three hundred miles distant.

'What's happening?' he demanded of a NASA specialist aboard the carrier, but that man could give no definite explanation: 'Fuel problem, apparently.'

'Isn't he going to land here?' Pope asked.

'Splash down,' the NASA man corrected, and he said the words so mechanically, as if using the right terminology was important, that Pope wanted to slug him.

'Is he going to splash down here?' he asked, emphasizing each word, but before the NASA man could respond, the radio crackled: 'USS *Intrepid,* prepare to recover.' The *Intrepid* was 250 miles away! Shepard had landed almost on target. So had Gus Grissom, while Glenn's landing had been marvelously good. This one was a fiasco, and as the minutes passed with nothing in the sky, John Pope stood by the railing of his carrier and came as close to cursing as he ever had.

Why did we have to be the ones they cheated? he asked himself again and again. He had practiced how he would greet Carpenter when he came aboard: 'Good afternoon, Scott. Some distance from Pax River.' For two days on the trip out he had been unable to remember Mrs. Carpenter's name, although he knew her well, and the papers given him did not state it, so he had TWXed the Cape: 'WHAT NAME MRS. CARPENTER?' and they had replied 'RENE,' and then of course he remembered.

He had planned to end his greeting with: 'They assure us Rene is fine.' It would have been a nice touch.

And now it was all down the drain. The minutes passed and the surface of the Caribbean remained unruffled. No boats were launched, No helicopters left the deck. The great carrier rolled almost imperceptibly on the bosom of the sea, and John Pope became more and more outraged.

When the radio announced that the *Intrepid* had made a good, routine recovery and that Carpenter was in fine shape despite his misadventure, Pope's confusion reached an apex: he was wildly furious at having been robbed of an experience he had planned for, but he was also torn with longing: God, I want to fly again! I want to test every plane in the world. The Moon . . . He bit his lower lip until the pain startled him: The Moon. I know every crater on the Moon. He remained by the ship's railing, tears of desire flooding his eyes, and then he stormed down to his cabin, where with trembling fingers he typed out a dispatch to a friend at BuPers in Washington:

> I'm informed that before NASA selects its first contingent of astronauts trained in science, it's going to enroll a special group of six with intensive flight-test experience. I fulfill their specifications as to age, weight, height, combat duty and flight-test. I seek permission to apply and will clear personally with my commanding officer, Admiral Crane.

To his surprise, the admiral flew personally to the *Tulagi,* where in the flag quarters he delivered a message from the Navy brass which astonished Commander Pope:

> 'John, I gave you bad advice at Jacksonville, and I apologize. When I cautioned you then against becoming an astronaut, I was thinking selfishly only of the Navy. I failed to realize how immense this space

thing was, and how vital it's going to become in the future to the Navy's interest.

'NASA is going to pick six men in the special draft, we're told, and it's of maximum importance that at least two of them be Navy men. I know that the Army is grooming some of its likely candidates and the Air Force is frantic. They feel space belongs to them and that they've been short-changed. We have to get in there fighting. We've got to put our best men forward, and we all agree that you're our prime candidate.

'The head of the selection committee is an Air Force astronaut you may have known at Edwards. Deke Slayton. This gives them a leg up, but they assure me he's very fair. You know anything about him? Well, study up. Find out what he likes to drink, what planes he flew, everything, because his veto is fatal. I suppose you know he was scheduled to take the flight that Carpenter took. Heart trouble scrubbed him. I wouldn't blame him if he were bitter about it. But he's the man you have to satisfy.'

Admiral Crane arranged for Pope to be relieved of duty aboard the *Tulagi* and flown to New York, where a selected group of Navy and civilian types briefed him and seven other Navy applicants on how men of promise conducted themselves when applying for important assignments. A psychologist stationed at Annapolis identified the body signals which indicated whether a man was a hard driver, or, God forbid, a born loser.

'Lean forward from the knees, not the waist. Always look as if you were prepared to step into a major task or belt someone right in the nose. Do not cock your head. It indicates indecision. If you have an unusually dark beard, shave twice a day, but never, never use powder. Real men use soap.'

He specified some fifty signs which other men check for when seeking prime movers, and the young Navy men listened, but they remembered longest the less highly structured advice given by an Annapolis man who had left the Navy to become head of a large corporation:

'Men of substance, and that's what the committee will be looking for, wear socks which reach to the knee. There's nothing worse than to see an executive showing ten inches of bare leg. Not one of my assistants has a pair of brown socks or brown shoes. The work of the world is done by men who wear neatly polished black shoes.

'And for God's sake, if they ask you to dinner, which I'm sure they will, remember three things. Do not drum nervously with your fork or spoon. Pick them up only to eat with, then put them down. Second, if drinks are ordered, don't ask for wine. Men drink whiskey, never rum, that's for exotics, and gin only in martinis. Third, it can be very effective if you eat English style, knife in right hand, fork in left. It lifts you out of the ordinary.'

A football coach had been invited, not from Annapolis, whose teams were pretty awful, but from one of the Big Eight universities, which took education seriously:

'I've talked with men who were on the earlier selection committees and they have the widest possible interests. Look at the great job they've done. Sixteen choices, sixteen winners. And they mean to extend that record. So try to create the impression that you're rugged, that you can respond constructively to pressure. For Christ's sake, don't stand with your hands on your hips. Window dressers do that.

'But on the other hand, and this is important, don't come at them like gangbusters. They're not looking for gorillas, they're looking for executive types who can take charge of a mission valued at billions of dollars. They know you're brave or you wouldn't be in the final draft, so you don't have to impress them with your heroism. They don't want heroes, they want competents.

'Now, this is funny for me to say, a football coach, but watch your language. Speak in complete sentences. Because in your training you'll have to do an immense amount of reading, a lot of writing. You can use test-pilot lingo, but don't use a lot of *er*'s and *uh*'s, because there will be men in the group just as good as you are in flying planes who can also speak English.'

From New York, Pope and the others flew down to Houston, where they were registered under assumed names in the Rice Hotel. Since there would be four days of intensive interrogation and medical checking, the candidates were advised by means of a printed sheet on their pillows to get a good night's sleep, and Pope did.

He awakened early, determined to make a good impression on the committee, and after shaving, called his wife to assure her that he was in this to the bitter end: 'When I stood by the railing of that carrier, waiting for the sky to bring us its messenger, I knew I wanted to be an astronaut. I have never wanted anything so much. Pray for me, because this is what God intended me to be.'

When he walked briskly in to the committee, leaning slightly forward in his polished shoes and knee-length black socks, he was enormously attractive, in a manly sort of way, five feet seven inches tall, one hundred and forty-seven pounds, close-cropped brown hair, thirty-two strong teeth, and eyes with 20-20 vision. He could write well, knew astronomy at the professional level, and carried with him one of the best records ever compiled at Pax River, but when he looked into the eyes of grim-faced Deke Slayton he realized that during the next few days this committee was going to meet with more than a hundred young pilots as good as he, and he was terrified.

However, alongside the stern-faced military men on the selection committee, there was at one end of the table a man who looked more like a college professor. He was in his forties, perhaps, wore steel-rimmed glasses, smiled easily, and stood when Slayton introduced him: 'Dr. Stanley Mott, our resident brain.' Pope believed that his destiny rested in the vote of this sympathetic man, but then he saw with amazement the candidate who had preceded him, and his jaw dropped. The test pilot had lingered to speak with an Air Force officer on the board, and now saw Pope.

'Pope! They must be scrapin' the bottom of the barrel.' It was Major Randy Claggett, the Marine's favorite candidate and a man not at all overawed by the committee. When he clapped his old buddy on the back before sauntering from the room, Pope saw that he was not wearing knee-length black socks.

It was a gala night for the Germans in Huntsville: a local cinema had obtained a print of the new motion picture *I Aim at the Stars,* and everyone bought tickets because this was the film biography of their hero, Wernher von Braun.

There were rumors that the movie took unwarranted liberties with his life, and that in order to make it more appealing to female audiences, his well-remembered German secretary at Peenemünde was converted into a beautiful English spy, but it was also said that the popular German actor Curt Jurgens gave a sensitive portrayal of Von Braun himself. At any rate, the Peenemünde gang appeared in full force, hoping for the best and eager to show their children what the German rocket center had been like.

The program started with selections by the local orchestra, and young Magnus Kolff distinguished himself with a beautiful rendition of *Carnival of Venice,* which pleased his parents, who invited him to sit between them when the movie started, but he disappointed them by preferring to remain with the younger orchestra members.

The movie was a disaster. Hardly an item of engineering background was accurate. The set bore no resemblance to Peenemünde, and the incidents were so contrived as to be grotesque. The Kolffs looked in vain for any of the scenes they had known so well during their courtship, and other engineers were openly disgusted by the nonsense. Von Braun, fortunately, was not present to share the ignominy of this night, but all who were felt that their role in history had been denigrated or even burlesqued.

For example, the miracle of Dieter and Liesl Kolff's escape with the crucial papers was not even mentioned, and what was worse, a newspaper in the area reprinted an irreverent review of the picture which had appeared in an English newspaper: 'I Aim at the Stars, but Sometimes Hit London.' The Peenemünde people were outraged, and Mrs. Kolff told her son, 'A man as great as Von Braun, nobody should be allowed to make fun of him.'

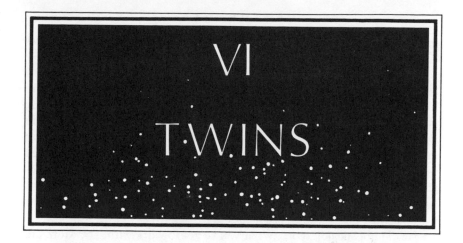

VI

T·W·INS

WHEN STANLEY MOTT TOOK HIS SEAT AT THE TABLE DURING THE first meeting of the selection committee and saw the list of the hundred and ten applicants for the six available spots in the astronaut program, he went immediately to the chairman and said, 'I think I must disqualify myself. I know one of these men.'

'Which one?'

'Number forty-seven. Charles Lee, Army test pilot. If he uses the nickname Hickory, I know him. He worked for me as gate-guard at Huntsville.'

'What did you think of him?'

'Real Tennessee hillbilly. Finest kid I ever knew. My wife thought the same about his wife, another hillbilly called Sandra. I told him to quit his guard's job and get himself an education.'

'Did he?'

'Yep. My wife found his wife a nursing job. He went to Vanderbilt. Graduated with honors.'

'That's the kind of man we're seeking. Stay here and share your opinion with us.'

'I won't vote when his name comes up.'

'If he's that good, you won't have to.'

So Mott had stayed, had studied each of the competitors, and had voted strongly for Randy Claggett of Texas and John Pope of Fremont, both of whom were accepted. His rugged testimonial on behalf of Hickory Lee enabled that young man to make the list also, but his three other choices were rejected.

After the six winners had been introduced to the public at a large press conference, NASA officials handed Mott a radical new assignment, but one which would give him great satisfaction during the next decade: 'You're a sensible man. Know a lot about engineering and science. We want you to look after the indoctrination and education of these young men. The way things are going, they'll form the backbone of our program some years down the line and we want them to be in top shape.'

The first thing Mott did was to check his impressions of the six new astronauts against the more technical knowledge of the psychiatrist who had supervised the analyses of the original hundred and ten, dismissing about thirty out of hand, and he found Dr. Loomis Crandall of a clinic in Denver a most engaging fellow. A chain-smoker, prematurely gray, he was in his early forties, a graduate of the University of Chicago with advanced work in Vienna and Rome and solid experience as an Air Force psychologist at Colorado Springs. His youthful energy, coupled with his gray hair, lent him exactly the proper combination of erudition and street smarts for working with brash young test pilots.

He did not speak jargon. 'What you've got to work with, Dr. Mott, are six of the most highly motivated young men in America. Look at their faces. Look at their records.' And he spread on the table six large photographs of the winners, each with a three-line summary:

> Randolph Claggett, 1929. Texas A & M. Major, USMC. Patuxent River.
> Charles 'Hickory' Lee, 1933. Vanderbilt Univ. Major, US Army. Edwards.
> Timothy Bell, 1934. Univ. of Arkansas. Civilian. Allied Aviation test pilot.
> Harry Jensen, 1933. Univ. of Minnesota. Captain, US Air Force. Edwards.
> Edward Cater, 1931. Mississippi State. Major, US Air Force. Edwards.
> John Pope, 1927. Annapolis. Cmdr., US Navy. Patuxent River.

Mott checked this list as Dr. Crandall recited his conclusions: 'Pope's the oldest, Bell's the youngest, the rest are nicely bunched. Homogeneous in most other ways, too. All Protestant. All from small towns. All married and all with at least two kids, except Pope. All from the Midwest or South.

'Now, that last point's significant. To have passed our strict surveillance, these men must have had a central tendency in their lives. Good behavior, bravery, a certain religious bent. The whole mix. And what do you suppose is the best name for that? Patriotism. Old-fashioned patriotism. And where do you find that these days? Mainly in the South. In the Civil War country. Mott, if you took one thousand of the men who really run the Army, Navy, Air Force and Marines, you'd find that seventy percent of them come from the South, which has only . . . what? Thirty percent of the population. Totally out of proportion, but that's because the heroic occupations have always appealed to the Southern man . . . and the Southern woman. Look at the list. Texas, Tennessee, Arkansas, Mississippi. And the chap who graduated from Minnesota was born in South Carolina. Went north only because his family was Swedish and they wanted him in Minnesota surroundings.'

Mott asked why the astronauts so far contained no Catholics, and Crandall had a prompt answer: 'What have we insisted on in these first groups? Training in math, engineering, science, test-piloting most of all. And what does test-piloting demand? Training in math, engineering, science. And what do the great Catholic schools emphasize? Anything but math, engineering and science. So up to now a young man trained in the Catholic tradition has simply not been eligible.

'Hell, I'm Catholic. I desperately wanted a Catholic in this batch, especially since none appeared in the first groups. But where to find one? Not at Notre Dame. Not at Villanova.' He pushed his papers back and said enthusiastically, 'We've got some great leads for a couple of hotshot Catholics in the next batch.'

Crandall emphasized the conspicuous fact that almost all the astronauts so far, and certainly all of this group, came from small towns. 'I've pondered this, and it can't be genetic, or a matter of aptitude. It must be a socioeconomic factor. Boys from small towns tend to live close to their parents. They're urged to take things seriously. Their families encouraged them to study, join the Boy Scouts, play games. These men, all of them, had character ingrained in them by the time they were ten.

'You can get that in the city, but more often you're led into other channels. Business. Manipulative professions like the one I'm in. Political management.' He paused. 'I'll tell you one thing, Mott, I'd hate to live in a country governed by these astronauts. Very conservative. Very unimaginative in any field outside their own. They're all Republicans, you know.'

But he also stressed what Mott already knew, that these men were determined to succeed. 'Every one is a superachiever, driven by the most profound determination to do things right. Cowardice, recalcitrance, the temptation to do sloppy work, all suppressed. Their capacity to do extra work is unbelievable, so if you're to be in charge of their education, don't fear to pile it on. These men will learn ten times as much as the average A student. Ten times as much as you or I could have mastered. These are super machines.'

When Mott queried him about one peculiarity shared by the six, Crandall grew expansive. 'The point you raise worried me at first. Twenty-two astronauts—twenty-two of the best young men in America and not an outstanding athlete among them. Why? Well, I did a lot of double-doming and came up with a batch of fancy explanations. "Boys with the amount of drive they have don't waste their time with games." Or maybe "Engineering and science require so much lab work, there's no time for daily football practice." Or perhaps "In athletics the motivations are all external. What the coach says. What the rules say. In the fields these men work in, the disciplines are internal." I had half a dozen other goodies, and when I discussed them with faculty members some of the teachers were rather pleased that in this most demanding of life tests, the superathletes did not do poorly. They did nothing. Blank.'

He raised his hands as if to confess his bewilderment, then broke into a cheerful laugh. 'Stupid me! I had overlooked one simple fact which explained it all. In each successive selection, we've picked smaller men. So they can fit into the machines we're building. If we had selected the really bright football linemen, and there are some, believe me, they'd have stood six feet four and weighed two hundred and fifty. One of those gorillas would require more space than two of our men like Grissom and Young. As a matter of fact, the engineers who build the machines wish we'd keep the maximum height something less than five-eight and the weight no more than one-sixty.'

Mott said, 'I seem to remember that John Pope did pretty well in football. Claggett, too.'

'They all played games,' Crandall conceded. 'And some were pretty good. But not one of the first twenty-two was what you'd call a superjock, and very sneakily I weasel back to my first guess. They weren't because men like these do not waste their time on sports, for the good reason that the goals they've set for themselves will not permit that extravagance.'

He made two other warning points. 'Astronauts by an enormous margin are first-born children. They've been pampered. They have powerful egos. Their parents may have driven them too hard, but they also loved them. These men expect to be cared for. Do not brush them off. On the other hand, no astronaut, regardless of the pressure we put him under, has ever developed a gastric ulcer. These sonsabitches know something you and I haven't learned. Work like hell all day, but turn it off at night. Eat a good meal and get a good night's sleep. So you don't have to treat them like china. These bastards are tough.'

He had more statistical analyses which he might have shared with Mott, but he felt that since the salient points had been covered, it was time to bring in a man with whom Mott would be forced to work in close tandem. 'I want you to meet Tucker Thompson, chief honcho for *Folks* magazine. He's primarily responsible for breaking the stranglehold *Life* had on the astronauts, and he's got to make good on these six or get fired.'

Before Mott could say 'I've already met Thompson,' the editor burst eagerly into the room, smiling enthusiastically, and Mott had an opportunity to inspect more closely the man with whom he would be working. He was tall, bronzed, about fifty, and when he extended his hand, his cuff disclosed an imposing link made of a large gold nugget. He wore a button-down collar and a tie of rich solid color, a pair of exquisitely pressed black trousers, an expensive white jacket and, of course, tasseled shoes. He was slightly bald, a fact which showed to good advantage when he smiled, for then his large face seemed enormous—a vast expanse of tanned skin, shimmering eyes and very white teeth.

'I'm Tucker Thompson,' he said, starting to step forward. But then he stopped, drew back, and pointed at Mott with a long forefinger. 'Hey! I know you. I met you in Senator Grant's office. You're . . .' He hesitated. 'You're Dr. Mott.'

He brought with him a set of the family photographs already taken by his magazine, and when he spread them on the desk, Dr. Crandall added an obvious point: 'Yes, I forgot to say. These young men were never afraid to marry the prettiest girl in town. No psychological hang-ups about the conflicting roles of husband and wife. Boom! They're in bed.' And with a pencil he identified the wives.

'Four normal. Two problems. The Swede Jensen married the Swede Inger. All-American, all-Americans. The Tennessee boy they call Hickory married a daughter of a Tennessee hillbilly, and every man should be so lucky. Outdoor type, has her own horse, her own used car. But when she dresses up! Get back in line, you guys.'

Mott studied Mrs. Lee's photograph and marveled at how far she had progressed from the rather awkward girl he had known at Huntsville. 'She was a friend of my wife's. Look at those steely eyes. That one can do anything she puts her mind to.'

'The civilian Bell,' Dr. Crandall continued, 'the lad so highly recommended by Senator Glancey, found himself a real doll, as you can see. Probably the best mother of the group.'

'She photographs like a million,' Tucker Thompson said. 'With or without the three kids.'

'Ed Cater, the Air Force man from Mississippi, married himself a woman who is most deceptive. Looks like Miss Confederacy but ran a mortgage firm before she married Ed. Bright as they come.'

'I don't see any problems there,' Mott said, adjusting his glasses. 'Except my own. Keeping my mind on the job.'

'The problems hit us with these two,' Thompson said, 'and if I'd have been on the selecting committee, I don't think I'd've allowed these two in. They damage our case.'

He pointed to the photograph of Debby Dee Claggett: loose-fitting blouse, sandals, blond hair somewhat awry, smoking a cigarette. 'Frankly, she looks blowzy. We had a board meeting to decide how we should play her. She's not an outdoor type. She's not a cover girl. And she has two real significant drawbacks. Two of her kids are by another man. He's dead, of course. They were legally married. And I find she has the habit of calling anyone she doesn't like, or likes a great deal, "that sonnombeech." '

Distastefully he turned Debby Dee's photograph face downward and in its place produced a real horror. 'Our makeup people decided to see what they could do with Debby Dee. What do you think?' In her improved version Debby Dee wore frills about her throat, dangling green earrings, a bouffant hair style, and a smile displaying more than twenty teeth, two of which had been filled with gold.

Nobody spoke, and after a while Tucker Thompson confided: 'When she saw the photo she said, "That sonnombeech looks like a Shanghai whore." We have a problem with Debby Dee.'

'What did your board decide?' Mott asked.

'We can play her two ways. Texas wholesome. We can claim her father owned a large ranch.'

'Did he?'

'Nobody knows where he is.' He coughed. 'Or what I proposed, we can stress the death of her first husband.'

'But you said his being the father of two of the kids was a drawback,' Crandall said.

'In our business you often take a weakness and make an asset of it. Throw it right in the public's face. We've been checking the record, and she seems to have behaved with extraordinary courage when her husband went down. We have some pictures. We can claim that Claggett was the closest family friend. Proposed immediately to care for the orphans, all that jazz. We convert a liability into an asset.'

'Your best bet,' Crandall said, 'is to play her as a windblown original.'

'Dangerous,' Thompson warned. 'Very dangerous. Because you never know how the American public is going to react to an original. Especially a female original. Now you take two all-time winners, Gertrude Stein and Amy Lowell. God, you couldn't get two zanier women than that, but we took them to our hearts. Now we sell automobiles with Picasso's portrait of Gertrude Stein. We might have the same phenomenon with Debby Dee, but we might not, too.'

'Can we prohibit her from saying *sonnombeech* in public?' Crandall asked.

'I'm not sure that Debby Dee will take correction,' Thompson said, and with this he turned to his last photograph, Mrs. John Pope, legal counsel to the Senate Space Committee. She appeared in office garb, a neat red skirt falling just below her knees, a white Peter Pan collar and a string of beautiful imitation pearls. Her hair was pulled back and fastened with a barrette, but it was her dark eyes which commanded attention.

'We saw her, you know,' Mott reminded the editor, 'in Senator Grant's office.'

'I remember. In an office she's great. But in our effort, she could turn out to be poison.'

'Why?' Mott asked. 'She fills your bill completely, I'd say. Small town. Attends church. Childhood sweetheart.'

'She's a time bomb, gentlemen,' Thompson said from long experience. 'What has *Life* discovered with its astronauts? On the day the flight takes off you want a news photo of the wife waiting at home, or maybe praying in church. The kids. The white picket fence. The distressed neighbors on whom she leans. If one of the sons has a skateboard, so much the better, but a bicycle's best of all. The daughter with a doll, not a teddybear. This tears at the heart, makes the space shot much more real than the pictures of the rocket blasting off.

'Now what the hell do we photograph if Astronaut John Pope takes off on a dangerous mission? His wife in her Washington office biting a pencil? She ought to be miles from Washington in some small town in a white house with a picket fence. And dammit, she doesn't have any children. Everything about this capable woman adds up wrong. And do you know what I fear? These damned professional women. During the flight, when we can't keep the ordinary press away from her, she'll say something. "Why aren't there any Colored in the program?" "When will they take women up the way the Russians have just done?" God knows what she'll say, but you can bet it'll be counterproductive.'

He tapped the handsome photograph with his pencil and predicted: 'That woman's a nuclear bomb. Planted right at the heart of my program.'

'The obvious story,' Mott said, 'is that this brave girl works in the very office, et cetera, et cetera.'

'In my business,' Thompson said, 'you're not to be too clever. Stick to the little house and the white fence. And do you know why? Two-thirds of our readers are women, and they instinctively despise bright young women like Penny Pope who hold jobs and keep their weight down.'

'Except for Debby Dee,' Mott pointed out, 'your first four are rather thin.'

'But they're also pretty. Like models. Women expect models to be thin. And none of them is contaminated by having a job.' With a broad sweep of his hand he indicated the entire gallery. 'If a woman is pretty, thin is beautiful. If she has an administrative job, thin is avaricious and mean-spirited. You tell me what to do with this one.' And he pointed accusingly at Penny Pope.

All such questions became vital to Rachel Mott when NASA employed her to act as a kind of cicerone to the families of the six new astronauts. She got the exciting assignment because of the excellent record being compiled by her husband, but everyone who knew her realized that she was perfectly suited for such a task. She was a mature forty-three, always well groomed, a fine housekeeper with children of her own, and a Bostonian with a strong sense of obligation.

When she and Stanley took up residence near the new space headquarters in Houston, she was distressed when Millard elected to remain in California with the young men of the surfboard coterie, but she was pleased to see how easily Christopher, now thirteen, adapted himself to life in Texas. What gratified her especially was the respect shown her husband by everyone at NASA, where he was recognized not only as the mentor of the new astronauts but also as one of the most brilliant of the permanent staff. It seemed that he moved from one important ad hoc committee to another, serving first as an engineer on some highly technical problem, then as a scientist on matters dealing with outer space.

His principal energy, however, was directed toward inducting the six young men into the mysteries of NASA, and within a week of their reporting to Houston he had them scheduled into a round of learning situations which resembled advanced work in some fine engineering university, except that the men had two hours a day of theory and ten hours of laboratory. This schedule would continue for about six months, after which they would move into specialized applications.

Such concentrated work left the wives free to follow their own obligations and interests, and this was where Rachel Mott's responsibilities began.

Tucker Thompson saw to it that the wives were photographed regularly at those occupations which would best represent the female half of the NASA effort. Since three of the women had strong church affiliations—with the most respectable denominations, not the Holy Roller type that flourished in the South—there was a fruitful opportunity for shots of a reassuring nature: Sunday School, picnics, suppers for old folk, standing outside the church with the other parishioners on Sunday morning. He was also very strong on family outings when the astronauts were in Houston and on Little League baseball games; he had a low opinion of basketball: 'Mostly a Colored game these days. Baseball is what our readers have faith in.'

Rachel saw the women at their more normal tasks, and although at first they had been suspicious of her, judging her to be a NASA spy, they came in time to respect her professionalism and her force of character. She was both sympathetic and persuasive and was never reluctant to express a strong opinion if she felt it needed. Her neatness, her command of English and her taste in clothes were impressive to these young women, who were equally attentive to their own appearances.

She had a hard time with Debby Dee, who was only six years younger and not disposed to pay much attention to what anyone presumed to tell her, but Rachel did not brood upon this failure, for she found the Texas woman far too brash for her taste and the Claggett children even less disciplined than her own. The Claggetts were not a family she would have sought out, and she was somewhat gratified when her husband reported that he was not having much success with Major Claggett. 'He finishes his work faster than others and he knows airplanes inside out, but he's very difficult to communicate with. Fends everything off with a joke.'

Like everyone else, Rachel found herself in love with the Swedes, Harry and Inger Jensen, for they were attractive, bright and extremely eager to please. 'Perpetual Boy Scouts,' someone described them, and Harry had indeed been an Eagle Scout. They were a pair easy to identify in that each had blond hair and a narrow triangular face. Their eyes were blue; they smiled incessantly; and they were in love.

She worried about the civilian couple, for they seemed to lack the harsh fiber that characterized the military families, even though Stanley assured her that Tim Bell was one of the hottest pilots private industry had so far produced. 'General Funkhauser of Allied Aviation does not recommend a man who can't cut the mustard. Look for the wife's good qualities, not her weakest ones.' The trouble with the Bells, as Rachel saw it, was that the husband was inordinately good-looking, while the wife had that baby-doll prettiness which often spelled danger. Since she photographed magnificently, and since her husband looked more like a hotshot test pilot than any of the other men, their pictures were widely distributed, and in time Mrs. Mott came to agree that despite their possible weaknesses, the Bells were a considerable asset to the program.

She found it easy to like the three pretty Southern wives, Cater, Jensen, Lee; they conducted themselves well, assisted whenever called upon, and seemed indistinguishable from the millions of resilient wives who had accompanied their husbands in ages past when the latter went forth with Julius Caesar to the frontiers of empire, or with Robert Clive to the pacification of India, or with Douglas MacArthur to his occupation of Japan. They were professionals, and since she had made herself one at El Paso and Huntsville, she respected them.

Gloria Cater, the one-time business woman from Mississippi, was a constant surprise, a combination of Southern ante-bellum beauty and a tough sense of self-protection. Inger Jensen was frail, talkative and great fun to be with. But the gem of the Dixie contingent, in Rachel Mott's opinion, had to be tomboy Sandra Lee from the hills of central Tennessee.

She had been extremely fond of this self-directed beauty and saw with approval that Sandy apparently assessed the NASA experience with neat accuracy. She could turn on whatever mood Tucker Thompson and his photographers wanted, then walk away untouched by the nonsense. Rachel enjoyed hearing her tell how Hickory had wound up an astronaut: 'My boy tore Vanderbilt apart. Straight A's. Earned a commission in the Army, then his wings, then a master's in aeronautical engineering at MIT, straight A's again.' But Rachel noticed that one could approach the Lees only so far; then the mountain couple retreated; they did not permit anyone to know them intimately.

Rachel felt her closest identification with Penny Pope, of Washington, for in this competent, self-directed woman she saw the kind of efficiency she tried to maintain in her own life, plus a high degree of personal charm which she herself had never been able to generate. Also, Mrs. Pope was obviously more gifted intellectually than the other five and therefore more rewarding to talk with on the few occasions when she left her duties with the Senate to visit with her husband. Rachel did not feel, like some other NASA personnel, that 'this Pope dame is a cool customer,' for she sensed the strong opinions and great warmth Penny was capable of, but she did know that the perfectly groomed young woman from the West was going to present problems quite different from those offered by the Southern belles. Rachel Mott liked Penny Pope, liked her enormously, but she also feared her.

'Well, what do we have?' Tucker Thompson asked at the beginning of the fourth week, when his magazine was preparing its initial presentation of the six wives. 'What I'm looking for is a theme to hand the American public, and especially the American housewife. Because these are "her girls" and we've got to keep them that way.'

'They're beautiful. Your photographers should have an easy time.'

'But we've got to show them as more than beautiful. We're after their collective soul, and in this game first impressions are fatal.'

'They're intelligent. There's not a dummy in the lot. Even Debby Dee Claggett is as sharp as a pin, in her own way.'

'Intelligence is a negative factor when you're trying to sell a group of women. One woman, like Oveta Culp Hobby, yes. The public can take pride in an exception. But not six. We're looking for the theme that will make America's heart sing. We do not have an easy job, Mrs. Mott, and I'd appreciate some serious help from you.'

'Start with the beauty, Tucker, but call it "the well-scrubbed American look," and then make a virtue of their diversity. Use Tomboy Sandra. Use cool, efficient Mrs. Cater, and contrary to your fears, I think you have a real goody in Mrs. Pope's quietly helping to make decisions that enable her hero husband to fly his dangerous missions. Unity in diversity is your theme, Tucker. Or maybe it's diversity in unity.'

There were several exhaustive meetings on the subject of how to present the wives, but in the end, it was Rachel Mott's ideas about the cover which prevailed: 'A small American flag in the center, blowing in the breeze, surrounded by the six wives shown in the most carefully chosen vignettes. Sandy Lee with an Indian sweatband around her head. Gloria Cater chewing an executive pencil. Penny Pope standing before a Senate eagle. Cluny Bell with her left hand framing her fragile face. Inger Jensen in an Eton collar being her adorable self. And Debby Dee Claggett—'

She stopped. How could the big Texas woman best be depicted? Tentatively she suggested, 'With a martini glass, a cigarette . . .'

'One thing for sure,' Thompson said, 'our psychological studies prove that in a circular picture, people will usually overlook the eight o'clock position. Lower left-hand corner. Debby Dee comes in at eight o'clock.'

The cover was a sensation, the handsome American flag surrounded by six of its most appealing daughters. As soon as customers started writing in for copies without printing so they could be framed, *Folks* ran off two hundred thousand and sold them for twenty-five cents each, and when the lot was gone and the six wives properly presented, Thompson had one of his secretaries summarize the mail:

> Most comment on: Inger Jensen, the one everyone would like to have as their daughter. Least comment on: Penny Pope, who struck readers as indifferent and why wasn't she with her husband? Most

liked: Debby Dee Claggett, who looked like the best mother in the lot. Consensus: An American bouquet the nation can be proud of.

Rachel Mott felt, with some justification, that she had played a helpful role in getting her six debutantes properly launched into the American social season, but on the day when Virgil Grissom and John Young made their historic first flight in the new spacecraft Gemini, she discovered that she was living in a fool's paradise. It was a tense moment in space history, when the fate of the national program hung in the balance and when the safety of two astronauts—not one, as before—was at stake. All NASA was on edge, and Tucker Thompson felt that this might be a good moment for the general press to see how the new wives reacted to the machine in which their own husbands would shortly be flying. He called Mrs. Mott: 'Rachel, where are the girls?'

'I believe four of them are watching the television at Gloria Cater's.'

'Marvelous. That'll make a great shot. But why only four?'

'Mrs. Pope's in Washington, as usual. And Inger Jensen's visiting her folks in Minnesota.'

'Damn! She's the most photogenic of the lot. That little-girl charm. Well, we'll go with what we have. Meet me at the Caters'.' He was about to hang up, but asked hurriedly, 'It's got a picket fence, hasn't it?'

When they reached the Cater home Thompson explained to the waiting newsmen the ground rules governing the interviews and photography: 'These women are under extreme tension. They've gathered here for mutual support. No harsh questions. Nothing at all about what would happen if the mission failed.'

Rachel should have gone into the cottage first to alert the wives, but she stayed outside to coach the women reporters on the personalities of the four wives, and this meant that Tucker got to the living room first. He almost fainted, for he found the women with their shoes off, playing gin rummy and drinking martinis, while the television droned on, with no one paying attention. Mrs. Claggett and the hostess, Mrs. Cater of Mississippi, were smoking cigarettes.

'Good God!' Thompson cried. 'A sacred moment in history. Men's lives in the balance. And you're playing poker.'

'Gin,' Mrs. Cater said.

'The press is out there. Reporters from all over the nation, all over the world. Get your shoes on.'

Sandy Lee took charge, and in her most efficient manner swept up the cards, hid the martinis and whisked away all sights of debauchery. Then, with the utterly disarming charm that she could turn on when needed, she went to the door and said quietly, 'Persons from the major wire services and two reporters from overseas may come in for fifteen minutes. Then we'll come out and meet with you for as long as you wish. Because this is a historic moment and we feel deeply proud to play even a minor part in it.'

With graciousness unbounded she escorted the five selected newspeople into the cottage, then smiled bravely at the sixty or seventy others as she closed the door and moved to where Gloria and Cluny and Debby Dee were staring at Walter Cronkite on the television screen.

The program for which the new astronauts had been selected was named Gemini because for the first time two men were to fly the spacecraft in a compartment so restricted that one man lay almost touching his partner and remained there immobilized for periods of up to fourteen days. When Dr. Mott actually inspected the capsule, he appreciated what Crandall had said about NASA's restraints on the height and weight of its astronauts; no two men of normal-large dimension could possibly wedge themselves into this confined space, and even highly trained men like the lean astronauts had trouble doing so.

Gemini was a form of exploration unprecedented in world history, and it demanded men of agility, bravery and enormous competence.

At the beginning of the six-month indoctrination, Deke Slayton, lean and mean, appeared before the astronauts with a stack of basic manuals and specific flight plans twenty-seven inches thick. 'By the time your name is called for a flight, you will have memorized everything in boldface and understood the rest.'

The basic manuals were like intricate games for grown-up children, in that each depicted in the most carefully analyzed form the operation of some one system of the Gemini craft: in one, colored diagrams showed the movement of electricity through literally miles of wiring; in another, the most elegant break-away drawings of the type developed in World War II to facilitate the repair of airplanes showed how the hydraulic system worked; in yet another, four cleverly printed sheets of transparent plastic lay one atop the other to allow the astronaut to see inside one of his rocket thrusters.

The fields of knowledge seemed endless, sixteen major concentrations of information, all of which had to be mastered, and regardless of which field the men attacked next, the same rule applied: two hours of intellectual discussion, ten hours of laboratory break-down, then two hours of comparing notes and ten more hours of tackling the problem physically.

From its earliest days NASA had followed a sensible program of requiring all its astronauts to study everything, but then to assign each man a field of specialization in which he was expected to become a top expert, familiar with the most arcane concepts and possible future developments. It was always an exciting time when these assignments were made, and one morning Deke Slayton appeared with a list: 'Claggett, because of your unusual knowledge of airplanes, structures. Lee, because you've already done a lot with electronics, the electrical system. Bell, because you specialized in aerodynamics at Allied Aviation, flight surfaces. Jensen, because you're small and tight, flight gear and survival mechanisms. Cater, because you've done good work on propulsion at Edwards, rockets. Pope, because of your doctorate in astronomy, navigation and computers.'

John noticed that whenever assignments of any kind were published, the same pecking order maintained, with Claggett at the top and himself at the bottom, and one day when he was alone in Dr. Mott's office he saw on the desk a list giving the names in the accustomed ranking and titled ORDER OF SELECTION. Since he was reading upside down, he had no time to decipher the typing which accompanied the list, but when Mott returned, he asked him bluntly, 'Why am I at the bottom of the list?'

'You weren't supposed to see that.'

'I didn't read it. Just saw the title and the order.'

After Mott put the list in a drawer he said, 'That's the order in which you were selected. There's no better airman around than Claggett. I suppose you know that.'

'I knew him in Korea and Pax River. The best.'

'The others have terrific records, Pope. This boy Bell, the civilian. He flew everything with wings and helped Allied improve every machine they ever made.'

'But why me at the bottom?'

Since Pope seemed bewildered by this ranking, Mott decided to level with him. 'It wasn't your flying. You're up there with the best. And certainly not your bravery, because in Korea and Pax River . . . well, you have the medals to prove that.'

'What was it? What's my hidden weakness, because I certainly don't know and I ought to.'

'Patterns,' Mott said, and when the young flier looked amazed, he added, 'You didn't conform to the patterns. You don't live with your wife. You have no children. Statistically you represented a gamble, especially your wife. NASA feels safer when unknowns like Claggett and Lee conform to patterns. Because then the numbers are in our favor. With you we were flying in the dark. I think you know that.' When Pope made no reply, Mott said, 'It surfaced in Korea and it certainly surfaced at Patuxent.'

'What surfaced?'

'That you were a loner.'

'What's that got to do with it? Seems to me, the main thing is . . . I was also good,' Pope said with that charming frankness which characterized the best test pilots. John Pope was one of the best fliers in the business; he knew it and was not hesitant about claiming his rights.

'That's why we chose you, John.' This sudden use of his first name, as if the discussion had entered a new and more confidential phase, mollified the astronaut, and he asked, 'Why were you willing to overlook the anomalies?'

And now this unusual word, so scientific and so exactly right in this context, relaxed Mott, and he broke into a laugh. Taking off his glasses, he looked at Pope, nine years his junior and one of the most capable men he had ever met, and said, 'We chose you because we knew that in the air you would prove to be one of the very best men on our roster. And you will be.'

'But on the ground, watch out.'

'Yes.' An embarrassed pause, then: 'Any chance you could persuade your wife to quit her job and move down here to Houston?'

'None.' Pope blew his nose, more to gain time than for any other reason, then said, 'Penny told me last weekend that she felt your wife was the person closest to what she's like. You must have faced these same problems.'

'Curious. My wife said the same about Mrs. Pope. "More like me than any of the others." But I never faced your problem, John, because my wife accepted the work I did. Some day I'll tell you about El Paso. And getting eased out at Huntsville. My wife stayed close.'

'Mine doesn't,' Pope said crisply, and without waiting for Mott to indicate that the interview was over, he rose and left the room.

The specialty he had been assigned delighted him, and had he had a free choice from the entire field, he would have elected astronomy and the new navigational systems, for he found them captivating. 'They drive my mind to its ultimate capacities,' he wrote his wife, 'and I feel constantly submerged. But damn it all, I'll work it out in the end.'

The heavy problem of field trips prevented him from becoming narrowly specialized in navigation, for the astronauts were required to jump about the nation and the world with an agility that left some watchers bewildered. In one three-month period Pope and Claggett were occupied with these trips:

> ... To Worcester, Massachusetts, the David Clark Company, to be fitted for two different kinds of spacesuits, plus an extra one for Pope in which he might walk in space.

> ... To Los Angeles, California, for a two-day meeting with General Funkhauser's men, who had won a contract to supply the controls in the capsule.

> ... To St. Louis, Missouri, the McDonnell Astronautics Co., to work on the spacecraft itself.

> ... To Cleveland, Ohio, to work at NASA's Lewis Center on the performance of jet engines and rockets.

> ... To Sunnyvale, California, the Lockheed Space Company, to check the progress of the Agena target vehicle with which Gemini would hook up in outer space.

... To Owego, New York, IBM, for familiarization with the new, smaller computers which would run the spacecraft.

... To Fort Apache, Arizona, to engage in a three-day survival test on the desert, finding food and water as they became available.

... To Canoga Park, California, Rocketdyne, to study the principles and controls governing reentry through the atmosphere.

... To Redondo Beach, California, the Ramo Corporation, to work on trajectory calculations.

Plus several more of the 319 industrial sites where components of the Gemini program were being assembled, including many of the foremost names in American business: Bell, Burroughs, CBS, Douglas, Engelhard Minerals, General Electric, General Motors, B. F. Goodrich, and on down the line.

Some of the excursions had special meaning to the fledgling astronauts, but each man seemed to identify particularly some visit which proved unique for him. Hickory Lee came back from the wild C-135 parabolic flights at Edwards Air Force Base ecstatic: 'By damn, they took me up there to forty thousand feet, flew damned near straight up, then turned the nose down, and in that swift change, Zoom! No gravity! I bounced around in the padded cargo space like a feather in a Texas tornado. Absolutely no gravity. For thirty-two seconds. Down we went, then up again in the parabolic curve, then over and down. We did it thirty-eight times and I came out bruised from ass to elbow. Them mats, they don't protect you no-how.' But for several days he kept talking about those moments of accidental freedom from the pull of Earth.

Some men found it difficult physiologically to adjust to the C-135 routine; all they got was an unmerciful pounding as the huge plane nosed down, and John Pope was one of these: 'I was probably free of gravity, as they say, but I barely knew it.' What imparted the sense of space to him were two much more mundane experiments, but in a way more sophisticated, since they depended upon simple perceptions of gravity.

'If you're like me and fail to catch the feeling in that bang-about C-135,' he advised the others, 'try that Langley Space Walk they showed us in the movies. Out*standing*!'

But his closest approach to a perception of null gravity came in a swimming pool, or rather a huge cubic tank installed at the new center in Huntsville, where in full astronaut's gear he was thrown into the water wearing just enough lead weights about his waist to achieve a neutral buoyancy: 'It was weird and kind of wonderful. Not real weightlessness, you understand, because if you stood on your head in the water, blood rushed to your head, because gravity still operated. But there was a marvelous sense of freedom. I loved it. Whenever I suited up and the crane dropped me into the drink, I thought I was a medieval knight being hoisted onto my white charger. But my lance was a monkey wrench. The world I was to conquer was outer space.'

The most dramatic expedition was Randy Claggett's to Johnsville, the Naval Air Center, just north of Philadelphia, where he was to undergo tolerance tests on the mammoth centrifuge. Using exactly the kind of whirling machine used to separate cream from milk, but on a larger scale permitting many more controlled variations, the men conducting the tests placed their subject in a pilot's chair and whirled him about at ever faster speeds until the required G was reached:

'One look at that sonnombeech and I wanted out. They strapped me in eyeballs out and said, "Can you take ten G's," and I said, "How in hell do I know?" and they said, "Well, you're gonna find out." It was kind of hairy, but I yelled, "I ain't feelin' no pain," so they yelled, "Here come fifteen big ones," and I had a little trouble focusin' my eyes, but when they yelled, "Think you could take twenty?" I yelled back, "Let me outa here," and they said, "You're the judge," and when I got out, the register marked sixteen G's. That's what I took.

'But they was this farm-boy sailor sort of standin' around and he volunteered to try the machine, and when they strapped him in they ran it to fifteen pretty fast and he grinned and yelled, "I kin take it," and they whomped him up to eighteen and asked if he'd like to go for twenty, and he shouted, "Why not?" and they gave him that and then told him that no one had hit twenty-one yet, and he said, "Give it a whirl," but he was spinnin' so fast the words kinda slipped outa the corner of his mouth, and they gave him twenty-one G's for about ten seconds. Dreadful pressure.

'When they stopped the centrifuge he jumped down as good as new, but he was kinda dizzy, I could see that. He started home drivin' his own car, but when I left the test area I saw him parked dead across the median strip, sound asleep. His brain musta been completely addled by the twenty-one G's, but when I took him back to the base the doctors never gave a damn. I often wonder what happened to that farm boy.'

The excursions, which never abated, were made doubly enjoyable when NASA acquired the use of several dozen T-38 two-seater supersonic Northrop jet trainers. These were sleek, exciting aircraft which could hit Mach 1.3 or better, and to leave a late-afternoon meeting at Cape Canaveral, hurry to the airfield and whip a T-38 through the sky to Houston in time for dinner was a delight.

Because the T-38 could carry two, Claggett and Pope, as two buddies from Pax River, often found themselves sharing a plane on some swift flight to a contractor's meeting or to the next field test, and one day they flew to Key West for a drill on parachute landings in water, since every emergency had to be anticipated. For three days the two pilots were hauled aloft in an old DC-3 and tossed overboard at a height of 9,000 feet. As they descended, slowly twisting in the Caribbean sunlight, they would make silent bets as to which powerboat on the waves below would get to them first. On the third afternoon, when the tests were over, they sped to the airfield, climbed into their T-38 and flew across the Gulf of Mexico to the haven of Ellington Air Force Base north of the Houston space center, landing just as the sun was setting behind the city.

To be young, to be at home in the heavens, and to have a T-38 at one's disposal, with airfields across the nation at which one could land for fuel or for a critical meeting, was to know the best of life. By no means was it recreation; the pilots had to do this flying to maintain their skills, and it was obligatory that they fly a certain number of hours each month, some at night, to qualify for the salary adjustments which meant so much to them. 'Hell,' Claggett said, 'me and Debby Dee, we couldn't live on my base pay. Without that good ole flight pay, our kids would have to live on grits.'

The flight they liked best was from Houston to Cape Canaveral, for this meant that they were headed toward the mystical site from which they would one day soar off into space, and with a kind of reverence, they approached the sandy spit on which the launching pads waited. 'This is for real,' Claggett cried one day as he took his T-38 far out to sea before landing.

Also, several of the most effective simulators were located at the Cape, and the astronauts never wearied of climbing into these extraordinary devices and going through imaginary flight procedures. NASA had developed a simulator for everything, Claggett said, 'except tying your shoes, and the minute that becomes important, presto, they're gonna have one.'

There was a simulator for launch, another for coming back through the atmosphere. There was one for the guidance system, another for the computers. There was an amazing simulator for aborting a flight, and a Rube Goldberg type, all angles and elbows, for landing on the Moon. There was a simulator covering every conceivable emergency, but the best of all was operated by a tall, mournful doctor in engineering from Purdue University who had a kind of Fu Manchu beard and whom everyone called Dracula.

His job was to anticipate disaster, to imagine the worst possible outcome of every step his astronauts would take and then to simulate the disasters they might encounter. Halfway into the launch on his simulator, power in three rockets would be lost and a set of highly sophisticated telemetry devices would register every mistake the agitated pilot made. Or just at the crucial moment the two main computers would blow, and every wrong move made by the pilot in the right-hand seat would be coldly registered. Engines would catch fire; the ablative shield would burn off; the drogue parachute wouldn't pull out the main; when Dracula was on the scene, playing his simulators like a violin, disaster was omnipresent.

And when the test flight was over, he would meet with the two pilots and read them his scorecard: 'At 00:01:49 into the flight compression was lost.' The bastard never said, 'I cut compression.' It was always an impersonal compression that acted poorly. 'The commander made two wrong responses before he hit the right one and the mission crashed. At 00:05:23 an exaggerated pogo began. Pilot attempted correction using procedure abandoned four months ago and mission crashed.' It sometimes seemed as if Dracula could never be content until the imaginary Gemini spacecraft plunged into the Atlantic, killing both pilots, but when real flight began and absolutely no crisis eventuated for which Dracula had not prepared his crews, the astronauts began to generate a real affection for him. But he was, as Claggett said, 'a real bastard,' which the Twins verified one morning.

Dracula was a genius at devising sight-and-sound spectaculars that exactly duplicated what the astronauts would see in the flight. Motion picture cameras displayed the heavens which would surround the men at a particular moment; the seasick motion of the descending capsule could be evoked with gimbals; noises were easy to duplicate—so that by the time Claggett and Pope had flown the various simulators for well over a hundred and fifty hours, they believed with some reason that space could hold no surprises for them.

In that mood they climbed into the main simulator one morning after it had been mysteriously shut down for three weeks, and as they listened to the countdown numbers coming over their earphones—7–6–5–4–3–2–1– blast off—they grew tense, as always, awaiting Dracula's next disaster.

But on this day the simulator was playing for real. It blew up. There was a terrible explosion, wild noises, with flame and smoke invading the capsule as it simulated lifting into the air atop its Titan rocket. To his credit, Claggett in the left-hand seat took every step calculated to diminish the consequences of the explosion, and in his right-hand seat Pope did what he could to control the fire. The flames, from whatever cause, were extinguished, so that the simulator, badly damaged, could be repaired and used again.

And then the two astronauts realized that it had all been faked. Dracula had devised a set of excellent motion pictures, a new sound system and a machine which would rock the simulator while giving off flame and smoke. At the debriefing the gloomy man droned: 'At 00:01:09 one of the main rockets exploded. Commander and pilot responded with all the right procedures except emergency control of oxygen, so the mission crashed.' When headquarters asked Claggett and Pope how they had reacted to the unexpected explosion, the latter retreated to his test-pilot training and said, 'I tried this and it failed. I tried step two and it failed. But step three proved effective.' Claggett was more direct: 'I was scared shitless.'

.   .   .

Senator Grant did not propose to do the Republican dirty work on the Space Committee for the Democrats Lyndon Johnson and Michael Glancey without getting something for his state in return, but when the time came to identify the quid pro quo he ran into difficulty. Eastland of Mississippi had cornered most of the easy plums controlled by the Senate, while Mendel Rivers of South Carolina commandeered so many posts and establishments that an admiral had once growled, 'Mendel, if we give you one more base, Charleston will sink.'

Of the NASA assignments, Johnson was taking care of Texas, and Glancey was protecting Red River with multiple contracts. Trying to combat such patronage crocodiles was difficult, but Grant was not powerless, and when he threatened revolt, the Democratic leadership had to consider ways to placate him.

'Norman,' Glancey said one morning prior to a committee meeting, 'Air Force and NASA both could use another airfield west of the Missouri, and we've decided to place it just north of your hometown. Very convenient when you get your own plane.' Glancey also persuaded General Funkhauser to locate a branch of Allied Aviation next to the industrial city of Webster, and Grant was mollified except for one additional boon in which he had a personal interest.

'Glancey, our astronomer at Fremont State has talked some well-to-do people into giving us a planetarium. His name's Anderssen, splendid scholar. I think it would be proper if this new bunch of astronauts reported there for their star studies.'

'Well . . . you know, Norman . . . we've been sending our men to Chapel Hill in North Carolina. They do an excellent job.'

'I'm sure they do,' Grant said crisply, 'but I'm equally sure Anderssen can do as well.'

Nothing came of this exchange, but Grant was so eager to have six astronauts walking on the streets of his college town that he returned twice to the matter, and in the end Glancey surrendered: 'I'll speak to NASA,' and when those officials said that although North Carolina was doing a fine job, they could see no reason why Anderssen at Fremont State couldn't do as well, the indoctrination was moved west. At his first meeting in the new planetarium the old man told the astronauts:

'When a man has studied the heavens for ten thousand nights he is entitled to make certain generalizations. Space is without limit or definition. There is no east or west, no north or south, no down or up, no in or out. It is truly boundless and must be respected as such. It cannot be measured or comprehended. All we can do is behave in accordance with its laws as we dimly perceive them.

'It is those laws I wish to speak about, and I need not exhort you to master them, for the day is not far off when you, and each of you, will be soaring in outer space, with the welfare of this nation and indeed of all mankind depending upon how you perform.

'This is a galaxy. [And he flashed on the heavens of the planetarium a stunning photograph of M-51, the Whirlpool.] There are about one billion stars in that galaxy, and about one billion galaxies in the universe as we are allowed to know it at this moment. That means that we may have as many as a billion billion different stars. I shall now increase the light so that you can write on your pads a billion billion. That's the figure one followed by eighteen zeros.

[He lowered the light and showed the astronauts a beautiful photograph of the galaxy in Coma Berenices known as NGC-4565, an elongated mass of stars and galactic dust.] 'If we could see our Galaxy, spelled always with a capital G, from a vast distance it would look like this, a collection of some four billion stars arranged about a central core. I want each of you to guess where our Sun, one of those stars, is situated within the Galaxy.

[He replaced 4565 with an artist's conception of our Galaxy as viewed from above, and with a flashlight-pointer indicated how the Sun stood far off to one side, well away from the vital center.] 'We are attached to a star of only average size, in a galaxy of only average size, far from the center of action where new stars are being born, far from those centers of the universe where new galaxies are being born. Never, never, young men, believe that we stand at the center of things, or even close to the center of anything.

'But the position we do occupy within our marvelous Galaxy is a magnificent one whose complexities will occupy you for the rest of your lives. I have spent sixty years, as a boy in Norway and an astronomer in this country, endeavoring to penetrate the mysteries of our planetary system, and I suppose I know as much about it as anyone living but I do not know its precise origin, or the construction of any component except Earth, always spelled with a capital E, or the mechanics which ultimately hold the system together, or its final destiny.

'I stand before you an ignorant old man terribly jealous of the astounding opportunity you have to explore our system and most eager to help you acquire the tools to accomplish that exploration. To perform your task, you must know the stars.'

The next thing he showed them, with the aid of special devices on the planetarium instrument, was the ecliptic, that arbitrary band of the heavens through which the Moon and the planets moved and along which the Sun appeared to move, and when this imaginary line was fixed in the men's minds, he threw upon it handsome streamlined interpretations of the zodiacal signs, immemorially ancient in origin, the signposts of the heavens.

'I have studied the zodiac in five different languages, and with every known mnemonic device, but a child's rhyme fashioned in England long ago remains the best help so far devised. It's printed in your material and I shall expect you to memorize it by tomorrow. I use it almost every night, and so will you.' And he recited the childish rhyme which helps astronomers organize their work, pointing with his light-wand to the curious collection of figures associated with the words:

> 'The Ram, the Bull, the Heavenly Twins.
> Next the Crab, and the Lion shines.
> The Virgin and the Scales.
> The Scorpion, Archer and He-Goat,
> Then the Man with the Watering Pot,
> And the Fish with the glittering scales.'

Having made the circuit once, he returned the heavens to Aries and cried, 'Now all together,' and like a group of kindergartners, the six astronauts recited the nursery rhyme.

Professor Anderssen was rigorous in demanding that the astronauts master the navigational stars situated along the ecliptic, for some of these would usually be visible, but they were not conspicuous, their names were unfamiliar, and they gave the young men much trouble: 'You simply must learn the easy ones by tomorrow. Spica, Antares, Aldebaran, Pollux, Regulus.'

When these were mastered he turned to the difficult ones, some scarcely visible to unpracticed eyes: 'Nunki in Sagittarius, easy to find in the group that looks like a Tea Kettle; Deneb Algedi in Capricornus, not easy to find. Hamal in Aries, very difficult to find. But the most difficult of all, either to find or say, this one in Libra, Zubeneschamali.'

He was having some difficulty with Randy Claggett, who gave the star names his own pronunciation. The Big Dipper became Ursula Major, Zubeneschamali was Reuben Smiley, and the important navigational star Nunki became Nooki. 'Am I correct in thinking, Major Claggett, that the word *Nooki* has sexual overtones?'

'Well . . . it means . . . you're getting some.'

'Then I think we'd better call that star by its right name, Nunki,' but when in oral review Anderssen pointed his wand at Sagittarius and asked Claggett to identify the principal star, he bellowed, 'Nooki.' For a brief spell the professor thought of disciplining the Texan, but he observed that Claggett was learning the stars faster than anyone else except Pope, who had a Ph.D. in related fields, so he tolerated him, and once when he was trying to teach the more difficult stars he shouted, 'Learn it! It's difficult! It's Reuben Smiley!' and the class applauded.

When the northern stars were mastered, he convened his students in the planetarium and told them something they would often refer to when they talked among themselves. He was proving to be an inspired teacher, one whose obvious enthusiasm brightened his subject; when he said that he had studied the stars for ten thousand nights he meant just that, three long nights of observation each week for sixty years:

> 'We have mastered, I think, the northern stars, the easy bright ones especially, and we have seen how fortuitous it was that God or nature placed Polaris at the precise spot where it would be most useful, at the North Pole. Now look at the South Pole and see how empty it is. Look at the entire southern hemisphere and see how few bright stars we have to guide us.

> [He allowed the sky to move slowly, majestically through three complete days, speaking a few words now and then to impress upon the men the emptiness of the southern regions and the obligation they faced of being just as familiar with these few helpful stars as with the more numerous and conspicuous ones of the north.]

> 'When I was a boy in Norway and had mastered the northern stars, as you have done, I used to stand on my hill and rage at the heavens, pleading with them to shift so that I could see the southern stars, which I knew to be hidden below the horizon. "Canopus," I shouted. "Come forth! I know you're down there. Southern Cross, let me see you!"

> 'Think of it, gentlemen. We seven are among the well educated, and not one of us has ever seen the stars that guide the south. Now we shall learn them, but I cannot convey how jealous of you I shall be when you leap into space and fly beyond the shadow of the earth and see in all their glory the southern stars which I have never seen.

> [Quietly he moved into his heavens the Magellanic Clouds which had so captivated the Portuguese explorer, the Southern Cross which had guided and delighted Captain Cook, the brilliance of Centaurus and the cold beauty of Canopus, second brightest star in the heavens.]

> 'I will expect you to know all the easy stars by tomorrow morning. Then we shall drop down to the difficult ones.'

And they were difficult: Achernar, Al Na'ir and crazy stars that not even Pope had ever heard of: Miaplacidus and Atria. But as Anderssen insisted:

'They're essential because at some crucial moment up there, it may be only this part of the heavens that you will be able to see, and if you do not know these stars, you will be lost.'

In his concluding lecture, when he was satisfied that his six students had learned in their 120 hours of assigned time more than he had known at the end of five years of study, he told them:

> 'You are prepared to identify the stars which will give you the data you need to navigate to the Moon, or Mars, or Jupiter. You must now move on to master the computers which will absorb these data and tell you exactly where you are. But in a larger sense, none of us will ever know where we are. We are lost in the stars, in our little Galaxy, among the billions of other galaxies that help to control us within a universe we can neither define nor comprehend. The steps you brave young men take with your marvelous machines will push back the veil of ignorance a little way, and then our concern will be with the newly revealed and greater ignorances which will dominate us until others like you, with their own machines and understandings, push their veils aside to reveal the new imponderables. How I envy you.'

Tucker Thompson was enjoying such a great run with the six astronauts that his magazine advertised his work as 'a better job than *Life*,' and the astronauts applauded this because according to their contract with *Folks*, each man stood to make about $23,000 extra income if the series was sold abroad. The fliers therefore worked closely with Tucker and encouraged their wives to do the same, but all of the women resented Thompson's invasion of their privacy, and he had some trouble getting them to do the things that the American public had a right to expect of their heroines.

Thompson had particular cause to worry about Cocoa Beach, the explosive town to the south of Canaveral which had once contained 2,600 people and would soon have many times that number. Never a pretty town, in the old days it had served as a winter resort for snow-birds who flocked south each December from places like Maine, Minnesota and especially Ontario. Those with wealth continued on to Palm Beach, a hundred and twenty-five miles farther south; only those on budgets parked their caravans at Cocoa Beach. The houses tended to be one story, frame, unheated and dusty, the stores two-storied and jumbled. There had been bars, most of which were shuttered during the summer, and living quarters for a small permanent population whose men commuted to jobs north along the coast to Daytona Beach or inland to Orlando.

Like Canaveral itself, the little town huddled on the outer chain of islands and expanded not like a lovely rose which flowered in all directions, but rather like a radish which elongated at each end but stayed the same in the restricted middle. Yet the town had a wild beauty, for to the east roared the somber Atlantic.

When the astronauts flew in to Cape Canaveral on duty assignments, which was constantly, austere bachelor quarters were provided in NASA buildings, but they preferred the livelier scene at Cocoa Beach, twenty miles to the south, and if they brought their wives along, which they often did, it became the custom for them to take rooms at a new and glossy motel called the Bali Hai, a name borrowed by many joints across the country from a popular song that was supposed to be tropical and sexy. This Bali Hai had been built by Canadians, who seemed always to have an uncanny sense of which Florida beach was going to become popular next, but it was run by a pessimistic married couple from Maine who had spent one winter too many among the snowdrifts of that igloo.

They were the Quints, 'named after the Dionnes,' they told guests who had never heard of the famous Canadian sisters, and in one way they were ill-prepared for the high nonsense that preempted their motel, for they were dour Yankees; but in another, they were a good choice, because in Maine they had spent their long winters studying wildlife and had learned that 'animals, four-footed or two-, are capable of damned near anything.'

The Bali Hai had three considerable assets: a white beach from which the husbands could plunge into the high waves of the Atlantic, a blue-tiled swimming pool shaded by palm trees in which the wives could disport, and a large dark bar in which both could celebrate. The walls of the Dagger Bar were tastefully decorated with daggers, swords, knives, sabers, cutlasses, krisses, poniards, stilettos, rapiers, machetes and dirks, most of them con- tributed by well-traveled patrons who had brought them home from foreign ports. The effect was quite stunning, a congenial bar with inviting tables surrounded by weaponry which recalled the violence of the world and reminded the drinkers of the violence which had sometimes threatened their lives.

About the room evocative objects hauled in from the Bahamas were placed: large clamshells, fishing nets, green-glass floats used by fishermen, and two gigantic stuffed swordfish. The Dagger Bar featured rum drinks with exotic names like Missionary's Downfall or Virgin's Last Stand and an excellent fish dinner for a flat three dollars including one free beer.

Each new group of astronauts was advised by those who had gone before: 'The scene is at the Dagger Bar. You'll love the Quints, gloomiest people since Cotton Mather. But those fresh oysters, all you can eat for fifty cents!' Tucker Thompson, anticipating that his crowd would want to lodge at the Bali Hai, checked the place out and satisfied himself that the rooms were clean and the drinks honest, but then he discovered something that sent icicles right up his spine: the Bali Hai was sometimes overrun by hordes of groupies who wanted to be where the action was, and since many of them were delectable and still in their teens, he could foresee disaster.

The Cocoa Beach groupies following space were identical with the girls of Europe who idolized bullfighters, those of South America who traipsed after race-car drivers, or those of Canada who chased hockey players. All societies appeared to produce a plethora of young girls eager for excitement and willing to break away from stable homes in order to seek it. And around the world they behaved the same: frequent the scene of action, haunt the popular bars, and jump into the right bed with practiced alacrity.

Rachel Mott, observing the phenomenon for the first time, was appalled by the undisciplined behavior of her sex; it was really quite shameless the way the girls threw themselves at the men, but when Tucker Thompson asked about it one night in the Dagger Bar while five or six toothsome girls, all under the age of twenty, were clustering around Randy Claggett, she admitted grudgingly, 'I've been quite shocked by these children. Where are their parents? But upon reflection, I've had to conclude that girls just like these probably haunted the camps where the gladiators trained, and on the day when the little men descend from another planet, a supply of our girls will be there to greet them.'

'Well, they've got to lay off my astronauts,' Thompson said, 'or we're going to look like fools.' And he showed the Motts his magazine's next week's issue, in which his long-range program for the Special Group was revealed. It displayed on the cover, in the neatest possible array, the new astronauts, each man looking right into the camera with chin set, eyes ablaze and hair cut short, Marine style. THE SOLID SIX cried the headline, and Thompson sat back highly pleased with his work.

'In our business,' he said, 'the battle's half won if you can label your product with a snappy title. The Brown Bomber made Joe Louis twice the man he would have been otherwise. The Lone Eagle—nobody ever did better than that. It made the public see Lindbergh, who was not an easy man to sell, as both aloof and particularized, almost human, you could say. I like that one they've started using for Brooks Robinson—the Glove. That's classy. And I liked the Velvet Fog, the name they gave Mel Tormé when they discovered he couldn't reach the hard notes. Saved his career. But the best they ever did was for that likable London heavyweight who came over here, to disastrous results. Phil Scott, his name was, and when he was knocked flat three times by punkos even before the big fight and all seemed lost, some clown gave him the name Phainting Phil, the Swooning Swan of Soho, and thousands paid to see him.'

'The Solid Six,' Mott repeated. 'It has a good sound, and they certainly look solid.'

'What we thought . . . and you understand, the final choice wasn't mine. The whole board wrestled with this one. Our thinking was that *Life* had pretty well preempted the field of glamour with their crews. Glenn, Borman, Shepard. That's a pretty classy group. Did you know that some people are now calling the original astronauts the Sacred Seven? Well, we couldn't replay that record, but we could identify our men with something patriotic and lasting.' He stopped to make an entirely different point: 'The lasting part is important. Because our boys are going to be on the scene for a long, long time. The Sacred Seven are dropping away like flies . . . private business . . . all that. It will be our boys who make the great Gemini flights, the ones who'll later fly the Apollos to the Moon.'

He drummed on the table, then looked past Rachel Mott to where the teenage groupies were still making a fuss over Claggett. 'We blow the solid bit if any one of our boys explodes in scandal. The newspapers are already fussing about the fact that we have an exclusive, and if they could blast us out of the sky with a juicy scandal, they'd descend on us like hungry wolves.' He stopped, looked at Mott and asked, 'Did I mix my metaphors?'

'You did,' Rachel said.

'Forgive it. Point is, Mott, I want you to talk with your boys.'

'Problem's not mine.'

'You bet your sweet ass it is,' Thompson said sharply. 'Excuse me, ma'am, but this is important. Mrs. Mott, here, is doing a great job with the girls. You keep the boys in line.'

He was so insistent and so irritated with Mott for not assessing the danger seriously, that he got in touch with his superiors at *Folks* and they called Senator Grant, who seemed to be the Senate spokesman for the space exercises, and he telephoned Cocoa Beach immediately: 'Mott, Tucker Thompson is dead right. It would be disastrous if scandal touched this program. You get those men straightened out. Pass the word.'

'Senator, I can't—'

His protest was not allowed. 'Those lads are your responsibility, Mott. Pass the word!'

Mott waited till all the men were at Canaveral, for he did not want to discharge this messy task piecemeal, and the delay proved almost fatal, for a persistent teenager from Columbus, Missouri, the daughter of a professor no less, forced her way into Randy Claggett's bedroom while he was working in one of the simulators at the Cape and was waiting for him, undressed, in bed when he returned to the Bali Hai.

Randy did not feel obligated to force the girl from his bed, or even to make her put her clothes back on, but when he told her at half past nine that he really must go down for some supper and that she could not walk down with him, she understood and used a fire escape. Tucker Thompson watched the way they came straggling in from two different directions, painstakingly unassociated, then met casually as if for the first time and sat together for a huge plate of oysters and two bowls of chili, and he was positive that his carefully orchestrated plan for his six astronauts was on the verge of destruction. Looking hastily about the darkened room to see if any newsmen had witnessed the sexual charade, he was relieved to find that all of them were absent, attending a briefing at the Cape regarding the impending second Gemini shot in which the popular Edward White was going to walk in space. But even as he took a deep breath he saw at a corner table a compelling young Japanese woman, not yet thirty, small, exquisitely framed, with becoming bangs, high cheekbones and just a hint of Asia in her eyes. Her complexion was that delicate coloring which appears on the finest celadon vases of the Orient, smooth and placid, and she seemed the kind of woman with whom any responsive man would want to discuss his troubles. Also, she wore that special combination of informal clothing which invited men to approach her table when she sat alone: a pleated blouse in handsome tan colors that matched her skin, a casual sweater thrown carelessly about her shoulders, a very wide belt emphasizing the smallness of her waist, a free-swinging skirt and Italian-style loafers with broad, blunt toes.

As soon as Tucker saw her, warning bells started ringing: That one is no groupie. She's for real. But what truly terrified him was the fact that from her corner, under the Malayan daggers which framed her lovely square face with its sensuous drooping mouth, she was watching with professional cynicism everything Randy Claggett and his teenage supper companion were doing and was occasionally writing in a notebook.

'Who's that?' Thompson asked.

'The woman in the corner?' Mrs. Mott asked. 'She's an accredited reporter from Japan. Well regarded in the profession. Did a stint with the *New York Times.* Got an M.A. with top grades from Radcliffe. Now writes for the *Asahi Shimbun,* biggest paper in the world, and is syndicated in Europe.'

'What's a Japanese doing at Cape Canaveral? Spying?'

'She writes beautifully about space. Has a real feeling for it. Has a pilot's license, I believe, and she did a lot of glider soaring in New Hampshire when she was at Radcliffe.'

'What's her name? She's not on my list.'

'Yes she is,' Rachel said with some embarrassment. 'She's the one we thought was a Japanese man. Rhee Soon-Ka. Rhee's the last name. When I went to meet Mr. Rhee—*voilà!*' And she pointed to the lovely young woman taking notes under the Malayan daggers.

'A Japanese!' Thompson growled. 'Emperor Hirohito would do anything to get even.'

'Tucker, take it easy!'

He could not. He had lost too many battles with the press not to recognize an enemy when he saw one, and knew intuitively that he would find himself, during the next decade, doing continuous battle with Madame Fu Manchu. 'You say she worked for the *New York Times?*'

'An exchange job, I believe.'

'The evil tricks she didn't learn in Japan, I'm sure she picked up in New York.' A flash of genius struck him: 'Do you think I could go over and strangle her right now?'

'Tucker! She's a woman doing a job. She doesn't weigh more than a hundred pounds.'

'A cobra doesn't weigh six.' He studied the intruder for several minutes, then rose abruptly and walked to her table. 'I'm Tucker Thompson, *Folks.*'

'I know,' she said in a lilting voice. 'Sit down. You're the one who keeps the six little Boy Scouts locked up.'

'It's our job to write about them.'

'You don't seem to have that one behind bars,' she said, pointing to Claggett.

'His niece, from Kansas.'

'Popes used to have nieces. Astronauts have pickups.'

'You write one word . . .'

'I intend to write about sixty thousand words.'

'You be careful . . .'

'It's your job, Mr. Thompson, to provide the American public with fairy tales. It's mine to provide the rest of the world with adult interpretations.'

'You be very careful . . .'

'I don't have to be. I'm not trying to sell anything. Tonight I'm taking notes on a most attractive young man, a most lecherous one.'

'Now, Miss . . .' He hesitated. 'What's your name?'

'Born Rhee Soon-Ka. In America, I use Cynthia Rhee.'

'As a Japanese alien, you could find yourself in a lot of trouble, Miss Rhee.'

'I'm Korean.'

'Just as bad. I have the power to cause you a lot of trouble.'

'Have you chanced to read my series on the Kremlin? I'm always in trouble. You get fine stories when you place yourself in harm's way, as your Admiral John Paul Jones so handsomely phrased it.' She spoke a beautiful, halting English, so carefully pronounced that it stung and infuriated, and she was not even trivially disturbed by Tucker Thompson's bluster.

'I wish you a lot of luck with your story, Miss Rhee,' he said as he rose to depart.

'And you will do everything possible to prevent me from getting it.'

'With my six astronauts, I will.'

'And they happen to be the very six about whom I am writing.' And without referring to her notes, she recited the names in order: 'Randy Claggett of Texas, wife Debby Dee. Hickory Lee of Tennessee and his wife Sandy. Timothy Bell of Arkansas and his wife Cluny. Harry Jensen of South Carolina and his pretty wife Inger. Ed Cater of Mississippi and his wife Gloria. And perhaps the most interesting of all, John Pope of Fremont and his ambitious wife Penny. You'll be reading about them, Mr. Tucker.'

When Thompson returned to his table he received the harshest shock of all, delivered by Rachel Mott: 'She's supposed to have said in the bar that in order to complete her research, she intended to sleep with every one of our six.' She paused a moment, then added, 'The Solid Six, as you describe them.'

The urgent meeting was held in Thompson's room at the Bali Hai, and although he had originally intended for Stanley Mott to carry the ball, he could not refrain from getting immediately to the heart of the crisis. 'Men, it's very simple. If you besmirch the name of *astronaut* with cheap sexual adventures, you endanger a program of vital importance to the nation and to the world.' The listeners could see that he was sweating, and as they wondered what he would say next, he added, 'Rumors are circulating. I myself have seen things that would have looked damned suspicious to a knowing reporter.'

He really did not know how to proceed past that point, so he shifted gears completely. 'You stand to lose a great deal of money, all of you, if this thing blows up.' And as soon as he uttered these words, he knew he had blown it. What lusty young man would quarantine himself from some of the most nubile young women in the world simply because a monetary contract was in danger?

Mott took over. 'Senator Grant just telephoned me. He's responsible for the funds you fellows spend in your T-38s. He's got to wangle through Congress the billion-odd dollars for your Gemini program.' He stopped and laughed at himself. 'How in hell do you say that word? I hear it four ways. Hard *G*. Soft *J*. Dictionary says it ends *-eye*. NASA uses *-ee*.'

Ed Cater said, 'Our radio station has an astrology program and they give it the hard *G* and the *-eye*.'

'I would despise taking my intellectual leadership from an astrology program. Forgive me if I call it Jem-in-ee.'

With the tension broken, Thompson adopted a different tone. 'Men, the Senate leaders, the NASA leadership, all of us want to see this program move forward in an orderly way. You know you're already being ticketed for future flights, ones of profound significance. Don't blow it by allowing some silly—'

He was interrupted by a hard, flat, unemotional voice; it belonged to John Pope. 'If you're talking about sex, say so.'

'That's exactly what we're talking about,' Thompson snapped. 'If you men allow yourselves to get mixed up with those groupies . . .'

Pope was inflexible. 'It's highly improper for you to come here and lecture us on such a subject. We're not Boy Scouts.'

'The public thinks you are.'

'Maybe that's because of what your magazine writes, Mr. Thompson.'

'We write what America needs to hear.'

'We're test pilots. Each of us had to decide long ago how we'd behave.

So far we've done a pretty good job, and frankly, we do not seek high-school counseling now.'

The words were so unexpected, and from a source so surprising, that Mott made no effort to respond; these were not the statements of some young astronaut, but rather the end-of-life reflections of a Socrates or a Voltaire. But Tucker Thompson was not silenced, because he was custodian of property rights which must be protected. 'Don't take this too lightly. There's a newswoman in these parts who's announced publicly that she's going to sleep with every one of you, then write a book about your performances.'

Some of the men gasped, but the effect Thompson sought was dissipated when the husky voice of Randy Claggett whispered, 'Get that girl's full name and address.'

When the NASA high command learned through its grapevine of the threat posed by Cynthia Rhee, they gave Tucker Thompson a clear directive: 'Get that Korean reporter straightened out,' but Tucker, remembering his first encounter with her, knew that he was not the man for that job. Calling Mrs. Mott to his room at the Bali Hai, he said, 'Ride herd on our Miss Kimchi.'

'Who's that?'

Impatiently Thompson explained: 'Kimchi is the smellingest coleslaw in the world, and the bitingest. It's Korean, loaded with garlic. And that Rhee dame is twice as obnoxious. You're to tell her what's what. She's to lay off our astronauts.'

Rachel laughed. 'What an unfortunate use of words, Tucker. Lay off.'

'It's your paycheck if she gets out of line.'

So Rachel went to the Dagger Bar, where Miss Rhee was sitting alone at her customary table in the rear. Walking up to her, Rachel said, 'May I join you?'

'Has Mr. Thompson ordered you to check on me?' the Korean woman asked with transparent insolence.

'He did just that,' Rachel snapped, grabbing at a chair and pulling herself up to the table. 'I've been informed that men at the bar heard you boast that you were going to sleep with each of our astronauts. What a vile thing to have said.'

To her surprise, the Korean woman lost all belligerence. Like an autumn sunrise a warm smile spread over her beautiful face and she placed her small, well-tended hands over Rachel's. 'Surely you must know that men always spread such rumors when they feel challenged by women who are brighter than they are.'

'Do you challenge them?'

'I certainly do. Men like your Mr. Thompson have been getting away with murder . . . the bullshit they write about the astronauts.'

'Do you have to use such words?'

'That word is the only one which describes what the men writers around here have been throwing into the wind.'

'And you intend to correct that?'

'I surely do.' She leaned back against the wall to study Mrs. Mott. 'You know, of course, that I'm extremely pleased to have you here at my table. I've been wondering how I might meet you.'

'Why?'

'You're just as much a part of my story as Randy Claggett.'

'I'm surprised,' Rachel said.

'Don't be. Your husband is a prime part of NASA, and to understand him, I must understand you.'

'And to keep you from wrecking things,' Rachel said, 'I must understand what motivates you.'

'I'm relatively simple. Fiercely oriented. Self-controlled. But never complex.'

'Tell me,' Rachel said, and the sincerity in her voice encouraged the Asian woman to confide:

'Because I was born at the right time, in 1936, I profited from the groundwork done by the great women journalists who preceded me. Simone de Beauvoir, Dorothy Thompson, and especially the three younger Americans of the postwar period. I have no illusions that I'm as good as they were, but I am their inheritor and I intend to send my profession forward, as they did.'

When Rachel said, 'Tell me about the three Americans,' Cynthia replied, 'A woman like you ought to know about them,' and Rachel said, 'There's a great deal I don't know.'

'The significant fact is, they're all dead. Each one killed herself at the extremes of her profession, and I suppose I'll do the same. Maggie Higgins worked herself to death in Korea. Dickie Chapelle proved herself braver than most men, parachuting behind enemy lines, submarining in dangerous waters, leading a patrol of Marines with flame-throwers, and finally blowing herself to fragments on a land mine in Vietnam. Nell Nevler, as you know, plunged to a shattering death when the Russian transport in which she and her Russian colonel were escaping plunged into the Kiev airport.

'They were brave women, brilliant women, who established new freedoms, who redefined how women could be employed. That they performed well in the 1950s enabled me to try my hand in the 1970s, and I assure you that I do not intend to be a lesser woman than they were.'

When Rachel probed as to what her intentions were with the Solid Six, Cynthia laughed. 'Who knows? When NASA launches a satellite, who can certify where it will head? Many have gone their own ways, to the consternation of your bright boys in Houston. Same thing happens when you launch a person with ideas at a target with emotional content. Who can anticipate?'

The two women reflected on this for some time, then Cynthia added what was perhaps the most relevant in all that she had revealed:

'In comparison with the women I've mentioned, I consider myself rather limited, but I do have one thing none of them did. I'm driven by a compulsive force you would not believe. You see, I'm a Korean brought up in Japan, where Koreans are treated like dirt. And that's a furnace which forges a special kind of steel—flexible . . . keen . . . indestructible. I'm like a sword of the Japanese samurai, whom I detest but also admire. Their swords cut to the quick of things, and I do the same.'

When Rachel looked up she saw Tucker Thompson approaching the table. 'And how are you two girls getting along?' And Rachel thought: What an unequal battle this is going to be! The Korean karate champ versus the Madison Avenue hack, but later, when she had watched how adroitly Tucker protected himself in the dirty infighting, she concluded that perhaps the duel would not be as uneven as she had thought.

John Pope's blunt defense of the right of his fellow astronauts to behave without supervision by NASA and *Folks* had several repercussions. The five other astronauts, knowing him to be a rather stuffy straight arrow who never dallied with the groupies, were impressed by his willingness to defend them on a matter of principle, and they appreciated this. They had already elevated Randy Claggett to the position of master pilot, and now they conferred on Pope the unannounced title of political leader. This gave him no added perquisites, only additional responsibilities, but when difficult problems arose, or confrontations with the high command, they expected him to make the first statements and then to defend them. It was not a position he sought, nor one that gained him ease; observed behavior among one's peers accounted for it, and a herd of cattle in a meadow or a flight of geese at sunset will make the same kind of election for the same kind of reason.

It was perplexing that the men accorded Pope this honor, for they did not especially like him; he was too rigid, too much an overage Cub Scout, far too much a loner. He did not drink or smoke; he quarantined himself from the groupies; and while the other astronauts lounged in the Dagger Bar, he was apt to be on the beach, running six or seven miles to keep the fat down. This separation of Pope from the rest did not mean that the latter conformed to the pattern of Randy Claggett, with his wild and sometimes crazy Texas ways. The normative astronaut was Hickory Lee: quiet, fearfully efficient, solid drinker off duty, quick to anger if his rights were trespassed, and average in almost every other human reaction. Pope and Claggett stood at the extremes; Hickory commanded the middle.

For two reasons the NASA brass were not happy with Pope's outspoken defiance of Stanley Mott and Tucker Thompson: they had carefully cultivated the myth that the astronauts were almost heavenly creatures—'a cross between Jesus Christ, Ulysses and Joe DiMaggio,' one writer had said —and they had profited enormously from it; they must preserve this myth unsullied; and they had entered into a contract with *Folks* whereby it and Thompson enjoyed special privileges, and to have him rebuffed so harshly was distasteful. So for some weeks, until it became clear that the Twins were not going to continue any rebellion which might endanger the great project of ultimately placing a man on the Moon, Pope and Claggett were looked upon with suspicion.

The astronauts maintained a careful balance between rigorous attention to detail and rowdy relaxation, and one afternoon, following an informal meeting with the press, five of them huddled around a corner table in the Dagger Bar, conducting a noisy debate concerning where, during a journey to the Moon, Earth's gravity ceased to exercise dominance and Moon's took over. Preposterous guesses circulated, after which Hickory Lee banged his beer glass and cried, 'Pope, you studied astronomy. Where is the break-even point?'

John did not know, but across the room he spotted Stanley Mott and invited him over to settle the debate, and after the answer was given— 220,000 miles from Earth, 19,000 miles from the Moon—Mott lingered to check on how his young men were doing, and he was pleased. But as he talked with the five he noticed that they were looking over his shoulder at someone who had just entered.

It was Tim Bell, the civilian, fresh from the barber, who had given him an especially sharp haircut. It made Bell, always studiously neat, seem even more handsome than usual, a fact which the young man was approving as he looked at himself in the mirror. Mott was perplexed when Claggett whispered, 'Let's give him the haircut routine.'

The five young men rose and walked casually across the room toward where Bell was admiring himself, and as Mott watched them go he felt pride in being associated with them. Slim of hip, broad of shoulder and slightly underweight, they created a trim appearance, and because of the press meeting, each was still dressed in a dark suit and crisp white shirt, with a sober tie knotted in a severe V that nestled neatly within the collar. What differentiated them were their shoes, each having chosen a style which best reflected his way of life. Claggett wore Texas boots, tall and limber. Harry Jensen had chosen French-style pumps with extremely thin soles. Pope, of course, preferred the 1920 wingtip decorated with little holes punched in the leather to make artistic patterns. And each of the others had his own unique wear, always highly polished.

What made them appear the same, like five clones of the one ideal astronaut, were their watches, each man wearing on his left wrist a chronograph, immensely big, heavy and expensive. It told local time, Greenwich Mean Time on the twenty-four-hour system, the day of the week, the month, the phase of the Moon, and served also as a stopwatch, lap timer and alarm clock. Hickory Lee said of his, 'I had more trouble learning how to work this monster than I did with advanced calculus at MIT.'

For one brief moment, as they passed from the shadowy darkness of the barroom into an aureole of sunlight coming through a western window, they looked as if nature itself were applauding their excellence, and Mott wondered if anywhere else in America there was assembled a more attractive group. But when he looked again they had passed on, and surrounded Bell as if they intended to beat him up.

'Bell!' Claggett said with a rush of emotion. 'We've decided to stand with you, no matter what.'

Ed Cater took him by the arm and said confidentially, 'At first we thought you might be a jerk, but you've shown us you can fly with the best. I'm going to back you all the way.'

Jensen said brightly, 'Call on me, Tim, whenever you need help. As for right now, you say the word and we'll move out.'

'What's this all about?' Bell asked nervously.

'That haircut,' Claggett said. 'We're ready right now to go in town and beat hell out of the man who gave you that haircut.'

Bell smiled weakly, suspecting correctly that the horseplay had something to do with his not belonging to the military.

Mott, watching the nonsense, experienced an intense desire to see his own son, who had elected a course so different from that chosen by these young gods, and that night he confessed to his wife: 'I've been doing a great deal of thinking, Rachel. About Millard and us. And the fact that we'd allowed his life style to drive a wedge between us.' His voice quavered and tears threatened.

'What is it, dear?'

'Working with these young men, day after day . . . It's made me hungry to see our boy. I don't give a damn how he's living or what other people think. He's our son, and I see now that we're obligated to stay with him, hell or high water.'

Rachel bowed her head to hide her own tears, then muttered, 'You may be right. What do you intend doing?'

'I've asked headquarters for permission, next time I'm in California. Three-day leave to visit with Millard.'

'To what purpose?'

'No purpose. No purpose in God's world. I just want to see him and let him know we love him.'

Stifled sobs prevented Rachel from speaking, but after a long interval during which she blew her nose twice, she laughed nervously, then said softly, 'It's strange, you know, speaking about how your work with the six men has affected you. I see their wives day after day, and I suppose I know everything that's wrong with every one of them. But do you know what? I'd be overjoyed to have any one of them as a daughter-in-law. I wish to God that Millard would marry someone like them.'

'Apparently that's not going to be, and frankly, I no longer give a damn. As Pope said the other morning, "We do not seek counsel from you." Millard's made a life decision and now we're the ones who have to adjust.'

'Even though we despise the decision?'

'Yes. We must keep in contact with our son. No matter what he does.'

During the next visit of the astronauts to check on progress at Allied Aviation, Mott slipped away, rented a car and drove to Malibu Beach, where with the help of a girl in a bikini he found the cottage occupied by Millard and a young man from Indiana named Roger. Millard, taller than his father, no glasses, very slim, very tanned, appeared to be in excellent health. He wore his hair much longer than did the astronauts and apparently he owned no socks, for during their entire visit together his father never saw him in any.

The son, supposing that his father had come to lecture him, was decidedly cool at first, while Roger was openly defensive, but as the afternoon passed with no lectures, the atmosphere eased, and by the time Stanley invited the young men to have dinner with him, they were almost eager to accept because they wanted to hear what had brought him to their cottage. At first the talk centered on the astronauts.

'Are they really as . . .' Young Mott did not know how to finish his question without insulting his father, and there was an awkward pause.

'As square as they seem?' Stanley suggested, and when the young men laughed, he raised three fingers and said, 'Eagle Scouts, word of honor. Millard, you would not believe how square these fellows are.'

'To what purpose?'

'Every time they go aloft they lay their lives on the line. One slip and they're dead. They need discipline.'

'They've had no accidents yet. Aren't you overplaying it?'

'The accidents will come. But they'll forge ahead. And one of these days they'll stand on the Moon.'

'As I said, to what purpose?'

Stanley Mott spoke very carefully. 'Because that's the job they've given themselves. That's their scene, as you say.' When neither of the young men spoke, he added, trying to sound casual, 'The way you men have worked out your own scene.'

Silence. So he added, offhandedly, 'I respect the astronauts' choice. I respect yours.' And before either young man could respond, he launched hurriedly into a recitation of what the astronauts had to know before they could participate in a space flight: 'Math, vector analysis, orbital mechanics, computers, rocket engines, the characteristics of three hypergolic fuels, digital systems, radio, television and another ten or eleven really tough fields.'

'You make them sound like geniuses,' Roger said. He had been unable to master algebra.

'Let me tell you a funny thing, Roger. What I've just recited are the basic fields. When they get through them, then they begin the hard work. Tracing out the particular systems of their particular spacecraft. The manuals, eight and a half by eleven, typewriter size, stand this high.' And with his hands he indicated a pile nearly two feet high, waiting for his listeners to absorb that staggering fact.

'The other day I saw two of the men running to a class, and they were on a slanting surface so that their heads were tilted to the left, and I had this crazy feeling: They better stop that or the knowledge will spill out their ear. They must have, right now, as much information in their heads as the human brain can accommodate. They must be among the brightest men on Earth.' He paused, then concluded: 'Maybe only squares would be solid enough to absorb so much without going nuts. Maybe they have to be square.'

The young men nodded, and Roger smoothed the expensive cashmere sweater he was wearing. 'Another round?' Mott asked, but no one wanted any further drinks, so the waitress brought the food, a delicious seafood salad with Italian garlic bread and iced tea.

As they ate, Millard said cautiously, 'Back there you said something about life styles.'

'Yes. I said I respected life styles.'

'I have a job, you know.'

'I didn't know.' He took off his glasses, wiped his tired eyes, and said, 'I'm delighted, Millard. What's it deal with?'

'Now that's odd,' Millard replied. 'You ask "What's it deal with?" as if the job itself was more important than the man doing the job.'

'Habit of speech, I guess.'

But Millard would not let his father off the hook so easily. 'If I told you that I had a job which sounded important. Computers. Plastic forms. Damned near anything mechanical. You'd be proud, and you could say offhandedly at the country club, "My boy Millard's into computers." Well, your boy Millard's into nurses' helper in a children's hospital. And so is Roger.'

'Damned good public service,' Mott said.

'We think so,' his son said defiantly.

'In the normal swing of events, what will it . . .'

'Lead to? Nothing, so far as I can see. It's a way of life for the present, and where anything leads to I haven't a clue.'

'Go with the flow?' Mott asked.

'Yes.'

This required no further comment, so after a while Mott said brightly, as if opening a completely new subject, 'Your mother and I are eager to maintain contact, Millard. If your work ever brings you back East . . . or vacations . . . you must stay with us. You, too, Roger.'

'You won't shoot me?' Roger asked.

'Why would you say that?'

'Because if I went home to Indiana, my father would shoot me. Especially if I took your son with me.'

'Four months ago I'd have shot you. But now . . .'

'What happened?' Roger asked, boring in.

'My work with the new astronauts. I'm sort of their den mother. They've moved me deeply. Made me see that six men could be six radically different human beings, although as you implied a while back, they seem at first like paper cutouts. So different.'

'And?'

'I saw human capacities, human variations if you will—I saw the whole ball game in a different light. And I felt driven to tell you so, Millard.'

'This is a very good salad,' his son said.

'Would you like to hear what my father said in those circumstances?' Roger asked.

'I would.'

'He's a minor official at the raceway. Very gung ho. When he heard how I was living he blew a gasket. Said if I ever let anyone at the raceway know what I was doing, he'd kill me. So I laughed and asked him, "Who do you think were the first two men I slept with?" And he damn near fainted when I told him, giving names, "Two of your best drivers." He screamed, "I'll kill them," but they were important figures at the raceway, so he didn't kill them. Father is very strong on killing people. His father was a leading figure in the days when the Klan ran the state.'

'What do young men like you . . .' Mott was embarrassed at having used such a cliché phrase, but he could think of no circumlocution. 'How do you envisage the future?'

'We don't,' Roger said.

'But Millard's mother and I—we look forward to gainful occupation till I'm sixty-five. Then forced retirement . . . then a reduced standard of living. Grandchildren to occupy us. One of us dies . . . we all die. An orderly progression, you might say.'

'A statistical one,' Roger said.

'Statistics surely govern your situation, too.'

The young men did not care to discuss the probabilities which dictated their lives, but throughout the remainder of this first evening they talked freely of their jobs at the hospital and of the kinds of work beachboys were able to get. Roger said, 'The post office employs a lot. If you can pass Civil Service.'

Stanley Mott spent two fascinating days with his son, discussing things he would never have imagined possible. As a straight arrow he could not approve of any deviation from the norm; indeed, a straight arrow was a man who defined the norm. But as a human being whose parameters of vision and understanding were being expanded by the expanding age in which he played a central role, he could appreciate the tangled drives, so unlike his own, which motivated these two young men.

'Do you find any satisfaction in what you do?' Roger asked on the last evening.

'Each day is a new beginning, an overwhelming challenge.'

'Like what?'

'You know, I didn't take my doctorate—an entirely new field—till I was forty-four. Celestial mechanics. That wakes a man up.'

'So what are you doing with it now?'

'NASA assigns me to one committee after another. Where I can apply what I've learned.'

'Like what?' Roger persisted.

'Would you really want to hear? I mean, listen for about an hour?'

'Test me.'

So Mott took a large sheet of paper, and with the exquisite line and lettering he had mastered at Georgia Tech in Drafting II, drew a schematic of the solar system, naming the Sun at the left hand and the Earth fairly close in, but not naming what he called 'the nine other wanderers.'

'Can you tell me how to name them?' he asked, and neither of his listeners could. So starting close to the Sun he printed the names: Mercury, Venus, Earth, Mars, Jupiter, Saturn, Uranus, Neptune, Pluto.

'That's only nine planets,' Roger said. 'You just said there were nine besides Earth.'

'I think of the collection of asteroids as a planet,' Mott said. 'One that broke into fragments, from one cause or another. They hide between Mars and Jupiter.'

When the young men finished studying the diagram, Mott said, 'What I'm engaged in is what we call the "grand tour." There used to be a time when young Englishmen of good family were not considered educated until they completed a grand tour of Paris, Geneva and Rome, with maybe a stopover in barbarian Germany. Long after the Moon shot is history, we propose to launch a single space vehicle which will take off from Florida, and move purposefully past all the other planets. Its course could be something like this.'

And with the most careful strokes of his pen, making never a mistake or a strikeover, he sketched a majestic itinerary, twisting and winding among the planets, sometimes turning in unexpected ways and leaping off into unexpected directions. When he finished his diagram he said, simply, 'If we're able to start this tour in 1970, we'll end it with our craft heading past Pluto and out to the remote stars of our Galaxy sometime about 1997. It'll wander among those near stars for about four million years, then leave for the remote galaxies, and after about two thousand billion years, it may get somewhere important.'

'You speak of it as if it was immortal.'

'It will be. No atmosphere to disturb it. No moisture to rust it. No burning fuel to clog the pipes. Only the perpetual journey.'

'How will you know it's still on its journey?'

Mott pointed to the single light that illuminated the cottage and said, 'It will carry a device which generates electricity from radioactivity. This will activate a radio that will send us messages . . . one-tenth of the power of that little bulb. But it will penetrate the billion miles separating us from Saturn as if that planet were next door. It'll require ninety minutes for us to receive the message, of course, and when the grand tour reaches Pluto, nearly five billion miles away, it'll take nearly four hours . . . electrical impulses coming to us at the speed of light, and when the craft reaches the edge of our Galaxy its messages will require thousands of years to reach us, but the messages will come.'

The young men contemplated this for a while, then Millard asked, 'But how does the spacecraft get its power to keep moving outward?'

'We start it with a good boost at Cape Canaveral. And we head it with great precision, so that every time it encounters a planet, it does so in a way to pick up energy from the rotation of that planet about the Sun—sort of like the last child at the end of a crack-the-whip—and this throws the craft sharply onward to the next planet in line.'

'You can schedule it so exactly?' Roger asked.

'Almost to the second,' Mott said. 'Almost to the mile.'

'And that's what you're doing . . . when you're not baby-sitting?'

'Yes.' And on a separate sheet of paper he drew a beautiful depiction of the planet Saturn, with its rings handsomely inclined and its ten known moons depicted, and what he now told the men paved the way for them to tell him things that concerned themselves. 'My task, and I'm low man on the totem pole working on this, is to bring our craft toward Saturn on this kind of heading on a specified day in, say, August 1981, when the exact location of Saturn and its moons has been determined.'

'You like to use the word *exact*, don't you?'

'If data can be known, they should be used.'

'And you know where Saturn will be?'

'Kepler and Newton taught us how to know.'

'And from a distance of a billion miles you're going to pilot your tiny craft so that it threads its way past the moons and the rings.'

'That's exactly what we're going to do.'

'How?'

'Newton once said that if he could see great distances, which he could, it was only because he stood on the shoulders of giants—the brilliant men like Kepler who went before him. We can solve the mechanical riddles of the Sun's system because some damned good mathematicians completed the basic work before us. We will lead that spacecraft here and here and here and here, and we will make not one damned mistake.'

He spoke with such fury, such iron-hard determination, that his listeners dared not make snide attacks on his beliefs, and after they had sat for some time in the near-darkness, Mott said, 'The grand tour requires an infinity of calculations—where every planet and every moon will be down to the minute and the second. Then we must work backward to a specific two-week period, and within each twenty-four hours we will have a launch window of exactly—there's that word again—four minutes and nine seconds. We're going to penetrate the remotest corners of the universe, and we have four minutes and nine seconds to do it in.'

No comment, and then he said, 'The point is, for Johannes Kepler to calculate the orbit of one planet required mathematical equations and solutions covering papers this high—ten years of solid work. With a good computer we do it in about seven seconds. What I'm doing has nothing to do with the Moon or Saturn. I'm building for the clowns who'll be trying things in the next century. And there will never be an end.'

He had no more to say, nor did the young men. The three of them sat there, looking at the incredible diagrams, listening to the noisy surf, and after a long while Roger said, 'At dinner last night you told us that you and your wife lived in a situation governed by statistics. The mortality tables say you'll live to age seventy-nine, then kaput. I refused to admit that Millard and I also fall into the middle of statistical predictions. We do.'

It was approaching midnight, and now Roger wanted to talk. 'At nineteen you're a young god. You can handle any breaking wave. Girls stop to look as you pass, and men too. Those are the golden years. Christ, you can do anything, write any rules. The good years are these, twenty to thirty-five. So many opportunities in so many fields, you get dizzy. Beach houses everywhere. Girls with convertibles. Men with high salaries. California sunshine. You cannot imagine how good these years can be. And no responsibility—except to pray that the nuclear bomb doesn't swoop down to wipe it all away before you've finished with your fun.

'From what I've watched, the numbers begin to tell at about forty, and at fifty you're a real statistic. I'll probably continue lucky and find someone to share a house with, and our salaries, too. Or maybe I'll escort women without husbands, women who can help me pay my bills. I'll have a steady job, I suppose, but I don't look forward to that, and if I'm still as strongly sexed as I am now, I'll have trouble finding partners, because I know I'll never be rich. I'm not built that way. But I'll get along. And at sixty, just like you, the numbers will overwhelm me, and God knows what I'll do. But I'll survive. And if I'm lucky enough to have found an excellent person like your son, we'll live where it's warm and collect social security. Then our problem becomes identical with yours, Dr. Mott. Find a place to live, enough to eat on, and an orderly burial when we die.'

To Stanley Mott's surprise, his son now said with quiet vigor, almost accusingly, 'Dad, you watch what happens to your godlike astronauts. I've seen a lot of retired Army and Navy people in this part of California, and I can tell you with certainty what it's going to be. You have six under your wing. Two will be killed young. Two will be divorced and marry girls twenty years younger. One of the others will quit the program, go into business, and become an alcoholic. And the other will do something of minor significance, then sit around and show the neighbors his scrapbooks. Why go through all the hassle today to accomplish so little?'

Mott had an instant response: 'And of the six, three will probably stand on that Moon. And that makes all the difference. Nothing, not time nor wrinkles nor scars nor divorce nor alcoholism, can erase that. They will have been there, and we will not.'

In the morning, when he had to return to General Funkhauser's meetings, he told Millard, 'The door will always be open. Bring Roger. You're a bright son-of-a-bitch, Roger. You won't be satisfied with beach life permanently.'

'Try me,' Roger said.

In the spring of 1964 Norman Grant found himself in good shape and his party in chaos: no Republican in the state of Fremont wished to run against him in the senatorial primary, but he could foresee that nationally his party might be sorely weakened if it split down the middle over the candidacy of Barry Goldwater of Arizona. Grant supported Goldwater and prayed that the stubborn Rockefeller liberals might see the light and halt their divisive actions.

'They can only damage us,' Grant told his long-time assistant, Tim Finnerty, 'and I'm beginning to think they mean to go through with it.'

'I'm more worried about Lyndon Johnson. That Texas cracker is a tough politician. He could win this thing going away, if we nominate Goldwater.'

'We're going to nominate him. Give the people a choice, not an echo.'

'Are you happy with that cliché, Senator?'

'We're going to win with it, if the Rockefeller people don't do us in.'

'Your problem, Senator, is your own election in Fremont. I think we're in trouble.'

'Trouble? We don't even have an opponent in the primary.'

'But we could be vulnerable in November. This could be a big Democrat year.'

Such talk made sense to Grant, for he had learned that a politician or an admiral should approach every battle as if it were the culminating one;

besides, as he said, 'If I've learned anything in the Senate, it's that Lyndon Johnson is a frightening opponent.'

So he began campaigning across Fremont in May and hit every major concentration of voters before the end of June. At the Republican convention he was a fortress of strength for Goldwater and a major irritation to the Rockefeller people, and when William Scranton of Pennsylvania made a belated run, spurred on perhaps by Eisenhower, he was remorseless in rejecting him. He spent much of the summer campaigning for Goldwater in other states, then hurried home to defend himself against a very strong Democratic senator from the Fremont legislature.

After only a few exchanges it became apparent that his early optimism was unfounded; his challenger knew far more about state conditions than he, and during one strategy session with Finnerty and his local aides, the Irishman slammed the cards on the table: 'Senator, if you go on this way, you're going to lose. Goldwater is an albatross around your neck. Stop defending him.'

'Barry Goldwater is my man, a fine decent man who could save this country.'

'Look at Hugh Scott in Pennsylvania. Faces the same race you do. He's smart enough never to mention Goldwater's name. Listening to him, you'd never know there was a presidential race on. Look at this literature. "No matter who else you vote for, pull the lever for Hugh Scott, a great American." Can I print up some of them for you, in the tough districts in Webster?'

'You cannot. Barry Goldwater is my candidate. I sink or swim with Goldwater.'

'I was afraid you'd say that, so I've been restructuring the last eight weeks. Hanley is killing you on local issues, and my polls show that you're barely holding your own. You can't match him where he's strong, so you've got to club him down where you're strong. National leadership. Patriotism. Space. Do you think you can get John Pope to campaign for you?'

'NASA forbids it. Absolutely.'

'That's what I was afraid of. So we bring Penny Pope back here. She's worked for you three times before. Strictly legitimate, and everyone in the state will remember that she's John Pope's wife.'

'Will Glancey permit it? Presidential election and all that?'

'I took the liberty of speaking with Glancey, and he and I both know that Goldwater's going to lose by a landslide, but without saying so, he let me know that he'd be happy having you back in the Senate. Penny's free.'

Penny Pope was proud to work for Norman Grant's reelection, for she had watched him at close quarters for more than a dozen years and had never found him doing a dishonest thing. 'He's straight out of the Ark, an antediluvian, the poor man's Barry Goldwater, but he has a backbone of steel. I love the man and want to see him get six more years.'

Finnerty asked her to appear with the senator in public as often as possible so that he might introduce her as 'that brave daughter of Our Fair State who helps run Washington while her brave husband, a brave son of Our Fair State, heads for the Moon.' No mention was ever made of the fact that the only thing John Pope had flown so far was the Cape Canaveral simulator and a borrowed T-38. But when Grant did finagle orders allowing Pope to land his T-38, with Randy Claggett in the back seat, at the new NASA air base near Clay, Finnerty had photographers present, and after the two astronauts were shown strapped into their seats, Penny was brought forward to hand them flowers.

She was also given the delicate task of explaining to the press why the senator's wife and daughter were not campaigning for him this year: 'Elinor Grant has had severe nervous headaches which quite incapacitate her, and Marcia, as you know, is busy with her work as dean of faculty at the university out West.' When one enterprising newsman flew to California to inspect the university and the nonexistent faculty, his exposé ran in several Eastern newspapers but appeared in no major paper west of the Missouri River and in none at all in Fremont.

'We got home free on that one,' Penny told Finnerty. 'Thanks for having muzzled the jackals.'

'I didn't threaten the press, just reasoned with them.'

To keep the lid on the Elinor Grant story, however, was much more difficult; Penny had to give sworn assurances that the problem was not acute alcoholism, as certain Washington papers had intimated when trying to explain her absences from the capital, but beyond that, Penny was not willing to perjure herself.

Mrs. Grant was drinking, but she was far from being a dipsomaniac; her problem was that the little men from outer space threatened more seriously than ever before to take over control of the country, and when Penny went to reason with her she found the woman as 'spaced out' as if she had been taking drugs. Her first question to Elinor Grant was: 'When did you first correspond with Dr. Strabismus?'

'Maybe ten years ago, maybe more.'

'Let's say it was ten years. That means you've received one hundred and twenty monthly special deliveries, all saying about the same thing. Don't you get suspicious?'

'The danger is very great, Mrs. Pope.'

'And in those ten years you've received not less than forty telegrams telling you that at the last minute the little men have refrained. Doesn't that get monotonous?'

'When they do land, Mrs. Pope, adventuresses like you are going to get their just deserts.' When Penny ignored this, she continued: 'Why do you come out here to flaunt your affair with my husband before the entire state?'

'Please, Mrs. Grant, let's just talk about your husband. He's in the midst of a very difficult campaign. He could lose, you know. And this nation needs him.'

'It does. It does. Norman's a real patriot and the country needs him.'

'So I come begging you to help this good man . . . forget your personal feelings. Your father was a notable servant in this democracy . . .'

'He was indeed, Mrs. Pope. Father was a saint, as big a hero in his way as Norman is in his.'

'I've often heard your husband say that.'

'I would not want to damage Norman's political career. I'm sure Father wouldn't want me to.'

'Then you must meet with the press. They're demanding it. They're beginning to hint at ugly reasons.'

'I couldn't meet the press.' But with unrelenting pressure, applied over more than a week, Penny Pope convinced the frightened woman that she must do so. 'It can be brief, but it can't be silly-silly, Mrs. Grant. You must answer their questions, but I would suggest this. You must not create panic in this nation. Dr. Strabismus takes you into his confidence about the arrival of the little men. But I don't think he would want you to circulate that news generally.'

'You're quite right. He always says that he will alert the world when the proper time comes.'

'He would be most unhappy, I'm sure, if you beat the gun before he gave you permission.'

'I'd never do that,' she promised, so one afternoon in early October she and Penny conducted one of the most carefully orchestrated press conferences of the entire national campaign. Elinor spoke of her husband's heroism, his commitment to honest government, and his considerable contributions to the space program which would soon place an American flag on the Moon.

Only once did she come close to breaking the fragile spell, when she alluded to the grave dangers hanging over America, but when the press bored in to ascertain which dangers, Penny interposed the word *Communism*—and Mrs. Grant gave a little speech on that subject. At a signal from Penny, Senator Grant happened into the room, kissed his wife for Tim Finnerty's cameras, then left for a rally in Webster.

Later that day, when Finnerty sought Penny's advice as to whether they should bring back the other enlisted men to wave the bloody shirt of naval heroism, she was inclined to advise against it. 'You can use a war only so long. This Vietnam thing is beginning to worry people, especially students.'

'Our party used the Civil War from the 1868 election through the 1908. That's forty years, and it gained them victory after victory. Norman Grant was an authentic hero and the theme isn't exhausted by any means.'

Reluctantly she agreed, but when she saw the three veterans in their uniforms she realized that unless the seams were let out, the effect was going to be comical. 'Old, I don't mind. Lends a sense of history. But tight is funny, and people will laugh.' Actually, when she got through with the three men they looked great, and when she sharpened their speeches to give them a more topical relevance, the effect was almost as strong as it had been during that pivotal campaign of 1946, and she told the men, during the last days when it looked as if Grant might win the seat for another six years, 'You've helped a really great man sustain a career that has strengthened this nation.'

She saw that Finnerty of Massachusetts and Penzoss of Alabama were touched by what she said, but that the black high-school principal, Gawain Butler of Detroit, was unmoved, and she was not surprised when the latter said, on the eve of the election, 'If Senator Grant wins, I would like to see him as soon as possible.'

'Why not stay over? There's no man in America he's more beholden to than you, Dr. Butler.'

Two days after the election, when the Republicans of Fremont were trying to decode what had happened to their man Goldwater while celebrating quietly the reelection of their senator, Penny Pope ushered Gawain Butler in to see the victor, and after the big man had adjusted his artificial leg and seated himself comfortably, he said, 'I'm sure you must think this is about a job of some kind, but it isn't. I'm doing very well, thank you, and there's even some talk that I might become a superintendent of schools, either in Michigan or California.'

'Congratulations,' Grant said with real enthusiasm.

'Yes, if you've used me to get elected to the Senate, I've used you to further my career in Detroit. To hear my wife talk, and she does, you'd think you made no move without consulting me.'

'Your wife's right. How many times have I called you?'

'It's not about jobs, and yet it is,' Butler said. 'It's about space.'

'Space? You mean the Moon and that?'

'I do,' Butler said quietly. 'I'd like to show you some pictures,' and from his briefcase, the imitation-leather kind favored by school administrators, he produced four glossy photographs sent him by NASA public relations. The first showed seven handsome masculine faces: Glenn, Slayton, Schirra and the other four from the first selection; Armstrong, Borman, Conrad and the six others from Group II; Aldrin, Cernan, Scott and eleven others from Group III; Claggett, Pope, Jensen and the three others from the Special Group.

'They're our boys,' Grant said.

'Thirty-six fine Americans,' Butler said. 'How much would you estimate it costs you to educate each of your boys, as you call them.'

'We have no figures, but someone gave an off-the-cuff guess of about three million dollars . . . each one.'

As he had practiced in his office in Detroit, Butler pointed casually at the determined face of John Pope: 'This boy's from your hometown, isn't he, Senator?'

'I had nothing to do with his appointment.'

'But he is from your town, and the government is paying three million dollars to educate him.'

'For a very special task.'

'A noble task, I do agree. But don't these photographs seem strange to you?' When Grant shrugged his shoulders, Gawain Butler said sternly, 'Not one black face among them.' The senator was stunned by the forcefulness of this complaint and said nothing, so Butler continued: 'We blacks comprise about twelve percent of the national population. There ought to be about four of our young men in those photographs.'

'We have a very careful process of selection. I'm sure that if . . .'

Butler was not listening. From his briefcase he produced another glossy showing the tense scene in Mission Control when a critical decision had to be made concerning a Gemini flight; it was the kind NASA took pride in circulating, for it indicated the intense concentration of some hundred men in short sleeves, grappling with the life-and-death crisis of a spacecraft two hundred miles aloft, where the blackness was intense and gravity practically null. Most of the men had crewcuts, which they believed made them look young and serious, and no one was smoking, although some were biting on pencils. They looked like the associate professors of some excellent engineering university who had just attained tenure, and they were all white.

'By proportion, Senator, we should have twelve or thirteen black faces in that fine snapshot. We have none.'

'I'm sure—'

'This nation has made space its major effort. Five billion dollars a year, maybe six, I'm told. Publicity, speeches, whole magazines given over to this program, and not a single black man participates. Why do you always cut us off from the best parts of our national life?'

The question came so from the heart, not only of this Detroit educator but also of the entire black community of America, that Senator Grant had to recognize its legitimacy. Why were there no blacks in this great enterprise which he had labored so strenuously to launch and keep on course? The ugly thought came to him that Lyndon Johnson and Michael Glancey were technically Southerners, so that perhaps their regional inheritance had manifested itself, but this was unworthy, because no senator or President had ever done more honest work on behalf of the blacks than Johnson, and no so-called Southern senator had employed black secretaries in his office sooner than Mike Glancey.

He wondered if the committee that selected astronauts was in any way contaminated, but then he visualized its chairman, Deke Slayton, as tough and fair a man as he had ever met, and said to himself: Deke would never permit such nonsense. If a qualified black came along, he'd grab him. Checking a folder in his desk drawer, he thought with satisfaction: Besides, he's from Wisconsin and we Westerners have no prejudices.

He rang for a servant and asked if Mrs. Pope was in the house. She wasn't, but the maid said she thought she might still be at headquarters, and in a few minutes Finnerty delivered her to the Grant residence.

'You stay,' the senator told Finnerty, and when the newcomers were seated, Grant nodded at Gawain Butler. 'Tell them your complaint.'

'It's not a personal complaint,' Butler protested. 'It goes far beyond that,' and once more he spread his photographs, after which Grant asked his assistants, 'How do you account for it?' and Mrs. Pope had to confess: 'The problem never came up.'

'And that's the problem,' Butler said. 'Nobody ever noticed that one of our nation's greatest enterprises was lily-white. Nobody gave a damn.'

He took from his briefcase three other photographs, not glossies this time, for they came from varied sources and not from a government public relations office. The three white people recognized the faces immediately: Jackie Robinson from baseball, Jim Brown the great football running back, and Oscar Robertson, perhaps the best basketball player who ever lived. 'If black men can excel in any job you give them, why wouldn't they prove capable in space?'

The problem was so real, and pointed so directly at the men running the program, that Senator Grant said frankly, 'Gawain, you hit me with something terribly important. I wasn't aware of this, and I propose to do something about it. Gather three of your best people and I'll have Mrs. Pope issue travel orders. Be in my office in Washington on Monday.' Turning to the others, he said, 'See that Dr. Mott is there, too.'

But if Grant had even the slightest suspicion that Dr. Mott was going to fudge the interview with bland excuses and easy promises, he did not know that tough-minded expert, for when the four black leaders were settled, and after they had made their protest in excellent fashion, he took over.

'I've served on three selection committees now, and we've striven desperately to pick Catholic or Jewish pilots, women pilots and, especially, black pilots. We've wanted to show men of good will exactly like yourselves that we were not bound by religion, sex or color. But when the final moment came to make the harsh choices, from about a hundred down to six, we knew that each of the persons we selected had to have these qualifications,' and he handed the committee mimeographed sheets listing these requirements:

B.S. degree in science or engineering
M.S. degree in science or engineering (advisable)
Military flight training
Test-pilot school
Advanced university training
Solid mastery of mathematics, physics, combustion engines, calculus
Service with a flight squadron
Test-pilot experience in at least two dozen types of aircraft

'It's very simple, gentlemen. You find me the young black men who have subjected themselves to training as rigorous as this, and I'll lead the battle for their selection.'

'For astronauts, maybe yes,' Dr. Butler agreed, twisting the condemnatory paper in his fingers, 'but how about the Mission Control people? Are we to be excluded from everything?'

Mott produced another mimeographed sheet, a long one this time, showing the educational qualifications of the men in Mission Control and a summary of the fantastic spread of special skills they had. On a large blow-up of a NASA photograph of the control crew at work, he pointed to one man after another, reciting his name and the great breadth of his education: 'Tom Fallester. B.S. Cornell. M.S. Cal Tech. Ph.D. MIT. Qualified in all branches of engineering relating to combustion engines. Six years' work at Lewis Center in Cleveland on rockets. Our expert during flights on fuel management and engine repair.' On and on he went, probing behind the white shirts and the grim smiles, explaining the arduous paths these notable men had followed in acquiring the manifold skills they commanded. In the entire group there was no one of whom it could be said: 'Tarnoff, here, had a good high-school education and one year at a teachers' college in which his work emphasized nothing special, but he is a likable fellow.' Tarnoff either mastered four or five fields of specific knowledge or he was in no way eligible for the team.

Stanley Mott was as distressed as the four black men to whom he was talking. 'I cannot even guess what the solution is, gentlemen.'

'Do the rest of the astronauts, those coming along . . . do they have to be so highly trained in test-piloting and the like?' The questioner was a black professor from Harvard.

'Each man in the capsule has to be qualified to take over,' Mott said without a glimmer of conciliation.

'But down the line?' the Harvard man insisted. 'Are scientists never going into space?'

'They are,' and Mott waved the list of qualifications for the Mission Control people. 'But they will have to be at least as well qualified as these men. There will be no place for a black man who played four years of basketball and took basket-weaving to remain eligible.'

At his suggestion the four-man committee, accompanied by himself and Penny Pope, visited with the faculties of five excellent universities, three with engineering schools, two without, and at the conclusion of this most revealing tour, Penny compiled this doleful summary for her Senate committee:

> We could not find in these five student bodies even one black man who was pursuing a course of hard, scientific training which would later on qualify him for astronaut selection. It was never a limitation of intelligence or ability that caused this state of affairs, for often

the black males had higher raw test scores than their white class-mates.

In this generation the gifted black student looks to business as his ladder leading out of the ghetto and to a top salary. His eye is not on the stars, it is on the board room, and at the conclusion of our tour, not one black member of our group could identify one black young man who was going to be eligible for selection ten years from now, nor even one who was preparing himself for an assignment to the Mission Control team. They do not take hard subjects.

Penny Pope's accurate summary may have satisfied the committee of black protesters, but it certainly did not satisfy Senator Grant, for when he received a copy he rang bells furiously, and that afternoon he and Senator Glancey met with Dr. Mott and his associates. Grant spoke first, using white-hot profanity, which he usually avoided:

'Goddammit, I want a black astronaut. I don't care if we have to lower standards to the third-grade level. I want to see a black astro-naut on our roster, and I don't want to be told it can't be done.'

Mott interrupted: 'At this point it cannot be done. Do you want to endanger an entire program?'

'The entire program will be shot to hell right here in Congress if you don't find us a black astronaut. Do you think we can go on disinher-iting over twenty million of our people? Barring them from a pro-gram on which we spend billions of their tax dollars? Let me tell you, if the public ever turns against your program, Mott, you are a dead duck. Now, when the next photograph is taken of Mission Control, I want to see at least four black faces in there.'

Stubbornly, Mott asked, 'Doing what?'

'I don't give a goddamn what they're doing. They can be knitting, for all I care, but I want them to be there. Don't you agree, Senator Glancey?'

It was agreed that before another year ended, there would be black faces in the control room, but finding them proved almost impossible, for reasons cited by the faculty and students of the five universities, but when Mott and his team really searched, they found at Wayne State University in Detroit an exceptionally well-trained young man who was gifted in meeting people, so although he lacked calculus and flying experience, he was given the job of liaison with the press, in which he performed superbly. Further search

revealed a young man in Alabama, another in California and one in Massachusetts with first-class scientific backgrounds, so that when the next photographs were released, that sea of radiant white faces was speckled more
realistically. Senator Grant took one of the pictures, circled the three faces
in red ink, and mailed it to his good friend Dr. Butler of the Detroit Public
School System: 'Dear Gawain, you challenged us to find them and we did.
Norman.'

The mishap in Scott Carpenter's Mercury flight, which carried him two
hundred and forty miles beyond Commander John Pope's waiting *Tulagi,*
reminded NASA that even the smallest error in calculation or execution
might drop its returning astronauts in some Central or South American
jungle, so it was obligatory that all astronauts practice surviving in that
terrain. Some trained in Costa Rica, some in El Salvador, but the Solid Six
were flown to the Amazon, and they were surprised at how near it was.

They left Cape Canaveral at 0800, landed at Miami Airport at 0845 and
took a Pan American non-stop to Manaus, Brazil, where they landed in late
afternoon at a fine, clean city eight hundred miles up the Amazon. Officers
of the Brazilian navy had launches waiting, and by 1700 that same day Pope
and his colleagues were boating on the world's greatest river.

The Americans could not believe what they were seeing, for in their
flights back and forth across the United States they had grown accustomed
to the Ohio, the Mississippi and the Missouri, no mean rivers, and the
marvelous Colorado, a source of continuing enchantment, so they carried
in their minds some concept of what a major river should be, but they were
unprepared for a real river like the Amazon.

'Look at the damned thing!' Claggett cried, and as the launch pulled
away from shore the men could barely see the other side. The Amazon was
not big, it was stupendous, a vast moving lake.

'Gentlemen,' the Brazilian officer said, 'on this bank you will notice the
line of discoloration, twenty feet up, running along the entire stretch of
river.' He interrupted to tell the astronauts he had received his education
at West Point. 'Now what do you suppose that line represents?' After some
irrelevant guesses were made, he said, 'That's how high the Amazon rises
every year in its early summer flood.' The line was incomprehensible,
twenty feet higher than where the launch rode the muddy waters.

'You have cliffs here,' Claggett pointed out. 'On the other side, the flood
must stretch forever.'

'It does,' the officer said, and the Americans looked across that fantastic
expanse, trying vainly to imagine what such a flood must be like.

'Technically,' the Brazilian said, 'we're not really on the Amazon. This
is the Negro, a jet-black network coming down out of Colombia and
Venezuela. A few miles east of here, the Solomon, bright yellow like his
mines. You won't believe what happens.'

He sped the launch downriver, pointing out to the men the dark color of the stream, and after a while they became aware that off to the right a really tremendous river was about to join, its waters angry from their turbulent trip down from the distant mountains of Peru and Ecuador. By itself it would have formed the largest river in the world; when it joined with the Negro it would be incomparable. Then the Amazon proper would begin.

'Watch!' the Brazilian said, and it was apparent that no matter how many times he had taken visitors to see the impending miracle, he was still as thrilled by it as he had been the first time, for from the south came the mighty yellow Solomon, while from the north came the huge, surly black Negro. They met, but they did not blend. Side by side for nearly twenty miles the two majestic rivers shared the same channel, each as separated from the other as if a wall had been erected between them. Yellow and black, they moved toward the ocean side by side, and even when the launches cut through them, again and again, the two rivers maintained their individuality, each carrying an immense load of detritus which gave it color, each pursuing its own course.

And then, as night began to fall, the Americans saw two sights they would never forget. Up the newly formed Amazon came a twenty-thousand-ton ship from Bremerhaven, Germany, its dark flag flying in the jungle breeze, its nose pointed toward Manaus. It was eight hundred miles from the ocean, yet it was steaming full speed ahead, secure in its knowledge that this vast river was as safe as the open sea.

'We're in middle Kansas,' Claggett cried, 'and here comes an ocean liner.'

Then the dolphin began to leap, blue, silvery beasts frolicking as if they were in the deepest Pacific, leading the ship homeward to its evening haven. Right off the bow of the launches the dolphin rose, twisting in air to spy upon the astronauts, then diving to the unplumbed depths of the Amazon. Six of the dolphin accompanied the launches back to Manaus, and as they leaped in the dying sunlight Pope told the men in his boat, 'Hey! They're an omen! Altair's always been my lucky star!'

'I don't get it,' Cater said.

'The constellation Dolphin. It protects Altair. You watch! We'll handle the Amazon.'

The men spent the next day sightseeing in Manaus, to which the governor of the state came to pay his respects. Tucker Thompson's photographers took many pictures of the ceremonies, after which the governor said, through an interpreter, 'Gentlemen, we have what I think may be a surprise for you,' and he led their motorcade to the center of the city, where a jewel of an opera house had been erected by the Amazon rubber barons in the closing years of the nineteenth century. Architecturally it was a gem, a Venetian dream in crystal and silver, and it contained many mementos of the great days when this little town had been a major metropolis.

'Caruso sang here, and Édouard de Reszke, and Adelina Patti. We had magnificent seasons, with stars from all over Europe coming up our river in German ocean liners. I'm told that Sarah Bernhardt played *L'Aiglon* on that stage, and Helena Modjeska was here, too. We were the Athens of the jungle.'

It was agreed that the Solid Six would be taken by launch sixty miles up the Rio Solimões, as the Solomon was spelled in Portuguese, there to be led ten miles up a minor tributary, from which local guides would take them five miles into the jungle and leave them. They carried with them nothing but knives, cloth that could be used as a mosquito net, and three radios that would broadcast their position constantly but not receive messages from the outside. If a man broke a leg, he would be rescued automatically, after three days.

The guide into the jungle was mestizo—Indian-black-Portuguese-Spanish—and he said nothing as he led the men into an area from which it would be unlikely that they could extricate themselves. Without saying goodbye, he turned to retrace the confusing path he had taken, but just as he left the group he looked at Pope, winked, and with his head indicated a tree heavy with palm leaves of a sort John had not seen before: '*Muy bueno, señor,*' he said in Spanish, and disappeared.

The seven men were now ominously alone, seven because they had with them a canny French-Canadian woodsman, master of many tricks, and it would be his job to instruct them in the wily arts of survival. His name was Georges, which the astronauts quickly transformed into Gorgeous Georges. He told them, 'Anything that moves, grab it. Anything that looks good to eat, let me smell it.' It was no longer a game; now seven hungry men without weapons had to forage and improvise for three days, and hope to come out alive.

By the close of that first day it was clear that the hero of this expedition was going to be Harry Jensen, the cotton picker from South Carolina, for this hard-grained little fellow had a score of ingenious ideas remembered from his boyhood days in the cypress swamps along the Little Pee Dee in his home state. He could divert a small stream and thus isolate a fish; he could set traps for any animals that might wander by; he devised a snare for birds and another for monkeys; and he said that if anyone spotted a python moving in, to call him.

He was witty, and persistent and lucky, and although he caught nothing that first day, so that the men went to bed hungry, on the second day one of his traps did snare an iguana, but since the others had not found a way to make fire, the astronauts had to eat it raw, which they did eagerly if not with pleasure.

Pope, remembering the signal thrown by the mestizo guide, asked the men what good the palm tree might serve, and Timothy Bell, who had lived on an Allied Aviation expense account and thus knew the better restaurants, said, 'A very expensive item is hearts of palm salad,' so Pope and

Jensen attacked the tree without knowing where its heart was or what it was supposed to look like.

The palm tree defended its secret stoutly, and the two men were in a drenching sweat by the time their small knives had hacked it apart, but when Jensen passed down the succulent baby leaves the astronauts tore into them, and one of the men said, 'With a Caesar dressing these could be delicious.'

'They're not too bad with raw iguana, either,' Pope said.

The late afternoons and nights were made unbearable by insects, whose stings were intensified by the constant rain of sweat that poured from every crevice. Hickory Lee, an outdoorsman, kept tasting the sweat on the heel of his left thumb, and said ominously, 'We're losing our salt at a dangerous rate,' and when the others made this most useful test they confirmed Lee's suspicion that their perspiration was turning acid.

Ed Cater, the Air Force major from Kosciusko, Mississippi, told the men of a story he had read about fliers in World War II being lost in the jungles of Guadalcanal: 'Two bad scenes, Jap snipers and any cut on the legs. You cut your shin in this climate, ninety-nine percent humidity, it never heals. Just rots away.'

'How soon?' Claggett asked.

'Maybe six months.'

'Good. We'll live till Christmas.' Claggett's humor never riled his companions.

He was a loud Texan, but he was also the best pilot in the group and the one most likely to survive any ordeal. Now he said soberly, 'Let's suppose our radios go on the blink. All three. We're in this jungle and we don't know a damned thing more than we do right now. How in hell do we get out?'

The astronauts looked instinctively to Gorgeous Georges, who demurred: 'That's your job.'

'The important thing,' Jensen said, 'is to sit quietly for about an hour and figure everything you do know.' And he led the group in an analysis of its situation.

They said they knew they were in Brazil, but he would not allow that. 'If we crashed in a Gemini capsule, we wouldn't know where in hell we were.'

'We'd know we were in South America.'

'Granted.' Jensen made it a kind of game, twenty questions, with him the moderator. They did not know they were near the Amazon River, but the humidity and the thickness of the jungle made it likely they were close to some body of water. They knew that so far, at least, what water was available was potable, and they knew they could subsist on hearts of palm for some days; at least it stifled the belly pains.

Gradually they concluded that the imperative thing would be not to guess where the larger body of water was, nor in which direction safety lay, but the construction of a signal which could be seen from search planes. They could not clear the jungle to do this, but they could fasten large white flags made of their cloth to the tops of trees.

'And how do we get up there?' Bell asked, and Jensen replied, 'Simple, you haul your ass up or you die.'

'Can we be sure that search planes will be looking for us?' Bell asked.

'As sure as the sun will rise tomorrow,' Jensen said. 'That's one thing we must never doubt. Their radar will tell them about where the capsule went down. America will never let us rot here. They'd launch a thousand planes if necessary. That we must never doubt.'

Cater said he'd read a story about a naval pilot downed in the waters off Guadalcanal in World War II, right under the nose of Japanese shore guns, and how planes of the Army Air Corps, as it was called then, fought an entire day to save that one flier. 'And they did,' he said.

'But was it a true story?' Bell asked.

'I think it must have been,' Cater said.

When the three days were over, and the radios vectored the rescue teams to where the hungry astronauts were waiting, their faces scarred from mosquito bites, Cater said, 'Jensen, I don't know whether you can fly an airplane or not, but if I'm in one that has to crash in a jungle, I want you as my copilot.'

It was a tense moment, for the four other astronauts shared Cater's assessment of the young fellow, but Jensen reverted to a gag Army men had used when starting their flight training. Spreading his legs as if working the rudders in a trainer, he grabbed an imaginary stick with both hands and cried in horror, looking hard to his right, 'Sir, sir! How do you pull this thing to make it go up?'

When the bone-tired astronauts reached their quarters in Manaus, Cater cried, 'My God! It can't be!' But it was. Sitting on a bar stool in the lounge was petite Cynthia Rhee, her impudent eyes laughing at them, who had trailed her subjects down the length of Florida and across the Caribbean to the confluence of the Negro and the Solimões, where the Amazon began.

'I had to see how you looked when you came out of the jungle,' she said in her lovely accent. 'You look awful.' She touched Cater on the cheek. 'The bites, do they hurt?' She stared straight into his eyes as she said this.

'After you get a certain number . . .'

'Who assumed control at the bad moments?' she asked.

'Guess,' Cater said, falling onto a stool.

'I think maybe Jensen from South Carolina.'

'Now why would you say that?' Cater asked.

'Because he would know swampy land. South Carolina has many swamps.'

'You still have all your marbles,' Cater said, and Cynthia turned her attention to Claggett.

'You promised at Cocoa Beach to tell me about your early days,' she said.

'Work comes first,' Claggett said, reaching for a beer.

'Perhaps the most important work you'll do outside the flight,' she said to all the men, 'is talk to me. Because what you're doing is very important, and you don't want it immortalized in the bullshit this man peddles.' And she pointed to Tucker Thompson hurrying in to protect his charges from this dangerous slant-eye, as he called her.

Despite Tucker's efforts, she succeeded in leading Claggett to his room, where they engaged in love-making so wild and varied that Randy finally asked, 'Does the Japanese government give you kids graduate courses?'

'I'm Korean,' she said as they lay exhausted after an especially vigorous engagement. 'You don't even know where Korea is, do you?'

Claggett smiled. 'It's part of China, somewheres. Japan invades it every twenty years.'

'Why are you Americans—even you bright ones—why are you so ignorant of the rest of the world?'

'The rest of the world is that flea-bitten jungle out there.'

This made her quite angry. 'Do you know that Korea is divided in half. Communist and free?' She jerked the bedclothes up to her chin and glared at her stupid American.

Very quietly Randy droned like a briefing officer: 'You take off at Fukuoka on the island of Kyushu. It's a short hop across the Korean Strait to Pusan. Then Taegu, Seoul, west to Inchon, then Kaesong and a hard flight northwest to Pyongyang, where the heavy antiaircraft waits. Then up to the Yalu River and down the east coast to Hungnam, where all hell breaks loose. Then down to K-22 on the Sea of Japan . . . where I fought the Russians and the Chinese for one hellishly cold winter and dreamed of a beautiful Korean Jo-san I had fallen in love with at Pusan.'

Cynthia Rhee said nothing. With the sheet tucked under her chin, she gazed at Claggett for some moments, then leaned over and kissed him. 'I apologize. I should know by now not to ask questions before I finish my research.'

'Can you reach me a beer?'

Deftly she knocked the cap off by wedging it against the bedstead and the wall, marring each. 'I learned that during the weekends at Yale. But if you were in Korea, then you know how the Japanese despise us. I could take a machine gun to every damned Japanese in the world.'

'But you went to college there.'

'I was born there. And my parents were treated like cattle. I have this burning hunger to show the Japanese . . .'

'Don't fight your battles in my bed. Lie down.'

They made love through the night, talking intermittently about Korea,

NASA, the jungle. Never before had Claggett met such a woman, one so delicately lovely yet so sternly driven. Usually she was far ahead of him in her shrewd analysis of the astronaut program, and her witty observations on the other men of the Solid Six were startling in their perceptions. 'If I were Deke Slayton . . .' she began.

'You know Deke Slayton?'

'It's my job to know everybody. So if I were Slayton organizing a Gemini flight, I'd want you as commander, and guess who as pilot? In the right-hand seat?'

Claggett guessed Jensen, but she said, 'Wrong. On land he's fantastic. He'd be sensational managing a department store like Macy's. But upstairs I'd want John Pope. Not a pleasant man, but very capable.'

'You don't cotton to the straight arrows, do you?'

She knew the term. In fact, she knew all the terms and their accurate definitions; she had made herself into an astronaut and intuitively she knew how they functioned. 'Pope would get the capsule down when you blanked out—and that's what counts. Getting the damned capsule down. Pacific . . . Atlantic. Desert . . . jungle. Let's get the damned thing down.'

As they left the room to join the others for the short flight back to Cape Canaveral—primitive Amazonian jungle to the Moon craft in one short day—Claggett asked, 'Is it true what Slobber Lips Thompson told us? That you said you intended sleeping with all of us? As an act of research?'

'Randy, do I ask you "Is it true that on your first Gemini flight you became so excited that things came apart and you wet your drawers?" Shouldn't people with a fondness for each other take certain things on faith?'

'Well, did you say it?'

'No. Did you wet your pants?'

'Yes.' And they kissed for a long time.

No one in America, not even the NASA high command, followed more assiduously the country's adventures in space than Dr. Leopold Strabismus, president of Universal Space Associates and chancellor of the University of Space and Aviation, for he knew in his bones that massive changes were under way in American life and that space was only a fragment of the whole. He suspected that the present surge of interest would finally transform itself into something quite unexpected, and it was necessary for him to be ready for whatever did happen.

His original USA flourished, with more than sixty thousand apprehensive citizens pouring money into his account and receiving in return his constantly improved explanations of what the little men were up to. Ramirez, with an enlarged budget, was able to contract with a Los Angeles printer for a monthly letter done on good stock, with an occasional color diagram explaining how the spaceships from distant planets maneuvered among the Sun's planets: one popular edition showed a cutaway of a space-ship itself. Strabismus drew the diagrams but used the newfangled appliqué alphabets printed on transparent cellophane for the lettering.

'Renewed subscriptions have increased forty-one percent since our use of color,' Ramirez reported to Dr. Strabismus, but the latter was no longer acutely interested in his first venture; the university was succeeding beyond his hopes. It still had no students or faculty, but its issuance of diplomas had multiplied tenfold. 'There's an insatiable desire for education,' he told Marcia as they lay in bed one night. 'And have you noticed that if a person is willing to pay three hundred fifty dollars for a master's degree, he's just as likely to cough up six-fifty for a doctorate.'

He and Marcia often speculated on what the purchasers did with their degrees, and just as his instincts had warned him to prepare the pamphlet which Senator Grant's wife had used to refute Dr. Mott when he tried to attack USA, so he now had his staff compile a reassuring publication about the university, which was sent in response to inquiries from any institution whose administrators were becoming suspicious that one of its faculty who offered as his proof of education a degree from USA in Los Angeles was committing fraud.

The pamphlet was a masterpiece, showing a complete faculty with distinguished degrees from all over the world, including Witwatersrand in Johannesburg, and a list of recent publications written by these scholars. Dr. Strabismus himself wrote the bibliography, and it included papers on splitting genes, synthesizing a new drug that would replace insulin in the treatment of diabetes, and a cost-time analysis of assembly work at a General Motors plant. His knowledge was so encyclopedic, and his interests so broad, that he was able to dash off these titles in correct phraseology without consulting any books, and as he dictated each one he thought: I wish I had time to write that paper. Now. It's needed: *Theory of Tumbling Bodies Entering Planetary Atmospheres with Application to Probe Vehicles and Australian Tektites.*

Once, when a full professor from the University of Wisconsin came out to investigate the credentials of an applicant who had landed a job using fraudulent degrees, Strabismus told him frankly, 'Your man's a fake. Fire him. His check bounced.'

'How do you get away with this, Strabismus?'

'In California, so many churches and colleges want to crank up that the state has little energy left over to supervise us, once we get started. We're free to do about what we want, so long as we don't steal state funds. We pay our registration fee, our yearly renewals. We keep our nose clean and we delude nobody.'

'How about this faculty list?'

'Does it hurt anybody? Does it fool anybody like you?'

'Don't you feel like a criminal?'

'I certainly do not. I've been bucking the system all my life, and I think

I've performed a useful service.' He was so frank that the Wisconsin man actually liked him, and they talked for a long time.

'Tell me, at Wisconsin do you detect the beginnings of a falling away from science?'

'We certainly do. The flood of money pumped by the federal government into the science faculties has caused a lot of resentment among the rest of us.'

'What's your field?'

'Humanities. And we're hurting. I'm philosophy, principally.'

Strabismus wanted to know his specialty, and when the visitor said the Nature of Truth, the president of USA surprised him with a flow of names associated with that subject and an accurate summary of the positions of many: Hobbes, Kant, Bradley, Brand Blanshard of Yale.

'You think the antiscience movement will continue to grow?' Strabismus asked.

'I do. I see it in my students, most clearly.'

'Tell me, are your young people big with tarot cards? I-Ching?'

The professor snapped his fingers and said, 'Strange you should ask that. There's a real movement toward the occult.'

'Astrology?'

'Very big.' The man from Wisconsin stroked his chin, then stared at the floor. 'It's quite confusing, really. In space we're having our greatest scientific triumphs. On the ground our young people are turning sharply away from science.'

'How much of it is mere youthful rebellion?' Strabismus asked. At this moment he heard his dean of faculty at the door. As she walked into the hall he called out and invited her to join them. 'This is Dr. Grant, my dean.' He brought her up to date on the science-antiscience rebellion and restated his question.

'Clearly,' she said, 'many young people rebel against science, any kind of order, just to gig their parents.'

'Excuse me,' the professor said.

'Gig their parents. Make them uneasy. More important, gig their professors.'

'You mean that if the university goes over heart and soul to science . . .'

'Then to hell with science,' Marcia said.

Success in charlatanism had produced subtle and pleasing changes in the administrators of USA: Dr. Strabismus was somewhat heavier from continued good eating; his beard was more neatly trimmed and his face more rounded and benevolent; in fact, he looked like a contented university president whose football team had just been invited to play in the Rose Bowl. Marcia's handsome face had lost its perpetual pout, for she was no longer angry at anyone, and her body had lost a good deal of its baby fat, so that while the president grew stouter, she grew slimmer, and she was so attractive, with her warm smile and her hair in neat braids, that when she suggested to the professor that he join them for dinner, he accepted eagerly.

'Tell me,' he asked over the wine, 'how did you two ever get involved in these rackets?'

'Did Leopold tell you who I am?' she asked. 'Senator Grant's daughter. I just grew tired of hearing his patriotic bullshit.'

The professor winced. 'So you're part of the rebellion?'

'I sure am.' When he asked if she had finished college, she said, 'Freshman year, almost. C-minus. You see, I got tired of your bullshit, too. You professors, I mean.'

'What do you foresee as the next big mania?' Strabismus asked.

'Something antiscientific, that's for sure.'

'I did most of the talking before. Now you tell us why *you* think that.'

The professor of philosophy said that when a democracy responds totally to an imagined outside threat, the way America did to Russia's Sputnik, the intellectuals quickly see that this is spurious and rebel against it, but in this particular case the situation was further confused by anxiety among college students over the military draft and among the lower middle classes by the fact that the nation was spending so much on space when things close at hand required attention. 'The blacks, you know, are quite opposed to the space program. They're cut out of it.'

'The blacks are cut out of everything,' Strabismus said. 'Do you know that in my Universal Space Associates, one of the hottest movements ever, I have not a single black enrolled, so far as I know. But in the diploma thing, quite a few put down their dollars for that degree. They believe the framed diploma will make the difference.'

As they spoke, Marcia turned on the television, and a news program refuted what they had been saying, for at a gala press conference officials of NASA were presenting the next two heroes who would fly in the Gemini program, and the junior member, who would sit in the right-hand seat, was Randy Claggett from Texas. He was most appealing as he smiled, gap-toothed, into the camera and allowed as how his success so far had been pretty much due to the support of his beautiful wife, Debby Dee, and their three fine children.

'One more step on our way to the Moon,' the spokesman said as the camera zoomed in on Randy and Debby Dee.

'There's a lot of fascination left in space,' Strabismus said. 'And it'll increase when they actually attack the Moon. But believe me, Professor, the drop-off is going to be sensational . . .'

'And you want to be in first when the next racket starts?'

'I do. The diploma thing adds nice extra money, but I doubt that it could finance our big building. You need something big, some big, swinging movement. All I know is, it's going to be antiscience, antispace. But what form it's going to take . . . I wish you could tell me.'

. . .

The five Earthbound members of the Solid Six were proud that Claggett had been chosen so early for a ride in space, and they haunted the control rooms at Cape Canaveral to follow his progress. The center had been redesignated Cape Kennedy in honor of the President slain less than two years earlier, but none of the professionals ever used that name; to them it would always be Canaveral.

They were living, as usual on their eastern trips, at the Bali Hai in Cocoa Beach, and when it appeared assured that Claggett and his teammate were going to make a success of their flight, Ed Cater suggested that they all drive back to the Dagger Bar for a celebration at which he and Gloria would provide the beer, and Hickory Lee the oysters. All the astronauts, especially those from landbound states, relished Florida seafood, particularly the oysters, because they could be consumed in great quantities without producing fat. As Claggett and his partner were now learning, even one extra ounce of fat in that Gemini capsule meant added problems, so that the young pilots had a phobia about pies and cakes: 'They can wait till we're retired.'

There were three routes by which a car could travel the twenty miles from the space center to the motel: it could stay on A1A and keep to the fringing islands, or it could come down the middle on Route 3 and make better time, or it could move sharply west onto the mainland and come speeding down U.S. 1, a well-kept double highway. The last way was longer but much quicker.

General Motors had presented each astronaut with a Corvette, and the men loved these sleek, swift cars. Lee, Cater and Bell drove theirs down A1A to enjoy the relaxing scenery along the shore. Pope and young Harry Jensen, having been held up by consultations with Dr. Mott, left late, and they elected to drive over to U.S. 1 and then to speed south to the town of Cocoa, then east on Route 520 to the island at Cocoa Beach.

It was a gala afternoon; everything was going right and their team was at last in the air, which meant that quite soon the rest of them would be entering space, too. Jensen, who was better with a car than Pope, led the way in his specially painted gray Corvette, and Pope, trailing in the aged Mercury convertible, which he still preferred, admired the manner in which the South Carolinian handled his car, never making a foolish move, always prepared to ease sideways, left or right, to enter a spot left open by the slower traffic. It was like flying, really, riding tail gunner to Harry Jensen.

Pope, peering ahead, spotted the heavy old Buick coming from the opposite direction when it was a good distance away, and casually muttered to himself, 'That one doesn't know how to drive.' As the big black car neared, he thought: He's weaving. Is his front wheel funny? Instinctively, Pope took maneuvers which would provide him maximum escape room if the Buick really was in trouble, and noticed with some dismay that Jensen was not doing so.

Then he uttered a wild cry as the Buick leaped across the median strip and plowed directly into Jensen's Corvette, knocking it clear across the roadway in such a manner that Pope had great difficulty maneuvering his Mercury past the two tangled cars. Only his moments of anticipation saved him.

When he elbowed his way through the crowd he found the driver of the Buick unscathed and very drunk. Harry Jensen was so completely mashed he was barely recognizable through the blood and scattered brains.

Restraining himself from killing the murderer, Pope spoke to no one, returned quietly to his Mercury and sped off before the police arrived, for he had work to do. He roared down U.S. 1, spun his car east on Route 520, then swiftly south on A1A, grinding his wheels into the parking lot of the Bali Hai.

He did not run through the entrance lobby, but as soon as Cynthia Rhee saw his ashen face she knew something terrible had happened, and she supposed it had to do with Claggett's flight: 'John, what is it?' Because he had come to think of her as a member of the team, he grabbed her left arm and pulled her along as he sought for Cater and Lee in the bar. When he saw them, he beckoned them into a corner and said bluntly, 'Harry Jensen's just been killed.'

'How?'

'Drunk driver came across the median on U.S. 1. Wiped him out.'

'You sure?'

'Brains across the highway.'

'Oh Jesus!' The two men who had intended to host the party stood silent for a moment, then Cater said, 'Where's Tim Bell? See if you can find him, Hickory.' And when Bell joined them, shaking and pale, Cater said, 'Anybody know where Inger is?'

'I saw her at the pool,' Bell said.

'We can't tell her there,' Cater said.

'I'll take her to her room,' Cynthia suggested, but Cater grabbed her firmly: 'I think not.' The men knew that Jensen and the Korean girl had been sleeping together at odd opportunities and they suspected that Inger also knew.

Cater went to the pool, and in his gentle Deep South drawl, said, 'Inger, we're having a blowout tonight, and Harry said he'd be a bit late. The girls are dressing . . .'

When she reached her room she found the three astronauts waiting— Pope, Bell, Hickory Lee—standing very straight, their distress clear in their eyes as they looked at her.

'Oh God!' she gasped.

'On the highway,' Cater said. 'Totally wiped out.'

'Oh God!'

In her presence Cater went to the phone and called Deke Slayton: 'This is Ed Cater. Astronaut Harry Jensen has just been killed in a highway accident on U.S. 1 between the Cape and Cocoa Beach. No word of this must be sent aloft to Claggett. Call the police for verification.'

Miss Rhee had alerted the other wives, and now they streamed into the motel room, composed, tight-lipped and beautiful. Sandy Lee, the tough-minded girl from Tennessee, took command, ordering the men from the room. Cool, determined, she pushed the other women away when they wanted Inger to lie down, said brusquely, 'Walk it off, kid.' When the phone started to ring she answered the first two calls, then left the receiver off the hook. She would not allow the others to turn on the television, but she did order drinks and suggested that Inger have a Jack Daniels straight.

Through that long night the five women sat together, talking, now and then laughing as they recalled some scandalous thing that had happened to them, weeping more often. And in the course of the night each woman called Texas to ask about her children. At about two-thirty Inger said, 'If she wants to come in, let her.'

And Debby Dee found Cynthia Rhee in a corner of the Dagger Bar, transcribing notes. The men stayed in the bar, drinking, except that Pope and Cater ducked out to accompany the police to the morgue to identify the corpse, but this they could barely do, for Jensen had no face.

When Randy Claggett splashed down after his Gemini flight, the first thing he heard aboard the rescue carrier was that his good buddy Harry Jensen had been killed by a drunk driver, and as soon as he returned to Canaveral he stormed into the police station, demanding to know who the killer was. He learned that the man had accumulated six citations for drunken driving and had once caused a woman to lose a leg. His license had not been taken away because his lawyer pleaded that 'it would be unfair to deprive this fine young man of his means of earning a living.' He had never gone to jail; he had never been penalized; he just kept driving that big Buick when he was dead drunk, and nobody gave a damn.

'Fifty thousand people killed a year,' the police chief said. 'We have good reason to believe that more than half are because of drunk driving.'

'Can't you do anything?' Claggett asked in seething anger.

'Automobile people won't let us. Whiskey people won't let us. And the courts abuse us if we arrest them. I've arrested your man three times. Told the judge he was an accident looking for a place to happen.'

Randy studied the dossier: Melvin Starling, 28. Married. Arrest 1: Drunk driving. Arrest 4: Drunk driving hitting a woman. Arrest 6: Drunk driving. He pointed to that last entry: 'That was only three weeks ago.'

'America wants it that way,' the policeman said, folding the file and jamming it into his desk.

·   ·   ·

And then a familiar miracle of military life occurred. Older officers—Army, Navy, Air Force, Marine, it made no difference—who had lost their wives began flying in to Canaveral to talk with Inger Jensen and take her two children on picnics. Younger officers not yet married, who had served with Harry at some remote base, turned up to see how she was doing, and three men who had tested planes with him at Edwards stopped by.

It was as if signals had been flashed through the military establishment: 'One of our women has been left a widow with two kids.' In other walks such a woman with two rambunctious flaxen-haired children might be at a serious disadvantage where remarriage was concerned, but in the military a young woman with children became especially attractive, as if she brought with her a ready-made family. So like white corpuscles hastening toward a wound to purify it, officers unmarried or widowed leaped forward to protect Harry Jensen's widow.

To the surprise of the five astronaut families who vetted the suitors, she would have none of them. Bundling her children into a secondhand station wagon bought with Harry's insurance, she started across country to a small college in Oregon, where she had been offered a job as librarian. When Debby Dee kissed her goodbye, the big Texan woman said, 'You're a horse's ass, Inger, but God, I love you,' and the little Swedish girl replied, 'It's as if he was in the seat beside me. He'll always be.'

When Stanley Mott's younger son, Christopher, was arrested for selling marijuana to grammar-school students in suburban Washington, his father spent three nights, after daylong meetings of his committee on the Moon, pleading with police and district attorneys not to send his boy to a house of correction, and on the afternoon of the fourth day, during a heated debate on whether the surface of the Moon might be composed of deep dust into which a landing vehicle might sink never to be seen again, he leaned forward onto the table, collapsed, and slipped sideways to the floor.

When Rachel Mott was informed, she was sure it was a heart attack, but after NASA doctors had examined him they assured her that it was mere exhaustion: 'Even geniuses have to rest some time. Keep him in bed. Don't let him worry.'

As soon as word of his collapse circulated among the Solid Six, now Five, each of the astronauts wrote personally to Mott, attesting to their appreciation of what he had done for them, from the days of the selection committee to his supportive work at the time of Claggett's flight, and the five wives did the same with Mrs. Mott, but the most surprising outcome was a personal visit to the sickroom by Cynthia Rhee: 'I'm here for two reasons, Dr. Mott. To express my hopes for your speedy recovery, for you are a good man and you're needed, and to see firsthand what penalties a scientist pays for his dedication to space.'

'How can you afford to spend so much time on one story?'

'I submit something almost every week. The paper gets good return on my modest expense account, believe me.'

'Am I your story this week?'

'You are. "Overworked Scientist Collapses on Way to Moon." Everyone in Japan will be able to visualize that.'

'Engineer, not scientist.'

'So there we have the first conflict. Since you always resented your below-the-salt status as an engineer, now that you've become a real scientist, you refuse the title. Out of intellectual pique?'

Wrapped in his bathrobe, Mott adjusted his eyeglasses and smiled. 'You may be right, but I'm an engineer, always will be.' He laughed outright. 'Know what a really fine engineer told me when I came to work for the old NACA? "Scientists dream about doing great things. Engineers do them." '

It was surprising how men of all caliber, and many women, were willing to talk freely with this remarkable Korean woman. She was almost thirty now, 'all nonsense flushed away' as she once said to Rachel Mott, and everything about her seemed to disqualify her for the arduous task she had undertaken: she was too small to wrestle with the crowds that surrounded the astronauts, too pretty to be taken seriously. Her English was delightful to hear, with its occasional mispronunciation of l, r and f, and she had never learned to control her fiery temper; but she had a charming way of throwing herself upon the mercy of listeners, a woman without sham or pretense who wanted to delve into problems of intense mutual concern. Nothing derailed her, not abuse or scorn or outright refusal to answer her intrusive questions. As she had told Rachel one night at the Bali Hai: 'Gigantic things are under way, supervised by little men, and the world requires to know all aspects.'

'I should like to tabulate the forces that brought you down,' she said as she sat beside Mott's bed. 'Jensen's death. I think you were like all of us. We saw that heavenly boy with his fairy-tale princess of a wife as the perpetual youth, gallant . . . so goddamned gallant.' After pausing to bite her lip and keep back the tears, she continued to bore in. 'So you must have seen Jensen as the son you never had . . .'

'I have two sons.'

Without altering in any way her tone of voice, she said, 'Of course. But one is a California homosexual, the other a Washington drug pusher.'

Mott did not attempt to fight back. On these two difficult confrontations he had made his peace, but he did ask, 'Is it necessary to print that?'

'To print it? Maybe not. To know it? Absolutely,' and she digressed to explain her attitude toward data. 'Have you ever studied the ceramics of Korea? Probably the greatest in the world. Our potters never try to make a perfect vase, flawless in all dimensions. They allow the clay to manifest itself, to work out its own destiny. And how do they achieve that unmatched celadon finish? They don't apply it as a celadon color. They underglaze, one subtle shade after another. Pale colors you are never allowed to see. And they follow this patient ritual because they learned that if they go in some bright morning, all eager to create a masterpiece, and simply brush onto their vase the celadon color, it will always remain just that, as long as the vase exists. But if they start way back and apply first a slight gray, then a green, then a shadowy brown and finally the pale yellow, when the time comes to place the real yellow, it rests upon a pulsating base which will enable it through the next five hundred years to become whatever shade of exquisite celadon the passing fancy requires. That way you get a piece of crockery that dances and breathes and lives it own life.

'I work like a Korean potter. I underpaint, ridiculously. I must know how you felt about Jensen's death, and a thousand other things, so that when in my book I present you as my scientist—forgive me, my engineer —the underpainting will be so generous that your portrait will vibrate for five hundred years.'

'You have a long perspective.'

'No, a very long perception. You seem sometimes to forget that you and your glorious young men are engaged in an adventure that will command public interest for at least five centuries. You're not in America in 1965. You're in the books of world history in 2465. And if dedicated people like me do not tell your story accurately today, do you know how the books of 2465 are going to tell it? "On 12 April 1961 the heroic Russian cosmonaut Yuri Gagarin became the first man to enter space. Much later some Americans followed." And that will be the summary of your whole ambitious program unless writers like me engrave the real story honestly.'

'Must you speak of my sons?'

'Millard and Roger had no restraints when I interviewed them on Malibu Beach.'

'You went to that trouble?'

'And I have the statements of the three major policemen in Christopher's case. I never cared much for you, Dr. Mott, till I saw for myself how much you love your sons.'

'Why was I repulsive?'

'Because in my little world I saw you always in your companionship with Tucker Thompson, and that is a very shabby setting for an honest gem.'

'I read your story in the German papers about the death of Jensen. It wasn't much different from what Thompson wrote for his rag, except his pictures were better.'

'Wait! Wait, Dr. Mott! For current publication I can write pure bullshit with the best of them. To pay the rent. But I certainly shall keep the B.Q. very low when I write my book.'

'B.Q.?'

'Bullshit Quotient. We try to keep it as low as humanly possible.'

'Then it's true, you are writing a book?'

'All newspaper people are writing books. Mine will be short, and I hope poetic, and I believe it'll be the one that will move into the next century, because my underpainting will be very solid. The old Korean potters will be proud of me for observing their rules so rigorously.' Then, in a preamble to the penetrating questions she was about to ask Mott, she did some revealing underpainting on herself: 'Did you ever stop to think, Dr. Mott, that for really great ceramics, the ones that sing, you must go to Korea. Japanese work is heavy, uninspired, often very ordinary. Because they don't know how to sing, and we Koreans do.'

His second visitors from the Bali Hai were equally surprising. Randy Claggett and John Pope came cautiously into the sickroom, obviously bursting with pride and carrying a heavy bundle stuffed into a paper shopping bag.

'How you doin', Doc?' Randy asked.

'No strain, no pain.'

'What happened? Everything hit you at once?'

'You could not possibly explain it better. Let it be a warning, you young tigers. Everybody has a limit.'

'We came to buck you up, Doctor. Deke Slayton told us yesterday and we hopped a T-38 to come up and give you the good news.'

'I can see it in your faces. You fly the next Gemini?'

'Two down the line, but we get the one heavy with science, a lot of extravehicular activity.'

'The man in the right-hand seat is the one who leaves the capsule and walks in space?'

'Yep,' Claggett said. 'Pope goes out, and if I still like the look on his ugly face, I let him back in.'

'And if you don't?'

'We're paintin' his ass in radioactive fluorescent, and for the next hundred years amateur astronomers will be able to follow him orbit after orbit.'

Mott was as excited as they were about the projected flight, the first in which the entire crew would be composed of the astronauts for whom he was responsible, and then he had to laugh. 'I'll bet Tucker Thompson is going ape.'

'That he is,' Claggett said. 'Has his men photographing Debby Dee and Penny like mad, in hopes we'll crash and he can play up their heroic sorrow the way he did with Inger Jensen. Christ, did you see what he did with that one?'

The three men discussed Inger for some moments, and Mott learned that she had arrived in Oregon, where she could escape memories of NASA. 'She won't be single long,' Claggett said. 'I warned Debby Dee last night. "If that Swede is still around next autumn, out you go, babe, and in she comes."'

Now Pope broke in. 'Tucker's in a state of schizophrenia, and you better get out of bed real soon to straighten him up, Dr. Mott.'

'What's the problem? I should think he'd be overjoyed, an entire trip controlled by two men on his payroll.'

'That part's fine. Last night he told everyone at the Bali Hai, "We'll teach *Life* how to cover a space flight." But what eats him is the fact that of the six available wives—five, now that Inger's out—he gets for his exclusive the two he likes least.' And Pope counted on his fingers: 'He'd love to have Gloria Cater and that Mississippi charm. Or Cluny Bell and her sultry come-at-me, tiger. Or everybody's favorite rags-to-riches hillbilly, Sandy Lee. He could do wonders with any two of them. But what does he get? Debby Dee, who calls NASA brass "them stupid sonnombeeches," and Penny Pope, who insists on staying in Washington with no white fence and no kids.'

Claggett was laughing. 'I heard him tell Cater last night, "Well, we have to work with what we got." But we came on a different mission, Doc,' and he began to fumble with the shopping bag, taking from it a stack of books whose covers were lurid and torn. 'You take space too seriously, Doc. That's why you're flat on your ass and we're up and about. Now, the proper trainin' for an astronaut, or for someone like you who works with astronauts, is not all that calculus shit you bother your brains with, but some good old science fiction of the kind that got me and Pope started.'

'I never wasted my youth on that crap,' Pope protested.

Mott pointed out that of all the engineers he had known, practically none had bothered with science fiction, whereas almost all the scientists had. 'Why is that?' he asked his two visitors.

'I think you were always preoccupied with how to do it,' Pope suggested. 'The scientists were always far out, setting goals to try next.'

'How did you get hooked, Randy?' Mott asked.

'Those wonderful sexy covers. I didn't give a damn about science fiction, but I always hoped that the gorillas from outer space were gonna rip the rest of the clothes off and go at it. Month after month I longed for the miracle, but it never happened, and after about six years I was bright enough to see that they were connin' me, so I began to read the stories for the content. And they were very good.'

He had brought eight books, three anthologies with sexy covers, five full-length novels with covers featuring the anomalies of outer space, and as he passed them over to Mott, he spread the sexy items on the bed and said, 'It's always perplexed me. We speak of women as the weaker sex. But have you noticed these covers and the ads in the magazines? The men are always dressed to the hilt to protect them from the sun and the dust and the frozen snow, and the women are nearly naked. Look at these cosmonauts! Every inch of their body covered to ward off radiation. The women, hardly a stitch on.' With his hands on the anthologies he said, 'When I first joined my Marine squadron I thought, "These must be the brightest officers in the world. They all read the Sunday *New York Times*," and I was a dumb stiff from Texas, so I figured that if I wanted to keep up,

I'd better read the *Times* too, but then I found that all they read was the glossy magazine section, to see the naked women in the ads. Fifty science-fiction magazines don't give you half the naked women that a good issue of the Sunday *Times* does.'

'How am I supposed to read these?' Mott asked. 'Any special order?'

'There sure is, and I have 'em marked. Please read 'em in order, because then you'll get the drift. But I'm gonna read the first one aloud, so that you get started right.' And from one of the anthologies he began to read in his strong Texas voice a story much loved by sci-fi fans.

It was called 'To Serve Man,' and dealt with porcine visitors from outer space who arrive mysteriously on Earth with two inestimable boons: a way to neutralize all weaponry, so that perpetual peace can reign, and an unlimited free food supply, so that want will be eradicated. They also introduce better systems of government and one gentle innovation after another for the betterment of man.

The Earth is ecstatic, all except one suspicious computer expert who keeps trying to decipher a handbook one of the Earth's defensive men has acquired surreptitiously from the spacecraft. Day after day, as the rest of the world applauds the swinelike intruders, he labors at his task of breaking their code, and after many futile leads he succeeds in at least interpreting the title of the manual, *To Serve Man,* and with this reassurance the Earthlings accept the benevolent visitors at face value, realizing that a millennium has arrived.

But just as the hero of the story and his associates are entering the spacecraft for an exploratory trip to the distant planet from which the strangers came, the computer expert rushes out to warn them: 'It's a cookbook.'

'I like that!' Mott cried, and Claggett said, 'I thought you would.'

'Who wrote it?' Mott asked, and Claggett said, 'A favorite of mine. Damon Knight. You'll find other yarns by him in the anthologies.'

In the ensuing days Mott made his acquaintance with that gleaning of elegant stories crafted by men like Asimov, Bradbury and Leiber. Two of the shortest stories illustrated why their authors were deemed masters of the genre. The first was by Robert Heinlein and depicted a loud-mouthed drunk in a sleazy bar near a field from which a spacecraft is about to take off for some far planet. The man has suspicions about this particular experiment and a generally jaundiced view about exploration in general. 'Columbus Was a Dope' was the name of the tale.

The bore rambles on and on, reciting the pitfalls of space and the senselessness of further adventures, and nothing much seems to be happening until two glowing paragraphs at the end. The bartender throws one of his glasses into the air and watches approvingly as it drifts very slowly downward. Then he tells his listeners that working in one-sixth gravity has done wonders for his bunions, which had been killing him on Earth. The bar is on the Moon.

Mott was enchanted by the skill displayed in such stories, but the one which made the most lasting impression was by an Englishman living in Ceylon, Arthur C. Clarke, of whom even the astronauts who did not like sci-fi spoke highly. It was most adroitly told: a Jesuit priest is on an inter-planetary probe in what appears to be A.D. 2534, and he is much perplexed by the impact of science on his religion, but at last he reaches the environs of the Phoenix Nebula, whose central star exploded about 3500 B.C., becoming a mighty nova.

Of course, several planets near the star were consumed by fire, but at the far edges of what had been the star's planetary system—as far away as Pluto is from our Sun—one small planet had survived extinction. All life on it had been burned away, as life on Earth must some day be, but the rocky structure of the planet had survived, and when the exploring team reached the surface, they found that the people who had lived there thousands of years before, and had foreseen the extinction of their society, had compiled a record of what life had been like on their especially congenial planet. By means of tapes and maps and diagrams buried deep where fire could not touch them, they explained to those who they were sure would visit their homeland one day what a splendid, vibrant life they had enjoyed: the great cities, the accumulated knowledge, the happy lives. And the picture of their society was so enviable that the Jesuit wondered why God, in order to send His planet Earth a signal in the year 4 B.C., had set ablaze this great nova so that its light might guide three wise men to Bethlehem, while this remote planet with a civilization much more advanced than Earth's had had all of its living forms of life scorched away.

With real avidity Mott read Claggett's recommendations, and almost never was he disappointed, for the chaff had been winnowed away, leaving a core of stories that would have graced any imaginative literature. He was especially impressed by the writing of a man whose name he had never heard before, Stanley G. Weinberg, who during the 1930s had produced a small collection of stories which had lifted science fiction out of the swamp of little green men and naked ladies.

He wrote of the impending exploration of Mars with subtlety and almost love, populating the planet with creatures facing the real problems their inhospitable climate would create; these were stories in the great tradition of Petronius and Boccaccio, and Mott wanted to know more about him. He had started writing, the brief notes said, only when an inescapable death loomed, and he was allowed only eighteen months in which to report his vision.

When Mott read this his eyes filled with tears, and since he was alone he made no effort to halt them; he was thinking of Harry Jensen, that golden child who had been so carefully nurtured by his society for some great task and who had been struck down so senselessly by one of the worst manifestations of that society. He calculated the investment society had made in Jensen from the day he entered the University of Minnesota, through the airplanes he cracked up in flight training, to the heavy cost of his work at Edwards and on to the millions spent on him in NASA. But the greatest loss was what he might have contributed to the NASA program—he would have been one of the best—or to the American society later, because he and Inger stood for something. He could be a rowdy child, this Jensen, and he was not above ducking out for a quick weekend with Cindy Rhee in an Oklahoma motel, but he was a man and his loss was inconsolable.

Dead Jensen, wandering Millard in California, brittle Chris in trouble with the police, he loved them all. He wanted to grapple them to his heart, and through his tears he prayed for others: God, watch over Claggett and Pope, for these are good men.

Mott's recovery from his breakdown coincided with the completion of his reading, and when Claggett and Pope returned to pick up the books, he told them, 'It was fun, this course of study you set me. Are you interested in my reactions?'

'Blaze away,' Claggett said, imitating a machine gun. 'Shoot 'em down.'

'First the negatives. Some of your best writers sound like real fascists. I suppose you know that.'

'Some of the critics have been saying so,' Claggett conceded.

'And some of them really despise women.'

'So do some astronauts,' Claggett said. 'So do some bullfighters.'

'And they despise the world they're forced to live in, this imperfect Earth.'

'Don't we all?'

'And all of them except Weinberg— You know, Claggett, I thank you for bringing him to my attention. That man had something.'

'I guessed you'd like him. I find him too sentimental. My type is more "Bang-bang, let's atomize the planet Oom." '

'I was about to say they're all extremely militaristic. Real gunslingers.'

'A lot of good men are. Look how easy it is for the National Rifle Association to maintain membership.'

'And they have almost no patience with the less fortunate. They're elitist.'

'So were you, when you sat on the selection committee.'

'Worst of all, they're strongly antidemocratic. Their first choice would be a one-man dictatorship, a Hitler or a Mussolini or a Stalin, cleaned up a bit. Second choice would be a benevolent king. Our kind of democracy would be far, far down the line.'

'Science fiction is popular,' Claggett said, 'because a whole lot of people are beginning to think along those lines.'

'Final negative, the novels particularly, and many of the stories, are no more than good American westerns rewritten. Instead of a cowboy loving his horse, you fellows love your space machines.'

'No comment.'

'But the virtues of these books,' Mott said, touching them with his fingers, 'are many, and I can see why fellows like you, Claggett, find such enjoyment. They're very well written. Wonderful touches. Strong insights. You know, when you brought these books in here I expected juvenile junk. But these are well done, at least as good as some of the novels I used to read when I had spare time.

'And to a gratifying degree, they all had something substantial to say. They really grappled with ideas . . . concepts . . . the things about to happen. In that respect they were damned refreshing. But now let's get down to the nitty-gritty.'

'Yes,' Claggett said, 'I knew all you've said so far twenty years ago.'

'These men were far out on the frontier. They saw things that not even the NACA engineers at Langley were ready to accept as impending realities. I'm stirred by how clearly the best of these writers could visualize what was about to happen. Nothing we've been doing the last six years went unanticipated.'

'That's why I was so excited by these smoke dreams,' Claggett said. 'I was far out in space, and my teachers were futzing around with one hundred miles up. I've been one hundred miles up and it's not even a beginning. The Moon? Nothing. Send me to Mars. That's the first real step. These men were doing my thinking for me.'

'But in the midst of this praise we have to remember one thing. These men had a free ride. They never had to lay their lives or their reputations on the line. Men like me did not have that indulgence. We had to get a specific instrument weighing a given number of pounds to a given altitude and bring it back with all its telemetry functioning. We have to bring you two back with your telemetry in order.'

'But the books were fun, weren't they?' Claggett asked.

'They were. But I suspect it was only a childish sort of fun.'

'Isn't that the spirit we're trying to keep alive?' Claggett asked, and when he grinned the gap between his broken front teeth appeared as if in the face of a delighted child reading one of Edgar Rice Burroughs' books about the glamorous princesses on Mars.

Gemini, the flight of the Twins, was best seen as a provisional program halfway between the exploratory one-man flights of Mercury and the culminating three-man flights of Apollo. It had five obligations which had to be discharged before the more important Moon flights could be attempted: 1) to prove that two men could survive extended flights; 2) to compile information on the effect of weightlessness; 3) to prove that man could walk in space and perform specific operational tasks of importance; 4) to demonstrate that one spacecraft could rendezvous and dock with another; and 5) when these jobs were completed, to bring the capsule down very close to the designated rescue ship.

Each of these desiderata had been handled more or less successfully by one or another of the previous Gemini flights, but the tour planned for Claggett and Pope would endeavor to bring them all together in one master demonstration. It would, for example, cover sixteen days of fairly constant experimentation. The spacecraft would seek out and dock with two different target ships left orbiting in space from previous docking attempts, Agena-A in low orbit, Agena-B in one much higher, and when docking was completed with the latter, the Agena's rocket would be fired in an attempt to soar higher than man had ever gone before. John Pope would spend seventeen hours walking in space, doing repair jobs on the two Agenas. And Claggett vowed that he would bring his Gemini to splashdown within a quarter of a mile of the USS *Tulagi* waiting west of Hawaii.

The important flight had another overtone of which the two astronauts were especially aware. The six tremendously exciting flights of the one-man Mercury so far had been conducted by astronauts from the original Sacred Seven, while the two-man Gemini had been dominated by men from the charismatic Second Group—Armstrong, Borman, Lovell, Young—with some help from three of the Sacred Seven, Cooper, Schirra and Grissom. The adventurous work had been handled by the old-timers, and many thought that it should continue to be.

But Dr. Mott had argued strenuously, before his attack, that the less-dramatic men from the Solid Six should also be given a chance, along with a few from the Third Group, like Buzz Aldrin and Mike Collins. Randy Claggett had performed well in the right-hand seat of one flight, which had accomplished almost nothing because of parts failures, and his report on that mission was already a classic:

> Commander and pilot had accumulated a total of seven hundred hours in simulators and were as well prepared as they could normally have been. But at Allied Aviation in Los Angeles the people responsible for assembling the fuel tank ran into bad luck. I found that Mr. Bassett, who was responsible for the nonflammable lining, caught cold and was not on the job when the lining was inspected. His assistant, Mr. Krepke, was well prepared to stand in, but his wife went into labor pains three days early and he left. *His* assistant, Mr. Colvin, was in Seattle that day, consulting with Boeing, so the job was left to Mr. Swinheart, whose regular responsibility was the electrical wiring, and because he was so concerned about doing a good job on the lining, which he did backward, he forgot to check the wiring. *His* assistant, Mr. Untermacher, was absent that day because his eleven-year-old son was playing in a championship Little League game, so no word was passed to his assistant, a Mr. Sullivan, whom I did not see.
>
> As a result of the unfortunate omissions, the lining of the fuel tank was not secured and the electrical wiring was not given the final

inspection which would have shown even a high-school science teacher that the control switch would not work when activated. For these good reasons the three-hundred-million-dollar flight could not go forward, and only because the commander had iron balls did the crew land safely in the Pacific.

The crew for this culminating flight had been put together with studied care. Randy Claggett was a known factor, an unflappable test pilot who could bring to safety a seagull with two broken wings, and John Pope had the most reliable and solid record in the corps. He said little, always did twice as much as was required, and would have been voted by his fellow astronauts as the man they would prefer to have in the cockpit as their copilot, always assuming that it was they who sat in the left-hand seat. If the Solid Six could field a team with every chance of success, this was it, and everyone was pleased with the choice except Tucker Thompson, who had not even yet decided how to play these two difficult wives, Debby Dee and Penny. Debby Dee had stated that she would not come to Cocoa Beach and eat those sonnombeechin' oysters at the Bali Hai, while Penny said quietly that she would of course stay in Washington and follow the launch on the television set in her office.

Before the flight could be launched the two astronauts had to master one final skill, a most beautiful and intricate exercise, and the scholars whose job it was to drill them in it now appreciated the fact that NASA had required superior intelligence in the men who would go into space. Claggett and Pope would be required to project themselves into universes which could be perceived only intellectually.

Dr. Mott, in charge of this indoctrination, called the two men out to those vast salt flats surrounding Edwards Air Force Base, where he started with a simple two-dimensional experiment. Placing each man in a Jeep, with Pope well in front and Claggett trailing off to one side, he instructed them over headphones: 'Pope, maintain your heading without deviation in direction or speed. Steady fifty mph. Claggett, keep your eyes left and watch Pope's Jeep until you have a sure sense of what it's doing. Then accelerate to sixty-five mph and calculate a straight line that will carry you to a point where you feel sure you'll intercept him.'

They did this a dozen times, until Claggett became expert in calculating in his head the trajectory which would probably enable him to intersect; also, he could identify in advance the spot where the intersection would occur. In fact, he became a human computer, feeding into the kinesthetic part of his brain the relevant data and almost intuitively getting the answer.

Then Pope was placed in the pursuing Jeep, and in somewhat longer time than it had taken Claggett, he, too, converted himself into a computer.

'You're really quite remarkable,' Mott told them. 'You've acquired a very subtle coordination of eye, hand and foot for seeing, for steering and for acceleration. Both of you, in your last runs, achieved rendezvous in a straight line. But nothing you've learned on these salt flats applies in space.

'Because when you transpose this problem into space, you add the complicating factor of altitude, and everything you've learned changes. If you try by your own physical perceptions to bring your Gemini into rendezvous with your Agena, you'll fail every time. Oh, you can make a coincidence. You can come quite close. But at that moment you'll be in an entirely different orbit—you going one way, Agena another, and you'll pass slowly, beautifully, just out of range.'

He took the astronauts back to Edwards, and on a very big blackboard, drew a diagram which magically unlocked the system; it was a perfect demonstration of how one intelligent man can convey to another arcane facts that might never be comprehended without the aid of a drawing: 'This big circle is the Earth. This is its center. This first blue circle outside the Earth is your initial orbit in Gemini. This red circle farther out is the orbit of Agena-A. The green circle way out is the orbit of Agena-B. Now watch.'

From the center of the Earth he drew radii, not too far apart, which intersected the four circles: Earth's surface, Gemini orbit, the two Agena orbits, and with a very heavy line he emphasized on each circle the distance between the radii.

'The crucial fact to master is that the farther away from Earth you move, the slower your vehicle goes. When you're a hundred miles up in this blue circle, your speed will be about seventeen thousand five hundred mph. In the red circle, at two hundred miles, about seventeen thousand two hundred fifty. And the Moon, which is also a spacecraft far off the diagram, has an orbital speed of only two thousand three hundred mph. Remember, if you stay low, you go faster. But also, if you stay down here in the blue circle closest to Earth, the total length of an orbit is much shorter. So if you stay low, you gain two ways, speed and distance covered.'

He paused, reviewed what he had been saying, and added, 'I want you to burn this diagram into your brains. Because successful rendezvous depends upon understanding it.'

After they had analyzed every aspect of it, and had imagined themselves in their Gemini above the Earth but well below the orbits of the two target craft, Mott resumed. At the points where the left-hand radius cut the three circles he placed little magnetic simulations of the three spacecraft, and began his extraordinary explanation: 'Let's say that I am Agena-B way up here, Dr. Stanhope is Agena-A in middle position, and you two men are Gemini close in. You want to make rendezvous with me, all of us traveling at eighteen thousand miles an hour. What would you normally do, Claggett?'

'I'd eyeball it, calculate where the point of interception was, and burn my engines to get to it.'

'In other words, you'd burn your fuel to ascend toward Agena-B?'

'Sure.'

'Completely wrong. Look at the diagram. If you climb, you slow down as you move into a higher orbit. You're bound to wind up far, far behind your target and then waste fuel trying to catch up. By going faster, you actually go slower.'

'That sounds insane.'

'Let's take another example. You're in the same orbit as Agena-B, but trailing. How will you catch up?'

'I'm afraid to give you a sensible answer.'

'To catch up, you slow down. Drop into a lower orbit, where you acquire a faster speed, and you gain rapidly on your target in the higher orbit.'

'I can't believe it,' Claggett said, but Pope, who had continued his study of astronomy and celestial mechanics, cried, 'Hey! At the lower orbit, we'd be on the circumference of a much smaller circle.'

'Right,' Mott said, 'and going faster, to boot.'

'I'll take that on faith,' Claggett said. 'But how in hell do I ever get hooked up with that flyin' sonnombeech? If I burn toward it, I always miss.'

Mott clapped his hands. 'Randy, you've learned the big lesson,' and he drew other diagrams to illustrate the mysterious relationships of two hurtling spacecraft on near but different orbits, and Claggett asked, 'How will I ever find the proper orbit?' and Mott replied, 'You never would, not in a million years. But the computer will.'

The next maneuver that Mott proposed for his pupils was most complicated: 'Randy, you're in Gemini down here and you must intercept Agena-B up here. Don't go for the target. Burn straight ahead. Go faster to go slower.'

'Doc, I understand that part. But what in hell do I do next?'

'As you move to a higher orbit, your speed will begin to drop off, and believe it or not, if you obey the figures your computer will be feeding you, you'll bring your Gemini right in behind the target. The computer will time it so that when you're about a hundred feet apart, your speeds will be identical, and so will your orbit. Then your twelve-year-old son could dock the two vehicles, because you can make the Gemini move a quarter of a mile an hour faster than the Agena, ease it into a docking.'

Claggett and Pope looked at each other, and the former said, with his bright Texas grin, 'Like the pretty girl said in *My Fair Lady,* "I think I got it." '

'I believe the professor said that,' Mott said. 'And to protect you,' he added, 'we always time the docking so it occurs in the daylight part of the orbit.'

'Real thoughtful,' Claggett said.

'So think about the orbits tonight. Memorize the diagram. And keep telling yourself, "To go faster, I must go slower." '

Next day he placed them again in their Jeeps, taking them to a remote part of the salt flats, where he had marked three concentric roadways. 'Claggett, you're in Gemini orbit on the inside track. Pope, you're Agena-A next out. I'll be Agena-B farthest out. If we all start from the same radius, Gemini will drift far ahead, so Claggett must start from behind you.

'Remember, there's a specific speed associated with each orbit. You, Claggett, on the inside, have to drive at sixty mph, Pope at fifty-five, and me at fifty. When I tell you over the headphones "Burn engines," accelerate to sixty-five, but as you drift outward toward Pope's orbit, your speed will decrease well below Pope's, say to fifty. And that should put you in perfect position right behind him, which is what we want, isn't it?'

Under radio communication the three Jeeps started forth, and when they were in position Mott instructed: 'Claggett, burn engines, but when you have speed, try moving directly up at Pope, in the old way.' In three attempts, using the system that would have worked on land, Claggett failed miserably, so on the fourth try Mott suggested: 'Now try it the way we talked about. Burn straight ahead, pick up speed, then drift quietly up to Pope's orbit.'

With exquisite precision Randy Claggett accelerated to sixty-five mph, drifted up, slowed down as he had been taught, and with a final adjustment, matched his speed to Pope's in a perfect intercept. 'It can be done!' he shouted over the intercom, so for three hours the Jeeps moved back and forth in obedience to the new rules, until both Claggett and Pope could achieve rendezvous and docking while moving either up to a slower orbit or down to a faster.

For two days the men repeated these maneuvers, after which Mott astonished them by saying, 'Now you must forget everything I've taught you, because in space you're not on a flat surface where ordinary rules apply. You're in space, where eyeballing a problem does no good at all. The Russians have tried five times to make rendezvous and have failed every time, even though they show us photographs of their spaceships only a few leagues apart. They were on different orbits and they might as well have been ten thousand leagues apart, for they were never going to meet. Today when we go out to the circles, Claggett, you must imagine yourself not going across a salt flat to catch Pope, but on a diagonal right up into the sky, and your eyes will not be reliable judges of where you are.'

'What do I rely on?' Claggett asked.

'The computer. I'll be your computer, talking to you over the headphones.'

And when Claggett was seated in his Jeep, with the headphones adjusted, he could hear Mott's metallic voice feeding him instructions, and

rendezvous became so easy it was magnificent, a subtle adventure in nine
or ten different dimensions.

At the close of three additional days of drilling his two astronauts,
Computer-Mott said with some pride, 'You men will complete a perfect
rendezvous.'

But Randy, who became an automobile when he was driving or a plane
when flying, had a gut premonition which warned him that he still lacked
some vital understanding, and he asked, 'Doc, suppose that with all I know
personally, the on-board computer goes out.'

'You have a backup.'

'And suppose it goes out. There I am, bare-ass in space. Can I, with my
own intelligence, eyeball it carefully and achieve rendezvous?'

'Not in a million years.'

'Jesus! Those computers better work.'

'No sweat, because the duplicate computers in Houston can send you
the required data.'

'And if it's my bad day, and the radio goes out, too?'

Mott studied this for some time, forming diagrams in space with his
fingers. 'Knowing you, Randy, you'd make one futile try, then another, then
another. And when you realized that since they failed, all the rest would
fail, you'd bellow "Aw shit!" and drift off into space . . . permanently
. . . forever.'

And it was only then that the two astronauts appreciated the delicate
symbiosis of man-machine-computer that would enable them to make this
flight and this rendezvous.

At 0415 on Tuesday morning the two astronauts were awakened in the
isolation quarters, where extra precautions had kept them from contamination by colds or measles, for if they came into contact with either, the
sixteen-day flight might have to be aborted. Dressed in slacks and T-shirts
they had a carefully evaluated breakfast calculated to produce a minimum
of urine and fecal matter.

When the time came for assistants to dress them, and they climbed into
the ingenious underwear with its arrangements for handling urine and
bowel movements, Claggett studied the condom-like affair that fitted over
his penis and was reminded of the story about how Winston Churchill had
rescued the honor of the Allies at the meeting with Stalin at Teheran:

> 'Stalin wanted to throw a psychological scare into the Americans,
> so he said to Roosevelt in private, "Our greatest need to keep the
> morale of our fighting men high is rubbers. We just don't have any."
> And Roosevelt told him grandly, "We'll send you five hundred

thousand. What size?" Without blinking, Stalin said, "Sixteen inches long. Our standard size."

'Roosevelt confided that night to Churchill that Stalin was throwin' darts, but good old Churchill never blinked an eye. "Make 'em up and send 'em. But stamp each one, in English and Russian, *Texas medium.*"'

Claggett told his dresser that for his urine-catcher, 'my motorman's friend' he called it, he would take a Texas super, and the dresser said, 'You do that, my bucko, and you'll be lying in piss the whole flight.'

At dawn the two astronauts, fully suited, climbed with help into a waiting white van, which moved quietly past lines of people who had come to see the launch and across the marshes where alligators spawned, to the rim island where the majestic Titan rocket waited on end, with the almost minute passenger capsule on top.

The entire assembly reached 109 feet into the air, and seemed enormous as the first rays of the sun broke upon it, but when the waiting spectators, two hundred thousand of them, focused on only the capsule, they were aghast at how trivial it seemed, only nineteen feet long and ten feet across, outside measurements. Thus in flight, 82 percent of the total vehicle would break away and plunge into the sea.

The two men and their helpers moved with utmost precision because of a peculiarity of this flight: since they desired to make rendezvous with two different Agenas parked long ago in two different orbits, trajectory specialists like Dr. Mott had had to calculate to the second the proper moment for blast-off at Canaveral so that the Gemini capsule would reach the precise altitude (116 miles straight up) at the precise speed (18,000 miles an hour) at the precise moment (85 minutes 16 seconds after takeoff). Also, the relative position of the second Agena had to be cranked into the data, and when this was done, it was found that Claggett and Pope had a window for proper takeoff of only nine seconds, which meant that all things had to come together properly for ignition within a nine-second interval, and if for any reason it was missed, the astronauts would have to wait another eleven days.

As a matter of fact, at the final briefing Dr. Mott, sitting with his charts and his computer, had said, 'The optimum allows us a window of exactly two seconds, within the endurable nine. If we miss the two, we can still go, but we'll have to waste a lot of fuel to correct.'

If one remembered the endless delays of the early rocket flights, the sad disappointments of men sitting alone in their capsules atop some giant rocket for hours at a time, and the repeated postponements of the same rocket, so that no flight seemed ever to take off within hours of the time planned, the probability of getting this rocket off within a two-second window seemed remote.

An elevator carried the men up the gantry, alongside the glistening body of the rocket and onto the walkway that provided entrance to the capsule, and now the endless hours of stimulation paid off, because had the two men seen their prison for the next sixteen days cold turkey, and realized that they would have to lie side-by-side in that minute space for all those days, they might have panicked, and once a man allowed himself even to think of claustrophobia, he would be incapacitated. The space was so unbelievably cramped that when the astronauts were suited up in those bulky white Eskimo outfits, they lay literally touching, even pressing upon each other, in their narrow couches.

Claggett, as commander, slipped into the porthole first, adjusted himself to the sloping bed conformed in a soft, sturdy material to his particular body, then gave the signal for Pope to ease himself into the right-hand seat, and when all the elbows and knees and hips were adjusted, the two men occupied a space shockingly smaller than a very narrow single bed, and much shorter, too, for heads and toes exactly touched the limits of the capsule's interior. Men had been fitted into a specific contour for a specific mission to answer a specific question: Can two healthy men survive and work in such surroundings for sixteen days?

The hatch was closed and bolted shut. The bodies were eased this way and that. The quiet voice of fellow astronaut Mike Collins as CapCom started the countdown, and the two-second window approached.

'You have ignition,' CapCom said steadily. 'You have lift-off,' and it was good that he told them, for the men in the capsule atop the mighty rocket could barely feel the moment of firing, so smooth were the engines with their 430,000 pounds of upward thrust, sustained for moment after moment.

'Gentle as a baby's kiss,' Claggett reported, and then, with unbelievable persistence, the powerful engines kept thrusting upward, ever more powerfully, until at last the astronauts realized they were truly on their way to space.

Now the first stage of the rocket shut down, and for tantalizing seconds —hours it seemed—the rocket continued its climb in silence, but then the powerful second stage blasted off with 110,000 pounds of thrust, and this force acting on the relatively frail Gemini produced a sudden impact of seven full G's, so that Pope was jammed back into his contoured couch.

'Sayonara!' Claggett cried into his mike, and everyone in Mission Control realized that this was a phrase of farewell, elegantly appropriate, which Cindy Rhee had taught him.

'Houston!' Pope broke in. 'We have pogo.'

'We see it, Gemini,' CapCom said. It was a tradition that when astronauts were cooped in their tiny quarters, hundreds of miles from anything and thousands of miles into an orbit, only one person on ground must be allowed to communicate with them lest there be confusion in commands or a babel of voices, and that one person must be a fellow astronaut, preferably one who had already flown. Each flight tended to have four CapComs, coming on at intervals, and it was a second tradition that the

CapCom maintain a steady volume, a steady emphasis, a kind of bland streetcar-conductor tone, so that no accidental excitement be transferred across the vast spaces.

'How much pogo?' CapCom asked quietly.

'Vibration pronounced,' Pope reported. There was nothing that could be done to alleviate the bone-shattering pogo-stick leaping of the vast machine; it was as if a monster accordion player were activating the Titan rocket and its Gemini capsule.

And here was an anomaly of NASA. With the best brains in the world, it was as yet unable to prevent pogo or even to determine exactly what caused it. The violent, shaking contractions had appeared in the first Gemini flight and had continued through the tenth. Now it was assaulting this flight, and all the brilliance of NASA could not diminish it. The men could only hold tight and hope that it would go away, and after a while it did.

'Stand by for engine shutdown,' CapCom said. He was the final link in a tremendous chain of persons and machines around the world. At Mission Control in Houston hundreds of highly skilled men traced every item of the flight with their computers and charts. At radio stations in Australia, Spain, Madagascar and across America men listened to signals which assured them that this Gemini was sailing serenely, and on all the oceans ships kept silent watch.

Also, in the headquarters of every one of the 319 private companies that had supplied parts for the flight, men waited on call to provide immediate analysis if one of their parts failed to function, and in some ways they were the most expert of all, because they had made the parts and were intimately familiar with them.

Finally, at each of the many simulators in Houston or Canaveral or the other sites across America, men familiar with their operation waited in case it was necessary to visualize just what was going wrong in the capsule. At a signal, they would jump into the simulators and feed in data which would place them in a jeopardy imitating the one aloft.

When Ferdinand Magellan explored the Earth's oceans he and his men traveled alone in their frail ships, out of touch for years with their supporters in Spain, but when Claggett and Pope sought to explore the oceans of the upper sky they had immediate call upon about four hundred thousand assistants, and at times it was difficult to determine who was doing the exploring, Claggett and Pope or the men like Stanley Mott on the ground who fed them their information and their commands.

When pogo stopped, as mysteriously as it had begun, shutdown followed and the time came for Claggett to detonate the explosives which would separate the Titan rocket from the capsule, and after checking with Houston, he did so at the exact second dictated by the computer that was masterminding this intricate flight. There was a shattering explosion, a ripping away and a violent change in acceleration, after which the little capsule floated serenely into a nearly circular orbit, 116.7×164.6 miles above the surface of the Earth. Somewhere ahead lay the first target, Agena-A.

Now began one of the most curious experiences of mankind in recent decades. Agena-A was locked into its own secure orbit, which it had been following blindly, coldly for more than a year, and it was the job of this particular Gemini to enter that orbit, to fall in line behind the target, and slowly overtake it, thrusting the nose of the Gemini into the tail of Agena-A and making a lock, all at a speed of 18,000 miles an hour. It sounded difficult, but it was made immeasurably more so by the fact that an added dimension of complexity had to be taken into account.

At 00:02:21:36 into the flight (days-hours-minutes-seconds) Claggett informed Houston: 'I see the little stinker,' and Mike Collins at CapCom said quietly, 'We find you thirteen miles below and twenty-two miles ahead,' and Pope responded, 'Our computer says exactly the same.'

Coolly, as if he had performed the feat a hundred times, which in a sense he had, Randy made a series of the most delicate adjustments, which brought his spacecraft gently upward, at 18,000 miles an hour, until it found the orbit Agena-A was following. Deftly he edged the massive Gemini forward until it was close to the speeding target.

'Houston,' Pope said triumphantly. 'Would you believe it? At 02:22:07 into the flight we've made perfect rendezvous.'

'Proceed to dock,' CapCom said, and then a miracle of space occurred. The Gemini, traveling at an incomprehensible speed and weighing 8,400 pounds, edged inch by inch up to the Agena, weighing 1,700 pounds and also traveling at fantastic speed, and with the delicacy of a surgeon sewing together a torn heart, Claggett brought the two craft together and made a secure lock. The secret was simple: if both craft were flying at the same basic speed, docking was as easy as moving a car into a garage, for the relative speed could be kept to two or three miles an hour.

They docked and undocked three times to prove the practicality of this maneuver, and then Claggett told Houston: 'I want the right-hand seat to make the dock next time,' and CapCom, a new man now but an astronaut, agreed: 'Roger.' And Pope, with his heartbeat showing a slight increase on the monitor at Houston, eased his Gemini into position, then edged it forward, and made a perfect rendezvous. The pathway to the Moon was open; men could take two or more vehicles into space and rendezvous them, if their computers could place them in the right orbit at the right time.

For this very long flight the astronauts had agreed to keep their watches on Houston time, CST, and as this first long day ended after its flawless takeoff within the two-second window and the even more gratifying docking with Agena-A, the men went to sleep. Their craft was within two miles of Agena, but round and round the Earth they sped, these two massive vehicles, making a complete circuit of a twenty-four-hour Earth day of sunrise-sunset-sunrise every hour and twenty-six minutes.

And as they lay there, sleeping fitfully, they became indeed twins. If one rolled over, the other did also, because neither wished to breathe in the other's face. They had to plan every action so that it would not interfere with the man in the next couch, and even when one had to relieve himself, he did so with his face less than a foot from his companion's. And this would continue for sixteen days.

By the third day the Twins had adjusted rather well to their cramped quarters. Everything movable had been stowed, sometimes in the most ingenious way, and often the men gave thanks to that genius who invented Velcro, the miracle fabric with a million fingers that enabled them to attach pens and compasses and data books arbitrarily to any spot on the interior surface which had been covered with Velcro. The capsule looked like a room in the dollhouse of a very careless child.

They had almost no trouble with null gravity, except that they had to be extremely careful when they ate, lest crumbs float permanently about them. Liquids, if spilled, formed beautiful droplets, or if in large quantity, globules the size of a fist. But even in these first days they began to appreciate what Dr. Julius Feldman, their expert on health in space, had told them: 'The most dangerous part of weightlessness, especially in a Gemini capsule, is the fact that you don't exercise your legs. Let them remain motionless long enough and your muscles will atrophy so badly that they'll be too weak to support you when you try to walk after splashdown.' To prevent this, he had provided bungee cords, a device into which they could slip their feet and against which they could exert extreme pressures, thus providing the exercise the legs were not otherwise getting. Fortunately, such vigorous effort also diminished the likelihood of embolisms forming in the legs.

For the astronauts flew flat on their backs, day after day, with not nearly enough headroom, considering the couches and gear, to permit walking about. But they were able to climb out of their heavy suits, with extreme difficulty, taking about forty minutes to do the job, so that they flew in loose garments in relative comfort. It was interesting for one man to watch another emerge from his suit and stow it painfully under his couch. 'Hello, Chrysalis,' Claggett greeted Pope after one such exercise, and the latter broke into laughter as he said, 'I was thinking about those poor soft-shell crabs in the Chesapeake. Penny and I gorged on them when I was at Annapolis. The poor things struggle like this to get out of their shells, and as soon as they succeed, some cook plops them into a hot pan and sautés them.'

'How do you and Penny hack it, you in Houston, she in Washington?'

'We're a Navy family. Lots of good people live like us.'

'She's mighty good people. When she first stayed with us on Solomons Island, I found her a mite aloof.'

'I find her that way myself, sometimes. She holds down a complex job, you know?'

'She has class. She has mighty class. She's gonna be somebody one of these days.'

'She's somebody now. Randy, have you heard anything about Inger Jensen?'

'Two kids, Army pension. What else do you need to know?'

'How long was Debby Dee a widow before you married her?'

'Six months, eight months.'

'I hope somebody like you comes along for Inger.'

'I'd like to come along for that one. But I don't think I was such a catch for Deb. In many ways I'm a complete horse's ass.'

Pope did not ask in what ways, for he often felt the same way about himself.

On the sixth day Pope's time of testing approached, for he was required to climb into a special suit, strap cumbersome gear to his back, leave the capsule, and retrieve from the flank of Agena-A a dosimeter (dose meter) which had been left there a year earlier to monitor the amount of radiation accumulated by men voyaging in space. While walking, he would be attached to the mother craft by an umbilical which would bring him oxygen and he would carry a small kit of tools with which to work on the Agena.

It required more than an hour, with constant help from Claggett, to don the suit, and an unexpected fifteen minutes to wrestle open the door to the hatchway from which he would exit, but before this could be completed, Randy had to get into his spacesuit also, for once the hatch was opened, it would remain that way, which meant that the capsule would afford no oxygen. Both men would be in space, the difference being that Randy would remain inside the shell of the capsule.

This preliminary part of the exercise required much more time and energy than Pope had calculated, because in the simulators on Earth, things had gone rather more smoothly, and for a simple reason: the simulator existed in one G, so that by merely leaning an elbow against something, one gained stability; but in null gravity, if one pushed his elbow against a wall, even slightly, one sent his body spinning across the room and he could not stop his aimless flight until he succeeded in grasping something, which was why every astronaut who returned from space told those who debriefed him: 'More handholds. More footclamps.'

At last both astronauts were suited and the hatch opened. Outside waited the boundless reach of space, that colorless, weightless, formless medium in which the universe exists with all its stars and galaxies and mighty conformations as yet unknown to man. How majestic it was, how inviting, and as Pope hesitated in the doorway, he was like an infant about to leave the womb which had been so pleasant and enter the world which would be so infinitely more exciting.

To the east, as he calculated his position, although this term meant little, blazed the incredible Sun, wasting energy at a rate which must imperil it after another fifteen or twenty billion years, poor fated thing. It stood at the margin between Capricornus and Aquarius and thus obliterated Pope's guardian star, Altair, and its bright associate Vega. To the west, or away from the Sun, shone the dark night with the glorious winter constellations in view: Orion, the Lion and the one that watched over this flight, Gemini. No astronaut who went into space would know more about the stars than Pope, and now as he prepared to walk among them he greeted them as if they had always been his counselors, and took quiet delight in the fact that he would see those southern constellations which his first professor, Anderssen of Fremont State, had never been allowed to see: 'I'll say hello for him to Achernar and Miaplacidus.'

Most impressive of all, below rode the planet Earth, its features ascertainable when in daylight, barely suggested when its spinning carried one-half the surface into darkness. How big it seemed at times, how small now as Pope looked down upon it from a distance: 'Hey, Randy. It really is a planet.'

'Jump, you chicken.' And he was off into space.

He moved with all four extremities slightly extended, like a falling parachute diver, but he did not fall, for there was no gravity to command him, or rather, as he had phrased it to himself so many times: There is gravity from every item in the universe, even my wife's teacup exerts its gravity upon the Galaxy Andromeda, but it doesn't factor very much. Of course, the Earth's mass, slightly less than two hundred miles distant, continued to exert enormous gravitational pull, but it was so delicately counterbalanced by the centrifugal force generated by the spacecraft's forward velocity that Pope was effectively free of any detectable gravitational effects.

He was aware that he had started the EVA (Extra Vehicular Activity) rather tired, so he moved cautiously in his approach to the waiting Agena, and he supposed that when he reached the monster he would find time to rest, but when he got there he found himself confronted by an entirely new problem. There was nothing he could grab hold of, and when he endeavored to fasten himself to the huge, slippery target he merely drifted about, bruising his knees and elbows as he struggled vainly to hold fast.

After a half-hour of this he was sweating so furiously that his face mask began to steam, so he slowed down, but then he remembered that he was supposed to detach the dosimeter from the Agena and bring it back to Earth, so he moved awkwardly along the hulk till he reached the three bolts holding it. And then he faced a new problem, for when he took from his kit the special monkey wrench and fitted it to one of the nuts, he found he could accomplish nothing. If he applied pressure to the wrench handle, hoping thus to apply torque to the nut, he found that since he had no purchase, it was he and not the nut that revolved. No matter how simple the task he attempted, whenever he exerted force in one direction, his body flew off in the opposite.

For twenty minutes he tried vainly to perform the planned task, and accomplished nothing. Tears of frustration came to his eyes and fogged his visor, and all the joy of walking free in space was dissipated; what was worse, he was becoming so dangerously debilitated that he must in common prudence pull himself back to the capsule before he became so totally exhausted that Claggett would have to undertake the impossible task of maneuvering an inert mass.

'I'm coming in,' he told his partner.

'You're scheduled for thirty-four more minutes.'

'I'm coming in or you'll have to come out and get me,' and when he reached the hatchway to the capsule he was much too tired to climb in, and he rested there for nearly half an hour until he recovered his strength.

'It's no picnic out there,' he said when he got his helmet off in the repressurized capsule.

'Next time better luck,' Claggett said. As commander of this flight he refused to accept defeat on any point, but he also knew that Pope had been near collapse.

He devised an interesting amusement for the next flight walk. When the astronauts accumulated a body of refuse, including bags of urine, they vented it through an ingenious system of locks, and in doing so one morning —Houston time, because in this orbit a kind of morning occurred every hour and twenty-six minutes—some of the ejecta had smeared Claggett's window and he complained about it so constantly that on the spur of the moment Pope said, 'I'll go out and give it a wash,' which was what Claggett had intended.

This time the space walk was a huge success, for it pertained only to the Gemini itself, which, being the last in the series, had been modified by McDonnell to provide some sixteen extra handholds and footclamps. Now Pope had something to wedge himself against so that he could use the flattened expanse of his body to counterbalance the return thrust of whatever he was working upon, and in this way he was able to apply torque without having it spin him around. Also, by moving himself to the opposite side of the craft, he could give Claggett's window an effective cleaning.

That night the two men talked at length with Houston to see if anyone could devise some way that would enable Pope to retrieve the dosimeter, and CapCom said quietly, 'Dr. Feldman is most eager for you to retrieve it. Data are badly needed on the accumulation of radiation in space,' and Pope replied, 'Give me some guidance,' so three astronauts hurried to the deep swimming pool at Huntsville, and after suiting up and applying weights to their belts, achieved the sensation of null gravity and went underwater to work on a mock-up of the Agena hull. They suggested that Pope try establishing leverage by hooking his left foot in a hold he had overlooked, by approaching the nuts from a different angle, and by keeping his belly, one leg and one elbow disposed so as to distribute his weight differently: 'We think this will allow you to apply torque.' He went to sleep at what they had agreed to call night, swearing to Claggett, 'If I have to use my teeth, I'm going to loosen those bolts,' but Claggett had a better idea: 'I think we stowed a tiny can of oil somewhere in here, and I want you to go over one hour early and soup 'em up.'

Next morning the two men dressed extremely slowly, allowing no perspiration to accumulate, and then they opened the hatch with a minimum of effort, and Pope, taking very slow breaths to control his respiration, left the capsule carrying almost nothing except the tiny can of oil, which he applied to the bolts before returning to the capsule. He did not try to climb back in, but simply held on, drifting across Africa and Australia, to whose communicators he spoke.

'I feel great,' he assured Claggett, and when the latter handed him the tool kit, he set off for the Agena with real enthusiasm. Positioning himself astride the huge craft as the Houston men had advised, he found that by grasping it with one foot, one knee, one elbow and gut, he could achieve a kind of leverage, so that when he began to twist the lubricated nuts, they moved and not he.

'Semper fidelis!' he called to Claggett as he unbolted the dosimeter, stowing it carefully in a pouch attached to his belt, but when it worked free, one bolt fell away . . . well, it certainly didn't *fall* away, for there was no gravity to attract it, but it slid out of his control and moved away from the Agena, impelled by his futile attempt to retrieve it, and there it drifted like a minute planet, circling the Earth at an altitude of 149.3 miles above the surface, 4,108.9 miles above the molten center.

Six days had now passed, and the next three were spent uneventfully discharging tasks which had been set by the ground experts, especially the space scientists. This series required the most exact timing, collection of data and attention:

. . . Study the effects of weightlessness on neurospora to see if any genetic damage is done by extended voyages in space.

. . . Make 149 photographs of different Earth terrains using the Maurer camera.

. . . Make 36 photographs of gegenschein, the faint nebulosity which appears opposite the Sun in certain conditions.

. . . Investigate the L-4 and L-5 equilibrium points of the Earth-Moon system to determine whether clouds of particulate matter have collected as predicted by LaGrange in 1772.

. . . Check UHF-VHF polarization as it affects radio transmission through the atmosphere.

. . . Accumulate data on frog-egg growth in space.

. . . Do bioassays of body fluids, which meant urinating into a special bag. (But this study failed because Claggett broke his bag twice. The medics were sure he did it on purpose.)

On the tenth day they rose early, stowed every piece of movable gear, fastening pens and cups to the walls with Velcro, against the violent shock which they would soon receive. Checking with Houston, they reassured themselves that Agena-B, the one with ample fuel and good engines, was about twenty miles behind them, so they speeded up sharply in order to fall back, and as soon as they attained a higher orbit, the Agena, below them, started moving ahead. When it was well in the lead, they slowed down so that their relative speed would increase, and sure enough, they came right in on target, making a docking so perfect they could not feel the join.

'Houston, we're ready for fire.'

'Everything is go,' CapCom said, and with that vote of confidence, Claggett fired the powerful main engine of the Agena, which the Twins were facing, and for a full twenty-nine seconds a wild explosion of fire and flying fragments engulfed the capsule as the men felt six G's knocking them about. At an additional speed of 469 miles per hour, the whole assembly shot away from Earth until it reached an orbit of 748.3 miles, higher than any man had gone before.

'Holy cow!' Claggett cried into the mike. 'Houston, that was some sleigh ride.' And then, with the world listening, he added a most unfortunate afterthought: 'If God was a golfer and made an approach shot like that with a niblick, He would be cheering.' Thousands of religious listeners felt that he had blasphemed, and NASA would spend hours and days denying that that had been his intention. 'God is not a golfer,' one of the journals said in harsh rebuke, and Thompson would have difficulty preventing Claggett from responding, 'Well, if He is, He made a great niblick shot on that one.'

Pope was more restrained, and his enthusiastic words were piped eagerly into the worldwide communications system, to be heard instantaneously in the very parts of Earth about which he was speaking: 'Oh, how magnificent the Earth is from here! I can see its edge as it starts on the way back. The line between night and day down there is as clean as a knife edge. Oh! Oh! There's Africa exactly as it should be. And the oceans are blue and I see Asia coming up. Oh, the Himalayas. You should see the beauty of our Earth.'

It was his casual, tourist photographs, more than two hundred of them made at this great height, that first showed the people of Earth what their planet looked like and what majestic colors it commanded, and the precious thing it was. And at the apogee of their flight, when the Agena was shuddering into permanent orbit, Claggett cried to all the Earth: 'I wish we could go on forever.'

The Twins landed in the Pacific Ocean, 781 yards downstream of the *Tulagi,* where they had been ordered to land sixteen days and 7,000,000 miles ago, and at the debriefing the men voiced only two complaints. Pope: 'Claggett took country music on his tapes, and I never again want to hear women singing through their noses.' Claggett: 'John took what he claimed was Bach and Bartok, and I don't never want to hear no more of that spaghetti music.'

The Claggett-Pope flight was so successful in every detail, except the collection of urine, that the Gemini program was allowed quietly to phase out. It had served its purposes splendidly, and its cost of $1,147,300,000 had been amply repaid, for Gemini proved that men could survive handsomely in zero G if they exercised their legs, that they could take two monster craft aloft and join them as gently as if they were baby carriages, that they could walk in space and complete tasks if, like Archimedes, they could only find a fulcrum, and that a trip to the Moon was only an extension of the flight that Claggett had contemplated when he cried, 'I wish we could go on forever.'

And then the goodies began falling into the laps of the Twins. They addressed a joint session of Congress, had ticker-tape parades, were sent to seven foreign countries as ambassadors and counterthrusts to Yuri Gagarin and his cosmonauts, and were offered free automobiles and enticing real estate deals. But what was really significant, having proved their professionalism, they found it much easier to get T-38s when they wanted them, and in these sleek, swift jets they sped from one part of the country to another, making practical suggestions for the Apollo program that would soon carry them to the Moon.

The Greek word is *hubris,* the central theme of the great tragedians. It designates that pride and insolence which infuriates the gods and causes them to strike men down at the height of their success. Hubris had invaded the NASA program, and on the afternoon of 21 February 1967, when three astronauts were running through a routine drill in their capsule atop a Saturn rocket at Canaveral, an unguarded electrical wire threw a spark into the pure oxygen of the cabin, and the resulting fire cremated the men.

The surviving Solid Six were at the Bali Hai when this occurred, and as the news spread through the community the families clustered automatically together, and Penny Pope was flown to the Cape in a NASA plane, and the ten young people sat in the Dagger Bar—the Claggetts, the Lees, the Bells, the Caters, the Popes—reflecting on the inexorable movement of which they were a part, while in a corner Rhee Soon-Ka sat, unobserved, taking notes, for this was the kind of day she had long anticipated: as a modern Aeschylus, she knew what hubris was.

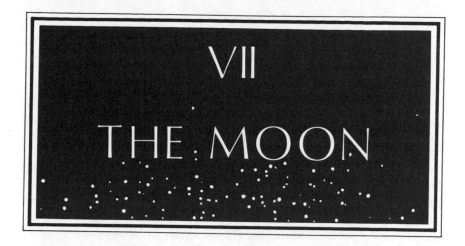

VII

THE MOON

ONLY ONCE DID THE FOUR FAMILIES SO INTRICATELY INVOLVED IN America's space program meet together in one place at one time, and that occurred in the Longhorn Motel in a dusty suburb of Houston, Texas, during the climactic July in 1969 when astronauts finally walked on the Moon.

In preceding years, of course, the men had met one another but never in concert. For example, Senator Grant had known John Pope as a boy in his hometown and had helped get him into Annapolis; he had often consulted with Stanley Mott, sometimes on personal matters; and he had twice summoned Kolff to his Washington offices for reports on what was happening in Alabama, but he had never seen the three together.

No one of the wives had ever seen all of the other three, not even Penny Pope, who might have been expected to. She had certainly met with the senator's wife, for the two women had grown up in the same town, and she'd had many occasions for meeting Rachel Mott, but she had never gone down to Alabama to meet Liesl Kolff, who had never ventured into Washington. In fact, the only wife Liesl Kolff knew was Rachel Mott, whom she loved like a younger sister.

The families should have met a few days earlier at the Cape Canaveral launch of Apollo II; the four men had of course been there to discharge official duties, but two of the wives, Elinor Grant and Liesl Kolff, had preferred staying home. The meeting between Stanley Mott and Dieter Kolff, after seven years of strained separation during which each man had concentrated on his own unique problems, was an emotional one, for Dieter, in a surrender of his old prejudice against manned flight, ran forward to embrace the man who had saved him. 'Stanley, what an hour of triumph for you!' Mott clasped the engineer and said, 'The triumph is yours, old fellow! That day I found you in Germany you promised: "I'll send a rocket to the Moon." And in a few hours we'll be there, your rocket and my man.'

The bitterness returned, and Dieter said, 'Not my rocket. It won't get there. You chose the other solution, the wrong one.'

Mott, not wishing to reopen that old wound, asked brightly, 'Where's Liesl?' and Dieter said, 'She was afraid to come.'

For many years Liesl Kolff had wanted to see the installations in which her husband spent so much of his time, but she had been apprehensive of participating in the gala celebrations which attended the launch in Florida: 'I'd be out of place. All those expensive wives in their expensive clothes.' Now, with an opportunity to visit Houston, the very center of space activity, she still demurred. She would have preferred Boston, where her son Magnus had been offered a summer job with Arthur Fiedler and the Boston Symphony Pops, with the promise that if he passed rigid tests, he would be given the position of second trumpet for the winter season of 1970 and those to follow. Magnus had known of his mother's dilemma and over the telephone from Boston had told her: 'Go to Texas, Mom. You can see me anytime the next ten years. I'm determined to win the permanent job.' On the night when the astronauts were supposed to land on the Moon he would face his major test: solo part in Stradella's lyric Concerto in D Major for Trumpet. 'Please, Mom, go to Houston with Father.' She complied, and was delighted with the Longhorn Motel and the respect shown her husband.

Senator Grant had been ordered by President Nixon to be in Florida for the launch and now in Texas for the landing, and for a very solid reason. As one White House staffer pointed out: 'The damned Democrats have been trying to steal this show for years. Kennedy, Johnson, Glancey. You're our top Republican in the program, Norman, and the President wants you to be damned visible.' The young man had added, 'They'll make it a highly social affair, with lots of photography and television. Be sure to take your wife.'

On the Florida trip Grant had been unable to persuade Elinor to come along; she insisted upon staying home, and for a very good reason: on the Monday before lift-off she had received from Dr. Strabismus an urgent telegram informing her, and a select handful of other $72 subscribers, exactly what was happening:

Do not be alarmed if the tottering American government tries to place a man on the Moon. This has been orchestrated by those Visitors who infiltrated NASA seven years ago, as I warned you at the time. Ordinary American scientists could not possibly have solved the difficult problems involved in a Moon shot. The Visitors could.

Our informants within the Visitor ranks assure us that very secure colonies have been established by them on the dark side of the Moon, away from our telescopes, and that when our men try to land, every assistance will be given. This will ensure that the attempt will be successful, because the Visitors want us to be preoccupied with the Moon while they finalize their assumption of power in Washington. These are critical days, but do not be deceived by the Moon landing. The really important event will be the impending takeover in Washington, London, Rome and Tokyo.

Elinor had felt that she could probably help the nation most by staying in Clay to cooperate with the Visitors, so she missed the excitement of the lift-off, viewed by more than a million people lining the Florida roads, but when the White House itself telephoned to urge her to attend the celebrations in Houston which would accompany a successful Moon landing, she had to listen. Calling the headquarters of USA in Los Angeles, she asked Dr. Strabismus whether in his opinion it would be permissible for her to leave home on the eve of the Visitors' takeover, and he said it would be all right, for they had assured him that it would be peaceful. So she joined her husband at the Longhorn Motel.

Rachel Mott was still shepherding the wives of her astronauts, but since the emphasis would now be on the families of the men about to attack the Moon, she had free time to be with her husband, and she needed the semivacation. She had been spending long hours with her son Christopher, who seemed to thrive under the relaxing Florida sun. He had been suspended from the University of Maryland for grades that were abominably low, but she felt sure that the stabilizing influence of family life would enable him to resume his studies. She wanted him to accompany her to Houston, but he had preferred staying in Florida, where he would be attending anti-Vietnam rallies in Miami.

When Penny Pope brought her senators back to Washington after the hugely successful launch of Apollo 11, tough-minded Mike Glancey took her aside. 'This is top secret, but President Nixon's insisting that Elinor Grant attend the Moon-landing celebration at Houston. She's as crazy as a bedbug and it's your job to see she stays undercover.' When Penny protested that she was not a baby-sitter, Glancey growled, 'This time you are. There would be hell to pay if European newspapers got hold of the fact that a leading member of our Space Committee had a fruitcake wife who was peddling state secrets to little green men.' It would be Penny's job to keep Mrs. Grant isolated until either the shot succeeded or the little men took over.

At half past eleven on this dramatic day, when the temperature outside was a boiling ninety-six, the four couples sat down to lunch in a reserved corner of the Longhorn bar. Two televisions had been brought in at Senator Grant's request so that he and his guests could listen to both Walter Cronkite and John Chancellor, and after two rounds of cocktails, which John Pope and Liesl Kolff refused, the euphoric lunch began with large plates of Louisiana oysters. Liesl refused these, too, having been indoctrinated from her earliest days in El Paso with the belief that one could eat oysters safely only in months containing an r.

Liesl Kolff was in some ways the most interesting of the group, for with a stubborn peasant sense of destiny, she had allowed a varied experience to modify her very little. As a girl she had been destined to be fat, and she was, a roly-poly woman in her early fifties composed of three rather shapeless globes: a large head with fat cheeks, a very large torso ill hidden by an inexpensive flowered dress, and an extremely large bottom which protruded strikingly. She wore heavy-rimmed glasses that accented the fullness of her face; she had been told often that if she chose glasses with no rims, she would look better, and she had tried this, but she was essentially clumsy and after she had broken the rimless glasses twice she threw them away: 'Chust one trick by the doctors to get our money.' She confessed to her son Magnus that in the rimless glasses she had looked better, 'but I got no time for vanity. These other glasses, you could chump on them, they don't break.'

'I understand you didn't want to come,' Senator Grant said as they waited for the chicken salad.

'I didn't,' Liesl said.

'But this is a triumph for your husband.'

'He has many triumphs. Today is also a triumph for my son. His first.'

'And what has he done?'

'Tonight he plays the Stradella, a trumpet concerto, with the Boston Symphony.'

'Your son? How old is he?'

'Twenty-two.'

'Isn't that delightful! Elinor, Mrs. Kolff's son is only twenty-two and he's playing trumpet with a famous orchestra.'

Elinor smiled indulgently without making any comment; she felt quite detached from this assembly, for she faced problems that they could not remotely be aware of, and furthermore, she had learned that whenever the senator praised some young person who was behaving well, he intended it as a rebuke to her for having allowed their daughter Marcia to behave, as he always put it, 'so poorly.' As for herself, she considered Marcia an outstanding success, to be dean of a major university at such a young age. She nodded slightly to Mrs. Kolff, as if to say, 'I'm pleased that you've found some satisfaction in this country. You look as if you needed it.'

Despite her aloofness, Mrs. Grant did now and then steal a glance at Mrs. Pope to see if this brazen creature would betray in any manner the fact that she was sleeping with the senator, but the adventuress was a wily one who disclosed nothing. Mrs. Grant deemed it outrageous that her husband would have the effrontery to bring this woman to Houston, and she felt sorry for Commander Pope, who seemed a fairly decent young man, which was to be expected, since he was the son of Dr. Pope the druggist. Penny Pope, she never forgot, came from one of the poorer Clay families, one without distinction, so her immoral behavior was no surprise.

At about the time the salad was served, excitement on the television stations began to escalate, for it was apparent that the astronauts were preparing the dangerous and thrilling descent to the Moon, so the diners ignored their food, except for Mrs. Kolff, who was hungry, not having had the oysters, and talk turned to the miracle of receiving television signals across a space of 238,000 miles.

'They could come from 238,000,000 miles,' Kolff said simply. 'As long as it's a straight line, no mountains, no planet to interfere, an electrical signal will go forever.'

When Senator Grant challenged this, Kolff put down his fork and asked, 'How much electrical power to send a radio message, Moon to Earth?' Everyone but Mott and Pope made extravagant guesses, whereupon he went to a bridge lamp and turned on a sixty-watt bulb, which competed poorly with the light from the two televisions. 'One twentieth of that bulb will do it well,' he said.

Discussion raged about this claim, and Kolff had to bring in Dr. Mott for assistance: 'Yes, one of these days we'll have a radio at Saturn, more than a billion miles away. With power much less than that light bulb, it will send us messages, quite easily. It's like Kolff says, if a straight line is uninterrupted by mountains or other interjections, the signal goes on forever.'

'Is what we're seeing from the Moon instantaneous?' Grant asked.

'Not at all,' Mott said. 'When Pope here speaks to the man in the capsule, 238,000 miles separate the two men. And since an electrical impulse travels at the speed of light, it requires 1.3 seconds for Pope's voice to reach the Moon. When Mike Collins up there replies, it takes another 1.3 seconds for his voice to come back to us.'

'And if we ever go to Mars, like they keep telling us, what time lag?'

'I don't have the exact distance to Mars . . .'

'About two hundred million miles in the most likely configuration of orbits,' Kolff interjected, and Mott bowed in his direction.

'That'll require eighteen minutes up and eighteen back down.'

'Can we send men to Mars?' Grant asked Mott, but before the latter could respond, Kolff broke in: 'Of course! I could build a rocket which would carry a man safely to Mars. Next year.'

Grant, who knew that some 450,000 different Americans were engaged in supporting today's Moon shot, did not appreciate the German's saying that *he* could get to Mars; it would require more than half a million men, more than twenty billion new dollars.

But such calculations were made meaningless by events at the Moon itself, for the astronauts Armstrong and Aldrin were preparing to break loose from their mother ship and drop down to the surface of the dead minor target.

'I still can't believe it,' Grant said. He was fifty-five now, a handsome older man with a grave worried countenance, graying hair and the stable professional look that one acquires after long years of service in Washington. He had been very close to the space program, one of its pillars, but he had usually been required to provide vast sums of money for projects he did not really understand, and now he was faced by a moment of triumph which was totally incomprehensible, with Dieter Kolff telling him that soon other men would be on Mars. He was almost as confused as his wife, except that her adventures cost thousands of dollars; his, billions.

Seven of the eight people picked at their food while Liesl Kolff asked the waiter for a second helping of salad. 'You can have mine,' Elinor Grant said generously. 'I haven't touched it.'

It was two o'clock, Central Standard Time, 20 July 1969 when the dishes were cleared away and an ice bucket filled with bottles of beer was brought in. Dieter Kolff took the caps off two bottles, handing one to his wife, but she refused: 'The Americans make their beer too weak, too sweet.' Grant summoned the waiter to see if he could fetch any German beer. 'Mexican is good,' Liesl said. 'Or Filipino. Or even Danish.' The motel had some Tuborg and she was content.

Penny Pope was on the telephone to Senator Glancey's office in Washington, and between long pauses she shared information with the people in the room: 'Things look unbelievably good. Maybe within the hour.'

Now the tension mounted, and Grant kept revolving an empty ginger ale bottle in his two hands, staring at first one television screen, then the other. The images were excellent and he said, 'Damn, we do some things right. Look at that.'

As the landing module began its descent, the actual approach to the Moon after all these years of travail, Penny Pope went to stand with her husband, who better than the others could understand the significance of the moment, and she took his hand. Mrs. Kolff did the same with her husband, recalling the years when his optimism alone seemed to keep the Peenemünde men working on their great dream. Mrs. Mott wanted to go to her husband, too, but she could not, for Mrs. Grant held her by the hand, assuring her in a low voice that what was happening on the television screens, which she refused to look at, was trivial compared to what was about to happen in the world generally. 'You have no idea, my dear, but I feel assured that men like your husband who know so much will be of extra value when it all happens.'

'When what happens?'

'You'll see.'

Mott stood beside Senator Grant's chair, sipping idly at a beer that was growing increasingly warm. 'This is almost unbearable. I helped plot the trajectories, and to see them come alive. You know, this is really quite extraordinary. Those men will land precisely where we planned three years ago.'

'This is a great day for America,' Grant said, and before his eyes flashed the other days that he remembered: the Japanese fleet bursting out of the dawn to destroy MacArthur; Gawain Butler, that gallant man fighting off the sharks; the morning when Senator Taft led him into the well of the Senate to be sworn in, his own senior senator having been called away by death; death, yes, the assassination of John Kennedy, a man he had never much liked, a dilettante but one who caused little harm; the resounding triumph of Richard Nixon over Hubert Humphrey, a clown really, the latter, a man in no way entitled to be President; and often among the images the face of good old Mike Glancey of Red River, a Democrat but a man you could trust and not at all like Lyndon Johnson, whose Presidency had been such a mishmash.

'This nation has its great days,' Grant said, clasping Mott's hand.

Now silence filled the afternoon. Even the televisions seemed to halt out of respect for the tremendous moment at hand, and then came the news that reassured the world: 'Houston. Tranquility Base here. The Eagle has landed.' For just a second no one spoke, then two of the men, Grant and Mott, showed tears of exultation, and to everyone's surprise Dieter Kolff leaped up and down like a maniac, shouting first in German, then English, 'It is done!'

'Oh my God,' Grant mumbled. 'The risks we took.' He pointed to one of the televisions and asked no one in particular, 'Do you realize the risks we took? The whole world watching?'

John Pope started the real celebration by kissing Penny, who had tears in her eyes, and she turned to kiss Senator Grant, whose fortitude she had so often witnessed. 'We did it,' she cried. 'In our bumbling way we did it.'

It would be six and a half hours before the astronauts actually left their module to step upon the Moon, and everyone was prepared to wait for the historic moment, so the dishes were cleared away and fresh drinks brought in, with three bottles of Tuborg for Liesl Kolff. Many telephone calls were placed by Penny Pope, with the senator saying, 'Charge them to the committee. This is one day in a century.'

One call was to Skycrest, Colorado, where Millard Mott and his friend Roger were running a health-food store, which would scarcely have survived except that the young men had two profitable sidelines, cheese-and-wine parties and a fine selection of classical records. They were elated with the Moon shot and Roger told the senior Motts, 'You'll never know how proud of you Millard is. He's a champion, you know.'

Penny reached Magnus Kolff in Boston just before he was about to go on stage, and he told his parents that he was a celebrity this night, because the other musicians knew that his father had helped build the rocket that did the trick. 'When the doorman called me to the phone he said, "Houston Spacecraft Center calling" loud enough for the others to hear. I am so happy for you, Father.' He spoke in English, his parents in German.

Mrs. Grant placed only one call, to Dr. Strabismus, who told her, 'Everything is stable. Our colony on the dark side of the Moon is standing by to give every assistance. They'll see that our men succeed.'

John Pope spoke frequently to Mission Control, where excitement crackled on the telephone; it was a triumph for so many men, and one of them said, 'Tell that old son-of-a-bitch Stanley Mott that he was on the beam when he sponsored lunar-orbit rendezvous.' And when Pope relayed this message, Mott asked Penny if she could get the NASA base at Langley in Virginia. When she did, he talked with the engineers there who had inducted him into the world of space and thanked them.

Grant took a dozen calls, one from President Nixon but none from his own daughter in Los Angeles, and when the furor quieted he asked the Kolffs, 'How did your son learn the trumpet . . . so young?'

Liesl Kolff answered, eagerly, 'In America you want people to learn. Mrs. Mott, here, she taught us English at El Paso. No charge. When we move to Huntsville, first day they give out band instruments. How old was Magnus? Four maybe, he took one.'

'But we had trouble,' Dieter said. 'You might say the big decision, when he wanted to do funnies with the football band. I put my foot down. "You do not do funnies with Beethoven." He wanted to cry.'

'How were you able to make him see things your way?' Rachel Mott broke in.

'You tell him once, he don't listen,' Liesl said. 'You tell him twice, he shouts at you. So you don't tell him a third time. You get a hammer and smash his trumpet.'

Dieter laughed. 'It belonged to the school. We had to pay for it. Magnus was so ashamed, he said a truck ran over it, his fault.'

'We got him a better one, and with it he joined our little orchestra. Then University of Alabama. Then Munich for one year. Now Boston, maybe forever.'

'You must be very proud,' Rachel said.

'We are,' Liesl replied.

Grant turned to the Motts. 'Weren't you having a little trouble with your son?'

'Both of them,' Rachel said. 'And not just a little.'

'In what respect?'

Stanley Mott was hesitant to speak of family troubles, but his no-nonsense wife was not, and appearing almost prim and an epitome of rectitude, this forty-nine-year-old New England woman said, 'Life styles, I think. Our eldest son—' She corrected herself. 'Our elder son seems not to like girls. He's living with a young man about his own age in Skycrest, Colorado. They run a shop featuring health foods.' And before anyone could comment, she added quite firmly, 'We've made our peace with Millard. He's a fine, gentle boy and we have no doubt he'll be the same kind of man.'

'He's twenty-six,' Mott said.

'I think of him still as a boy,' Rachel said, and her husband added, 'It's a shock when your son exhibits traits that you, well . . .' He stopped in confusion, then blurted out: 'We're lending him the money to get his store started, and I for one am proud of what he's been able to accomplish. He's well spoken of in the Skycrest community.'

'Young Christopher's troubles are more serious,' Rachel said. 'He's been arrested for selling marijuana.'

'Drugs?' Liesl asked.

'I'm afraid so. Tell me,' Rachel asked, throwing herself, as it were, upon the mercy of her audience. 'How do you keep your children out of trouble in this permissive society?'

'There is a vast difference,' Senator Grant said as he watched the televisions. 'When I was a boy in Clay, every element in the society was supportive. The police were friendly. Sunday School teachers wanted us to do the right thing. Our football coach was an admirable figure, and I remember one day when I sneaked into the poolroom to see for myself what infamous things were going on, and two of the town roustabouts took me aside and said, "Norman, you're supposed to grow up into a fine man. Maybe marry the judge's daughter or something like that. You're not meant to be in poolrooms. Now get out." '

'It's not that way any longer,' Rachel Mott said. 'Right now our son's in Miami chanting "Ho, ho, ho! Ho Chi Minh!" '

Senator Grant turned from the televisions. 'He's what?'

'It's a childish nonsense. They think it's funny to make us older people angry.'

'But what's the Ho Chi Minh nonsense? Surely your son is not . . .'

'They want the war in Vietnam to end. They insist we get out.'

'That's government policy,' Grant snapped. 'That's not for puling children to determine on their own.'

'Christopher's no child. He's nineteen. He's terrified of the draft.'

Grant rose. 'When we faced a much more terrible enemy, two of them, my generation volunteered. You did, didn't you, Mott?'

'The Army picked me up,' he said evasively, not wishing to admit on this night that he had not been in uniform.

'How about you, Pope? You volunteered, didn't you?'

'I was playing football, sir. Still in high school.'

'But in Korea?'

'I was already in uniform, sir, but I did a lot of combat flying over there.'

'You certainly volunteered for the German side, didn't you, Kolff?'

'I fought on the Russian front,' Dieter said, not caring to explain that it took four Nazi detectives to find him in the fields of southern Germany before the Army could throw him into uniform.

'In time of crisis,' Grant said, 'men rally to the support of their homelands.'

'Millard, out in Colorado, denies it's a crisis. He told us in his last letter that he's sure the whole thing is contrived.'

'Contrived!' Grant snorted. 'When the Congress of the United States . . .'

'That was his major point,' Rachel said. 'Congress has not had the courage to declare actual war. Millard says it's all a political game, an avoidance of reality.'

'Your Millard had better watch out, Mrs. Mott.'

'He says it's what he calls a ploy. A way to get the children of the poor to defend the privileges of the rich without disturbing business as usual.'

'He sounds like a Communist.'

'He tells us that most of the young people in Colorado think the same way. Two of his friends have escaped to Canada. To avoid the draft.'

'Escaped? America's no prison. If they ran away to Canada, they did so because they're cowards. President Nixon and Congress have laid out certain plans, and it's the duty of all citizens to obey them.'

Stanley Mott, not wishing this argument to proceed any further, asked, 'In a time of wildly changing mores, what can a parent do to keep his children stable?'

'Sometimes,' Liesl Kolff said, 'sometimes you have to take a hammer and smash the trumpet.'

More than six hours had passed since the module Eagle had landed on the Moon, and the two astronauts who occupied it had rested fitfully in order to be at maximum alert when the time came to leave their secure pouch and, like baby kangaroos, venture forth to leap about. During this interval, experts had congratulated NASA for having adopted the simplest and safest mode of approaching the Moon, lunar-orbit rendezvous rather than a direct shot from Earth, with all the massive construction that would have required, or Earth-orbit rendezvous, with its added complexity. The science consultant for ABC-TV had said:

> 'The genius of this flight was the man who pleaded with NASA to reevaluate procedures and study afresh the difficulties of other modes and the essential rightness of this one. We do not know that man's name. Most likely he was a committee, but even in committees it takes some one person with insight and courage to urge upon his companions the right course of action, and then to defend it against challenge. So as we wait for our astronauts to venture forth upon the Moon, let us salute the organizational genius responsible for the decision that enabled them to get this far so easily and so correctly.'

'He's speaking of you, Mott,' Senator Grant cried.

'Me and a dozen others.'

'Was it an argument difficult to win?'

Mott was about to make a grandiloquent statement concerning the protracted debate when he chanced to look in the direction of Dieter Kolff, one of the men he had been required to oppose most vigorously, and he saw two things: that Kolff was moody and depressed at this moment of triumph, and that it would be most ungenerous to expatiate upon his defeat. Let it go at that.

Now, as 2200 approached, a miracle almost beyond comprehension occurred. In the landing module resting on the Moon one of the astronauts positioned a television camera so that the movements of the other man could be photographed and sent to Earth, which meant that all the world would be able to see, almost as it happened—plus the 1.3 seconds it required the signal to travel the 238,000 miles at the speed of light—an event of supreme historical importance. It was as if cameras had been aligned on the *Santa Maria* to catch the landing of Columbus, or under the apple tree to chronicle the moment when Isaac Newton conceived his theory of gravity, or in the fires of Moscow in 1812 to record the second when Napoleon decided to turn back. The world would visibly participate in the dawning of a new age, the Exploration of Outer Space.

The door to the module opened. A figure clothed in cumbersome white slowly backed down the short ladder, reached the last rung, and felt tentatively with a booted foot. Firmly, confidently, the man left the security of the ladder and stepped safely upon the Moon. Lunar dust did not envelop him as some had predicted, nor did the granules burst into flame as others had warned.

And then over the radio, so incredibly far away, came the human voice, as clear as if the speaker were in the next room: 'That's one small step for man, uhh, one giant leap for mankind.' Later, NASA would amend it into the form it would take in history books: 'One small step for a man, one giant leap for mankind.'

Seven of the eight people in the motel room at the Longhorn burst into applause, and each man kissed his wife in sheer jubilation. For Dieter Kolff, depressed as he appeared to have been, it was a mighty victory, for his rocket had behaved just as he had predicted. For Senator Grant it was a triumph of his careful planning and unwavering leadership. For Stanley Mott it was vindication in his protracted struggle to get NASA to adopt lunar rendezvous. And for the Popes it was a double victory: John's demonstrations in Gemini 13 had sped the day when the Moon trip became viable, and Penny's faithful shepherding of her committee had kept the vast project on track. She had helped supervise the spending of some $23,000,000,000.

'We've shown them!' Grant exulted. 'We've shown the Russians!'

'They did it so effectively,' Pope said in admiration of his fellow astronauts, and the celebrators wanted to know what Armstrong and Aldrin were really like. Liesel Kolff said, 'I wonder how that Michael Collins feels, all alone out there.'

'That's his job,' Pope said. 'If I'd been chosen for this flight, that would have been my job.'

'Isn't he lonely?'

'I spent sixteen days with this much space between me and my commander.' He held his hands eight inches apart. 'I'd have been glad for a little loneliness.'

'Look at them!' Grant shouted. 'Look at those American boys on the Moon.'

Toasts were proposed and there were general congratulations, after which Elinor Grant, smiling at the vanity of these seven unaware people, excused herself and went to bed. Liesl Kolff had now had six Tuborgs, and she, too, departed, unsteadily. Rachel Mott, sensing that the men would celebrate for a long time, preferred to go to bed, but Penny Pope, who felt herself a part of the great adventure, remained behind, throwing beer bottles into a wastebasket and ordering some more sandwiches and pretzels from room service.

When things had quieted down, and the four men were comfortable in their chairs, they listened to a remarkable broadcast by a correspondent in Spain:

> 'It was early Sunday evening in Spain when word of the Moon landing was broadcast to the nation, and shortly thereafter a Father Tomás Uruzippe, a Jesuit scientist of note, came on the radio to assure the citizens of Spain that the Pope had been kept aware of all developments, that he had given the Moon mission his blessing, and that walking on the Moon in no way transgressed Biblical instructions. And now I quote Father Uruzippe's words as he closed his homily to the nation: "I repeat that the Pope has been kept fully informed by the American government of its plan to send men to the Moon, and His Holiness has found no reason to protest. I assure you again that everything is all right and in accordance with Biblical teaching." '

'I should think that would be very comforting,' Senator Grant said, but then he caught sight of one of the astronauts pogo-sticking across the lunar surface, and he said something which proved extremely discomforting to two of his listeners: 'Well, we've certainly shown the Russians. Now we can turn to other things.'

At one in the morning John Pope had to leave for Mission Control, where he would put in his next stint as communicator, so Penny departed with him, and after further celebration of this historic moment, Senator Grant trailed off. Now Mott and Kolff were left alone with the two televisions:

KOLFF (with real anxiety): Did you hear what he said? 'Now that we've shown the Russians, we can turn to other things.'

MOTT: Battle fatigue. He's worked very hard to achieve this victory.

KOLFF: It all ends tonight, Stanley. And it's your fault.

MOTT: Don't throw guilt at me. I feel none. Look at those celebrations.

KOLFF: The circus will soon be over. The dancing bears will retire. And we can turn down the lights.

MOTT: Quit? No. We already have eight or nine more shots on schedule.

KOLFF: But the steam goes out of the calliope. I'm so worried about this night. Now that we've shown the Russians, the accountants will move in. The grand adventure.

MOTT: Maybe a society can absorb only so much. Maybe it has to pause to catch its breath.

KOLFF: One part of society is allowed to pause. Senator Grant has finished his job. He's exhausted intellectually. I'm not surprised at that. 'Now we can get on with more important things.'

MOTT: Wait a minute. He didn't say it that way.

KOLFF: But he meant it. Bring the men back to Earth. Tackle the problems here.

MOTT: Do you know what my own son wrote in his last letter? 'Science runs wild in our society. It sponsors great boondoggles.'

KOLFF: What are these *boondoggles?*

MOTT: Moon shots. What you call circuses.

KOLFF: I'm sixty-two. Two more years, I must retire from the battle. And it breaks my heart to think that I leave with everyone in retreat.

MOTT: Now that's a silly statement. I'm not in retreat. I'm looking forward to the Mars shot, the exploration of Jupiter and Saturn.

KOLFF: The things you speak of are niggardly. Less than they should be at this time in man's intellectual history. We should be bursting at our seams, men like you and me.

MOTT: I am. Have you been following the discoveries of Penzias and Wilson? The Bell Laboratory people?

KOLFF: Of course. That's what makes me so uneasy tonight. We should be building on what men like them have found.

MOTT: I am. If they're right, and the sounds they hear are echoes of the Big Bang which occurred at the start of things, we can begin to assemble a logical theory of the universe.

KOLFF: But not unless we move forward on every front. We must have our instruments in the sky, our minds down here working on the data. We're in an age of fabulous discovery, Stanley, and that damned Moon has nothing to do with it.

MOTT: It's a first step. An exciting one.

KOLFF: But now do you confess the folly of your decisions?

MOTT: I do not.

KOLFF: Watch what happens. When those men climb down off that Moon we'll make gods of them.

MOTT: We should. They're the Columbuses of our day.

KOLFF: And we'll let it go at that, our job is done. Let's get on with other more important things.

MOTT: A little hero worship never damaged a long-range program.

KOLFF: That was your first error. To send men instead of machines.

MOTT: No! Glancey was right. Americans understand men. They can't identify with your machines. And without emotional identification, we have nothing.

KOLFF: My machines could have startled the world.

MOTT (pointing at the television): My way worked. Look at the celebrations.

KOLFF: And what does it leave you with? A program that you can build on?

MOTT: You heard them. Even in Spain they're celebrating.

KOLFF: And in the morning, what will we have left? The capacity to place useless men on a useless Moon. While the Russians forge constantly ahead in the real tasks.

MOTT: Wait! Wait! Don't you think the Kremlin is biting its nails now in frustration? Who in Paris will give a damn for Yuri Gagarin when Neil Armstrong rides down the Champs-Elysées?

KOLFF: Mere exhibitionism.

MOTT: Let me assure you, exhibitionism counts . . . among nations. I'll let you in on a secret. Washington has alerted me to be ready to honcho a tour of the Moon astronauts to sixteen major nations, once they get out of quarantine. That's what your circus produces.

KOLFF: But the noble task . . . it lies sidetracked.

MOTT: What is your noble task?

KOLFF: We live within a universe. Our petty lives are spent within its constructs. Our nations rise and fall in accordance with its limitations. We know almost nothing about it, and it's our obligation to know.

MOTT: The information may not be knowable.

It was now toward four in the morning, and although each of the men was exhausted by this long, eventful day, neither wanted to break this exploration, for it dealt with the remaining years of their lives: the things they would be attempting, the hopes they would be passing along to others, and it was Dieter Kolff, the inheritor of those stubborn Germans of the Raketenflugplatz in Berlin who had first dreamed seriously of how to throw great machines toward the stars and of those even more stubborn Prussians at Peenemünde who had actually tried to do it, who sustained the clearest vision of the future, but before he could elaborate upon that future, he was interrupted by two figures who passed through the Longhorn bar without seeing him. One was Cindy Rhee, coming back from celebrations at Mission Control, and she was accompanied by Ed Cater, whose wife, Gloria, had stayed at headquarters. They formed a stunning pair, she in one of those exquisite gray-tan Korean dresses that dropped in a straight line from a point just below the neck, he in blue California shorts and matching T-shirt, and when they came to the parting point, from which she should go to her room and he to his, he suddenly caught her in his arms, lifted her high off the floor and kissed her ardently where her neck joined her shoulder. When he put her down she grasped his hand and they walked dreamily toward her room.

KOLFF: Your astronauts attend to the simpler problems . . . and leave the universe to us.

MOTT: Whenever I see one of the young men, I think of Harry Jensen. You didn't know him, Dieter, but he was a young Scandinavian god . . . out of the sagas.

KOLFF: I'm so sad in this moment of celebration. So many of the things we dreamed of at Peenemünde are decaying into insequentiality . . . *(He tried to pronounce* inconsequentiality *again, fumbled it and stopped.)* Would you mind if we spoke in German? Well, you continue in English, but I want to express myself accurately.

MOTT: Go ahead.

KOLFF: At any moment in intellectual history things arise which must be attended to. Who determines the ought? Not governments, not self-appointed individuals. Only the vast sweep of human knowledge. Copernicus felt this and so did Dr. Harvey with the bloodstream. The Russians felt it long before we did and that's why they got to the Moon first. *(Mott raised his eyebrows.)* Yes, in our celebrations we'll try to forget that they got there first, landed first, got samples first, photographed the far side first.

MOTT: Don't exaggerate. Russia's like Spain and the New World. We're like England. Spain may have got here first, but it was England that did something important about it.

KOLFF: You don't call South America important?

MOTT: Not really.

KOLFF: We're very arrogant tonight, aren't we?

MOTT: I sure am. My team set out to do something extremely difficult. We chose the one right way to do it. And we succeeded. If you want to do something different, you find your right way. But don't complain about mine, because for its task it was perfection. Let's order more beer.

KOLFF: I'm pleased to see that you're capable of emotion. I'm not. Not when the cause is so spurious.

MOTT: What would you have us do?

KOLFF: Very simple, Stanley. Cancel the rest of the Apollo shots. Fire all the astronauts. Assemble the hundred brightest astrophysicists, give them a minimum budget, and tell them to get on with it.

MOTT: With what?

KOLFF: The study of the universe. If we apply ourselves diligently for the next hundred years, we can solve all the great riddles.

MOTT: Like what?

KOLFF: The origins of the universe. Its probable life history. The specific role of our Sun and its planets. The origins of human life. Even things like when the next ice age will overtake us. You know, of course, that when it comes, fifteen or twenty thousand years from now, the ice will obliterate New York. And later, when it melts, the oceans will ride completely across Florida. It's matters like that we should be addressing.

MOTT *(with some irritation):* Dieter, have you ever seen my office? What do you suppose faces me on the wall every time I look up? A marvelous photograph of the Galaxy 4565 . . . twenty million light-years away. That's where my imagination lives. That's where I want to go eventually . . . in my mind.

KOLFF: Then why are you fooling around with the Moon?

MOTT: Because Senator Glancey taught me that I'll never get where I want to go unless I take the taxpayers along. We move one step at a time, and the Moon's our first big one.

KOLFF: And maybe the last. Maybe we've done our one great thing tonight. We may have to pass the torch along . . . Do you have the French word *gonfalon?* We may have to hand it to others.

MOTT: What others?

KOLFF: Japan? Germany? Russia?

MOTT: Are they capable?

KOLFF: People make themselves capable. *(Many minutes of silence followed.)* I go to bed tonight sorely worried. I see my adopted nation on the wrong course and I must soon retire from the battle. Goodnight, Stanley, in your hour of erroneous triumph.

A week later, while the world still reverberated with cheering, it was Mott's turn to be worried, because the mail sent down from Washington included a letter from Alberta, Canada:

Roger and I decided to close our shop in Skycrest and take refuge in Canada. We cannot submit ourselves to the draft for a war that is so terribly wrong and being fought on principles so terribly corrupt. We could both register at the University of Colorado and thus escape the draft, but we cannot avoid danger in that spurious way and watch young men with less money being sent to do our dirty work for us. I hope that my action will not bring discredit on you, at a time when you have a right to savor your triumph.

MILLARD

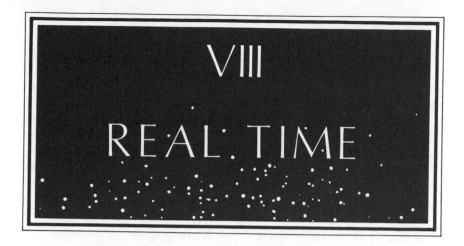

VIII

REAL·TIME

THE RETREAT FROM SPACE WHICH DIETER KOLFF PREDICTED OC-
curred more swiftly than even he had expected, and with much greater
severity. NASA's budget was slashed from five billion dollars a year to four
and then to a mere three; experts in various fields were laid off; and there
was talk of closing down some of the centers where exploratory work was
being conducted.

What was even more surprising, trips to the Moon became routine, so
that often the general public was not aware that one was under way, and
people grumbled about wasting money on the collection of 'more Moon
rocks, when we already have enough.'

Astronaut Randy Claggett, himself from Texas A & M, brightened the
gloom by circulating a joke on his alma mater:

> 'Seems the geology department at Texas Aggies was miffed because
> the University of Texas got Moon rocks to study and they didn't.
> So a NASA scientist, thinkin' to halt the complaints, went into a
> barnyard, picked up a handful of rocks and give 'em to the Aggie
> scientists to analyze. Seven months not a word, then a neatly typed
> report: "There are many aspects of these rocks we cannot explain,
> but we can state one thing for certain, that cow really did jump over
> the Moon." '

Randy also reported, in his Texas drawl, the results of the visit of two
astronauts to a community in Iowa, an offshoot of one founded in Illinois
by Wilbur Glenn Voliva, the apostle of a flat Earth. This group sustained
the hopes of people across the country, and in Europe, too, who longed for
the simpler world of A.D. 1300. When Randy handed the present leader of
the community a series of splendid color photographs showing an Earth as
round as an orange with the blue oceans held in place by gravity, the
gentleman studied the evidence for a long time, then said, 'If a man wasn't

a trained observer, he might be deceived by this picture.' When Randy pressed the true believer, the man growled, 'I never said it wasn't a circle.' Five days later the Iowa community circulated a learned paper explaining why, from a certain distance, the flat Earth might look somewhat rounded: 'It's a matter of parallax.'

When Randy took his own flight to the Moon, he provided some much-needed levity by reporting the progress of his Apollo in terms that gave the newsmen some trouble, because when he ran into momentary difficulties, he told Houston: 'It was pretty ginchy there for a moment.' When crumbs from the dehydrated meals hung suspended throughout the capsule, he reported: 'Things are gettin' pretty grotty up here.' Another time they were 'scuzzy,' but when he said that the fuel problem was getting 'just a bit grunchy,' Houston had to warn him to speak English.

When he surveyed the Moon while his two companions were on the surface exploring it, he told the world: 'It looks like General Sherman marched acrost it with a legion of boll weevils,' and he irritated some patriots by exclaiming: 'We ought to send an expedition to the back side of the Moon and find the highest mountain and name it Von Braun, because he put us up here.'

He was refreshing, and when the flight ended, reporters were more interested in him, alone in the capsule, than they were in the other two men who had actually walked on the Moon. When they asked him how he felt, circling the Moon alone, he replied, frankly, 'It was real scuzzy.' NASA, recognizing a popular figure when they had one, sent him on various public relations tours, and his face became familiar: a thin, puckish cowboy with an attractive gap between his big front teeth and a propensity for the outrageous statement, as when he told a Denver audience: 'Travelin' in a space capsule is no more dangerous than travelin' Route 85 to Colorado Springs in a car on a Saturday night when the beetpickers is out drunk.' Statistically, of course, he was correct.

But he could be extremely sharp when required, and he delighted the science community at Boulder with an erudite joke: 'Seems there was this hotshot geologist at Stanford, great authority on earthquakes. Predicted that all of California west of the San Andreas fault would disappear into the Pacific on 6 June 1966—that's 6-6-66—and when he woke up that morning he found that everythin' west of the fault was still standin', but everythin' east of it had vanished. Looking at his calculations, he said, "Damn, I got my sign wrong." '

When speaking to these same scientists, he said, 'We're now moving into fields of constant speculation with experts in all areas acomin' at us with their theories. Most of them, I find, have a correlation of 1.0 if you take only one instance.' There was a moment of silence, then some of the audience began to chuckle, and as explanations spread, the whole room began to applaud, for they appreciated his adept statement that if a scientist uses only one cause-and-effect instance, he will invariably produce a correlation of 1.0. Indeed, a gentleman in Boulder had recently been guilty of just that blunder; in an attempt to explain the influence of sunspots, he speculated that they dictated the behavior of the recently discovered Van Allen belt, which was certainly correct, if data from only the year 1968 were studied.

When Claggett met privately with technical experts at the various contractors' offices, he was a source of much stable information, and three different corporation presidents inquired quietly if he would be interested in joining their firms: 'The space program is running down, Colonel Claggett. You must see evidence of that. We'll be moving into fascinating new areas, and we'd be proud to have you aboard.'

He always said, 'I'm a Marine. I'd never fit in.' But when he and Debby Dee were alone with John Pope and Penny, they discussed with sharp attention the future of their strange profession.

'How do you see things, Penny?' Claggett asked one night in the Dagger Bar.

'Retrenchment all along the line.'

'How many more Apollo missions will Congress stand for?'

'We started with a budget that would cover us through Apollo 20. I'm sure they're going to knock off two of them. They may even cut us back to Apollo 17.'

'You think that'll be the last?'

'I do.'

'Damn! I coulda been in line to command 18. Take you along, John, like Gemini.'

'One thing I know,' Penny said. 'The next flights must carry scientist-geologists. The public insists on that. You should see the complaints that hit our office.'

'Well, the scientist and me, we go down on the Moon. John tends the store upstairs.'

'Would you accept that?' Penny asked her husband.

'I'd walk if I could even get near the Moon.'

'I have heard one rumor,' Penny said. 'Apollo 18 would have a good chance of Congressional support if you landed on the dark side of the Moon.'

'Don't say that!' her husband interrupted with some irritation. 'Everybody uses the phrase *the dark side of the Moon*. It isn't dark at all. It gets exactly as much sunlight as the side we see. It's just that it never turns that face for us to check.'

'Everybody in Washington calls it *the dark side.*'

'Everybody's wrong. They often are. And we can't call it *the unseen side,* because both we and the Russians have photographed it.'

'What should we call it?' Penny asked. 'The far side?'

'No! The other side. We must no longer describe everything in the planetary system from our parochial perspective.'

'Well, however you call it, if you could focus Apollo 18 on what we in Washington still call *the dark side,* you'd be able to enlist strong support from the scientific community . . . and from the general public, too.'

'That's not a bad idea!' Claggett cried, opening another beer, but Pope was setting up a diagram with two bowls, one large, one small.

'There's one knotty problem. On all previous missions we've had direct radio communication. Canaveral is here on Earth. Your men, Randy, were here, on the Moon. If we'd had telescopes strong enough, we could have watched you, and you us. But,' and he accented this word so heavily that Randy put down his beer, 'when we land Apollo 18 on the other side of the Moon, which my wife insists upon calling *the dark side,* though why I can't imagine, look what happens.'

He asked for a piece of cellophane, with which he made a lunar landing site on the other side, and now straight-line communication was impossible: 'Radio waves from this landing site can't penetrate the solid Moon, that's for sure. And we know they have to travel in a straight line, so they can't bend around the edges of the Moon. So, Randy, if you and your scientist do land down here, and let's say you stay four or five days, which is now possible . . . during descent, work, ascent, when anything can go wrong, you have no contact with Earth, no support from NASA.'

Claggett reminded the wives of the remarkable job done by Houston when Apollo 13 got into trouble because an oxygen tank ruptured: 'Only the ground computers and the brilliance of the NASA staff, with an assist from the contractors' men, got those astronauts back alive. Wonderful orchestration of talent. But without radio contract, three dead ducks.'

'What excites me about a mission to the other side,' Pope began, but Penny interrupted: 'Oh no! You do not spend four or five critical days with no communication.'

'We can have communication. That's the beauty of it. Debby Dee, let me have two oranges,' and when he had placed them in carefully selected orbits about his Moon, he explained: 'One of the satellites will always be in communication with my capsule, with Claggett, on the surface of the Moon, and with Houston down here on Earth. Beautiful.'

'Can it be done?' Penny asked.

'We're doing it now, on Earth, with our communications satellites. With these Moon orbiters in position . . . maybe we'll need three to assure constant coverage . . .'

'How will you get your three oranges into the proper orbit?' Penny asked.

'You take them up as baggage, and when the computer gives the signal, you toss them out, one by one. And there they stay, like three good little oranges.'

'You think we could sell it to Congress?' Claggett asked.

'Congress says it's dead set against anything beyond Apollo 17, but Norman Grant might be attracted to this . . . a noble swan song . . . John

Pope, a kid from his block.' She mused on this and said, 'Randy, I think you have a fighting chance.'

'That's all I need.' He took a deep swig of beer and said, 'You know why I'd like to make one last trip with your ugly husband? Because the capsule on the Apollo is big enough, we could enjoy the trip. Room to move around. And when you go to the john, you don't do it eight inches from the face of your partner. You go into a corner. You cannot imagine how refined that would seem after our Gemini flights.'

Tucker Thompson was worried. The Quints, who ran the Bali Hai motel, had warned him that the *Life* people, who owned the exclusive on all the other astronauts, had been snooping in corners, asking questions about Randy Claggett, Debby Dee and the Korean reporter Miss Rhee, and this could only mean trouble. 'What do you think they were after?'

'Well, it's general knowledge here in Cocoa Beach,' Mr. Quint said, 'that Claggett's been shacked up with this lady for some time. *Life* must've heard it. I suppose they want a scandal to discredit you *Folks* people.'

'But why Claggett? Hasn't she . . . well . . . hasn't she been rather . . . peripatetic?' When the Quints looked at each other quizzically, he added, 'Moving around a bit? From bed to bed?'

'She's been studying the field,' Mrs. Quint broke in to say. 'I like her. She's a fine, responsible girl.'

'She's thirty-five and I wish I could strangle her.'

'When a pretty woman pays her bills, doesn't raise hell in the bar, and attracts customers because she's so amiable,' Mrs. Quint said, 'I can excuse almost anything.'

'Not meddling around with my boys.'

'Tucker,' Mrs. Quint asked, 'how old are your boys, as you call them?'

He took from his pocket the small card on which his secretary had written in minute script the salient details of the Solid Six. 'They do run into the later thirties.'

'And early forties,' Mrs. Quint said. 'I was reading an article about John Pope. Intellectual leader of the group, they called him. He's forty-four.'

'Has Miss Korea been fooling around with Pope?'

'Stalwart John? No, while the others are upstairs with her he's out jogging. Our good seafood cooking, it puts weight on most of them, but good old Pope runs off every extra ounce. You hear the great crack Claggett made about him? "Give Pope a pair of water wings and stick a Roman candle up his ass, he could tow Apollo to the Moon." '

'Claggett is a loud-mouth,' Thompson said huffily.

'He's the first to admit it.'

'What can we do to avoid a scandal?' Thompson asked, and when the Quints vacillated, he warned: 'You know, you could be big losers in this, too, if things go wrong.'

'A good scandal never hurts a bar. What I'd really appreciate, some Miami gangster come in here and mow down four members of the opposition. This bar would make money for the next ten years.'

'NASA could put this joint off limits, Quint. No more astronauts attracting the customers.'

'I wouldn't like that,' Quint said.

'Then you figure out a way to put a brake on Madame Egg Foo-Yong.' He had also fallen into the habit of calling his little adversary Madame Fu Manchu, the Dragon Lady and Three from Column B.

'She's not an easy woman to discipline,' Mr. Quint said, and suddenly Mrs. Quint turned to stare at her husband as if he had opened new windows.

'Maybe you better move her out,' Tucker suggested.

The Quints did not solve the problem; Tucker himself did by the simple device of getting Claggett and Debby Dee dispatched on a foreign good-will tour, shepherded by a reporter from *Folks* and a functionary from the State Department, who sent Washington a chain of ecstatic cables:

> Recommend you send Claggetts every country in world. He tells jokes to kings and prime ministers. She beams and visits hospitals. Have developed a routine in which he is a Tex-Mex astronaut coming home after eleven months on the Moon, she pregnant. Very ribald, very funny.

Cynthia Rhee stayed behind at the Bali Hai, and when Timothy Bell flew in to Canaveral for some hours on the simulators, she quietly moved in with him, for she needed some specific quotes on how it felt to be the only civilian amidst a group of gung-ho military pilots.

'Wait a minute!' he exploded in near-anger. 'I'm no second-class citizen. Don't ask me questions like that.'

'You're giving me a good answer, right now, Tim.'

'Well, keep in mind that the first man to step on the Moon was a civilian. Neal Armstrong was no military type. A civilian test pilot just like me. Claggett may have been the first of our group to get to the Moon. I'll probably be the next.'

'Rumor says you will be, Tim.'

'Have you checked out the big brawl between Aldrin and Armstrong over who would be first out of the capsule? Aldrin raised hell when NASA decided it would be best if a non-military type took the big step. Buzz said it denigrated the whole military component. Made them out a bunch of warlike killers.'

'That's why I asked the question, Tim. I wanted to hear your gut responses. Not the ones you recite so glibly at press conferences.'

He became so agitated that he left the bed and stalked about the motel room naked. Then he stormed back, climbed in, and grabbed her by the shoulders. 'Of course I feel the difference sometimes. They form a kind of gang that I can never enter. The fact that I earned so much more than they do because I was a civilian test pilot, that gigs them, too.'

'Do you feel any difference in . . . shall we say . . . competence?'

'I could fly any one of them right into the ground.' He hesitated. 'Any one but John Pope. I suppose you know he's the best.'

'NASA thinks Claggett is.'

'And so do you, I suppose.'

'I don't evaluate. I thought maybe young Jensen was the best of your lot.'

'But not rock-hard like Pope. Not inspired like Claggett.'

'How do you locate yourself, Tim?'

'I'll make two flights. Sensationally good. And I'll become president of some company building airplanes.'

'Allied Aviation, maybe?'

'You said it. I didn't.'

'Is that your ambition, Tim?'

'It's my training. When I'm through with NASA— Wait a minute. Put it that when NASA is through with me, I'll have had an education that not forty men in this world have had. Frank Borman, John Pope, a handful of Russians. I have been taught everything. Six Ph.D.'s, seven. I'd have to have an IQ of 31 not to have mastered a universe of knowledge. I'll put it to some constructive use.'

'And Cluny? What happens with her?'

'She has three wonderful children. She fits in anywhere. Test flying, business, NASA—whatever I do, she blends in. She'd be sensational as the wife of a corporate president.'

'Do you love her?'

Timothy Bell reflected on this for a long time, not as to the facts, but as how properly to present them. 'I was a junior at the University of Arkansas. Spring of the year. Heavy schedule of laboratory work because I took all the hard courses. It was about quarter to six and I was kind of soul-bleary coming out of the lab, and I saw this girl in a pale blue-and-white dress, like Southern girls favored before the Civil War, and I was knocked dumb. I just stood there as she went by, then I started running after her, and she said her name was Cluny, and my three laboratory courses, they went straight to hell. And after a while she said, "Tim, we must do things right. Tend to your grades first," and I did and we were married that summer. And when I think of her now she's always in that pale blue-and-white dress.'

'And she's still that little girl?'

'Yes. She'll always be.'

· · ·

In Washington, Penny Pope campaigned furiously for the money to fund one more Apollo mission, and she had the full support of NASA, which commissioned Dr. Stanley Mott to help in the lobbying, but thoughtful senators like Proxmire of Wisconsin could find no justification for redundant visits to well-known terrain, and the appeals failed. The House was even more opposed to an Apollo 18 because the NASA scientists were unable to demonstrate what new truths might be unfolded, so Dr. Mott retreated, leaving the aborted mission in Penny's care.

When she sat before her committee, reporting her failure, she gained no sympathy, and even Senator Glancey, a tired old man now, said, 'I think we've run our course. It's been an honorable one and let's let it stand at that.' But she was persistent, and introduced a new idea which attracted strong support from a few senators and respectful attention from all:

'It would be pusillanimous of us to terminate these explorations without seeing the far side of the Moon. If we explore only the easy near side, we leave the job half done. We can go to the other side, make comparisons, and lay the groundwork for everything that will follow later on. I believe we have a moral imperative to finish the job.'

When her own Senator Grant objected that any such expedition would have to do its work without radio communication with Earth, a fact which condemned her proposal, Penny borrowed two water carafes and duplicated the demonstration her husband had devised:

'You're entirely correct, Senator Grant, radio communication in a straight line from the far side of the Moon is an impossibility. We remember that from Frank Borman's tremendously exciting Christmas flight around the Moon when we had that painful radio silence. But what we can now do is this. Take three devices with us into lunar orbit . . . these three glasses . . . and drop them out here . . . here . . . and here. They will relay radio messages exactly the way Comsat relays messages now from one part of the Earth to another.'

When one of the senators asked, 'If you need three radio stations at the Moon, will you be asking us to fund an extra Apollo to carry them there?' she apologized: 'I'm so sorry, Senator. Sometimes I don't explain things well. The kind of satellite I'm talking about will be little larger than a volleyball.'

'But if every inch of space is already taken, where will you be able to store three of them?'

'That's easy. In the lunar module.'

'And how will you launch them?'

'We'll have an explosive bolt. At the proper signal it blows open a hatch cover. The satellites will be spring-loaded, and at the proper signal they'll leap out and be on their way.'

'How can such little things have their own propulsion?'

'They won't need it. They pick up the same propulsive speed as the Apollo from which they're launched.'

'How do you know so much about these things, Mrs. Pope?'

'Because it's my job to know,' she said with a smile. 'And remember, I've been working with this committee since 1949,' and the senator asked, 'Are you a Republican or Democrat? I mean, how have you been able to hold on through all the changes?'

'By my fingernails,' she said.

'But what you just said, it'll work?'

'I'm assured it will.'

'By whom?'

'By the best brains in this country,' and in subsequent meetings she brought before the committee a succession of excited scientists who explained how they were only on the verge of comprehending the Moon and its place in the celestial system.

'Won't that always be the case?' one of Senator Proxmire's supporters asked. 'Won't you forever be coming before us and begging for just one more exploration. Will it ever end?'

'No, sir. Because the pursuit of knowledge never ends.'

'Then why should we . . .'

'Because we Earthlings are in the position that Europe was in 1491. They knew half the globe—Europe and Asia—but nothing about the other half, the Americas. It would have been perilous and craven to have stopped there, when the richness of the Americas—'

'There's no richness on the Moon. We know that.'

'In understandings, it's a gold mine. And we've only begun to exploit it.'

The scientist, an astrophysicist from the University of Chicago, asked an assistant to bring before the committee a rather large globe sixteen inches in diameter, unlike any they had ever seen before. Indeed, only within the last few years had the making of such a globe become possible:

'I helped Denoyer-Geppert in Chicago put this together. It shows the complete Moon, both hemispheres. And I want to assure you that if you were to authorize a mission that landed on this unexplored side, its intellectual returns could be tremendous. Let's look at this well-defined area of maximum interest.

'Here we have the Sea of Moscow 30° north of the lunar equator. On the equator we have the fascinating crater Mendeleev. Down here the beautiful medium crater Tsiolkovsky and over here, forming a handsome triangle, Gagarin . . .'

'They're all Russian names!' one of the senators said.

'That's the whole point,' Penny broke in. 'We have much work to do to catch up.'

This was not entirely true, even though it was a sensible reason to place before the senators. Starting in 1962, the Americans had launched four Rangers in rapid succession to photograph the Moon, and all failed miserably: on one, the command system went haywire; on another, the television system broke down; and in two instances, the craft missed the Moon entirely, for they never left Earth orbit.

The Russians, in the meantime, had succeeded in sending their Luna spacecraft behind the Moon and photographing it in some detail, once in 1959, later in 1965, and again in 1966. It was they who uncovered for the world a vision of what the other side was like, and because of their priority, it was they who had the right to name the features.

But the Russian photographs were of poor quality and haphazard siting; it was really the later American orbiters which had provided the serious photographic mapping of the other side, so that the Chicago professor's new globe showed Russian names on American photographs. It had been a good joint exploration, but because of American tardiness, the other side of the Moon would be forever Russian.

'We scientists believe that if an Apollo 18 could land within that triangle of Mendeleev, Tsiolkovsky and Gagarin— ['Who in hell was Tsiolkovsky?' a senator asked. 'The father of us all,' the Chicago man said. 'He established the scientific principles of space flight in 1883.'] If we could land in that triangle, we could produce miracles.'

Penny lined up fifteen scientists to testify that an Apollo 18 flight to the other side was not only practical but obligatory, and gradually the senators began to agree with her that to leave a major exploration of the universe half-completed was imprudent. Dr. Mott, testifying for NASA, assured them that an Apollo 18 would be no more expensive than any of the preceding flights: 'Less so, really, because the exploratory work on the instruments we would want to use has already been done.'

'How much would the three orbiting satellites for radio transmission cost?'

'About ten million dollars each. They'd have to be foolproof, you know.'

Now a fire of enthusiasm swept the scientific community, and support for a shot to the far side began to pour in, until Congress was forced seriously to consider what Penny Pope, the counsel for the Senate committee, called 'our magnificent farewell to the Moon.' In April 1971 the final launch was authorized and some eight thousand men and women across the nation rushed to resuscitate earlier plans which had been lying dormant, and in Houston, Deke Slayton informed the press that Apollo 18 would be crewed by one of the most interesting three-man teams in the history of flight: 'Flight Commander Randy Claggett of the Marines. Command module Pilot John Pope of the Navy. Lunar module Pilot Dr. Paul Linley, Professor of Geology, University of New Mexico, with a civilian pilot's license. Dr. Linley, a graduate of DePaul and Indiana with a doctorate from Purdue, is our first black astronaut.'

NASA, relying upon the 17,000 close-up photographs taken by lunar orbiters, drafted a large-scale map of the Mendeleev-Tsiolkovsky-Gagarin triangle, from which technicians constructed small papier-mâché mock-ups which the three astronauts could carry with them until they were as familiar with that portion of the Moon as they were with their own backyards. The simulator chief, Dracula, instructed his clever photographers and lighting experts to make television shots of the area as the astronauts would see it from their spacecraft, and these he fitted into the cameras of his landing simulators, encouraging the men to fly mission after mission into this arid rocky area.

One curious technological device enabled Dracula to produce simulations of striking effect: when a good camera had taken a well-resolved photograph of hilly terrain, or even slightly bumpy land, a computer could look at that photograph and imagine how *another* camera *might* have photographed the identical scene *if* it had been stereoscopically placed in relation to the first. When the two photographs were developed and placed side by side in a stereopticon viewer, almost identical with the ones that had enchanted tea parties in the 1890s, features leaped from the flat surface, and one could see Moon rocks looming up ahead and craters and rilles.

'Watch what happens when we make a movie that way,' Dracula said with an evil leer to his assistants, and without warning the astronauts, he cranked his stereoscopic films into the Moon-landing simulator just before Claggett and Linley entered it to run through their landing one more time. Suddenly, as they approached the crater Gagarin, they saw ahead not a photograph of rocks but the actual strewn surface coming up to meet them with boulders and giant depressions. It was uncanny.

Claggett and Pope took an instant liking to Paul Linley. He was younger than they and slightly smaller, but he was lean and wonderfully coordinated. He had starred as play-making guard on DePaul's championship five, going head-to-head with men almost a foot and a half taller. As a black he had run into some rough experiences when he served as a geologist in the Texas oil fields, but his obvious willingness to mix it up with all comers quickly established his integrity, and during NASA field trips to the arid wastes of Arizona, which had always been used to familiarize astronauts with the probable surface of the Moon, he demonstrated more raw endurance than either of his mates. NASA at last had a black man, and everyone was proud of him.

But he had much background information on the lunar module to catch up on, and his study hours tended to keep him up night after night till eleven at least. He was married, had three children, but his wife realized that his obligations were too intense to permit much family life, so she stayed in Houston with the children while he thundered about the United States from one simulator to the next: in Houston, landing; at Canaveral, taking off; at MIT, managing computers. He wrote his wife: 'I'm spending so much of my life in simulators at Allied Aviation, I won't know what real living is when I see it. But I'll always recognize your ham and lima beans, and by damn I wish I had some now.'

For Claggett and Pope, on whom the heavy burden of managing this unique flight would rest, the last months of 1971 and all of 1972 formed a period of the most intense concentration. Day after day they analyzed the terrain south of the Sea of Moscow, naming objects as small as a tennis court, constructing road maps that Pope could follow from aloft while Claggett and Linley pursued them on the surface, and gradually, as directed by a team of nineteen lunar specialists convened from NASA staff and fourteen major universities, they focused upon the exact site on which the module would land—

'You got a name for your craft yet?' Mott asked.

Claggett pointed to Pope. 'He's flyin' it alone when we're down on the Moon. It's his baby.'

'*Altair,*' Pope said without hesitation. It had been Altair since that October night in 1944 when he first saw that perfect star in his borrowed binoculars. It was Altair when he followed that star over the night skies in Korea. It had been Altair during indocrination in the planetarium at Fremont State. He and the star were one, and now he would take *Altair* aloft among the stars.

The NASA people were astounded when they asked Claggett what he would be naming the lunar module. '*Luna,*' he said. "The Russians got there first with their Luna, let's pay them respect.'

Considerable opposition was voiced to this radical selection, but Mott and the other NASA types found that Claggett was immovable: 'I'm riskin' my ass in it. I'll name it.' Pope supported him, but gave the NASA people an easy escape: 'Luna's always been the poetic name for the Moon. We don't have to mention Russia.'

'That's okay with me,' Claggett said. 'I'll know and you'll know and nobody else needs give a damn.'

Rachel Mott found an appropriate quotation from Virgil, 'Through the friendly silence of the Moon,' and Claggett said that's exactly what he had in mind. Soon the press was handed the details: 'Apollo 18 composed of the command module *Altair* and the lunar module *Luna* will take off for a landing near the crater Gagarin in early 1973 with the crew Claggett, Pope, Linley.' The astronauts named were studying eighteen hours a day.

· · ·

Whenever the astronauts relaxed in the Dagger Bar, they called upon Paul Linley to perform a vaudeville act, which delighted the customers and even caused the newsmen to applaud. With the most beguiling body movements he walked into a space between the tables and announced himself as the head cheerleader of the Albuquerque Technological Institution, and with a riotous zoot-suit vocabulary, explained how there had been racial tension at good old ATI, where the eleven basketball players were black and the twelve cheerleaders white:

> 'Problem solved by our pres-ee-dent, Lucullus Beauregard of South Carolina, a wily cat who suggested that I be assigned to the cheer-leading squad and his nephew Robert E. Lee Beauregard to the basketball team.'

He then gave a demonstration of how Robert E. Lee, five feet ten, defended against Kareem Jabbar, seven feet two, but quickly he turned to his own performance as cheerleader, at the end of which he enlisted everyone in the bar to help him spell out the victory howl of Albuquerque Technological Institution.

He started briskly with 'Gimme an A'—at which everyone bellowed '*A*.' 'Gimme an L.'

By the time he reached the spelling of *Technological,* he lost all control, throwing in frenzied K's and Q's. Abruptly he stopped to tell his audience, 'President Beauregard warned me that I had to spell it right at least one time in four, and when I asked why, he said, "Because my faculty can't spell it either, and I want 'em to learn." ' When he launched into *Institution* he quietly transformed himself into a wizened old man, calling feebly, 'Gimme another of those damned T's,' until toward the end he slipped out a white wig, jammed it on his palsied head, sank to the floor, and whispered, 'Gimme that good old final N.'

When he rose exhausted, he gasped, 'Next time I'm gonna be cheer-leader at Yale.'

CBS wanted to televise the whole performance, but Tucker Thompson vetoed that in a hurry: 'Can't you see his act has racial overtones?' And Linley said with a straight face, 'I often wondered about that.'

It was Dr. Mott who first noticed that Captain Pope was doing rather more work than necessary, or at best prudent, considering the problems of health. When he saw John hunched over a desk at eleven-thirty one night he asked, 'What's up?' and he found that Pope had been writing out on small sheets of flimsy but fire-resistant paper procedures which he would put into effect in every conceivable type of emergency.

'But they're all in the handbooks,' Mott said.

'I want them up here,' Pope replied, tapping his forehead.

'You can't burden yourself with that much detail.'

'That's why I'm writing them down.'

'But they are written down.'

'Not till I write them.'

Mott asked Dr. Feldman if he had noticed Pope tightening up, and Feldman said, 'He's always tightened up. That's the definition of a straight arrow.'

'Is it necessary?'

'He thinks so, and that's what matters.'

'Well, I—'

Feldman interrupted: 'The time can come in any mission when one man's right actions will make all the difference. Iron will. Coupled with the proper hours in the simulators. Those little pieces of paper are Pope's simulators. Let him go.'

But Mott observed a growing testiness in the astronaut, and when he reached Houston he suggested that Pope be summoned back from Canaveral and be given some rest and recuperation. The wisdom of this recommendation was so obvious that NASA directed Pope to join Timothy Bell in an inspection of work being done by Allied Aviation in Los Angeles: 'And we suggest that instead of flying a T-38 west, you travel by commercial airline and get some relaxation.' Pope, acknowledging at last that he might be approaching battle fatigue, counterproposed that instead of flying, he and Penny drive across country, something they loved to do, and NASA assented.

When Pope informed the crowd at the Bali Hai what he and Penny were about to do, Tim Bell asked to ride along, but John demurred: 'Three on a honeymoon, never works.'

'But I'd bring Cluny.'

'Would she want to spend that much time?' And with the perception that marked most of what Pope did, he added, 'You remember, the Mercury's a convertible.'

'If it rains, you put the top up, don't you?' Bell argued so persuasively that Pope told him to go ahead and phone Cluny to see if she was interested, and Bell described the trip so glowingly that she flew in to join them. Twisting her pretty head this way and that as she tried to visualize what the five hurried days would be like, she had the good sense to decline: 'I'm sure I wouldn't like it.' But when she saw her husband's disappointment, she added, 'But you go, Tim.'

'It's a kind of honeymoon for the Popes. They won't take me alone.'

'How will you go if I don't come along?'

'I'd fly out later in a T-38.'

'Alone?' She had an intuitive fear of this sensitive plane that had already killed two other astronauts, and her apprehension showed.

'I enjoy flying that plane,' Bell said honestly, for the swift courier was a joy when handled with respect.

'No. I'll drive out with you,' she said, and her husband, trying to be fair, said, 'You know the Popes have a convertible.'

'I'd like that.' And so the trip was arranged, but when Penny heard the details before flying down from Washington to join the safari, she asked over the phone, 'Are you sure, John, that you want to take her with us on so long a trip?'

'The Bells are fun. He's a prime mover.'

'I know he is. But I wonder if she'll fit in.'

Cluny certainly did not fit into the Mercury convertible, or any other. If the top was down, she insisted on riding front seat so the wind wouldn't blow her hair, but if it was raised, as it tended to be when late afternoons grew cool, she wanted a window halfway down so she could breathe, then complained that her hair was still being blown.

Things had started badly on the first day, for the Popes wanted to leave Cape Canaveral at 0400, as usual, but thanks to Cluny's unwillingness to rise early, they could not start west until 0900, by which time John had expected to be three hundred miles on the way.

She absolutely demanded that they stop for lunch, and by six she was whining that 'if we don't find a motel soon, we might never find one.'

'Haven't you ever slept in a car?' Penny asked.

'Certainly not!'

'Try it, you'll like it.'

Cluny interpreted this correctly as a flip attack upon her, and while she did not complain to her husband, he knew that she had tensed up and would soon become unmanageable, so he supported her plea that they find a motel, and quickly.

Since it was only 1730, John pointed out, accurately, 'We have four more hours of driving, Cluny.'

'And no motel when we stop.'

'We always find something.'

The statement terrified her, for she could visualize them knocking about some grubby Alabama town and settling at last upon a dirty boardinghouse or a totally unacceptable hotel. 'I want to find our place while it's still light,' she said firmly, so to John Pope's disgust and his wife's amazement, he pulled into a clean, modern motel that satisfied all of Cluny's demands. It was 1733—half past five civilian time—and they had covered 316.3 miles instead of the more than twice that which the Popes were accustomed to do in a day.

They ate a leisurely dinner, each bite of which gagged Penny Pope, who warned the Bells as everyone went to bed, 'Tomorrow, 0400. Sharp.'

This was agreed, but in the morning it proved impossible for Cluny to rise, shower, dress, make up and fix her hair till 0730, and then she refused to start until she had her cup of hot coffee: 'It's uncivilized to travel on an empty stomach.' Their caravan hit the road at 0814 and John Pope was livid.

It was the business with the map that started him plotting as to how he might escape from this disaster. When he and Penny roared across country it was their delight from time to time to use lesser roads and to make excursions to spots they had always heard of but never seen, and they never allowed their headlong flight to prevent them from enjoying themselves.

Now, although they were only in western Alabama when they should have been leaving Mississippi, Penny wanted to see Mobile and its bay, important in the War of 1812 and in the Civil War. Normally, if John had been driving, she would have been riding shotgun with the map on her knees, and she was expert in identifying alternate roads of promise: 'Turn left at the fork. Looks like a great trail beside the river.' Quite often she would have made a disappointing guess, so she would cry, 'Let's try the next road to the right. It's got to get us back to Route 10 one way or another.'

On this day, because the top was down, Cluny Bell sat beside John as he sped the Mercury along minor roads, so it was she who held the map, and this was a disaster. For the wind made it difficult to keep the map in order, and when John did show her how to fold it, she could make absolutely nothing out of east or west, north or south. Once when he demanded in a hurry to know whether he must turn right or left at the next crossroads, she wailed, 'How do I know?'

'It's on the map,' he said curtly, and when she proved incapable of even guessing where they were, he grabbed the map abruptly, consulted it for less than five seconds, jabbed at it with his finger, and snapped, 'There. It's very clear.' She did not break into tears, but she almost did.

It was curious, thought Penny in the back seat. American culture is based on the automobile, and any young man of promise is going to own one and want to travel great distances in it. Consequently, any young woman of aspiration should expect to spend most of her vacations in a car, probing into unfamiliar corners. She is not required to know how to drive —Cluny doesn't—but she will certainly be expected to read the road map while her husband drives, and if she can't, or if she's abnormally slow in giving him help, she's bound to cause trouble. Therefore, you'd think that colleges which train the bright young women who're going to marry the bright young men who are going to own the Cadillacs that roar back and forth across this continent would teach the girls to read maps. None do. They teach a hundred other useless things, but never a word about the one that will cause the greatest friction.

'Can't you see where the road joins Route 65?' John asked plaintively.

'The map is going north,' Cluny said, 'and we're going south.' And it was only when she said this that John realized she was powerless to imagine how the map worked, or how one intuitively corrected for east and west regardless of orientation, or how one extrapolated information or calculated distances. The totality of America lay unfolded on Cluny's knees, and she was unable to decipher a single element of it.

'Better give the map to Penny,' John said compassionately.

'I never wanted it in the first place.'

'If we drove a couple of hours after supper, which I like to do,' John informed his passengers, 'we could probably reach the Mississippi . . .'

'I think we should start looking for a good motel pretty soon,' Cluny said, and again the battle was joined. This time Penny supported her husband in his desire to reach the Mississippi, but Cluny created such a scene of petulant anxiety that her husband had to support her. They stopped at 1723, an ungodly hour when three hundred miles could be added to the log, and although Pope laid down the law at dinner—'We leave tomorrow at 0400 or we'll never reach California'—they actually left at 0752.

What was more infuriating, when they stopped for lunch Cluny spotted a hairdresser's, and before anyone could stop her she had left the group and dropped in for a quick set to repair the damages caused by the windy convertible. She reappeared fifty minutes later, and at 1730 that afternoon began to whimper about a good motel, so they stopped.

As was customary on such cross-country trips, John Pope awakened at 0330 and did the isometric exercises which kept him trim, but as he did so, Penny wakened, too, and after lying silent for a few minutes, she whispered, 'This trip is a disaster. And it gets worse every hour.'

'I have never struck a woman . . .' He did not finish his statement, but he did turn on the light, and when he saw their clothes lying on the floor, waiting to be jumped into, and the minute hand of his chronograph climbing toward 0400, he turned and looked intently at his wife.

It was she who spoke: 'We could, you know.'

'It's the only sensible thing to do,' her husband said.

In a flash they were out of bed and in their traveling clothes. 'How much money have you?' John asked.

'In traveler's checks I have—'

'I mean cash.' Between them they could scrape up $143.55, of which they must withhold $20 for gasoline to be purchased before places would be open to cash their checks.

They took the $123.55 and placed it in a motel envelope, which they addressed 'The Bells, Room 117,' and this they intended jamming under the door of their companions' room, but at the last moment John felt that some statement was essential, so on a clean sheet of paper he wrote:

Dear Tim and Cluny,

Obviously this isn't going to work. Here is all the cash we have. It will get you to the nearest NASA installation. See you at Allied Aviation.

All the best,
Penny and John

As soon as they were safely on Highway 10, roaring west toward Louisiana, John at the wheel, Penny with the map across her knees, they broke into joyous song:

> 'Bring me my Bow of burning gold:
> Bring me my Arrows of desire:
> Bring me my Spear: O clouds unfold!
> Bring me my Chariot of fire.'

No reference to this incident was ever made by either of the two astronauts. Tim Bell realized that his partner Pope had faced a problem and had done what was required, honestly and without hesitation; in a similar circumstance he would probably have done the same. At Allied Aviation the two men worked together effectively, and once or twice they caught sight of Penny Pope performing her inspections for the Space Committee. The two couples did not dine together, but when they met at the hotel provided by Allied, they were reserved and courteous.

They could not escape having a goodbye lunch with General Funkhauser, who was in charge of Allied-NASA relations, a two-billion-dollar windfall for his company. He was expansive as he presided in the company dining room.

'This is abalone,' he said in his attractively accented English. 'In Germany, I had never heard of it. And this is Oregon duckling, which I hadn't heard of either.' He spoke revealingly of what Allied proposed to do about an instrument of radical new design that could walk on the Moon. 'One-sixth gravity permits us to do wonders. Better than an automobile. Lighter than a baby carriage. Hermann Oberth always told us, "Your imagination must live, yes, in one-sixth gravity." '

There was an embarrassing moment when he asked the astronauts how they were returning to Cape Canaveral, for Pope said bluntly, 'Penny and I are driving.'

'Can you take so much time away from Washington?' Funkhauser asked. He had been especially solicitous of Mrs. Pope, anticipating the day when her committee might want to investigate the Allied-NASA contracts. They were honest, he felt sure, but they were also very favorable to the company, and if they were ever reviewed by the Senate, he knew that he would be expected to defend them, since senators listened to generals.

'And you?' Funkhauser asked the Bells.

'I'll ask your secretary to get us a Transportation Request from the NASA office. Fly back commercial.'

'You cannot leave Allied on a commercial plane,' Funkhauser snorted. 'You and Mrs. Bell will fly back in my jet.' And it was so arranged.

On the return trip in the convertible—never less than seven hundred miles a day—the Popes discussed their ungallant behavior toward the Bells, and whereas John was inclined to feel ashamed, his wife refused to be apologetic. 'We have only so many trips across this great country. To allow two of them to be ruined would be craven.'

'But one of these days I may have to fly with Tim.'

'He'll think more of you for your courage in handling this problem.'

'And I'll be more attentive to him, after treating him so badly.'

'John! Stop blaming yourself! You and I do fine work for this nation. More than any other couple I know. We're entitled to get up at four and drive till ten, if we want to.'

They always preferred the eastbound trip, for then in the early evening they could watch the new stars rise from the horizon and climb toward the apex. It was exciting to see the summer stars coming at them in grand array: Vega, Deneb, Altair.

'It's very strange,' he told Penny as they climbed through the Rockies. 'Every chart advises the beginner to identify these three stars in relationship to each other. I can never find Vega. Not until I see those four little stars to the north. Head of the Dragon. Whenever I spot that parallelogram I know where I am.' She could not even see it.

Capricorn appeared and the Great Square of Pegasus, and John wanted to drive all night, to see the stars climb up at him as he had come to know them on the plains of Fremont, and the battlefields of Korea, and the hilltops at Boulder. 'We wouldn't have to drive too long before the blazing constellations start to appear,' he told Penny.

'Why not?' she said. It would be about three hours before Capella and the Pleiades and the Bull, so John suggested that they drive off the main road and catch a couple of hours sleep, and in the high country they found a meadow set down between tall peaks, and there they slept, huddled under coats, John in the front seat, Penny in the back.

They had no trouble in waking, and when they resumed their trip eastward at three in the morning, Orion and the Twins and the Dog were preparing to greet them, and as night faded and the Rockies gave way to vast and empty plains and the brilliant stars left the heavens, John said, 'Why don't we push right on to Fremont?' They did, arriving there exhausted in late afternoon.

Dr. Pope hurried home from the drugstore, and the Hardestys came from across the railroad tracks for a celebratory supper, but the younger Popes were too tired to enjoy it. They went to bed early, but at 0400 they were in the convertible heading east across the Missouri River, and as they sped once more into the path of the morning stars Penny caught a slight glimpse of what it meant to be an aviator or an astronaut.

'You fly toward the stars, don't you?'

'And sometimes away from them, but always in relation to where they are,' and for the first time she sensed what the ancient Assyrians had known and the men at Stonehenge and Albert Einstein: that man and all his doings and his Earth and his Sun and his Galaxy are held in interlocking responsibilities which operate beyond the farthest reaches of the mind.

John Pope was working at Cape Canaveral on a computer to be used in the next flight, and Penny was in Washington organizing a meeting of the Space Committee, on the day when Tim Bell, returning from a contractors' meeting in Wichita, flew his T-38 into a radio tower in Cincinnati, where he was stopping for fuel. His plane exploded and burned so furiously that it could almost be said there was no corpse.

Word was flashed to NASA headquarters in Houston and from there immediately to Cape Canaveral and to the Space Committee in Washington, so that John and Penny heard the desolating news at about the same time. Each could guess what the other must feel, but Penny could not know that the local command had directed John to rush down to Cocoa Beach to inform Cluny Bell of her husband's death.

'I don't think I'm the man,' Pope said.

'It can be no one else,' the administrator said, for in NASA it was obligatory that a fellow astronaut be the one to inform a widow of tragedy. No clergyman, no reporter, no sobbing woman television star and no front-office administrator would do. An astronaut had died in line of duty, and another astronaut would carry the fatal news.

A police escort was assigned to lead him south to the Bell cottage before any news flash could alert the widow, but when John heard the sirens wailing he pushed the Mercury ahead, and signaling to the men, he yelled, 'Turn those things off when we reach the Beach.'

'Roger,' one of the policemen said, and they entered the little town in silence; but knowing persons could guess that some tragedy had occurred, and wives started telephoning to be sure it wasn't their husband.

Pope signaled for the escort to leave him when he approached the lane on which the Bell cottage stood, and he parked his car some distance from it. Leaving the convertible, he walked slowly toward the front door, saying to himself, 'Pull it together, buster.' And he tightened his gut.

He knocked on the door, and when he heard sounds inside—children playing and the movement of feet—he wanted to flee in terror, but he muttered again, 'Not now, you bastard.'

The door opened. Cluny, with curlers in her blond hair and an apron about her waist, took one despairing look at Pope, then asked, 'Is it Tim?'

'It is, Cluny.'

For one endless moment she stood there, no expression on her face. Then she slowly collapsed, as if all the muscles and joints of her body had been removed. Pope caught her, and for a few seconds she rested in his arms.

'Mommy, Mommy? What is it?' a child asked.

John felt her strength returning, and he watched as she left him and went to her three children. Gathering them to her, she started to speak, but no words came, and she turned pitifully to Pope, who took the children from her. When she saw them leave, as if they were permanently departing, she realized what a terrible blow had struck these little ones and she uttered a penetrating scream.

At this moment Tucker Thompson walked into the room, and with a sensitivity and control that amazed Pope, took over. Quietly he assured Cluny that everything would be handled as she directed; he helped her to a sofa and asked if she wanted some brandy, which he had brought with him. He then attended to the children, telling them honestly, 'Your father will not be here. You must take great care of your mother,' and he placed them beside her.

'Pope,' he snapped at John, who stood bewildered, 'we've got to get her out of here before the press gets the word. Is your wife down here?'

'She isn't. But Debby Dee is three blocks down the road.'

'Walk. Don't run. Have Deb prepare everything, and I'll be there with Cluny in five minutes.' When John left, Tucker was gathering the children's clothes.

Penny flew down, of course, and so did the other husbands and wives. It was a somber funeral, with the four young astronauts in their military uniforms and medals. General Funkhauser came to pay tribute to Allied Aviation's finest test pilot, and administrators from NASA paid their astronaut high honor. Tucker Thompson irritated some of the press by keeping them away from Cluny Bell and the children, but he was in no way obtrusive, insisting that even the *Folks* photographers operate from a distance; since he had provided them with high-powered Japanese telephoto lenses, they had no difficulties.

And when the funeral was over, and the lease on the cottage terminated, and the wreckage of the T-38 removed from the field at Cincinnati, the same miracle that had embraced Inger Jensen when her husband died came consolingly to Cluny Bell. Divorced test pilots and widowed military aviators started dropping by Houston to see how Tim Bell's three kids were doing, and after one such visit Debby Dee Claggett had a long talk with Cluny: 'Marry the sonnombeech. Don't be like Inger, wasting your life in a library somewheres. You got a lot more to take care of than books.'

Cluny was vulnerable, and alone, and very beautiful, and it did not matter if she was flighty and could not read a map or a bank statement. She and her children needed help and they needed it now. Not six months had passed before she took Debby Dee's advice and told an Air Force major she would marry him. The family moved back to Edwards, where she remembered many people from the days when Tim Bell had tested planes there, and where her new husband would be doing similar work for the next four years.

The essence of any NASA job was travel, and Stanley Mott was working with Boeing in Seattle when he received urgent instructions to fly immediately to Miami, where Mrs. Mott would meet him in the public terminal. When he hurried up to her she was in the company of a tall man in his fifties, who said, 'Hello, Mott. I'm Harry Conable, lawyer.'

'For what?'

'For your son Christopher. He's been caught with a very unsavory group. Almost a ton of marijuana.'

'Oh my God!' Mott had been aware for some years of the ugly drift into which his younger son's life had fallen, one damaging incident after another, starting in grammar school and continuing through the unsatisfactory half-year he was in college. There had never been any one act which by itself indicated criminality, but taken together they gave evidence of a young man sadly disoriented and heading for big trouble. During one miserable four-month period he had associated himself with a neo-Nazi group in Maryland and had been photographed in white robes without a hood, burning a cross on the lawn of a Jewish residence near the university, and from that escapade he disappeared into the desert in Arizona, where he underwent paramilitary training for soldier-of-fortune recruitment against the new black governments of Africa.

In all of this sorry rebellion against his parents and their society Chris had avoided serious confrontation with the police, but now a prison sentence loomed, as Conable explained: 'The magnitude of this operation can't be ignored. The government thinks the marijuana came into Florida by small speedboat from Mexico. At any rate, it found its way to Miami, probably brought here by your son and two others, and now it's in a federal warehouse.'

'Is it considered a drug? I mean in Florida?'

'It sure is.'

Mott retrieved his baggage from the conveyor and walked soberly to Conable's car, listening attentively as the lawyer spelled out his plans for the trial: 'I can't advise your son to plead guilty, although I'm sure he is.'

'Why not?' Mott asked. 'If Christopher has done this criminal thing . . .'

'Because I believe his relative youth—he's only twenty-one Mrs. Mott tells me.'

'Twenty-two,' Mott said.

'I think we can prove something like stupid involvement with older men.'

'Was that the case?' Mott asked.

Mr. Conable was driving, his eyes straight ahead, watching for the turnoff from the airport where he would deposit the ten-cent toll. 'Your son is a very difficult type, Dr. Mott. Two more years of this, he's going to be a criminal.'

'Oh God.'

'In the long run it might be best if we let him go to jail now. I could arrange a short term, I'm sure. Might scare the hell out of him.' The Motts did not respond to this, so he added, 'But I have a low opinion of Florida jails. I think we must get him off if we possibly can.'

Next morning he took them to see Christopher in the lawyer's room at the jail, and when the Motts saw their handsome son and visualized him as a young instructor in some good college, tall and straight and clean, they lowered their heads. Chris was not repentant: 'Mary-Jane's no drug. This country is off its rocker.' He would make no concessions, refused to cooperate in his own defense. Stanley Mott wanted to shake him, Rachel Mott longed to take him in her arms—but seeing the anger in his father's eyes, the love in his mother's, he rebuffed them both.

The judge, witnessing the same recalcitrant behavior in court, listened patiently to the arguments of Mr. Conable, then sentenced the young man to six months in jail.

The Motts rented a car and drove north to the Bali Hai at Cocoa Beach, where they sought consolation with their NASA friends. Mr. and Mrs. Quint said that they saw a good many families in Florida with sons like Christopher: 'And there isn't a hell of a lot you can do about them.' They told of friends of theirs who had a son who began to steal cars at the age of nine. Couldn't keep his hands off them. Parents tried and tried to reason with him, so did the judges. One morning at six he came to this motel, stole the car of a man from Wisconsin, drove up the highway at a hundred and ten, and killed himself.

'And you know,' Mrs. Quint said, 'not a soul in this town mourned that boy's passing, not even his own parents. We were just glad he didn't take some innocent person to death with him.'

The Motts were hiding in the Bali Hai, trying to comprehend what had happened to Christopher, when NASA called from Washington with news of an assignment that would determine the general emphasis of Dr. Mott's obligations for his remaining years with the agency: 'We want you to familiarize yourself with the Mars project and become our contact with the media.' Mott was elated, for this was a logical step toward his permanent interests, the outer galaxies. For some years NASA scientists had been endeavoring to photograph the planet, and no mission evoked a deeper emotional response among professional astrophysicists. From the days of the Assyrians the somber red planet had tantalized astronomers, and Mott could recall vividly how as a boy he had devoured Percival Lowell's remarkable 1906 book *Mars and Its Canals*.

'You know that Professor Lowell is the brother of Amy, the one who wrote poetry and smoked cigars?' his mother had said when she found him reading the advanced book.

Mott had been no child genius; like his astronauts, he had matured slowly but with great sturdiness, but as soon as he saw Lowell's intricate maps of what he called 'the canals' he began to suspect that the whole design was nonsense. Later, when he learned that Lowell had mistranslated the Italian astronomer Schiaparelli's word *canali* (which the latter had used to mean *channels* that might have been cut by rivers or casual floodwaters) into the much stronger word *canals,* which would have had to be cut purposefully by sentient beings of some kind, he knew that Lowell was spouting nonsense.

Nevertheless, he asked the Newton librarian to borrow Lowell's later book from the Harvard library, *Mars as the Abode of Life,* and read with disbelief as the author constructed a fantasy world of agriculture and oases and cities and canals thousands of miles long bringing water down from the melting polar ice caps. He decided then, on the basis of everything else he read, that Mars was probably uninhabited, and when he found a chance to look at the red planet through a Harvard telescope, he was satisfied that his first judgment was correct. Mars was a dead planet, and when his schoolboy friends offered him their copies of the Edgar Rice Burroughs yarn about the beautiful princesses who inhabited Mars, he said, 'No, thanks.'

He had been amused, that time in the hospital, to find that about half the science-fiction tales brought by Claggett dealt with missions to Mars, the ones most worthy of study being those by Jules Verne and Arthur C. Clarke. Most of them had described the beings living on Mars, even the poetic masterpieces of Stanley G. Weinberg, but the dazzling photographs from Mariner 4 showed him a bleak and barren terrain, and he concluded that the writers had been indulging in the lovely, forgivable dreams of childhood.

He was excited when the NASA high command told him: 'Mariner 4 did brilliant work, but it was merely a fly-by. Took only what shots it could catch on the wing. Mariner 9 will be an orbiter. Photograph the entire planet in high resolution.' And when he reported to the launch pad at Canaveral and saw the sleek, powerful rocket with the rather small spacecraft perched atop, he wondered at the skill of his associates in building a device which could transmit photographs over a vast distance. Depending upon where Mars and Earth were in their respective orbits, this distance could vary from as much as 249,000,000 miles to as little as 34,000,000. For this shot the mileage would be 75,000,000.

It was a hot morning at the end of May when the rocket fired and the Mariner soared high over the Atlantic to a trajectory that would carry it, after one hundred and sixty-eight days, to Mars, and as it disappeared high in the heavens, its trail still blazing, Mott thought: Our astronauts are rather glib in stating they're ready to take the next Apollo to Mars. I wonder if they make adequate calculations? For a trip to Mars the spacecraft would have to be bigger, but that presents no problems, because in space an object weighing fifty tons moves at the same speed as one weighing fifty ounces. But up and back at the present state of the art, plus time to explore the surface, might take as long as three years, and I wonder if three men could survive with only dehydrated food and a bungee cord to exercise their legs?

While the Mariner was on its lonely way to the planet, he had more than five months to acquaint himself with the elegant system whereby the photographs would be returned to Earth, and when he dug in at the Jet Propulsion Laboratory in Pasadena he found that he had to unlearn a great deal of what he thought he knew. Marvin Template, a twenty-three-year-old bearded wizard in blue jeans, became his teacher:

'Knock the words *camera* and *photograph* out of your mind. I don't like to use either because they confuse thinking. With us it's *scanner* and *picture*. The scanner bears little relation to a camera. It's a device which points at a subject, breaks it down into little squares. They're called *pixels,* from picture elements. The scanner detects with its magic eye the relative value from perfect black to perfect white of each pixel.

'It can differentiate 256 gradations of grayness from 000, which is total black, to 255, total white. And how does the scanner send its judgment to us down here on Earth? In binary computer language, each "word" consisting of eight bits, 0 or 1. Thus a pixel might be reported as having a gray value of 227, and we would receive something like 11100011.

'At top speed the scanner can send us 44,800 of these bits every second. Yes, I said second. During its entire stay aloft it'll send us 350 billion bits of information at the relaxed rate of 29,900 bits a second, day and night.'

Mott, having learned a great deal about computers at Cal Tech, was prepared to accept Template's bizarre figures, but he did want to see a mock-up of the scanner that could perform these miracles, and when he had one in his hands he could scarcely believe that an instrument so small and so insignificant in appearance could do so much. It resembled a tiny one-gun turret on a battleship; a protruding eye, a traverse gearing, a lot of connecting wires, and it could be activated by radio over a distance of 75,000,000 miles. After he had taken the practice scanner apart and reassembled it, he felt that he had a preliminary knowledge of what was about to take place.

But it was what happened to the flood of information when it reached California that enchanted him, and he spent the better part of four months receiving data from other spacecraft and transmuting the bytes (groups of eight bits) into pictures, always under the meticulous supervision of Marvin Template. Once Mott said to him, 'Considering what you do, Template, somebody gave you a most appropriate name.'

'That's just what we do down here. We set up a template, 832 pixels by 700 and this becomes the base on which we construct our picture, 582,400 pixels in all.' With a battery of sophisticated machines he demonstrated the miracles he could perform using these data:

'As each byte for this pixel arrives from Mars, the machine will apply the appropriate amount of grayness. And watch! As we fill in the empty spaces, the picture begins to grow, like a flower coming into bloom at the edge of a marsh.'

The process was quiet, mysterious and wonderful, a blank sheet of paper springing to life as if some master artist were slowly applying his brush in the creation of a masterpiece, but what Template could do with the finished work astounded Mott:

'Now the wonder-working begins! We have this completed picture, but if we find that our scanner has not used very frequently the dark degrees 000 to 048, or the light ones from 241 to 255, we can direct it to ignore those outer edges and redistribute the remaining 193 good numbers along the entire scale of 000 to 255. This makes the central values much more discriminative.

'But that's only the beginning. With the purified data stored in our system, we can play the game of *What if?* What if the scanner was tilted to one side so that all values above 55 were skewed toward the dark end of the palette? We command the computer to unskew them, and we get this improved result.

'What if the scanner saw everything three levels too bright? We tell the computer to make the correction. What if the right-hand edge of the scanner consistently gave darker values than proper? We lighten up only that edge. And best of all, what if we are interested only in the central block of 40 pixels by 40? We can direct the computer to hold those values, ignore all others, and distribute these 1,600 little squares across the entire 000–255 spectrum, and we get a close-up that really shows something.'

When Mott made himself familiar with what this amazing device, half in the heavens, half in California, could produce, he spent hours at the receiving console, playing God with the data being sent in by different satellites, and he became quite proficient at the game of *What if?*, cutting away unwanted pixels, intensifying others, and rebuilding whatever portion of the universe the scanner had been studying.

And just when he had convinced himself that he understood what was about to happen at Mars, the JPL men reminded him of a phrase he had often heard but never really comprehended: 'You can't play *What if?* if you're operating in real time.' He asked what the men meant by *real time,* and they explained:

'We'll get data from Mars in two forms. When it comes directly to us as the scanner picks it up, that's real time. Or the scanner can acquire such a flood of information, it can't possibly transmit it instantaneously, so it puts it on tape and later on, when we're not so busy, we signal the tape to unload what it's accumulated. That's delayed time. Handling a project becomes a nice problem in adjusting our use of real time and delayed time.'

Mott saw the fallacy in this: 'But if it takes a message from Mars six minutes and forty-four seconds to reach us, we can never operate in real time.'

'Wrong. Real time means that you handle the data as soon as it comes under your control. You're not expected to be a psychic genius, anticipating what's going to arrive. If we ever get to Saturn, the time required for receiving data will be about ninety minutes, but if we go right to work, we'll still be in real time.'

It's much like a human life, Mott reflected as Mariner drew ever closer to Mars. A man spends his youth accumulating data, billions of bits, and some he must handle in real time, some he stores in his computer for later inspection. And balance in life consists of handling in real time those problems which cannot be delayed, then recalling more significant data during periods of reflection, when long-term decisions can be developed. And as we grow older we recall great segments of experience, deriving such lessons from them as our personal computers are able to decipher.

He built an imposing analogy, quite beautiful really, until he almost broke into tears: But what in the name of mercy had happened to Christopher? That he failed to accumulate the data? Or lacked the skill to recall and reorganize it when needed?

In his grief he compared Chris with his other son, Millard, a fugitive in Canada: Very confusing data had flooded in upon Millard, but damn it all, he had organized it, and concluded: 'I'm thus and so and that's it'— and he's handled himself as well as I have. But then his thoughts reverted to Chris, and he was sitting with his hands over his eyes when Template, about the age of his sons and already the master of profound knowledge, asked, 'Are you sick, Dr. Mott?' and Stanley wanted to cry out, 'I am sick at heart,' but he merely shook his head, so Template said, 'I want to show you what else we can do . . . quite miraculous,' and he took Mott to a new machine:

'This one works with a special scanner that sends us three distinct indications of value for every pixel. That means, for a complete picture, it sends us 13,977,600 bits in about 5.2 minutes.

'What it's doing is sending us a color picture, but we can't be sure what color. So we say that one of the sets represents the red portion of the spectrum, one the yellow, and one the green. We could use any three other colors, but these give us good results. And when we print the three color sheets and combine them . . . *"Voilà!"* '

He showed Mott a dazzling color picture of the Earth as seen through the eye of a scanner and corrected by Template in his game of *What if?* It was so majestic, so much a sphere whirling in distant space that no one could see it without acquiring a deeper reverence for his planet, and he recalled Claggett's experience with the flat-worlders in Iowa: 'If a man wasn't a trained observer, he might be deceived by this picture.'

Template said, 'The colors we finally select aren't arbitrary. We look at the object visually through our telescopes to determine what the color seems to be. We use the spectroscope to establish an objective definition.' He hesitated, then chuckled. 'And we guess a lot. But in the end we balance out the three sets of values, and as I said, *"Voilà!"* '

When Mariner 9 reached Mars on 13 November 1972, the NASA men were appalled by what the incoming photographs revealed, for they revealed nothing. Mars was engulfed in a vast planet-wide dust storm which obscured everything. The fragile little craft had negotiated millions of miles, only to be defeated by howling storms more comprehensive than any the Earth knew. For nearly two months Mariner obediently kept watch on its obscured planet, producing nothing, but in mid-January the dust began to settle and it looked as if this flight might produce results.

'Tomorrow,' Mott assured the press, and when they reminded him, 'You said that before,' he said, 'This time Mars will cooperate. It's calling in its storm clouds.' And next day men watched in awe as the data began to filter in and the top row of pixels assumed their designated shades of gray.

Volcanoes began to emerge, three times higher than any mountain on Earth, and great deep canyons that could have reached from Boston to San Diego, hiding the Earth's Grand Canyon in one shallow rift. The scarred face showed where asteroidal fragments had bombarded the surface in times past, and the desolate, cruel beauty of the vast plains reinforced Mott's doubt that anyone in recent times had lived there, or grown vegetables or tended cattle.

The pictures that mysteriously effloresced from the pixels were forbidding yet magnificent, and as they glowed from the machines the planet Mars seemed to enter the laboratory, and the enchanting speculations of the Italian Schiaparelli with his *canali* and the American Lowell with his canals vanished the way dew departs with morning sunlight. Long shelves of romances dealing with Martian kings and battles slipped into honorable retirement, making way for the detailed maps and geological surveys of actual rocks and strata that would now replace them. The old Mars was dead, a splendid new one was being born.

The effect on Mott could not have been predicted. He had taken man's exploration of the Moon in stride, because his long speculative apprenticeship at Langley had prepared him for its reality, and the other events of the 1960s had borne no surprises, since he had anticipated such accomplishments back in the 1950s. He had come within a few weeks of being the first to throw a satellite into orbit, and everything after that followed inevitably. 'Of course men will walk on the Moon,' he had assured Rachel years ago, so that when it happened it was an aftermath. Besides, the Moon was only a few hundred thousand miles away.

But to travel to Mars, 75,000,000 miles distant, to penetrate its secrets with a scanner, and then perhaps to go to Saturn, nearly a billion miles more distant, and see its surface, too, and its many moons, was so grand an accomplishment that he was awestruck. This was man knocking on the door of infinity, and he was honored that he had been allowed to be even a humble part of it.

Unhappiness over his sons, the deaths of the two astronauts with whom he had been associated—even these defeats could not diminish the triumph of sending that small messenger to Mars and receiving in return such a wealth of mind-shattering information. On his way back from the JPL to the motel he looked at the stars and felt them to be infinitely closer; they were no longer dots of light gleaming at immense distances; they were now real burning entities, incandescent torches scattered through the Galaxy, and some, like the Sun, perhaps had planets, and of those random planets —billions of them in space—one or two, or a million or two million, might have sentient beings living on them.

'You out there!' Mott called to the stars. 'We have taken our first steps!'

In later years Dr. Strabismus often referred to the moment when he first caught a clear vision of the path ahead, and he spoke of it in the exaggerated rural illiterate lingo he had cultivated beginning in 1976:

> 'It was a misty day in December 1972. I was a-drivin' home from visitin' the sick and the road was long and dusty, so I turned on my radd-eeo and there I hear this voice a-comin' at me and it was the voice of God, speakin' through the agency of a minister-man from Georgia, and it spoke of revelation and salvation, and I knowed then it was a-speakin' personally to me.'

What Leopold Strabismus, president of the University of Space and Aviation, heard that morning was the syndicated broadcast of a radio minister who spoke with fantastic speed for his allotted time, during which he solicited funds four times, and the man was so effective, so overwhelmingly convincing in his sincerity, that Strabismus was captivated. For several weeks thereafter he sought out these religious services on the radio, studied the charismatic ministers on television, and even drove long distances across Los Angeles to hear the better local evangelists in person.

He would sit in the back of their mean storefront churches and mutter to himself, 'With proper management, this man could have himself a temple,' and he would devise the strategies whereby this could be accomplished. What impressed him most, however, was the fanatic loyalty he witnessed in the congregations; these people, hungry for leadership and moral direction, gave not only their money but their whole affection to the ministers, and Strabismus realized that the two forces taken in union—pastor and flock—represented a burgeoning power in American life of which he had been ignorant.

He had known, of course, that established religions like Methodism and Catholicism exercised power in the American system, just as the Orthodox rabbis of his mother's religion exerted leadership among the Jews of New York, but he had not realized that congruent with these known religions ran this substratum of storefront belief, and of the two types he suspected that the latter was the stronger.

In later days he would tell his congregations that his conversion occurred on that dusty road from San Bernardino; it actually took place in a religious palace on the edge of the Watts section of Los Angeles, for after some weeks of exploring the alleys of California religion he wanted to see the glittering highways, and this search took him to those varied temples and basilicas and grand pantheons built by the clergymen who knew how to collect major tithings from their congregations. He was stunned by the grandeur of some of these temples, but the one that commanded his attention over the longest span was this affair near Watts.

It was administered by a tall, thin, very attractive black man who called himself the Mighty Spirit and who preached while clothed in a long ermine robe paid for by the ladies of his congregation. He was a powerful orator specializing in the Books of Daniel and Revelation, but he attracted Leopold's attention and even affection because of the lawsuit which the government had brought against him. As the story unfolded, it concerned two middle-aged black women schoolteachers who claimed they had been defrauded by the Mighty Spirit, and they had a persuasive case, Strabismus thought, as he sat in court, listening to the charges:

'Our mother is seventy-nine years old, stricken with arthritis. She can't walk easily and putting on her clothes is a misery. The Mighty Spirit told her that he could cure her, so she gave him all her money and he wrote out the directions for what she must do to be saved: "Go to the Greyhound Bus Station in Los Angeles. Take an even-numbered bus to Long Beach. Enter the Greyhound Station there and drink water from three different fountains, saying the Lord's Prayer after each drink. Come home on a bus with an uneven number. Go to bed. Pray before you fall asleep, and in the morning you will be cured." '

Strabismus whispered to Marcia Grant, who had accompanied him to the courthouse, 'They may get him because he put it in writing?' and she replied, 'It's damned ingenious, whatever.'

The judge explored in some detail the minister's behavior in this case, the amount of money taken from the mother of the schoolteachers, and the degree to which the old woman had obeyed the prescription. Satisfied that here was a case of most palpable fraud, Strabismus sat silent as the defense attorneys, one white, one black, called Mrs. Carter to the stand.

'Did you follow the instructions given you by the Mighty Spirit?'

'Yes, sir, I did.'

'You got on the bus going to Long Beach.'

'Yes, sir, even-numbered.'

'And you drank from three different fountains.'

'Yes, sir, I did.'

'And you got aboard another bus and came back to Los Angeles.'

'Yes, sir, odd-numbered.'

'And what happened?'

'When I woke up next morning I could walk, just like he said.' And when she pointed to the Mighty Spirit sitting in court in his white ermine robe, the minister's supporters broke into cheers which the bailiff could not silence. The Mighty Spirit rose from the accused's chair, spread his arms wide, and shouted, 'I forgive them, for they know not what they do.'

'That was some trial,' Strabismus said as he drove Marcia back to their university, and from the manner in which he returned to it again and again in subsequent days, it was clear to Marcia that he had been deeply moved.

He was forty-seven, about two hundred and ninety pounds, handsomely bearded, deep of voice, and he could visualize himself in robes, bringing direction and meaning to the lives of others. In ermine? No, that was for blacks, who handled the wilder manifestations with an aplomb no white man could muster. In red, perhaps? No, the best was still solid black. But wait! In an Episcopal church once, at the funeral of a friend of Marcia's, he had seen an elderly minister in a robe of beautifully tailored wool, not black, not brown, but rather, a delicate tan-gray.

'What color do you call that?' he had asked Marcia.

'I think the stores call it fawn.'

'It's quite effective.' Yes, he could imagine himself in a fawn robe.

He was so disturbed about the present and the future—so confused might be a better description, he thought—that when he reached the university he asked Elizondo Ramirez to report to him on the finances of their various USA operations, and the Mexican assistant placed the figures before him:

'Universal Space Associates is plugging along. Normal subscriptions stay high. Special gifts have tailed off since you don't travel so much, but we're making a steady $185,000 a year and could do better if we applied ourselves. But, Dr. Strabismus, all I can do is service new mail subscriptions. Only you can bring in the special gifts.

'The University of Space and Aviation? Maybe we've reached a plateau. We do very well with our Ph.D.'s at the new price of $750, but only average with our M.A.'s at $400. I've tried pricing them at different levels and $400 seems about right. I don't think we can take it any higher.

'What I did not anticipate was the very good business we've been doing in selling copies of UCLA, Southern Cal and Stanford diplomas, with a very nice business in University of California at Berkeley. We just print them, fill them in, and sell them, no granting of degrees or anything else.'

Ramirez did not consider himself a forger. He referred to himself as a printer with imagination, but this was not accurate either, for he himself did none of the printing; he simply knew where to get it done. He had discovered that a good many practitioners of one kind or other, even doctors and dentists, liked to have an extra certificate on their walls, and he had uncovered this excellent printer in the valley who could copy anything. Together they had located four diplomas from the four most prestigious universities in the region, and by blanking out the names of the recipients, they had a stack of fine-looking pieces of paper on which a woman with a smooth handwriting could incribe the names of purchasers. The diplomas were priced at twenty-five dollars each, thirty for Stanford, and sold about two hundred a year, which, as Ramirez said, 'gives us some extra pin money.'

His genius manifested itself in an operation about which Strabismus had been ignorant until it began to pour in the money; modestly Ramirez credited the idea to pure luck:

'I love basketball, especially at UCLA with those great teams John Wooden turns out, and one night I read in the paper about how this fine colored center was ineligible because of his grades and it occurred to me, "Why don't he take make-up classes at USA?" And before the year was out we had more than two hundred fine university athletes enrolled in special classes, Oregon to New Mexico. We never saw them. They never saw us. Their coaches just sent us the papers and we signed them. But I'll tell you this, Strabismus, if we could of had half those cats on our campus at the same time, we could of won the NCAA going away.'

The various operations, Ramirez concluded, were bringing in about $255,000 yearly, 'and with this big building paid for, we have the space to branch out and do much better.'

It was interesting that not one of the principals in this operation sought money for himself. Neither the space report nor the university was ever used to collect funds for the personal gratification of Strabismus, Marcia or Ramirez. They lived simply, drove modest cars, avoided expensive clothes, and usually ate in the restaurants of the lower middle class. Each year they saved more than 60 percent of what they took in, holding it in banks against the day when they might want to make some major move, and even their most jaundiced critic could not accuse them of personal cupidity. To look at Elizondo Ramirez on the street you would have thought that he worked at some taco stand, and it would have been inconceivable to picture Marcia Grant as the daughter of a well-to-do United States senator. They were marking time, all of them.

But when Elizondo and his ledgers departed, Strabismus addressed the real problem which agitated him: 'Marcia, I've made up my mind. You've got to get the abortion.'

She was thirty-three and not likely to become pregnant again if she allowed herself to be robbed of this child, and she loved Leopold, big, conniving fraud that he was. For five painful weeks she had argued against the abortion, citing one good reason after another, and he had countered with reasons of his own: 'Marcia, I have this persistent feeling. Something big is going to turn up. We mustn't be saddled with an illegitimate child.'

'You could easily marry me.'

'I don't see that, either. Look, Marsh, we're not the marrying kind. We're gauged to a much different track.'

'Home and children aren't so different. Millions of people are able to handle homes and children.'

'It's not for us, Marsh. I want us to simplify our lives. Get things organized for whatever's going to happen.'

He was so insistent, and upon principles which he could not explain or she understand, that in the end she consented to the abortion. Assuring her that this was a simple operation without risk, he drove her to the home of a man known in the community as Dr. Himmelright, and there she met one of the most despicable men of her experience. It was not his ghoulish profession which annoyed her; it was his manner.

Himmelright had been born in England, and whether he had ever graduated from anywhere could not be ascertained. On his wall he displayed diplomas, but she recognized two as the handiwork of Elizondo Ramirez. He spoke in an Oxford accent, quite charmingly, and apparently did a good business, for Leopold had had to accept whatever appointment Himmelright had free.

He tried to put Marcia at ease: 'We call this little deal, quite painless, you know, "Knocking Little Willie off the wall." ' He chuckled at his joke, then showed Marcia how she must lie down. 'What we're doing,' he said in a professional whisper, 'is taking out the crib but leaving in the playpen.' This joke pleased him immensely, and he laughed for nearly a minute.

As he fumbled among his instruments he said, 'Considering the over-population in Africa, what you're doing, Mrs. Strabismus, may be a very wise thing. And Asia's worse. Every fourth child born in the world is Chinese, and a woman came running in here the other day in tears. Said I had to operate right away. This was her fourth child and she didn't want no Chinese baby.' This quite captivated him, and when he turned to face Marcia he was grinning so broadly that he seemed quite awful, and before he could touch her she leaped from the couch and ran from the building.

Strabismus had gone for a cup of coffee to steady his nerves and it was some hours before he could locate her. She was wandering aimlessly along the streets back of the university, and at first she would not get into his car. When she did she neither cried nor made a scene. She simply sat there, quite erect, her hands folded on her pregnant belly. 'It's Christmas and I'm going home.'

'To Clay? That would be impossible.'

'I want to go home.'

'From here in Los Angeles it looks possible. But think of it from the Clay end. Think especially of your father.'

And when she did think, and saw her cuckoo mother and her pompous father, she realized that Strabismus was right. She could not go home, so she allowed him to drive her slowly back to Dr. Himmelright, who made no more jokes.

Stanley Mott, striving to attain some sense of what the universe was, sat perfectly still on the bank of the Tennessee River, south of Huntsville, Alabama. Keeping arms and legs motionless, he endeavored to move not even his eyes, for he wished to experience the sensation of a body at complete rest, and at last he achieved this. He was as still as a human being could be; indeed, he might as well be dead except for the inescapable functioning of autonomic systems like breathing and heart beating.

I am motionless, he said to himself at last, and he kept this posture for ten minutes, thinking of nothing. Then his brain insisted, recalling data he had memorized at Cal Tech:

But at this moment I'm sitting on a piece of Earth at 34° 30' North, which means I'm spinning west to east at a rate of about 860 miles an hour. At the equator, because of the larger bulge, 1,040. At the same time, my Earth is moving through its orbit around the Sun at 66,661 miles an hour, and my Sun is carrying itself and its planets toward the star Vega at something like 31,000 miles an hour.

Our Sun and Vega move around the Galaxy at the blinding speed of 700,000 miles per hour, and the Galaxy itself rotates at 559,350 miles an hour.

And that's not all. Our Galaxy moves in relation to all other galaxies as they rush through the universe at a speed of better than 1,000,000 miles an hour.

So when I sit here absolutely still I'm moving in six wildly different directions at an accumulated speed of . . . (he could not add the figures in his head) maybe two and a half million miles an hour. So I can never be motionless. I'm traveling always at speeds which are incomprehensible. And it's all happening in real time.

He considered these demonstrable facts for some moments, then concluded:

And perhaps the universe itself is hurtling toward some undefined destination at a speed which could hardly be stated, perhaps to clear our space for a better universe which will supplant us, while we rush off to some new adventure.

When he rose and felt his limbs moving only inches, he thought: What a trivial journey we make. Inches under our own power, two and a half million miles with the universe. But ours is the journey that counts. Our slow inching along to understanding and control. When he headed back to his car, he calculated that he was walking at a rate of perhaps 2.3 miles an hour, hardly worth noting in comparison to the speeds he had been dealing with: And yet, for millions of years of our existence, that's about the best we could do. It got us where we are, and that's not trivial.

When Claggett, Pope and Linley were only three weeks from takeoff, with the lunar terrain south of the Sea of Moscow engraved on their brains and the procedure for placing the three radio satellites in orbit memorized, their mission encountered a snag that almost destroyed it. John Pope was the first to hear about it.

Claggett said one night at the Bali Hai, where they were staying as they spent time in the Canaveral simulators, 'Johnny partner, Debby Dee and me's gettin' a divorce. I'm marryin' the Korean.'

'Come at me slow. You're what?'

'It's all settled. Deb knows. Cindy knows.'

'But does NASA know?'

'None of NASA's business.'

'It certainly is. They've got millions tied up in this flight. Billions.'

'What the hell is a few billion dollars? I'm talkin' about a private, personal affair.'

'There's nothing private, Randy. If this thing breaks, they'll take you off the flight, for sure.'

'So what? We got backups. They can move Lee into my seat.'

'They can hell.'

Pope did not inform NASA of this impending disaster, although for some time Claggett thought that he had: 'That damned Straight Arrow Pope. Always thinks he's running a Sunday School.'

It was Tucker Thompson who got wind of the domestic scandal; the Quints of the Bali Hai advised him that Debby Dee had flown in from Houston, found Randy and Miss Rhee in bed and had raised hell, 'and without getting out of bed Claggett told his wife, "Babe, it's finished." '

Thompson, better able to visualize the catastrophe that threatened than even the participants, went directly to Claggett. 'Randy, you can't do this.'

'I've already done it.'

'The American public won't let you. My magazine won't let you.'

'To hell with your magazine. I won't say to hell with the American public, because it's treated me pretty good. And I'll bet they won't give a damn.'

'Randy, you're not thinking straight.'

'Deb won't have any trouble findin' a new husband.'

'That's not the point, son.' He was sweating. He had visualized Apollo 18 as the glorious culmination of the *Folks* involvement, with two of his astronauts aboard and that fine black geologist adding spice to the photographs. He would show Claggett striding across the dark side of the Moon, Pope manfully at the controls, Debby Dee waiting in Texas, and that pretty black chick, Doris Linley, behind a white picket fence, waiting loyally for her man. Now it could all go down the drain, with *Time* and *Newsweek* ridiculing the operation.

Unable to convince Claggett of the gravity of what impended, he hurried to Pope's room at the motel. 'John, this could be a disaster. Really, I don't . . .' He collapsed onto a chair, where he sat mopping his forehead.

'Randy can be stubborn, you know.'

'But this is so unlike an astronaut. The American public will not tolerate him chucking a fine home-loving American wife and running off with Madame Slant-Eye from Column B.'

'From what Randy told me, it's all settled. Even Debby Dee has agreed.'

'Nothing's settled! Believe me, when Glancey and Grant hit this town, Randy Claggett is going to shiver.'

'I don't think he shivers easy.'

But when the two senators, accompanied by Dr. Mott from headquarters, appeared at the Bali Hai, discussions took a much different turn. These three did not plead, they came harshly to the point:

GRANT: You're jeopardizing fourteen years of our work, young man, and we can't allow it.

GLANCEY: Just because you get hot pants for some Japanese broad.

GRANT: You seem to forget that the American public has invested great sums of money and interest in you. You're not merely Randy Claggett. You stand for something.

MOTT (*gently*): A large part of NASA's future rides with you, Randy.

GLANCEY: One asinine gesture on your part, Claggett, the whole structure could collapse. You ditch your wife for some Japanese broad . . .

GRANT: It speaks to what an astronaut is all about. We've spent fourteen years carefully cultivating the image of what an astronaut is supposed to be . . . what his wife is supposed to be . . . and divorce simply does not fit into the picture as we've constructed it.

GLANCEY: Divorce would shatter the image. We can't allow it.

GRANT: An astronaut means something specific to the American public. Tucker Thompson can instruct you on your responsibilities in that area.

MOTT: Do I need to remind you, Randy, of how painfully we labored to get this mission authorized?

GLANCEY: The infinite trouble we had in slipping it past Proxmire?

MOTT (*persuasively*): If this story broke now, Randy . . . Damn it all, man, I've babied you fellows along for nearly a decade. This is your apex . . . our apex. You and Pope, two from the same class.

CLAGGETT: I see no reason why anything I'm doin' should endanger things.

GRANT: Well, everybody else can.

CLAGGETT: Lemme finish. Hickory Lee's been to the Moon. He can move into my seat with hardly a hair of change, so if you feel that my actions . . .

MOTT: We can't shift the crew around three weeks before launch.

CLAGGETT: Three weeks? You shifted Apollo 13 three days before takeoff.

GLANCEY: And look at the bad luck it had. We can't afford any more disasters, not at this stage.

GRANT: The bottom line, Claggett, America's space program cannot absorb a divorce.

CLAGGETT: It's gonna get one.

This first interview was much rougher than a conciliator like Mott would have wanted, much less conclusive than a hard-liner like Grant had hoped for, and when the three negotiators realized what a difficult man they had to deal with, they altered their strategy. In another room they tackled the Korean newspaperwoman, and that also was a mistake:

GRANT: Young woman—

CYNTHIA: I'm thirty-seven.

GRANT: Are you aware that you could be deported?

GLANCEY: Do you know what moral turpitude is?

CYNTHIA: Something you thin paint with?

GLANCEY: Don't joke with me, you tart.

GRANT: Because you lied on your visa application, you can be deported.

CYNTHIA: Proceedings would take months. By that time I'd be married, the wife of an American hero.

GRANT: You'll be in jail.

MOTT: Miss Rhee, the senators are serious. You imperil a project they've worked on for years.

CYNTHIA: It's a noble project. I've worked on it, too.

GLANCEY: What do you mean?

MOTT: She's writing a book.

CYNTHIA: Chances are it'll be remembered as the true account of this period.

MOTT: I must explain. This woman is a distinguished writer in Japan . . . in Europe. Held in very high regard.

GRANT: Why do we need a foreigner to write about our astronauts?

CYNTHIA: Because you won't allow your own writers to write about them.

GRANT: *Life* magazine? Tucker Thompson? Hundreds of reporters? The Korean woman broke into a disrespectful laugh, and her interrogation collapsed in shambles. It was obvious that she could not be scared, but there was a chance she could be reasoned with:

MOTT: Will you, for the welfare of a great mission, leave for Japan?

CYNTHIA: Doesn't that sound ridiculous, even to you? Newspeople flying in from all over the world to see this launch. Me flying out.

MOTT: I have a ticket for you. Won't you fly with me to New York? Pan Am has a reservation all the way to Tokyo. Or TWA, if you prefer.

CYNTHIA: Of the two, I would much prefer Pan Am.

GRANT: Thank God.

CYNTHIA: But since I have no intention of flying anywhere, neither airline can be of interest.

MOTT: Please? For the good of a great venture?

CYNTHIA: No.

The three men, having accomplished nothing except the disruption of training procedures, retired to their rooms at the Bali Hai, went to bed, and early next morning motored up to the launch area, where they asked NASA officials to bring the three astronauts before them:

GRANT: A serious problem threatens to disrupt your flight.

CLAGGETT: Lemme speak. I've already cleared this with these two.

POPE: Linley and I see no problem.

LINLEY: That's right.

GRANT: Well, the American people . . .

CLAGGETT: I don't think they care a whistle.

GRANT: Young man, do you have any idea at all of the flak that hit us in the Senate when those fellows in Apollo 10 called their spacecraft Charlie Brown and Snoopy?

GLANCEY: I received hundreds of protests from taxpayers: 'We don't pay our hard-earned dollars for some clown to jump around the sky like a comic strip.'

GRANT: Can you imagine what'll hit us if *Time* and *Newsweek,* not forgetting the *New York Times,* break it to the world that the man in charge of the flight has abandoned his American wife for a Japanese?

CLAGGETT *(shouting):* Why don't you get your facts straight? She's Korean.

GLANCEY: That's no improvement.

MOTT: It could be disastrous, Randy. For this flight. For all later flights.

CLAGGETT: Ain't no later flights lined up.

GLANCEY: Will you help us?

CLAGGETT: What you ask, no.

Curiously, it was Navy-tough Norman Grant who produced the line of reasoning which finally made sense to the three astronauts, and he presented it in a conciliatory, almost fatherly way:

GRANT: You know, men, this flight wasn't our idea. Glancey and I, we didn't want it. I even fought against it. It was you who wanted it. Your wife, Pope, she brought us the clinching arguments. Glancey and I and the others, we went way out on a limb for you men. Dark side of the Moon. Culminating scientific experiments. You persuaded us. Now don't walk away from us. Damn it all, it wouldn't be manly.

CLAGGETT *(after a long silence):* What do you want?

GRANT: Something extremely difficult. But something only you can handle. Tell him, Mott.

MOTT: We want you to tell Miss Rhee to fly with me to Kennedy Airport in New York and quietly take Pan Am's round-the-world flight to Tokyo . . . or to Korea, if she wishes.

CLAGGETT: She won't do it.

MOTT: She will if you ask her.

CLAGGETT: I can't do that.

No one in the room spoke. Six men—three older, three younger, but all widely experienced from the battling cloakrooms of the Senate to the far reaches of space—sat and pondered a problem of the most complex dimension. Finally it was Straight Arrow Pope who broke the impasse: 'All things considered, Randy, I think they have a point.'

What Claggett told Cindy in the upstairs room at the Bali Hai was not revealed to the others, but at eleven o'clock that morning an Air Force jet from Patrick Air Base a few miles south of Cocoa Beach took off with two United States senators, a high NASA official and a Korean newspaper-woman. It flew directly to Kennedy Airport in New York, where it was brought in ahead of orbiting planes and was met by a State Department limousine, which whisked the passengers not to Pan Am and not to TWA, for they flew out at dusk, but to a BOAC plane waiting at the terminal at the far end of the runway.

There Miss Rhee was hurried aboard, while the three astronauts at Cape Canaveral resumed last-minute training on the simulators.

Of course, when BOAC landed at London, Cindy strode swiftly across Heathrow Airport, caught a plane to Montreal, and secretly slipped back into the United States along a dirt road southeast of Sherbrooke. Hurrying to Florida, she climbed into a jumpsuit tailored from gray linen, donned a Greek sailor's cap, and took her place unostentatiously among the people who lined the highway overlooking Cape Canaveral. There she watched as Apollo 18 carried two of her special astronauts, Claggett and Pope, toward their appointment with the dark side of the Moon.

As the magnificent craft soared majestically into the air, the last of its glorious breed, she circulated among the watchers, taking careful note of where they were from and how they reacted to this historic moment. It was important, she believed, that their behavior be recorded in real time.

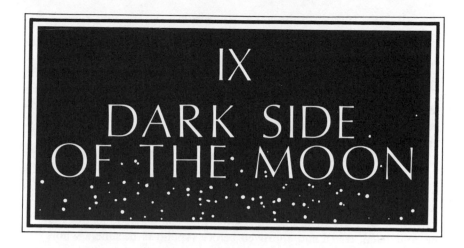

IX

DARK SIDE
OF·THE·MOON

WHEN IT WAS DECIDED, BACK IN 1961, TO LAUNCH THE PREDICTED
Apollos from Canaveral, the engineers and scientists of America
faced a tantalizing problem. The vehicle would be so massive, 363 feet high,
which was longer than a football field, that if it were assembled in one place,
say Denver, it would be so big and weigh so much—3,150 tons—that it
could not possibly be transported across the country. It would have to be
built at six separate locations and brought to Canaveral for final assembly.

The original plan had called for this assembly to take place in the open,
at the launch site itself, but even a cursory analysis of this proposal uncovered its dangers. Dr. Mott had served on the review board and had helped
draft the condemnatory report:

> One must remember that the Apollo will reach the Cape in six huge
> parts, with thousands of air- and water-tight connections still to be
> effected. Even one rainstorm would be disastrous, and in the five
> months required for assembly the local weather bureau estimates
> that we will encounter not less than sixteen rainfalls of varying
> strength. More important, the winds here are incessant, forty- and
> fifty-mile gales being common and 130-mile hurricanes not uncom-
> mon. The smaller parts would simply fly away. Undercover assem-
> bly is obligatory.
>
> We confess that the problem of moving the completed Apollo,
> weighing some 6,300,000 pounds, will present a problem which
> should be attacked immediately.

The first problem was solved majestically. Beside a canal into which
barges could come bringing the components, a stupendous white cube was
built, rising from the Canaveral swamps like some modern-version pyramid,
preposterously big. Silent, isolated in the landscape, an abiding symbol of

the space age, it became the mammoth barnlike building in which the Apollo complex would be assembled, and square though it was, it rose in the air almost as high as the needlelike spire of the Washington Monument. The face of the cube to the east contained doors half again as high as a football field is long; the covered interior provided a work space of 130,-000,000 cubic feet. In many respects it was the largest building in the world, and it had been completed at breakneck speed.

In it, six extremely complicated machines would meet for the first time; none would ever have been in proximity to any other, and not until they were intricately fitted together, with each bolt and wire in one component interfacing with its mate in another, could the spacecraft be said to be in existence. One workman had calculated that some 22,000 joinings had to be completed, tested and approved before Apollo 18 became a whole.

The constructors of this giant machine, working in six widely separated sections of the nation, required 30,000 different complex documents to ensure congruent fittings from one manufacturer to the next. The massive Stage I was put together in Louisiana by Boeing; the powerful Stage II was built in California by North American; Stage III, containing the crucial single engine which would send the spacecraft toward the Moon, once it got aloft, was built in a different part of California by Douglas. And the instrument unit, built by IBM in Alabama, was so huge and complicated that one traditional engineer said, 'That had to be built by some kid with an Erector set.'

Those four basic parts comprised only the rocket, but the process was the same for the two craft in which the astronauts would actually fly. Their command and service module was built in Downey, California, by an independent branch of North American and was broken down into two intricately related parts: the command module in which the men lived, and the service module which kept most of the gear out of the way. The astronauts considered this a single unit, the CSM, and spent days in its simulator, for upon it they must depend. The lunar module in which two of the men would drop down to the Moon and fly back to the orbiting CSM was built on Long Island by Grumman.

It was a preposterous way to construct one of the most intricate machines ever devised by man, for no one could predict whether the system would work until the six pieces—seven, really—were assembled in the waiting cube on the Florida swamplands. As Randy Claggett said irreverently, while orbiting his first Apollo when his companions were walking on the Moon, 'Here I am tooling along in a machine with four million different parts, each one supplied by the lowest bidder.'

And how did NASA bring these widely separated items together at the Cape? The instrument unit was placed on a barge on the Tennessee River, sent north to the Ohio River, then floated down the Mississippi, and around the southern tip of Florida to Canaveral. Stage I followed the same route, starting at New Orleans. California forwarded its segments two ways: by

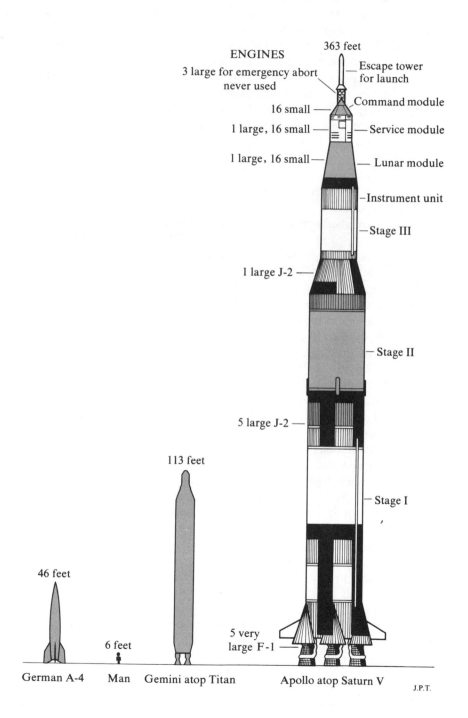

ENGINES

363 feet

3 large for emergency abort
never used

Escape tower
for launch

16 small — Command module

1 large, 16 small — — Service module

1 large, 16 small — — Lunar module

— Instrument unit

— Stage III

1 large J-2 —

— Stage II

5 large J-2 —

113 feet

— Stage I

46 feet

6 feet

5 very
large F-1 —

German A-4   Man   Gemini atop Titan   Apollo atop Saturn V

J.P.T.

ship through the Panama Canal and by a huge Boeing Stratocruiser converted into what NASA people called our 'Pregnant Guppy'; its belly could accommodate a completed Stage III.

In fact, NASA was in the transportation business with a fleet of five full-time vessels, one Pregnant Guppy and innumerable T-38s.

Claggett's Apollo 18 was scheduled to lift off on 23 April 1973, and as soon as the time was announced, Randy endeared himself to the press by saying, offhand, 'What a lucky date for us. Shakespeare's birthday. If he was alive today, he'd write a play about it. "The still-vext Bermoothes." '

'That's from *The Tempest,* isn't it?'

'It is.'

'How do you happen to know that?'

'They learn us things at Texas A and M,' and on the spur of the moment he told the reporters of an elderly man who taught Freshman Lit: 'He said, "It don't matter whether you remember anythin' else, but please, each year, remember that April 23 is the birthday of one of the noblest minds that ever existed, and pay him homage." Some smart ass—'

'Scrub that!' Tucker Thompson cried.

'Some wise guy said, "But I thought everyone knew Sir Francis Bacon wrote the plays," and the old gentleman never batted an eyelash, just said, "Then for the love of God celebrate Bacon's birthday, but at least once in your narrow, cornfed lives, pay respect to someone bigger than you are." And he took us all to a saloon and treated us to ale, which he said was what Shakespeare drank.'

The six components had to reach the assembly building four months prior to launch, and it was an exciting Christmastime when the barges came up the canal and the gigantic airplanes dropped down with their precious cargoes. Engineering teams from each contractor's home office arrived for extended duty at Canaveral, responsible for seeing that their part of the system functioned, and for three months the meticulous work proceeded as the disparate units were introduced one to the other and fitted together.

In February, Senator Grant and his committee factotum, Penny Pope, visited the assembly building to compile figures for presentation to the Senate budget officials, and for the last time in the Apollo program they watched the intricate labor being done in the assembly building. Grant was not unhappy to see the vast program grinding to a halt. It had been necessary in its day, to remind the Russians and the rest of the world that America was still competent, but the last few missions had been merely flourishes, and he knew it. However, this farewell flight, to the other side of the Moon, was going to be a dandy: 'We're going out with an appropriate bang.' He then handed the press a statement containing statistics collected by Mrs. Pope:

In mounting this tremendous effort to overtake the Russians, our nation has not stinted, and when we observe this vast assembly of buildings, what we see is the imaginative effort a free nation can make when it feels itself under the gun. Cost of the land, 140,000 acres at $72,000,000. Cost of the shell of this magnificent building in which we meet, $89,000,000. Cost of the equipment inside, $63,-000,000.

Look at that supertractor on which Apollo will be carried to its launch site, $11,000,000, and we must have an extra for backup. Total cost of ground installations alone, $800,000,000. Number of persons working here, 26,500. Number of high-powered experts needed to supervise the forthcoming launch, 500 here, another 1,500 in Houston.

The statement then dealt with support systems elsewhere in America and around the world, relying on such estimates as local officials could provide:

Number of radio ships dispersed around the world, four. Number of communications aircraft in flight during an Apollo mission, five. Number of ground stations in various foreign countries, thirteen. Number of eligible target ships positioned in various oceans, seven. Total number of men and women involved one way or another in this mission, 450,000. Total number of men who will finally stand on the Moon, two.

However, despite the staggering cost, this senator is more than pleased with the results of our national effort. He is especially gratified by the caliber of astronauts who will fly this final mission. He has known Captain John Pope, USN, all the latter's life and considers him one of the finest young men our nation has produced. His commander, Colonel Claggett of the Marines, has already flown three times in space, with outstanding results. But he is particularly honored that the third crew member is the nephew of a man he had the honor of serving with at the Battle of Leyte Gulf, Dr. Gawain Butler, Superintendent of Schools in Mesa County, California. As our first black astronaut, Dr. Paul Linley occupies a proud niche in our program.

His final paragraph summarized this thinking, and although Mrs. Pope urged him to soften it, he refused, reminding her: "You're loyal to your husband, as you should be, but I must be loyal to the nation as a whole.'

It is appropriate now for the United States to wind down this extremely costly adventure, which was amply justified in 1957 when Sputnik invaded our skies but which has trailed off into mere exhibitionism. We've reached the Moon. With this daring voyage we shall explore its dark side. Now we must direct our attention to equally pressing problems here on Earth.

In mid-February the experts in the vast assembly building reported: 'All okay'—and this became the signal to initiate an operation of ponderous elegance, one which always caused gasps of approval from the hordes of visitors allowed to watch from a safe distance. The gigantic doors of the building drew aside, 456 feet tall, to reveal, standing erect inside in the darkness, a gleaming white masterpiece, heavy at the bottom but tapering to a delicate point 363 feet in the air. The simplicity of the streamlined exterior, each surface honed smooth, belied the extreme complexity within, and often at this moment of revelation watchers applauded.

Through the vast doors they could see that the Apollo had been assembled attached to a massive gantry, both structures resting on a heavy metal base supported by pillars which kept them well above the floor, and now the tremendous supertractor—each of its four sets of what should have been normal cleats being individual tractors of gigantic size—moved from its waiting place outside the building, up a gentle gradient, and right into the heart of the building. There it eased its way under the waiting spacecraft, activated its hydraulic lifts, and tenderly assumed control of the entire mighty structure, Apollo and gantry alike.

At that moment even the workmen cheered, but now a most difficult problem arose. Tractor-plus-Apollo-plus-gantry weighed 18,480,000 pounds —9,240 tons—and how could such a burden be moved three and a half miles across Florida swampland?

> 'What we did was call in the best roadbuilders in the world, and they said, "Simple. You build a road wider than an eight-lane superhighway. You go down nine feet, line the bottom of your trench with big rocks, then seven feet of aggregate, then eight inches of pebbles. Cost? We can do it for about $20,000,000." '

Gingerly, the massive tractor and its precious cargo edged its way out of the assembly building, down the incline and onto the waiting roadbed, where its four corner tractors, each carrying more than 2,000 tons, ground into the surface and inched its way along.

It required a crew of fifteen to operate it at a speed of not quite a mile an hour, but when it came out into the February sunlight, moving purposefully like some majestic dinosaur, watchers cheered as the great thing went past: 'It moves fast enough to do the job.'

Slow, vast, creaking, grinding its massive cleats into the especially hard pebbles imported from Alabama, it carried on its back the soaring white Apollo nestled into the even taller launching gantry that would keep everything in order until the moment of launching: 'There she goes! Destination Moon!'

As gently as if it were carrying the child Moses along a canal of rushes, the supertractor moved out toward Complex 39, where the launch would be made, and as it passed majestically through the Florida sunshine, three men watched with special interest, for they would ride inside the capsule mounted at the top; they would guide this exquisitely beautiful thing to the other side of the Moon. 'The last and the best,' Claggett said.

John Pope, still amazed by the actual size of this giant, whispered, 'It's a privilege to be associated with it,' and Claggett reminded him, 'You named it, son. There goes your *Altair.*' This would be their home, their responsibility, the last noble bird of its breed, and they watched with love as it crept along. 'It wants to fly,' Randy said. 'Twenty-five thousand miles an hour, not crawl at twenty inches a second.'

After it had traveled three very slow miles, the importance of the top eight inches of pebbled rock and sealer became evident, for now the crawler was required to take a smooth curve to the north, and if the surface had been concrete, or macadam, as originally planned, the twisting of the cleats would have torn the road to pieces. As it was, the tremendous torque pulverized the top pebbles, but the metallic beetle inched ahead.

When it reached the approach to Pad A, from which the rocket would be fired, it faced a five-degree ramp up which it must move to the launch position, and now a score of computers, pumps, hydraulic systems and controls sprang into operation, lowering the front end of the crawler and raising the back so that an absolutely level platform was maintained.

When the climb up the ramp was completed, the crawler delivered the great Apollo with its gantry to the proper point, lowered it onto its stand, then backed slowly away as if it were some fairytale bullfrog who had saved a princess. Job done, it retreated groaningly back across the marshes, never again to bring a gleaming Apollo from its place of birth.

Among the 450,000 persons who were more or less directly responsible for the success of Apollo 18, including the Australians, Madagascans, Spaniards, Guamanians, Antiguans and Ascension Islanders who manned stations at their various locations, was a crew-cut Colorado farm boy from the little village of Buckingham in the drylands. An astronomer since his ninth birthday, when an uncle gave him Japanese binoculars and the Norton *Star Atlas,* he had won a scholarship to the agricultural college at Fort Collins, where like so many of the support team, he had graduated with honors.

His name was Sam Cottage, and his parents, immigrants from the German settlements along the Volga River in Russia, had worried about what kind of job their son could land with only a degree in astronomy, but he surprised them by quickly finding work at the Sun Study Center in Boulder, where high in the clear air of the Rockies, he studied the Sun. It was his responsibility, four times an hour, to focus his sixteen-inch solar-patrol telescope, with its special filter and obscuring disk, to see if any flares had arisen anywhere on the visible side of the Sun or along its perimeter, throwing disturbances a hundred thousand miles into the air; and then, through a restricted lens and carefully darkened eyepiece, to record patiently any spots which might have appeared on the surface of the Sun itself. Special attention had to be paid to regions that might conceivably erupt later into major flares which would produce what astronomers called *solar proton events.*

The United States government judged it profitable to keep Sam Cottage at such work because the significance of sunspots was just beginning to be appreciated: they caused northern lights, which sometimes halted radio transmission; they seemed to disrupt the Earth's magnetic field; and what was of great importance now, they had the capacity to launch a particularly vigorous flare which would discharge a dose of radiation so powerful as to be lethal to any human being caught unprotected. That was why Dr. Feldman, NASA's medical expert on radiation, had been so eager to have Claggett and Pope retrieve that dosimeter from the flank of Agena-A during their Gemini flight: 'We needed to know how much radiation accumulates during a long flight.'

Astronomers had to be consulted before the schedule of any flight could be fixed, because only they could say that the timing within the sunspot cycle was favorable. Spots had been meticulously counted since the year 1843, when astronomers first became aware that they varied within an eleven-year cycle, and these cycles had been numbered, so that Apollo 18 would lift off during the fading years of Cycle 20. This cycle had begun with a marked low in 1964, had achieved a below-average peak in 1970, and was now in swift decline, but as Cottage's office warned NASA:

> Even in the latest stages of a cycle, there is always a possibility of an unexpected solar proton event which might cause you to abandon a mission if it were still on the ground or terminate it if in flight, but Cycle 20 has been notably less violent than Cycle 19, which produced a heavy concentration of flares in 1957. We judge you can proceed with your plans for Apollo 18 with some feeling of security, but we shall maintain a close watch on the Sun's behavior.

So each day young Cottage compiled four reports on what the surface appeared to be doing, and at the close of day helped prepare a summary to be distributed to interested observers throughout the world.

In his spare time Cottage pursued advanced studies with a man who knew as much about the Sun as anyone on Earth, a soft-spoken Ph.D. named Jack Eddy, who worked atop a spacious hill outside Boulder in a research unit operated by a consortium of American universities. Cottage had been advised by one of his superiors: 'There won't be many advancements in our field for a young man who has only a B.S. degree. You're bright. Get your master's and then a doctorate.' He was now working with

Eddy, through the University of Colorado, for his master's, and he was struck by the imaginative work his professor had done in reconstructing the life history of the Sun through the last three thousand years. As Sam told the coed from Wyoming he was dating:

> 'This guy Eddy is fantastic. He's reviewed every study ever made about the Sun since we've had writing, and even some like tree rings that don't require writing. There was this guy Maunder at the end of the last century who claimed that in the late 1600s sunspots almost disappeared for a period of seventy years. People laughed, but Eddy proved that Maunder was right. That was the age of bitter cold on Earth. Glaciers edging down.

> 'The Maunder Minimum was a real thing. I suppose in the centuries ahead we'll have other minimums, but right now I'm trying to predict what will happen from year to year, and I'm getting nowhere.'

He had an affinity for mathematics, and under Eddy's guidance, had compiled mounds of data which he ran through the computer, satisfying himself but not others that over long stretches of time the Sun's activity balanced out and that a minimum of energy here was corrected by an abundance later on. He was convinced that the significant cycle was really twenty-two years and not eleven, for during the first half the magnetic character of sunspot regions followed one pattern, reversing during the second half. He was also much impressed by studies from Germany indicating that a superior cycle of eighty-eight years might be operating, but whatever he did, whatever theory he followed, his statistics showed that Cycle 20 was grossly aberrant and could be brought back into balance only if a major proton event erupted in these dying days of its existence.

Daily he gazed at the Sun's impassive face, trying to deduce what was happening there, but he could discover nothing, so he returned to his piles of data with what was almost anger, for he knew they were hiding information, if only he could unravel it.

In some irritation he telephoned Dr. Eddy, but found him unavailable; he was at Kitt Peak in Arizona pursuing his own studies. So Sam was left alone with his data, and late one night he left his work and wandered to the dormitory where his Wyoming girl friend slept and rousted her from bed by throwing pebbles at her window: 'No matter what cycle I use, eleven years, twenty-two or eighty-eight, I keep reaching the conclusion that we're due for a really major event.'

'Why don't you report it?'

'Because no one would believe me. I haven't a single solid fact to go on, only theories.'

'Ask Eddy what he thinks.'

'He's in Arizona, dammit. I've called twice but he's on a field trip.'

'Your problem will wait till he gets back.'

'Wait? Do you know what a real major event can be? A region on the face of the Sun fifty times bigger than the entire surface of the Earth. It explodes. In thirty minutes it can throw masses of material a hundred and fifty thousand miles out into space. In less than an hour it sends forth enough energy to supply every electricity need in the United States for a hundred million years. That's titanic.'

'And dangerous?' the girl asked.

'Our atmosphere protects us. But if you were in an airplane very high, real danger.'

'And astronauts, like Apollo 18 maybe?'

'Deadly.'

So during the last weeks of March, Sam Cottage watched with extra care his Sun's behavior, but when nothing exceptional occurred he put that month to bed with a reassuring summary:

> All solar activity low during past 24 hours. Only small subflares. Magnetic field has been only mildly disturbed. General activity should remain low. Potential for major events low. However, it could increase if new Region 396 should amalgamate with neighboring regions.

Two committees had been convened, the first composed of scientists to determine what instruments Apollo 18 should carry to the Moon in order to acquire data that would help explain the genesis of that satellite and perhaps the universe. They began their discussions on a sober note:

> 'On earlier explorations, the astronauts could place the instruments, point their antenna toward the Earth, and expect that radio signals would carry the data direct to our stations in Australia, Spain or the United States. And they were correct. As of last week our Moon stations were sending us nine million separate bits of data every day, throughout the year. We are getting to know the Moon as well as we know Rhode Island.

> 'But from the other side we can have no direct contact. Everything will depend upon the two or three satellites we place in orbit about the Moon. If they fail, we fail. To state it another way, if they fail, the whole Apollo 18 flight fails.'

NASA brought in communications experts, who promised that the three proposed satellites would be at least as reliable as the other devices they were gambling on, and with this assurance they reached a most sensible decision:

> 'Since experiments initiated by previous Apollo missions have succeeded much better than we had a right to expect, with every instrument functioning four times longer than predicted, it is essential that we receive the same kind of data from the other side of the Moon. We recommend these duplications:
>
> 'A suprathermal ion detector to measure the mass and energy of any gases on or near the lunar surface.
>
> 'A solar-wind spectrometer to measure the flux and energy of atomic particles from the Sun, an experiment of greatest significance.
>
> 'A lunar-surface magnetometer to measure fluctuations in the magnetic field at the Moon.
>
> 'A passive seismic experiment to measure lunar vibrations from whatever source.'

They then turned to a series of experiments specifically designed for the new side of the Moon: using a device that sent radio impulses into the body of the Moon to see whether any ice or water existed below the surface, and conducting a fascinating experiment which might help to decide a furious lunar debate: Are mascons merely impacted meteors, suggesting that the Moon had a cold origin, or are they submerged lava flows, indicating a hot origin? Ten years earlier the word *mascon* did not exist; it meant *mass concentration* and referred to mysterious but ordinary-looking locations on the Moon where the force of gravity noticeably increased. Obviously, something unusually heavy lay hidden below the surface, and it was given the name *mascon*. The scientists wanted to know about the mascons on the other side.

Dr. Mott was a member of the second committee, which had perhaps the more exciting assignment: to select the spot on which Claggett and Linley would try to land, for it was imperative that a location be chosen which would yield a rich variety of rocks and afford good terrain observations. The two astronauts attended every meeting because they must become familiar with the area they were to explore, and as they studied the new maps, constructed from data supplied by the Russians after their successful photographic flight to the far side in 1959 and by the American flights of the 1960s, they realized that almost every site they might want to explore carried a Russian name—so awarded because the Russians had got there first. Claggett asked, 'You mean, whenever anyone goes to the back of the Moon, he'll be using Russian street signs?' And when the committee members nodded, he said, 'Now I understand why Senator Grant was in such a sweat to catch up.'

Landing a spacecraft on the Moon presented unusual problems, as the astrophysicists explained:

'You will be faced by the same constraints as the earlier Apollos. You must bring your module down a very narrow corridor. If the Sun is below 7°, your landing area will be in shadows so deep you won't be able to distinguish dangers like big boulders. If the Sun is higher than 25°, landing is quite impossible, for you lose shadows, and without them you cannot ascertain what lies ahead.

'The ideal is a space only 4° wide—12° to 16°—because then the Sun behind you acts like a helpful flashlight, pointing out the dangers.

'Of course, if you reach your desired landing spot too late, so that the Sun is high and blazing, quiet simple. You just speed farther ahead to your alternate landing site, and as you approach the terminator line, you find yourself once more just where you want to be, 12° to 16°.'

When Paul Linley heard these very exact limitations, comparable to those restricting the capsule when it tried to return to Earth, he said, 'From our takeoff spot that day we fly 238,848.7 miles and have to land at precisely 70 hours, 37 minutes, 45 seconds after takeoff, and right in relation to the crater Gagarin.'

'And don't be a minute late,' Claggett said, 'or the damned Sun will be too high in the heavens.'

It was only then that Linley appreciated how that requirement of sunlight and shadow on a remote valley on the other side of the Moon determined when, four days earlier, Apollo 18 must ascend into the air at Cape Canaveral. 'We climb into this machine weighing 6,300,000 pounds,' he wrote to his wife, 'and we fire engines producing 7,500,000 pounds of thrust, and we're restricted by minutes and seconds. Space flight is an exact science.'

When the two committees submitted their reports, NASA was highly pleased, because everyone now saw that Apollo 18 promised exciting rewards, a worthy capstone in every respect. But when it dawned on people that this would probably be the last Apollo that would ever fly, engineers from all over America came to the Cape to see it standing in majesty beside the ocean at Complex 39.

Two carloads of engineers from Langley Field drove down non-stop—nineteen hours—to see the splendid thing they had visualized years before, without having had a reasonable clue as to how it would ultimately be effected. Dieter Kolff had government orders to fly to Canaveral, but he preferred to ride, so he organized an expedition from Huntsville of old Peenemünde hands, nine of them driving straight through in thirteen hours, to see the glorious rocket they had built, and when they stood looking at it, Kolff said, 'When this goes, we've launched fourteen of our Saturn-Apollos, and not one has failed. We've gone to the Moon and we could have gone to Saturn. Look at it!'

He stayed at the Cape to supervise the final touches to his masterpiece, the last in a proud series, and sometimes when he wiped dust off the giant, as engineers will do, he grieved that of all the men who had pioneered this great machine, not one had ever ridden on its high nose: A group of American boys who weren't born when we started work. They get to go and we don't. He prayed that the culminating flight would be a good one and that it would bring further honors to Von Braun.

One evening as he ate alone at the Bali Hai a handsome Oriental woman in a gray linen jumpsuit asked if she could sit with him, and although he expressed his astonishment at her daring, she drew up a chair and introduced herself as Rhee Soon-Ka from *Asahi Shimbun* of Tokyo: 'Could I ask a distinguished German scientist a few questions?'

Dieter was flattered, and they talked for many hours, for she had a knack of guessing what a man like him would want to speak about in these days of beautiful tension.

'What kind of man was Von Braun?' she asked.

'He never betrayed anyone who worked for him.'

'Or anyone he worked for?'

'All of us who reached Huntsville alive, we owe it to Von Braun.'

'When the rocket lifts off, in April, what will you think as it soars into the air?' She spent almost an hour on this question: the things that could go wrong, that had indeed gone wrong with the many failures of the A-4 at Peenemünde; the emotions that overcome a man when a long-sought goal is attained; his feelings toward his fellows who joined the Russians in 1945; the relative costs of an A-4 and a Saturn V.

She took few notes, for she suspected that she would use very little of what Kolff was telling her, but she needed his insights to provide a solid underpainting for what she would write, and it was almost dawn when she asked, as good reporters often did, 'What would you like to tell me that I haven't asked?' and he said, 'You know it's all wrong? Pointed in the wrong direction?' and she said, 'I've known that all along. It's exhibitionism. Little boys showing off.'

They discussed this for some time, and finally Kolff asked, 'What do you see in them? The way they live and die?'

And now she wanted to talk, for this had been a night of enrichment. 'They are so small. Herr Kolff, have you noticed how small these wonderful young men are?'

'They have to be, to fit into our capsules.'

'But the rest of America's heroes are so tall, so huge.' She stopped speaking and drummed on the table for some moments. 'I've been developing a theory that whenever a nation elects great giants as its heroes, it's doomed. Tall Prussian cavalrymen. Those pathetic Swiss guards at the

Vatican. The huge gladiators of Rome. And the ridiculous sumo wrestlers of Japan.'

'I have little regard for giants,' Kolff said.

'In America it's all monstrous football players and hyperthyroid basketball players.' She became quite excited. 'I was in the Atlanta airport when a basketball team, the Boston Celtics, I think—they came through as a team, and I had to look up like this to see them. Those gods, those great muscular gods.' She laughed nervously. 'It was quite revolting, really. America and Japan both electing their heroes by weight. Both societies doomed.'

She spoke more on this subject, analyzing it from various angles, and concluding, 'I think Europe may be saved because they make heroes of little, ordinary men like soccer stars and bicycle racers. They have sense enough to look at Goliath and his Philistines with suspicion. They see the merit in normality, and I think that's why I'm so infatuated with the astronauts. They're so little and so ordinary and so very brave.'

Kolff had not thought of this before, having accepted the government's decision to select small men for the capsules, but he found that he liked the idea, for he had never been able to see merit in a man simply because he was seven feet tall or weighed two hundred and seventy pounds.

They sat quietly for a while, both weary from the long night's talk, then Kolff said, sighing, 'When you're a young man, you imagine that when you grow old and fill a position of responsibility, all discussions will be like this one tonight. Instead, we waste our time in trivialities. I am indebted to you.'

'On the contrary.'

On 3 April 1973, Sam Cottage, working at his telescope in Boulder, spotted on the receding western limb of the Sun at a point 10° above the solar equator, a new collection of sunspots and he duly noted them: 'Region 419, horseshoe shaped. Below average in luminosity.' And that evaluation was forwarded to numerous stations around the world.

As always these days he asked himself as he filed his report, 'Could this be the big one?' but the modest appearance of 419 forced him to answer no.

On 4 April the collection of spots had moved closer to the extremity from where it would move around to the invisible side of the Sun, and Sam needed to be sure how many days would pass before it reappeared at the eastern limb. His calculations would have surprised some who thought they knew the Sun well.

Because the Sun, like all other visible stars, is gaseous and not a solid, it rotates on its axis at sharply different speeds, depending on how far from the solar equator a spot is. It is as if Ecuador had a day of 22 hours, the United States 24 hours, and Greenland 27 hours.

At its equator the Sun requires only 26.7 days to complete a revolution, but at any point approaching a pole, it takes 32.1 days. Region 419, which stood just north of the equator, would make its circuit in 27.6 days, which meant that it would be out of sight for at least 14.

On 5 April, Cottage caught his last glimpse of 419 as it disappeared, and although the amount visible was minimal, he thought he detected in it substantial variations from what he had seen previously, so after filing his routine reports, he went to headquarters and said, 'I caught just a glimpse of 419 as it went around the bend, and I thought it had become more active.'

'Damn,' the manager growled. 'Fifteen days and we'll see nothing. It could come back at us on the east limb a full-fledged terror.'

'All we can do is guess.'

The manager sat clasping and unclasping his hands. 'Twenty years from now we won't be so powerless. We'll have monitors up there checking all sides at all times.' He left his desk in some agitation, looked at various photographs, then shook his head. 'Cottage, the Sun is the single most vital item in our universe . . . to us. And we know so little about it. The only star among the trillions that we can study close up, and we practically ignore it.'

He stomped about the room for additional minutes, then stopped abruptly and snapped, 'You want me to issue an advisory, don't you?'

'I'm very nervous, sir.'

'But have you any hard evidence?' He answered himself: 'None.' Then he asked, 'What was this eighty-eight-year cycle you mentioned the other day?'

Cottage outlined his nebulous theories, but even as he voiced them he had to acknowledge how tentative they must sound. The manager, apprehensive himself about the dying gasp of Cycle 20, wanted to find substance in the young man's ideas, but could not.

'Sam, do you agree that we have no justification for issuing an advisory?'

'I do.'

So none was issued.

Nine days before the flight was scheduled, the three astronauts were placed in quarantine to protect them against germs, especially colds and measles, which might be brought to them by others, and in this time they went through daily drill in the simulators. Pope, as the most methodical, shuffled his three-by-five single pages made of a very high quality fireproof French paper, summarizing and indexing ninety-six different contingency sequences covering every emergency for which he would have any responsibility, and although he knew these procedures by heart, he kept cutting the pages arbitrarily, as if they formed a deck of cards, and rattling off the steps he would have to take if *that* accident occurred. For example, the first paper

reminded him of exactly how high and how far down range the rocket ought
to be at crucial stages during the first two hours:

APOLLO 18 LAUNCH EVENTS

Time H M S	Event	Altitude	Velocity MPH	Miles Down Range
00 00 00	First motion Lift-off	182.7 feet	914	0.0
00 02 40	Jettison Stage I	8.2 miles	1,798	2.7
00 08 56	Jettison Stage II	111.5	15,516	887.9
00 08 57	Stage III engine ignited	111.1	15,492	888.4
00 11 24	Stage III engine shut down	116.9	16,131	1,113.6
01 26 28	Decision to go to Moon	119.6	17,432	1,997.8
01 35 08	Stage III engine re-ignited	123.2	17,422	3,481.9
01 40 50	Stage III engine shut down	200.5	24,247	2,605.0

At this point *Altair* will still have 236,245 miles to go before ignition for
lunar orbit. That'll take us 60 hours, 36 minutes, 7 seconds, or 60.61 hours.
We'll start out at a speed of 24,247 mph and constantly diminish to 1,398.
That'll give us—and he worked the small circular slide rule he had bought
in Japan during his Korean duty—an average made-good speed of 3,898
mph.

When Claggett saw what Pope was up to, he asked, 'You proposin' to
replace the computer?' and Pope said, 'If I have to,' and Randy said, 'Don't
lose them slips of paper.'

On 20 April, three days before lift-off, Region 419 reappeared almost coyly
on the extreme eastern limb of the Sun, as if it were a high-school-freshman
girl peering around a corner in her first modish dress. Cottage, staring with
the keenest interest, could detect nothing, but when he alerted the manager
that the region was again visible, three experts crowded into the telescope
area to compare judgments.

'Lots of regions on the Sun more active than that,' one old-timer said.

'Granted,' the manager said, 'but is there any evidence of significant
change?'

'None,' Cottage said. 'If you'll compare photographs of fifteen days ago,
you'll see it's less active now.'

'Thank God. Anything could have happened on that other side.'

. . .

The astronauts went to bed on the night of 22 April with such a wealth of information that only young men in the finest physical condition could have hoped to keep it in order and available. Claggett, for whom this would be his fourth trip, told the NASA people who dined with them, 'In raw data to be handled, if Gemini was indexed at 1.0, my Apollo flight was 2.3, but this one, to the other side of the Moon, it's got to be 3.3. This is really complex.'

They were wakened for breakfast at 0400, and Deke Slayton with five other NASA officials was surprised when Claggett lifted his glass of orange juice and toasted: 'To William Shakespeare, whose birthday we celebrate with a mighty bang.' Slayton helped them dress and accompanied them to Complex 39, where a score of searchlights played on the waiting rocket and nearly a million spectators gathered in the pre-dawn to watch the last flight of this majestic prototype as it headed for regions doubly mysterious.

Despite NASA's unhappiness with the inaccurate description *Expedition to the Dark Side of the Moon,* this had become the popular designation, and more than three thousand newsmen and women waited in and around the grandstand erected on the far side of protective lagoons, five miles distant. Automatic cameras, emplaced in bunkers around the Complex, would ensure excellent shots of the historic moment.

By elevator the astronauts rode 340 feet in the air, walked across a bridge to the White Room, and with hardly a pause, proceeded directly to the capsule. Without ceremony, Claggett eased himself into the left-hand seat, and while he adjusted his bulky suit Dr. Linley awaited his turn, assuring Deke Slayton, who had picked him for this flight, that he would surely bring back rock samples which would answer some of the questions about the Moon's structure and perhaps its origin. Then he slipped into the right-hand seat, after which Pope eased himself into the one in the middle.

When the men were finally in place, strapped flat on their backs to the seats specially molded to their forms, the critical moment of the countdown arrived. In a bunker below, Dieter Kolff looked stolidly ahead, assuring himself that his final Saturn would soar as planned. At 00:00:00 he saw a blinding flash of fire and felt the ground tremble, as 28,000 gallons of water per second gushed forth to quench the flames, and another 17,000 gallons protected the skin of the machine. From this deluge the rocket began to rise.

Inside the capsule the three astronauts barely felt the lift-off, and Linley, who had not flown before, said, 'Instruments say we're off,' and Pope, busy with check sheets, tapped the geologist on the arm and nodded.

At this moment, when it was assured that Apollo 18 would be successfully airborne, control passed from Cape Canaveral, whose engineers had done their job, to Houston, where Mission Control had hundreds of experts prepared to feed information and instructions into the system:

HOUSTON: All systems go.

APOLLO: We're getting ready for jettison.

In less than three minutes the huge Stage I had discharged its obligation, lifting the entire burden of 6,300,000 pounds eight miles straight up, and now it was useless; indeed, it was worse than useless, for it constituted dead weight and had to be discarded before Stage II could be fired. So Claggett watched as automatic switches—he had more than six hundred above and about him—blew Stage I away, allowing it to fall harmlessly into the Atlantic some miles offshore. With satisfaction, Pope noted that all events so far had adhered to his schedule.

Since Apollo 18 developed no pogo, these first moments of flight were extremely gentle, no more than a G and a half developing, but when Claggett ignited the five powerful engines of Stage II, the rocket seemed to leap upward from an altitude of a mere eight miles to a majestic 112 and to a velocity of more than 15,000 miles an hour. The flight was on its way.

Now Houston began to feed in data, all suggestions being delivered by a team of three CapComs, and it had been agreed that Hickory Lee and Ed Cater would conduct most of the communication. Lee was speaking:

HOUSTON: Okay, Apollo 18. You must be doing everything right.

APOLLO: We were happy to avoid pogo.

HOUSTON: Sometimes our engineers develop real smarts.

APOLLO: Pope speaking. This craft is sure roomier than Gemini. I can hardly wait for the signal to run about.

HOUSTON: You stay put, Bunny Rabbit.

Now Claggett jettisoned Stage II with its five massive engines and Apollo was powered by only the single strong engine in Stage III, the one that would be burned once to insert the vehicle into orbit around the Earth and once more to thrust Apollo into its course to the Moon, after which it, too, would be discarded. But of course the system as a whole would still have the smaller engines in the modules, and after Stage III was jettisoned, about three hours into the flight, these smaller rockets would control until the landing capsule returned to Earth.

At the 84-minute mark a conversation of immense importance began:

HOUSTON: All systems say go.

APOLLO: We read the same.

HOUSTON: We're ready to make the big decision.

APOLLO: No opposition here.

HOUSTON: It's go for the Moon.

APOLLO: We read 17,432 speed at an altitude of 119.6 miles.

HOUSTON: Roger. Fire at 01:26:28. And you'll be on your proper trajectory.

With everything set for a long, leisurely drift to the Moon, the men turned to an exercise that was fundamental to the flight but which might have terrified one not accustomed to space. The components of the vast machine had been packaged in a way that would provide the best aerodynamic surface for climbing through the dense atmosphere, and this required that they be packaged in what one might call an upside-down position; Claggett called it ass-backwards. But now, since frictional drag in space was negligible, one shape was as good as another for drifting through the reaches, and it was advisable for the astronauts to take their monstrous machine apart —massive pieces drifting independently at nearly 18,000 mph—and reassemble them properly, at which time the cumbersome unnecessary portions would be jettisoned and allowed to fall back and burn up in the atmosphere.

'Wish me luck,' Claggett said as he began this preposterous maneuver, and when the parts had been separated and the command and service modules, as a single unit, had been turned completely around, he edged them gently against the lunar module and docked them. Then with great skill he pulled his entire package away from the useless Stage III and watched as it started its swift descent to destruction. The astronauts were alone in the small vehicles that would deposit them on the Moon.

But there was one further obligation. As the tricky maneuver ended, Claggett and Pope did something that no former astronauts had ever done: with the most careful timing they fired the explosive bolts, knocking open the hatch cover and allowing the three spring-loaded communication satellites to eject from the Apollo. Utilizing the same forward thrust that their mother ship had, they would in due course reach a position near the Moon, but much too high and too speedy to attain orbit. At that time Claggett would send a radio signal which would activate a small retrorocket in each satellite, causing it to drop dutifully into its assigned position around the Moon. There it would serve as the vital connection with Earth when the astronauts were working on the other side.

'Now we can go to sleep,' Claggett said, for it would be a slow, methodical, totally supervised trip that Apollo 18 would engage in for the next sixty hours. Claggett would play country music on his tape machine, Pope the symphonies of Beethoven when it came his turn. Dr. Linley monitored communications with Houston and took note of the NCAA basketball scores as CapCom Cater read them off. On the second night, to coincide with prime-time television in the States, Dr. Linley activated *Altair*'s television camera and relayed to Earth a fifty-minute program depicting life aboard the spacecraft. Claggett told some rather dreadful Texas jokes, mainly about his uncles, but the highlight was an exposition by Pope of the consequences of weightlessness. He showed how a spill of water formed a globule, how one man would sleep with his head in one position, his companion upside down relatively, and the special problems of eating and drinking in space. To delight the children he added, 'Going to the bathroom isn't simple, either.' He used the word *urine* and showed how it was expelled from the capsule, and then he asked Linley to carry his camera behind his, Pope's, head, so that the children could see the absolute welter of switches the astronauts had to memorize. He stressed the device which had come late in the space program, a kind of metal bar behind which each switch hid, protected against accidental activation. With a grand sweep he brushed his left arm across one bank of switches and showed how such a careless gesture would leave the switches undisturbed.

He then took the camera and asked Linley to explain the heart of the system, the computers which stored the data necessary for such a flight, and as the scientist detailed the amazing amount of information the computer held, Pope said, 'In a few minutes Colonel Claggett is going to fire an engine for eleven seconds, no more, no less. How does he know when and how long to fire? The computer tells him, and after he fires it, we'll be on dead target to the Moon.'

Claggett felt the program was getting somewhat professorial, which was bound to be the case when Pope was in charge, so he took a bite of cracker, producing large crumbs, which hung in the capsule. 'Catch the crumbs,' he yelled at the other two. 'That's how we do our housework up here. Catch the crumbs, you limeys. I'm Captain Bligh.' And he held the camera while Pope and Linley tried to capture the errant bits.

On the next day things sobered considerably, for the men of *Altair* were about to attempt something never tried before, a walk on the other side, and as the Moon loomed ahead, enormous in their small windows, they could identify areas where the earlier Apollos had landed, and they felt momentary remorse that they were not headed for any of the sites they had memorized as beginning astronauts. But when they swung around the edge of the Moon and saw for the first time the strange and marvelous mountains awaiting them, they gasped with delight.

Flight plan called for them to make many orbits of the Moon before actually descending, and in this waiting period they talked with Hickory Lee in Houston:

APOLLO: Things couldn't look smoother.

HOUSTON: Who wrote Claggett's lines for the television show?

APOLLO: Joe Miller, two hundred years ago.

HOUSTON: The show was an enormous success. Editors liked Pope's explanation of weightlessness.

APOLLO *(Claggett speaking):* So did we. I never understood it before.

HOUSTON: Could you see any debris from previous landings?

APOLLO: None. And we really searched.

HOUSTON: That's hard to believe. When you drop to lower orbit, of course . . .

APOLLO: Our landing spot is in darkness now, but what we can see of the lighted area looks reassuring. Totally different from the Earth side. Many, many more craters.

HOUSTON: We want you to make four sunlight passes.

APOLLO: You can be sure we want to.

HOUSTON: Any glitches?

APOLLO: None whatever. Fingers crossed, but this has been a perfect mission so far.

. . .

There was a glitch. Sam Cottage, monitoring the Sun on the morning after lift-off, saw with interest that Region 419 had maintained its horseshoe configuration, with signs indicating that a sunspot big enough to see with the naked eye might be developing, but there was no indication that a solar proton event might erupt. His summary that day informed the world and NASA scientists:

> Region 419 produced several subflares. New spots are appearing in white light. Region exhibiting mixed polarities. Geomagnetic field likely to remain unsettled. Region likely to produce moderate flares.

But on the next day, as the astronauts were preparing their approach to the Moon, Region 419 subsided dramatically, so that the summary contained nothing to alert the NASA scientists that anything of importance might be impending.

However, Cottage could not sleep, and during the hours when Claggett and Linley were preparing their descent to the Moon, he was alone in his workroom, reviewing all the data regarding Cycle 20 and the behavior of Region 419, and the more mathematics he applied to what was before him, the more apparent it became that if his theories were correct, Region 419 must soon erupt as a major flare.

He had nothing to work on except his correlations, but in the morning he carried them to the manager and said, 'Here I am again. Statistically, everything would balance out if 419 did go bang.'

'We're not gypsies telling fortunes.'

'All right, disregard my figures. What do you think?'

'It's a troublesome region, but dammit, we don't have enough here to warrant an alert.'

And again none was issued.

On 26 April, as the two astronauts were making their final decisions regarding a descent to the Moon, Sam Cottage did not leave his watching post for lunch, because a routine event was occurring on the Sun which, although it involved no specific danger, did produce a period of maximum risk to the two men who would be walking on the Moon. Region 419 was moving from the eastern half of the Sun's visible surface to the western, and this made it triply threatening. First, because of solar rotation the paths followed by energetic atomic particles thrown out by the Sun are curved, so that those originating on the western half are more directly channeled toward the Earth and Moon. Even a truly massive flare on the eastern half would do little damage, for its ejecta would curve outward and away from Earth, to be lost in space. Second, the travel time for deadly particles originating on the western half is much shorter than those coming from the eastern, so that the likelihood of their overtaking the astronauts before they could seek shelter was much greater. Third, solar-flare particles reaching Earth or Moon from the western side are just more energetic than those from the east.

The most threatening single position for a flare is twenty to forty-five degrees west of the Sun's central meridian, and that was the ominous area into which Region 419 now entered.

When Sam missed his lunch, his girl friend appeared with a sandwich and watched the Sun with him. "I was jittery yesterday,' he said. 'Took all my data to the boss and showed him nothing. He told me we weren't gypsy fortunetellers, and he was right. Look. It's a calm Sun. Region 419 is transiting from east to west in an orderly fashion. This time we're going to escape, but I'm still convinced that before Cycle 20 ends, there has to be a bangeroo.'

'Lucky for the guys up there it skips us this time,' she said.

'Why, are they on the Moon?'

'Not yet. But I heard the broadcast from Houston and they're on their way down.' She hesitated. Seeing that he was bleary-eyed and nervous, she said, 'Why don't you take a walk with me over to the library? You could use a break.'

'I want to see this thing vanish off the western limb.'

'How many hours?'

'Six more days.' Then he broke into a laugh and surrendered. 'All right, off we go, but only for an hour.'

At about the time that Sam Cottage was going to the library with his girl, Claggett and Linley were slipping through the chute that carried them into the landing module, and after they had satisfied themselves that everything was in readiness, they signaled Pope that he could cast them loose, but he was so busy verifying the check lists that governed his solitary command of the capsule, that he asked for more time: 'I've got three more pages. I want this place to be locked up when you pull away.'

'We want it, too,' Claggett said over the intercom. 'Something to come home to.'

At the conclusion of his meticulous checking Pope cried, 'Randy, it's everything go. Contact Houston.'

So the word was given; the computers aloft and their mates in Houston concurred, and the Luna broke away to start its descent to what Tucker Thompson had told his readers was 'the dark and dangerous chasm in which unknown forces threaten the life of any trespasser.' Dr. Mott, reading the report in *Folks,* growled, 'The basic forces are identical with those which govern Brooklyn. Only the landscape is different.'

It certainly was. As the Sun began to illuminate regions farther and farther into the hemisphere, Claggett and Linley could see a Moon very different from the Earth side they had once studied so assiduously. Here there were no vast seas, no multitude of smooth-centered craters, no rilles leading out in tantalizing patterns. This was a brutish Moon composed of great mountain ranges, valleys perilously deep. The Earth side had been known for twenty thousand years and mapped for three hundred. Grammar-school children could make themselves familiar with their side, but only scientists studying the Russian and American photographs could say that they knew much about *Luna*'s chosen landing spot.

With unmatched skill, Claggett brought the lander right down the middle of the corridor—enough Sun to throw shadows that identified every hillock—and as the long delicate probes which dangled from the bottom of the landing pads reached down to touch the Moon and alert the astronauts to turn off their power, lest they fly too hard onto the rocky soil, the final conversation with Houston took place:

LUNA: Everything as ordered. God, this is different.

HOUSTON: We read perfection. Soon now.

LUNA: No signals from the probes. Could they be malfunctioning?

HOUSTON: You're still well above the probe level. All's well.

LUNA *(Claggett speaking):* Too busy to talk now. Drifting to left. Too much.

LUNA *(Linley speaking):* No strain. Straighten up, dead ahead I see it.

LUNA *(Claggett speaking):* I can't see a damned thing. We're tilted.

LUNA *(Linley speaking):* You are tilted. Left. Five degrees.

LUNA *(Claggett speaking):* I thought I was. There, that's better. Houston, I see now. All is copacetic.

LUNA *(Linley speaking):* Perfect landing.

HOUSTON: Great job.

As gently as if he were parking a large car at a supermarket, Randy Claggett had brought *Luna* to rest at the extreme far edge of the Sun's rays. Ahead lay darkness, soon to be converted into dazzling sunlight; behind lay the areas which had been bathed in sunlight but which would later pass into the terrible cold and darkness of space where no atmosphere reflected light.

LUNA: We've had a close look through the windows. Same only different.

HOUSTON *(Ed Cater as CapCom):* You must get some shut-eye.

LUNA: We want some.

HOUSTON: All systems shut down?

LUNA: All secured.

HOUSTON: We'll waken you in seven hours. Egress in nine.

LUNA: That's what we came for.

So eager was Sam Cottage to see what his Sun was going to offer the morning of 27 April that he unlimbered his solarscope an hour before dawn, then spent his time nervously waiting for the great red disk to appear over the flatlands to the east. For about an hour after sunrise it would be fruitless to take photographs, for the Sun would be so low in the east that a camera would be unable to penetrate effectively the extreme thickness of atmosphere. Later, when it stood overhead, the thickness would be at a minimum and good photographs would become possible. Even so, he studied the Sun through its blanket of haze to see whether any conspicuous event had happened overnight.

Against the possibility that he might have to issue an alert, he spent his time reviewing the data on radiation; the present thinking of the world's experts was summarized in *The Rem Table* (Roentgen Equivalent in Man), from which sample lines read:

100-150 Rems	Vomiting, nausea but no serious disability.
340-420 Rems	All personnel sick. 20% deaths within 2 weeks.
500-620 Rems	All personnel very sick. 50% deaths within 1 month. Survivors incapacitated about 6 months.
690-930 Rems	Immediate severe vomiting, nausea. Up to 100% fatalities . . .
6,200 Rems	Total incapacitation almost immediately. All personnel dead.

These data, of course, referred to 'an unprotected white male,' and the dosage could be dramatically reduced by various kinds of protection: 560 Rems striking an unprotected human drop to 400 if he wears his astronaut's suit; to 128 if he can get back inside the lunar module; to 26 if he makes it to the command module, with its solid sides and ablative shield; and to an inconsequential 7 if he stands behind the stone wall inside a well-constructed house.

When Cottage had digested both sets of figures he concluded: That's why they keep people like me on watch. Early warning. If the man's caught unprotected, he's dead. If we can get him back inside that command module, he survives.

In the fading darkness, while he waited for the blazing appearance of the Sun, he thought of himself as an ancient Aztec priest on the highest altar at Tenochtitlán waiting in darkness for the return of the life-giver, and he thought: They knew what they were doing. They knew where the power came from.

When light filled the room Cottage walked nervously about, stopping now and then to study the remarkable series of photographs taken on 23 February 1956 showing several stages of the greatest solar flare ever recorded. It would have generated, Cottage estimated, a total dose of more than 2,000 Rems as measured on the Moon.

Now came the Sun, this all-powerful agency, this source of light and heat and life and continuance which most men accepted so casually and understood so poorly. Sam, unusually captivated by the power of his star, stared at it naked-eyed as it rose orange-red, and paid his tribute:

> What a powerhouse! I still don't believe it. During all the billions of years you've been in existence you've thrown into space six million tons of matter every second. And you can go on doing it for another ten billion years without using up even 1/100th of 1% of your mass. Please, please restrain yourself for three more days.

While Cottage was pleading for days of grace, Hickory Lee from Houston was trying to awaken his two astronauts with a persistent 'Luna, Houston. Luna, Houston.' And when he succeeded he warned them not to skip breakfast; then he confirmed schedules as they opened the hatch on the lunar module and lowered their ladder.

Randy Claggett's style was to be irreverent about everything: marriage, fatherhood, test-piloting or engaging Russian MiGs in Korea, but when he felt his heavy boot touch the surface of the Moon and realized that he was standing on a portion of the universe which no one on Earth would ever see, not even with the most powerful telescope, he was overcome with the solemnity of the moment:

LUNA: Nothing could prepare you for this moment. The photographs weren't even close. This is . . . it's staggering. An endless landscape of craters and boulders.

HOUSTON: And not a dark side at all?

LUNA: The Sun shines brilliantly, but it's sure dark in spirit.

As soon as Paul Linley joined him on the surface, a curious transformation occurred: up to now Claggett had been the skilled test pilot in command, but here among the rocks of a wildly unfamiliar terrain, the geologist assumed control, and he reminded Claggett that their first responsibility was to collect rocks immediately, lest they have to take off in a hurry. Placing the scientific instruments and doing the systematic sample collecting could come later.

Only when the emergency bags were filled with rock samples and stowed aboard did the two men proceed to perform an act which seemed miraculous when it was flashed by means of the orbiting satellites to television watchers back on Earth: at an opening in the base of the lunar module they opened a flap, activated a series of devices, and stood back as a most bizarre creation started to emerge like a chrysalis about to become a butterfly. It looked much like a frail shopping cart that had been run over in some truck accident, compacted and twisted, but as it came into sunlight, its various parts, which were spring-loaded, began to unfold of themselves: four wheels mysteriously appeared, a steering handle, a tonneau with seats. Like a child's toy unfolding at Christmas, a complete Moon rover materialized, with batteries strong enough to move it about for three days or eighty miles, 'whichever comes first,' as Claggett reported to Houston.

When the rover stood clear, the astronauts did not leap into it for a gambol across the Moon; in fact, they ignored it as they went about the serious business of unloading and positioning the complex of scientific instruments which would make this journey fruitful for the next ten years. In each of the preceding Apollo missions, men had placed on the Moon devices which were expected to send messages to Earth for up to a year, but they had been so beautifully constructed, with so many sophisticated by-passes if things went wrong, that all of them were still functioning long after their predicted death. 'Sometimes we do things right,' Claggett said as he emplaced the instrument which would measure the force of the solar wind.

'You seem to have the wires crossed,' Hickory Lee cautioned from Houston. 'Red to red.'

'I had it ass-backwards,' Claggett said, and Lee had to remind him: 'We're working with an open mike.' Prior to every flight, NASA officials had warned Claggett that since what he said would be heard by millions or even billions of people around the world, he must censor his ebullient speech, and this he promised to do, but occasionally a test-pilot phrase crept in and NASA shuddered, for the men in charge knew that every vulgarism would bring thousands of protests and even questions in Congress: 'How could you men who stood closer to heaven than men have ever stood before use such language?' And Mott, listening to the exchange, knew exactly what Claggett would reply: 'Senator, it was a serious moment. Houston was right. I was about to muck up the whole experiment because I did have the wires ass-backwards.'

When the eight separate scientific devices were placed and the antenna which would relay their findings were oriented so that the satellites could intercept their transmissions, the two men were ready to send test signals.

HOUSTON: We read you loud and clear.

LUNA: Voltages in order?

HOUSTON: Could not be better.

LUNA: We're going to rest fifteen minutes.

HOUSTON: You earned it.

LUNA: Then we start on Expedition One. Seven miles to the reticulated crater.

HOUSTON: Roger. Are you checking your dosimeters?

LUNA: Regular.

The astronauts gave this much-used word its Mexican pronunciation *reg-u-larrrr,* with heavy accent on the last syllable, which made it a fine-sounding statement: not good, not bad, nothing out of the way, just regularrrr. If someone had asked Claggett what kind of test pilot he had been at Pax

River, he would have said, 'Regularrrr,' flipping his right palm face-up, face-down. 'Nothing special. Regularrrr.'

After their rest, taken to avoid perspiration or heavy breathing which might consume too much oxygen, the two men climbed into the rover with Dr. Linley at the controls, for the machine was his responsibility, and as the rover pulled away, Houston received a remarkable message:

LUNA: Linley speaking. Please someone inform my uncle Dr. Gawain Butler, who would not allow me to drive his used Plymouth, that I am now chauffering a jalopy with a sticker price of ten million clams.

HOUSTON: Obey all traffic signs.

Each trip had been constructed with almost every minute accounted for; the men would work incessantly, searching for specific things that would illuminate the history of this other side. The distances to be traveled had been carefully studied, for a basic consideration had to be the point of safe return, that point so far removed from the module that if the rover broke down completely, the astronauts could still hike back, taking into account exhaustion and oxygen supply. On previous flights six miles out had been the limit, but Claggett and Linley were in such superb physical shape, and their traveling gear had been so improved, that seven miles was being authorized.

This carried them to one of the most interesting small craters on this side, one whose flat central section was so reticulated like a mud flat in August that the astronauts had named it the Giraffe Crater. When they climbed a small mound at its edge Linley gasped with pleasure, and informed Houston that it was even more exciting than they had supposed when studying photographs.

LUNA: Magnificent. We have a whole new world here.

HOUSTON: Better change that to Moon.

LUNA: Corrected. We're going down on foot to collect samples.

HOUSTON: Too steep for the rover?

LUNA: We think so.

HOUSTON: Roger. We'll follow you with the television camera.

LUNA: We're going left. To get those rocks that look yellowish.

It was truly miraculous. The two astronauts left the rover and descended gingerly into the crater, but as they went, technicians in Houston sent electronic commands to the television camera mounted on the side of the rover, and obediently it followed the progress of the men. Its electrical impulses were dispatched by a special antenna on the rover to one of the waiting satellites, which reflected them to collecting stations at Honeysuckle in Australia and Goldstone in California, where they were transformed into television pictures for commercial stations. And the linkage was so perfect that operators in Houston were able to point the camera and activate it rather more meticulously than a man could have done had he stayed in the flimsy rover.

. . .

At the Sun Study Center in Boulder, Sam Cottage turned the cranks which moved his solarscope into position, brought the hydrogen-alpha filter into the optics in order to obtain the most sensitive view of activity on the Sun, and waited for the great star to lose its redness so he could get a clear look at its face, and when he did so he saw that Region 419 had reached the precise spot from which it could create the maximum danger. It had edged across the mid-line at which it would have stood closest to the Moon but still remained close enough to deliver a powerful shot, and it had entered the ultra-dangerous western hemisphere from which extra-powerful discharges were possible.

With every minute successfully negotiated, the possibility of danger diminished, and Sam was pleased to see that 419 remained quiescent; however, for his morning summary he did consult his charts to make an estimate of the size of the region, and was surprised at his figure: 'Region 419 is now 63 times larger than the entire surface of the Earth.'

Before filing his report he looked back to verify the astonishing size of this disturbance, and as he did so he saw the area expand significantly: 'Jesus, what's happening?'

He reached backward for his telephone, but his attention became riveted on that distant battleground where primordial forces had reached a point of tension that could no longer be sustained. With one mighty surge, Region 419 exploded in titanic fury. It was no longer simply a threatening active region; it was one of the most violent explosions of the past two hundred years.

'Oh Jesus!' Cottage gasped, and while he fumbled for the phone, figures and delimitations galloped through his head: Sun to Moon, less than 93,-000,000 miles. What we see now happened 8.33 minutes ago. But radiation travels at speed of light, so it's already hit the Moon. Oh Jesus, those poor men! Rems—5,000, maybe 6,000 total dose? And in the brief seconds it took for him to pick up the phone, two thoughts flashed across his mind: What else might have happened during the eight minutes it took that flash to reach here? and *God, God, please protect those men.*

He spread the alarm, but by the time his superiors could alert NASA, two other observatories and three amateurs in the Houston area had already reported that a gigantic solar proton event was under way.

HOUSTON: *Luna, Altair,* do you read me?

ALTAIR: I read.

HOUSTON: Why doesn't *Luna* answer? *Altair,* can you see *Luna* at this point?

ALTAIR: Negative.

LUNA *(breaking in):* I read you, Houston.

HOUSTON: There seems to have been an event on the Sun. Have you checked your dosimeters?

LUNA: Uh-oh!

HOUSTON: We read your telemetry as very high.

LUNA: So do we. Dosimeter is saturated.

ALTAIR: Confirm. Very high.

HOUSTON: We now have confirmation from different sources. Major solar event. Classification 4-bright, X9 in x-ray flux.

LUNA: What probable duration?

HOUSTON: Cannot predict. Wait. Human Ecology says two days, three days.

LUNA *(Claggett speaking):* I think we may have a problem.

HOUSTON: The drill is clear. Return to lunar module. Lift off soonest. Make rendezvous soonest.

LUNA: We do not have data and time for lift-off. We do not have data and time for rendezvous.

HOUSTON: Our computers will crank up and feed you. What is your ETA back at lunar module?

LUNA: Distance, seven miles; top speed, seven miles. Yield, one hour.

HOUSTON: How long to button up?

ALTAIR: Am I to drop to rendezvous orbit?

HOUSTON: Stand by, *Altair.* We'll handle your problems later.

ALTAIR: Roger. Wilco.

HOUSTON: Repeat, how long button up, *Luna?*

LUNA: Abandonin' gear, twenty minutes.

HOUSTON: Abandon all gear. *Luna,* there is no panic, but speed essential.

LUNA: Who's panickin'? We're climbin' out of a crater, rough goin'.

HOUSTON: Manufacturer assures rover can make top speed eleven miles per hour.

LUNA: And if we break down? What top speed walkin'?

HOUSTON: Roger. Maintain safe speed.

LUNA: We'll try nine.

HOUSTON: We're informed nine was tested strenuously. Proved safe.

LUNA: We'll try nine.

Now the Sun reminded Earthlings of its terrible power, for it poured forth atomic particles and radiation at an appalling rate, sending them coursing through planetary space and bombarding every object they encountered. Wave after wave of solar-flare particles and high-energy radiation attacked the Earth, but most of this was rejected by our protective atmosphere; however, enough did penetrate to create bizarre disturbances.

. . . In northern New York a power company found its protective current breakers activated by huge fluxes of electrical power coursing along its lines, coming from no detectable source to disrupt entire cities.

. . . An Air Force general, trying vainly to communicate with a base one thousand miles away, realized that the entire American defense system was impotent: 'If Russia wanted to attack us at a moment of total confusion, this would be it.' Then he smiled wanly. 'Of course, their system will be as messed up as ours.'

. . . Taxi drivers in Boston, listening to the radios connecting them with their home offices, received instructions directing them to addresses in Kansas City.

. . . A world-famous pigeon race between Ames, Iowa, and Chicago launched 1,127 birds, with a likelihood from past experiences that more than a thousand would promptly find their way home. But since all magnetic fields were in chaos, only four made it, bedraggled, confused and six hours late.

. . . People in Florida reported seeing the aurora borealis for the first time in their lives, and in northern Vermont the display was so brilliant that people could read by it.

. . . And in Houston the knowing men in charge of Apollo 18 assembled quietly, aware of how powerless they were. The mission controller and Dr. Feldman looked at the dosimeter reports and shuddered. More than 5,000 Rems were striking the Moon. Very calmly the controller said, 'Give me the bottom line.'

Dr. Feldman ticked off on his fingers: 'Highest reading we've had is 5,830 Rems,' and a NASA scientist said, 'Absolutely fatal,' but Feldman continued his recital: 'If, and I repeat if, 5,830 strike a naked man, he's dead. But our men have the finest suits ever devised. Enormous protection. Plus their own clothes. Plus the most important aspect of all. It isn't radiation that might kill them. It's the outward flow of protons from the Sun. And they will not reach the Moon for another fifty minutes.' He ticked off his last two points: 'We rush our men into their Moon lander, where they find more protection. Then we rocket them aloft to the orbiter with its heavy shield.'

Throwing both hands in the air, he shouted, 'We can save those men!'

The controller summoned his three CapComs and said, 'No fluctuation in voice. No hysteria at this end.' To the hundreds gathering, he conveyed the same message: 'I want all ideas and I want them quick. But only the CapComs are to speak with the astronauts.'

Turning to the chief astronomers, he asked, 'Could this have been predicted?'

'No,' they said. 'Closing months of a quiet cycle. It should not have happened.'

The controller wanted to say, 'Well, it did. Six thousand Rems.' But he knew he must betray neither anxiety or irritation. 'Now it's our job to get them home safe.'

By the time Claggett and Linley reached their rover and turned it around, they no longer bothered with their dosimeters, because once the reading passed the 1,000-Rem mark, any further data were irrelevant. They were in trouble and they knew it, but they did have a chance if they did everything right.

For nearly an hour their rover crawled back toward the waiting lunar module, itself attacked by the solar outpouring, and the two men wanted to talk about their predicament but could think of nothing sensible to say. So they took refuge in trivialities: 'Men have absorbed large doses of this stuff, haven't they, Linley?' and the scientist replied, 'Every day, in dentist's offices,' and Claggett asked, 'Do those lead blankets they throw over you do any good?' and Linley said, 'We could profit from a couple right now.'

And then Houston heard raucous laughter coming from *Luna*. It was Linley: 'Hey, Claggett! Did you see those medicals they threw at us last week? Said that a man with black skin had a 23.41 better chance of repelling radiation than one with white skin. Hot diggity! At last it pays to be black.'

Then Claggett's voice: 'Move over, brother, so I can sit in your shadow.'

Alone in *Altair,* John Pope carefully shuffled his summary sheets until he came to one bearing the elegant printing he had learned at Annapolis: RADIATION PRECAUTIONS, and when he had memorized his instructions to himself, he took down the massive volume of additional advice and went through each line, so that by the time his two companions reached their module he would be as prepared as any man could be. Like them, he felt no sense of panic, only the added responsibility of doing the right thing in an emergency.

HOUSTON: *Altair,* have you cranked in the data we sent?
ALTAIR: Affirmative.
HOUSTON: You have the drill on turning the CM around so the ablative shield keeps facing the Sun?
ALTAIR: Affirmative.
HOUSTON: Execute immediately rendezvous has been established.
ALTAIR: Will do.
HOUSTON: What is your dosimeter reading now?
ALTAIR: As before.
HOUSTON: Excellent . . . your reading is much lower than *Luna*'s. You're going to be all right.
ALTAIR: All ready for rendezvous. Get them up here.
The CapCom, up to this point, had been one of the older astronauts, a

man with a stable, reassuring voice, but the NASA command felt that it would be advisable to use in this critical situation someone with whom the men upstairs were especially familiar, and Hickory Lee took over:

HOUSTON: This is Hickory. All readings are good. *(This was a lie; the dosimeter readings were terrifying. But it was not a lie, either; the prospects for an orderly rendezvous still existed.)*

LUNA: Good to hear that Tennessee voice. We can see the module. ETA fifteen minutes.

HOUSTON: I will read lift-off data as soon as you're inside. You don't have a pad available now, do you?

LUNA: Negative. Pads not a high priority aboard this bone-rattler.

LUNA: Linley here. We have terrific rock samples. Will salvage.

HOUSTON: Appreciated, but if transfer takes even one extra minute, abandon.

LUNA: We will not abandon.

HOUSTON: Neither would I. What's that? Who? *(After a pause): Luna,* Dr. Feldman is here. He asks, 'Dr. Linley, is your voice sort of drying up?'

LUNA: Affirmative.

HOUSTON *(Dr. Feldman speaking):* Imperative you swallow spit.

LUNA: Fresh out of spit. Send orange juice.

HOUSTON *(Lee speaking)*: Dr. Feldman says, 'Dr. Linley, keep your mouth moist.'

LUNA: Mouth! Be moist!

Mission Control in Houston had received, in the past hour, a flood of additional men rushing to emergency posts, each determined to get the two astronauts into the slightly better environment of the lunar module and headed for rendezvous with *Altair.* But when they saw the shocking data from the dosimeters they could not be sanguine; this was going to be a tough ride, a very tough ride.

HOUSTON: Park the rover close to the module.

LUNA: Roger.

HOUSTON: Inform me the moment Claggett steps into the module. I will start reading data for check. Nothing is to be done without full check.

LUNA: I have always been one of the world's most careful checkers. Call me Chicken Claggett.

HOUSTON: Give me the word.

As soon as Linley stopped the rover, Claggett dashed for the module, climbed in, and started taking down the instructions Hickory Lee transmitted. Since NASA could not wait for an ideal lift-off time, when *Altair* would be in maximum position to achieve rendezvous, schedules had to be improvised for second best, and when Linley saw that his commander would be occupied for some minutes, he welcomed the opportunity to return to the rover to rescue the precious cargo he had collected at the reticulated crater. He had been sent to the Moon to collect rocks and he proposed to deliver them, but as he heaved aboard the second batch, he seemed to tremble and reached for a handhold that was not there.

LUNA: I think Dr. Linley has fainted.

HOUSTON: Inside the module or out?

LUNA: Halfway in.

HOUSTON: Drag him in, secure all and lift off immediately.

LUNA: I have only partial data. He's in. You can do wonders in one-sixth gravity.

HOUSTON: Lift off immediately.

LUNA: I am using Runway 039. Ain't a hell of a lot of traffic on it. John Pope, coming from the Earth side of the Moon, which was now in darkness, used the sextant as a telescope to spot the module, and when he had it fixed he reported to Houston: 'Everything regularrrr,' but he had already heard that Linley was unconscious and that Claggett would be making the complicated maneuvers alone: 'If anyone can do it, he can.'

LUNA: Linley out cold.

HOUSTON: Have you completed your check? And his, too?

LUNA: Shipshape.

HOUSTON: It's go.

LUNA: You ready up there, *Altair*?

ALTAIR: Three orbits should do it.

LUNA: Here we come.

And then, as Pope watched and the world listened, Randy Claggett, working alone, lifted the lunar module off the surface of the Moon and brought it six hundred feet into space.

HOUSTON: All readings correct. One hell of a job, Randy.

LUNA: I feel faint.

HOUSTON: Not now, Randy. Not now. You dare not.

LUNA: I . . .

HOUSTON: Listen, Randy. Hickory here. Hold the controls very tight.

LUNA: It's no good, Houston. I . . .

HOUSTON: Colonel Claggett, hold tight. You must not let go. You must not let go.

LUNA *(a long silence, then a quiet voice):* Blessed Saint Leibowitz, keep 'em dreamin' down there . . . *(A choking sound)* . . .

John Pope, who had heard this conversation, stared at the module through his sextant, saw it waver, turn on its side, sort of skid through space, and descend toward the Moon with fatal speed.

HOUSTON: Hold on, Randy. You must not let go. Randy, you must not let go. Randy . . .

ALTAIR: *Luna* has crashed.

HOUSTON: Location?

ALTAIR: East of landing. Mountains.

HOUSTON: Damage?

ALTAIR: Obliterated.

HOUSTON: This is Hickory. *Altair,* climb to orbit.

ALTAIR: Negative. I must stay low to check.

HOUSTON: I'm talking with Dr. Feldman. He asks, 'Is your voice sort of drying up?'

ALTAIR: Obliterated. My God, they were obliterated.

HOUSTON: Hickory here. *Altair,* you must ascend to orbit. You are wasting fuel.

ALTAIR: I will not leave until I see where they are.

HOUSTON: You've already told us. East of landing. Mountains.

ALTAIR: I will not leave them.

HOUSTON: I think he turned off his mike. John, John, this is Hickory. It's imperative that you proceed to orbit and prepare to ignite engine. John, John, this is Hickory.

For two orbits John Pope flew alone through the intense radiation being poured out by the errant Sun, and each time when he headed directly toward the Sun he realized the heavy dosage he must be absorbing, for his dosimeter was running wild, but when he slipped behind the Moon, putting that heavy body between him and the Sun, he knew that he was reasonably safe from the extreme radiation.

On each pass he stared for as long as he could at the site of the crash, and although he was at an altitude from which not much could be seen clearly, it was nevertheless obvious that the astronauts' suits had been ripped by the crash and that death must have been more or less instantaneous, and he chanted to himself:

> 'How different death is there. No worms to eat the body, no moisture to corrupt. A thousand years from now, there they'll be, the first, the only. When wanderers come from the other galaxies, there our two will be, immaculate, unburied, waiting for the resurrection, all parts intact.

> 'Oh, Randy, how I loved you. Warring together in Korea. The mock fights over the Chesapeake. The flights across the country, you pilot out, me pilot home. Those sixteen days in Gemini, with you drinking nothing but orange juice and farting in my face. The hours of simulation. Drinking beer with Debby Dee.

> 'Jesus, Randy, it can never happen again—but it happened once.'

In hurried consultations NASA agreed that they would explain these two orbits of silence as a radio blackout caused by the Sun flare, which had now reached catastrophic proportions. Astronomers all across the world were focused on it, and scores of photographs were showing television viewers just how titanic the explosion had been, so that John Pope's temporary silence must not be construed as anything untoward. Without discernible agitation, Houston asked all its stations to try to make direct contact with Pope, and a welter of international voices sped toward the drifting *Altair.* Pope listened dully, but snapped to attention only when a familiar one echoed:

HONEYSUCKLE: This is Australia. *(Or-stry-lee-uh, the voice said)* Calling *Altair.*

ALTAIR: Aren't you the man who watched over Claggett and me in Gemini?

HONEYSUCKLE: The same.

ALTAIR: I remember you pronounced it Jimmin-eye.

HONEYSUCKLE: How else?

ALTAIR: I love your talk.

HONEYSUCKLE: Houston is eager to speak with you.

ALTAIR: I'd like to speak with Houston.

HONEYSUCKLE: Everything roger?

ALTAIR: Copacetic.

HONEYSUCKLE: Good on you, Cobber.

The hearty voice with its cheery brightness brought Pope back to attention, and when Houston reached him again, he was ready to talk:

ALTAIR: *Luna* crash confirmed. They bought the ranch.

HOUSTON: Any possibility of survivors?

ALTAIR: Negative. *Luna* completely fractured.

HOUSTON: Hickory speaking. John, we want you to go immediately to orbit.

ALTAIR: Roger. Wilco.

HOUSTON: John, during the blackout we calculated every mile of your way home. It looks good.

ALTAIR: I'm ready.

HOUSTON: It will be obligatory for you to get some sleep. Will you need sedatives?

ALTAIR: Negative. Negative.

HOUSTON: Can you stay alert for the next six hours?

ALTAIR: Affirmative. Six days if we have to.

HOUSTON: Six days you'll be in a feather bed. Now, John. Do you read me clear?

ALTAIR: Affirmative.

HOUSTON: And you understand the burn sequence?

ALTAIR: Affirmative. Repeat, my mind is clear. I comprehend.

HOUSTON: You're going to have to do everything just right. Exactly on the times we give.

ALTAIR: I intend to.

HOUSTON: And if there is anything you do not understand . . .

ALTAIR: Lay off, Hickory. I intend to get this bucket safely home. You take it easy. I'll take it easy.

HOUSTON: God bless you, Moonshiner. Bring it down.

ALTAIR: I intend to.

As methodically as if he were in the seventeenth hour of a familiar simulation, Pope ran through his check lists, took note of his fuel supplies and when the firings were to be made to correct his course so that he would enter the Earth's domain correctly. When all was secure, so far as he could control, he said quietly to Houston, 'I think it's go all the way,' and at the signal he fired the rockets which inserted him into the orbit that would carry him about 238,850 miles back to the safety of the Pacific Ocean.

He now faced some eighty hours of loneliness, and from the left-hand seat the capsule seemed enormous; he was surprised that anyone had ever felt it to be cramped. Aware that he had been motionless for a long time while Claggett and Linley had been active on the Moon, he began to worry about his legs, and for two hours he banged away on the newly provided Exer-Genie, which produced a real sweat.

He then turned on his tape, listening to Beethoven's joyous Seventh, but remembering how Claggett had objected to what he called spaghetti music, he found it distasteful. Instead, he routed out some of Claggett's tapes and listened to hillbillies singing "D-i-v-o-r-c-e," which not even his longing to see Claggett again could make palatable. When CapCom Ed Cater came on from Houston to ask if he wanted to hear the news, he said curtly, 'No!' So Cater said that Dr. Feldman wished to ask a few questions.

ALTAIR: Put him on.

HOUSTON (Dr. Feldman speaking): Are you experiencing any dizziness?

ALTAIR: Negative.

HOUSTON: Any excessive dryness in the throat? Any spots in the eyes?

ALTAIR: Negative.

HOUSTON: Any blood in the urine?

ALTAIR: Who looks?

HOUSTON: I do. And I want you to. Report as soon as you check.

ALTAIR: Will comply.

HOUSTON (Cater speaking): Your favorite shrink says it's very important he talk with you.

ALTAIR: Shoot. He may know something I don't.

HOUSTON: Crandall is here.

ALTAIR: I remember him. Joe Rorschach.

HOUSTON: He says, 'Only reason you're up there is because he passed you.'

ALTAIR: Ask him if he remembers Claggett? Toward the end of the test Crandall showed us that blank sheet of white paper, and guys like me said,

'Outer space' and 'The face of the Sun,' and stuff like that, and Claggett took one quick look and said, 'Two polar bears fornicating in a blizzard.'

HOUSTON: Open mike.

ALTAIR: That's why I said *fornicating*. You remember what he said.

HOUSTON: Dr. Crandall says, 'Claggett was stable all the way.' *(No comment)* And he says it's imperative that you remain stable. You have much work to do, coming up.

ALTAIR: I'll do it.

HOUSTON: This is Hickory. You're doing just fine. But we want you to sleep regularly, John. We want you to listen to the news.

ALTAIR: Hey, knock it off. I'm not depressed. There's nothing wrong with me.

HOUSTON: For sure there isn't, John. But you ate nothing yesterday.

ALTAIR: I was vomiting.

HOUSTON: You refused to listen to the news. You cut me off and you cut Cater off.

ALTAIR: I'd like to talk with Cater. I always like to talk with Cater.

HOUSTON: Cater here. We're not kidding, John. Thirty-six hours from now you have three men's work to do. When you give me the word, I want to go over four special check lists with you.

ALTAIR: You mean one-man emergency reentry?

HOUSTON: It could be a little tricky, you know.

ALTAIR: I figured that out a year ago. I have it programmed on my papers.

HOUSTON: You really are a straight arrow. But we can't just let you drift along up there for all these hours . . . well, alone.

ALTAIR: Plans called for me to be alone over the Moon for about this length of time.

HOUSTON: Roger, but things were different then.

ALTAIR: They sure were. Excuse me.

He refused to speak any further, but when Hickory Lee came on again they talked freely about the familiarization trip to the Amazon:

ALTAIR: If I put this bucket of bolts— Remember how Claggett used to describe his test planes? If I land this in the Amazon jungle, I'll know how to live on hearts of palm and raw iguana.

HOUSTON: They wanted to ask you if anyone had taken any alcohol aboard?

ALTAIR: Do they want me to take it or not take it?

HOUSTON: They thought it might calm things, but I told them you never touched the stuff.

ALTAIR: Roger. I had this wild-eyed football coach who preached that the worst enemies a young man could have were cigarettes, booze, fried food, refined sugar and girls. And I was dumb enough to believe him. I've continued to avoid the first four.

HOUSTON: Penny's here at Houston with us.

ALTAIR: She's not putting on a big act, I'm sure.

HOUSTON: She's with Debby Dee.

ALTAIR: I would expect her to be. Tell her I'll see her May second.

HOUSTON: You're due to land May first . . . remember?

ALTAIR: Hawaii, May first. Houston, May second.

HOUSTON: They'll probably fly her out to Hawaii.

ALTAIR: Negative! Negative! She wouldn't want to come anyway.

It seemed as if the entire nation, and much of the rest of the world, was watching as John Pope prepared to bring his *Altair* back to Earth. Prayers were said and cartoonists hailed his solitary effort; television provided meaningful analyses of his situation, and various older astronauts appeared on the tube to share their estimates of what the real danger points would be. All agreed that a practiced hand like John Pope, who had tested scores of experimental planes and engaged the enemy in combat over Korea, was not likely to panic at the necessity of doing three men's work. The highlight of the return trip came on the last full day, when Hickory Lee was serving as CapCom:

HOUSTON: *Altair,* our double-domers have come up with something everyone here thinks has merit.

ALTAIR: I'm listening.

HOUSTON: They think it would be good for the nation, and for you, too, if you would turn on your television camera and let the people see what you're doing.

ALTAIR: I wouldn't want to leave the controls and move around.

HOUSTON: No, no! Fixed focus. *(A long pause)* It was our unanimous opinion . . .

ALTAIR: You suggesting this to keep my mind occupied?

HOUSTON: Yes, I recommended it. Strongly.

ALTAIR: You usually know what you're doing, Hickory.

HOUSTON: Tomorrow can be a very demanding day.

ALTAIR: What could I say on television?

HOUSTON: You have a thousand things to say. Read your emergency notes. Let them see.

ALTAIR: Does Cater concur? He's a solid citizen.

HOUSTON: We present it to you together.

ALTAIR: The hours pass very slowly. They are very heavy. *(His voice sounded weak and hollow.)*

HOUSTON: That was our guess. *Altair,* set up the camera. Make some notes. Get your ideas under control, and in forty minutes we go.

ALTAIR: Does Dr. Mott approve such a scheme?

HOUSTON: He says it's obligatory. It will bring you all together.

ALTAIR: Roger.

At nine o'clock on the night of 30 April, prior to the time when Pope would make an important course correction, he turned on the television that stared down at him from a holding place on the bulkhead just aft of his right shoulder, and no more effective spot could have been found, for the camera did not reveal his full face, but it did display most of the capsule, especially the welter of switches and devices which confronted him.

He could not bring himself to use the pronoun *I,* so he fell naturally into the *we,* and this produced a riveting effect: 'We are bringing this great spacecraft back to Earth after an abbreviated visit to the other side of the Moon.' It was clear to everyone who saw the missing seats whom he meant by *we.*

'Dr. Linley should be in the right-hand seat, over there. And our commander, Randy Claggett, would be riding in the middle seat. He brought us to the Moon. It was my job to bring us back.'

Then came the most dramatic segment: 'When we lifted off from Cape Canaveral our two spacecraft, this one and the one going down to the Moon itself, weighted 17 tons empty. We carried 35 tons of fuel, just for these two little machines. We had to know where 40 miles of electrical wire ran, in and out. We had to memorize how 29 different systems worked, what every one of them did and how to repair each of them. Look, we had 689 separate switches to flick off and on. We had 50 separate engines to speed us through space. And we had, I believe, more than 4,000 pages of instructions we had to memorize, more or less. No one, I'm sure, could memorize that much.'

Although it was not looking at his features, the camera gave an excellent portrait of an astronaut: smallish, slim, shirt sleeves, short hair, strong, firmly set jaw which flexed now and then, showing muscles, small hands which moved masterfully, a sense of competence and a startling command of detail: 'I have a diagram here of the spacecraft as it was when we started out on what will be a 200-hour voyage. Here it is, 363 feet in the air. In the first two minutes we threw away the entire Stage I. Its job was to lift us into the air, and when that was done, we didn't have to use the escape tower, fortunately, so we dropped it off at three minutes. It had no further purpose. Stage II was finished after eight minutes, and down it went. Stage III, which sent us off on our way to the Moon, lasted for about two hours, then we got rid of it. The lunar module had two parts, one we left on the Moon on purpose. The other was supposed to rejoin us, but as you know, it didn't. If it had, we would've dropped it, too.

'So that leaves us only these two small parts, the service module, which carries all the things that keep us going, and tomorrow we'll throw that away. That'll leave this little portion I'm sitting in, and we'll fly it down through the atmosphere backward, to fight off the heat. It will be 25,000 degrees outside tomorrow, but we won't even feel it in here.

'And then a drogue parachute will open, a little one, and it will pull out a bigger one, and we'll land west of Hawaii like a sea gull coming home at the end of the day, and ships will be waiting there to greet us.'

He then turned and looked directly into the camera. 'Some years ago a hundred and ten of us, all test pilots, volunteered to be astronauts. Six of us were lucky enough to have been selected. Harry Jensen, perhaps the best of us, all round. He was killed by a drunken driver with God knows how many previous accidents. Timothy Bell, the only non-military man among us, flew into a radio tower. Randy Claggett, who was a legend long before this flight, got hit by a wayward Sun. That leaves Hickory Lee of Tennessee and Ed Cater of Mississippi, and me, and if the three of us could persuade NASA to send us to Mars in a craft as good as this one, we'd lift off tomorrow.

'Mankind was born of matter that accreted in space. We've seen dramatically these past few days how things far off in space can affect us deeply. We were meant to be in space, to wrestle with it, to probe its secrets. I'd like especially to say to Doris Linley that her husband was coming home with a multitude of secrets and new theories, and we feel his loss most grievously. The world will have to wait till next time, Doris!'

He turned back to his console with its 689 separate switches, and he let the camera run, ignoring it as he went about his work, and after a while on Earth they stopped transmitting.

The men at Houston who were guarding his welfare had been prudent in asking him to make the television broadcast, for he awakened on the morning of 1 May relaxed and eager to start his last demanding tasks, and although he was now approaching an operation which had previously proved exacting for three men, he neither brooded about it nor sought to avoid thinking about it.

When the time came for his stripped-down craft to plunge into the atmosphere at the tremendous speed generated by a return from outer space, it would have to hit that semi-solid layer, upon which all life on Earth depends, at exactly the right angle. If it came in too directly, pointed straight at Earth, it would encounter so much opposition, it would burn up almost instantly, and if it came in at too shallow an angle, it would fail to cut into the atmosphere at all and would become like a stone that boys skip across a pond of water: the craft would bounce once, twice, five, six times, and go careening off into space, flying endlessly, never to be seen again, and when the limited supply of oxygen vanished, the man would lie there in his couch, unbroken, unsullied, uncontaminated, moving through space forever.

Pope checked the approach once more: No steeper than 7.3° or we burn up. No shallower than 5.5° or we bounce off. This means hitting a corridor 27 miles in diameter at the end of 238,000 miles at a speed of better than 24,000 mph. Let's hope our computer's working.

Laymen, when they first heard of this delicate problem of reentry, often asked, 'If you come in too shallow and bounce off, why not turn around and make a second try?' and they were shaken by what astronauts told them: 'You won't believe what we do just before we try to reenter.'

John Pope was now preparing for this remarkable act of faith. With about ninety minutes before scheduled splashdown, he consulted his computer and fired rockets briefly to make the final small correction in his orbit. When the computer confirmed that his capsule had responded correctly, he activated explosive devices which blew off the service module, blew it right off into space, where it would burn up as it entered the atmosphere. This left him without any support system, any large supply of fuel, any of the instruments he would require for extended flight. If he missed the proper angle at reentry, he could do nothing to correct it, for all the impedimenta of flight would have vanished with the explosion. He was alone and almost powerless in a speeding vehicle heading for near-destruction.

He had rockets left for one life-saving maneuver; he could turn the capsule around so that it flew backward, presenting the big curved end with the ablative material to the incredible heat.

HOUSTON: Lee here. You never looked better, Moonshiner.

ALTAIR: Things going so well I've got my fingers crossed.

HOUSTON: This is your day, Moonshiner. Bring her down.

ALTAIR: I intend to.

With quiet confidence he slammed into the atmosphere, and even though he had been warned many times that it would be tougher than Gemini, he could scarcely believe it when it happened. Great flames engulfed the capsule, wiping out the sky. Huge chunks of incandescent material, 25,000° hot, roared past his window, reveling in the oxygen they were finding for their flames. More colors than a child has in a crayon box flashed past, and at one break in the tremendous fireworks he caught a glimpse of his trail, and he calculated it must be flaming behind him for five hundred miles.

It was impossible to tell Houston of the great fire; the heat was so intense that all radio communication was blacked out; this was the flaming entry that astronauts had to make alone, and the flakes of ablated material became so thick that he felt sure that everything was going to burn up, but the interior temperature did not rise one degree.

The flames stopped. He could feel the G's slacking off as the capsule was braked, and when he activated the drogue parachute, he felt with satisfaction and almost joy its first sharp grip.

USS TULAGI: We have you in sight, *Altair*. Three good chutes.

ALTAIR: Quite a reception committee you arranged. All the Roman candles.

USS TULAGI: Looks like you're going to splash down about six-tenths of a nautical mile away. Perfect landing.

ALTAIR: That's what I intended.

The NASA high command was outraged when they learned that the intrusive Japanese newspaperwoman Cynthia Rhee intended being present at Arlington when Marine Colonel Randolph Claggett was to be buried, as it were, and Dr. Stanley Mott and Tucker Thompson of *Folks* were sent to her hotel in Washington to try to dissuade her from attending.

In the cab on the way, Thompson said, 'I'd call it the biggest surprise of my life. The way this Debby Dee has risen to the occasion. Hard drinker, hard talker, you'd have expected her to louse up the whole procession, but what does she do? She comes on like Melanie in *Gone With the Wind*. Perfect picture of genteel Southern womanhood.

'I've been through nine NASA tragedies now, and no astronaut's wife has played her role better than Debby Dee. It would be disgraceful if that goddamned Dragon Lady showed up to ruin the funeral.'

Thompson had proved twice that *Folks* knew how to handle the funerals of its astronauts, once in the Jensen case, once when Tim Bell flew into the tower; he knew where to catch the young widows to evoke the awful loss, how to photograph the kids, the minister at the graveside, and he better than most sensed what a jarring note it would be if Debby Dee were confronted by her dead hero's mistress: 'I wouldn't blame her if she swatted Madame Butterfly right in the kisser, but I would sure hate to see it photographed. Especially by *Life*. They'd drive us into the ground with a shot like that.'

He explained, when the cab neared the hotel, how diligently he had worked to keep the threatening scandal out of the press. 'You got a man like John Glenn, a winner like John Pope, they stand for something. People make fun of us for cultivating the Boy Scout image, but dammit, that's what this nation wants. This man Pope, bringing that Apollo back alone, that's heroic. Give me two million bucks, I could elect him President.'

In Cynthia's room, an inexpensive one rented by the day, Mott spoke first, and in his gentlest voice: 'This is terribly embarrassing . . .'

'Not for me,' the Korean girl said softly.

Thompson then launched his campaign, as unctuously as possible: 'Now, Miss Rhee, we know how you slipped back into America . . . illegally . . . and we know where you came over the border . . .'

She moved a step nearer her tall adversary, a porcelain hand grenade ready to explode. 'Mr. Thompson, don't talk like a fool.'

Tucker sucked in his gut. If it was to be warfare, he was prepared with some salvos of his own. 'You show your face at this funeral, Madame Butterfly, out you go . . . right on your ass.'

'Why?' she asked brazenly.

'Because the senators do not want a scandal.'

'Don't they have one already?' When Dr. Mott looked bewildered, she said, 'I mean your young farmer, Sam Cottage. I've been talking with him about the warnings he tried to issue, but I suppose your spies have told you that.'

'Rumors,' Thompson said. 'We've already looked into the Cottage case.'

'You hope it's rumors. You hope there's nothing in writing.'

'Miss Rhee,' Thompson said in a fresh attempt at conciliation. 'When

America has two bona-fide heroes like Claggett and Pope, you wouldn't want to . . .'

'I am attending the funeral,' she said firmly.

'Then Senator Grant is going to order you arrested.'

'What for? Hundreds of people slip across the border from Canada . . . and Mexico, too.'

'I'm warning you that he's going to hit you with the heavy stuff. Like being a prostitute.'

She laughed. She had been a world-ranging newspaperwoman, and that was all. True, she had traveled with the six astronauts exactly as she had traveled in Europe with Fangio and the other racing drivers in order to catch their unadorned stories, but if any senator tried to expel her on trumped-up charges, she would create a real scandal. 'A great man lies dead on the Moon. I loved him, and it matters very little who knows it. Because one day I shall write about him, and his widow will thank me.'

Thompson grew furious. 'For you to appear at Arlington . . . Scandal sheets are just waiting for something like this.'

'It will be very difficult for you to stop me, or for your senators, either.'

Dr. Mott felt he had to speak. 'This is a solemn moment, Cindy. I've always aided you, when I could. Now I'm begging you to stay away.'

'Impossible. Because I'm being escorted by John Pope.'

'Pope?' Thompson yelled. 'Have you been messing around with Pope, too?'

'During the flight to the Moon, Randy told John— I'll let him tell you. He'll be here shortly.'

Within a few minutes Pope entered, accompanied by Penny, and as soon as they saw Mott and Thompson they could guess what was happening. Pope said, 'We've come to take Cindy to the ceremonies,' and Mott protested: 'Senator Grant and Senator Glancey expressly asked that she be kept away.'

'I believe I was Randy's best friend, and I'm prepared to say who—'

'John,' Mott interrupted, 'you could make some people very high in NASA most unhappy.'

'This is the funeral of my friend. The nation is honoring a sensational man, and I know he'd want Cindy to attend.'

'How can you know such a thing?' Thompson asked, red of face.

'Because on the flight to the Moon he told Linley and me, "Soon as I get back to Earth, I'm chucking NASA and the *Folks* contract and marrying the Korean." When we argued against it, especially Linley, who'd seen a lot of interracial marriages fail, Claggett said, "When I was flying in Korea, I shacked up with this Jo-san—" '

'What's a Jo-san?' Penny asked.

'A Korean whore,' Thompson interjected, and Pope stared at him venomously: 'You use that word again, Thompson, I'll take you apart. I met Claggett's Jo-san. Two years of college. Caught up in the war. Impossible to live, so she took a job slinging hash for the American flyers and Claggett fell in love with her. Told Linley and me she was the best loving he'd ever had, and he was mortally ashamed he hadn't married her. Told us he didn't want to lose happiness twice, so he was going to marry this other Korean woman,' and he bowed toward Cindy.

'Mrs. Pope,' Thompson pleaded. 'Can't you bring some sense—'

'I can vouch for what my husband has just said because after you men and my two senators put the arm on Randy not to leave Debby Dee before the flight, he took me aside in the committee room and said, and I quote with great accuracy: "Tell your boys they win now, but when I get back they can all go fuck a duck." '

Thompson gasped. 'Are you in this with your husband?' he asked weakly.

'I sure am. And so is Debby Dee, it may surprise you to hear. I had the decency to warn her over the phone that John was determined to escort Cindy, and she said, "Bring the slant-eyed sonnombeech along. I think Randy would've had a lively time with that one." '

'Pope!' Tucker Thompson shouted. 'I warn you, the big men aren't going to like this!' and Penny said, 'My husband's a big man now, and I'm his wife, and we're taking Cindy right into the front row where she belongs.'

'Your senators will fire you if—'

'I work for my senators,' Penny said. 'I do not allow them to dictate how I behave.' And when Debby Dee arrived, mascara running and blouse awry, Penny took charge. 'Debby Dee, this is Miss Rhee,' and Debby Dee said gently, 'I suppose you could say we've already met . . . through a third party.'

Tucker Thompson charged right into battle. 'Mrs. Claggett, do you want this woman at your funeral?' And he jabbed an accusing finger at Cindy.

'I invited her,' Debby said. 'Wouldn't I look cheap as hell if I disinvited her?'

Before Tucker could launch his moralities, Senator Grant entered, bearing on his arm the beautiful widow of Dr. Paul Linley, a tall ebon-faced woman of thirty. His voice choking, he said, 'I encouraged my dear friend Gawain Butler to place his nephew in our NASA program. So in a sense I feel responsible for his death.'

'And for his chance to prove his heroism,' Doris said, and Penny, comparing the two widows, thought: How wonderfully American they are. Debby Dee, rock-hard from deepest Texas; Doris Linley, survivor of the Detroit ghettos. Which one made the greater journey to get here? And although she knew it was exhibitionistic, she could not restrain herself; dashing across the room, she embraced them and for just a moment there were tears which could not be contained.

After the stately ceremonies with the seventeen-gun salutes and the muffled drums, Debby Dee, a blowzy woman of forty-seven, who had maintained a gracious, solemn posture for Thompson's cameras during nine heartbreaking days, grabbed Doris Linley's hand and growled, 'Let's get the hell out of here and find some beer.' They drove in their government limousine to Penny Pope's Washington apartment, where with John and Cindy Rhee they guzzled beer through the night.

'Randy Claggett was one of the world's basic men,' Debby Dee said, 'and I was privileged to know him. Good times and bad, he was one hell of a man.'

'What was it like, Deb, when you were widowed the first time?' Cindy asked, and after this had been explored for more than half an hour, she wanted to know how they had lived at Pax River.

'Ask them,' Debby Dee said, pointing to the Popes, and for two hours they reminisced about the days at Solomons Island, the old cars, the Pax-Jax-Lax routine, the dogfights above the Chesapeake.

'What was it like?' Cindy asked Doris. 'I mean, his being black and not a military man?'

'Everything Paul did, and he did so much, he started way behind. Black boys always do. But he caught up fast. At the end he was as good as any of them.' And she looked to Captain Pope for confirmation.

'In brains he was better than most,' John said. 'In courage no one surpassed him.' When he tried to visualize Linley, all he could see was the irrepressible comedian leading cheers for Albuquerque Technological Institution, and he had to subdue a smile, but after a while he said, 'For sixty-six hours and seventeen minutes he was my seatmate in space. None better.' Then he walked across the room and kissed Doris.

When the night was almost gone, Cindy said, 'I loved him in a different way. The symbol . . .'

'If there was one thing Claggett wasn't,' Debby said, 'it was a symbol. That sonnombeech was basic.'

'He was *the* astronaut,' Cindy said. 'Not Glenn, not Shepard, not you, John Pope. He spent more hours in space than any other man, and I watched him. He approached a spacecraft as if he owned it. Once he said as he left for the sixteen-day flight with you, Pope, "Well, let's see how we fly this bucket of bolts." '

Debby Dee wiped her eyes, and later, in her hotel room, Rhee Soon-Ka started her manuscript about the Solid Six:

> They took a dark stone and stood it in a dark place, publishing to the world that Randy Claggett was dead. But we who knew him were convinced that his spirit still stunned and startled and confused the ribbon clerks, as always.

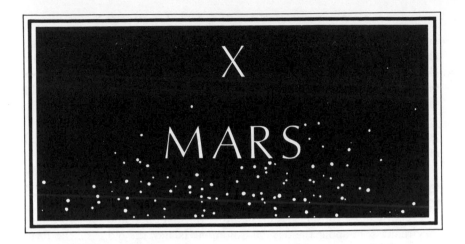

X
MARS

THE NATIONAL EXCITEMENT OVER JOHN POPE'S HEROIC ODYSSEY
lasted eleven days, and then the nation awakened to the fact that never
again in this century would an American walk on the Moon. The enchantment of Apollo vanished, the glory of the astronaut dimmed.

Dr. Loomis Crandall, the Air Force psychologist who had helped select
the various groups of spacemen and who knew more about them than any
other official, compiled a condescending summary which infuriated Mott:

> Our sensible astronauts, correctly assessing the national mood, are
> resigning from the program, seeking employment in business, but
> most often merely drifting from one public relations job to another
> for the good reason that they have no basic skills except calculus and
> astrophysics.
>
> True, John Glenn has gone to the Senate and Frank Borman to an
> airline, but the typical astronaut is Ed Cater, who left NASA to front
> for a real estate developer in Miami, then to an insurance company
> in New Orleans, and now to a used-car dealership in his hometown
> of Kosciusko, where his wife has become a partner in a dress shop
> and earns more than he does.
>
> Nine of the finest we had are dead. All the living comported them-
> selves with a heroism and dignity of which we can be proud. But we
> can also be disappointed, for they produced no national spokesman
> for space, no poet of the skies like Saint-Exupéry of France. They
> were in effect red-hot test pilots who transformed themselves into
> red-hot spacecraft pilots—and nothing more. In this limited re-
> sponse they reflected the national attitude toward space.

When Mott finished reading, he stormed into headquarters, eyes blazing
behind his steel-rimmed glasses, a small, wiry man whose most sensitive

nerves had been abused. When he found Crandall in the administrator's office he bored right in: 'Let's take an equal number of graduates from the Harvard School of Business, from Cal Tech, MIT and Notre Dame and let's compare records. Glenn a senator. They tell me Schmitt of Arizona might make it next time. Borman at Eastern Airlines. Anders an ambassador. Young men doing wonderful things way beyond their age qualification. I'll put my astronauts up against any group you assemble, Crandall, including an equal number of Ph.D.'s in psychology, psychiatry, psychoanalysis and psychosometric voodoo.'

'Stanley,' the administrator interrupted, 'Crandall's only writing a report.'

'Well, I don't like it. I do not like to see the great work done by this agency denigrated. If our program is grinding to a halt, it's not because it was a bad program, but because we stopped too soon.'

In this fighting mood he trudged up to the Capitol to defend NASA in one more public hearing, and normally he would have been the quiet, self-effacing scientist on whom Congress had come to rely. But on this morning a senator from North Dakota had asked why NASA lagged so far behind private industry in certain learned fields, and Mott almost lost his temper:

> 'NASA is private industry, Senator. We make nothing. We're a grandiose procurement agency, one of the best this world has ever seen. We've spent more than fifty billion dollars since I came aboard, without a single case of fraud or embezzlement or malfeasance. The nation has never had to apologize for our behavior, and although I can give you a dozen examples where in my opinion we chose the wrong contractor, you cannot give me one where we awarded that contract fraudulently. I would be proud if all government operations could say the same.'

Yet, even as he defended his agency Mott realized it was beginning to retreat from its days of grandeur, and he told his young assistants, 'We ought to be taking bold new steps in space, dispatching spacecraft with and without men to probe the farthest frontiers. When we do this, philosophers will face new complexities and be forced to explain them to the public.' At a conference of astrophysicists at Purdue University he warned:

> 'Within the last few years we have made discoveries which stagger the knowing mind. Arno Penzias and Robert Wilson have identified the residue reverberations of the original explosion which set our universe in motion. Maarten Schmidt has made brilliant deductions about the speed at which distant galaxies travel. Hawking at Cambridge asks awesome questions about quasars, pulsars and black holes, and I believe we must rethink all our basic concepts.

'How will the general public react? Three precedents provide some guidance.

'Copernicus kept his new knowledge largely to himself, and when the Church objected to his conclusions, he stifled them. His immediate impact was nil, but his ultimate effect on morals, theology and individual comprehension was profound.

'Giordano Bruno flaunted his radical theories, irritating Catholics and Protestants equally. He agitated society by pointing out the consequences of scientific discoveries, and in the end, was burned at the stake to refute his astronomical heresies.

'Charles Darwin's work produced so many shattering implications that he was rebutted immediately, and since his theory of evolution abused religious sensibilities, it aroused intense opposition which has not yet abated.

'I believe that the speculations we have awakened regarding the ultimate nature of the universe must disturb our generations as profoundly as Darwin's theories affected his. Whenever we stand on a threshold, as we do now, we must inescapably bring into question positions held previously, and when such revision involves the origin of the universe, we find ourselves on inflammable ground and must anticipate vigorous rebuttal.'

Mott had always been a religious man. His father, after all, had been a Methodist minister, and young Mott had been raised with the Bible as a constant presence. At one time he had been able to recite from memory the names of the books of both Testaments, a skill which he found useful in later years when he wished to locate a quotation, but he had also known their content rather thoroughly, and this, too, had been significant, for it prevented him from slipping thoughtlessly into a cliché 'scientist-as-atheist' position. When his father's ministerial friends railed against Darwin's theory of evolution, he was never contemptuous in his attempts to defend it, and if they pressed, 'But do you believe in God?' he was always able to answer without dissembling, 'Yes, I do.'

But he also believed, without even the smallest nagging question, that mankind evolved in much the same way that the Sun had evolved from primordial matter, and he believed this because when he inspected the heart of existing galaxies, including our own, he could watch stars evolving from great clouds of matter. This was fact, not theory, and he could conceive of no alternative. He supposed that when religionists abused Darwin and proposed an instant, godlike creation, they were merely saying what he was saying, but in a more poetic form, and therefore he felt no sense of opposition to his father's affirmation of *his* belief.

But he also believed without any reservation whatever that this universe

of which he and his Earth and his Sun were a part had come into being—
that is, in its present form—about eighteen billion years ago, with the Earth
assuming its existence and shape about four and a half billion years ago.
When his father's friends insisted that the Book of Genesis was the accurate
statement, he was able to agree: 'It's a poetic version. It says about the same
thing I've been saying, except that its word *day* is best understood to mean
a vast geologic era.'

If debaters tried to make him deny that the billions of years required
for the formation of Sun and Earth ever existed, and if they argued that all
the magnificent galactic structure came into being a mere six or seven
thousand years ago, with geological strata and dinosaur bones hidden in
place like some jolly theological treasure hunt, he refused to argue. 'Possible
but not likely' was all he would respond.

The real question in this debate had been posed by his father: 'If I
concede, Stanley, that the universe did begin with your big bang eighteen
billion years ago, tell me what set that bang in motion?'

'Science has no answer to that.'

'Was it not God?'

'I think so. Or some force mysteriously like God.' But when his father
smiled in philosophical relief, his son insisted upon adding, 'The big bang
could not have taken place 4004 B.C.'

'Fair deal,' the elderly minister said. 'I'll give you your billions of years
if you'll give me my God.'

Once while vacationing between meetings he listened to a park ranger
on the rim of the Grand Canyon describing to some tourists how that trivial
stream, the Colorado River, had through the ages cut the gorge from one
level of rock to another until the masterpiece stood revealed, and after the
ranger ended his talk and went back to his office, Mott remained on the rim
speculating on the beautiful accident by which the United States had acquired parks like this Grand Canyon and Yellowstone, and he silently
congratulated those social pioneers who had fought the battles for succeeding generations: This canyon is totally unspoiled. Somebody deserves a lot
of credit. And he could envisage someone like himself, three hundred years
from now, standing on the edge of a canyon on Mars and saying, 'That
NASA gang, whoever they were, who reached here first, they did very little
to destroy what they found,' and if he was proud of what his team had done,
he was even more proud of what they had not done.

He had barely formulated such thoughts when a tall, awkward, flaming-
eyed man stepped out of the crowd who had been listening to the park
ranger's description of how the canyon had evolved, and shouted for attention:

> 'These park rangers, government employees, have been getting away
> with murder for too long. Standing here on government property
> and spreading lies that contradict Holy Scripture. Telling us yarns

about how that little river down there took a hundred million years to sculpture this magnificent canyon. You know and I know that that's a lie. That's a damned lie, and one of these days, mark my words, park rangers like that are going to be held to account.

'This noble canyon was born about five thousand years ago, no more, when God sent the planet Venus scraping along the edge of the Earth, building mountains and cutting gullies. You can look at that canyon and know in your hearts it can't be a million years old. And a hundred million? That's laughable. It was cut down when men like Moses and Jeremiah were living on this Earth, and it is not the handiwork of some puny little river; it is the handiwork of God.'

He orated with fiery eloquence for nearly half an hour, holding Mott and the other vacationers captivated by his bold assertions, and at the end of his argument he cried, 'Let's have a show of hands. How many of you know in your hearts that I'm right and the park ranger is wrong?' To Mott's surprise, more than half the listeners voted that the Grand Canyon of the Colorado could not be more than five thousand years old.

Wherever he went these days the world seemed to be divided into two groups, the few who had followed the deeper researches of the astrophysicists and the many who appeared to long for a simpler universe, one with fewer speculative aspects, and this feeling intensified as the year 1976 approached, for across the land people yearned for a return to the simplicities of 1776.

His son Millard was a case in point. When President Ford, following his pardon of Richard Nixon, offered a meager and grudging pardon to the young men who had fled to Canada to escape the draft, Millard crept back to the Mott home under the most humiliating circumstances, even though, as he told his father, 'everyone now concedes that men like me and Roger were right to protest. America knows that Vietnam was a horrible mistake.'

Roger had refused to accept America's reluctant forgiveness and had elected to remain in Canada. When Millard told his parents of their separation, he burst into tears, and for the first time the older Motts realized what a deep human attachment their son had felt for Roger, and they were surprised the next day to learn that Millard was now living with a young man named Victor, who ran what was known as a 'head shop' in Denver. They did a big business in astrology books, tarot cards, the I-Ching, and cheese-and-wine lectures by gurus from India who explained to the college students in the area how society ought to be organized.

After Millard flew back to Colorado, Rachel Mott studiously tidied the apartment: the Mondrians were straightened on the living-room wall, the classical records were alphabetized again, excess books were placed in a corner to be given to the community college, and various unnecessary things which had accumulated were thrown away. When she finished getting all things in place, she sat on her bed and looked once more at the loving Axel Petersson figures carved in wood, and said to her husband, 'Talking with Millard about his Roger and Victor was exactly like listening to a headstrong daughter who has divorced her banker husband and is living with an architect. It's very difficult to keep values straight.'

'Especially for people in their late fifties,' Stanley said.

While brooding about his sons he idly thumbed a science magazine, and came upon a startling proposal by a scientist named Letterkill: 'We should position in outer space a gigantic radio telescope whose distance between its two elements would be ten astronomical units. That would give us a base line of 900,000,000 miles.'

His imagination ablaze, Mott started drawing diagrams at top speed, then explained the basic principle to his wife: 'It's magnificent! The problem of parallax carried to the ultimate. You know how a range finder on a battleship works? You have this very long base line, say ninety feet. The longer the better. And they have two small telescopes, one at each end. And the difference in angle between how each looks at the same target can be converted into precise distance. Boom! Your big guns fire, hit the target and sink the enemy, all because you used parallax intelligently.'

He proceeded to explain that earlier astronomers had determined star distances through clever applications of parallax: 'On December 20 they took a photograph of the star Sirius. On June 20, when the Earth had moved halfway through its orbit and was as far away from its December position as possible, they took another photograph of the same star, using the same camera. Parallax revealed that Sirius was 8.6 light-years away.'

He said that astronomers had already devised a vast radio telescope, one leg in California, the other in Australia, with each taking a 'photograph' of some heavenly body at exactly the same moment, so that the differential in angles could determine distance: 'But now what this fellow Letterkill proposes is to place a huge radio telescope atop a rocket and fire it a billion miles into space, and lock it there. Then fire the other half of the telescope out into space, a billion miles in the opposite direction. What a fantastic base line we'd have. Rachel, we could see to the outer edges of the universe.'

His excitement grew at such a pace that he telephoned Huntsville, even though he suspected that Dieter Kolff would be asleep, and when the drowsy man came on the telephone, he asked, 'Dieter, read about a man who has just made a dazzling proposal and I want your reading on it. Could we build a giant gossamer telescope in two parts? Throw one by rocket about a billion miles out into space and fix it there in orbit? Then throw an exact duplicate a billion miles out in the opposite direction? I think he recommends an angle of about a hundred and twenty degrees and . . .'

'You have a base line of enormous length.'

'Something like ten astronomical units.'

'And you could penetrate beyond the farthest known galaxy.'

'Is it practical?'

'We could do it tomorrow.'

The two men talked for about an hour, with Kolff always bringing the discussion back to the two activating rockets, which he was prepared to build if NASA wanted to bring him back from retirement, and Mott speaking always about the gossamer construction of the telescopes: 'You understand, Dieter, we use no metal except in the frame for the radio eye. Everything is gossamer. Whole telescope would weigh, what? Less than three thousand pounds?'

When the call to Huntsville ended he could not sleep, and as he pored over Letterkill's proposal, the thought came to him that this might well be the same man who had planned to make the Wallops Island rocket device the first satellite into space, and at four in the morning he had an operator track this Letterkill down at the Lewis Center in Cleveland: 'Are you the fellow who came up with that brilliant proposal at Wallops Island? Excuse me, I'm Dr. Stanley Mott, who supported you at that time.'

It was the same Levi Letterkill. A man who has one good idea is always apt to have another, but his proposal for a telescope with a base line of ten A.U.'s did not get immediate attention, because later that morning, about 0830 Washington time, the Miami police called to inform the Motts that their son Christopher was in jail again, this time on a very serious charge of bringing cocaine in from Colombia.

When Christopher Mott went to trial in Florida on the charge of smuggling cocaine from Colombia to the street value of $3,000,000, as they said in the newscasts, his parents defended him in anguish. Nearing sixty and unwavering defenders of all that was good in American life, they flew down to the muscular town of West Palm Beach, across the Intracoastal Waterway from the real Palm Beach, and sat for three days in a grubby courtroom while the state's attorneys wove a web of damning evidence against their son.

The Motts presented a sorrowful picture as they listened to the ugly facts they had tried so diligently to ignore through the preceding years: a middle-aged couple who had always tried to appear respectable—Rachel, her Grecian hairdo severely in place, her tailored suit neatly pressed, her firm mouth never quivering; and Stanley in his blue-black pin-striped suit, white shirt, foulard tie and steel-rimmed glasses. They looked like an executive family from Bethlehem Steel or IBM, but since the trial took place so near to Cape Canaveral, the papers emphasized their membership in the NASA family.

Christopher was twenty-five years old now and no longer entitled to consideration as an unknowing youth, but as he sat with the defense lawyers he seemed so slim and frail, so close to what a young man of his age with an assistant professorship at some college like Bates or Bowdoin should look like, that Rachel sometimes had to bow her head to keep from weeping, but then fresh evidence of his behavior would echo throughout the courtroom, and she would ask herself: How could this have happened? What in God's name went wrong?

At the end of each day's testimony she and Stanley returned to their glossy motel near the big shopping center, and it seemed to her that this was the other face of Cape Canaveral: up there the huge rockets soaring off into space with cheers and hundreds of technicians monitoring the flight and the young heroes in the capsule; down here, only a few miles away, a confused young man in a courtroom attempting to defend himself against a society which had almost encouraged him to become a criminal.

The songs of his day, the patterns of dress, television's idealization of the illiterate rowdy who disrupts the classroom, sleazy newspaper stories and the dreadful pressure of one's peers, all had conspired to put her son on trial, and she and Stanley had been too preoccupied with society's business to combat the destructive influences.

'We never worked for ourselves,' she whispered as the damaging second day ended. 'It was always for the Army, for the Germans at El Paso, for the Alabama rural children, even now, for the families of the astronauts. We've not been selfish, Stanley.'

'I may have been,' he said mournfully as he sat on the motel bed casting up the accounts of his life. 'You tried to warn me in California when I was studying so hard. We know that's when Millard started running with the wrong crowd and Chris began his undisciplined behavior. I feel the guilt almost unbearably.'

On the third day the case went to the jury at eleven in the morning, and shortly after lunch the seven men and five women brought in their verdict of guilty on all counts. The judge announced that because Christopher's parents had to leave Florida quickly, he would sentence their son two days later, and they spent most of those days at the jail talking with Chris and giving him what belated support they could.

When Rachel heard the sentence—five years in jail—she almost fainted, but then joined her husband and the defense lawyers in a plea that her son be remanded to a minimum-security prison where the likelihood of abuse and sodomy would be diminished. The judge listened attentively, said that he could not accept the insinuation that Florida jails were out of control, and denied the request.

When the President suggested that John Pope make a world tour to allow other nations to see what an engaging hero America had produced, the NASA medical staff demurred on the grounds that he had undergone a grueling experience and deserved rest, but Pope said, 'I'll go if I can be routed through Australia. I'd like to thank that fellow at Honeysuckle. He was very important to me—twice.'

So Pope flew to Europe, where the papers made much of his determination to visit the Australian voice that had helped save him, and Down

Under newspapers kept track of how many days it would be before he reached Australia. The American ambassador flew from Canberra to Sydney to welcome him, then flew him in an American plane to receptions in rowdy Brisbane, staid Adelaide and gracious Melbourne, with a final stop at the American embassy in Canberra, where a large assembly waited to greet the hero.

He was courteous as always, explaining several times that his wife, Penny, would normally have accompanied him, except that this time she was kept in Washington by her duties with the Senate. The Russian ambassador gave a small party for what he termed 'the American cosmonaut and a very brave man,' and then Pope called it quits.

'I came here to see the Australian communicator at Honeysuckle, and it's time we got to it.' The U.S. ambassador agreed, and next morning a car and driver were provided to take Pope to the concentration of huge radio dishes hidden among the hills south of Canberra. These formed the system whereby Houston kept in touch with its satellites when they were over the Indian Ocean and the western Pacific, and Pope was awed by their size, their complexity and the beauty of their setting.

'This must be one of the most attractive features of the space age,' he told the Australian manager, and before he entered the low buildings where the messages were processed in a bank of computers, he walked among the trees and flowers that made the place a garden.

'Appropriately named,' he told the Australians, then he stopped suddenly to watch two kangaroos feeding in a grassy swale. 'They really do hop along on their hind feet,' he said, and his guides had to tug at his arm. 'McGuigan's waiting,' they said, 'and some press people want to talk with you later.'

So reluctantly he left the Australian woodland with its enchantments and entered the working area of the communications center, where wires from the great hemispherical dishes pointing to the invisible satellites delivered their messages. McGuigan, a tall, thin, hipless Australian with a barbarous accent, stepped forward eagerly to meet the man with whom he had talked in both Gemini and Apollo.

'Hello, Pope. Glad you made it back.'

'Thanks to your help.' They talked for some minutes, most amiably, and then Pope said to one of the managers, 'I guess I've got to go through with it,' and the manager shrugged.

'Call the staff together, please,' Pope said, and while the local workers assembled he inwardly asked forgiveness for what as a guest he was now required to say.

On almost every important American space shot, the Australian workers had waited till the last crucial moment, then threatened a strike for higher wages. For a spacecraft to try to negotiate the vast corridors of heaven without any contact over half the surface of the Earth was unthinkable, so always NASA had to surrender to the blackmail, but Pope also knew that once the higher wages were agreed to, the Australians provided the best communications in the entire network. On one occasion men left the picket line, and under the most adverse circumstances, walked miles into the arid backlands to repair a communications link to ensure that the American spacecraft passing over the Indian Ocean could maintain its communication with Houston.

When the crew was assembled, Pope said quietly, 'All astronauts realize what a profound debt they owe you wonderful communicators in Australia, and especially this superb crew here at Honeysuckle. On two occasions Mr. McGuigan here provided me with assistance beyond the call of duty, and I should like to hand him two medals, placed in my care by the American government. The first is to him personally. The second is to him as representative of your excellent crew.' As he handed over the medals and listened to the cheering, he wanted to add, but didn't: 'That's till the next time you strike, you lovable sonsabitches.'

After the crowd dispersed, the manager said, 'The press is in the other building,' and Pope had a second chance to observe the rugged beauty of this unusual place. He was therefore in an amiable mood when he entered the press room to find five journalists awaiting him, four from Australia, one from Japan. He could see only Cindy Rhee, beautiful like the flowers outside, dressed in somber colors and staring at him with those dark, slanted eyes.

'I have wanted to finish my story,' she said as she took his hand.

'You came all the way here from Tokyo?'

'I wanted to see the last of my astronauts in a real setting. With his own kind. At Honeysuckle.'

'This is Captain John Pope,' one of the managers said. 'You're all aware of his accomplishments.' In answer to the Australian questions, John lied: 'We've never had anything but the most amiable relations with your stations. They've been invaluable links in our chain of communications, and I particularly can testify . . .' He saw Cindy smiling sardonically, and then he remembered the night at the Bali Hai motel when Claggett told the gang how the Australians at Honeysuckle had threatened a strike before his first Apollo flight. 'I wanted to go down there when the flight was over and cut their balls off,' Claggett had said, and Pope had watched Cindy copying his words in her notebook. Now she was copying his, and smiling.

'I asked especially to come to Honeysuckle,' he continued, 'to pay my respects to Mr. McGuigan. I couldn't always understand his accent, but I sure could appreciate the warmth of his interest.'

When the press conference ended, the managers started to walk Pope back to his embassy car, but Cindy interposed, saying, 'I've a rented car. I'll take him back,' and before anyone could protest, she had ordered the American car to return empty to the embassy compound while she led Pope to her Volkswagen.

'I have a room in a village toward Mt. Kosciusko in the Australian alps,' she said, and they drove for more than an hour through parklands that sometimes teemed with kangaroos, large, tawny beasts that played along the roadway. 'I've written my book,' she said, 'but it can't be completed without your story, John.'

'Mine's easily told. Three of us went up, one of us came down.'

'But why did you go up? When, on those great flat plains of Fremont, did you first visualize yourself in the heavens?'

'Did you take the trouble to visit Fremont?'

'I visit everywhere. I visited Honeysuckle last week to be sure I would know my way around.'

'But why?'

'John, you and the others, you're real . . . don't you realize it? You're immortal. Four hundred years from now they'll read about you the way we read about Magellan today.'

She said this so simply, and with such conviction, that he could say nothing, nor did she, and after passing through a village he asked, 'What did you mean by *real?*'

'Well,' she said as she looked directly at him, her hands almost off the steering wheel, 'there's Randy Claggett, one of the best men this century will produce, and then there's Timothy Bell, a pathetic bombast.'

'Are you going to say that? He's dead, you know.'

'He was always dead, and I shall say so.'

'You're remorseless.'

'So is the truth.'

She drove to an inviting country inn whose sign announced that it sold Toohey's ale, and since it was not yet dusk they sat in the garden with their tea. Slowly, at first, he began to talk; then words rolled out unimpeded, as if he had hoarded a universe of impressions which he must now share. He spoke of things close to the heart of space, things he had never before been able to verbalize, not even in those long debriefings conducted by the super brains of NASA.

'They kept asking how I felt, alone in the command module flying home, and I kept feeding them the answers I knew they wanted, expressed in words I knew they would accept. Responsibility. The job I was assigned to do. Training in the simulators quite adequate. Plus a lot of real guff about loneliness. But would you like to hear the truth?'

'That's why I'm here.'

'The module was a very small place. Like from here to here. When I was alone, how did I feel? I felt roomy. Free to spread out. At last I had all the space I needed, and to confess the truth, I was rather relieved.' He laughed at himself for having revealed his anti-heroism, but then he stopped. 'The others? Even in the roominess their ghosts crowded in upon me.'

They talked till dinner was called, and all through the meal, and afterward in the parlor decorated with brightly colored English hunting prints, a great outflowing of evaluation, and when the time came to go to bed, there was a brief moment of embarrassment, as if Cindy expected him to suggest that they sleep together, or as if he expected her to. It passed when he banged on the desk bell and asked the manager, 'Can you show me to my room?' Cindy followed them upstairs and accompanied him to his door, where she said, 'Goodnight, John. Let's continue at breakfast.'

They spent the entire next day lounging about the inn or walking its flower-strewn grounds, but always talking about space, and when they passed members of the hotel staff he could hear them whisper, 'That's John Pope, the one who brought the spaceship home. He's rooming with the Japanese newspaper girl.'

By the end of that day it seemed as if everyone in Australia knew what he was up to, plus many of the people in Washington. Senator Grant, receiving a flow of confidential messages from NASA, did his best to keep their content hidden from the committee counsel, but before long one of the secretaries felt that Mrs. Pope should really know how her errant husband was behaving: 'He's shacked up with that Korean babe.' With a forced smile Penny said, 'Occupational hazard,' and no more.

When cables began pouring into the embassy in Canberra, demanding that Pope be found and escorted personally to his major speech in Sydney, the embassy tracked down where he was hiding and telephoned to reprimand him, but he would accept no calls, so the woman running the inn brought him the messages in person: 'I'm afraid the fat's in the fire, Captain Pope.'

'It's been there before,' he told her, and to Cindy he said, 'We seem to have whipped up a storm.'

As if they both realized that this probing interview could never be repeated, the mood and the willingness having been lost, they spent that last day at the core of the space experience, and Pope found himself saying strange things which he would never have divulged to another:

'Claggett from the South and me from an area where there were no blacks, yet we had the standard prejudices. 'Niggers smell funny,' Claggett insisted, 'and bein' cooped up in that tight module ain't gonna be fun.' So I pointed out that this would be my problem, since it was my seat which jammed against Linley's.

'Well, Paul was about the most fastidious man I ever knew. Cleaner than an elk's horn in autumn. Me? After a couple of days without proper washing I began to smell like fermenting turnips. Just before we reached the Moon, I asked Paul, 'Do I stink?' and he said, 'You sure do.' And all three of us busted out in laughter because we all knew that he was the one who was supposed to smell bad.'

Cindy took notes constantly, then bored in with her harsh questioning: 'Pope-san, do you think of yourself as mature?'

He bit his lower lip. 'I guess I've always been a plebe at Annapolis.'

'The others were simply oriented, too. Claggett, Jensen. From the day of their births they were intended—'

'I use that word a lot. *Intended.* I intended to do certain things, in certain ways. I believed that manhood consisted of stating your intentions and fulfilling them.'

'Did you ever fail?'

'No,' he said, and then he shivered. 'I'm not sure how to answer that truthfully. As a boy I dreamed of going to Annapolis. Our senator, Ulysses S. Gantling—get the son-of-a-bitch's full name—promised me an appointment, but at the last minute he reneged. I was left with nothing.'

'What did you do?'

'For two days I cried. Thought my heart would break. Then I began to curse him, which I never did before, and I've never cried or cursed since that second day. You know the rest.'

'You enlisted in the Navy for spite. Practically tore it apart till you got sent to Annapolis . . . second in your class. You got everything you wanted, didn't you?'

'Nothing I didn't work for.'

'Was Penny the first girl you ever kissed?'

'The only one, really. I've been remarkably happy with Penny. When you look at the six of us, only Hickory Lee has a marriage as good as mine.'

'How about Harry Jensen? Inger is a dear.'

'Compared to Penny, Inger is a piece of fluff.'

'Will you ever go into space again?'

He left his chair and stalked about the room, wondering whether he ought to speak to this strange woman about a subject so personal that he had not even discussed it with Penny. 'Have your spies told you that NASA is fed up with me?'

'I've heard rumors you're in the doghouse. Ed Cater dropped a hint in his last letter.'

'Does he write to you?'

'Of course. We were very dear friends. Always will be.'

'What gossip was he selling?'

'He said, if I remember correctly, "Straight Arrow Pope surprised us all by disobeying the brass twice. When Claggett died he refused to leave the scene. And when Claggett was buried he insisted upon taking you to the funeral." He said he supposed your days were numbered.'

'You know more about this than I do,' he said with some petulance.

'That's my business,' she said.

He was tempted to show his irritation, but instead he broke into a smile. 'When Claggett flew with me in Korea, I could never understand how he could love Debby Dee working in Japan and at the same time his little Jo-san at our air base in Pusan. I didn't know you then.'

She shrugged her shoulders, her warm amber-gold smile irradiating the parlor. 'You're worth knowing, Pope-san. Another time, another age . . .' She looked down at her note tablet and made a promise: 'You and Penny have something very precious, and I shall try to depict you both as you actually are. And if I can achieve that—'

They were interrupted by the sound of some man bustling into the reception hall and loudly demanding to know where this damned John Pope was shacked up with his Korean popsie.

It was Tucker Thompson, rushed out by NASA, the State Department and *Folks* to protect their shared investment in Astronaut Pope. He looked awful. 'They shoved me aboard an Air Force jet at Dulles. Flew to Los Angeles. Fifteen minutes to board Pan American, then non-stop across the Pacific to Auckland. Australian airline to Sydney. Same one to Canberra, and excuse me if I fall flat on my face.'

'You exhausted hero,' Cindy said. 'Have a drink.'

'And what do I find? America's favorite Boy Scout shacked up in a cheap—'

'Let's start with one understanding, Tucker. We have not been shacked up. We've been talking.'

Tucker looked with amazed delight at the two, then broke into a wide grin. 'You stay with that explanation, Pope, and I hope to God you can peddle it. But if *Time* gets hold of the truth, we're dead ducks. And I mean all of us.'

Pope swung him around. 'I told you. We came here to talk.'

Thompson brushed Pope's hand away and fell into a chair. 'In 1960 I sold the hard-shell Baptists in Texas on the line that John F. Kennedy was a sweet, simple-hearted Irish spalpeen who sang "Mother Machree" and would take no orders from the Pope. Maybe I can sell this. That a red-blooded American hero and his almond-eyed Dragon Lady . . .'

Pope came extremely close to belting Thompson in the mouth; instead he reached out and embraced him. 'Tucker, an hour with you is better than a year in the sewers of Middle America. I love you.'

'Stick to your story, son. It'll draw more comment than the truth.'

'It all matters so very little,' Cindy said. 'You took six American boys and the girls they married when they were young, and you wove a fairy story—' Her voice broke and suddenly all her bravado vanished. She started to cry, and when she found Pope's hand she held it close to her lips. 'You were all so very small,' she whispered. 'You never told the world that, Tucker. That they were such ordinary little men. Not big and heroic at all, not with wide shoulders and heavy jaws. God, they were heroic in their age, and whenever the Moon rises red in October they will be remembered.'

Several fine books would be written about the astronauts—Mailer, Collins, Wolfe, to name the best—but if you want to know how it really was inside the men inside the capsule, the book to read is the one by the Oriental newspaperwoman Rhee Soon-Ka. She was a Korean, but to irritate her Japanese enemies she adopted an American name, Cynthia, and to irritate the American establishment, which she despised, she titled her account *The Golden Midgets.*

Any average wife who might have heard of Mrs. Pope's reaction to her husband's Australian escapade with the Korean newspaperwoman would have been dismayed that a self-respecting woman would allow herself to be so abused, and so publicly. It would be three more weeks before Captain Pope returned to the States, for he was obligated to tour New Zealand and then fly to South America via Fiji, Tahiti and Easter Island, and during this waiting period Penny Pope conducted her normal work with the Space Committee, often dealing with matters which affected her absent husband.

She never alluded to his misbehavior, and when Senator Grant tried to comfort her, she rebuffed him: 'Captain Pope knows what he's doing. We've always trusted each other.' But if she would allow no one to mention the matter, she herself speculated constantly on how she must behave when John returned, and she found herself limited by restraints which other wives might ignore.

For she was not an average wife. She was a Navy wife, and that made a huge difference; from the first day of their courtship she had been prepared to stay at home for long periods while her husband served on some distant ocean; she was prepared to supervise the moving from place to place while he was in Japan or Germany; and she had always known that if she and John had children, it would be her responsibility alone to care for them during his long absences.

Those, of course, were the housekeeping details, and like many Navy wives, she never complained; Navy wives since the days of Darius and Xerxes had anticipated such absences, but there was also an emotional component of this problem, and this was a subject about which the wives rarely spoke among themselves.

Their husbands tended to be absent during the very years when their sexual drives were strongest; when they finally became stay-at-home admirals, they were in their fifties, when absences would have been easier to handle. So the Navy wife always knew that her lusty man was stuck in some foreign port at a time when his desires, and hers, were greatest, and she preferred not to be told what happened at such times. Indeed, she blanked out this portion of her married experience and was usually none the worse for it.

Penny had tried to be an ideal Navy wife, and although her work in Washington had prevented her from living with John at his various duty stations, she had visited him whenever practical and had known with favor the wives of many of his associates. Once when she was visiting with the Claggetts at Solomons Island, Debby Dee had observed: 'It's really as if John was the civilian married to Penny, who's in her own Navy.' And that was often the way it was: he would have some free time but she would be occupied with her Washington duties, and she never pried into how he spent his freedom.

She knew from her Patuxent River days that Navy families were usually too busy to permit much hanky-panky when the husbands were ashore, and she was constantly surprised at how capably the wives adjusted to all difficulties; there were very few Navy divorces, and when one did occur, the separating partners quite often found some other Navy type to marry, as if they knew that it was they and not the system that was at fault.

The one constant peril faced by the military wife was not infidelity, it was alcoholism, for the officers' club was always open, booze was cheap, loneliness was a constant spur to heavy drinking, and there were always older women on the bottle who sought the companionship of younger wives. Penny had watched a dozen older women become flaming alcoholics, and she had heard rumors of several celebrated cases in which the wives of top generals and admirals were habitually attended by junior officers whose job it was to see that the dipsomaniac did not create a scandal or fall headfirst down a flight of stairs. Since Penny drank only an occasional beer, this major pitfall presented no danger.

Most of all, her attitude toward marriage, and particularly Navy marriage, had been determined by her husband's character. As a plebe at Annapolis he had been a straight arrow, always near the top of his class, always dating only her. At Pax River he had occupied bachelor quarters to save money, which he turned over to her. In Korea, according to Claggett, John had avoided the airfields where the pretty little Jo-sans waited table and slept in the officers' quarters. He had never gone ratting about the countryside with Hickory Lee, and when this Korean woman invaded the Bali Hai with the avowed intention, some said, of sleeping with the entire contingent, she had been assured by the other wives that her husband would have nothing to do with her. Now both Debby Dee Claggett and Gloria Cater, eager to believe that the idol had crumbled, sent letters using the same rowdy phrase: 'Join the club!'

A subtle change took place in Penny's attitude. She still trusted John, but she also had to consider her self-esteem. She was three years shy of fifty, the occupant of a position of some importance and looked up to by the women graduates of good colleges who aspired to better jobs than typing. She represented something, and it was galling to think that she had been so poorly used, and in public. Her resentment caused her to look unsentimentally at the ramifications of her life, and what she saw evoked even deeper indignation.

When she attended public Senate hearings she noticed how many of the heavy-drinking old men found it impossible to follow arguments, frequently falling asleep in the midst of testimony. She marked the ones who grubbed servilely for every passing penny, yearning to sell their votes to any likely bidder, not even waiting to arrange the most profitable deal. When she compared these bumbling fellows with the best women appointees to federal positions, she was startled by the difference, and when she started to study the House members she knew, she was even more distressed, for here she saw public servants accepting money from Korean lobbyists, pursuing wildly deviant sex behaviors, and voting like idiots, while able women languished as mere assistants.

Her standards of comparison were high, for she had worked closely with three first-class politicians: Lyndon Johnson, who could contrive anything if it gave Texas and his private bank account a slight edge; Mike Glancey, who was perhaps the best man she had ever known, but whose vote was always negotiable on the principle of 'You scratch my back, I'll scratch yours'; and good, faithful Norman Grant, a man of impeccable integrity who did the same swapping of votes, but on a slightly higher level. These were good men and they served their nation admirably, but it was quite clear to her now that America produced an equal number of good women who were held contemptuously down.

She had for some years been listening carefully to the arguments of certain liberated women who had been addressing these problems, but she had never been attracted to their cause. Germaine Greer, the Australian, she found too harsh, Bella Abzug too abrasive, and Betty Friedan far too lacking in feminine qualities; and sometimes she suspected their logic, for without fanfare she had acquired one of the good jobs in Washington and she supposed that other women could do the same. But when Gloria Steinem and a woman with the fascinating name of Letty Pogrebin began analyzing situations exactly like her own, she began to listen more attentively, and she saw that women were discriminated against in scores of situations, that they were compressed by society into certain cliché molds, and that the consequences were nearly as damaging to the men as to the women they subjugated.

She became painfully aware of these matters when Tucker Thompson returned breathlessly from Australia to coach her in how the good people at *Folks* expected her to play the role of the insulted wife. 'Mrs. Pope, in Australia we had a near-miss. I flew all the way to Canberra. Christ, that's a big country, and I suppose you know what I found. Scandal about to erupt all over the place. NASA is fed up with your husband, and *Time* and *Newsweek* are sitting on the story, just hoping for a break that'll allow them to level a real blast.'

'What's holding them back?'

'Your husband is a national hero. How would they play it? For laughs? I don't think they'd dare. As a hard sex story? I doubt it. Now, if we get in first with a style-setter, we can pull their fangs.'

'What does your magazine recommend?'

'That we take the bit in our teeth, run the flag up the pole, and show a spread of you welcoming your husband home after his triumphal tour.'

'Would I be kissing him, did your editors think?'

'Yes. The important thing is to set the pattern. It would be dreadful if this affair got out of hand.'

'Isn't it already out of hand?'

'Not unless you make it so,' Thompson said firmly. 'This is a national problem, Penny. NASA's reputation at a time of budget review. The whole shmeer.'

'It would be quite easy for me to kiss my husband,' Penny said, 'because I love him.'

'God, if we could only work a quote like that into the story. But it would raise more questions than it answered.' Then, for the first time, he began to suspect that this dangerous woman whom he had never liked was toying with him. 'You do intend to cooperate, don't you?' he asked hesitantly.

'It would be undignified to behave otherwise,' she said.

'You mean that?'

'Of course I do.'

'Could I have more coffee?' He was perspiring, and after a deep swig of java he said expansively, 'It's downright remarkable, Penny. The NASA selection committee picked six families, out of a hat as it were, and they got six all-time winners. How many other American girls would have behaved better than you six? Death, disappointment, threats of divorce, now scandal, you kids were champions.'

'We intended to be,' Penny said, borrowing her husband's favorite phrase.

'It's been an honor to be associated with a girl like you.'

'I'm forty-seven.'

'We never mention that in the articles. To our readers you're all still girls, well dressed, well behaved. I'm terribly proud to have known you girls, Penny.'

'You keep speaking as if it were all past.'

'It is. Space is a dead duck. If I were an evil man, I'd play this Pope versus Pope thing for high scandal—the end of the epoch, the fond farewell to a group of symbols. I could write that story now, no strain. And it would be one hell of an exit.' He shook his head as if regretting that he was no longer working for a Hearst newspaper with its huge headlines. Then he said, 'But I love you kids as if you were my own family. This is my swan song, too, you know. Yep, retired against my will next month. And I refuse to sully something I've loved. Penny, let's go out in style.'

'What is the proper style?' she asked.

'The American wife, loyal, trusting, forgiving. We don't want to show you in your office this time. We've done that and it always seemed harsh. What I have in mind is a small house somewhere—'

'What I have in mind, Tucker, is my office, with an American flag in the corner, as always, and the big photograph of Johnson, Glancey and Grant, the architects of our space program.'

'But—'

'I am just as much a part of NASA as my husband, and in some ways, I think, even more important, because I helped keep the whole damned thing running.'

Thompson saw instantly that he was venturing into waters far too deep for him to negotiate. This office bitch was going to behave just as he feared she might: *Give me a hundred Alabama cheerleaders any day, twisting their pretty asses in the sunlight, to one girl who got straight A's in college. The cheerleaders know how to act in any situation, and the damned college girls never learn.*

'I'm afraid what I had in mind won't work, Mrs. Pope.'

'I'm sure it won't.'

'You better pray that *Time* and *Newsweek* don't start running with this story.'

'They have my office number.'

He was about to leave, but he could not allow one of his Solid Six to dash headlong into danger. 'Please, Mrs. Pope, we've had a tremendous run with this story. Gemini . . . Apollo . . . your husband's heroics . . . Claggett. Jesus Christ, don't throw mud on Claggett.'

Lowering her head, she said in a whisper, 'You wrote in one of your stories about how Randy and John had flown together in Korea, then tested planes at Pax River, then shared a Gemini phone booth for sixteen days. And of how John had to leave him dead on the Moon. It was very strong writing, really.' She looked up at him. 'Do you think I'd do anything to sully those relationships?'

'I don't think you would.'

'Of course I'll cooperate. Bring your photographers. But it will have to be in my office.' When he groaned, she said, 'You're a master with words, Tucker. Spin one of your fables. The modern wife who does two things superbly—runs her office, loves her man.'

'I don't think it'll play in Peoria.'

He decided not to try the John-Pope-and-his-loving-wife-Penny story, for he saw that it contained far too many time bombs, but as he was about to leave, distressed by his failure to manipulate Mrs. Pope, she suddenly caught his arm and forced him back into a chair.

'You've done me a great favor, Tucker. Up to one minute ago I never gave Betty Friedan much time. I simply did not like her style, but everything you said fortified the basic thesis in her *Feminine Mystique*. Writers like you, and your magazine, are major forces in creating the myth of what an American woman should be. The little house, not the office. A white jumper, not a business dress. The forgiving wife, not the woman who feels herself humiliated.'

'Penny,' he broke in, 'it's no longer something I worry about with *Folks.*

To hell with *Folks,* they've said to hell with me. But I beg you, don't divorce—'

'Who said anything about divorce?'

'You said you were humiliated by John's behavior in—'

'Of course I am. I'm humiliated by what he's done to me. But I'm just as humiliated by what you and your magazine would like to do. The fake posing. The fake quotations. Tucker, you're on your way out. John's on his way out of NASA. I may be on my way out of my job as counsel to the committee. Let's all go out with a bang. Here's the one quote from me you're authorized to use in your wrap-up: "Mrs. John Pope said, when apprised of her husband's juvenile performance in Australia, 'I'd like to kick his ass from Canberra to Tahiti, then hand him a NASA medal for acting like a perfect Boy Scout.'" And I want you to run it with the photograph of me kissing him beneath the American flag in my office with this caption: "All is forgiven. He's the only Boy Scout I have."'

'I wonder if we could get away with it?' Thompson mused. 'I wonder if there's some way I could imply that you said "kick his ass from Canberra to Tahiti" without actually saying it?'

'Use it as I said it,' Penny snapped, 'because that's the way I'm going to say everything from here on out.'

Disgusted with this modern woman, he started to stamp out of her office, but one more danger signal flashed. 'Maybe you haven't heard, but your husband has cooked up a story that all he and the Korean Typhoon did for three days was talk. Please, if that's going to be his version of three days in the sack, let him get away with it. Don't laugh at him in public.'

'Did he say that?' she cried, and when Thompson nodded she gave him a huge kiss. 'Tucker, you are adorable, corrupt, stupid, even a little evil . . . but downright adorable.'

When her husband landed at National Airport with two suitcases of medals and mementos, Penny was there to greet him. On the tarmac he said, 'I'm sorry, Pen, if I caused you embarrassment. But I had to talk. It was important that I get it on the record with someone who understood.'

'Why couldn't you have talked with me?' she asked, tears of joy filling her eyes.

'You were always so busy.' He corrected that: 'I was always so occupied with things that didn't really matter.' Arm in arm they walked toward the waiting cameras.

Like an ultra-sensitive barometer that monitors the atmosphere, predicting when the hurricanes will strike, Leopold Strabismus followed every nuance of the national mood, and long before Senator Grant realized that the space age had stumbled to a conclusion, he had detected the change, and with the termination of the Apollo program, he realized that he must alter his strategies or suffer loss. Accordingly, one morning in the summer of 1976 he woke, pulled down the bedcovers, pulled up the nightgown of his sleeping partner, slapped her roundly on the bottom, and said, 'Out of bed, Marcia! We're getting married!'

She was thirty-seven that year, still slim and beautiful with her pouting look and her feline skills, and she had about given up on the possibility that Strabismus would ever marry her. Still, she had a good life. They continued to make substantial profit from the menace of little green men and a small, steady income from the sale of diplomas, so that she had her own Mercedes and a secretary to look after her affairs. Ramirez still ran the general office with imagination and things were prospering, which made this sudden proposal of marriage a shock.

'What's eating you?' she asked.

'The handwriting is on the wall, my lovely.'

'Investigation? Police?'

'No, the turn of the wheel. The awakening of the public.'

'What are you talking about?'

'I've had a kind of vision, Marcia. The kind I had at Yale when I saw as if in revelation that California was the promised land.'

'I don't want to leave California.' She shuddered. 'Could you imagine us living in Fremont or Nebraska?'

'We get married today. And we make California twice the home it ever was before.' When he jumped out of bed and grabbed the trousers of a business suit reserved for trips to wealthy donors back East, Marcia saw that his eyes were aflame with enthusiasm.

'What is it, Leopold?'

'Goddammit, get your clothes on. This is for real.' And when they were dressed, he led her outside to a roadway from which she could see all of the fine building that housed their university, and she could feel him almost trembling as he divulged his plans: 'We have enough money right now to build the two wings I used to speak about. One here. One there. Not little wings, big ones.'

'To what purpose, please tell?'

'Religion.'

She said nothing, but in the protracted silence she could imagine what her brilliant companion could do with this volatile subject. She imagined him behind a pulpit—big face, beard, huge imposing body draped in a robe of some kind, thundering voice—and she knew instinctively that he would excel. She could visualize the university building expanded into a cathedral, with hundreds of cars parked in front, and devoted followers, and the money rolling in even more generously than before. It was quite clear, given the nature of her man and the nature of California, but it had to be done correctly, because the competition was terrific. Running a bogus university was easy, because not many manipulators sought to operate in that specialized field, but the religious arena was brutal, and unless one could invent some special allure, success was not assured.

'What religion?' she asked.

'I've been thinking about that for the last two months. I'd like to keep USA. It's a good set of initials. How about Universal Spiritual Association?'

'Every word is wrong. The U must be United. Start from there.'

'You may be right. What's wrong with Spiritual?'

'Sounds too much like spiritualism. Too restricted.'

'You may be right again. How about Salvation? I plan to hit very hard on salvation.'

'I like that. I like it, Leopold. Hold on to that.'

After discussing for some time the appropriate word for A they could agree on nothing, so they drove to one of the storefront churches where the seedy minister was willing to forgo the legal waiting period and predate the marriage certificate to 1973, which he said a clerk at the courthouse would register as of that year for an extra ten dollars. They then returned home and telephoned the Red River Bible University: 'Reverend Hosea Kellog? This is Dr. Leopold Strabismus, president of the University of Space and Aviation in Los Angeles. I've heard of your good work, Reverend Kellog, and my university would like to award you with a Doctor of Laws if you would give me a Doctor of Divinity. This is extremely important to me, and I'd appreciate it if the date could read 1973.'

It was arranged, and Strabismus asked Ramirez to prepare an especially ornate diploma for Dr. Kellog, and with the same plate but different lettering, to print up one for Strabismus from the University of Western Dakota in the fields of Hebrew, Greek and Latin. With these and other impressive documents framed on the wall behind his head, he was qualified to decide what branch of theology his new church would sponsor, but before he printed up any materials, he had long discussions with his wife.

'We had to get married,' he said, 'because I plan to stress morality. This country is hungry for a revival of the old-time spirit, Marcia.'

'Hadn't you better send those two girls from Texas packing?'

'That's a possibility, but the important thing was to have you up front for people to see. I plan to use you extensively. Senator Grant's daughter. Play up his heroism in World War II.'

'And what else?'

'A rejection of scientific atheism—Darwin's evolution from apes, geology. All that rot.'

'But we've done very well with science. The pamphlets . . .'

'That's all finished. We'll keep the university, that's a gold mine. But we'll let someone else handle the little men, because flying saucers have run their course. Believe me, Marcia, the new field is old-time religion.'

He told her that he had been much impressed by a Southern television preacher who had mounted a campaign against what he called 'atheistic humanism,' and although neither Strabismus nor the minister seemed to have a very clear concept of what this was, it made a splendid target, and when Leopold reached home he took four or five books from the Los

Angeles Public Library and within a week made himself an expert on atheistic humanism.

'It's the mind-set of smart-ass librarians who corrupt our young people with their immoral books. It's the beliefs of college professors who seek to destroy this nation. It's what makes the editors of the *New York Times* and the *Washington Post* soft on Communism. It's what's wrong with this fine country, and people who subscribe to it have got to be rooted out of our national life. A lot of generals in our Army are secret humanists, and they've got to be identified before they destroy our armed forces.'

In the days when the two wings of his temple were being erected he began to speak like an illiterate Southern farmhand, using phrases like: 'Nukelar warfare,' 'Old Tessamint religion,' 'Socialist subsidation of infamy,' 'Dimunition of our power to defend ourself,' and 'Irrevelant big-city argaments.'

At New Haven he had twice written Ph.D. theses for laggard scholars in English literature; now he habitually used 'Jesus wants you and I . . .' and 'We wuz lost in the wilderness of sin.' But what made his oratory especially effective was his new pronunciation of old words; for example, it was always *'God's luuuv'* in three long-drawn syllables. It was *hisse'f,* and *shouldn't auter,* and *evoluushun.*

He adopted this usage because he knew that people who craved an old-time doctrine were intuitively suspicious of university types and big-city editors and hotshot television announcers; they yearned for the simplicities of rural life and believed that only a man who was close to the untutored farmlands of their remembered youth could be trusted. They thus became not only a part of the national swing away from learning; they became with their cash contributions a leading factor in the movement. The nation, as if surfeited with the marvels of space and medicine and science and sophisticated social analysis, seemed hungry for anti-intellectual preachment, and Leopold Strabismus was eager to provide it.

He saw immediately that to be effective he must have access to television, but he knew he should move cautiously. 'Marcia, I want you and Ramirez to scout every corner of this area and find a radio station that we can buy cheap. I don't care where it is or what its power. Buy us a station.'

They found a fifty-watter, a dawn-to-dusk affair in the hills back of Los Angeles, and because the Reverend Dr. Strabismus spoke from it with great passion during all daylight hours, using the same taped sermons over and over, with no apologies, it became a sensation: 'Why do I have to stop deliverin' God's message at sunset? Why am I forbidden to bring you the word of the Lord when the sun goes down? Because the atheistic humanists who run our State Department have entered into a corrupt deal with Mexico . . .' He heaped special scorn on Yale University and Stanford as centers of the humanism that was destroying our nation.

With sizable funds collected from his radio ministry, he was able to acquire a real twenty-four-hour radio station, which he threw open to the electronic ministers across the nation, and through the cooperation of these gifted orators he at last found an opening on television, where his bulk, his beard and his fiery oratory gained immediate approval. His income, after only twenty months of his ministry, was $300,000 a year.

Marcia, who was one of the factors in his success—for she sat beside the pulpit whenever he preached, giving testimony when called upon—identified the one weakness which might destroy his effectiveness: 'Leopold, one of these days the newspapers have got to discover that your real name is Martin Scorcella and that you're Jewish. That could create quite a scandal.'

'Half-Jewish,' he corrected. 'And I'll handle it the way Fiorella La Guardia handled his problem, which was just like mine, Italian father, Jewish mother. He said nothing about it during six elections. Let all the voters think he was Catholic. When he was finally challenged and some smart-ass newspaperman asked, "Why did you hide the fact that you were half-Jewish?" he said, "Half-Jewish ain't enough to brag about." When they find out about me six or eight years from now, I'll be so firmly established they can't touch me.'

'People who take religion seriously, they could be very disturbed. The way the Jews crucified Jesus and all that.'

'I've thought about it, Marcia, and I think I have the perfect answer. I'll say, "Yes indeed, I was born a Jew, like St. Peter and St. James and Jesus Christ Hisse'f. But like them, I seen the true way, hallelujah, and became a Christian, and I will not rest until every Jew on this earth acknowledges his error and, like me and St. Paul, converts to Christianity." And you can bet that'll hold 'em.'

He first attracted statewide attention because of his television program *Chimp-Champ-Chump,* in which he savagely attacked the theory of evolution. He was especially effective because in his New Haven days he had produced three graduate theses on the Darwinian theory which had required him to master the details of this controversial subject. He was, indeed, better informed on the theory than most of the professors who defended it, and when he poured his scorn on Darwin and his atheistic humanism, he was more amusing than the average vaudeville show.

He asked Marcia and Ramirez to scout the animal trainers in Hollywood for a likable monkey, and they came up with a chimpanzee named Oliver, whom they dressed in short satin pants and big white shoes. He appeared with Reverend Strabismus seated at a desk under the handsomely lettered sign CHIMP-CHAMP-CHUMP, and he took a liking to Leopold's beard, which he pulled frequently. He had the attractive gift of listening attentively and smiling when Strabismus talked to him, and of nodding aggressively whenever the Reverend made a telling point. He was a delightful animal, and viewers up and down the state applauded whenever he appeared.

'I love this little animule,' Strabismus bellowed. 'Look at him, he's as cute as a button. It's a privilege to call him my friend, but I do not want to call him my grandfather. There ain't a shred of evydence in ever'thin' that Charles Darwin ever wrote that proves to me or to any sensible man or woman that this here monkey was my ancestor, and there is ever' evydence in the Bible that he was created as an animule and me as a human bein' with God-given intelligence and immortality.'

Chimp-Champ-Chump became such a popular show that it led the movement in California to ban the teaching of evolution outright, or at least to require the parallel teaching of Biblical genesis. Wise science teachers, sensing the shift in public opinion, accorded more time and emphasis to creationism, as they called it, than to the much-ridiculed theory of evolution, and a generation of California students was beginning to believe that Darwinism was a fraud perpetrated by atheistic humanists, because Reverend Strabismus and the other preachers who shared his television show said so.

Strabismus muscled his way onto the national scene by his imaginative campaign to force rangers in national parks to stop saying in their lectures that places like the Grand Canyon had evolved through billions of years, when it was known from the Book of Genesis that they had been created within the passage of one week. Whenever listeners reported that federal employees were supporting evolution during their public talks in national parks like Yellowstone and Glacier, he moved in furiously to combat their heresies.

But now the nation's leading scientists began to take his attacks seriously, and there was a countereffort. Men at Harvard, Chicago and UCLA felt obligated to inform the people that America was going to make an ass of itself in the eyes of the world if it engaged in a know-nothing persecution of science, and they had begun to make some headway when Strabismus and a score of his associates launched a frontal assault, charging the professors with being atheistic humanists and Communists.

The confrontation became ugly when Reverend Strabismus, in a widely repeated harangue, invited his listeners to join him in a great crusade: 'It ain't my doin'. It's the work of devoted Christians back East. They call theirselves the Righteous Rulers, and under their inspired leadership we are gonna drive the money changers outa the Temple. We are gonna defeat ever' United States senator who supports the atheistic humanists. We are gonna drive from ever' campus in this nation perfessers who teach Communistic evolution. We are gonna cleanse our library shelves of ever' book that contains filth and un-American teachings. And we are not gonna halt until we bring this nation back to God.'

When the response exceeded his hopes—hundreds of thousands of dollars streaming in through the mail—he told Marcia, 'I think we got somethin' important started, somethin' much bigger than you and me foresaw.' He was now talking rural illiterate, even in his private life.

. . .

Senator Grant suffered no ambivalence about his role in space. He had bombarded NASA with the credentials of Gawain Butler's nephew and had watched with pride as that young man became the nation's first black astronaut. He had delighted in the early behavior of Captain John Pope, a lad from his hometown who had become rather difficult after his historic solo flight. Nevertheless, he had gone personally to President Nixon, urging that Pope be sent around the world as an ambassador of good will and 'to remind the Russians who's still ahead.'

But as for any future NASA spectaculars, or for providing federal funds for such escapades, he was rigorously opposed: 'We had three men who fought this battle when the honor of our nation was exposed, Lyndon Johnson, Michael Glancey and me. The first two did their work honorably, and are now dead. I feel myself to be their surrogate, and I am satisfied that if they were still living, they would vote with me against any enlargement of the NASA commitment.'

He never ranted against NASA, nor did he attempt to lead any kind of open crusade; he merely voted consistently in favor of cutting the budget for space, telling anyone who asked about his activity, 'We've proved that we can do anything we put our minds to, and now we must address more serious problems.'

Much of his attitude stemmed from the fact that he was up for reelection in 1976, and like a cautious politician, he endeavored to sense the national mood, which had shifted markedly and now opposed any further adventures in space. As one farmer said during a campaign meeting in Calhoun, 'There's damned little plowing to be done on the Moon and a great deal down here.' Blacks objected to further expenditures; young people who had opposed the war in Vietnam now turned their animosity toward science in general, so that when Grant surveyed his electorate he found almost no constituency for space.

'It's a dead issue,' he told Finnerty. 'Let's take credit for everything we've done so far but avoid questions about the future.' He asked Finnerty to schedule John Pope, as a local hero, for meetings across the state, knowing that the astronaut would not be able to speak out publicly in his behalf, but would consent to being photographed with him.

What worried Grant in this campaign was not space, but the deplorable spiritual condition of the American people: 'Here it is, the two hundredth anniversary of our republic and we find ourselves powerless even to mount a national birthday celebration.' The grand designs which had been discussed since 1969 for a world fair, immense parades, exhibitions and innovative enterprises in theater, sports, publishing and television had all collapsed; a great nation, one of the gleaming hopes of mankind, was celebrating its triumphs in virtual silence, as if it were ashamed of itself.

'The reason,' Grant mourned, 'is that 1976 happens to be an election year, and we Republicans started out trying to make capital of the celebration, as a kind of jubilee honoring Richard Nixon's eight years in the White House and paving the way for Spiro Agnew's eight years to come. Well, that part of the plan collapsed with Watergate, so we decided to make the Bicentennial a celebration of the new Republican leadership. Totally the wrong thing to do.

'And the Democrats were just as venal. Publicly they gave lip service to a grand national holiday, but since we would manage it, they wouldn't vote a dime. So because of election politics, we're celebrating one of the noblest days of our history in craven silence. How contemptible.'

He was also deterred from taking any major stance that might attract too much attention by his wife Elinor's sad deterioration, and only the kindness of the local press prevented her behavior from becoming an election scandal. She had given her entire personal inheritance to Dr. Strabismus to support the good work he was doing in California, and if the senator's staff had not stopped payment on certain checks and recovered others she had forged, the Grant name would have been badly sullied.

Elinor, far better informed on the perils facing the nation than her husband, had complained to reporters that Norman was starving her and keeping her imprisoned: 'It's very much like Bluebeard. Here I am a captive in a castle.'

'But we were free to come here to see you,' a woman reporter said.

'Yes, but you can't imagine what would happen if I tried to leave when you do.'

'Let's try. Let's the five of us go downtown for lunch.'

'I wouldn't dare. There are spies everywhere.'

'You mean, the senator employs spies . . .'

'Not only the senator,' she said darkly.

When the editors read such reports they decided that Norman Grant was stuck with a whacko, and out of respect for his heroism in the war and the good work he had done subsequently, they decided to suppress the story, but they continued to express interest in the deportment of the senator's daughter out in California. In news reports written with extreme delicacy and utilizing all kinds of ingenious innuendo, they referred to her association with the notorious fraud Leopold Strabismus and his diploma mill:

> Marcia Grant, daughter of Senator Norman Grant (Republican—Fremont), longtime personal friend of Strabismus and now his wife, serves as his dean of faculty with the degree of Ph.D. conferred upon her by her own institution. What her role is other than the collection of fees is difficult to ascertain, since the university appears to have no faculty. Repeated demands to meet with at least one professor have been rejected by Dean Grant on the grounds that her staff was

far too busy correcting examination papers, written presumably by students who also do not exist.

Careful investigations in Sacramento have revealed that the state of California accredits several degree mills like the Strabismus USA on the grounds that 'They do very little real harm and everyone knows their degrees are spurious.' When we asked why the state condoned such open fraud, we were told, 'If we attempted to discipline the fake universities, then we'd be expected to do the same with the bogus churches, and defenders of the First Amendment would climb all over us. In this state you can have any religion you like, any university, and this office can do nothing about it.'

It was curious, really, that in the heat of a senatorial campaign the Democrats made so few attacks on Norman Grant's private life, but as Tim Finnerty told his staff one night, 'In the American system everyone knows that men are incapable of disciplining their wives, their daughters or their sons. If you start to raise hell with Grant, where do you stop?'

The senator was grateful for this courtesy, but the deportment of his women caused him deep concern, for he believed that if he had been a better husband and father, Elinor and Marcia would have developed more normally, and never was this feeling more intense than when Penny Pope flew west to help in his campaign, for then he saw a local girl, much like his daughter, who with far fewer advantages had become a leading Washington figure. At forty-nine she was tough-minded in committee meetings, self-directed in her personal life, and a most attractive wife to a national hero. Grant had seen the reports submitted by State Department people who had chaperoned John and Penny Pope on their triumphal tours to foreign countries:

> John Pope is a winner wherever he goes, modest, self-effacing, a most likable hero. He meets kings and presidents with an attractive reserve and addresses public gatherings with skill and good sense. A winner all the way. But wherever we go, Penny Pope steals the show. She dresses immaculately, tends her appearance and is refreshingly frank in whatever she says. In diplomacy, she's worth ten battleships.

Penny was never loath to heckle Grant about his retreat on space, but she did so only in private, and was especially careful never to speak as John Pope's wife but only as counsel to the committee: 'To hear you talk, Senator, one would think that America had quit the space race. Look it up. How many satellites do you think we have up there right now? Year after year? Going round and round and sending us billions of messages?'

'I know from our committee that a lot of work keeps going on. But we have no Apollos. Skylab's ended, so we have nothing big up there.'

From her briefcase she took a NASA publication, *Satellite Situation Report,* and with a delicate finger pointed to a line of figures: 'Every item that has ever been shot into space has been given a serial number, starting with 1. What do you think the Russian Cosmos that went up the other day was numbered?' And she showed him—9,509.

'Good God! Why don't they bump into each other?'

'Different altitudes. Different orbits.'

'Who put them up there?' he asked, and she reminded him of the wild variety of nations that had the capacity to do so: 'Spain, India, Czechoslovakia, Italy, Netherlands and, of course, the United States and Russia.'

'We have 2,116 American objects sending signals right now,' she said. 'Russia has 1,205.'

When the senator borrowed the report he spotted an ominous column: 'What's this "Inanimate Objects—6,078" and most of them Russian?'

'They've run out of electrical power. Send no messages. Just go round and round in timeless beauty.' She pointed to Catalogue Number 4041: 'That's the little craft that carried Armstrong and Aldrin down to the Moon in 1969. When they came back to Apollo 11 they jettisoned it. Read Footnote 9.' And Grant read: 'A manned spacecraft which successfully landed on the Moon, after which it went into perpetual selenocentric orbit.'

'What's selenocentric?' he asked.

'Selene was the Greek goddess of the Moon. Around the moon forever.' She laughed. 'Senator, the other night in Webster you spoke as if we'd abandoned space. We're just beginning to use it.'

When Penny spoke with such authority, Grant could not help speculating on what his life might have been had he married such a woman, one who was stable and judicious. There had been talk in Nixon's first administration of bringing Grant into the Cabinet in one of the really good positions, perhaps even Defense, and because of his winning margins in Fremont, there had even been suggestions that he go on the ticket as Vice-President to forestall Rockefeller, but he had been painfully aware of his vulnerability because of his wife and daughter, and when he confided his fears to the Nixon advisers they quickly saw that he was prudent, and talk of any high-visibility position evaporated. As one of the California mafia said, 'We have hundreds of men in this country who would make damned fine senators but lousy national leaders. And Norman Grant of Fremont is perhaps the outstanding example.'

With a wife like Penny Pope, he mused, anything would have been possible.

But whenever she campaigned on behalf of Senator Grant and listened to his oratory, Penny realized what a soggy, pathetic politician this particular

Republican had become. He stood for nothing. He represented no vital force. He had no vision of the future. And he ran on the simple program of patriotism and the fact that he answered his constituents' mail within forty-eight hours.

His life had known two apexes: when he steered his destroyer escort right at the heart of the Japanese fleet, and when he lined up with Lyndon Johnson and Michael Glancey to lead America into the space age. Everything since had been downhill, and now he presumed to ask the voters of his state to return him for another six years of futility. Penny was ashamed to be part of his team.

'Now wait,' Finnerty said one night in June after they had arranged a rousing campaign rally in Calhoun. 'Norman Grant represents this state almost ideally. Look at the federal funds he's brought in—the installations we'd never have had otherwise. And the service he gives his constituents.'

'I'll grant the last. No senator takes more visitors to the Senate dining room. But his ideas . . .'

'They're adequate. Look at what happened to Fulbright. Rhodes scholar, wonderful orator. He has ideas galore and no Senate seat. Grant plays it safe.'

'Grant does nothing, Tim. You came to my office seven times in the last few years—make that a dozen times—bewailing his refusal to vote for good projects.'

'Penny, he's infinitely better than the Democratic opposition.'

'Conceded. He won't be a disgrace, the way that lumphead would, but he's no ornament, either.'

'Few senators are.'

Her face-to-face meetings with Grant were depressing. He was only sixty-two, but he seemed a worried old man long past any constructive act, and the behavior of the women in his family prevented him from being impressive even with his dark suits and silvery hair. He was a hollow shell, and what was worse, he reverberated rather loudly: 'We must turn our attention to more serious matters. We must cut the budget and increase our military power. We must get chiselers off the taxpayer's back and take drastic steps to control crime in the streets. If you return me to Washington, my first priority will be to lower taxes without impairing our ability to defend ourselves.'

And then he would parade onto the stage, in their historic uniforms and medals, Tim Finnerty, Larry Penzoss and Gawain Butler, who would relate the facts about his heroism and solicit votes for this great American.

'Tim,' Penny said after the Webster rally, 'you really ought to knock the heroism bit in the head. You fellows look plain silly in those faded uniforms,' but Finnerty pointed out correctly: 'It's what's kept him elected for thirty years, going on thirty-six.'

Tucker Thompson, still searching for one last good story about his Solid Six, arranged for Captain John Pope to fly out to Benton for the rally on

November 3, when it was clear that although President Ford might be in trouble, the reelection of Norman Grant was assured. Pope, still a charismatic hero, came onstage, kissed his wife, and in defiance of NASA rules, said a few words asking the voters of his home state to send a great patriot and a foremost figure in America's space supremacy back to the Senate.

Penny, like a good wife, posed with her left hand in her husband's right, but the camera caught her looking with extreme uncertainty at Senator Grant, who was shaking hands with a group of women voters. Tucker captioned the picture, the last his magazine would run of the astronauts:

> She had threatened to kick his butt from Canberra to Tahiti, but in the end she supported him enthusiastically when he campaigned in the successful reelection bid of Senator Norman Grant.

When Penny saw the picture in the magazine she was alone in her office, and she could not restrain herself from muttering—using profanity, something she rarely did:

> 'That sonnombeech Tucker! Male chauvinist pig! He knows it was me campaigning for Grant, and John only flew out to help me. But he's got to write that John was doing the work and I flew out to help him. Penny, this sort of bullshit has got to stop, and you're the only one to stop it.'

In this period of emotional turmoil regarding his sons, Stanley Mott took refuge, as men will, in his work, but here also he was confronted with confusion, for in his studies of the planets which he was obligated to conduct for NASA he found himself always oscillating between engineering and science. As an engineer he wanted to build bigger and bigger machines with ever more sophisticated capabilities, regardless of the specific use to which they were put; but as a scientist he longed to send small, precise machines into bold new adventures of the mind: There's a universe out there we've only begun to perceive. And if we had the courage, we could be living intellectually at the heart of it.

His indecision was marked by the two books he kept near him: the first, an engineering marvel by a physics professor at Princeton; the second, a summary of the scientific knowledge of space by a much different kind of professor in London. Whichever book attained ascendancy at the moment persuaded him to move in that direction; he had become a pendulum.

The Princeton book was Gerard K. O'Neill's *The Colonization of Space*, in which an engineering job of immense dimension—the assembling of a gigantic machine in orbit to be occupied by thousands or even hundreds of thousands of workers and explorers who would spend most of their lives there—was considered by many to be practical. The beauty of O'Neill's proposal was that work on it could be started now. Rockets like those built by Dieter Kolff, hundreds of them a month, could certainly carry the materials into low Earth orbit. Construction devices already in being at Houston and Huntsville could bind the parts together, while gossamers of enormous dimension could bring from the Sun all the energy needed to operate such an enterprise.

All that would be required to build such a station would be $1 followed by 27 zeros—a billion billion billion dollars—and that posed problems. Of course, enthusiasts argued that it could be shaved to a mere billion billion, but Mott doubted it.

Yet he was captivated by the boldness of the concept and convinced himself that before long some nation was going to break O'Neill's grand design down into manageable parts and build itself a space station not for hundreds of thousands of settlers but for eighty or a hundred, and that nation would acquire an advantage in world control which might never be overcome by other nations less adventurous: From such a station you could beam down the energy of the Sun, making petroleum obsolete. You could control the weather, making rain fall where needed and preventing it from falling elsewhere. You could devise new forms of life, construct new combinations of material, conduct researches into the nature of the universe.

And whenever he reached that point he stopped, for he could hear the Germanic accents of Dieter Kolff: 'But you can do all that right now with unmanned probes, and for one-thousandth of the cost.'

The London book was an extraordinary affair, C.W. Allen's *Astrophysical Quantities,* compiled by a retired professor of astronomy at the University of London and offering in 310 pages a summary of everything known about the structure of the universe, with hundreds of tables and thousands of footnote references indicating where the data could be verified. It was the handbook of any Russians, Japanese, Pakistanis, Germans or Americans who addressed themselves to the mysteries of space, and Mott referred to it almost daily.

It was a book of beautiful simplicity, for it started with a compact list of those constant values which govern existence, then summarized what mankind knew about the atom, and moved purposefully outward to the structure of the Earth, the other planets, the Sun, the fellow stars, the Galaxy, the distant clusters of other galaxies, and on to the infinite reaches of the universe. Even to read the table of contents was an adventure of the mind.

Mott found special pleasure in the first section, that list of immutable laws so painstakingly uncovered by investigators in so many different centuries and so many different countries. Pi was 3.14159265 . . . , which Mott had memorized as a boy, and not some other value. There was a Planck constant governing energy, an Avogadro number giving the number of molecules in a standard volume of gas, a Faraday in electricity and a Stefan-Boltzmann constant in radiation.

To consult this list was a humbling experience: Damned few of the great constants were discovered in America. We build on the work done by men overseas.

On the other hand, when Mott turned to the later chapters of the handbook, the ones that concerned him, he found that much of the pivotal work had been done in America, as if our people had assembled the wisdom of the world and applied it to daring new concepts. Harlow Shapley initiated the studies which determined the size of our Galaxy; Carl Seyfert identified new types of galaxies; Edwin Hubble derived the constant that governed them; and Maarten Schmidt extended the definitions.

For Mott to look even casually into *Astrophysical Quantities* was like a lover of literature browsing in the *Oxford Book of English Verse;* every page had its own resonance. Here stood Isaac Newton and Max Planck and Albert Einstein and Ejnar Hertzsprung. Here stood the gateway leading into the heart of the universe, and whenever Mott laid the small green-bound book aside he felt refreshed.

It was a curious book, the work of an old man who had loved his subject, and the edition that Mott owned, the third, carried this extraordinary preface:

> It may be anticipated that yet another revision will be justified after a lapse of about seven years and preparation for this should begin at once. The author would like to negotiate with anyone willing to cooperate.

When Mott first read this invitation to become co-author of an established best seller, he idly considered applying, but quickly broke into laughter: All I'd be required to know would be atomic physics, spectrum analysis, radiation, geology, subatomic particles, astronomy, photometry and the whole crazy field of astrophysics. Damn! Wouldn't it be great to be eligible?

The whole set of his mind was toward science, but whenever he was tempted to go too far down that road, he could hear old Crampton in the wind tunnel at Langley: 'Scientists dream about doing things. Engineers do them.' And he would turn to the more practical jobs at hand: What can we do now? And this would throw him back onto Gerard O'Neill's space station, a version of which America could have been building right now.

His day-to-day work with NASA focused on a managerial problem faced at one time or other by most big operations: 'How do we hold our key personnel together in a time of retrenchment?' With the Apollo program wiped out and no clear mission to replace it, cutbacks were inevitable and firings had to take place. When he visited Cape Canaveral he found Cocoa Beach in a state of shock: the Bali Hai motel had only two waitresses instead of the eight who had served the astronauts and their friends in the roaring 1960s, and Mr. and Mrs. Quint sat mournfully with Mott in a darkened corner of the once-lively Dagger Bar: 'Homes that people bought for nineteen thousand dollars ten years ago, you can pick hundreds up for nine thousand dollars each. We lost thousands in population, stores and bars shutting down the way they are.'

When Mott asked if they thought they could keep the Bali Hai open, they were gloomy: 'We have a better chance than most, our good beach, and people know us. One Apollo shot a year would keep us prosperous. But that's all gone, and we just don't know.'

'But you are going to try?'

'Resort type of business, maybe. Catch the snow-birds as they drive south for the winter.'

'I wish you luck. This place is a part of American history.' He could hear the vanished astronauts; he could see Cynthia Rhee flashing into the bar like a comet in low orbit; most of all he could see the three young men he had admired so much when he supervised their activities: Bell the proficient civilian; Jensen the dream kid who typified the perfect astronaut; Claggett the tight-jawed doer, the clown, the best young man he had ever known, flawed but magnificent. They died, and now Canaveral was dying, too. When he left the Bali Hai to drive down to Palm Beach to visit his son in jail he saw the mournful signs: HOUSE FOR SALE. ANY REASONABLE OFFER.

It was the same wherever he went: the great, proud bases from which man had conquered space were retrenching, and some were on the verge of extinction. Personnel were being fired at an appalling rate, but it was not until he reached California on his inspection that he appreciated the real problem facing NASA and the nation, for at both Ames and the Jet Propulsion Laboratory he heard the same story: 'We can cut back. We can fire people. But how do we maintain a basic capacity to spring back into action if we're needed in a hurry?'

That was the headache. How does one preserve a cadre of intelligence and skill? What manufacturing jobs do you assign them to in the downswing? And most important of all, how do you keep the infrastructure vital so that it can be quickly expanded in time of need? Automobile companies, military units, big retail stores all faced that problem, but never so acutely as NASA did in these painful years, because each man it fired carried with him some unusual and vital skill that could not easily be replaced.

Mott listened as supervisors described the men let go at JPL: 'Henderson knew more about computer enhancement than anyone else on the block. He could take data and make the whole thing sing. If a war came along, he'd be invaluable to the military, but what can he do working the salary list at Sears Roebuck? Ondrachuk knows more about metal stress than any of us. A very cautious man. But how can he use such knowledge teaching in junior high school, supposing he gets the job?'

There was an even deeper problem: 'Henderson and Ondrachuk had learned how to work together. They'd evolved a jargon which extended to fifty other experts, each with his own peculiar field. In a pinch we could probably find men as good as they are, but without the accumulated jargon. And what's worse, keep them out of the program for three years and they'll have lost the jargon. They won't have kept up with their fields, no matter how much they study. Space is a hands-on experience. You have to do it to learn it.'

Sometimes at night he trembled to think of the intellectual capacity his country was squandering . . . dissipating to the four winds . . . ignoring at a time of no-crisis and perhaps destroying against the day of great-crisis. But a democracy worked that way, by fits and starts, by dynamic response to felt emergencies, then slothful indifference when the emergency dissolved. However, when he reached the Lewis base near Cleveland and found that the creative engineer Levi Letterkill had been let go, he perceived the problem not in the abstract but in fiercely human terms.

'You can't fire Letterkill. Call him right now and get him back on the job.'

'We had to let him go. Quotas.'

'I don't give a damn about quotas. Letterkill is twice as bright as I am, and this country needs him.'

'We don't. Not in this shop.'

'You think you don't. But let me tell you about this man. In 1957, well before Russia put Sputnik up, he devised a way for the gang at Wallops Island to put one of our little machines into orbit. You know what he came up with last year? A radio telescope with a base line ten A.U.'s long. We need this man.'

'Not here, we don't.'

'If he goes, I go.' He had thrown out a challenge which the Lewis people jumped to accept. They called Washington and said that they refused to be overridden by some headquarters has-been; then Mott took the phone and said calmly, 'If Letterkill is fired, I have to be fired, too.' There was a long silence, then a conciliatory voice: 'Is this a conference call? Are you both listening? Mott, why don't you see if Huntsville could find Letterkill a place?'

When he reached Huntsville he found them in a frenzy of retrenchment, too, but with urging from Washington he persuaded them to take Letterkill into their think tank, where bold ideas were generated, and Mott thanked the administrators profusely.

That evening he dined with the Kolffs up on Monte Sano, and after supper, as he and Dieter and Liesl sat on the front patio overlooking the city, they told him the wonderful news: 'Always when I was working at Peenemünde I loved to borrow classical records from Von Braun. He loved music. The records were Polydor, the best ever made, no scratch. And I used to dream that the day was coming when I would be a big manager like Von Braun and I, too, would be able to afford Polydor records. Beethoven, Brahms, Wagner. Now look!'

He returned to the living room and turned on his record player; soon sounds of heavenly clarity filled the night with music Mott could not identify, but quite soon Dieter was back with one of those handsome album jackets of Deutsche Grammophon with the golden-yellow cartouche across the top: VIVALDI. CONCERTO IN A FOR TRUMPET AND ORCHESTRA. *Magnus Kolff with Herbert von Karajan and the Berlin Philharmonic.* Holding the jacket on his knees, Mott listened to the brilliant trumpet sounds as they filled the room behind him, making it a noble symphony hall.

'Is it too loud?' Dieter asked.

'No. I like the reverberations.' After a while he said, 'You must be very proud, Dieter.'

'I am. It's better to me than all of Von Braun's Polydors.' Then he explained: 'You understand, of course, that Polydor merged with Deutsche Grammophon. It's the same company, really.' When Mott turned the jacket over he found a photograph of young Kolff, twenty-nine years old, his German-American face smiling, his left hand clasping his trumpet.

'How do we keep the team together?' Mott asked.

'We had the same problem at Peenemünde. Hitler blows hot, lots of work. He has a negative dream, fire everybody. He has a positive dream, the A-4 will win the war, our staff triples. Vietnam and Watergate, America has a bad dream.'

'How did Von Braun handle it?'

'When General Funkhauser came along to find volunteers for the front, he hid people in barns.'

'Did you hear that Congress gave Funkhauser a medal last month?'

'I saw the papers. He deserved it, Stanley. He did one hell of a job in this country.'

'He got me my job with NASA. It was NACA then. I wonder where I'd be if he hadn't intervened?'

Kolff laughed. 'I know where I'd be if Liesl hadn't stopped him from intervening. I'd be six feet under in some German potato field.'

'What should NASA do now?'

'Hide its best men in a barn. Wait for Hitler or whoever to have a better dream.'

Mott received advice that was more specific from Senator Grant when he visited him in the Senate Office Building: 'I've resigned from the Space Committee, Mott. Made my small contribution and turned the job over to younger men. When we had astronauts up there—Glenn, Armstrong, Claggett—the whole nation throbbed with excitement. Today, what? Total indifference. This Mars thing you're about to do. What's it really mean to the man in the street?'

'It could be our most significant accomplishment in space.'

'Don't you believe it. If no men are involved, it's merely an exercise.'

'But men are involved, sir. The comprehension of the entire world . . .'

'That comes later. Much later. In books that men like you read. Not in real life.'

'What would you advise NASA to do?'

'Cut back to the bone. Close down three-fourths of your installations. Go ahead with your inexpensive shots that explore the planets. Keep the scientists happy, but don't try to occupy center stage.'

'What about preserving our cadre? In case of a national emergency down the line?'

'That's the military's problem. I've done some studying of my own. Every really competent man NASA's fired has gone either to the Pentagon or to the air-space industry and got a better job. The capacity is kept alive, but in a different set of buildings.' When Mott tried to counter this argument, citing the preeminence of civilian control, Grant cut him short: 'Why do you suppose I quit the Space Committee? To take a more important job on military affairs. That's where the action's going to be.'

Again Mott tried to interrupt, and again Grant forestalled him: 'Look at your own group of astronauts—the ones you brought in and coddled. Three dead. That fine man Cater back in civilian life. John Pope from my hometown about to resign. Only that chap from Tennessee . . . what's his name?'

'Hickory Lee.'

'Only one left. Too limited in outside experience to land a good civilian job. Well, we need caretakers.'

'How far should we cut back, Senator?'

'I was rather startled the other day when our committee counsel, Mrs. Pope—you know her—told me how many satellites we already have in the air, and the good purposes they serve. Keep them up there. Add to them. Improve the new models and be sure they function. Work hand in hand with the military and you'll find enough to do. But drop the idea that you're some superagency, some Manhattan Project inventing the atomic bomb. You're the Department of Agriculture now, a service agency with a limited budget. Learn to live with it.'

'Did you say that John Pope was leaving the program?'

'He's bright. He can see we're at the end of an epoch.'

'What's he going to do?'

'I don't know. He has an able wife with a good job to tide him over till he makes up his mind.' Grant grew hesitant. 'You know, I suppose, that the high brass at your shop is displeased with Pope. His arrogance when we talked Claggett into postponing his divorce . . . the bit about that Japanese newspaperwoman at Claggett's funeral. And I don't need to specify the Australian foul-up . . . the high brass . . .'

'I'm fairly high brass,' Mott said coldly, 'and I find no fault with Pope.'

'Neither do I! Look, he's from my hometown. I'm indebted to him. He campaigned for me. But . . .'

He walked Mott to the door. 'The days of wild blue yonder, the science-fiction bit—that's all finished, Mott. Now we address ourselves to practical matters.'

Senator Grant was correct; John Pope had concluded that he would do better if he resigned from NASA. 'It's this way, Penny, I'm forty-nine. They're not ever going to send me up again. Nothing to send me in.'

'They surely have some kind of job for you, an outfit that big.'

'Sure, pencil-pushing in some third-floor office. I'm not the type.'

'You can do anything you put your mind to, John. I've watched you.'

'That's true, but it has to be something of significance. Now, if they wanted me to study a completely new field—for a new kind of flight, that is—I'm their boy. But that's passed. The whole establishment is chairborne now, and there's really no place for me.'

'John, I see the budget. It's enormous even now. A lot of work to be done . . .'

'I've been in space. I've been to the Moon. If the flight program has ended, I can't spend the rest of my life at a desk.'

'What will you do?' They were in her apartment in Washington, where the activity of a great nation throbbed with vitality, and to hear him talking as if life had somehow ended was distasteful, an evaluation she allowed to creep into her voice.

'I'm still a Navy captain. I can always go back.'

'John, the best you could do in the Navy is more pencil-pushing. They don't want an old-timer like you, respected though your record would make you.'

'Look, I'm still one of the real pilots around.'

She burst into laughter as she poured him a ginger ale. 'John, those young tigers at Pax River wouldn't know what to do with you . . . or me.'

They thought about this for some time and after a while John turned on the television, but Penny immediately turned it off. 'We must talk about this, John. The Navy's no solution. It's trading a NASA desk job for a Navy desk job, so who's ahead?'

'Who has to be ahead? I could teach astronomy at Annapolis, maybe.'

'No, if you're going to make a break, make a big one.'

'Like what?'

In their dilemma the Popes became just another NASA family faced by unemployment because a great program was winding down, and like the other perplexed experts, they wandered off into many different possibilities.

'John, have you ever considered us both moving back to Clay? We'd have a decent pension. We could—'

'We could what?'

'You could go into politics, maybe.'

'I'd never touch it.'

'You could get elected, you know.'

'I am not a politician.'

He refused to discuss that possibility any further, turned on the television and watched a football game, but next day when he went to Navy headquarters in the Pentagon he received a jolt: 'John, the Navy would always find a place for you, but you've been away so long. You're definitely age in grade.' This meant that in the normal flow of a Navy's man's career, someone like John Pope ought statistically to be much further advanced than he was; his lagging on the promotion ladder meant simply that the Navy no longer expected him to become one of its senior admirals. He was tagged, indelibly, as a loser.

'But in aviation . . .'

'You're a champion, John. No doubt about it. But you've converted yourself into a civilian.'

'Sir, I could certainly . . .'

'I can't think of a commander who would feel easy having a national hero your age, your reputation, under him. It would be quite out of balance.'

'They tell me Yeager's being promoted to general. I'm due for admiral.'

'Yeager stayed in the chain of command. You didn't.'

'How about Patuxent River?' Before the admiral could respond, Pope added with obvious enthusiasm, 'I sometimes think they were the best days I ever had. Did you know that Claggett was there with me? Hickory Lee did a stint there, too, while he was in the Army.' The admiral listened with respect, tapping his fingers, as Pope recalled the glory days when he was a hotshot lieutenant commander, probably, and gradually the fire subsided. 'I suppose I would be overage for Pax River. But those were damned good days.'

'Believe me, John, you'd make a terrible mistake trying to come back in.'

He was not wanted. There was no way that the Navy could feel comfortable with a front-line civilian hero like John Pope on its administrative hands, and when he left the Pentagon it was with the solid knowledge that retreating to the blue uniform was not a possibility. Penny had been right, and when he reported to her apartment this time he was prepared to listen.

'You feel it's the end of the line at NASA?' she asked.

'Definitely. I'm through there, whether I want to admit it or not.'

'And you're through at the Navy?'

'I'm sure that's what they were trying to tell me.'

'How about business? Claggett told me that six different firms wanted to lure him away from NASA.'

'That was Claggett. He could sell anybody anything.'

'Well then, I have a surprise for you. Behind your back Senator Grant and I have been doing some logrolling. The State University of Fremont invites you to join its faculty.'

'As what?'

'Professor of Applied Astronomy.'

John leaned back in his chair, hands to lips, and tried to visualize the job, and gradually a big, relaxed smile came over his lean, tough face. 'That I would like.' Then he asked, 'You coming, too?'

'Much of the year. Yes, I know just the house we must buy.'

'What do you mean by *much?*'

'I have work here I want to finish up. At the committee. What with Glancey gone and Grant out, I'm needed.' She moved about the apartment, straightening chairs, something she did only when inwardly confused. 'And there's been some loose talk about appointing me to one of the federal agencies . . . maybe even a judgeship.'

'You'd be damned good, Penny. If they make a solid offer, grab it.'

'I'd have vacations. You'd have vacations. I'm sure it would work, John, but on the other hand, if you wanted to find something here in Washington . . .'

'I think I've had Washington.'

'I think you're right. I have this strong feeling that you ought to get back to your home soil. Dig in for the hard work that lies ahead.'

'Like what?'

'Who knows? You're not fifty yet. You have twenty-five good years ahead.'

'Penny, the most important aspect of this making decisions . . . it's difficult to say.' He seemed to choke on his words, then blurted out: 'You know I love you—more than flights, more than anything else.'

'That's hard to believe . . . sometimes.'

'But we always seem to be you here, me in Korea. You here, me at Pax River . . . or the Moon.'

'You trained me to be a Navy wife, John. You did a great job.'

'So it's still you in Washington, me in Fremont?'

'During these good years of our lives, yes. But we can handle it.'

'I intend to,' John said.

To honor John Pope's return to his hometown, the citizens and the university united in organizing a gala celebration worthy of a national hero, but the community itself was far from united on anything else; in fact, it was riven into warring segments.

Religious fundamentalists who believed in the literal truth of every word in the Old Testament had some time before launched a crusade in the state of Fremont to expunge from the school curriculum, elementary through university graduate work, any reference to Darwin's theory of evolution, and the movement might have died under the scorn of editorials and expert testimony had not the Reverend Leopold Strabismus of the United Scripture Alliance of Los Angeles seen the situation as a heaven-sent opportunity to lead a publicity campaign against godless humanism: 'We have a state-wide arena, Marcia. We have a new area which has never heard our preachments before. And I think we can command a national audience.'

He therefore moved into his wife's state with great force: tents for rural meetings, sound systems to amplify his thundering voice, choirs to provide music, and local enthusiasts to keep the excitement moving. Fremont had never seen the like, and people who normally might not have bothered with a revivalist's meeting flocked to hear Dr. Strabismus excoriate science, Communism, false prophets and Yale University. It was an excellent side show, at first, but it quickly degenerated into a searing attack on the general intellectual establishment.

The most popular member of the Strabismus troupe was not Strabismus himself, huge and hefty in his white suit, nor his very attractive wife, who nodded vigorously when he made his major points, but the appealing little animal, quite tame now and hungry for applause and bananas, who participated in the lectures as Chimp-Champ-Chump:

> 'Do you good folks really believe that this here monkey was your grandfather? Do you accept the teaching of the atheistic humanists at Yale University that this here monkey lived two million years ago, breeding a nest of half-animals, half-men, when the Bible itself says God made this Earth about six thousand years ago, and we have proof to prove it?'

His assault became so powerful and his logic so persuasive that the voters of Fremont placed a referendum on the ballot so that the citizens of the entire state could vote on whether Genesis was correct or Darwin, whether God was supreme or some Communist atheistic humanists at Yale University.

Men and women defending each point of view stormed into the state, and the air was filled with acrimony. In a rousing revival for rural communities in the western half of the state, Strabismus spelled out the goals of his campaign:

> 'I got me on'y five points, and they're taken straight from the Bible. First, in no tax-supported institution in this state, elementary school through the university, can anyone teach Darwin's atheistic theory as a fact. Second, in every institution, God's creationism has got to be taught as the fact that all sensible people believe. Third, we have got to erase from our textbooks any reference to millions and billions of years. This Earth came into bein' about six thousand years ago, and that's that. Fourth, we have got to stop talkin' about dinosaurs and the like as havin' lived a very long time ago and died out for some confused geologic reason. They died in the Flood, that's how

they died. Five, we don't want no more geology of any kind pollutin' our kids' minds.'

When the full force of his crusade was appreciated and it was seen that his side had a chance of winning the referendum, scholars from other states and textbook publishers from New York and Boston streamed into the state to try to restore reason, but they were powerless to quench the firestorm he had ignited.

He based his persuasive reasoning on two books which a Mississippi clergyman of some erudition had brought to his attention. The first was by Philip Gosse, an English writer, who argued simply that there were fossils, yes, and there were dinosaur bones, and there were geological strata, and everything was exactly as Darwin and the geologists described it. The secret was that in the year 4004 B.C. God had created the world exactly as Genesis said, and had hidden all these bits of evidence in the rocks and in the dinosaur bones as a kind of temptation to man's intellectual presumptions. Gosse explained everything in such simple and beautiful terms that Strabismus said, 'No further discussion is necessary. The record is exactly what the atheistic professors at Yale say. It has to be, because God placed it there on the day of Creation.'

The second book was extremely useful when arguing with people from the universities who had a smattering of knowledge. It was George McCready Price's *The New Geology,* which Marcia Strabismus sold for ten dollars a copy, to those who sought the truth. It was a formidable essay, well founded in scientific jargon and difficult to rebut. Its major thesis appealed to all who suffered from the tyranny of science, and when Strabismus translated this into his own terms it made a persuasive argument:

> 'These here scientists try to tell us that fossils found in rocks always grow from primitive forms to complex forms like you and me. And to prove this they show us that the primitive forms always appear in the earliest rocks, and the complex forms in later rocks. But how do they date the layers of rock? You stop right now and tell me how they date the layers of rock.
>
> 'They do it by seein' that primitive forms are in what they call the older layers. And the complex forms in the younger. Don't you see that they's arguin' in a great big circle. It's jest like a boy tellin' his girl, "You ought to kiss me because it's Valentimes Day, and Valentimes Day became special because that's when girls kissed boys."
>
> 'That's crazy reasonin' and the boy knows it, and the scientists know it, and they's pullin' the wool over the eyes of the public. I say it's time to stop.'

Several professors of geology volunteered to debate Strabismus, but he would meet them only in his tent, where the choir, the charm of Mrs. Strabismus, the cheers of his supporters and the antics of Chimp-Champ-Chump put the scientists to rout.

Leopold Strabismus was a most formidable adversary, much better educated than most of his opponents, and as the time for voting in the referendum approached, it became obvious that the citizens of a great state were going to throw evolution, geology, anthropology and paleontology out of the state curriculum. Two hundred years of the most painstaking accumulation of data and understanding were to be tossed overboard.

Why did Strabismus pursue this campaign so frenetically and with such diabolic effectiveness? He made no money from the crusade, since everything that reached him in the nightly collection was spent on rentals of the tent and the sound system. He could not have done so because of ignorance of the subject matter, for he had written Ph.D. theses on both evolution and Devonian geology. And he certainly did not act from deep religious conviction, for he had none.

He was driven by two great compulsions: a desire for power, and a longing for revenge against the academic community which had refused to accept him on his own dubious terms. Sooner than most, he had sensed that America was becoming surfeited with science and longed for simpler explanations, and very early in his crusade he had discovered that people in the hinterlands enjoyed listening to attacks on places like Yale University and institutions like the *New York Times*.

But most of all, his antennas, those remarkably sensitive probers of the national consciousness, reported to him that America was preparing itself for a major swing to the right, and he proposed to help lead that swing.

What were his own inclinations? His Italian grandparents would have been Christian democrats had such a party existed in Mount Vernon, and his Jewish grandparents were still avowed socialists. His parents on each side had softened these beliefs, becoming standard Democrats who voted now and then for really good Republicans like General Eisenhower and Jacob Javits. In the normal unfolding of events, Martin Scorcella should have been a moderate liberal, which is exactly what he was until his expulsion from New Haven.

Then he began to wonder, falling into the habit of telling jokes on himself in public: 'I came from a family of eleven Democrats, but I learned to read.' And what did he read? Eugene Lyons, Igor Gouzenko and, especially, Ayn Rand, and gradually he came to see that liberalism with its state-social approach was horribly wrong.

His next decision was vital, one often made by brilliant young men since the days of Greece: If society is rotten, I shall manipulate society. He had started with little green men, moved on to the founding of a bogus university and now to a religious temple, but what not even his wife Marcia had detected, he planned soon to surrender his basilica in Los Angeles and acquire several thousand acres in the suburbs to house a temple and a real university based on the Bible. In the meantime, he had the Fremont plebiscite to win, for he hoped that if he could encourage even one state to outlaw evolution, a groundswell would develop, and as its champion in state after state, he would inevitably become a man of considerable power.

When the vote was counted, the people of Fremont had elected to rescind most of modern science, and the educators of the state began the painful process of weeding out from their libraries any books which spoke well of Darwin, geology or dinosaurs. The task was easier than it sounded because avid citizens volunteered for the job, and there was a general cleansing.

It was into this heated atmosphere that John Pope returned, and there was general apprehension when the university announced that its most beloved professor emeritus, Karl Anderssen, who had taught John Pope his astronomy, would give the major address at the celebration. Anderssen was now a very old man and there was cause to fear that he might ramble on, and a possibility that although he had not participated in the fight against Strabismus, he might speak unguardedly and open old wounds. The officials were relieved, therefore, when Anderssen said, 'I'll give my speech honoring John in the planetarium.'

'The place is small enough,' the president of the university assured his board, 'so that the rabble can't force their way in.'

They convened at eight in the evening, the intellectual cream of the community, many of whom had voted to outlaw evolution and geology, but they were not fanatics and they wanted to hear what the old man had to say.

'Tonight is the twenty-second of June 1976, and when the lights go down we shall see the heavens as they are outside this planetarium. Now, I'm going to turn the sky-clock back 922 years. It is again June 22 in A.D. 1054. The sky looks almost the same as it does tonight, a few planets in different positions, but that's about all.

'I'm going to speed through eighteen days, and here we have the heavens as they appeared at sunset on the night of 10 July 1054. Let's go to midnight in Baghdad, where Arabic astronomers are looking at the sky, as they always did. Nothing unusual. Now it's 11 July 1054, toward three in the morning. Still nothing exceptional. But look! There in the constellation Taurus!'

In the silence of the planetarium the audience watched in awe as an extremely brilliant light began to emerge from the far tip of the Bull's horn. It exceeded anything else in the heavens, infinitely brighter even than Venus, and increasing in brilliance each moment.

'It was a supernova, in the constellation Taurus, and we know the exact date because Arabic astronomers in many countries saw it and made notes which confirmed the sightings in China. Indians in Arizona saw it and marveled. In the South Pacific natives marked the miracle. And watch as daylight comes in 1054! The new star is so bright it can be seen even against the rays of the Sun, which was not far off in Cancer.

'For twenty-three days, the astronomers of Cathay and Araby tell us, this supernova dominated the sky, almost as bright as the Sun, the most incandescent event in recorded history. No other nova ever came close to this one. Look at it! Challenging even the Sun! And watch how it commandeered the night sky, this flaming beacon.'

He allowed his planetarium to run rather slowly, re-creating the cycle of those twenty-three unequaled days, when watchers throughout the world had been stunned by this miracle. By day, by night, it filled the planetarium so that John and Penny Pope could see each other in its radiance, and the faces of all around them. And then, on the evening of the second day of August 1054 the great new star diminished, fading with a speed more precipitous than that with which it had arisen, until Taurus looked as it had for a thousand years and would look for a thousand years thereafter.

'Why do I tell you these things on the night we honor our cherished son John Pope? For one simple reason. This great star, which must have been the most extraordinary sight in the history of the heavens during mankind's observation, was noted in China, in Arabia, in Alaska, in Arizona and in the South Pacific, for we have their records to prove it. But in Europe nobody saw it. From Italy to Moscow, from the Urals to Ireland, nobody saw it. At least, they made no mention of it. They lived through one of the Earth's most magnificent spectacles and nobody bothered even to note the fact in any parchment, or speculate upon it in any manuscript.

'We know the event took place, for with a telescope tonight we can see the remnants of the supernova hiding in Taurus, but we have searched every library in the western world without finding a single shred of evidence that the learned people of Europe even bothered to notice what was happening about them.

'An age is called Dark not because the light fails to shine, but because people refuse to see it.'

Never had NASA's planning been more delicate. In the great orbiter mission to Mars in 1971 there had been no attempt to land on the planet itself, and since the Mariner remained aloft, taking from a distance those remarkable photographs which delighted the scientific world, there was no worry about safe landing sites. But on this flight the Viking was going to land on the actual surface of Mars and send its photographs from there. In 1971 Mars had been 75,000,000 miles away. This time it would be 199,000,000, and that, too, made a difference.

But what gave the exploration a touch of elegance was the time chosen for the landing. Starting back in 1961, when the trip was first contemplated, with little apparent chance of success at that time, skilled mathematicians had laid out a timetable which could deposit the machine on Mars at three o'clock Eastern Daylight Saving Time on the afternoon of the Fourth of July 1976. This daring, intricate, wonderful, imaginative feat would thus serve as capstone to our nation's two-hundredth birthday.

Year by year NASA leaders had asked their experts: 'Are we keeping to schedule? Will it land on the Fourth of July?' In 1975 they began asking monthly, and after the Viking was launched in August of that year, they checked week by week. Now, in the centennial year itself, with the landing date looming ahead, they verified their figures daily, and always they received the same answer: 'We're on schedule to land at three in the afternoon on the Fourth of July.'

Since the government lacked any other spectacular event to use as the highlight of its two-hundredth birthday, the politicians fastened upon the Mars landing as the apex of their celebration. President Ford would make a nationwide broadcast congratulating the scientists who had achieved this miracle. The three television networks would relay photographs as they reached the Earth. And the entire world would celebrate with us this exquisite intellectual victory. Thousands of Americans in all parts of the nation geared their lives to bringing this stupendous adventure to a successful conclusion.

The NASA high command asked Dr. Stanley Mott to fly out to the Jet Propulsion Laboratory in Pasadena to ensure that there would be no housekeeping glitches in a performance that would be watched by millions, and when he arrived three weeks before the Fourth he was pleased to find that leading scientists were gathering to study the data Viking would be sending back; engineers worked around the clock to keep the spacecraft on target; the Landing Site Selection Team would choose the exact spot for touchdown; the Image Processing Team would determine which of the thousands of photographs would be released to the media; the Inorganic Chemistry Team would analyze the data sent down by sensors; the Surface Sampler Team would concentrate on the actual composition of the planet; and at least three teams would try to collect any evidence which would prove that life had previously existed on Mars . . . or that it did now in some minute, unfamiliar form.

It was a dazzling concentration of brilliant minds, made more so when NASA flew in a group of distinguished civilians, not connected with the project but deeply interested in Mars, to conduct a seminar establishing an intellectual framework in which to understand the landing. Jacques Cousteau, lean and magisterial, spoke of the inner forces which goad men to explore, whether on Mars or in the ocean deeps. Ray Bradbury, the science-fiction giant, exploded into poetry to convey his feelings, while crippled little Philip Morrison of MIT, one of the sublest brains in the world, shared his reflections as Viking sped silently into orbit.

On the third of July, with President Ford preparing his notes to inform the world that we had landed on Mars and with television cameras crowding the room in which Dr. Mott and his men would make their scientific disclosures, a small group of NASA scientists, the ultimate wizards of this project, studied the latest close-up photographs of the site chosen for landing six years earlier and were shocked by what the scanner was revealing.

'We can't land in that nest of craters!'

'Look! The President of the United States is standing by. All those television cameras are waiting out there.'

'I don't give a damn. You can't land a fragile machine in terrain like that.'

'You don't give a damn for the President of the United States?'

'I didn't say that, but as a matter of fact, in this situation I don't.'

'What do you propose?'

'Slip the landing a few days. Look around for a better site.'

'Slip? Dammit, you can't slip!'

'I just did. Landing tomorrow is absolutely impossible. We must find a safer site.'

A sickening pall settled over the room, for these men knew the disappointment such an announcement must entail. They appreciated the abuse NASA would receive for having botched a mission of such importance, with the whole world watching. There was brief discussion as to who would announce the postponement, and a committee of three was chosen: two project scientists and Dr. Mott from headquarters. The grieving men took deep breaths, after which the one who had made the decision said, 'Well, let's get on with it.'

The formal announcement caused a dull mutter of resentment through the briefing hall, for these hundreds of reporters and television crewmen had traveled long distances to participate in this triumphant moment, and they were not pleased with the three men who gave them the bad news.

'So your whole delicate schedule is shot to hell?' one belligerent asked.

'It is,' the leading scientists admitted, but when the questioners reached Dr. Mott, they found him unwilling to concede a single point. Sitting primly and wearing a formal jacket while the others were in shirt sleeves, he parried all the castigations:

'We cannot land on July 4, which is a deep disappointment. But I feel confident from the new photographs that we will land on a better and safer spot on July 21 or even 20. That's a delay of sixteen or seventeen days, and in the long history of man's exploration, what did it really matter whether Christopher Columbus sighted his New World on October 12 or two weeks later?'

'If he'd delayed two more weeks,' a newsman growled, 'his crew might've lynched him.'

'We've spent years of effort and millions of dollars to bring this effort to the verge of success. An adventure like this has never before in the history of the world been attempted, and we must not endanger it at the last minute by trying to land in the middle of a plain of rocks.'

'Will your next site be any better?' a science writer asked.

'We're not guaranteeing anything, but this mission is so difficult, we've got to have as many factors as possible in our favor. We know that the July 4 site is no good. We hope the next one we select will be.'

'Why didn't you see that the present site was no good three weeks ago? Save us hauling out here on a no-go mission.'

'Three weeks ago we had to rely on photographs taken from a distance of several thousand miles. Now we have close-ups and radar probes, and I can tell you, that makes a difference. But if at the last minute on July 21 real close-ups show that site to be a bummer, we'll back away from it, too. Gentlemen, scientists grope for information, and when we get it we must obey its dictates. That's what science is.'

So this big day, the day of national celebration, passed ignominiously. President Ford filed his notes. The television crews went home, and second-guessers around the world explained how the affair should have been handled. But at the end of two weeks the NASA scientists concluded that everything was in their favor, so on 20 July men like Cornell's Carl Sagan and Hal Mazursky, the superbrain, bit their lips, and white-haired Jim Martin crossed his fingers and gave the signal to detach the small lander from the bigger orbiter which had brought it safely across so many millions of miles.

One of the young scientists gripped Mott's arm and whispered, 'It's got to work.' And when the signal reached Earth confirming that the lander had broken away neatly, the young man sighed and whispered again, 'I knew it would work.'

For two painful hours the NASA men checked indicators as the frail lander drifted down through Martian space, and then, when it began to descend precipitously, tension rose and in the disciplined silence excitement multiplied: 'Viking is 300,000 feet aloft . . . Viking is 74,000 feet from landing . . . Viking is at 2,600 feet . . . Viking is approaching Chryse in perfect attitude . . .'

The room fell silent; men could hear each other breathing. Then across 199,000,000 miles came the steady, unemotional signal: 'Viking has landed. All systems go.'

Men leaped into the air. Some wept. Jerry Soffen, project scientist for the adventure since its inception, shouted, 'After fifteen years . . . Mars!' Mott, overcome with emotion after having just witnessed the defeat of science in the Fremont plebisicite, danced with Carl Sagan in celebration of this tremendous victory.

Man had reached the planets. He stood challenging the entire solar system to reveal its secrets. Even the ramparts of the Galaxy were now approachable, and where this vast adventure into space would end, no man could predict. The landing on the nearby Moon had carried trivial significance compared to this, for the Moon was a dead appendage to planet Earth; Mars was a planet in its own right, and now it was being revealed as scarred, arid and lifeless.

The young fellow who had whispered at the moment of maximum tension now studied the first incoming photographs and again gripped Mott's arm. 'Damn it. Damn it to hell! A barren waste. If only it had shown a palm tree, we'd start planning a manned flight tomorrow. This way, we'll forget it by September.'

Mott, hearing this gloomy prediction, knew it to be true, but only insofar as the immediate future was concerned. And he felt he must correct the young scientist: 'In this work we build slowly. That photograph which is so disappointing to you . . . it could set the mind of some young Japanese ablaze. Or some schoolboy in Massachusetts.'

He stood apart, trying to recall the days when he had been such a schoolboy: 'Maybe the most important book I ever read was that ridiculous affair by Percival Lowell. It was totally wrong, but it set my mind working. Look! Seventy short years after he published it, here we are on Mars. And if I helped get us here, he helped get me started.' He moved in close to study the new photographs as they evolved in real time, and they showed no canals.

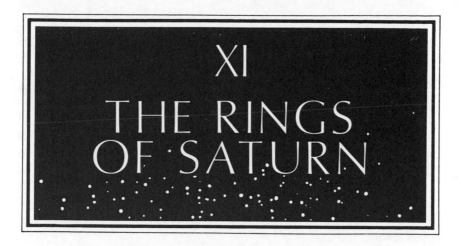

XI
THE RINGS OF SATURN

S TANLEY MOTT WAS IRRITATED. BY TRAINING AND PREDISPOSITION HE
should have been concentrating on the farthest edges of space, but
because of the various scandals in which his sons were involved he was
prevented from attaining any of the major positions in NASA management.
However, his unusual combination of skills—practical engineer plus vision-
ary astrophysicist—made him respected as a counselor in the varied activities of the agency.

Recently he had been assigned to analytical work in land-based aviation,
a task which might occupy him for many months. 'A terrible waste of
talent,' he grumbled to Rachel when the decision was announced. 'I've
always been the one who pushed for daring new explorations. Now I'll be
wasting my time at places like Boeing or Lockheed, and it hurts.' He glared
at his photograph of NCG-4565 and longed to be back in space.

But Mott had always been a devoted workman, and after he had spent
three weeks researching America's efforts in aviation, he became obsessed
with a desire to do a first-class job; his friends had to listen as he explained
his new enthusiasms: 'You forget that the first A in NASA stands for
aeronautics. In the past our agency made sensational contributions to flight,
and now that our space effort is in eclipse, it's only natural that men like
me should be reassigned.'

He pointed out that the country was in grave danger, again: 'You forget
that at three critical periods of our history America lagged far behind
Europe. In 1915, when the old NACA was established. During the period
after World War I. And in the closing years of World War II when the
English and the Germans were experimenting with new designs and new
engines. You know what I think? I think we're behind again.'

He startled listeners by arguing: 'Our aviation industry seems determined to repeat all the errors our automobile makers made. Lagging in
inventiveness. Not enough emphasis on research. Making no effort to build
the small aircraft the world needs. Resting on our duffs because we have

our marvelous Boeing 747.' But he attracted serious attention only when he revealed that the world's best small commercial carrier was now made in Brazil; the best medium-range, in Europe. 'NASA should do everything possible to excite advanced thinking—a helicopter that could fly forward at three hundred miles an hour, a plane that could take off and land in very short space, better jet engines, better everything.'

He was opposed in such a program by men in Congress and NASA who preached the doctrine that 'if an idea is commercially profitable, commerce should pay for its development and not the federal government.' It was the intention of these men that all of NASA's great aeronautics centers with their wind tunnels be sold to the big aviation companies so that they, and not NASA, could take charge of experimentation and the creation of new ideas for flight.

They had a certain logic in what they said, Mott had to concede. If a commercial company made a lot of money through adapting a NASA discovery, then that company should pay the freight; but even so he found himself arguing strenuously against these men:

> 'It seems to me that four of the wisest laws ever passed by the United States Congress were these: The Homestead Act of 1862, which gave away Western lands in order to settle the area and build a great free nation; the Morrill Act of the same year, which gave away lands so that each state could have its own agricultural college, producing excellent universities like Texas A and M and Oklahoma State; the GI Bill after World War II, providing free education for men who served their nation; and the act which gave free land to the railroads so we could build a vast transportation network to bind the country together and free land to build airports so that we could fly into a new age.
>
> 'There are certain fundamental things a nation should do to keep the creative pot stirring, and the energetic sponsorship of new technical ideas, advanced education and the creation of better modes is one of them. If the nation does not continue to sponsor experimentation in aviation, I fear it will not be done, and our marvelous industry, which earns us so much money, will languish as our automotive industry has.'

In vocal defense of this idea, he lectured at industry centers throughout the nation, and one day in January 1979, after a visit to NASA contractors in Denver, he hopped aboard the incredible commuter plane that flew in and out of the highest Rockies—'mountain goat with wings'—and landed at Skycrest, where the taxi driver delivered him at the shop run by Millard Mott: 'You'll find it's the center for the in-crowd. President Ford and his gang haunt the place when they drive over from Vail.'

Mott entered unannounced, and stood by the doorway for some moments appraising the store and liking what he saw. It was clearly a ski shop featuring the most expensive gear from Austria and a cadre of attractive young clerks who doubled as instructors for Easterners who wanted to try the slopes. Finally a brash young woman who should have been in school spotted him, hurried over, thrust her lovely face toward his, and asked brightly, 'Buster, can I sell you a pair of super skis? Only four hundred and fifty dollars?'

'You're confusing the men and the boys,' he said.

'Can you even ski?' she asked.

'I came in here to escape the snow. I hate it.'

'Have a beer,' and with that she went to a small refrigerator, produced a can of Coors, and knocked back the aluminum cap. 'What's your racket, buster?'

'I'm Millard's father.'

'Oh, wow!' she yelled, leaping up and giving him a kiss. 'You're the man who sends boys to the Moon when they've been bad!'

'When they've been good.'

'Millard,' she shouted. 'Your old man's here!'

Millard appeared from an inner office, a handsome young man of thirty-six who looked to be in his middle twenties—no fat, blond wavy hair. He was dressed in a Tyrolean sweater which looked as if it had been extremely expensive and a pair of pale blue après-ski lounging pants. He paused for a moment, recognized his father, and hurried over, extending his right hand, which Stanley grasped enthusiastically.

'You have some installation here. Is it paid for?'

'You know what you taught us. "The only thing to buy on credit is your casket." ' Millard laughed, led his father to the inner office, and confided: 'I borrowed like hell. Paid interest like you never saw. And the place caught on. I'm hiring another girl next week.'

'The two you have out there don't hurt business, I'll bet.'

'They're a rascally pair.' He leaned back in his chair and said, 'Dad, you never seem to get any older. How do you do it?'

'Your mother's a fabulous cook. A health nut. I see you're not gross.'

'How's Chris?' The question came much earlier than Stanley had intended, but he had to answer.

'He survives. Not even the jailers have much influence on him. He lives behind a wall, impenetrable.'

'When he gets out, could I offer him a job? Skycrest's a curious place. You find your own level. The mountain air clears things for some people. The saloons mark the end for others.'

'Chris would incline toward the saloons, I fear.'

'How dreadful. You see him, I suppose?'

'Whenever I go to Canaveral.'

Stanley found that what the taxi driver had said was correct: Millard's was the center for the in-crowd, for in the course of the morning he met three leading Republican politicians who had followed President Ford to nearby Vail and the presidents of two major corporations. The girl clerks treated them all with rowdy disrespect and the men responded. It was a lively scene, but Stanley noticed that one young clerk, a man from the Air Force Academy, quietly pushed merchandise on everyone who entered the shop. 'You ought to make him your partner,' he said to Millard.

'I have a partner. He'll join us for lunch, and I assure you, he'll be a surprise.'

Millard took his father to a chalet where nine of the prettiest girls Stanley had seen for some time, dressed in abbreviated winter costumes, served a severely limited menu: 'I'm Cheryl, from Montana. You can have shirred eggs with chicken livers, or a beef bourguignon at an outrageous price, or a very fine bacon-and-spinach quiche. Believe me, take the quiche.'

'There'll be three of us.'

'Three quiches?'

'I think we better wait for my partner.'

'Okay. Two beers?'

Stanley concluded that in Skycrest, one bought something, and quickly, or one was tossed out of town.

'The girls are all drop-outs from college. Vassar, Texas, Berkeley. You can staff a restaurant here in fifteen minutes.'

'What happens to them?'

'Some of them— Oh, here he is,' and Stanley looked up to see a handsome young man approaching, deep-set crevices in his cheeks, a touch of gray at his temples, and he thought he had met him before.

'I'm Roger, Mr. Mott. We met in California some years ago.'

'Roger from Indiana!' Mott remembered him well: the rejecter of amnesty.

'He served three years in Leavenworth for refusing the draft,' Millard said, almost proudly, 'and now he's back. Thank God, he's back.'

On the plane from Denver to Los Angeles, Mott wrote to his wife:

> I left in confusion, Rachel, but also with a sense of profound happiness. Roger is out of jail, bearing the marks of his confinement with dignity, and Millard has given him half-ownership of the shop on the grounds that Roger had served his sentence for both of them. They've built themselves a fine small house in Skycrest, where I met many of the leaders of this nation, for our son is a respected member of the mountain community. Once, after a visit with Millard and one of his friends, you said it was like having a daughter who had left her banker husband and was living with an architect. Well, the daughter is back with her husband and I simply did not have the courage to ask what had happened to Victor, the architect. But I

would be a liar if I refrained from saying that one sensed in the house and in the shop a presence of love.

The reason that drew Stanley to Los Angeles this time was not aviation, but a disruptive crisis in space. A decade ago, when he was occupied with other matters, the NASA high command had spent a great deal of time and intelligence trying to devise some major operation which would replace the Apollo program, and belatedly they recognized the validity of Dieter Kolff's persistent argument that what America needed was not something on the Moon but a floating platform in Earth orbit from which other vehicles could be launched for high-orbit work.

But NASA went one step beyond Kolff's prescription. Its spacecraft would be manned by astronauts who would bring it back to Earth for repeated re-uses. America would thus have a kind of inexpensive flying bus that could shuttle back and forth between Cape Canaveral and outer space.

As soon as Mott heard of this decision, he put his finger on the real problem: 'We've proved we can take off, maneuver and land. But what did we land? Only a minute percentage of what we took up. And it was wrapped in protective material which ablated away as it came through the fires of the upper atmosphere. No way we can ablate a whole aircraft and then use it again.'

When he heard the proposed solution—to glue onto the leading edges of this Shuttle small, individual tiles of a new material which would withstand the heat of reentry and could be used again—he was aghast: 'How many different tiles will you require?'

The answer was 31,689, and no two would match. As a scientist he was satisfied that such tiles could be manufactured and that a glue could be fabricated which would hold them in place, but as an engineer he could not believe that anyone in his right mind would come up with such a complicated procedure; however, those who made the decision defended it: 'Mott, we can't use an ablating material. You pointed that out. We've got to have something that stays put and can be reused. So what can we use? A special copper alloy would be great, but if you covered the Shuttle with three inches of copper, there isn't a rocket in the world that would lift it off the pad or brakes strong enough to stop it rolling when it landed. So what are you left with? We invent some new material, a new adhesive . . .'

'But why 31,000-odd titles?'

'Because the Shuttle will be a living, breathing, moving thing. Its various parts will interact, and if you simply plaster our new material over its face, hundreds of feet wide, inches thick, the first creaking motion in the structure would crack the protection and make it break off in huge chunks. By using the tiles, we build in 4 × 31,000 joints . . . well, somewhat less because the edge of one tile makes its joint with the edge of another. You figure it out. But one hell of a lot of joints. And they give, not the whole fabric.'

When Mott had a chance to inspect the new material these men had invented he was enchanted; a piece four inches square and an inch thick weighed about as much as a tiny box of safety matches, less, really. They glued a tile one inch thick onto his left hand and then applied a blowtorch to the outer facing, thousands of degrees hot, and the area exposed to the flame glowed a sullen red, then a white hot, but no heat came through the tile to his palm. Any structure protected by this tile could come crashing down through the atmosphere without burning up.

However, the fitting of the tiles to the Shuttle surfaces became, as Mott predicted, a task of infuriating complexity. A company in California had to produce 31,689 different, individual tiles minutely conformed to a particular spot on the Shuttle, and then apply each tile by hand in the most meticulous manner. Four different specifications were used in providing the outer facing of the tiles, depending upon how much heat each would be expected to absorb, and five different kinds of adhesive were needed to affix them.

Furthermore, when the finished Shuttle was transported from California to Canaveral for its launch, a horrendous number of tiles worked their way off, which meant that if this had been a real flight, the Shuttle and its two-man crew could have burned up.

So now the Shuttle was in Florida and the manufacturer of the tiles was in California, which necessitated a cross-country operation of the most complex nature. The fitters in Florida would make exact templates of the tiles they required and indicate what type of material must go into that tile, and with what surface. These specifications, with the template, were then flown to California, where highly skilled workmen, jewelers really, fashioned each tile to minute tolerances, whereupon it was flown back to Florida, tested for its waiting slot, and returned to California if even one edge or one thickness was out of line. Nearly twenty thousand times this intricate procedure had to be exercised, until an engineer like Mott shuddered. He could not imagine, not even late at night when he had had an extra beer, how such a solution had been accepted by his colleagues.

'Didn't they have any engineers on the board?' he asked his wife in frustration, and she countered: 'What you mean is, why didn't they have you on the board?'

As a good soldier, and a man furiously jealous of NASA's reputation, he never criticized the morass into which his beloved agency had fallen, but he did often speculate as to why the process of selection and verification, at which NASA had been so spectacularly successful, had this time gone awry, and in the end he had to conclude that it was that remorseless devil which haunts able men: hubris. The NASA scientists, bloated by one success after another—the Moon, Mars, Jupiter—had come to believe that they could do anything, and they saw nothing preposterous in a plan which called for the hand manufacture and hand application of 31,689 different tiles. They had overlooked the fact that *hand-applied* meant that individual men and women, hundreds of them, would have to work years on end doing the applying, and that when they were finished, half the tiles would fall off. An experimenter can determine the ultimate security of a process only by doing it and recording the outcome.

A week's delay turned into a month and a month into a year, and budgets exploded as men had to be paid for the extra work. Mott cringed as ABC-TV ran frequent specials deriding the Shuttle, and he grew actually nervous—had to take an antacid to quieten his stomach—when he was required to testify before Congress as to how this awful boondoggle had occurred.

But grimly he defended NASA, became its major spokesman in testifying both to Congress and to the press that the Shuttle would fly and that it would provide America with the space vehicle it needed. He said this so often and in such public places that he came to believe it. He defended the Shuttle before Rotary clubs, at universities, on television, and with great stubbornness among his colleagues at Houston or Huntsville.

'The Shuttle is aerodynamically even better than we've been saying. The tiles are a minor problem which an improved adhesive will solve. The lift-off system is the best we've ever had, believe me.' He refused to concede a single weakness, and it became obvious to his associates that at the age of sixty-three, when retirement faced him, this stubborn, able man had adopted the Space Shuttle as his final contribution to NASA. As an act of will power, which his associates had often seen him exercise in the past when difficulties arose, he would force this vehicle to fly, come back through the atmosphere, and fly again.

When a space expert from the *New York Times* heckled him about the cost and time overruns, he invited the learned gentleman to have a beer with him at the Dagger Bar. 'Every criticism you offer makes sense. The overruns have been distressing, but remember that if you crank in the inflation factor, we've spent very little more than we predicted we would back in 1971. And as to the changes, I'd like to share a story with you.

'Some years ago I met a man who had handled paper work on the Navy's PBY-5A. You may remember the original PBY, marvelous old warhorse, a seaplane that landed on the ocean to rescue downed fliers. Well, someone had the bright idea to make it amphibian, land on water if necessary, but also on land. Now, that doesn't double the complexity, it quadruples it.

'This fellow told me that after the manufacturer had made the plane absolutely foolproof and after the best brains in Navy procurement had approved it, and it was accepted by Navy aviators and was flying in combat, 536 different alternations were necessary before it was first-class. That's the nature of experimenting with a new idea. You do the very best you can, and when it's perfected in every detail, you make 536 alterations. With the Shuttle, we're at 421—but we're working.'

His present job was to fly out to a remote site in the California desert where scores of technicians were fabricating the final series of tiles, the ones which curved around a bump in the Shuttle or nestled into a corner, and he could scarcely believe the intricacy of the task. Even a simple square tile, ABCD, would have markedly different slopes from A to corner B, to corner C and to corner D, while the diagonal slope from A to C would not resemble the slope from B to D. And specifications might call for any one of four mixtures in the basic material, any one of four different finishes, and any of five different glues for attaching it to the Shuttle. It was an operation of preposterous complexity and he was ashamed of the engineers who had devised it. But when he gave press interviews he defended NASA against all criticism:

'This Shuttle will take off in March of this year. It will orbit the Earth for three days, exactly as planned, and America will be astounded by the beauty and skill of its performance. Obviously, we're entering a new age and I assure you it will be one of endless promise.'

But, when he was alone in his motel, unable to sleep, he would imagine what was going to happen to America's space program if the Shuttle floundered on its initial launch or turned to flame on its attempted reentry, and he could visualize the unbroken chain of disasters: ridicule in the press, sententious I-told-you-so reviews on television, pontifications in the editorials and, worst of all, direct abuse in Congress. He could see himself testifying before the Senate, with no defenders like Mike Glancey to protect either him or NASA. And then the heartbreaking images would cascade: Huntsville closing down; Wallops Island, where he had spent those wonderful days discovering the nature of the upper atmosphere, once more a bleak stretch of sand; Houston diminished; JPL, home of wizards, a warehouse.

Be there! he would pray, for he, more than almost anyone else in America, appreciated the dreadful burden of significance the Shuttle would carry on its maiden flight: Be there! Get up high and get down safe. At dawn he would finally fall asleep, but even then he would dream of tiles breaking loose at an altitude of 550,000 feet and a temperature of 25,000° and he would wake sweating, but this continual terror he shared with no one. He had been chosen spokesman for the Shuttle and he would serve that role, a man whose unblemished performances in so many different fields gave him credibility.

Professor Pope taught his astronomy classes at Fremont State as if he were training groups of future astronauts: 'You live among the stars whether you think so or not. Like ships adrift at sea, you identify your place on Earth through your relationship to the stars, and when you leave Earth and enter the air, your plane directs itself in obedience to the position of the stars. I insist that you know where the stars are and how they look, so that you can know where you are.'

His students spent a good deal of time in the planetarium familiarizing themselves with the heavens, and he was particularly eager to have them know the difficult southern stars which most of them would never see: 'If your plane captain gets lost and lands you in Australia rather than Woonsocket, I want you to be able to find your way back to Fremont State by following the stars,' and he taught them Canopus, Achernar, and Acrux.

He was a taskmaster, really, but the students indulged him because of what he had done when alone among his stars; also, he made the work fun, for he told them of how Randy Claggett had massacred the heavens, and whole generations of students at Fremont State came to believe that the North Star lay in Ursula Minor and that the proper names of Betelgeuse and Zubeneschamali were Beetle Juice and Reuben Smiley.

But occasionally moments of unexpected emotion took possession of the classroom, and then the laughing students remembered that they were studying with a real astronaut. One day a farm boy from downstate who had studied the heavens the way Pope had done as a boy and had even built his own telescope, polishing the glass like Galileo, said, 'Professor Pope, my Norton *Star Atlas* doesn't show three of the stars you have on your list. Navi, Regor and Dnoces.'

Suddenly Pope choked. He twice tried to speak but could not, and the students were powerless even to guess what was the matter, but then he controlled himself. 'At dusk on 27 January 1967 we were giving our first manned Apollo a shakedown. Something went wrong, and Grissom, White and Chaffee burned to death. There were three spaces in the heavens where navigational stars were needed but had not yet been named, so we called them Navi after Ivan Grissom, Regor after Roger Chaffee, and you'd never guess how we honored Ed White. He was Edward Higgins White II, so we reversed the Second, and I think that name's the best of all.' He stopped to let the students check the positions of these three important stars, and identify their constellations: Navi in Cassiopeia, Dnoces at the far tip of Ursa Major, and Regor to the south in Vela.

Then he said, 'As long as Americans venture into outer space, they'll be guided by the spirits of Grissom, White and Chaffee.'

One morning a girl student said, 'There's always been a lot of speculation about the last words of Colonel Claggett on your Apollo 18 mission. The real text has never been divulged, so far as I can find out. What did he say?'

'It was a garble,' Pope evaded. 'You know, that tremendous flood of radiation. It wiped out transmission to Earth.'

'But you must have heard the words. You weren't on Earth. You were right there.'

Pope considered this for some moments. He had always deemed Claggett's message, which he had heard so clearly, to be a privileged communication, and on this morning he persisted in that opinion, refusing to answer the girl's question, but that night, as he worked in the planetarium arranging the stars he would show the next day to explain the motion of the planets, it occurred to him that nothing was served by keeping Claggett's last words to himself. They represented his dead companion, so next morning at the close of class he answered the girl: 'I've never revealed what it was Randy said when he knew that he was about to crash his module and die on the Moon, but I see no good reason to keep the secret any longer. I shall tell you merely his words, and let you unravel their significance. What he said was, "Blessed Saint Leibowitz, keep 'em dreamin' down there." ' And he walked from the lecture hall.

The students scoured the campus trying to find clues to this remarkable sentence; the words *blessed, saint* and *Leibowitz* formed such a contradictory conjunction that they could make nothing of them, but one freshman boy had a buddy addicted to science fiction, the way Claggett had been, and this one solved the mystery in a moment. Next day the freshman raised his hand to inform Pope that he had the answer, and when Pope bent over his desk, the lad whispered, 'Walter Miller.' Returning to the front of the room, Pope said:

'Many believe, as Claggett did, that the best science-fiction novel ever written is a strange book by a man named Walter Miller. He called it *A Canticle for Leibowitz*. It takes place around A.D. 3175. The world has been shot to blazes by nuclear warfare, and in a great revulsion against science, like the one we're witnessing today, all libraries, laboratories and research materials have been destroyed. Scientists have been torn apart . . . Actually, people live in caves, with no electricity, no medicine, no books.

'North America has disintegrated into warring feudal states and life is unutterably bleak, but in one corner of New Mexico a group of dedicated monks, let's call them, has secretly kept alive the tradition of an all-wise scientist who had once lived in that area, a saintly man named Leibowitz. The most precious document in this sequestered civilization? A revered scrap of paper from Leibowitz's laboratory. Unquestionably authentic, it has not yet been decoded. It reads:

> Pound pastrami
> Can kraut
> Six bagels
> Bring home for Emma.

'From that shred of cryptic paper the culture of the entire western part of the United States will be re-created. I commend Leibowitz to you. Randy Claggett placed us in his hands when he died, and I'm sure the Blessed Saint would not be surprised to find that the state of Fremont had voted to outlaw all books dealing with evolution and geology, because that's what happened in exactly this part of America in his lifetime. Say A.D. 2010.'

In February 1981 the pressure on Stanley Mott, as spokesman for the Space Shuttle, became intense, because each trivial delay, unavoidable in an operation of this complexity and magnitude, became an occasion for reporters to bewail anew the failure of the entire concept. Thousands of sarcastic words were written about the tiles, and one enterprising woman reporter burrowed through the entire history of NASA, dredging up every instance of failure and asking in bold headlines, HAS NASA LOST ITS TOUCH? Doom and catastrophe reigned, and when two men were actually killed because they ventured into the wrong chamber at the wrong time to breathe pure nitrogen, Mott himself began to wonder if this great enterprise might be snake-bit, but he kept his apprehensions to himself.

In public he remained the stout defender, and when he flew down to Canaveral to see the majestic machine in place on the launch pad, even his most secret doubts were brushed away and he told the press in complete honesty, 'This thing will fly. It'll open a new age of space exploration.'

When the date for launch was fixed, Friday at dawn, 10 April 1981, he moved to the Bali Hai, where the Quints entertained him and the other NASA personnel with great meals and much good talk. Former astronauts Cater and Pope flew in for a reunion with Hickory Lee, who would serve as CapCom at the Cape before handing control over to Houston, once the launch was successful.

When all was in place and prognostications were positive, Mott almost relaxed, but his engineering background warned him that things could still go wrong. Those damned tiles could break away, leaving the great ship vulnerable, so he did not rest easy on the evening before the launch.

He rose at two on the culminating day, looked out at the dark sky and muttered, 'Thank God, it isn't raining . . . or blowing.' Things looked very good, all down the line, but when he and two others from NASA headquarters got in their car to drive north to the launch site, a distance of only a few miles, they encountered a traffic jam of awesome proportions, and when they finally inched their way to where a policeman stood, he said, 'I'm powerless. Maybe a million people descending on us. All those who missed the Apollo shots want to catch up.'

At 0500 his car was surrounded in every direction by impacted vehicles and it seemed unlikely that he would even get to Canaveral, let alone the launch site, but he took solace in the fact that from where he was immobilized he would be able at least to see the distant launch, but then traffic

SPACE · 564

inched ahead, and as the time for launch approached he found himself in a depression behind trees and tall buildings, without any chance of even seeing the shoreline where the Shuttle waited.

'We're going to miss the whole show,' he said resignedly to his partners, and one who had a transistor radio kept him advised as to the swift passage of time. It was a fiasco, the last in a long line, and Mott wondered again: Is this whole thing snake-bit?

Then came the good news! There would be a slight delay in the launch because of minor trouble with one of the five computers, and this might give them just enough time to break through the jam and get to the launch area. At this moment a larger car with several NASA personnel came rushing by with a police escort, and some of the passengers recognized Dr. Mott: 'Fall in behind!' And the chain of VIP cars drove across lanes, across lawns, and made it into the launch area.

It was a bright, perfect Florida morning made notable by that dazzling white spacecraft poised at the edge of the Atlantic. Mott and his men were in the stands closest to the launch, but even so, they were five and a quarter miles away, a distance dictated by the requirements of safety; if the rocket went wild, it would probably miss an area so far removed.

It seemed to Mott that everyone he had ever known was there to watch as America resumed its assault on space: past administrators who had fought budget battles, past engineers who had devised the great machines, past scientists who had charted the way to the stars, and good friends from Congress who had supervised the whole. But some of the best were missing: Lyndon Johnson, who had maintained such a steady perspective, was dead, and so were Mike Glancey, who had done the yeoman work, Wernher von Braun, whose boyhood imaginings had made it possible, and John Kennedy, who in a time of national malaise had had the courage to utter the magic words: 'I believe . . . before this decade is out . . . landing a man on the moon and returning him safely to Earth . . .'

But after the greetings ended, the empty minutes began to grow very long, and people began to fret, and old doubts resurfaced. One scientist tried to brighten the gloom by telling of the television network, one of those best informed on space, which had built itself a Shangri-la kind of headquarters from which to observe this launch: 'Must have spent ten thousand dollars. But they built it facing the wrong way. When the crew got here from New York they said, "Hey, we can't see a thing but swamp." We lent them a big crane, picked their building up, and swung it around the right way. They can screw things up, too.'

By 0900 it was obvious that the launch was not going to take place; the obstinate fifth computer refused like a petulant child to talk with the other four, so the gruesome announcement had to be made: 'The launch is scrubbed.'

Now the vast collection of cars reversed itself and the traffic jam back to the Bali Hai was even more tedious than the earlier one, but when the cavalcade finally reached there and disappointed men filed into the Dagger Bar, a phone call awaited Dr. Mott: 'Can you please come over to the press room at the Hilton? Two television crews would like to interview you.'

He looked about the bar, spotted Pope and Cater in disgusted isolation and asked them to join him—'Let's show a brave face to the slobs'—and they came eagerly. Several critics said later that it was by far the best show in the whole misadventure: 'It allowed us to see a real-life reflective scientist and two forthright astronauts who were not bright-eyed kids.'

Mott conceded nothing, and John Pope also demonstrated firmness in his support of the program, but it was salty Ed Cater from Louisiana who again and again brought the discussion back to practicalities: 'I've had more trouble with my Oldsmobile Toronado than they've had with the Shuttle. I'd fly in it tomorrow if they'd invite me. It can do so many things our Apollos couldn't do. I've walked on the Moon, it's fun, but now we have to tend our housekeeping chores. That Shuttle will take off Sunday morning like gangbusters, and if I know John Young, and I flew with him for a hell of lot of hours, he'll land it in California like a careful farm wife bringing in a basket of eggs.'

Mott, Cater and Pope spent the rest of that day in the Dagger Bar talking of past times and secretly keeping their fingers crossed. At nightfall Hickory Lee joined them, and they invited no one else, for they were the professionals, the ones with their necks on the line, and they prayed passionately that their bird would fly.

Mott could not sleep Friday night, and on Saturday, after another long day in the Dagger Bar, he wondered if he ought to take some sleeping pills, but the thought of lying in bed inert while the Shuttle took off was too depressing, and he lay awake till two, when he dressed, got in his car, and with three NASA passengers, fell in behind a police escort that whisked them right into the launch area. In the dark, while women filtered in to tend the refreshment stands, he met with his associates and assured them: 'This bird is going to fly. It's going to amaze America.'

At dawn the excitement was intense, and when the final countdown started on the radio Mott found himself breathing at an intolerable rate, and he thought: I hope those fellows up there are taking this easier than I am.

A roar! A flash of immense light! A thunder coming across the empty swampland! And then the slow, purposeful rise of the huge machine, an explosion of mist and fire as water rushed in to dissipate the extraordinary heat, and finally the Shuttle soaring majestically into the air.

Stanley Mott almost collapsed in his canvas chair. His energy had been drained away as if a siphon had been injected into his guts, and he could not speak, for he knew that now the real agony was beginning, never to end until those two men brought that spacecraft back to Earth with its tiles intact, and even as he was experiencing the first pangs of this uncertainty, a television commentator was announcing: 'When the doors to the bay opened, the astronauts could see that several tiles were missing.'

He flew with several others out to Los Angeles and then by a small NASA plane to Edwards Air Force Base in the desert, where he assembled with other scientists and a group of former astronauts. Two television stations asked if he would make himself available for interviews about the missing tiles, but since he could not risk displaying his anxiety in public, he declined, and he heard one announcer say, 'High officials of NASA have refused to comment on this perilous condition.'

Early on Tuesday he arose, cut himself while shaving nervously, and drove out to the vast stretch of flat, empty desert on which the Shuttle was supposed to land, and when he was confronted by the actual strip, waiting there in real time, he felt his knees grow weak: Please, God, bring it down safely. He shivered to think of how the critics would howl if there was a last-minute catastrophe.

He knew from briefings that just about now Young and Crippen would be making their final decision far above the Indian Ocean; they would cross Australia and speed toward California, descending as they came. In a few minutes they would begin to penetrate the heavy atmosphere at Mach 24.5, when the heat would become so intense— The loudspeaker interrupted: 'Columbia has now entered the zone of silence. Heat is so intense that radio communication becomes impossible.' Oh, Jesus, Mott prayed, keep those tiles in place.

This was the moment which the men aloft and those monitoring them below had to take on faith. When men have ventured toward the stars it is not easy to come back to Earth.

Mott almost stopped breathing. The men around him grew silent. What was happening up there? Then came the joyous, rattling sound of a human voice, no excitement, no panic: 'This is a great way to come back to California.'

Then one of the ordinary planes keeping watch in the sky sent television shots of the great spacecraft coming back, the first ever to fly its way home intact. Men began to shout, for they could see the Shuttle as it appeared in real time. It came to Earth like an everyday commercial airliner winging in from Australia, and Mott cheered as if he were a child at some game.

And finally the electric moment came when the beautiful machine triumphantly touched the gravel, settled down like an eagle returning to its nest, raced along the runway, and braked to a halt. Never had a major exploration ended so well when so many had expected it to fail.

Mott looked around for something to sit on, for he was afraid he might faint.

On the day after the Shuttle landed in California, Rachel Mott received in her Washington apartment a surprise gift from Huntsville. It came from the Kolffs and contained a handwritten note: 'Please can you call me and give me some advice? Dieter.' When she opened the package it contained two records produced and played by young Magnus Kolff; both were by an ensemble, which he had organized, called the Boston Brass, consisting of eleven of the top brass players from the Boston Symphony plus five men from other orchestras. The first record contained four classic pieces which Magnus had transcribed from the shorter ones of Vivaldi, Schumann, Beethoven and Brahms, and the rich sustained notes cascaded out with the joy these men had shared in playing music when they, and not the violins or the soloists, were the stars. Rachel could not detect when Magnus played, for he did not give precedence to the three trumpets, and certainly not to himself.

The second record was going to prove the more popular, Rachel predicted, for it contained Christmas carols played with a sweet verve that was bewitching. On the second side Kolff, who served as director of the group, had run out of carols and had filled in with three short pieces that Rachel had loved as a child before her tastes became refined: Handel's Largo from *Serse,* the Bach-Gounod *Ave Maria,* and the wonderful *Agnus Dei* of Bizet, which one rarely heard these days but which Caruso had sung with such overpowering effect.

She played both records twice, delighting in the rich tones that young Kolff's men had produced, and then she called Huntsville to determine what problem the older Kolff might have. The message astonished her:

> 'Rachel, I'm delighted it's you. I trust your judgment. It concerns my grandson Wernher. Magnus' boy. Did you get the records? Aren't they splendid sound? He conducts the group, you know.

> 'The problem is this. Magnus lives here in Huntsville, and young Wernher—named after Von Braun, as you might guess—well, the boy's old enough for serious studies now and Magnus thinks we must send him to Germany for his education. So do I and Liesl. What's your opinion? . . .

> 'Why? For a very good reason, Rachel. There's a fierce movement in Alabama to stop the teaching of evolution, geology, everything in science. A minister named Strabismus is leading a crusade and all decent teaching must stop. I think no boy of promise should be denied access to the full range of science. How could Von Braun have invented the rocket if—'

She broke in: 'Dieter, send your grandson to Germany immediately. If America insists on retreating to the dark ages, we may have to educate our brightest children in China and Germany. Sneak them out to discover the real world, then sneak them back in to keep learning alive.'

'That's exactly what I told Magnus. Young Wernher could be a new

Von Braun. He could be a bank clerk. How did I ever produce a boy who can play the trumpet like an angel? Who knows? But the boy must have a chance to know the truth, whatever he becomes.'

Liesl Kolff, sixty-five now and somewhat bewildered by the tenor of things in Alabama, came on the phone to ask, 'You think we're right, Mrs. Mott?'

'Send him on the next plane, Liesl. The safety of his soul is at stake.'

'Will you have Dr. Mott call us, please? I'm still an old German. I like to hear it from the man.'

When Stanley returned home and learned how his wife had advised the Kolffs, he was distressed and called Huntsville immediately: 'Dieter, I think Rachel gave bad advice. I see no reason to send your son to Germany. America is a free republic and its citizens are allowed to do any crazy thing they want. Like trying to rescind geology.'

'How do we refute such nonsense?'

'With data. With logic. With new developments. We protect science with science. Just as we protect faith with faith.'

'But they're starting to pass laws, Stanley. Our Wernher will not be allowed to learn the truth.'

'They pass laws, and then we knock them out, and they aren't laws any longer. I have great faith in this nation.'

'Millions of people had great faith in Germany, and look what happened.'

'Keep the boy in school, Dieter. Give him good books to read. And this summer, if you can afford it, send him to Germany . . . for a visit . . . to see for himself . . . to check on what they're teaching there. He'll come home better for it.'

When he hung up, Rachel asked, 'Was I hysterical? Am I wrong in fearing that the Neanderthals will win?'

'I'm sure they'll try, and I'm sure people like us will fight to knock them back.'

'Will we succeed?'

'We've been succeeding for the past six million years—with setbacks now and then of a thousand years or so.'

The three most dangerous airports in the world were in southern Florida: Miami, Fort Lauderdale just to the north and Palm Beach International. The chances of death here, if one's plane took off or landed after dark, were grotesquely greater than at an airfield in some backward country like Burma or rural Indonesia.

The Florida airfields had the best electronic equipment, the best-trained air controllers and big, broad landing strips, but still the danger mounted. Partly it was because the landing strips were so spacious; with tarmac going off in all directions, they constituted a temptation.

Smugglers, attempting to bring into the States huge cargoes of marijuana or smaller, more valuable ones of heroin or cocaine, loaded their small, illegal planes, often stolen from private owners, in Colombia, Ecuador or Mexico and flew them north at sunset. Keeping low over the Gulf of Mexico to avoid radar detection, they approached the western shore of Florida in darkness, dipped across the peninsula and came roaring in without lights, permission or radar assistance to land secretly at one of the big southern Florida strips.

How did they land? By sheer luck, hoping that the runways would be wide enough to accommodate them, no matter how they approached, trusting that no big commercial planes were landing or taking off. One airline pilot who had flown against the Japanese Zeros at Guadalcanal said, 'Landing a plane at Fort Lauderdale is the hairiest thing I've ever done in the pilot's seat. Radar gives you clearance. The field lies dead ahead. But what you don't know is whether some smuggler is choosing that minute to land his stolen plane down the middle to where the fast cars are waiting.'

Practiced travelers who knew of the clandestine landings refused to fly into or out of these airports after sunset. A German businessman who lived half the year in Palm Beach because of the advantageous exchange, said, 'In Berlin we have the Baader-Meinhoff Gang, sixteen or seventeen people who make life hell for the rest of us. But over here you have sixteen or seventeen hundred trying to use the airports after the sun goes down. They're the real revolutionaries.'

In June 1981, when the nights were shortest and therefore least helpful to the smugglers, a pair of daring aviators held secret sessions in West Palm Beach with a gang of resolute ground men whom the leader of the smugglers, Chris Mott, had met when serving time in the local jail. His plan was bold: 'Jake and I know a field in Louisiana where we can lift a Lear jet without too much trouble. We've had four dry runs to see if we could make it, and the owner is so damned careless we could take it out in a tractor trailer. He runs a fish-canning business, chowder and the like.

'Jake and I will fly it directly to a place called Las Cruces north of Medellín in Colombia, where our people will load the Lear with the biggest haul in the history of the Caribbean. We calculate that with a good wind we can make it straight in to this airport. We'll land about 0230, a good confusing time. Jake says he can bring it west-to-east, keep it off to the southern side away from the airport buildings, and you fellows will be waiting on Route 98 just off the tarmac, and of course you'll head straight for Orlando, where John will be waiting with a legal plane, at the far end of that runway.'

It was a neat plan, one that required timing and skill and not a little courage, for the flight from Las Cruces to Palm Beach just about represented the range of the Lear jet they proposed to steal. Jake, the pilot, said he was prepared to take the risk if the several ground crews would provide the fast cars, the legal plane at Orlando and the outlets in New York and

Boston. But the central courage, the hard brains of the planning, lay with Chris Mott, who, at the age of thirty-one, was fire-hardened and prepared for the all-or-nothing hazard: 'There could be eleven million dollars in this, and we take our risks evenly. The guys in Colombia, they get only six cents on the dollar unless we can sell the stuff in the big cities. Jake and I get peanuts unless you men succeed. And you get nothing unless we get the stuff to Palm Beach. *Comprendo, amigos?*'

Two of the couriers drove Jake and Chris to Baton Rouge and then southwest to Plaquemine, where a man named Thibodeaux had a packing plant and a sleek brown Lear jet with extra-large tanks. After the drivers of the car stole a large truck, which they placed across the roadway to forestall pursuers, Jake and Chris moved swiftly to the unguarded Lear, opened the locked door with a skeleton key, and slipped into the pilots' seats. Checking all systems with extreme care, Jake satisfied himself that the jet had sufficient fuel to get him into Mexico, where a dozen clandestine fields operated, then switched on the ignition.

It was imperative that once the engines roared into life, the takeoff proceed without a moment's delay, so while the various systems hummed with life, Jake checked one last time: 'Looks good, old buddy.'

'Take her up,' Chris said, and with a deep breath Jake applied power, heard the engines respond beautifully, and moved swiftly to the far end of the little runway. With a breathtaking U-turn to the right he reached takeoff position, poured on the gas, and roared down the runway. It was a perfect escape, and as soon as the plane was well into the sky, the two men in the automobile were speeding west to the safety of Lafayette, where traffic would absorb them.

In Colombia it was Mott who took charge. In jail he had learned Spanish, anticipating the day when his cloudy operations might require that language, and he dealt boldly with the brigands who controlled the heroin-cocaine market, offering them what funds he had collected in the States and assurances of a much heavier payoff if the smuggling succeeded. At first the Colombians were disposed to protest the relatively small amount of hard cash they were receiving up front, but when Chris railed at them, showing them his own empty pockets and reminding them of the great risks he and Jake and the others in the States were taking . . . 'Where do you suppose we got this plane? We heisted it, right off an airfield in Louisiana.' And he showed them an American newspaper he had purchased while waiting in Mexico so they could read for themselves about the daring robbery at Plaquemine. Fortunately, the account carried a photograph of the stolen plane and a description of its number and brown-painted body.

'Leave the jet with us,' the brigands suggested. 'One million, two million dollars.'

'What would we fly in?' Jake asked, but before the Colombianos could even reply to this stupid question, Chris stepped in: 'Fools! You could sell the jet for maybe two hundred thousand. We're talking about eleven million.'

Iron-hard, he kept everyone in line. He had brought less money than the brigands had expected and now he was taking out of the country a plane on which they might have made a substantial profit, but he convinced everyone that this was the only way. For one bad moment he suspected that the brigands might try to kill him and Jake and sell the jet to some South American customer, but he forestalled them by drawing his own revolver and indicating to Jake that he must do the same. Nodding to the heroin providers, he backed slowly to the Lear, sent Jake in ahead of him, waited till the engines coughed, then dashed in, slammed shut the big door, and waited breathlessly as Jake took the jet down the rough runway and into the air.

'I thought they might have a machine gun somewhere.'

'I'd've headed this beauty right into the trees,' Jake said. 'They'd have found themselves with zilch.'

'And we'd have been dead.'

'Sure, but we'd have had the laugh on those bastards.'

The load was so extremely bulky—bales upon bales of marijuana plus the smaller cartons of the heavy drugs—that there was scarcely room to move if one sought a drink of water or any of the beer in the packing company's icebox, so Chris stayed in the copilot's seat, staring at the dark waters of the Gulf as the sun disappeared. Their route would take them over the western end of Cuba and onto the Florida peninsula south of Naples, and as night fell Chris asked, 'You feel confident we can drop low enough to confuse the Cuban radars?'

'That's my job,' Jake said.

'If they did have a machine gun, and they got you,' Chris said, 'I was going to take this baby up. Or die trying.'

'You've never flown a plane.'

'I've watched you.'

'Could you land this baby? If anything happened?'

'I could sure try.'

Jake asked him ten or fifteen questions and was startled by the cleverness of Mott's responses. 'Maybe you could get this tub down. Wouldn't be worth much after you did, but you just might make it.'

'Our boy in Louisiana will get his plane back just about as good as when he lost it, won't he?' Chris asked. He was always fascinated with possibilities, with alternate ways of doing things, and he was known among his fellow convicts, in jail and out, as the man to have with you if the risks were great.

'What's your old man really do?' Jake asked as the Lear purred over the water.

'He's a mahoof with NASA. You know, the outer-space stuff.'

'What's he think about your operation?'

'Distressed.'

'You tell me once you had a brother?'

'He's an interior decorator.'

'For real?'

'I think he runs a bar in Denver, but he's an interior decorator.' They flew in quietness for about fifteen minutes—one hundred miles covered by the jet—and then Chris added, 'Millard, that's his name, he wrote to me while I was in jail—offered me a job. I think Pop got to him, suggested it. I'm sure as hell good old Millard didn't want me around. I didn't bother to answer.'

They slipped across Cuba without incident, edged their way up the western coast of Florida keeping very low, then darted inland south of Fort Myers and headed west-to-east for the spacious airport at West Palm Beach.

They came in low, as planned, saw the lights of the town, looked for the southern edge of the strip, and came roaring down just as another private jet lifted into the air for a flight to a meeting of a corporation board in Chicago. The two powerful jets, one brown, one a pale blue, smashed head-on eight feet above the ground, exploded, and fell in a blazing tangle.

The six men in the five fast cars who waited on Route 98 watched in awe as their precious cargo vanished in the intense flames. One driver suggested: 'We better get out of here. The cops might . . .'

'Jesus,' another said as he and his partner crept back to their car, 'eleven million bucks!'

The NASA high command was one of the most compassionate in government; for decades they had worked with high-strung scientists and for years with sensitive astronauts, and they appreciated the psychological tensions to which their personnel were vulnerable, so when tragedy struck in Florida they knew the Motts needed help. But by an unlucky chance, while dispensing sympathy they had to require Mott to confront an additional blast of bad news, and they decided to tackle the problem directly.

'Stanley, this is one hell of a time for me to say this, but you know your obligatory retirement takes effect on the last day of this year.'

'I've been aware of that,' he said dully. 'For some years . . .'

'But we appreciate enormously the way you defended the agency during the bad days with Shuttle. You were a man to be proud of.'

'Look!' Mott snapped. 'I'm retiring. Let's not make a big deal of it.'

The administrator did not alter the level of his voice. 'We wanted you to know that even when you do retire . . . well, we'll still want to call on you for consultations. You have a decade of hard work ahead of you.' Mott nodded. 'And to prove our appreciation, we want to headquarter you in California . . . work with the press on the Voyager 2 fly-by of Saturn in August.'

When Mott showed obvious relief at this unexpected good news, the administrator breathed more easily, and smiled approvingly when Mott spoke: 'You understand, Clarence, I've been preoccupied with Shuttle. I haven't kept up with all the great things the Voyagers have already accomplished.'

'We're aware of that. But a man like you, fresh to the program, enthusiastic, might provide just what the press needs to make this operation sing.'

'I would like that. I'd like a chance to catch up.'

'And, Stanley, we think you ought to take Rachel along. Get her involved.' Mott could not respond—the past weeks had been horrible—so the two men just sat there, and after a while Mott said very quietly, 'It's thoughtful of you to suggest that, Clarence. You know, she had to identify the boy's body from dental fragments.'

This assignment to Pasadena's Jet Propulsion Laboratory would be his final job with NASA, not out among the shadowy galaxies, but at least with the great planets, so he and Rachel packed their car to the brim, and during the long drive west talked and rediscovered each other. They stopped at Clay to chat with Professor Pope, then on to Boulder to consult with the Sun Study people, and into the mountains to visit briefly with Millard in his ski shop, where to their amazement his partner told them, 'Some of the Skycrest businessmen are thinking of running your son for mayor!'

By the time they reached California the dull ache of their son's death had somewhat diminished; the wonderful therapy of driving across America had asserted itself once again, and Stanley was eager to leap into the middle of preparations for the fly-by. Both he and Rachel were caught up in the euphoria which permeated the place. There were no loose tiles here, no soul-searching, for this was the kind of meticulous preparation and supervision that NASA had always done so well. There were no sleepless nights over Saturn.

Each morning he and Rachel met with the sixty or seventy experts responsible for the mission, and as soon as he began assembling technical details for the press, he fell under the enchantment of this last great planetary exploration, and he appreciated the sadness with which some of the men worked: 'You should stress, Mott, that this is our culminating effort. When Voyager 2 leaves Saturn it will head for Uranus, arriving in January 1986; then to Neptune, August 1989. After that, there'll be no more probes, no more landings. The American effort to explore the planets will have ended . . . for this century.' So the nation's fantastic adventure in far space was ending just as his personal career was drawing to a close; whenever he looked at the marvelous duplicate of the spacecraft, he felt as if he were seeing himself, and he prepared his materials with special reverence:

> In 1967, fourteen years ago, a band of visionaries saw that if they could launch the right kind of vehicle into space at the right time with the right velocity, it would fly in a beautiful arc to Jupiter,

where the gravity of that giant could be used to whip the vehicle on toward Saturn. Indeed, these far-seeing men argued that it would be possible to fly within a few thousand miles of the great rings of Saturn and to decide once and for all what they were composed of and what they signified in the grand design of our universe.

The data of this bold dream still amazed him: straight-line distance from Earth to Saturn, about 1,000,000,000 miles, depending on where the two planets happened to be in their respective orbits; distance of the actual route to be flown, 1,400,000,000 miles; time required for the trip, four full years less eleven days; average speed during that time, about 40,400 miles an hour.

Ten years ago he had asked those early gnomes with their primitive calculators, 'But what can you see if you do get to Saturn?' and they had jolted him with their answer: 'We'll cram onto our vehicle eleven subtle instruments, the like of which the world hasn't seen before. Special scanners to provide us with pictures. Devices to measure radiation, magnetic fields, plasma particles, cosmic rays. We'll do spectroscopy, and photopolarimetry, and all kinds of radio science. Things you don't even know about yet.'

They had shown him a mock-up of the spacecraft, and once again he was startled by the realization that even though it would be flying through space at enormous speed, there would be nothing in space to impede it, so it could have wonder machines dangling from it at any desirable attitude or spot: 'Looks like a flying bedstead.' And they countered: 'Four of our complex devices aren't attached yet.' And he asked, 'Where will you put them?' They replied, 'We'll hook them on anywhere.'

The magnetometer had captivated Mott, for it symbolized what science could achieve in this radically different environment. When he first saw the contraption it was a forty-foot length of filmy epoxy glass resembling a spiderweb and not much firmer. A breath of wind would disturb it. He was perplexed by a rather heavy instrument attached to one end, for obviously the web could not support it, but he watched as men from JPL coiled their gossamer into a tight package, storing it in a canister like ones that hold tea and placing the heavy magnetometer on top. Far out in space the top of the canister would be blown off, the spring-loaded gossamer would uncoil, and Voyager would have a long rigid arm supporting the Earth-heavy instrument. It was quite miraculous, but the inventor assured Mott: 'In space that gossamer arm'll be as rigid as a steel beam here in California.'

'But how do we get the commands from Earth to the spacecraft?' Mott had asked in those early days, and the project manager had explained: 'We'll build three maximum-efficiency computers into the craft, and while they're still on Earth we'll fill them with instructions—roll after roll of the most intricate things to do. "Point your scanner the other way." "Switch your focus from the star Canopus in Carina to Deneb in Cygnus" "Increase the speed of your read-out." "Take away the blue filter and move in the red."

'When the computers are crammed with instructions, we establish a radio link from them to the ground, but it's not like a telephone. Not a bit. Because of the vast distance, it takes our radio instruction—traveling at the speed of light—eighty-seven minutes to reach Saturn, and takes Saturn's answer eighty-seven minutes to get back. What does this mean? I say in the telephone, "Hello, who's there?" Then I wait three hours to hear you say, "Stanley Mott."

'So we construct a special language of about 1,300 words and we transmit those, and each word cues the computers to set a prearranged sequence of events into operation. Dr. Mott, how many radically different commands do you suppose we'll be able to send our spacecraft?'

'You mean, from JPL to Saturn?'

'Exactly.'

'You have 1,300 command words, I suppose each one controls . . . what? Ten . . . fifteen functions?'

'We can send 300,000 different, specific orders.'

Mott had stared at the man for almost a minute, trying to absorb this astonishing fact, and slowly, as if he were a child in school, he repeated salient data: 'After four years of remote travel, after a billion and a half miles on the road, with a system that requires an hour and a half to exchange one word . . . you can deliver 300,000 intricate orders?'

'Yes. With a likelihood of success. By that I mean, the craft will receive the new order and be in working condition to obey it—90.3 percent.'

From time to time during the following years Mott had been in touch with what the people in charge of Voyagers 1 and 2 were doing: 1972–1976, building the spacecraft and their various appendages; 1976–1977, frantic simulations to be sure things would work; 20 August and 5 September 1977, two perfect launches; 1977–1979, four hundred experts biting their nails; 5 March and 9 July 1979, glorious arrivals at Jupiter; 1979–1980, more nail-biting; 12 November 1980, triumphal photographing of Saturn by Voyager 1 . . .

Now, in the anxious interval before 25 August 1981—the hoped-for arrival time at Saturn of Voyager 2—his job was to check with the mavens at Jet Propulsion to ensure that usable photographs would be supplied to the hungry media, and he said to Rachel, 'You must see what these miracle workers can do.' When he took his wife to the laboratories, one of the men directing the overall flight told her, 'We threw this baby into the air four years ago with every intention of getting it into position to take the Earth's best pictures of Saturn. You see on the wall what Voyager 1 accomplished last November.' As Rachel studied the dazzling photographs, he said, 'When those rings come into closer view, we'll do even better.'

'How can you be so confident?' she asked, and he said, more quietly now, 'I'm positive we'll deliver the camera to the door of Saturn. What happens when it peeks through, that's Template's headache.'

When Mott heard this familiar name he cried, 'Rachel you've got to meet this character. If NASA has a verified in-house genius, Template's it.' And when the Motts reported to that man's cluttered office, Stanley said jovially, 'My wife is hoping to see some really great pictures. What can I promise her?'

'Mrs. Mott,' the enthusiastic young fellow cried, 'you're going to see a miracle. When we started with Mariner 4—back at the dawn of the space age, you might say—'

'It was only 1964,' Mott reminded him.

'Like I say, at the dawn of exploration. Our equipment then could deliver to Earth about six bits a second. This time, 44,000 bits a second! Think of it—44,000 clear, distinct pieces of information come at us each second from 1,000,000,000 miles.'

'You feel confident it'll still produce good pictures,' Rachel asked.

Template ignored the question, which he deemed irrelevant; his burning interest was in the process he and his associates had devised, not in the end results. 'Mrs. Mott, Mariner 4 required an entire week to send us 21 lousy pictures, exciting in that primitive time, but lousy. This baby will bring us 18,000 photographs in a jiffy. Right here in River City, I'll receive 184,-000,000,000 bits of information from Saturn. Enough data to keep the scientists of the world guessing for ten years.'

'I was told,' Mott said, 'the chance that Voyager would get from launch in working order . . . 90.3 positive. What's your prediction that the cameras will work if they do get there?'

'I still prefer the word *scanner*. My guess—97, 98 percent you'll get a batch of the world's greatest photographs, and some we'll convert to color.'

With such assurances from men who knew what they were talking about, Mott proceeded to supervise arrangements for the hundreds of press people who would soon be flooding JPL, for realization had spread that this might well be the last close-up the Earth was going to have of the nearer planets during this century. All major foreign countries were sending observers: fifty-two different foreign newspapers, seventy-one magazines, nine television crews from Germany, Japan, Great Britain and France, plus all the regulars from the United States. Many of the world's leading astronomers were planning to attend, and Mott saw with pleasure that John Pope's name was among them.

As the days neared when Voyager 2 would make its closest approach to Saturn, Pasadena became the intellectual capital of the world, for men and women were about to see a close view of this magnificently complex planet. Excitement was intense and debate heated, for this was one of the great moments in man's speculative history, when he would stand face-to-face with a celestial object which had captivated his imagination from that night more than a million years ago when someone cried in awe, 'It moves among the fixed stars!' and which had tantalized him even more when telescopes revealed that it was surrounded by a congregation of exquisitely beautiful rings.

Soon it would be revealed. There would be a brief hello, a respectful nod there in the timeless freezing wastes, then a photographic salute, and the endless departure. Fragile moment in time, hallowed by those hesitant guesses of Galileo— 'It seems to have horns, but my scope was not powerful enough to make sure'—this would be an instant of supreme importance to the scientists gathered here, but of little significance to the majority of the world. One astronomer well into his seventies said,

> 'Don't worry about that, Mott. I had my graduate students look into the experience of Copernicus, Kepler and Newton. Now, you've got to admit those men changed the history of the world. But when they were doing their work and announcing their discoveries . . . how many of their contemporaries even knew it was being done? How many could comprehend its significance?

> 'My bright young men concluded that perhaps three percent of the citizens living in their towns knew they were doing something that might be important. One-fiftieth of one percent could have understood what it signified.

> 'With television and our good magazines, a few people will know about our visit to Saturn, but of one thing you can be sure. As in the case of Copernicus and Newton, everyone who ought to know will know, and the reverberations of these next few days will echo through eternity, reappearing from time to time in manifestations that would astonish you.'

The final two days of waiting were as pleasant as any that Mott had known, for scores of his honored associates flew in to exchange greetings of great warmth. Carl Sagan was there in the flush of his enormous success; Bradford Smith, with his cool assessment of the images that were already arriving; John Pope, keeping somewhat to himself—the masters of this little world of knowing men and women.

'Here's a close-up of Titan, men, and what a hell of a lot of speculation goes down the drain with this one.'

Titan, largest of the Saturn moons, was the only one in the entire solar system with an atmosphere comparable in any way to Earth's and of a size sufficiently large and solid to warrant speculation that living beings might inhabit it. In science fiction it was already a populated center of extreme sophistication; in reality it was a gaseous concentration not much denser than water, and as one disgruntled astronomer said, 'If people are living there, they've got gills that can handle methane-hydrogen.'

A flood of color pictures was constructed, and even men who knew Saturn well gasped at the beauty of those heavenly rings, perhaps the most stunning sight in the planetary system; inherent in whatever force created that intricate halo was the artistry of a Michelangelo or a Picasso, for it was a work of art, as Mott explained in his briefing:

'The rings are very wide, but extremely thin, perhaps not more than half a mile. They're composed of ice chunks varying in size from BB shot to cubes as large as a boxcar. They're kept in place by gravity, of course. Saturn is an immense giant who draws things to him, but they're also kept in line by disciplining satellites which patrol the edges.

'How did the ice form? Speculation is infinite, but I incline to support the theory that elements which should have coalesced into a moon failed to do so, but you'll hear more about that at the roundtable tomorrow. I will give you one piece of reassuring news. We've run Saturn through the most advanced computers available to us, and we find that chunks of ice in varying sizes circulating around a planet like this will remain ice, in stable condition, for not less than five billion years, which covers the probable age of Saturn. You see, there is nothing to sublimate them, nothing to abrade them. They just circulate for five billion years.'

The part of the fly-by that Mott enjoyed most came when the newest pictures, corrected and enhanced by Template's wizards, were flashed on a large screen while a panel of the world's greatest astronomers made their original, free-wheeling guesses as to what these new data signified. Now these cautious scholars could not spend months in their laboratories running checks and eliminating ideas that were physically impractical. Now they stood alone on the frontier of thought, parading their ignorance, illuminating the room with their intuitive brilliance. For a brief, beautiful moment in time they and Saturn were co-conspirators regarding the great mysteries of the universe, and sometimes the room became electric with ideas that would reverberate for years to come; a few would prove accurate; others would be knocked quickly apart; none would have been useless.

Great Saturn, wreathed in icy glory, seemed to move majestically through the room, but not in awe-filled aloofness. These men were living with the planet, wrestling with its secrets, and once when Template posted a peculiarly mottled view of one of the moons, Brad Smith blurted out: 'I've seen a pizza that looked better than that.'

On the last afternoon as Mott was leaving Von Karaman Hall, where the convocations were held, he was accosted by a group of astronomy students from nearby universities who had come with their professors to participate in the fly-by. 'Are you the Dr. Mott who did those four seminal papers back in the late 1950s on the nature of the upper atmosphere?' Mott was delighted that young people should remember who he was: 'You know, I did those papers long before I had my Ph.D.'

This surprised the young people, who asked if they could talk with him, and after a while he was joined by an elderly professor from Stanford. Then the students spotted John Pope as he was leaving the hall; they cornered him, and there they sat in the fading sunlight, three older men of proved reputation, some sixteen young scholars beginning their careers, all abrim with excitement about a massive planet and a little spacecraft a billion miles away.

'If I were a teacher, how could I explain to my students that although Saturn has a density much less than that of water and only a gaseous structure, it doesn't just drain away?'

Some of the students laughed, but the old professor stopped them. 'That's one of the profoundest questions in astronomy, and unless your students appreciate its complexity, they'll never comprehend the easier difficulties. Start this way. Look at a globe of the Earth in good colors, and spend about a week trying to understand why the oceans do not, as you say, "just drain away." It's not easy to answer that question.'

'How do you answer it?'

'You know, I'm familiar with every equation in the book, and I know all about gravity and the tides caused by the Moon, but I'm damned if I can give you an articulate explanation.'

'How do you handle it?'

'Years ago I told myself, "You idiot! Anyone can see they do stay in place." And I accepted that.'

John Pope volunteered: 'In the Navy when we tried to identify men who had the capacity to become really good navigators—we needed hundreds of them—we'd put them all in a room and show them a globe, just like the professor said. And we pointed to where they were at that time, that meridian, and we said, "You know it's four o'clock here. Look at your watches. And we also know it's only three o'clock in the next time zone, and two o'clock in Denver, and one o'clock in Los Angeles and eleven o'clock in Hawaii." We took them all around the globe and showed them that we were ahead of every other place. But then we said, "But you know from news broadcasts that London is actually five hours ahead of us. Yet we just proved we're nineteen hours ahead of London. How can those two contradictory things be true?" We let them stew in this for a while, the way we had stewed when we began, until one of us said, "Isn't it clear that somewhere you have to institute an international date line?" When you reach there, this silly round robin ends and you start with new definitions.'

'That's brilliant,' one of the students said enthusiastically, taking mental notes.

'You haven't heard my point,' Pope said. 'We would stand at the front of the room and watch the faces of the plebes. Some of them, when their minds grasped this magnificently simple solution, lit up like light bulbs. They could become navigators. Others sat in absolute perplexity. They would never make it. They could become good gunners, or aviation experts, but they'd never make navigators, because you either understand the international date line or you don't, and if you don't, I'm powerless to explain it to you.'

Lights went on in several faces. 'Why didn't someone explain it that way before?'

They asked Pope what he had experienced in space for which he had been intellectually unprepared, and without hesitation he said, 'Gravity was nothing. We were prepared for that. And we expected the reimposition of gravity when we neared the Moon. But what blew my mind was the fact that when we left the shadow of the Earth and before we reached the shadow of the Moon, we had sunlight twenty-four hours a day on one side of our trajectory and perpetual night on the other side. I had somewhat anticipated this, but even so, I had not realized that almost all the stars in the sky would be permanently visible. There they were, an entire sphere, except for a region around the Sun. It was quite awesome to me, but when I pointed it out to Claggett, he said, "The Galaxy would be in poor shape if they weren't there." '

'How did you occupy yourself? Coming back down to Earth?'

The old professor would not permit this question. 'You must break the habit, in your thought if not in your speech, of saying "up to the Moon" or "back down to Earth" or "up to the stars." There is no *up* or *down,* no *above* or *below.* There is only *out to* and *back from* in reference to the center of the Earth. If you use the plane of the Galaxy as reference, we're clearly off the central axis, but whether we're up or down, who knows? I don't even like the phrase *out to the edge of the universe.* We may be the edge, so that everything we see exists between us and the opposite edge. More likely, the edge is everywhere, for I think that space is without direction or definition. You can't express it in words, I suppose, but you must induce that concept among your students, for otherwise they can never become astronomers.'

'Look!' one of the girl students cried. 'Saturn itself!' And there in the sky in close conjunction with blazing Jupiter and Venus, the ancient planet appeared, its magical rings not visible to the unaided eye, but its mysterious beauty magisterial. The old men who would be quitting their studies soon and the young who would be taking over stared at the planet with only a little more comprehension than that possessed by the Assyrians four thousand years earlier.

'Bits of ice no larger than those you use in a cocktail shaker. They don't melt in five billion years. We could use some down here.'

'Over here,' the old professor corrected.

His last big job for NASA completed, Mott slept that night without nightmares, and while shaving next morning he understood why: The Space Shuttle carried men, and that made us cautious. Voyager 2 carried only the minds of men, and they can be adventurous. A ray of sunlight coming through the window and throwing a shadow across his bed made a rude cross, and he cried, 'How profound the legend of Jesus is. His body died on the Cross, and that signified little, either to Him or His world. But His mind, what He thought, triumphed and reverberated forever.'

When he turned on the news he got instead an early-morning religious program, and a man he knew well was orating: 'This is Reverend Leopold Strabismus of your United Scripture Alliance.' Mott listened with attention as the preacher spelled out a splendid theory of salvation and the restructuring of a broken life; it was generous, loving and curiously reassuring. In exaggerated Southern accent Strabismus offered a sounder doctrine than most psychiatrists, and he did so with a personal conviction that won even Dr. Mott, for some of the things he said about the love that parents ought to feel for their children were directly applicable to the Mott family.

He spoiled his sermon, Mott thought, by two errors: he appealed four times for contributions, which Mott's father would never have dared, and in his peroration he shouted that what his listeners must do to attain salvation was to turn their backs on godless science and atheistic humanism and come back to the clear, simple teachings of Jesus. He then repeated three times the addresses of those California legislators who would be voting on his bill to drive the teaching of evolution and geology from state-supported schools.

Since Mott had some hours before his plane left, he thought it might be profitable to inspect what Strabismus called his United Scripture Alliance. Remembering roughly where it was, he reached the building once occupied by the University of Space and Aviation. He discovered it to be occupied by Mexicans, who explained: 'Reverend Strabismus sold us the building. We use it as our Chicano Center.' When Mott asked where Strabismus functioned, the pretty Mexican secretary said, 'He has a big church out in the country,' and she handed him a nicely printed map showing the route to the United Scripture Alliance and a message: 'All who seek the Light of God will be welcome.'

The map led him to a handsome mesa north of Pasadena, where Strabismus, with the large funds contributed by his radio and television audience, had built a series of structures which delighted the eye, for he had chosen the best architects in the region and had urged them to be daring and inventive. Dominating the area was the Temple of USA, a bold and comprehensive designation, and around it stood eleven low, strong buildings of the University of Spiritual Americans. The first building, however, which one encountered on entering the grounds, pertained to both the temple and the university: the Office of Perpetual Giving.

Mott went in and asked the very attractive young woman serving as hostess whether he might speak with Reverend Strabismus.

'I'm so sorry, sir, but he's not in California.'

'I just heard him on television.'

'That was taped. He leaves us eight pre-recordings whenever he goes on a trip.'

'Where is he? If that's not secret information.'

'Heavens, no!' the woman said with a disarming smile. 'He's meeting with the President today, then flying to the big campaign in the state of Fremont.'

'What's the campaign about?'

'A group of determined atheistic humanists is trying to overturn the law we passed some years ago.'

'The one that outlawed the teaching of evolution?'

'Yes.'

'I'm a school-board member, and I have reason to think that we have on our staff teachers who are humanists . . . who are teaching evolution subversively, as it were. Have you any literature that might provide me with ammunition?'

'We have indeed!' and she led him to a library room in which some dozen pamphlets and three more-substantial books were available to the inquiring public. Mott chose three pamphlets explaining how to launch local campaigns against teachers, elected officials and college professors suspected of being humanists, and a book called *How to Detect a Humanist.*

'That will be four dollars,' the hostess said.

'I thought the pamphlets were free.'

'Nothing is free.'

'How's the campaign in Fremont going?'

'It's a real struggle. They've done a disgraceful thing. Dredged up a former professor named Anderssen, so old they have to lift him onto the platform, and he rants about freedom of the mind.'

'They'll do anything,' Mott said, and as he left he reflected on the sardonic fact that the Temple grounds lay in an area marked by the historic observatory on Mount Wilson, from which the early photographs of galaxies had come to set minds ablaze; the California Institute of Technology, where some of the most unorthodox thinking in the world had taken place (speculation on the nature of the universe); and those centers of error, UCLA and USC. And he thought: Strabismus ought to cleanse his own backyard. All those scientific humanists down there staring at Saturn.

Stanley Mott was in for a shock when he watched Reverend Strabismus in action during the agitated campaign in Fremont, for the popular clergyman was even more rotund than before, a bearded three hundred pounds, and certainly more urbane and relaxed. He did not shout like some Old Testament prophet, nor did he display any animosity toward the atheistic humanists he was striving to eliminate from public life. He was reasonable, intelligent and persuasive, with uncanny skill in touching exposed nerves of national life. And he was remorseless in his hammer blows against science:

> 'Are you any happier because men claimed they walked on the Moon? Are your bills at the grocery store any lower? Are your children any better-behaved? Are you pleased that these crazy doctors in London can make babies in test tubes? Or that abortionists are free to run rampant in this here land? Are you safer in your homes because some knee-jerk liberal wants to take away your right to have your own gun?

> 'Where has evolution and fossils in the rocks and Pleistocene-Meistocene got you but into deep trouble? I'll tell you where science has got you—into the pigpen with the other animals.

> 'But I bring you release from all that. I tell you what you know in your hearts, that there's only one true way. Throw out these evil humanists. Get rid of their corruptin' textbooks. Bring God back into the schools and make this a decent country once again.'

Mott was surprised to learn that Reverend Strabismus and his wife were staying at the home of Senator Grant, up in Clay, and he followed the evangelist from town to town until the entourage of speakers, singers, trumpet players and Chimp-Champ-Chump reached the college town. The senator, hearing that Mott was in the neighborhood, invited him to dinner one night, and the occasion could have become an icy one because Mott launched right into the fatuities of the campaign.

'It's amusing that I should be here,' he said in his precise way. 'I mean, in this particular house. Because some years ago the senator gave me a commission in this very room. "Go out and see what that rascal has done to my daughter." I went, and I saw a brilliant young man making—'

'Please!' the senator interrupted, and with a nod of his head toward a largely inert mass sitting opposite him, he indicated that nothing must be said about the little green men of the past that might agitate his wife.

'How did you make the transition, Reverend Strabismus, from science fiction to religion?'

'God called me.'

'Did God also call Jim Jones of Guyana? And Reverend Moon?'

'Individual persons turn sour in every calling. Look at the mad scientists of fiction.'

'Yes, but my mad scientists are in fiction. Dr. Jekyll, Dr. Frankenstein. Yours occur in real life.'

'You asked me how I made the transition. In response to the heart cries of the American people. They were sick with a great malady, Dr. Mott, one caused by you scientists.'

'You're an extremely brilliant fellow, Strabismus. I've studied your record since those days at New Paltz and—' Again Senator Grant indicated that nothing must be said which would upset his wife, so Mott changed his tone abruptly. 'In public you speak like an illiterate hillbilly. Here you sound like Socrates . . . or better, Savonarola.'

'I have what you don't have, Dr. Mott. An acute sense of what the American public seeks. The vote in this state will prove it. They seek assurance from a simple man. They seek clarification, simplification, a return to historic ideals, the safety of the religion their grandfathers knew, cleansed of Darwin and Einstein and all that rubbish. They seek security, and they know instinctively that this comes from simple men like me, not atheistic scientists like you.'

'I suppose you know my father was a Methodist minister.'

'You've strayed a long way from his teaching.'

'I sometimes think I'm carrying it forward. Don't you see, Strabismus, if the things we're discovering are so extraordinary, so infinitely wonderful, isn't it likely that the force which created them was Himself a scientist?'

'Don't refer to God as force. He is God, exactly as the Book of Genesis states.'

'That's what my father taught me to believe.'

'Then why, in brazen disobedience to God's statements, do you teach children lies about dinosaurs and geology and evolution?'

'Because the record is before me . . . in the rocks . . . the relationships.'

'On the day of Creation, God placed those fossils in the rocks. He laid down the layers of rock to instruct us.'

'I refuse to believe that God is a trickster.'

'He is a Creator whose intention we are not allowed to penetrate.'

'You claim that He spent His energy putting together this jigsaw puzzle —the fossil fish high in the mountains, the dinosaur bones in a hundred varied locations, the geological strata. Isn't it infinitely grander to believe that He started everything with a mighty bang, let's say eighteen billion years ago, and then allowed His grand design to work itself out . . . according to the rules inherent in what He threw into the universe?'

'Once you start down that road, you find yourself with evolution and the claim that my Chimp-Champ-Chump was your grandfather.'

'You prefer to believe that God was a jokester?'

'He was the Creator. He began everything on one glorious day.'

'But if the entire record of the Earth drives us inescapably back . . .'

'You've lost your battle, Dr. Mott. And we've won. Regardless of how the referendum goes next month in Fremont—I mean, even if your forces of evil do revoke our law forbidding evolution—we've won the battle. Why? Because our people dominate the committees that select schoolbooks for California and Texas, and what the big states do, the little ones will have to follow. Atheistic science is being driven right out of our textbooks. Soon you won't dare show a fossil or a dinosaur, and you won't be able to preach your atheistic evolution. So what does it matter what a state like New

Mexico does? The corrupt New York publishers must print their books for sale in California and Texas, and that means they have to print them according to what we say. Your kind of science is dead in these two big states, which automatically makes it dead in New Mexico and Vermont, too.'

'So if I wrote a science book that showed fossils and spoke of dinosaurs roaming this area thirty million years ago . . .'

'It would be obviously false, because the world did not exist thirty million years ago. It couldn't have. It was created not more than six thousand years ago with the dinosaur bones and all that in place.'

'Is it true that your people have halted all geology lectures in the national parks?'

'A national park is a national schoolbook, and what we teach children in California we certainly teach their parents in Yellowstone and Grand Canyon.'

'Not long ago I put a little boy on an airplane for his summer vacation in Germany. His parents insisted that he learn honest science, not the mishmash you're prescribing. Do you fear the day when our best young people will have to flee to Europe to get a real education?'

'Dr. Mott, we have a committee right now compiling a dossier on the evils done to this nation by Rhodes scholars who came home with corrupt ideas. Fulbright of Arkansas, Sarbanes of Maryland, Carl Albert of who knows where, this man Bradley of New Jersey. If you ask me, I think they're all Communists. So you tell your boy who went to Germany to mark his ways, because when he comes back here, we're going to watch him.'

'Do you ever suspect that you're becoming the Jim Jones of the mind? That your ultimate effect—'

'Gentlemen,' Senator Grant interrupted. 'We're getting nowhere with this debate. Dr. Mott is a distinguished scientist, Reverend Strabismus is a leader in this nation. I believe there's room for both.'

'We need scientists to invent new medicines,' Strabismus conceded. 'Build better airplanes. But not to dabble in ultimate things like Creation.'

'That's where the trail ends,' Mott said.

The talk now turned to Mrs. Grant, who broke her long silence. 'I'm so pleased to have Marcia with us again. Is California very hot?'

'Probably the best climate in the world,' Marcia said. She was forty-two and almost radiantly beautiful; standing with her husband on a platform, she presented the reassuring image of a supportive wife whose sole interest was the promotion of his good work. She obviously enjoyed her role, and now spoke enthusiastically about it. 'You know, Dr. Mott, Leopold and I live very simply. We do have that imposing temple that you spoke about, but things like that and the university are built with funds placed in our hands by a believing public. We spend very little on ourselves.'

'The private airplane?'

'It belongs to a generous businessman who supports our work.'

'Your Mercedes?'

'We do move about.'

'How did you handle your old building? The one you were in when I visited you?'

'We sold it to a Mexican church for one dollar.'

'Is that true, Strabismus?'

'We're very strong in the Mexican community because of that. One dollar, when we might have sold it for one million.'

'Dr. Mott,' Mrs. Grant protested, 'you keep asking the Reverend difficult questions. You must stop.'

'I shall.'

'I've known Reverend Strabismus for many years now, even before Marcia knew him. And he has always been a bringer of light.' She reached out to touch his arm. 'If you ask me, it was only his tireless statesmanship that prevented the Strangers from taking over our government, although I was assured by their messengers that Norman would be kept on in government.'

Mott looked straight ahead, but then the senator said something which jolted him: 'From what the voters in Fremont tell me, I'm afraid we went too far too fast with the Moon business.'

'In your evangelism the other night, Strabismus, you said something about NASA "claiming to have reached the Moon." What possibly could you have meant?'

Instead of trying to defend himself, Strabismus leaned forward eagerly to explain. 'A lot of people in this country believe we never got to the Moon. They believe it was all a government hoax, and I was speaking to reassure them.'

'So you gather all the mind-weary dissidents—the anti-everythings—and you build a great constituency. And one day you'll find yourself the new Jim Jones . . . but in a more devastating arena.'

In a frail voice Mrs. Grant said, 'I wish we could retreat from all of this unpleasantness about schoolbooks and monkey grandfathers and women's rights and people who want to take away our guns. I wish we could erase it all and go back to the simpler life I knew in this house with my father. Reverend Strabismus, you must rescue that simpler life for us.'

In the brief silence that followed, Mott reflected that this good woman had seen space and been repelled by it. As the wonder-machines leaped into the air at Canaveral, probing ever outward, extending the dimensions of the comprehensible universe, she had intentionally contracted the perimeters of her world, making it ever smaller and easier to control. And he concluded that all persons are obligated to wrestle with the universe as they perceive it, and those who are terrified by the prospect retreat to little corners from which they seek to destroy the machines doing the outward probing and the men who manage them.

Senator Grant had perceived space only as a battleground on which to humiliate the Russians, who had done their best to humiliate us, and when that struggle was resolved, with Americans on the Moon and the Russians flopping about a hundred and ten miles above the Earth, he had retired from the great adventure. Indeed, he had turned his back on space and had voted against any major new appropriations. John Pope had performed better than anyone still living, but once he attained his limited objective, the Moon, he had retired to obscurity. Ed Cater had flown his two flights with distinction, but had retreated to a real estate office in his hometown. Lovely Inger Jensen had given her husband to the program and then fled to the sanctuary of a library in Oregon. Mott's own sons had been engulfed, but good old Debby Dee had guzzled her gin and handled space as easily as she had mastered her husband's rusted Chevrolets.

And how had he, Mott, met the challenge? Always he had tried to extend the frontier, first in Germany, where he knew he must rescue those Peenemünde men or see America go down the tubes, then at Wallops Island, where he had explored the farthest atmosphere, then in the Apollo program, and finally at the doors of Saturn. He had made an honest effort, but listening to how Reverend Strabismus was marshaling the nation against his principles, he suspected that he might have been fighting the wrong battle.

Dieter Kolff was wrong, he said to himself as the others chatted. He believed that with a rocket big enough, man could do anything. But he failed to protect himself against the frightened people who would always want to destroy the rocket. I suppose that's the historic failure of the Germans. They worship the machine but not the man who runs it. Maybe Strabismus is right. Keep the citizens ignorant. Burn the books that might distress or agitate them. Convince them that the truth lies elsewhere than in the questing human mind.

His reflections were broken by Mrs. Grant, who said, 'I think it's so wonderful, Reverend Strabismus, that you and Marcia will be able to vacation in Sweden after the vote.'

'Uppsala has been very good to me, Mrs. Grant. In all my literature I've referred to the happy years I spent there. Now I'm taking my wife to see those hallowed halls.'

'The real reason for our going,' Marcia divulged, 'is that Leopold is endowing a chair at Uppsala.'

'In what subject?' Mott asked, his mouth agape.

'The Strabismus Chair of Moral Philosophy,' Leopold said.

In the early spring of 1982 Penny Pope, working diligently in the Senate on the problems of NASA and refusing two superior appointments suggested by the new Reagan administration, reached two important decisions which she longed to discuss with her husband, so she arranged for herself a trip to NASA installations in the West, then telephoned John at the university, suggesting that he fly to Washington and help drive the Buick back to Clay. 'I know it's an imposition, John, but I enjoy nothing in life more than riding with you when we have a chance for long talks.' Since he felt the same way, he leaped at the invitation, arranged substitutes for his classes, and breezed into her apartment ready to go. They had dinner that night at a Chinese restaurant, went to bed early, and awakened at 0400 the next morning. Within ten minutes they were in the car, heading west over the mountains on Route 50.

They covered their customary seven hundred miles that first day, but the driving was not what commanded their attention; a long, passionate conversation did:

PENNY: I've been keeping an eye on Senator Grant. He's senile.

JOHN: Wait!

PENNY: I'll not wait any longer. He's senile.

JOHN: Like what?

PENNY: Like he can't follow a conversation. Like he gives the same speech on every occasion, regardless of the question.

JOHN: Those criteria would classify half the Senate as senile.

PENNY: But he could do so much good with his seniority.

JOHN: He's got a good record. He can get reelected as often as he wishes.

PENNY: He's not got a good record. He gives Reagan no creative assistance.

JOHN: I doubt if Reagan wants any. Grant votes the straight ticket, and that's all that's required.

PENNY: So much more, so very much more . . .

JOHN: Norman Grant will never supply that. He was never inclined that way. Your senator is a place-filler.

PENNY: He was a glorious leader in the space movement.

JOHN: Some men have only one contribution. Look at the astronauts who made only one flight. They still counted.

PENNY: But we can't settle for mere place-fillers. The times deserve something better.

JOHN: We could do worse.

PENNY: I've concluded that Norman Grant has got to go.

JOHN: You concluded?

PENNY: I'm a citizen. I'm a voter in his district. Yes, I concluded.

JOHN: And whom are you backing to beat him?

PENNY: You.

JOHN (almost driving off the road): That's fatuous.

PENNY: Not at all. Before you say another word let me get the facts on record. Barring a precious handful, John, you're much abler right now than most of the senators. Birch Bayh knew his way around, but he's down the tube. Strom Thurmond may be the ablest manipulator on the floor. I could name half a dozen other really powerful men who do a fantastic job. But the grand average? John, men like you and Hickory Lee surpass them in every direction. Grant must go, and you must challenge him in the primaries.

JOHN: Let me lay it out clear and strong. I'm not a politician. I'm not ambitious along those lines. I doubt even if I have the capacity. But the overwhelming fact is that Norman Grant got me into Annapolis. He saved my life the way he saved the lives of those three men who come back each year—

PENNY: John! Don't speak of those obscene men in their bulging uniforms. They're a disgrace to American politics.

JOHN: So if Grant saved my life—

PENNY: He did nothing of the sort, John. You were appointed to Annapolis because you did such a great job as an enlisted man.

JOHN: He saved my life. He sponsored me. I helped him get elected, and I owe him a debt forever. I will not run against him.

PENNY: Will you grant me one thing? That he's become a doddering old fool?

JOHN: I will not. He's a United States senator and worthy of the dignity.

PENNY: He's a busted record, and the cracks are echoing like dynamite explosions.

JOHN: I could never make a move against Norman Grant.

The conversation continued along these obdurate lines through Ohio and well into Indiana, with Penny marshaling a wealth of evidence proving Grant's deficiencies and John refusing to concede that the man should be defeated in that spring's primary.

JOHN: You're crazy if you think any insurgent can knock Norman Grant out of the box. The whole Republican party would rally to his defense.

PENNY: The Republican party is like any other party. It goes with the winner.

JOHN: The primary is ten weeks off. When does a challenger have to submit his nomination—a couple of weeks from now, isn't it?

PENNY: Tuesday of next week.

JOHN: And you think you're going to find some sacrificial lamb . . . How much money do you think you can collect to fight the power that Grant would have?

PENNY: Money, nominations, petitions—they all fall into place the minute you say you'll run. John, I've been testing the waters.

JOHN: In Washington, not Fremont.

PENNY: Most of Fremont that counts is in Washington. And they know to a man that Norman Grant is finished. He's run his course, John. He's a dodo. He's a plum ripe for picking.

JOHN: Let's stop this right now. Under no conceivable way in the world will I make a move against a man who's been my friend. You learn that in the astronaut program, and you learn it deep.

PENNY: We'll discuss it tomorrow in Illinois.

It was not until they were leaving Abraham Lincoln's state that she launched her most persuasive argument. She was driving at the time and they'd had a nine-o'clock breakfast of pancakes and sausage, a murderous meal except when one was driving all day without lunch.

PENNY: You're a military man, John. I want to talk strategy, not tactics. If you don't make your move now, some other good Republican will. He'll get his foot in the door, and by the next election in 1988 he'll be unbeatable. Your grand opportunity will be gone.

JOHN: I've told you before, I will not—

PENNY: Listen to my most important point. By 1988 Norman Grant will be a basket case. Anyone will be able to beat him, if he doesn't retire before then. The decision has to be made this year, to protect your position in 1988.

JOHN: As long as Grant wants the seat—

PENNY: Let's suppose you're right. Let's suppose that Grant is unbeatable this year. The strategy is to establish yourself as his inevitable successor. You do that by challenging him now. By conducting a high-level campaign. I'm positive that you can win even this year. In 1988 it'll be a lead-pipe cinch.

JOHN: Let Grant make the decisions. My sense of honor will not allow me to—

PENNY: If the Republican committee came to you?

JOHN: I'd have to tell them no.

PENNY: John, I think you underestimate yourself. You're an authentic American hero. Everyone in the country knows you.

JOHN: Everyone in America doesn't vote in Fremont.

PENNY: Everyone in Fremont loves you. You have an enormous capital to draw upon. You're electable. And you sit here and fritter away—

JOHN: Why are you so concerned about a Senate seat?

PENNY: Because I'm a patient in that dreadful Washington hospital.

JOHN: What do you mean?

PENNY: I'm infected with the incurable disease. Capitalitis.

JOHN: I've suspected this for some time. You don't want to come home?

PENNY: They made a study some years ago. One hundred ex-senators. Some had been defeated in primaries, some in the general, some had withdrawn voluntarily. But of the hundred, ninety-three were still in Washington, one thing or another. One of the men from Phoenix said it best. 'Me go back to Arizona? Are you nuts?' When you're in Washington you see the wheels go round. And sometimes you can give them a nudge.

JOHN: Then why don't you accept that judgeship they keep talking about?

PENNY: It was the Carter administration that did the talking. Glancey convinced them I was a Democrat.

JOHN: What are you, really?

PENNY: In 1982 I'd be dumb if I wasn't a Republican.

JOHN: You know, Penny, when NASA got the six families together that first time at Cocoa Beach, I had a strong feeling that you and I had the best marriage of all. I love you very much. More every year as we grow older. You have a lot of pizazz.

PENNY: I'm so proud of you I could burst. You've really hewn your log to a very straight line, John. Ain't many like you, kiddo. That's why I want to see you senator.

JOHN: Impossible.

Their incessant arguing slowed down their driving, so they slept that night in eastern Missouri, where they had Mexican food, made some phone calls, and went to a movie, but as they drove through the early morning on the last day, Penny returned to her basic theme:

PENNY: John, I'm asking you for the last time. Will you declare for the United States Senate?

JOHN: I cannot.

PENNY: This is dreadfully serious, John. I must repeat. Will you run?

JOHN: No.

She swung the car abruptly off the main highway, sought a gas station, and went inside to make a series of phone calls. When she returned, a handsome, strong-willed lawyer of fifty-five, well versed in the ways of Washington, she announced calmly as she swung the car back onto the road: 'I have asked my people to inform the papers and the television immediately. I'm entering the Republican primary for the Senate.'

Captain John Pope, USN (retired), slumped in the right-hand seat of the Buick as it sped toward the Fremont state line and wondered what he should say. If Penny had authorized her people to release the announcement, she would not be deterred now, and his mind twisted and turned, trying vainly to hit upon the right comment. That he would support her, there could be no doubt; she was his wife and he was extremely proud of her accomplishments. He knew her to be one of the best women in America, forceful but loving, hard as nails where principle was concerned but gentle in her personal relationships, and very bright. Both Glancey and Grant had told him at different times, 'Pope, your wife is just as important to our space program as you are. Because she knows where the bodies are buried.'

And yet, as a man of honor he would have to make his apologies to Norman Grant, and if asked, state in public that he knew Grant to be a splendid citizen and a good public servant worthy of reelection. It was going to be a difficult spring in the state of Fremont during the Republican primaries.

His mind then turned to the matter of living arrangements, and he concluded that practically nothing would change—he would remain in Clay and she in Washington, or wherever. They were a Navy family, accustomed to prolonged separations, and he knew they could hack it, as enlisted men said when unpleasant jobs lay ahead, for they always had. And then, smiling quietly as he glanced sideways while Penny roared down the highway, chin forward, he thought of the perfect thing to say: 'Penny, when I flew Gemini with Claggett, I sat in the right-hand seat. I can do so again.'

They arrived in Clay at eleven in the morning, and Penny drove directly to the home of the man who had been working quietly in behalf of John Pope for Senator, and there John received a lesson in practical politics, for a committee of nine awaited Penny's arrival. They had before them some sixteen nominating petitions covering all parts of the state, and all signed on behalf of John Pope, who was refusing to run. The chairman's wife had carefully typed in a Mrs. before the original candidate's name, then, following it: (Penny Hardesty).

'That's illegal as hell,' John exclaimed. 'They signed for one person, and you change it to another.'

'Not without permission,' the chairman said. 'We spent all last night calling every signer and getting permission to switch.'

When he looked at Penny, standing erect in the doorway, smiling, neat, suit presentable after three days of travel, he had for the first time a fleeting suspicion that she might really carry this thing off, and when he left the meeting, alone, to report to Senator Grant at the big house on the edge of town he received another jolt—two, in fact.

The first concerned Mrs. Grant, who appeared at the door to let him in. She did not recognize him, even though he was probably the best-known man in town and one she saw frequently, and when she led him toward her husband's study it was as if she were in an unknown house. She asked him if she could count on his support in the referendum regarding evolution, which was a pernicious theory destructive of human dignity, and he did not bother to remind her that the vote had been taken months ago and that her side had won.

The second shock came after Senator Grant had listened courteously to the explanation of how Penny had come to file for his seat and why Pope had told her that he could not in decency oppose a man who had done so much for him, who had been, indeed, a kind of father.

Grant laughed almost raucously. 'Pope! You miss the whole point. Penny's not got a chance of beating me this year. But she'll get her name known. She'll show the central committee she's a real contender. I think the world of that girl, and in 1988, when I certainly won't run again, she'll be in the front row. The very front row. And unless this nation falls to hell, she'll be United States Senator from Fremont. You go out there with my blessing, John, and give her every support. Because when I do step down, six years from now, I'll want somebody good in my place, and she's the one I'd choose.'

Exactly what Penny told me in Illinois, Pope thought. But I'd better not tell Grant she'd had him figured out so neatly. Also, there was the unsettled question: Did Penny mean it when she said so vehemently that Grant could be defeated? Was this primary to be the real thing?

There was another election which intruded before the Fremont primary. In the Colorado ski resort of Skycrest, the business promoters, the shopkeepers and the lodge managers wanted a shift in the political governance of the place: 'We have special needs which require special solutions. We're not dryland farmers raising Herefords.' By common consent they settled upon Millard Mott as their level-headed candidate: 'He knows business. He knows what it is to pay taxes. And look what he's done with his own shop.'

In a town that had once been mainly Democratic, the conservative Republicans offered Millard as their candidate, and although there was minor talk about the way his brother had been killed in Florida, it was agreed in the community that this should not be held against him. Also, the fact that he lived with this chap Roger, who had been a draft dodger, was ignored. Nor did the opposition make much headway with the charge that Millard had himself been a Canadian goose: 'Didn't he fly north?'

'He did, but everyone knows the Vietnam war was a shitty affair. Maybe he was just brighter than us stupid sonsabitches who went.'

He was elected by a huge majority, and at his thank-you party, catered by Roger and the college girls at the ski shop, he promised Skycrest: 'What everybody wants—more services, more police, more ski patrols, better roads and lower taxes. I hope somebody here will tell me how to do it.'

In June 1982 Professor John Pope heard with pleasure that NASA was thinking of assigning his friend Hickory Lee, last of the Solid Six, to command the fourth flight of the Shuttle. He would carry it to heights not attempted before, where various scientific instruments would be placed in orbit and checked during an extended extra-vehicular activity. The Shuttle was now a workhorse, and Lee would join that restricted group of astronauts who had flown in three radically different types of craft—in his case, Apollo, Skylab and Shuttle. None had flown in four different types, and as the program was working out, none ever could.

A much more personal surprise came on a bright morning when Senator Norman Grant, in the heat of his campaign for renomination to the Senate, announced that he would hold a press conference at noon sharp, and he telephoned Pope to ask if he would attend. John supposed that the surprising closeness of the primary, with Penny doing much better than predicted, had frightened the senator into a last-minute spurt, and that Grant was going to ask him for an endorsement.

Penny was in the southern part of the state, where she was amassing unexpected support, but he was able to reach her by phone: 'Darling, the damned pullets have come back to roost. Senator Grant is pressuring me for an endorsement.'

'We decided long ago you'd give it.'

'I'll have to. I'll simply have to. But it'll be very guarded. And, darling, I'll fly out to Calhoun this afternoon, Phil will take me in his plane. I'll appear on the platform with you tonight, and I'll speak. If you want to win this primary, I want you to win it, too.'

'I do want to win. And I do want your help.' Then she said brightly, 'Don't you see, John? If Grant feels he needs your endorsement, he knows he's in trouble.'

Satisfied that he had cleared this ticklish problem with his wife, Pope went to his university office, where a tough politico from Webster was awaiting him: 'Professor, does your wife really want to win this primary?'

'She sure does!'

'She's not just goin' through the motions?'

'Penny never goes through motions.'

'My wife is a trained nurse.'

'What's that got to do with the primary?'

'Plenty. She works with doctors. She listens.'

'Where's she work? Sit down, please.'

'She works in Webster General. But one of her doctors, a Dr. Schreiber, is a specialist who flies about the West on heavy missions.' He paused to allow this to take its effect, then said, 'Three days ago he flew here to Clay Municipal.' Another pregnant pause. 'His patient was Senator Grant's wife.'

'What about her?'

'She's in dreadful shape, according to the doctor. He treated her sickness and wouldn't say anything about that. But he did talk about her other behavior. The forgery. Signing the senator's name to a check. She's pumping money into the Strabismus crusade, the one in Alabama against Darwin and abortions and all that.'

'Forgery? Why would she commit forgery?'

'I don't know why. All my wife knows is that Senator Grant had to intervene to prevent the police—'

'Why did you come here to tell me this?'

'Because it makes Grant vulnerable. If your wife wants to really puncture that bag of wind . . .'

Pope did not lose his temper. This man was suggesting behavior that neither of the Popes would countenance or even remotely consider, but John had learned that politics produced all sorts of aberrations and the honorable man or woman looked at each as it was presented, accepting those that stood within limits, rejecting those that were outside the pale of decent behavior. Rising and placing his arm about the visitor's shoulder, he said quietly, 'My wife and I appreciate your interest, but this isn't the kind of private information that she would use. Thank your wife, and I hope you both continue to support Mrs. Pope.'

It was now forty-five minutes before the press conference, and Pope needed to clarify his thinking as to what exactly he could say in support of the man he still held to be a notable citizen, and this was difficult, for the campaign had proved that Grant really was doddering, lacking in focus and without any clear vision of the future. There had been a most painful night in the capital city of Benton, where the senator and Penny were to debate major issues; before the session Penny learned that Tim Finnerty was bringing Gawain Butler from his important job in California and Larry Penzoss from Alabama, and she went directly to Finnerty's hotel to confront him.

'Surely, Tim, you're not trotting out those miserable uniforms again?'

'They're the heart of his campaign. Voters love them.'

'Tim, that day is past. Believe me, if you three clowns get up on that stage—'

'The other two are not clowns. They're considerable heroes. Their stories—'

'Will make people yawn.'

'Why are you protesting? If it's a bad idea, as you say, you profit.'

'Nobody profits. Tim, if you do this, I'm going to have to rebut. I'll have to point out how silly the whole thing is.' Her jaw firmed. 'And I will, believe me, Tim, I will.'

The debate had not gone well for the senator, but Penny remembered that he was always best in his closing statements, when he drew upon patriotism, heroism and love of country to make telling points, the only ones that would be remembered when the night was over and the serious discussion forgotten. And sure enough, at the beginning of his peroration he signaled Finnerty, who marched out with Butler and Penzoss in their old uniforms. Unfortunately for Grant, the city of Benton contained three colleges, and students in the audience began to laugh, one black activist shouted 'Uncle Tom,' and suddenly the stage became a place of ridicule, and the heroic memory of those days adrift in October of 1944 seemed as remote as the Battle of Thermopylae.

Grant was confused. He had encountered student opposition during the bad days of Vietnam, when values were contorted, but now these young people were laughing at him and Gawain Butler and the heroic days when all values hung in the balance, and it was shocking. His opponent, Mrs. Pope, seemed to have tears in her eyes, and it was she who spoke:

> 'Students, stop that laughter. These four men, Senator Grant and his crew, were sensational heroes. The safety of our nation depended upon them, and I for one salute them. But I suspect you are right in believing that the day is past when we can rely only upon old

memories . . . old ideas . . . old ways of doing things. We need fresh spirit, fresh drives. Please try to get these conflicting good things straight in your mind. This nation needs some straight thinking.'

In her hotel room later that night she confided to her husband: 'I'm not proud of what I did tonight. What I should have done was machine-gun those little bastards for making fun of a profound idea. But I must say that I warned Finnerty not to carry his broken jugs back to that pathetic pump.' Tears came to her eyes. 'I was so sorry for Norman Grant. Did you see the shock on his face? He was facing a new generation, a whole new set of decades, and he hadn't a clue. John, he hasn't a clue and it will be God's mercy if I defeat him.'

Reluctantly, Pope left his office, and walked slowly to the campus building in which the press conference was to be held, still unsure of what he should say in view of the fact that later in Calhoun he was going to neutralize it. But when he entered the building and saw Norman Grant, big and handsome and very American, his heart went out to him: Best man this town ever produced. I'll help him win one more time. Penny can afford to wait.

But when Grant took the podium and adjusted the microphones, Pope received a shock: 'I am sorry that my talented opponent, Penny Pope, could not be here this morning. She's at work lambasting me in the southern part of the state, but I'm most pleased that her husband, our great hero John Pope, is with us.'

There was applause and someone nudged Pope, getting him to stand, and as he rose to acknowledge the cheers he thought: In for a penny, in for a pound. What a lousy pun.

'I've asked you here this morning,' Grant continued, 'to inform you that personal matters of the most urgent kind make it necessary for me to withdraw from the primary campaign. Those who know me will understand that this action does not come from fear of my worthy opponent, because I have faced others just as resolute. I am retiring from the fight for personal reasons which I can no longer ignore.

'I am relieved in this moment of great stress to know that I leave the field to one of the ablest people in America and one of the finest associates I have ever had, Penny Pope. We have worked together for thirty-six years, and no one in America is better qualified to give her a character reference than me.

'Mrs. Pope, you've won the Republican primary. Without question you'll win the November general, in which you'll have my fullest support. Astronaut John Pope, go out and help your wife get elected. She's worth it.'

When Pope finally reached his wife in a small town near the Kansas border, her first words were: 'John, get hold of Tim Finnerty before he leaves town. I want him for my campaign manager.' And when she was senator, she would want him as her chief of staff, because that crazy, Democrat, liberal, Boston-Irish-Catholic manipulator knew how the Senate operated and where the votes were. He had almost succeeded in making Norman Grant a first-rate senator; with better material, he might have better luck.

Stanley Mott was retired now, sixty-four years old and covered with the honors that came normally to a man of his competence; he had four honorary doctorates, awards from six learned societies, and invitations from across the country to speak on issues confronting the space program.

In his final days with NASA he had helped supervise two tremendous achievements: the launching of the Shuttle and the Voyager 2 fly-by of Saturn, and of the two, he had no hesitation in concluding that the latter was the more important, for it threw the mind of man forward to new horizons, and he had not interrupted when Dieter Kolff telephoned from Alabama:

'See what I told you, Stanley? The future of man in space is to build ever more capable machines and ever bigger rockets to launch them. We can go anywhere, you and I, and we don't need astronauts to clutter up the hardware. You devise a whole new family of instruments, marvels that can do anything. I'll build a new family of rockets that will land on Uranus and Neptune, and we can do this before we die.'

But he had also listened when Grant called from Clay:

'See what I told you, Mott? Practically no one noticed the Saturn thing. No men in the machine. But that Shuttle business with those two fine young men at the throttle . . . [Mott interrupted to remind Grant that John Young had been fifty-one.] Did you see how the world ate that up? Man is still the measure of all things, Mott, and you better remind your old buddies at NASA of that fact.'

Mott did not need to be reminded by Grant of the added value NASA received from a launch when men were aboard, and he conceded that years ago when he championed Kolff too strongly, NASA had been correct in disciplining him. Man is the measure of all things, he admitted to himself, but it matters greatly what he measures.

He worried about such matters because he had been nominated to receive the gold medal awarded occasionally by the three major scientific societies of the nation, and this obligated him to make a speech of some significance at the acceptance ceremonies. His whole thrust was toward the immaculate nature of science, especially since certain groups in many states were trying to outlaw it in their schools, and he knew well what he wanted to say in that respect, but he was deterred by things that Senator Grant and Reverend Strabismus were preaching: that man can absorb only so much abstract science, after which he reverts to a kind of childhood simplicity in which he rejects everything.

Are we the ones who are at fault? he asked himself. Have we failed to bring the world along with us? Why did Mrs. Grant retreat into her cocoon, denying everything that her husband stood for? Why does Strabismus receive such thundering approval when he turns the clock back? Stanley felt that the answer lay not in Mrs. Grant or Reverend Strabismus, but in men like himself who had blindly pursued their own narrowly defined interests while ignoring the vast, sloppy, stumbling universe of people who could not keep pace with the discoveries.

But he would make only limited concessions. The brilliant men and women of his age were pushing back the frontiers of knowledge, and if the general public was unable to keep up, that was a political matter; it must not be allowed to be an intellectual damper on the exploration itself. The Church had muzzled Copernicus, threatened Galileo and burned Bruno, but the truth about the position of the Earth in the planetary system had not been stifled. Today in America the television Ayatollahs and the Neanderthals in the Senate could force states to deny the palpable truths of science, and they could force that knowledge underground in some quarters, but they could not destroy the facts themselves. The Earth did revolve about the Sun; it was created about four and a half billion years ago; and dinosaurs had roamed the Earth in the periods cited.

More important to the present day, quasars and black holes did exist and they commanded the mind to explain them. As Mott said tentatively in the opening paragraphs of the speech he was preparing:

I am satisfied by all the evidence that reaches me that the mind of man stands now in much the position it stood at the beginning of the Copernican age. Ahead of us lies one of the world's major explosions of knowledge. Year by year the frontiers of the universe will be pushed ever outward by discoveries and interpretations which will dazzle the mind and force it to fashion new interpretations.

What our recent developments will produce in their train, not even the boldest of us can predict, but I am impressed by the fact that in 1938 President Roosevelt assembled the brightest scientists in America to the White House to help him envisage the things he might have to adjust to in the future.

'I want you to tell me what to expect,' he begged, and after three days of intense speculation these men, whose job it was to anticipate the future and who commanded more keys to that future than any other group, failed to predict atomic power, radar, rockets, jet aircraft, computers, xerography and penicillin, all of which were to burst upon the world within the next few years. They knew about the exploratory research, of course, but they could not believe it would produce functional products so soon. I assure you that if tonight you assembled an equal group of our most learned men, they would not anticipate the simple wonders which will engulf us by the year 2000.

His speculations were brought down to Earth when he learned, in his Washington office, that the Reverend Strabismus, in conjunction with several other religious leaders, had decided to launch a major campaign against homosexuality in American life and especially in public office. 'God created Adam and Eve, not Adam and Steve' became the battle cry, and they had decided to test their power in the Colorado ski community of Skycrest, which had just elected a notorious homosexual as mayor.

They would dispose of him, they said, as a warning to San Francisco, and they would do so by means of a recall referendum, an agency of policy they were finding to be of great value, since with television coverage they could persuade the American electorate to ratify anything. Mott felt obligated to fly out and assist his son, but he was little prepared for the vilification he would face. The campaign was horrible, with much citation of Leviticus 18 and 20, especially verse 13 of the latter. When Mott first heard Strabismus thunder on these texts he was shaken, for his father had taught him to take the Bible seriously:

'If a man also lie with mankind, as he lieth with a woman, both of them have committed an abomination: they shall surely be put to death.'

He pondered this for some days during the fiery debates when the clergymen tried to purify American politics, and he was so perplexed that he retired from the struggle, unsure of his moral position. His son Millard seemed a fine man in all respects save his sexual orientation, and Stanley had almost persuaded himself that a decent public life of service and the good report of one's neighbors counted more than an arbitrary condemnation by men like Reverend Strabismus, but this bald statement in the Bible lent great force to their preaching, and he was confused. Perhaps Millard was as evil as they claimed.

Sorely troubled, Mott borrowed a Bible and studied the whole of Leviticus carefully, and when he was finished he knew what he must do. He carried the Bible with him to the big meeting at which all five of the charismatic ministers were arrayed on the platform, and after several vain attempts he reached a microphone where the television cameras focused on him:

> 'Each of you clergymen has preached against my son, Mayor Mott, and I want to ask if you indeed support the teaching of Leviticus 20, verse 13, in which homosexual men are condemned to death. [Two of the ministers said yes, it was an abomination. Strabismus hedged.] Well, gentlemen, are you aware that this same chapter of Leviticus says that anyone who curses his father shall be put to death? Are you prepared to execute that sentence?

> 'Are you familiar with the last verse of your chapter? It says that anyone who appears to be a witch shall be put to death. Are you prepared to relight the fires of Salem? To resume burning old women who mumble?

> 'Are you aware that the same chapter directs you to execute every man and woman who has committed adultery? Has any one of you committed adultery? Are you ready to be executed? Do you honestly believe that everyone in the state of Colorado who has committed adultery should be stoned to death? How many in this audience tonight have committed adultery? Should you all be killed?'

His words created a firestorm in the hall, with Strabismus shouting that it was unfair to quote partially from the Bible, and members of the audience shouting back that it was just as unfair for him to quote it partially in support of his harsh ideas. The affair got out of hand when three college girls got to the microphones and said that they had committed adultery with leaders of the Skycrest community and were prepared, if pressed, to reveal names.

Next day several citizens appeared on the streets with big A's emblazoned on their chests and the challenge *Execute me.* One girl carried a sign: I AM A KNOWN WITCH. BURN ME.

The ministers ended their crusade with a huge meeting at which they announced that Skycrest was the new Sodom and Gomorrah, which surprised no one in Colorado, but which did send a ripple of altered vacation plans through the rest of the nation. The referendum to unseat Mayor Mott failed, but even so, the ministers considered their expedition a valuable experience. In their much larger campaign in California they would not stress Leviticus, Chapter 20, so heavily, for they had found that it could be turned against them.

When he returned, battle-fatigued, to Washington, Mott spent some days with his wife just listening to music, and one afternoon, at the end of Verdi's

Requiem, he said, 'Of all the couples we knew—the Peenemünde gang, the NASA people and even our Solid Six—I think you and I were the happiest. Thanks to you, we kept our lives simple, cleaned up. I appreciate that, Rachel.' They sat in silence for some time and then he broke into laughter. 'Guess what I'm going to play next?'

'You wouldn't dare!' It was the String Quartet in A Major by Luigi Boccherini, and whenever her husband forced her to hear it she blushed. But now as the limpid, formless notes came tumbling out, as if from a mechanical hurdy-gurdy, she had to laugh at herself.

At Wellesley she had fallen under the spell of a forceful woman teacher of music history who believed that the only European music worth listening to started with Palestrina and Purcell and ended with Handel. Vivaldi had been her special love, and a whole generation of Rachel's contemporaries had considered this amiable composer's *The Four Seasons* somewhat superior to Beethoven's Ninth and infinitely more elevated than Tchaikovsky, who did not even figure in the professor's syllabus.

Rachel had always kept with her a handful of Vivaldi records, which she cherished, and even when her husband discovered in program notes from the Boston Symphony that Vivaldi had dashed off some four hundred and twenty concerti, composing them sometimes of an afternoon, she refused to admit that much of the man's work was trivial or even tedious: 'The best of Vivaldi is the best of European music.'

Somehow she conceived the erroneous idea that Luigi Boccherini had been a contemporary of Vivaldi's and therefore commendable; in a record store she had chanced to see an album containing the String Quartet and had bought it eagerly. To tell the truth, when she got it home she found it somewhat banal, but since it came from a composer of the approved period, she forced herself to like it and endeavored to make her husband do the same, but as always, he looked things up in his encyclopedias and found that Boccherini was not an early composer at all, but a man who worked side by side with Joseph Haydn and was considered even then a facile hack: ' "Haydn's wife," the critics of that day called him, Rachel. Here, look at it for yourself.'

She had been outraged, first by her husband's unkindness in disclosing the fraud, then by her own gullibility. Boccherini became an ugly word in the Mott household and the cause for much hilarity, and it was used to puncture Rachel's Wellesley pretensions. But one Christmas, Stanley gave his wife as a present a magnificent German recording of the flawless minuet from the Boccherini Quintet in E Major, and it became one of their favorites: 'Our sentimental masterpiece. We play it to each other when we think we're in love.'

In retirement, Stanley also suggested that they bring that wonderful woodcarving by Axel Petersson in from the bedroom to the living room, where it could establish the humanity of the Mott household, and whenever Stanley saw that little wooden man with the jutting jaw and the low-

brimmed hat dancing with his wooden wife he felt good, and he loved
Rachel a little more.

Rachel agreed that their marriage was perhaps the most satisfactory in
their group, but she had a high regard for John and Penny Pope: 'I'd almost
say they were the best, except that they had no children. The joy and the
anguish of having sons and daughters . . .' She never once allowed even a
fugitive thought to stray across her mind that perhaps it would have been
better if doomed Chris had not been born: 'We had years of delight with
that boy. Where he got off the track, who can say?' She never went to his
grave in Florida, but he was in her thoughts constantly; as for Millard, she
chortled when he beat back the attempt to unseat him. 'My son the Mayor,'
she called him when she spoke with her friends, and she was happy that
he was back with Roger, if that's what gave him contentment.

She was pleased when Stanley read portions of his science speech to her,
for she realized that he was endeavoring to summarize a lifetime of experience and she applauded his conclusions:

'When the mind of man ceases to thrust outward, it begins to contract and wither. So with civilizations. In the fifteenth century Spain
and Portugal established new worlds and divided continents between
them, but in the sixteenth century they faltered in their willingness
to pursue vast goals, and one might say they withered intellectually
and even economically. They allowed other nations to take up the
joyous burden of developing new ideas, and from this decline they
never recovered.

'I am terribly afraid that in America's reluctance to proceed with the
exploration of space we are making the Portugal-Spain error. It is
not enough to initiate an action. One must also develop it to its
ultimate capabilities.'

She was delighted with his adept use of postwar Japan and Germany as case
histories of defeated nations which had been almost destroyed but which
by clever application of scientific advances had emerged rather stronger
than the victors.

'What's the secret, Stanley?'

'When you rebuild starting from scratch, you adopt only the most
modern concepts. This means those countries whose factories weren't dy-
namited are burdened with old-fashioned ways. They must fall behind.'

'Would you recommend that countries like England and the United
States blow up their factories every thirty years?'

'The world would be a much better place if we did . . . periodically.'

'Why don't we?'

'We wouldn't have to blow them up, actually. Not if we had the courage to gut them and start over. But we'd never be able to persuade our people to do that. So we wallow along with our outmoded ways and watch the defeated nations surge past us—in dozens of aspects.'

'Who would lose if we did revolutionize production, our way of doing things?'

'It's uncanny. You can see a hundred examples in history of nations that were destroyed, almost wiped out, who came storming back with renewed vigor. It's like pruning a tree. The novice never believes that you improve the tree by cutting it savagely back.'

'Yes, but who suffers?'

'The middle class. You, me. The very rich rarely suffer. The poor go on as usual. But when a currency goes sour, it's people like us who suffer. People on retirement pay. People who own a little property or goods. In fact, our class can be wiped out.'

She thought about this for some time, then asked, 'Is it proper to wipe out a whole class? So that the larger welfare can be helped?'

'I can't answer that. All I know is that nations which have allowed their middle class to be wiped out haven't suffered much at the time and have come back stronger than ever as a consequence.'

'You believe in the integrity of an idea, don't you?'

'I suppose that's all I believe in.'

'How about religion? As an idea, that is?'

'Quite necessary. As the adjudicator. It was the best-educated nation in the world, Germany, that lost its way most completely. It had brains galore, but no one to blow the whistle and cry, "This is wrong." Science could serve that role, but it never does. Politics certainly never does. Society requires some agency larger than itself to blow the whistle. My father taught me that.'

'Granted, but then what do you do about Reverend Strabismus and his ilk?'

'I think you bear with them. Admit that if society did not yearn for them, they wouldn't achieve the power they do. And hope that like Savonarola, they pass quickly without doing too much damage.'

'When will the present crop halt its damage?' she asked.

Mott left his writing desk and paced about the room. 'Giving it to you cold turkey, as the astronauts say, I think we're in for a very bad time for the rest of this century. I expect to be called before the Senate one of these days for having been subversive—'

'Good God, on what grounds?'

'Any they see fit to legislate. I expect to see book burnings one of these days. And families might begin to think like the Kolffs. Sneak their children out to some foreign country to learn forbidden subjects, then sneak them back in to keep learning alive.'

'When I told Dieter that, you said I was hysterical.'

'I've been wondering if maybe you weren't right. And if I think so, I'm morally obligated to say so. While I'm still allowed free speech.'

'I want to read your talk before you deliver it. To discuss possibilities in private is one thing. To do so in a public speech, quite another. I don't want my husband to sound the damned fool.'

'I'm not really concerned about what people in 1982 think. How an individual reacts to any stimulus is his own problem. I want this to be on the record for 2002. I want men and women then to know that I was scared silly by the nonsense and that I tried to do something about it.'

As shadows fell they played Vivaldi, looked lovingly at the Axel Petersson dancers, saw their patron saint Mondrian on the uncluttered walls, and tried to decide which of the good Washington restaurants they would dine in that night, for it was their fortieth wedding anniversary.

And just when Mott had adjusted to his retirement, conceding that the productive period of his life was past, he received two short-term assignments which gave him joy, for they enabled him to rush back into the heart of the great adventure. The first invitation came from Fremont State University, where Professor John Pope was doing final editing on the first eleven chapters of an important treatise he was writing on aviation and space:

> I'd be honored, Stanley, if you would take in hand the final three chapters. They need the expertise and understanding which only you can provide. Please say yes.

When the heavy package arrived at the Mott apartment in Washington, Stanley opened it with the keenest anticipation, for it obviously represented an intellectual outflow from the space program, and this was important.

Mott had never been one to justify the vast NASA program because it had provided stick-free Teflon frying pans to housewives or Velcro hold-fast fabrics to vaudeville performers, enabling them to appear in funny breakaway costumes. Again and again he refrained from testifying to the Senate that our explorations in space were vindicated by things like telecommunication satellites or the miniaturization of medical devices. He deemed it cheap to retreat to such sophistry when the noble adventure could be justified within its own terms: man had thrown back the perimeters of ignorance and darkness by quintillions of miles and centuries of years, and that was adequate justification.

But even when defending this austere intellectual position, he appreciated the parallel development of industrial products—especially computerization—and the application of space science to things like agricultural analysis and ocean prediction. He was pleased to know that John Pope, perhaps the brainiest of the astronauts and one of the most experienced, was putting his training to use.

CIRCADIAN DISORIENTATION
by John Pope, Ph.D.

The subject matter of this book is simply defined. Three times in recent years I have been ordered to fly nonstop from Capetown at the southern tip of Africa to London on the western edge of Europe, and because I stayed generally within the same time zone, I arrived at my destination only as tired as the very long flight demanded. Actually, since I sleep well on planes, I reached London quite rested and able to go immediately to work at the American Embassy for nine hours, then to the theater, and finally to a formal dinner.

During this same time period I was ordered three times to fly nonstop from Tokyo to New York, a flight of about the same duration, but because I was crossing ten time zones, my pineal gland secreted melatonin so abnormally that it required me four to five days to bring it back into balance. I therefore arrived in New York exhausted and disoriented and was insecure until my circadian orientation reasserted itself.

This book explores the phenomena cited, drawing upon animal experiments, the accumulated experience of airline pilots who make flights across time zones, and especially the reports of American and Russian astronauts who repeatedly crossed twenty-four time zones in ninety minutes.

The word *circadian* is derived from the Latin *circa diem* or *about a day* and refers to the mysterious twenty-four-hour rhythms which control all brain outputs—behavioral, autonomic or neuroendocrine —of all animals or humans who live on Earth with its twenty-four-hour alternation of light and darkness. We must assume that were our day only ten hours long, as on Saturn, our circadian responses would correspond to that timing.

Our specific problem is: What causes circadian disorientation when we cross time zones? And what can be done about it?

Mott leafed through the manuscript hurriedly to ascertain how Pope with his astronomical training had attacked the problem, and he saw with interest that John speculated that flying from New York to Tokyo was more troublesome than flying the same distance in reverse order:

It may be that when we fly from east to west we are flying *against* the motion of the Earth. Perhaps we fight against this dislocation, adjusting to it incrementally. But when we fly west to east, we are flying *with* the motion of the Earth and are seduced into accepting its domination, continuing to accept it long after we have ceased our flight. A simpler explanation might be that most people find it more difficult to get up early than to get up late.

He was halted in his skimming by the fascinating case histories of race horses flown practically nonstop from breeding farms in Delaware to race tracks in New Zealand and Australia:

> At both the Christchurch and Melbourne race tracks where I conducted my studies, I found that trainers had to be extremely careful with imported American horses, keeping them in artificially lighted surroundings which conformed to the day-night timing of their Delaware homeland for at least three weeks. Gradually the electric lighting became synchronized with the real lighting outside, at which time the horse could step out into his new environment with no apparent disorientation.

Pope was best in his careful analysis of two kinds of space travel, Gemini-type low orbiting, in which an Earth-oriented time zone was crossed every three and three-quarter minutes, and the far thrust into outer space which could be conceived as flying an immense distance within roughly the same terrestrial time zone. One of Pope's trenchant paragraphs amused him:

> We must remember, in evaluating these data, that only thirty human beings in world history have experienced travel of this second type: three men each in Apollos 8, and 10 through 18, and each man an American. No Russian so far has ventured into outer space; each of that country's daring cosmonauts has been confined to low Earth orbit, so their experience does not yet impinge on what we are discussing here.

Finally Mott came to the missing chapters for which he would be responsible. Chapter XII: *Travel to Mars;* Chapter XIII: *Travel to Proxima Centauri;* Chapter XIV: *Travel Outside the Galaxy.* When he saw the titles and visualized what must be said to enflesh them, he felt that surge of excitement which had overcome him when General Funkhauser inserted him among the geniuses at Langley: 'I'm being granted a second life . . . a second time.'

With an almost adolescent ardor he plunged into the three subjects, accumulating a bewildering array of technical studies and applying to them his own imaginative analyses. When three Americans blasted off from Canaveral for their journey to Mars, say in the year 2005, when that great surge of energy which marked the 1960–1970 epoch was re-created by some driving force as yet unidentified, they would be starting on a journey of about 200,000,000 miles one way at a speed of 25,000 miles an hour, which would then be feasible. The trip would take about 330 days out, two months on the surface and 330 days back, or just about two years:

> If prudent, they will maintain their natural circadian rhythm, basing it on Central Standard Time at Houston and adjusting their schedules to it. Of course, they could establish over that period of time a circadian rhythm coincident with the Mars day of 24 hours and 37 minutes, but the slight advantage of achieving this would scarcely repay the effort.

It was when he attacked the second problem of sending humans out to Proxima Centauri, the flare star closest to Earth at 4.3 light-years or 2.52 $\times$ 10^{13} miles (25.2 trillion) that he realized the irreversible change which had come over him. He discovered it first when he looked at the books he had assembled, for he found among them a score of the best science-fiction works:

> Good God! That damned Randy Claggett made a sci-fi nut out of me. And look at my stuff! Each book is what they call *heavy metal,* the hard-core scientific prediction of the machines and processes for real space travel. None of the soft-core analysis of future civilizations. This is vintage Jules Verne, Arthur C. Clarke, Robert Heinlein. Daring men in a crate heading into the challenge of outer space.

As he looked at the collection he had to acknowledge what had happened to him: Engineers don't bother with this idle speculation. Scientists do. Which means I've become a scientist, against all my better instincts. And it was as a scientist, the new breed of astrophysicist who lived among the farthest galaxies, that he placed before him only one book, his bible, Allen's *Astrophysical Quantities,* and from its recondite data he began to construct the patterns that men would some day follow in adjusting to the problems of traveling for 4.3 years at the speed of light over a distance of 25.2 trillion miles to the nearest star.

> Circadian rhythms will be just as important a problem as time dilation, and how the space travelers organize their capsule universe will be significant. Suppose they go the route of suspended animation: they will have to reinsert their sentient bodies into a specified circadian system, for if they do not, they will find themselves disoriented to the point that they might not be able to function during the precise period of readjustment when maximum brain efficiency will be at a premium.

As he drafted the detailed flight plan to Epsilon Eridani, the fascinating star only eleven light-years distant (65 trillion miles) he could feel the reality of such proposed travel and its problems become not abstract intellectual puzzles but specific difficulties to be overcome, and one night he threw down his pencil and cried, 'God, how I wish I could live into the century that will accomplish such things!' But as soon as he uttered this lament he was ashamed of himself, and he turned off his desk lamp and went in the other room to join Rachel, who was sitting prim and quiet in a straight-backed chair listening to Pachelbel.

'I'm so damned grateful,' he said.

'For what?' she asked without moving.

'That I was permitted by fate, or chance, or God's planning to live into the age when aviation was invented—into this explosive period when men could go to the planets.'

'And to be a part of it all. That counts, too.'

'I was so damned fortunate.' His voice broke and for some moments he stood silent, listening to the intricate canon as if it were an orderly echo from outer space. 'We were lucky.'

When he had his three chapters outlined and the research material on which they must be based identified, he started writing with a desire to summarize all known knowledge about man's probable reaction to travel in space, and he had pretty well completed his two-year trip to Mars when his former superiors in NASA called with another short-term project, one which could constitute the capstone to his life's work: 'Stanley, we're being badgered from many sides to make an authoritative statement as to the possibility of life elsewhere in the universe. The UFO contingent is after us, the L-5 specialists, half a dozen religious leaders who demand that we state definitely that life can exist only on Earth, and lots of people who've seen *Star Wars* four times. If we convene a workshop with top-drawer participants, will you chair it in your customary non-hysterical way?'

Mott wanted to leap into the phone to grasp the speaker's hand, to say yes immediately, but caution warned him to find out more about the composition of the workshop.

'Only the best, Stanley. Nineteen—like Sagan, Asimov, Cameron of Harvard, Bernie Oliver of Hewlett Packard, John Pope of Fremont State. Maybe we can get Freeman Dyson of Princeton. Then we'll give you two dozen NASA experts for the technical reports. And we'll invite about two hundred official observers—Army, Air Force, church groups, the sci-fi wizards—and we'll hold three plenary sessions which the general public will be free to attend.'

For a long moment Mott could not respond: from his childhood days he had speculated on the possibility of extraterrestrial intelligence and at critical moments in his life had addressed the unseen beings as if they could hear him. But he had never made up his mind as to the probability of their existence, and this opportunity to clarify his thinking, and that of the scientific community, was a joyous one. At last he would be free to reach out to the ultimate horizons.

'You there, Stanley?'

'I'll take it.'

He went to work preparing several guidance papers to be circulated before the nineteen official members met, then hurried to the millionaire's estate in Vermont, now a study center belonging to Harvard, where the four-week session would convene. With almost childish pleasure he supervised printing the plaques used to identify rooms to be occupied by men he had known for decades: Ray Bradbury, Frank Drake, Kantankerous Kantrowitz, Gerard O'Neill of Princeton, Nobel winner Lederberg, small, ultra-brilliant Phil Morrison of MIT, who had written a book on the subject, and Riccardo Giacconi, who had a mind like a restive volcano. It would be a reunion of what Rachel affectionately called 'our crazies of the far out,' but they would not preempt discussion, because the two hundred observers would contain disputatious experts prepared to challenge anything. Conspicuous would be the Reverend Strabismus heading the group of churchmen; at one time he had known as much science as any of them and was indeed the only man in the group who had written two doctoral theses in the fields to be discussed.

It would be difficult to hold these intellectual stallions in rein, but Mott would try.

Before Mott could devote full attention to his new job he was diverted by a shocking interruption. Senator Grant, with the generosity which had marked his incumbency in Washington, waited until Fremont officials had certified the election of Mrs. Penny Pope as their new senator, then resigned. The state governor was free to appoint Mrs. Pope to the remaining weeks of his term, whereupon Grant rushed her to Washington to be sworn in as his replacement, thus ensuring her permanent seniority over other first-term members of the Class of 1982.

On the afternoon of the swearing-in Senator Pope asked Mott if he could report to her new office, and when he reached there he found the Popes and Senator Grant in sober discussion. After an unusually brusque greeting Penny said, 'I've asked you three friends to give me some hard advice. I've been assigned to the Space Committee and I wish you'd tell me, Dr. Mott, what NASA's program ought to be.'

Mott bowed formally to the new senator and said, 'America must pursue a set of clearly defined, practical goals in space.'

With impatience at such a wobbly answer she snapped, 'And what are they?'

'I can tell you exactly, but I did not want to seem pushy.'

'Please push. In as few words as possible.'

'Solar-polar mission to study the Sun.' He paused, expecting to be asked what that might be, but Senator Pope nodded, indicating that she knew.

'A mission to greet Halley's Comet.' Another nod. 'The great space telescope. Retrieval of rock samples from Mars and, before long, a manned mission there. Intense study of gossamer flight, ramjet flight, solar-powered flight. Certainly the establishment of a permanent station in space. And above all, continued research in aeronautics.'

'Are they practical? Given the present state of the art?'

Mott deferred to Professor Pope, who said, 'Each one could be done.'

'But could they be financed?' she pressed, and this time Mott indicated that Senator Grant should respond.

'In the present economy, we can't afford even one of them.'

'Not even the aviation studies?'

'Private industry should assume that burden,' Grant said, and Mott winced.

'Where did we use to get the money, Norman?' Penny asked. 'Those billions your committee and mine lavished on Gemini and Apollo?'

'That was an easier world,' Grant said with some sorrow. 'In those days we believed we could do anything. We're no longer that kind of people.'

Senator Pope leaned forward, bit on a pencil, and studied each of her advisers. 'I fear that what Senator Grant has said is true.' Mott gasped. 'I've been studying the budget . . . seen the immense cost of programs that can't be cut. I find no margin left for space.' Now Mott had to protest, but she cut him short: 'That is, beyond the housekeeping functions NASA is already performing.'

'That's hardly enough to justify a major branch of the government,' Mott said.

'Exactly,' the new senator agreed, and she looked at her old friend with a harshness he had not seen in her before. 'It's quite possible that NASA should be closed down . . . completely.'

'But you were our principal supporter,' Mott cried.

Senator Pope ignored this and asked Grant, 'What's your advice, Norman?'

Grant cleared his throat. 'I've never said this in public, and I didn't reveal it even to you, Penny. But before he died Senator Glancey told me, "Norman, I think NASA should be quietly buried in the Department of Defense." I think so, too.'

'Oh, no!' Mott protested. 'That would be entirely wrong. A reversal of all the good decisions Eisenhower made to get us started.'

'In his day he was right,' Grant said, 'and you remember that I spearheaded his program. But in our day the situation is totally changed. Mission, budget, public support and military need, all different. Dr. Mott, your agency should be dismantled. Aviation and communications to private industry. Shuttle to the military. Close down the rest.'

'And what happens to science? To the inquiring mind of man?'

'Universities can assume responsibility for that,' Grant said.

Stanley Mott was courteous to senators, but he was not awed by them; he had seen too many awful mistakes, and now, since these two seemed determined to commit a colossal one, he could not stay silent. 'If you do what you're suggesting, you commit the United States to second-class citizenship. We have problems of the most profound importance—'

With some asperity Mrs. Pope interrupted: 'If we do what you suggest, we'll go broke.'

'I'm amazed at your reversal of attitude,' Mott protested.

'If I could butt in,' John Pope said, 'and if you'll excuse the expression, I think the Korean newspaperwoman said it all in her book.' He nodded gravely to his wife, who glared at him, then smiled.

> 'A free nation is capable of surviving one challenge after another, as America proved so clearly in meeting her Depression, World War II, the creation of an atomic bomb and the flight to the Moon. But it will rarely respond to the same challenge twice, as it proved when it behaved so cravenly during the Vietnam war. It needs the excitement of change, new dangers to be overcome, new frontiers to be pushed back. With John Pope's return from the dark side of the Moon, America terminated her space episode and retreated to a quiet corner to conserve her resources until the next challenge exploded.'

Senator Pope nodded. 'We challenged the Moon, and Mars, Jupiter and Saturn, and we won. Now we must wait for the next great adventure. NASA has made its contribution.' And the meeting ended.

In 1975 NASA had explored the possibility of life in outer space in considerable depth, with many of the same experts on the committee, so they required no indoctrination, but the new members, especially those not trained in the sciences, did, and at the opening plenary session, with nineteen committee members present, and forty-three NASA contributors who would provide much of the detailed study, Mott laid down the ground rules:

> 'We are commissioned by our government to make a simple, clear statement as to the probability of life elsewhere in the universe. The outward circles from Earth, each of which must be explored, are the Moon, the planets, our Galaxy, the other galaxies, the quasars and black holes of recent definition, and anything that lies beyond.

> 'We are speaking always of two forms of life, what we might call the lowest possible level of reproductive existence and sentient beings

who might be much like ourselves. Let's keep those two goals constantly in mind.

'We start with certain demonstrated knowledge that our predecessor investigators could not have had. We know there is no kind of life of either category on the Moon. We suspect the same of Mars. We have good reason to believe that sentient life exists nowhere in the planetary system and certainly not on the Sun. It is highly probable that even the lowest imaginable forms do not exist on planets like Jupiter, Saturn and Uranus. So let's not have any serious proposals regarding humanoids coming at us from Mars or Jupiter. They're not there and probably never were.

'That throws us into our Galaxy and out into the other galaxies, and to keep our thinking in focus I have prepared this simple sheet, which I hope you will keep with you during our discussion. It lists twenty stars and other celestial objects, and indicates rather nicely, I believe, the specific problems we face in either traveling to those distant objects or exchanging messages with them. Please, please, as we conduct our discussions, keep these data in mind.'

The sheet he distributed was arranged in neat columns, as any work he did would be, and it contained startling information. Six of the more interesting targets were:

DIFFICULTIES OF COMMUNICATION

Celestial Target	Miles from Earth	Years Travel at 25,000 MPH	Years Travel at Speed of Light	Years Needed Send Message & Receive an Answer
STARS WITHIN OUR GALAXY				
Altair	93,850,000,000,000	428,544	16	32
Capella	276,000,000,000,000	1,260,000	47	94
Antares	2,110,000,000,000,000	9,630,000	360	720
OBJECTS OUTSIDE OUR GALAXY				
NGC-4565	117,000,000,000,000, 000,000	535,000,000,000	20,000,000	40,000,000
Quasar 3C-73	5,865,000,000,000,000, 000,000	26,000,000,000,000	1,000,000,000	2,000,000,000
Object 0Q-172	117,000,000,000,000, 000,000,000	536,000,000,000,000	20,000,000,000	40,000,000,000

In presenting the table he apologized to his science colleagues: 'I very much wanted to give these big numbers as powers of 10, but I was afraid this might prove difficult for our many lay participants. To acquaint them with the proper system, the star Altair, a member of our Galaxy, is 9.385×10^{13} miles distant, which is read 9 plus thirteen additional digits, most of them zeros.

'Because Professor Pope is with us, I've started with the star Altair, a name he made famous during his solitary ride. If you can get hold of an old Apollo, John, you can travel to your favorite star in 428,000 years, one way. And when you get there you can tell us about it, but your radio message will require 16 years to reach us, but even so, you're lots better off than I am. As those of you who have worked with me know, I have for some years been enamored of NGC-4565, and if I send a message there right now, you and I will have to wait 40,000,000 years for a reply. So let's not talk glibly about easy trips or quick message exchanges with celestial objects—'

'Unless,' one of the younger men interrupted, 'we travel by time warp.'

'Exactly! We'll discuss that tomorrow.' Mott said.

A NASA man laid out the conventional wisdom: 'Our Galaxy contains about four hundred billion stars. There appear to be something like one hundred billion other galaxies besides our own. That means that we may have as many as four followed by twenty-two zeros of stars around us. And each of those stars could have nine planets accompanying it, the way our Sun does, which would make thirty-six plus twenty-two zeros of planets, and if each planet had a dozen or more moons like Jupiter and Saturn, we have a fantastic number of locations on which extraterrestrial life might exist. But Dr. Kelly has something to say about that.'

Now came the first striking bit of speculation: 'Suppose we look at the forty billion trillion possible stars and begin to cut away to see if we can bring this number down to an understandable figure. In a hundred stars taken at random, seventy will be double, triple or more complex. Only thirty will be single stars like our Sun. There is good reason to assume that no double star or triple can have planets, for the close passage of such masses would quickly destroy any planets. So right at the start we cut our number of possibles by seventy percent.

'I want to call your attention to a remarkable analysis by Michael Hart, which I've mimeographed for you. Hart shows that if the Earth had been only a little closer to the Sun, a greenhouse effect would have occurred four billion years ago which would have made life as we know it impossible. And if the Earth had been only one million miles farther away from the Sun, runaway glaciation would have frozen the world shut. So we see that accurate placement of the planets we're looking for is also of vital importance.'

'Sir,' came a strong voice from one side of the conference hall; it was Reverend Strabismus in the first of his many interruptions. 'Why are you surprised at the accurate placement of our Earth? Surely God intended it to be exactly where it is. He took all your calculations into consideration.'

'Some agency certainly did,' the speaker said without halting in his explanation, 'and unless a similar accuracy was exhibited in placing all the other planets we're to discuss, life of any kind might be impossible.'

'Life would be possible anywhere if God willed it,' Strabismus said and sat down.

The speaker used half a dozen criteria with which to whittle away that huge number of forty billion trillion, and in the end he had his remaining number so small that he ended with a brief statement which awed his listeners: 'The factors which operate against billions of possible sites for human habitation are so tremendous that I could be persuaded that Earth is so astonishingly peculiar that sentient life has developed only here.'

'That's what we've been saying since the Book of Genesis,' Strabismus said.

'There's a minority report on that,' came a stern voice from the rear. 'I give my paper tomorrow at eleven.'

Mott now called on a man from Cal Tech, who developed an amazing theme, one which shone like a light in a dark valley once it was enunciated: 'We shall be talking about enormous spans of time, and it's essential that we keep one fact in mind. No matter how many or how few other civilizations we postulate, they must be scattered at random over vast ages. It is extremely unlikely that if a planet like ours exists in Andromeda, and has developed sentient beings somewhat like us—'

'They will be like us,' Strabismus interrupted, 'for they will have been made in the image of God.'

'It's extremely unlikely,' the man from Cal Tech continued, 'that they will be at the same cultural level as we are. The laws of chance dictate that they will be everywhere else. Perhaps they matured a billion years ago and are now in sad decline, unable to communicate even with themselves. Perhaps they're just beginning and won't develop radio communication for another four billion years. It took us that long. So in everything we do during these next weeks we must visualize a situation like this.' And he covered the board with a series of vertical chalk lines, some near the top, some toward the bottom, but almost none overlapping. It was like a forest of telephone poles scattered upright in the sky, each in its own ambience, each at a different height, unrelated to the others.

'Here's an inhabited planet in Andromeda, way up here on the scale. Here we are down here in the first blush of morning. Gentlemen, remember that although this Earth has existed for about four and a half billion years, and human beings for a few million, we've been able to send comprehensible signals into space for only about forty-five years. Suppose Andromeda had wanted to communicate with us two billion years ago. There was no one here to listen, and even a hundred years ago when people were here, they hadn't mastered the techniques of listening.'

space between the spectral lines of water's components, hydrogen and the hydroxyl radical. For that reason we call it the Water Hole, around which creatures of space will congregate socially the way animals in a prairie gather at their water hole.'

Strange, strange, Strabismus thought. If I'd settled down at either Yale or New Paltz, I could have been one of the scientists here today. I know more than any I've heard so far, except maybe Mott. He listened attentively as a different speaker elaborated: 'We've done much work at the Water Hole already. We've sent thousands of messages out, and we've spent many hours listening with our great ears at Arecibo, and based on those solid beginnings, men like Sagan and Oliver are proposing interesting new attacks. Everything we do is based on the assumption that somewhere other intelligences are ready, perhaps even eager, to communicate with us.'

On the third day a pair of Drake's students from Cornell explained to the laymen in the group the frightening equation covering the probability of life on some other planet in the Galaxy:

$$N = N_* f_p f_e f_l f_i f_c f_L$$

When it was placed on the blackboard the non-scientific members groaned, but the speaker quickly explained: 'This proves how arcane we can be. All it means is that the first N represents the number of civilizations in our Galaxy capable of communicating with us right now. That's the figure we must have to make our discussion reasonable. The second N is a figure we seek to make our discussion practical. N_* is a very large number representing all the known stars in our Galaxy. Some experts say one hundred billion, some say four. In our example I'll take four. The next six letters with their subscripts represent fractions, with each subscript standing for a crucial word or concept. When you multiply the very large number by the six fractions, you get a constantly diminishing number of possible civilizations. First fraction: the portion of stars which have *planetary* systems, and we heard yesterday that this fraction must be considerably smaller than one-half, more likely one-quarter. Second fraction: the portion of planets with an *ecology* able to sustain life, perhaps one-half. Third fraction: the portion of the eligible planets on which *life* actually does develop; the biologists believe it must be almost nine-tenths. Fourth fraction: what portion of those with life develop *intelligent* forms? Given enough time, we think it could be one-tenth. Fifth fraction: the portion of civilizations with intelligent life which learn to *communicate* outwardly, maybe one-third. Sixth fraction: that gripping question we discussed yesterday, what is the *longevity* of a technical civilization?

'We must evaluate this question of longevity with all the philosophical resources at our command. The only hard evidence we have is our own experience on Earth. Four and a half billion years old. Technically compe-

The concept was so challenging, and so concisely presented, that Reverend Strabismus asked quietly, 'We know that the universe could not have existed in the time period you suggest. The Bible explains all that. But do you think, Professor, that even today the kind of imbalance you suggest—one civilization up here, one down there, with no chance of communication—could that exist right now?'

'I'm convinced it does.'

'Thank you for making something clear which was not clear before.'

'I'm not sure the various applications are clear to me,' the Cal Tech man said.

With these conservative caveats the first day ended, and dinner was spent in furious discussion, with younger scientists warning that on the morrow they were going to tear the place apart with some contemporary thinking; these cowboys of outer space held a rump session starting at ten-thirty that night to lay plans for the presentations they would make regarding the future of space communication, when their radical new procedures would be applied.

The second day started like a typhoon in the Pacific, building intensity with each hour until entire island structures were endangered. A delightfully brash young man from MIT said, 'I want you to disregard all the frightening statistics Dr. Mott handed you yesterday in his golden sheet, because he refused to take into account time dilation. For you non-scientists that's a major consequence of Einstein's Theory of Relativity. It means this. That time aboard the spacecraft is radically different from time as seen by those who remain behind on Earth. If Professor Pope, whom Dr. Mott mentioned yesterday, should want to fly to the nebula in Orion, it would take *him* only thirty years of elapsed time, but the people on Earth would have spent thirty-one hundred years.'

Mott heard two science-fiction writers: 'We explained all that forty years ago. They're just catching up.'

Another main speaker said, 'I visualize travel by as many as four hundred persons in a single spaceship that accelerates to the speed of light within one hour, then moves into a time warp that will enable the crew to take the ship to any spot within the Galaxy within a mortal lifetime.'

'How soon do you think such travel possible?'

'By the year 2050, but incoming voyagers from the Galaxy might g here before we leave.'

Strabismus was delighted to hear such speculation, for it reminded h of those early days his Universal Space Associates peddled little green m 'I was right all along,' he muttered to himself, 'just ahead of my time.' old interests awakened, he listened with acute attention as radio exp predicted that if intra-galactic communication ever did reach Eart would probably arrive on the 1420–1662 megahertz band: 'This occupi tent to communicate forty-five years. Likely to blow itself into extinction at any moment. So the last gloomy fraction must be 45/4,500,000,000 or 1/100,000,000. Let's face facts and multiply our equation:

$$No.\ of\ Civilizations = 400,000,000,000 \times \frac{1}{4} \times \frac{1}{2} \times \frac{9}{10} \times \frac{1}{10} \times \frac{1}{3} \times \frac{1}{100,000,000} = 15$$

This means that among the myriad stars of our Galaxy, there are probably not more than fifteen with whom we could converse.'

When some had expressed awe at the small number, others at the fact that there might be even one other intelligent society, the speaker said dryly, 'Of course, that's just our own Galaxy. Since we know of one hundred billion other galaxies, there could be more than a trillion civilizations spread around out there. Enough to occupy us for a while.'

The two big fights that preoccupied the commission, one mind-expanding fun, the other so fundamental that it threatened to destroy the workshop, began on the fourth day. The first pitted the old-timers, who were pessimistic about the possibility of interstellar travel and communication, against the avid youngsters, who predicted both.

'We have the technological principles right now to fly a spaceship into the Galaxy,' one young man claimed.

'Of course we do,' a cautious old-timer agreed. 'And have you calculated the amount of energy needed to do such a job? I have. Enough to illuminate the United States for the next fifty thousand years.'

'We'll devise new systems of propulsion,' the young man said.

'You solve every objection I bring up by a "new this" or a "new that." '

'That's how we solved the objections you made forty years ago!'

Mott took no sides in this debate, but he had always attended to the quiet sardonic guesses of salty Freeman Dyson of Princeton, and if Dyson now argued that both communication and travel might be practical sooner than some thought, he was inclined to go along, but after one evening session, when debate had sizzled, he walked alone under the Vermont stars and acknowledged that he had for some time been harboring a thought which stunned him when said aloud: 'Perhaps we are unique. Perhaps we're the only planet that developed life. Perhaps . . .'

A voice hailed him: 'That you, Mott?' It was Strabismus. 'The ideas thunder at you like railway trains,' he said.

'That's why we hold these sessions.'

'Cold turkey? What's your personal guess as to how many others there might be?'

As they walked side by side through the starry night Mott answered honestly: 'I was just about to concede that Earth might be unique—'

'But you didn't?'

'No, Strabismus. I think all our fractions were far too conservative. My calculations permit about two million societies with whom we could inter-act.'

They looked for a light, and when they found a lamppost Strabismus took a scrap of paper from his pocket. 'My fractions are bigger, too. I come up with about a million.' He folded the paper, returned it to his pocket, and said, 'But these are figures for those in the know. The general population, it would only confuse them.'

'And you intend to keep them confused?'

'I intend to work with them as I find them.'

'You mean use them.'

'They want to be used.'

'We'll resume in the morning!'

Like many great conflagrations, the fundamental fight began with a fire so small that a child could have extinguished it, and when it started, no one could have foreseen its destructive potential. It centered on the fraction f_l, the portion of eligible planets on which life actually develops, for what started out to be a problem in biology quickly became a question of meta-physical and religious values. The scientist who presented the basic data used an unfortunate term; he said that life would evolve compulsively whenever the primordial soup had the right components, temperature, pressure and general surroundings, and he believed that these rules must prevail throughout the universe, so that the genesis of life was possible in billions of imagined situations.

The religionists and some of the lay observers found this phrase *primordial soup* wildly offensive and withdrew any conciliatory gestures they may have made during the first days of the conference. One fiery Baptist, the Reverend Hosea Kellog of the Red River Bible University, shouted, 'Man was placed on this Earth by the personal intervention of God, as a man entire, and not as a cauldron of bubbling chemicals.' Quickly the debate ran wild, leading to this improbable exchange:

'Are you claiming, Reverend Kellog, that God saves only those who accept Jesus Christ? And all the rest are condemned to eternal hell?'

'That's what the Bible says.'

'Does this mean that all Jews are so condemned?'

'Especially the Jews. They had a chance to accept Jesus and they denied Him. They stand condemned.'

'And all the people in Asia who never heard of Jesus? And all those in Africa? And all the Unitarians in this country, and the non-believers?'

'They are all condemned.'

'And the millions who died before Christ appeared? They could never have known Him. Are they, too, in everlasting hell?'

'They are.'

Even Reverend Strabismus found such doctrine too extreme, and he surprised the assembly by refuting it: 'My Bible preaches hope for all. I was a Jew but saw the light, and I'm convinced that God welcomes me into His heaven. But this does not mean that I condemn the other Jews in this assembly or in this nation who have not seen the true way. If God is big enough to have set in motion the kind of universe we've been describing, He's big enough to find a place in it for a handful of Jews and Buddhists.'

'Anathema!' shouted Kellog. 'I rue the day I granted you a degree in theology.'

Strabismus had far more friends in the hall than Kellog, and this condemnation of their leader was offensive, so a brawl erupted, and soon scientists were defending their right to exist, while Kellog's men condemned them anew. The affair would have destroyed the workshop had not Dr. Mott gaveled the contestants to order and then abruptly terminated the stormy session.

He had little on which to congratulate himself, for at seven the next morning his phone began to jangle, and in quick succession he had three agitated calls from NASA headquarters and a stern one from Senator Pope: 'You were sent there to keep those tigers in their cages, Stanley. Throw them some warm meat and bring this thing under control.'

'How did you hear about it?'

'*New York Times, Washington Post, Christian Science Monitor.* Front pages are full of it. Do you think you should terminate the workshop?'

'Never.'

'Then knock some sense into their heads. That's your job.'

He skipped breakfast, spending the time drafting a few concise notes which he hoped would quieten things, but when he stood at the podium he could see that the conferees were still eager for battle, and he knew he must conciliate them:

> 'Yesterday evening we witnessed an unfortunate manifestation of the ancient and unnecessary quarrel between religion and science, and the chair feels obligated to make a statement.
>
> 'I would remind my scientific brethren, to whom personally I owe so much, that whereas each arriving piece of new evidence supports the theory of an original big bang which launched at least this portion of the cosmos into being, no one, and I repeat no one, has provided even one acceptable scientific guess as to what agency activated that primordial bang. If our religious participants insist that it was God, their reasoning is at least as good as anyone else's, and I think better.
>
> 'Now I must remind my religious brethren, and I feel justified in using that familial word, since my father was a clergyman, that all available evidence does point to a very old beginning for our Earth and to an immensely old beginning for our universe. Even though I believe in God as firmly as I do, I simply cannot deny the evidence,

and I hold it to be the task of knowing men to reconcile the two points of view which erupted here last night with such violence.

'My conclusions are threefold, and because this question is so vital to this workshop and to humanity in general, I have taken the precaution of writing them down on this small slip of paper lest I misspeak myself on what is proving to be the heart of this meeting.

'First, society cannot exist without a referee to judge the good and evil of any proposed act. Without this constant guidance, encouragement, and censorship we must revert to barbarism, as we have seen societies do in our lifetime. Science has not the moral force to provide this guidance, nor has politics. Only an ethical system can do this, and our inherited ethical systems have been given the hallowed name *religion*.

'Second, I am not much concerned with the doctrinal debates and differences of religion, nor are many of my scientific brethren, but I am deeply supportive of the solid work religion does in helping to structure society. I would not wish to live in any community which lacked churches. I have sometimes phrased it this way: If I were an unmarried young man of twenty-four, sent by my corporation to a new job in its Detroit plant, there is no possibility whatever that I would go to a bar to find my wife, or to a dance hall. I would join a church, or associate myself with a library or college, because I would want to meet people who supported the same ideals I did. Most sensible citizens support churches, and therefore the religious impulse which creates them.

'Third, as a scientist who did not attain that august title till he was a mature man of forty-four, so that he did not accept generalizations easily, I cannot deny or obscure the accumulated evidence that piles up before me. Our scientific probes of Voyager II, the photographs it returned to Earth, told us the nature of the planet Saturn, and regardless what ancient religious texts claim in their poetic form, that is the nature of the planet and I am bound by that truth.

'I am told that last night Reverend Hosea Kellog of Red River Bible University and Professor Hiram Hellweiter of Indiana University came to blows during the heat of their debate. Such partisanship is understandable and certainly forgivable, for decisions of great moment confront us, and it is inevitable that defense of one's priorities should become furious. But in the quietness of this beautiful morning I ask you two distinguished gentlemen to embrace, as I embrace each of you.

'For all of us must grapple with problems of tremendous import, and we must strive together in harmony, not in destructive discord. We can now reach out to the farthest galaxies and peel back the layers of confusion which in the past have obscured our understandings. What shall we do with this new knowledge? We have seen that we can harness the hydrogen atom. But how will we utilize and discipline that capacity? And perhaps of even greater significance and peril, we can now move into the structure of the human gene to create new forms of life. How can we supervise the exercise of that terrible power?

'Finally, the time may not be far distant when we shall be summoned back to this hall to discuss in secret not the exploration of other galaxies but the steps in which America can utilize her stations in space in mortal warfare with some other power which has also learned how to function in this medium and is determined to use it to destroy us.

'This first assembly of great minds must not be divided. We must work as partners in our exploration into the structure of matter, into the workings of the human mind, and into society's chances for survival. If we divide, we can destroy ourselves. If we unite, we can bring order to a threatened Earth.'

When he sat down, the participants, most of whom sought the conciliation he represented, cheered, but he was so exhausted nervously that he could not resume conduct of the session and excused himself. As he walked unsteadily toward the rear of the hall he felt his arm being taken by Leopold Strabismus, who whispered as he led their way to the sun-filled lawn, 'Forget them for a moment. They're resuming where they left off last night.'

'I noticed that you stayed out of that fray, Leopold. Uncharacteristic.'

'I wanted to find out what the more sensible men like you believed.'

'All of us scientists are convinced that this Earth upon which you and I stand this afternoon was brought out of chaos four and a half billion—'

'There it is, Mott! You said it yourself. Brought out of chaos. Who brought it out?'

'That has never concerned me. It could easily have been God. Or the Primal Force. Or Divine Chance. I have no problem with that whatever.'

'There's the difference. Men like me want to nail things down.'

'So you halt the teaching of evolution? You put a stopper on geology?'

'The common man must not be confused.'

Mott pointed over his shoulder toward the noisy session. 'Practically every man in there, including you and me, is a common man, and for sure we were the sons of common men. If we can grapple with these questions, and one day solve the easier ones, why not the common man? You and I are the common man.'

And so the grand debate continued. It had started eons ago along the camel trails in Mesopotamia and in the barren highlands of Judea. Ancestors of Mott and Strabismus had chosen opposing sides in Assyria and at Stonehenge. These precise questions had been raised in the temples of Thebes and Machu Picchu, and in the ancient universities of Bologna and Oxford. Now they were being revived on a hillside in Vermont, and a thousand years from now they would still be debated on some other planet orbiting some other star in some other galaxy.

Von Braun, Wernher. Born Wirsitz, Germany, 1912.

Funkhauser, Helmut. Born Hamburg, Germany, 1896.

Butler, Gawain. Born Detroit, Michigan, 1921.

Glancey, Michael. Born Magnolia, Red River, 1904.

Strabismus, Leopold. Born (Scorcella, Martin) Mount Vernon, New York, 1925.

Thompson, Tucker. Born Columbus, Ohio, 1912.

Rhee, Cynthia. Born (Rhee, Soon-Ka) Osaka, Japan, 1936.

THE FOUR FAMILIES

Mott, Stanley. Born Newton, Massachusetts, 1918.
Mott, Rachel Lindquist. Born Worcester, Massachusetts, 1920.
    Millard, born 1943.
    Christopher, born 1950.

Pope, John. Born Clay, Fremont, 1927. U.S. Navy.
Pope, Penny Hardesty. Born Clay, Fremont, 1927.

Grant, Norman. Born Clay, Fremont, 1914.
Grant, Elinor Stidham. Born Clay, Fremont, 1917.
    Marcia, born 1939.

Kolff, Dieter. Born near Munich, Germany, 1907.
Kolff, Liesl. Born Peenemünde, Germany, 1916.
    Magnus, born 1947.

THE SOLID SIX ASTRONAUTS

Claggett, Randolph. Born Creede, Texas, 1929. U.S. Marine Corps.
Claggett, Debby Dee Cawthorn Rodgers. Born Laredo, Texas, 1926.

Lee, Charles 'Hickory.' Born Teacup, Tennessee, 1933. U.S. Army.
Lee, Sandra Perry. Born Nashville, Tennessee, 1937.

Jensen, Harry. Born Orangeburg, South Carolina, 1933. U.S. Air Force.
Jensen, Inger Olestad. Born Loon River, Minnesota, 1935.

Bell, Timothy. Born Little Rock, Arkansas, 1934. Civilian test pilot.
Bell, Cluny. Born Little Rock, Arkansas, 1937.

Cater, Edward. Born Kosciusko, Mississippi, 1931. U.S. Air Force.
Cater, Gloria. Born Kosciusko, Mississippi, 1931.

Pope, John. (See The Four Families above)

APOLLO 18

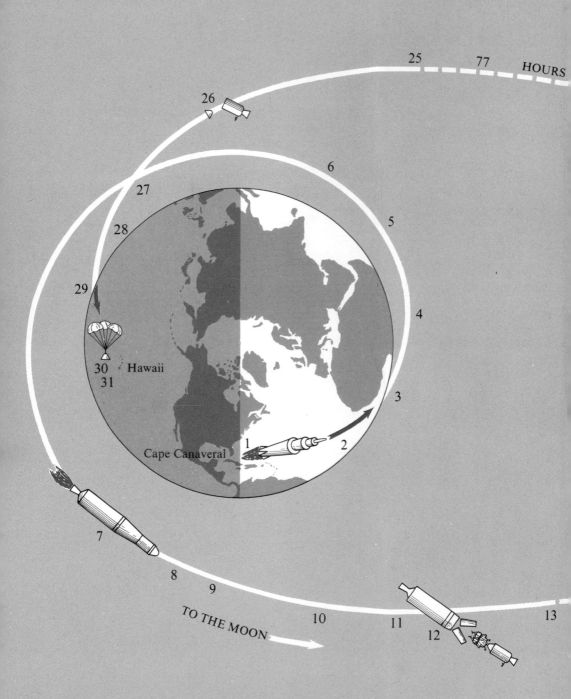

25   77   HOURS

26

6

27

5

28

4

29

3

30   Hawaii

31

1   Cape Canaveral   2

7

8

9

13

TO THE MOON

10   11   12

J.P. Tremblay